WV 100

Queen Elizabeth Hospital

UH00002738

This book is due for return on or before the last date shown below.

1 0 MAR 2011

2 2 AUG 2011

1 1 AUG 2015

1 2 AUG 2015

3 1 OCT 2016

D1349623

Evidence-Based Otolaryngology

Evidence-Based Otolaryngology

Editors

Jennifer J. Shin, MD
Harvard Program in Otolaryngology-Head and Neck Surgery, Massachusetts Eye and
Ear Infirmary, Boston, Massachusetts, USA

Christopher J. Hartnick, MD, MSE
Department of Otolaryngology, Massachusetts Eye and Ear Infirmary, Boston,
Massachusetts, USA

Gregory W. Randolph, MD
Department of Otolaryngology-Head and Neck Surgery, Massachusetts Eye and Ear
Infirmary, Boston, Massachusetts, USA

Section Editors

Pediatric Otolaryngology
Michael J. Cunningham, MD
Margaret Kenna, MD, MPH
J. Paul Willging, MD

Otology
Joseph B. Nadol Jr., MD
Steven D. Rauch, MD

General Otolaryngology
Jay F. Piccirillo, MD
Gregory W. Randolph, MD

Head and Neck Surgery
Jonas T. Johnson, MD
Gregory W. Randolph, MD

Statisticians

Sandra S. Stinnett, PhD
David A. Zurakowski, PhD

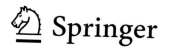

Jennifer J. Shin, MD
Harvard Program in Otolaryngology-Head and Neck Surgery, Massachusetts Eye and Ear Infirmary, Boston, Massachusetts 02114, USA

Christopher J. Hartnick, MD, MSE
Department of Otolaryngology, Massachusetts Eye and Ear Infirmary, Boston, Massachusetts 02114 USA

Gregory W. Randolph, MD
Department of Otolaryngology-Head and Neck Surgery, Massachusetts Eye and Ear Infirmary, Boston, Massachusetts 02114 USA

ISBN: 978-0-387-24447-1   e-ISBN: 978-0-387-49979-6

DOI: 10.1007/978-0-387-49979-6

Library of Congress Control Number: 2007921867

© 2008 Springer Science+Business Media, LLC
All rights reserved. This work may not be translated or copied in whole or in part without the written permission of the publisher (Springer Science+Business Media, LLC, 233 Spring Street, New York, NY 10013, USA), except for brief excerpts in connection with reviews or scholarly analysis. Use in connection with any form of information storage and retrieval, electronic adaptation, computer software, or by similar or dissimilar methodology now known or hereafter developed is forbidden.
The use in this publication of trade names, trademarks, service marks, and similar terms, even if they are not identified as such, is not to be taken as an expression of opinion as to whether or not they are subject to proprietary rights.
While the advice and information in this book are believed to be true and accurate at the date of going to press, neither the authors nor the editors nor the publisher can accept any legal responsibility for any errors or omissions that may be made. The publisher makes no warranty, express or implied, with respect to the material contained herein.

Printed on acid-free paper

9 8 7 6 5 4 3 2 1

springer.com

For Thomas Y. Lin,
because he's my favorite.
-J.J.S.

To my wife, Elizabeth, and children,
Marina, Nathaniel, and Eliza, who
shared their time and made this possible.
-C.J.H.

To my wife Lorraine and our children,
Gregory, Benjamin, and Madeline,
the joy of my life.
-G.W.R.

Foreword by Gerald Healy

The pathway to success in 21st century medicine will be lined by competent physicians practicing safe, evidenced-based, and cost-effective medicine. The foundation for this pathway must be carefully constructed by thoughtful investigation that documents sound treatment principles validated by acceptable measurement tools.

The physician of the 21st century will be asked to engage in a process that incorporates evidence-based education with a process of lifelong learning. The public, regulatory agencies, certifying boards, and payers will require this of every physician participating in our healthcare system.

The authors are to be congratulated for taking a bold step required to meet these demands in the specialty of Otolaryngology and Head and Neck Surgery. Even before the thousands of words in this publication were committed to print, a complex process was being planned by certifying boards that would require every certified physician to be engaged in an evidence-based process of lifelong learning and patient care. The payers are carefully crafting a "pay for performance" algorithm that will incorporate these same principles. This publication will help the otolaryngologist head and neck surgeon to better understand why a particular treatment is initiated, how it is evaluated, and how it can be changed by an ever-evolving validation system.

Generations of physicians have been trained with a different paradigm that allowed for immense variation in treatment. This is not a cost-effective, workable system going forward. It is the obligation of medical practitioners and educators everywhere to put the building blocks in place that will meet the new demands of 21st century healthcare. This publication is an outstanding step in that direction.

Gerald B. Healy, MD, FACS
Chairman, Board of Regents
American College of Surgeons

Foreword by K.J. Lee

As healers of the sick, we should be able to systematically and succinctly identify, summarize, and analyze the evidence regarding management of disease in our field. As clinicians, we have come a long way in establishing good diagnostic and treatment protocols for our patients. The methodologies used are based partly on published data and a great deal based on experience: "This is what I have always done for decades." The latter does not necessarily lead to poor outcomes, but the former does lead to improving outcomes.

This book, the brainchild of Jennifer J. Shin, Christopher J. Hartnick, and Gregory W. Randolph, encompasses evidence-based medicine and is the best on this topic I have come across in our specialty. It is well thought out, practical, and scientific. What is sorely lacking in our medical school and residency training is an emphasis on ethics. We need the ethics to treat every patient as a human being who has come to us for care, and not just as an opportunity for one (a) to learn from, (b) to practice upon, (c) to add to one's case studies for publication, or (d) to schedule tests and surgeries to produce revenue. Practicing evidence-based medicine will give doctors the scientific tools to treat every patient as if he/she were oneself or a member of their beloved family. Congratulations to the editors and contributors for this timely text.

K.J. Lee, MD, FACS
Surgeon, Teacher, Author, Lecturer,
National and International Health Policy Advisor,
Academy Leader

Acknowledgments

The editors would like to thank Ms. Kathleen Kennedy, Ms. Anna Getselman, Mr. Richard Schneider, and Ms. Judith Nims for their assistance with searching the literature and obtaining manuscripts. We would also like to thank Dr. Ying So, Ph.D., Senior Research Statistician SAS institute, for his assistance with Dr. Stinnett's chapter. We also would like to thank Ms. Paula Callaghan, Mr. Benjamin Rooney, and Mr. Brian Belval for their assistance with publication.

We invite you, our readers, to contact us if you have any questions or if you hope to see an additional topic included in future editions of this book. Please contact us at eborl1@gmail.com. Thank you!

Jennifer J. Shin, MD
Christopher J. Hartnick, MD, MSE
Gregory W. Randolph, MD

Contents

Section I   Introduction

Section II   Systematic Reviews in Pediatric Otolaryngology

Section IV   Systematic Reviews in General Otolaryngology

Section V   Systematic Reviews in Head and Neck Oncologic Surgery

Contributors

Manali Amin, MD
Department of Otolaryngology, The Children's
  Hospital, Boston, MA, USA

Shivan Amin, MD
University of California, San Francisco, CA, USA

Iee-Ching Wu Anderson, MD
The Johns Hopkins University School of Medicine,
  Otolaryngology-Head & Neck Surgery, Baltimore,
  MD, USA

Kian Ang MD, PhD
Professor and Distinguished Chair, University of Texas
  M.D. Anderson Cancer Center, Houston, TX, USA

Carol Bauer, MD
Division of Otolaryngology-Head and Neck Surgery,
  Southern Illinois University School of Medicine,
  Springfield, IL, USA

Mary Beauchamp, MD
Loyola University Medical Center, Otolaryngology,
  Maywood, IL, USA

Mark Boseley, MD
Massachusetts Eye and Ear Infirmary, Pediatric
  Otolaryngology, Boston, MA, USA

Thomas J. Brozoski, PhD
Research Professor, Southern Illinois School of
  Medicine, Surgery, Springfield, IL, USA

John P. Carey, MD
Associate Professor, Otolaryngology-Head and Neck
  Surgery, Johns Hopkins University School of
  Medicine, Baltimore, MD, USA

Grace Chan, MD
Harvard Medical School, Boston, MA, USA

Yen-Lin Chen, MD
Department of Radiation Oncology, Harvard Medical
  School, Massachusetts General Hospital, Boston, MA,
  USA

Wade Chien, MD
Harvard Program in Otolaryngology-Head and Neck
  Surgery, Massachusetts Eye and Ear Infirmary,
  Boston, MA, USA

Michael J. Cunningham, MD
Associate Professor, Department of Otolaryngology,
  Massachusetts Eye and Ear Infirmary, Boston,
  MA, USA

James Denneny, III, MD
President, American Academy of Otolaryngology-Head
  and Neck Surgery, Alexandria, VA, USA

Camille Dunn, PhD
Research Audiologist, Department of Otolaryngology-
  Head and Neck Surgery, University of Iowa, Iowa
  City, IA, USA

Marlene Durand, MD
Assistant Professor of Medicine, Division of Infectious
  Disease, Massachusetts General Hospital, Boston,
  MA, USA

Josh Finnell
Research Assistant, Department of Otolaryngology,
  Barnes-Jewish Hospital, St. Louis, MO, USA

Ramon Franco, MD
Assistant Professor Otology and Laryngology, Harvard
  Medical School Director, Voice Center, Massachusetts
  Eye and Ear Infirmary, Boston, MA, USA

Bruce J. Gantz, MD
Professor and Head, Department of Otolaryngology,
  University of Iowa Hospitals and Clinics, Iowa City,
  IA, USA

Richard Gliklich, MD
Massachusetts Eye and Ear Infirmary, Boston, MA, USA

Stacey Gray, MD
Department of Otolaryngology-Head and Neck
  Surgery, Massachusetts Eye and Ear Infirmary,
  Boston, MA, USA

Christopher F. Halpin, PhD
Clinical Associate, Division of Audiology, Massachusetts
  Eye and Ear Infirmary, Boston, MA, USA

James Hartman, MD
St. John's Mercy Medical Center, David C. Pratt Cancer
  Center, St. Louis, MO, USA

Christopher J. Hartnick, MD
Assistant Professor, Department of Otolaryngology,
  Massachusetts Eye and Ear Infirmary, Boston, MA,
  USA

Steven Hemmerdinger, MD
Clinical Instructor, Department of Otolaryngology,
  New York University Medical Center, New York,
  NY, USA

Jonas T. Johnson, MD
Professor and Chairman, Department of
  Otolaryngology, Pittsburgh School of Medicine, Eye
  and Ear Institute, Pittsburgh, PA, USA

Margaret Kenna, MD, MPH
Associate Professor, Department of Otolaryngology and
  Communication Disorders, The Children's Hospital,
  Boston, MA, USA

Merrill S. Kies, MD
Professor, Head and Neck Medical Oncology, M.D.
  Anderson, Houston, TX, USA

Walter Kutz, MD
Fellow, House Ear Clinic, Los Angeles, CA, USA

Ming-Yee Lin, MD
Department of Otolaryngology, Veteran General
  Hospital, Kao-hsiung, Taiwan

Saumil Merchant, MD
Professor, Department of Otology and Laryngology,
  Harvard Medical School, Gudrun Larsen Eliasen and
  Nels Kristian Eliasen Professor of Otology and
  Laryngology, Otology Service, Massachusetts Eye and
  Ear Infirmary, Boston, MA, USA

Ralph Metson, MD
Professor, Department of Otolaryngology-Head and
  Neck Surgery, Massachusetts Eye and Ear Infirmary,
  Boston, MA, USA

Joseph B. Nadol, Jr., MD
Walter Augustus Lecompte Professor & Chairman,
  Department of Otology & Laryngology, Harvard
  Medical School, Chief of Otolaryngology, Director,
  Otology Service, Massachusetts Eye and Ear
  Infirmary, Boston, MA, USA

J. Gail Neely, MD
Professor and Director, Department of Otolaryngology,
  Barnes-Jewish Hospital, St. Louis, MO, USA

James Netterville, MD
Professor of Otolaryngology, Associate Director of the
  Bill Wilkerson Center For Otolaryngology and
  Communication Sciences, Vanderbilt University
  Medical Center, Nashville, TN, USA

Kenny Pang, MD
Sleep Surgery Service Director, ENT Consultant,
  Department of Otolaryngology, Tan Tock Seng
  Hospital, Singapore

Randall C. Paniello, MD
Associate Professor, Department of Otolaryngology-
  Head and Neck Surgery, Washington University
  School of Medicine, St. Louis, MO, USA

Alison Perring
Southern Illinois University School of Medicine,
  Carbondale, IL, USA

Jay F. Piccirillo, MD
Associate Professor, Department of Otolaryngology,
  Washington University School of Medicine, St. Louis,
  MO, USA

Christopher Prichard, MD
Department of Otorhinolaryngology, Baylor College of
  Medicine, Houston, TX, USA

Melissa Pynnonen, MD
Department of Otolaryngology-Head and Neck
  Surgery, University of Michigan Health System, Ann
  Arbor, MI, USA

Mitchell Ramsey, MD
Chief of Neuro-Otology, Tripler Army Medical Center,
  Honolulu, HI, USA

Gregory W. Randolph, MD
Associate Professor, Department of Otolaryngology-
  Head and Neck Surgery, Massachusetts Eye and Ear
  Infirmary, Boston, MA, USA

Steven D. Rauch, MD
Associate Professor, Department of Otolaryngology,
  Massachusetts Eye and Ear Infirmary, Boston,
  MA, USA

Pamela Roehm, MD
Fellow, Department of Otolaryngology-Head and Neck
  Surgery, University of Iowa Hospitals and Clinics,
  Iowa City, IA, USA

J. Thomas Roland, MD
Associate Professor, Department of Otolaryngology and
  Neurosurgery, New York University Medical Center,
  New York, NY, USA

Rita M. Roure, MD
Department of Otolaryngology, New York University
  School of Medicine, New York, NY, USA

Jennifer J. Shin, MD
Harvard Program in Otolaryngology-Head and Neck
  Surgery, Massachusetts Eye and Ear Infirmary,
  Boston, MA, USA

William H. Slattery III, MD
Clinical Professor, Director, Clinical Studies, House
  Ear Institute, Associate, House Ear Clinic,
  University of Southern California, Los Angeles, CA,
  USA

Cristian Slough, MD
Department of Otolaryngology, Oregon Health and
  Science University, Portland, OR, USA

Roger S. Smith, DO, FAASM
Medical Director, SleepHealth Centers, Weymouth,
  Associate Physician in Sleep Medicine, Clinical
  Instructor in Medicine, Harvard Medical School,
  Boston, MA, USA

Michael G. Stewart, MD
Associate Professor, Department of
  Otorhinolaryngology, Baylor College of Medicine,
  Houston, TX, USA

Sandra S. Stinnett, PhD
Assistant Research Professor of Biostatistics and
  Bioinformatics, Assistant Research Professor of
  Ophthalmology, Department of Otolaryngology,
  Duke University Medical Center, Durham,
  NC, USA

Babar Sultan, MD
Department of Otolaryngology, Johns Hopkins
    University, Baltimore, MD, USA

Mark Syms, MD
Division of Neurotology, Department of Neurosurgery,
    Barrow Neurological Institute, Phoenix, AZ, USA

Jeffrey Terrell, MD
Associate Professor, Division of Head and Neck
    Surgery, Department of Otolaryngology, University
    of Michigan Medical Center, Ann Arbor, MI, USA

Richard S. Tyler, PhD
Professor, Department of Otolaryngology, University of
    Iowa Hospitals and Clinics, Iowa City, IA, USA

Mark Volk, MD
Department of Otolaryngology, The Children's
    Hospital, Boston, MA, USA

Regina P. Walker, MD
Clinical Associate Professor, Department of
    Otolaryngology-Head and Neck Surgery, Loyola
    University Medical Center, Maywood, IL, USA

Susan Waltzman, PhD
Professor and Co-Director of the Cochlear Implant
    Center, New York University Medical Center, New
    York, NY, USA

Randal S. Weber, MD
Professor and Chairman, Department of Head and
    Neck Surgery, University of Texas M.D. Anderson
    Cancer Center, Houston, TX, USA

Richard Wein, MD
Assistant Professor, Department of Otolaryngology and
    Communicative Sciences, University of Mississippi
    Medical Center, Jackson, MS, USA

David P. White, MD
Director Sleep Disorders Program, Sleep Medicine
    Division, Brigham and Women's Hospital, Boston,
    MA, USA

Lori Wirth, MD
Dana-Farber Cancer Institute, Boston, MA, USA

J. Paul Willging, MD
Professor, Cincinnati Children's Hospital Medical
    Center, Division of Pediatric Otolaryngology-Head
    and Neck Surgery, Cincinnati, OH, USA

David A. Zurakowski, PhD
Director of Biostatistics, Department of Surgery,
    Children's Hospital, Boston, MA, USA

SECTION I
Introduction

1 Introduction to Evidence-Based Medicine, Levels of Evidence, and Systematic Reviews

Jennifer J. Shin and Christopher J. Hartnick

OVERVIEW

Diseases of the ears, nose, and throat affect the vast majority of the world's population. In fact, otolaryngologic complaints are the most common reasons for adult and pediatric outpatient medical visits, and more than three million related surgical procedures are performed annually in the United States alone. Although medical and surgical developments have relentlessly advanced this field, the educational and explanatory literature regarding the evidence supporting those advancements has lagged behind. This deficiency is made more pronounced by burgeoning pressure from the academic medical community, third-party financiers, and members of the legal arena. Such growing responsibility to practice evidence-based medicine requires physicians to understand and critique the millions of articles that have been and continue to be published regarding the treatment of head and neck diseases. Time constraints and the overwhelming number of trials, however, serve as daunting obstacles for physicians who are now under such pressure to adopt an evidence-based approach.

Our text is comprised of systematic reviews that identify, summarize, and analyze the evidence regarding management of diseases of the head and neck in adult and pediatric populations. Sections on general otolaryngology, head and neck oncologic surgery, pediatric otolaryngology, and otology are all included. Although we adhere strictly to principles of evidence-based analysis, we have also developed a user-friendly format to maximize the accessibility of the content. We succinctly explain the contents and critique of the publications that guide management of otolaryngologic disease. Each systematic review provides "The Evidence Condensed" (© Shin, Hartnick, Randolph, 2003) and distills weeks of meticulous reading into portions that can be managed in minutes by busy clinicians and trainees.

EVIDENCE-BASED MEDICINE: WHAT IT IS AND WHY IT IS HERE TO STAY

Evidence-based medicine is defined as "the conscientious, explicit, and judicious use of current best evidence in making clinical decisions about the care of individual patients [1]." The appeal of evidence-based medicine is undeniable. Consider the following stark examples: Should a patient be treated with one drug "because it's what a colleague uses" when the patient could instead be treated with a drug that has been proven to result in decreased mortality as compared with placebo in randomized controlled trials (RCTs)? Given the choice, which option will health care insurers fund? If a physician were to be sued for malpractice, would he or she have a better defense if he or she "had used a treatment successfully during training" or if that treatment had been proven to have both efficacy and minimal morbidity in repeated high-level clinical trials with similar patients? It is because of the clear answers to these clinical, financial, and legal questions that the field of medicine has evolved toward the evidence-based approach.

In fact, as one author notes, we exist in an environment "whereby external pressures have changed clinical research from a cerebral pursuit to a necessity for practitioner autonomy and economic survival [2]." Indeed, evidence-based methodology has permeated day-to-day clinical practice. Clinical practice guidelines based on the best evidence available have been implemented in academic institutions and private practices around the globe [3–5]. Also, health care insurers consistently review and cite the published literature when evaluating new or even currently covered interventions. Otolaryngologists have frequently been asked to document treatment outcomes for third-party payers and managed-care organizations [6]. Furthermore, as of 2002, 42 states provided a process through which consumers could appeal denials of coverage by their health care plan to independent reviewers of the evidence [7]. Likewise, pharmaceutical companies face rigorous evidence-based review when attempting to justify the inclusion of their products within an institution's formulary. These changes are only the beginning.

This transformation will continue because there is also a concerted effort to push medical education toward an evidence-based approach. Medical residency programs have incorporated these concepts into their training programs, and academic institutions have actively recruited physicians who practice evidence-based medicine into teaching roles in their hospitals [8]. In addition, the editors of the *Journal of the American Medical Association,* a periodical with 365,000 subscribers, chose to feature a series of articles specifically designed to educate physicians on the principles and practices of evidence-based medicine [8]. Also, through an initiative of the U.S. Department of Human and Health Services Agency for Healthcare Research and Quality, twelve Evidence-Based Practice Centers have been established in the United States. These centers serve to educate current and emerging clinicians through evidence-based practice and research. Likewise, Centers for Evidence-Based Medicine have been founded in the United Kingdom and in Toronto, Canada. With this growing commitment of the medical field to the evidence-based approach, there promises to be a continually increasing need to conduct our practices on the basis of firm knowledge of the results of clinical trials. This need places an onus on physicians to base their management decisions on an understanding of the meaning and strength of the results of clinical trials.

CLINICAL DATA: THE CONTENT AND CREDIBILITY OF THE RESULTS

Evidence-based practice ultimately stands on three legs: clinical data, clinician judgment, and patient preference. For most physicians, the most daunting aspect of evidence-based medicine centers around the data. The data must be understood on two levels; both the content and credibility of published results are key. We'll begin with the former, the content of the results.

The Content of the Results. The content of the results is defined by the outcome measures used in the study. These outcome measures are critical, as they ultimately determine the clinical meaning of the results and the way in which they are numerically summarized and analyzed.

Clinical Meaning of Outcome Measures. The clinical value of results is influenced by the immediate relevance of the outcome measure. Some results can be measured directly, such as decannulation after tracheotomy. Some results, however, are harder to measure directly (i.e., improvement in nocturnal breathing after uvulopalato-pharyngoplasty) and a surrogate endpoint or representative parameter must be chosen in its place (i.e., respiratory distress index). Such surrogate endpoints should be directly related to patient-oriented outcomes in order to maximize the clinical value of the results [9].

The exactness of results also contributes to their clinical value. Some outcomes are clearly defined, with minimal room for error in interpretation (i.e., survival). Other outcomes, however, are less clearly delineated (i.e., throat infections). In a well-designed study, any potentially ambiguous outcomes are rigorously defined (i.e.,

each throat infection was documented and had ≥ 1 of the following: PO temperature >38.3°C, lymphadenopathy >2 cm or tender, tonsil/pharyngeal exudates, group A beta hemolytic streptococcus positive, antibiotics for proved/suspected streptococcal infection [10]). Precisely measuring an outcome permits the study results to be understood with complete certainty, maximizing their utility for a clinician attempting to apply them to his or her practice.

In some cases, additional tools are needed to ensure the exactness and accuracy of subjective results. Such tools are necessary when measuring quality of life. Quality of life is a broadly defined concept that encompasses how patients feel and function on multiple levels. Overall quality of life is affected by economic, emotional, spiritual, physical, mental, and other factors. A person's health status, or their personal condition because of bodily afflictions or lack thereof, is just one of these issues that affects people's well-being. As physicians, however, our main interest lies here, and thus we focus on that aspect of personal welfare that is affected by health status, or health-related quality of life.

When measuring health-related quality of life, investigators will ideally use a rigorously tested questionnaire, which is usually referred to as an instrument. A validated instrument has been tested to ensure that the following are true: 1) it measures what it is intended to measure (convergent validity, i.e., scores on a valid test of arithmetic skills correlate with scores on other math tests), and 2) it does not inadvertently measure irrelevant changes (discriminant validity, i.e., scores on a valid test of arithmetic do not correlate with scores on tests of verbal ability) [11, 12], 3) its scores are stable (reliability, i.e., a patient with the same disease impact will continue to have the same response), and 4) it is sensitive to change (responsiveness, i.e., a patient with a change in disease impact will have a changed score). Overall, this means that the validated instrument does in fact measure what it is meant to measure when it is administered to the correct population.

Instruments can be global or disease-specific [9]. A global instrument measures overall quality of life and may be used to determine the impact of many different diseases. Examples include the Short Form 36 (SF-36) and Child Health Questionnaire (CHQ). A disease-specific instrument, in contrast, is explicitly intended to measure the impact of one disease only. Examples include the Otitis Media 6 (OM-6) and Sinonasal Outcome Test 20 (SNOT-20). Often, both types of instruments are used in the same study to provide complementary data. By using these validated instruments, investigators strictly delineate the contents of their results.

Numerical Summary and Analysis of Outcome Measures. The outcome measures determine how the results are numerically summarized, as well as the type of quantitative analyses that can determine the statistical significance of the results. Every numerical outcome measure can be categorized as one of three types of variables, each of which is summarized and analyzed in standard ways. First, some outcome measures are like weight or oxygen saturation; these values are numeric with an inherent order and the incremental differences between numbers are equal. Values with these properties are defined as continuous variables and they are summarized in terms of means with standard deviations or medians with ranges. Continuous variables are analyzed using Pearson correlation coefficients, paired or independent *t*-tests, and analyses of variance [13].

Second, some outcome measures are like tumor staging or House-Brackman scores; they are categorical with an inherent order, but incremental differences between adjacent categories are not necessarily equal. To use the tumor staging example, a T2N1M0 parotid tumor is in a well-defined category. Such a tumor is also clearly less worrisome than a T4N3M1 tumor, because there is an inherent order to the staging. The difference between a T2 and a T3 tumor, however, is not the same as the difference between a T3 and T4 tumor, because incremental differences between categories are not necessarily equal. This type of variable is called an ordinal variable, and ordinal results are summarized in terms of medians with ranges or proportions and percentages. Ordinal variables are analyzed using Spearman correlation coefficients, kappa statistics, signed rank tests, Wilcoxon rank sum tests, and Kruskal-Wallace tests [13].

A third kind of outcome measure includes items like color or shape; they describe discrete categories with no order. A triangle, circle, and pentagon are clearly defined, but do not have an inherent order as no shape has more inherent value than the other. This type of measure is called a nominal variable, and nominal results are summarized in terms of proportions, percentages, and ratios. Nominal variables are analyzed with the following statistical tests: McNemar's, kappa, Fisher's exact, and chi-squared [13]. A dichotomous or binary variable is a particular type of nominal variable that has only two possible categories (gender, yes/no). Dichotomous data are often described in terms of an odds ratio, relative risk, or rate difference. A rate difference, also referred to as an absolute risk reduction, is a particularly useful measure, because it can also be used to calculate the number needed to treat. All of these terms, in addition to many others, are described in detail in Chapter 3, "English Translations of Common Statistical Terms and Study Designs."

Analysis of Diagnostic Testing. Four key concepts define the utility of a diagnostic test: positive predictive value, negative predictive value, sensitivity, and specificity. The positive predictive value is a measure of how much a positive test result can be trusted. This value defines how often a positive test result is correct; of values that test positive, it is the proportion of values that is actually truly positive. For example, the positive predictive value of a coagulation test for post-tonsillectomy

bleeding is 0.02 or 2% (see Chapter 4.D). This means that 2% of children who have a positive test result (i.e., abnormal coagulation test) will actually bleed.

Conversely, the negative predictive value is a measure of the truth in a negative test result, and defines how often a negative test result is correct. Of values that test negative, it is the proportion of values that is actually truly negative. For example, the negative predictive value of preoperative coagulation testing for post-tonsillectomy bleeding is 0.92 or 92% (see Chapter 4.D). This means that 92% of children who have a negative (normal) test will not bleed postoperatively.

The positive and negative predictive values are also influenced by the prevalence of disease, according to Bayes theorem. The concept underlying this theorem is that if a disease is more prevalent, then the positive predictive value is higher. Consider the following example: The test of looking at hairs on the floor is used to determine the hair color of the person who lives in a house. For example, black hairs on the floor mean that the person who lives there has black hair. This particular test result (black hairs on the floor) is very likely to be a true positive (the person who lives there actually has black hair) in China, where the vast majority of people have black hair (high prevalence). The exact same test result (black hairs on the floor), however, is more likely to be wrong (the person who lives there does not have black hair) in Scandinavia, where fewer people have black hair (low prevalence). Thus, the prevalence (pretest probability) affects the predictive value of a test.

Sensitivity and specificity are additional ways to measure the performance of a diagnostic test. Sensitivity is defined by the proportion of patients who truly have a disease that test positive for that disease. A high sensitivity means that a negative test result rules out the diagnosis. In other words, the false-negative rate is low. To better understand this meaning, consider how sensitivity is calculated: sensitivity = true positives/(true positives + false negatives). If the number of false negatives is 0, sensitivity is 100%. Also, because all patients who truly have disease must test as either a true positive or a false negative, if the number of false negatives is 0, then all patients who have disease must be true positives. Thus, in general, a high sensitivity also means that the screening test is a good predictor of those with disease. For example, the sensitivity of laboratory coagulation screening in identifying children who will develop post-tonsillectomy bleeding is 0.09, according to one study (see Chapter 4. D.2). This means that 9% of patients who will truly develop post-tonsillectomy bleeding will have an abnormal coagulation panel (positive test). The sensitivity is low, which suggests that a positive test may not be a good predictor of postoperative bleeding.

Specificity is the proportion of patients who truly are disease-free that test negative for that disease. A high specificity means that a positive result rules in the diagnosis. In other words, the false-positive rate is low. To better understand this meaning, consider how specificity is calculated: specificity = true negatives/(true negatives + false positives). Thus, if the number of false positives is 0, then specificity is 100%. Also, because all patients who truly do not have disease must test as either true negatives or false positives and if the number of false positives is 0, then all patients who do not have disease must be true negatives. Thus, in general, a high specificity also means that the screening test is a good predictor of those without disease. For example, the specificity of laboratory coagulation screening in identifying children who will develop post-tonsillectomy bleeding is 0.98 according to one study (see Chapter 4.D.2). This means that 98% of patients who will not develop postoperative hemorrhage will have a normal coagulation panel (negative test). The specificity is high, which suggests that a normal panel is associated with no bleeding.

A 2 × 2 table helps further illustrate these four key concepts of positive and negative predictive value, sensitivity, and specificity:

	Positive for disease	*Negative for disease*
Positive test result	True positives	False positives
Negative test result	False negatives	True negatives

Positive predictive value = true positives/(false positives + true positives) (also influenced by pretest probability, i.e., prevalence)
Negative predictive value = true negatives/(false negatives + true negatives) (also influenced by pretest probability, i.e., prevalence)
Sensitivity = true positives/(true positives + false negatives)
Specificity = true negatives/(true negatives + false positives).

The Credibility of the Results. The credibility of data is determined by the design of the study that produced them. Ideally, a study design ensures that only a truthful answer to the posed clinical question is obtained. A perfect study would show that an intervention (i.e., oral steroids) unequivocally caused an effect (i.e., regression of nasal polyps). A perfect study is flawless, and as such, is defined in terms of the flaws it lacks, just as a perfect test score is defined by the errors it lacks. Study flaws can occur because of chance (i.e., statistical probability) or confounding and bias (i.e., unwanted interference from ancillary factors). Both types of flaws detract from the quality of a study. We will consider errors from statistical probability first.

Susceptibility to Errors from Chance. A study may prove that a hypothesis is wrong, when in reality that hypothesis is right. Sometimes such an error occurs purely as a result of chance. There may be no human vice involved; it can just be bad luck. Consider the null hypothesis, which states that there is no difference between the groups being compared. In reality, this statement is often true, but even a well-designed study has a certain chance

of inappropriately rejecting it. With this knowledge, it is imperative to determine whether a reported result has a high likelihood of being the actual real-life result. If that likelihood is low, the study's results have low credibility.

To illustrate one type of error that may occur purely because of chance, consider a hypothetical study that determines whether the two sides of a penny are the same. In this hypothetical study design, the coin is flipped repeatedly to determine whether the outcome is all heads, all tails, or a combination of the two. If the penny has heads on both sides (i.e., there is no difference and the null hypothesis is true), then the coin flip study design is ideal. The flip outcome can only be heads, which will eventually lead to the conclusion that there are heads on both sides. In this scenario, there is no chance that the coin flips will find a difference when in reality the two sides of the penny are the same. Unfortunately, clinical trials are not as straightforward. With clinical trials there is such a possibility, where no difference is found, although in reality a difference is present. **Type 1 error** (the **alpha level**) is the probability that a study finds a difference when in reality no difference exists (i.e., the probability of rejecting the null hypothesis when in actuality the null hypothesis is true).

Next consider using the same study design in a different scenario, with a normal penny with a head side and a tail side. Using only coin flips, we might have flip outcomes of all heads or all tails. Such uniform outcomes would lead to the wrong conclusion about whether the coin has two heads, two tails, or both. In this scenario, the study could find that there is no difference in the two coin sides, even though in reality a clear difference exists. The same type of error may occur in clinical trials; it is possible that a study may find that there is no difference in outcome with or without surgery, when in actuality surgery results in a very different outcome. The probability that the study finds that there is no difference when in reality a difference exists (i.e., the probability of accepting the null hypothesis as true when in actuality the null hypothesis is false) is called a **type 2 error** or the **beta level**.

All is not lost, however, because there is still a possibility that a true difference will be accurately identified. The probability that a study will find a difference that actually exists is called the **power** of a study. Often, you will see power defined in the context of type 2 error as (1-beta). The power of a study depends on multiple factors, beginning with the sample size. One thousand coin flips that show tails are more likely to mean that the coin actually has tails on both sides, as compared to three coin flips that show tails. Therefore, a study's susceptibility to error from chance is partially controlled by the investigators. Power is also influenced by the alpha level (see above), which is by convention set at 0.05, or a 5% probability of inaccurately rejecting the null hypothesis because of chance alone. In addition, power depends on the magnitude of difference deemed clinically significant (the delta level); as the delta level increases, the power increases. Therefore, the same study may have a high power for finding a large difference in two populations but a low power for detecting a small difference. In addition, power depends on the final outcome measurements and a calculation of their variance. Because some of these measurements will not be apparent until the study is completed, investigators must rely on estimates when attempting to ensure that a planned study is adequately powered. Here, preliminary data from previous studies proves invaluable, because it provides those very estimates. Although investigators cannot control some factors, they need to estimate them in order to predict the number of patients necessary to achieve an acceptable power (90%) to detect a clinically significant outcome. In doing so, they increase the probability that their study will correctly reject the null hypothesis.

Susceptibility to Errors from Confounding and Bias. As previously stated, a perfect study is ideal because of the flaws it lacks. In a perfect study, nothing would get in the way of the examination of cause (the intervention of interest) and effect (the outcome of interest). This is real life, however, and sometimes things do get in the way. Sometimes other factors besides the intervention can cause the same outcome of interest. Furthermore, sometimes the way in which the intervention or its effects are made or studied can affect the measured outcome of interest. With this concern in mind, we will next discuss management of confounders, minimizing bias, and the use of a control group.

Sample size influences the power of a study.

To understand this concept, consider a coin flip example in which you are given a coin that has either two heads or one head and one tail. If you flip that coin twice and get heads twice, you have demonstrated no difference, but your confidence in saying that both sides are heads is quite attenuated by the fact that you only did two flips. This example is analogous to a low power study; the low number of flips (i.e., low sample size) gives low confidence that you would have found a difference in the two sides of the coin. Instead, if you were to flip that coin 10,000 times and get heads every time, then you could say with great confidence that there were heads on both sides, because it would be so unlikely to demonstrate no difference 10,000 times if one side was in fact different from the other. This example is analogous to a high power study; the high number of coin flips (i.e., high sample size) gives high confidence that you would have found a difference in the two sides of the coin.

A potential **confounder** is a factor that can cause the same outcome as the intervention of interest. A factor is said to be **confounded** with another factor if it is impossible to discern which of the two is responsible for the observed effect [14]. With **confounding**, a measure of the effect of the cause under investigation is distorted because of the presence of other potential causes of the

same effect [15]. In addition, the confounding variable may be associated with the intervention of interest, further complicating matters [16]. Consider studying the impact of antibiotics on post-tonsillectomy pain. Other factors besides antibiotics—such as surgical technique, anesthetic regimen, and use of steroids—may also influence postoperative pain, and could confound the results. When confounders are present, a singular cause and effect cannot be demonstrated. Therefore, a high-quality study will try to eliminate confounders or at least carefully account for them. Randomization is one way of carefully accounting for confounders, by ensuring that they are at least balanced in the two groups being compared. In fact, the first table in the results section of a well-reported RCT usually details potential confounders and demonstrates that they were distributed similarly in all of the groups that were compared. If such confounders are not managed properly, then no cause and effect can be demonstrated; the study's conclusions must then be limited to drawing correlations between the intervention and outcome. These correlations cannot be used as proof of the intervention's effects, although they may be used as just cause for further higher-level study in which confounders will be carefully controlled.

Study techniques can artificially push the outcome in one direction, preventing a neutral demonstration of cause and effect. **Bias** is simply an error in the technique of selecting subjects, performing procedures, measuring a characteristic, or analyzing and reporting data [14]. In clinical research, bias does not imply stubbornness or willful deceit as in colloquial speech, and many varieties of research bias have been described [15, 17, 18]. Bias can occur in many forms while performing a study. **Selection bias** occurs when study subjects are improperly chosen. For example, in a study of the impact of antibiotics on adult pain after tonsillectomy, choosing only stoic patients to receive antibiotics would bias results. Worse, if you were comparing this group to a control group that did not receive antibiotics, and only put timid patients in that second group, selection bias would be even more egregious. Another type of bias is **performance bias**. Performance bias occurs when there are inconsistencies in the care that is provided or exposure to other factors apart from the intervention of interest. Performing tonsillectomy with electrocautery in the group receiving antibiotics while performing cold tonsillectomy in the control group, for example, can bias results. **Detection bias** may also be present, where there is a partiality when assessing the outcomes. Perhaps the best-known form of detection bias is **expectation bias**, in which expecting a certain result can influence the result itself. Continuing with the antibiotics for tonsillectomy example, those in the antibiotic group might expect to have less pain than the control group. This expectation alone can actually result in less pain. This expectation bias can be eliminated by administering a placebo to the control group and blinding both patients and physicians.

Other types of bias may occur during the analysis, interpretation, and even publication of results. The compilation of data may be plagued by **attrition bias**, which results from an excess amount (>20%) of patients lost to follow-up. Using our ongoing example, if only 1% of the patients return to report their postoperative pain, the results from the other 99% patients could have easily outweighed the results from the returning 1%, so the real result remains unknown. In addition, bias may result from not including data from patients who withdrew from the study because of treatment failure. To counteract such bias, an intention to treat analysis is ideally performed. In an **intention to treat analysis**, results are reported in terms of the original treatment groups regardless of whatever happened to subjects subsequent to their enrollment in the trial. For example, in a trial in which patients undergo radiation therapy versus surgical resection for laryngeal carcinoma, the survival outcome for a patient who was originally treated with radiation should be included with the data for the radiation therapy group, even if that patient subsequently required surgical resection. When results are being interpreted, a **correlation bias** may occur when correlation is equated with causation. For example, in a retrospective study of survival rates in patients treated with or without chemotherapy, it may be that chemotherapy is correlated with worse survival rates. This does not, however, mean that chemotherapy causes death. It may simply be that chemotherapy was recommended in more advanced cases. Finally, bias may even occur in the publication stage. **Publication bias** in the otolaryngology literature has favored the acceptance and publication of reports of studies showing a difference in outcome in two groups, making it less likely that reports showing no difference between two groups will be distributed. Overall, bias can occur at multiple crucial junctures, and may be seen not only while performing the study, but also when its results are compiled and reported.

The use of a control group can be an effective way to thwart many of these biases. A control group is used to provide a measure of what happens without the intervention. This control measure allows comparison of the intervention group to a group that is ideally similar in every other way. Confounders that cannot be eliminated are at least balanced in each group. Likewise, patient selection, performance, outcome measurements, and analysis can be implemented in the same way in both groups to minimize bias. Ideally then, the addition of control subjects results in two groups that are the same with the exception of the intervention. If so, then the intervention is the only difference that can account for a difference in their outcomes. If the intervention is truly the only difference between the two groups, then a true

cause and effect is likely to be demonstrated. Therefore, the presence of a control is better than none. Also, in those controlled studies, the strength of the work is contingent on how well confounders and bias are accounted for and balanced between the two groups.

Managing all of these factors poses quite a challenge, however, and can be nearly impossible when the intervention has already been performed. It is because of this very reason that retrospective studies have inherent flaws; with retrospective studies, it is impossible to remove biases in selection, expectation, and detection, among others. In a prospective study, investigators can at least plan ahead to account for potential confounders and bias. They can arrange to use methods that minimize bias in selecting patients or collecting data. Even then, however, there may be potential biases or confounders that lie beyond the imagination of the study coordinator or anyone else for that matter. With this concern in mind, the randomized controlled study was born. Because patients are randomly assigned, confounders that are known or even unknown are likely to be balanced between the intervention and control group. Therefore, the management of confounders and bias is heavily dependent on the study design, which ultimately determines the level of evidence that a study provides.

LEVELS OF EVIDENCE: WHAT THEY ARE AND WHY SOME ARE BETTER THAN OTHERS

One of the challenges in reviewing the literature lies in bringing order to the assortment of articles that are relevant to each clinical query; approaches and results among articles may be similar or conflicting. The use of previously established levels of evidence for ranking published data helps readers understand the reliability of different reports. Using these levels also has the added benefit of providing guidance regarding the conclusions that can be drawn and the strength of recommendations made based on the reported data [2, 19, 20]. These levels and their implications are as follows:

Level 1 evidence includes RCTs or meta-analyses of RCTs. RCTs are the gold standard in study design, with randomization ideally removing unintended differences in the intervention and control groups before treatment. By using randomization to prevent bias in allocating patients to one group or the other, different results in the two groups may be attributed solely to either the intervention or lack thereof in the control group. Bias may be further minimized with this study type by blinding patients and caregivers to the type of intervention whenever possible. RCTs provide the strongest evidence for showing a direct cause and effect, and it is the best design to test the efficacy of the treatment in question. Recommendations based on RCTs are considered Grade A.

Level 2 comprises prospective studies with an internal control group or a meta-analysis of prospective controlled trials. In this type of study, plans are made before patient care begins. A predetermined research protocol is used to assign patients to an intervention group or a control group. Usually, this internal control group parallels the group that receives the intervention of interest in every way except for lacking that intervention. A premeditated standardized method of data collection is used to gather results. Without randomization, the investigator is responsible for regulating potentially confounding variables that may produce misleading results. In addition, conclusions of the study must be tempered based on potential confounders that could not be regulated. Recommendations based on prospective controlled studies are appraised as Grade B.

Level 3 includes retrospective studies with an internal control group or a meta-analysis of retrospective controlled studies. In this study design, the analysis is planned after patient care is already complete. For example, in a retrospective "case control study," records are reviewed to find subjects who had an outcome of interest (i.e., survival); these subjects constitute the "case" group. Then records are reviewed to find patients who did *not* have the outcome of interest (i.e., did *not* survive); these subjects constitute the "control" group. Ideally, this "control" group is matched to the "case" group as closely as possible except for the outcome (i.e., similar stage N0 oral cavity carcinoma with primary surgical treatment in both groups). The proportion of each group that was exposed to a certain intervention is then compared (i.e., neck dissection as part of initial therapy). This study design is prone to selection bias, so the investigator must minimize potentially confounding differences between the "case" and "control" groups to optimize the validity of the results. Recommendations based on retrospective controlled studies are also ranked as Grade B.

Level 4 studies are case series with no internal control group. With this type of study, the results of an intervention are reported in one group of patients without a comparison group; there is no report of a group that received either no intervention or a different intervention to place the results in context. It is purely a descriptive account, and as such, can only suggest correlations between the intervention and outcome. Alone, a study of this level cannot prove cause and effect, but it can document the potential for good outcome with a particular intervention. The most prudent use for this study design is to suggest hypotheses for higher-level study. Recommendations based on level 4 studies are considered Grade C.

Level 5 includes reports of expert opinions without explicit critical appraisal or on the basis of physiology or bench research alone. This designation is not meant to demean scientific research or the wisdom that follows from years of education and experience. In fact, it is because of the richness of these resources that medical advancements are initially conceived. With this potential, these opinions provide hypotheses that are worthy of higher-level study. Recommendations based on level 5 reports are deemed Grade D.

There are certain study designs that do not fall obviously into one of these 5 levels. After consultation with the Centre for Evidence-Based Medicine (the originator of the levels of evidence), we have leveled certain potentially ambiguous or controversial study designs in the following ways. In general, studies comparing preoperative results versus postoperative results for a single procedure could be level 2, 3, or 4. In order to be level 2, the study would need to be prospective and evaluate preoperative versus postoperative results in a selected subpopulation cohort (i.e., a population with a uniform disease process). For example, a prospective study of patients with chronic sinusitis who undergo sinus surgery, with prospective measurement of performance on preoperative versus postoperative quality of life instruments, would provide prospective comparative data from a selected subpopulation cohort, and constitute a level 2 study. In contrast, a prospective study of children who have undergone adenoidectomy for various indications, with prospective measurement of sinus-related quality of life instrument compared with population norms, would provide level 4 evidence (i.e., a non-specific population cohort with no internal comparative group). Retrospective studies with strong statistical and confounder-conscious comparisons between preoperative and postoperative results for a patient population with a uniform disease process (i.e., focus on tonsillectomy for sleep apnea specifically) were considered level 3. Meanwhile, retrospective studies with comparison of preoperative versus postoperative results for a procedure in general (i.e., sinusitis-related quality of life for all comers who underwent adenoidectomy, whether for chronic sinusitis, nasal obstruction, or suspicious mass) were considered level 4.

Although it might appear on first glance that only level 1 evidence should be considered acceptable, this idealized notion is not always practical, especially for a surgical subspecialty. Patients may hesitate to accept randomization to surgical treatment, and we frequently treat less-prevalent diseases, making it difficult to attain the sizable patient pool necessary to perform an RCT of adequate power. The truth is that not all otolaryngologic interventions can realistically be evaluated by level 1 studies. Therefore, if level 1 studies cannot be made available, level 2 studies must suffice. Likewise, if level 1 and 2 evidence cannot be achieved, then level 3 evidence is the best choice, and so forth. As one author summarized it, "Any grade of evidence is a valid platform on which to base decisions, but only to the extent that higher grades of evidence are unavailable [2]."

SYSTEMATIC REVIEWS: THE PROCESS AND THE APPEAL

The goal of a systematic review is to assess the literature critically to see if a particular clinical question can be answered through rigorous analysis of the available data. This type of review includes not only the detailed results of relevant clinical trials, but also an analysis of the validity of those results. A well-designed systematic review renders transparent the methodology of each of the studies included by focusing on the critical issues described above: the choice of outcome parameter, the chance of statistical errors, and the potential for confounding and bias. It differs in several fundamental ways from a traditional narrative review, and the next section addresses these concepts in detail.

A Systematic Review Differs from a Traditional Narrative Review. A systematic review differs in several key ways from a traditional narrative review. First, traditional narrative reviews often vary depending on the author. In fact, journals often solicit back-to-back narrative reviews to showcase two different opinions regarding management options (i.e., total versus hemithyroidectomy for low-risk papillary thyroid carcinoma). In contrast, a systematic review is designed to minimize personal predispositions. Reproducible methods are used to produce reproducible results, and at least two authors participate in each review to corroborate findings and minimize inadvertent bias.

Second, in a traditional narrative review, any variety of published articles may be cited—so in a worst case scenario, five low-quality studies that support a point may be showcased, leaving the reader unaware of 100 high-quality studies with opposing results. A systematic review, however, gives a guarantee of thoroughness: methodical searching techniques ensure that all potentially relevant data are considered, and the article selection process is explained in detail so that any skeptical reader can verify the thoroughness for themselves.

Third, a traditional narrative review typically reports results of relevant trials and whether they were statistically significant. In addition to these two features, a systematic review also gives an assessment of how credible any touted differences are, with emphasis placed on the most credible results.

Finally, a traditional narrative review provides a summary of the practice considerations of the author. A systematic review provides a summary of the published data, to whom they apply, and more so than a traditional narrative review, it empowers readers to make their own decisions based on knowledge of the strength of the data. Overall, a systematic review provides many benefits, and in order to obtain them, multiple methodical steps are involved. Next, we provide a brief explanation of those steps.

The Systematic Review Process.
1. Define a focused clinical query.

In a systematic review, well-defined methods are used to search and evaluate all published data on a focused clinical query [19, 21–23]. These focused clinical queries are stated in terms of a patient population, intervention versus control, and outcome of interest. Consider these examples: In children <18 years old with recurrent pharyngitis (patient population), does tonsillectomy (intervention) or no surgery (control) result in fewer episodes of sore throat (outcome of interest)? In adults with stage N0 oral cavity carcinoma (patient population), do supraomohyoid neck dissection (intervention) and modified radical neck dissection (control) result in similar survival rates (outcome of interest)? The narrow focus of each systematic review allows specific hypotheses to be tested, and defining that focus is the initial step in this process.

2. Perform a comprehensive search of the literature.
The next step in the process of systematic review is the identification of all relevant papers. First, before the literature search, meticulous inclusion and exclusion criteria are defined in order to provide a methodical, impartial means of article selection. Those inclusion/exclusion criteria are defined by the hypothesis developed in step 1. For example, inclusion criteria may require the presence of 1) a study population of children ≤18 years old undergoing tonsillectomy, 2) intervention with single-dose dexamethasone versus placebo, 3) measurement of the number of episodes of postoperative emesis, 4) follow-up time of at least 3 postoperative days. Accompanying exclusion criteria could be: a) children undergoing adenoidectomy alone, b) intervention with oral steroids, c) intervention with local injection of steroids, d) intervention with steroids and a second agent, e) outcome of subjective nausea only, without specification of episodes of emesis. These criteria are reviewed and approved by an expert in the field.

Next, a search strategy is used which is designed to include all potentially relevant studies. First, a computerized search is performed, mapping terms to subject headings and exploding terms so as to include all related subheadings. Second, using the inclusion/exclusion criteria, the first round of studies is selected. Third, the bibliographies for each of these studies are manually checked and any potentially relevant articles are reviewed to see if they meet inclusion/exclusion criteria. This step inevitably yields further articles, so fourth, the bibliographies of these new acquisitions are again manually checked. Fifth, this process is repeated until all appropriate articles have been identified. Finally, the technique and results of this search process are documented, allowing another investigator to duplicate the process.

3. Assess the quality of studies that meet the review's inclusion/exclusion criteria.
Once all of these relevant papers have been collected, the quality of each study's design is determined, even

before the related results are considered. This process is partially accomplished by determining the level of the methodology (see "Levels of Evidence" above). The quality is also determined by how well the methods minimize bias and control potentially confounding variables (see "Credibility of Results" above). The precision of outcome measurements and power of the given sample size and variability are also important (see "Content of Results" above). In addition, depending on the clinical query, other factors such as adequacy of follow-up time are also crucial. The highest-quality studies are identified for emphasis within the review.

4. Extract and analyze the results.

Once their quality has been determined, the results are analyzed. The outcomes of interest are extracted for the endpoints determined at the outset of the review process. In some cases, the outcome measures are similar enough, even in different studies, to allow pooling of the data. This statistical pooling of data can provide an estimate of the main effect of the intervention being reviewed. This pooling process is called meta-analysis, and usually incorporates the results of RCTs, yielding data that are representative of all of the included study populations [24–27]. Often, however, the data are not suitable for meta-analysis, because of inconsistencies in the outcome measurements or limitations of the study designs. When this is the case, no statistical pooling is performed, but data are methodically presented and a rigorous qualitative analysis is performed.

The Appeal of Systematic Reviews. With all of the meticulous steps involved, incorporating systematic literature reviews into one's practice can be a daunting task for the individual clinician, especially given the sheer quantity of medical articles peer selected for publication—approximately half a million registered on MEDLINE in 2002 alone. In fact, just tackling the plethora of recommendations on how to best search the literature and synthesize data can be a lengthy process, with multiple journal series and entire books dedicated to this subject alone [1, 8, 19, 28]. Therefore, individual clinicians are usually logistically unable to complete their own analyses of the evidence base for every clinical query within the myriad of diseases that they treat. Despite this, they are still responsible for maintaining their proficiency in these matters. Time constraints, together with mounting pressure from the medical community and third-party groups to adhere to evidence-based practice standards, make thorough, concise, unbiased reviews of the most relevant literature very desirable. In accordance with this, systematic reviews of the literature, often including a numeric meta-analysis of combinable data, have become increasingly paramount. In fact, the number of MEDLINE articles containing "meta-analysis" as a keyword or subject heading increased from 247 in 1989 to 739 in 1997 [29] to 1563 in 2002.

Performing just one systematic review of the literature relevant to a clinical query usually takes days to weeks, or sometimes months, with MEDLINE searches often yielding hundreds or thousands of potentially related articles that must be considered. This work is well worth it, though, as "the systematic review of the effects of health care is the most powerful and useful evidence available [19]." The potential insight gained from a *single* systematic review merits frequent selection for publication or presentation. In this book, we perform 111 of these systematic reviews. We use a process that allows us to address a wide range of queries for which there is a wide variety of quality and quantity of published articles. We have invested many thousands of work hours into in-depth searches and analyses of the literature regarding a range of otolaryngologic topics, but with each systematic review, we take a task that takes days and distill it down to a concise, consistent format that can be understood in minutes. Please see our explanation of this format in the following chapter.

REFERENCES

1. Sackett D, Rosenberg W, Gray J, Haynes R, Richardson W. Evidence-based medicine: what it is and what it isn't. BMJ 1996;312:71–72.
2. Rosenfeld R. Evidence, outcomes, and common sense. Otolaryngol Head Neck Surg 2001;124(2):123–124.
3. Farquhar CM, Kofa EW, Slutsky JR. Clinicians' attitudes to clinical practice guidelines: a systematic review. Med J Aust 2002;177(9):502–506.
4. Hoyt DB. Clinical practice guidelines. Am J Surg 1997;173(1):32–34; discussion 35–36.
5. Weingarten S. Translating practice guidelines into patient care: guidelines at the bedside. Chest 2000;118(2 Suppl):4S–7S.
6. Piccirillo JF, Stewart MG, Gliklich RE, Yueh B. Outcomes research primer. Otolaryngol Head Neck Surg 1997;117:380–387.
7. Sabin J, Granoff K, Daniels N. Strengthening the consumer voice in managed care: lessons from independent external review. Psychiatr Serv 2003;54(1):24–28.
8. Guyatt G, Rennie D. User's Guide to Medical Literature: Essentials of Evidence-Based Clinical Practice. Chicago: American Medical Association; 2002.
9. Stewart MG. Outcomes Research in Otolaryngology. Basel, Switzerland: S. Karger; 2004.
10. Paradise JL, Bluestone CD, Bachman RZ, et al. Efficacy of tonsillectomy for recurrent throat infection in severely affected children. Results of parallel randomized and non-randomized clinical trials. N Engl J Med 1984;310(11):674–683.
11. Campbell DT, Fiske DW. Convergent and discriminant validation by the multitrait-multimethod matrix. Psychol Bull 1959;56:81–105.
12. Trochim WM. Research Methods Knowledge Base. Mason, OH: Atomic Dog Publishing.

13. Stinnett SS. Statistical modules. In: Clinical Scholars Program, American Academy of Otolaryngology Head and Neck Surgery; 2004.

14. Dawson B, Trapp RG. Basic and Clinical Biostatistics. 3rd ed. New York: Lange Medical Books/McGraw Hill; 2001.

15. Cochrane Reviewers Handbook. 2001. www.cochrane.org, accessed December 18, 2007.

16. Hulley SB, Cummings SR, Browener WS, Grady D, Hearst N, Newman TB. Designing Clinical Research: An Epidemiological Approach. 2nd ed. Philadelphia: Lippincott Williams & Wilkins; 2001.

17. Sackett D. Bias in analytical research. J Chronic Dis 1979;32(1–2):51–63.

18. Hartmann JM, Forsen JW, Wallace MS, Neely G. Tutorials in clinical research. Part IV. Recognizing and controlling bias. Laryngoscope 2002;112:23–31.

19. Sackett D, et al. Evidence Based Medicine: How to Practice and Teach EBM. 2nd ed. New York: Churchill Livingstone; 2000:261.

20. Ball C, Sackett D, Phillips B, Haynes B, Straus S. Levels of Evidence and Grades of Recommendation. National Health Service Center for Evidence Based Medicine;

1999. www.biomedcentral.com, accessed December 18. 2007.

21. Juni P, Altman DG, Egger M. Systematic reviews in health care: assessing the quality of controlled clinical trials. BMJ 2001;323(7303):42–46.

22. Sterne JA, Egger M, Smith GD. Systematic reviews in health care: investigating and dealing with publication and other biases in meta-analysis. BMJ 2001;323(7304):101–105.

23. Rosenfeld R. How to systematically review the literature. Otolaryngol Head Neck Surg 1996;115(1):53–63.

24. Egger M, Smith GD, Phillips AN. Meta-analysis: principles and procedures. BMJ 1997;315(7121):1533–1537.

25. Egger M, Smith GD. Meta-analysis. Potentials and promise. BMJ 1997;315(7119):1371–1374.

26. Smith GD, Egger M. Meta-analyses of observational data should be done with due care. BMJ 1999;318(7175):56.

27. Sterne JA, Gavaghan D, Egger M. Publication and related bias in meta-analysis: power of statistical tests and prevalence in the literature. J Clin Epidemiol 2000;53(11):1119–1129.

28. Deeks JJ, Dinnes J, D'Amico R, et al. Evaluating nonrandomised intervention studies. Health Technol Assess 2003;7(27):iii–x, 1–173.

29. Rosenfeld R, Bluestone C. Evidence-Based Otitis Media. 1st ed. Hamilton, ON: BC Decker; 1999.

2 How to Use This Book

Jennifer J. Shin and Gregory W. Randolph

THE FORMAT

Our goal is to make evidence-based medicine—even with its heavy reliance on data, statistics, and analyses of clinical trials—as straightforward as possible for the average busy clinician or trainee. Therefore, we provide concise, consistently formatted synopses to maximize rapid accessibility of our systematic reviews. This format usually takes the form of a two-part layout:

1) The first part of this layout consists of a **concise text explanation** (usually 1–2 pages) that describes the data that is relevant to each clinical question. Within this description, there are three sections that describe: a) the methods of the systematic review, b) the results, and c) the clinical significance and suggested future reach directions. *A summary statement begins each section on the clinical significance and future research.*

2) The second part of this layout consists of **tables** that break down and highlight the key points of the relevant studies. The length of the data in tabular format depends on the number of studies that are relevant to each review.

In a select group of systematic reviews, the outcome measures are similar enough and the level of evidence is high enough to allow numerical pooling of the data. When this is the case, a third part is included in the layout for that clinical question. This third part details one or more **meta-analyses**, in which the data from all similar studies is pooled to provide an estimate of the main effect. These analyses include a description of the methods, the results, and a sensitivity analysis.

In addition, we assess the quality of the entire body of relevant data using a color-based rating system that can be understood at a glance. Further details regarding the format of this text, provided below, illustrate and describe our format.

THE PRINCIPLES

First and foremost, we adhere to the principles of a rigorous evidence-based approach. Procedures for systematically reviewing the literature have been carefully refined and are well described [1–4], and we have adhered to these guidelines: We pose focused, well-defined clinical queries, and then thoroughly scrutinize the literature electronically and manually. Unambiguous inclusion and exclusion criteria are utilized when selecting articles relevant to each systematic review. Each criteria-meeting article is then analyzed in terms of its study design and susceptibility to confounders and bias (please see Chapters 1 and 3 for further explanations of these terms). Finally, in addition to this discussion of the credibility of results, the content of the results is presented. These results are presented from each individual study, and if possible, they are also numerically combined.

In addition, we assess the entire body of data that are relevant to a particular clinical query. When doing so, we use a system based on the categories of consensus that have been used in the many previous and current editions of the clinical practice guidelines of the National Comprehensive Cancer Network, an alliance of 19 worldwide leading cancer centers [5]. The use of this system highlights two key aspects of the reviewed studies: the level of the evidence (as determined by the associated study design) and the consensus (or lack thereof) of the individual studies' results. Because we thought it was essential to denote both of these aspects, we chose to adopt a modification of this system, rather than simply use the system that grades an entire body of evidence A through D [6, 7]. Such a system focuses mainly on the levels of evidence available; whereas there is a clear designation for multiple studies of the same level with concurring conclusions, there is less emphasis on ratings for articles of varying levels and inconsistent conclusions. The color-based system addresses this issue and is further described on the subsequent pages.

Layout Part One: The Text

A brief text summary of the relevant data begins each review.

The Chapter Topic Is Shown Here

The clinical query for each systematic review is defined in terms of an intervention and outcome of interest for the patient population.

EVIDENCE METER: For use at a glance, the color indicates both the level and the consistency of evidence currently available to address this clinical query.

Green: There is high-level evidence with uniform results.

Yellow: There is either low–moderate levels of evidence with uniform results or nonuniform results but no major disagreement.

Red: There is major disagreement or only minimal low-level evidence available.

METHODS

The search strategy is described in detail, including the databases accessed, the subject headings or keywords used, and the dates included in the systematic review. Also described are the inclusion and exclusion criteria that ultimately determine which studies are selected. These criteria are determined at the outset of the search, and are designed to encompass all studies relevant to a particular clinical query.

RESULTS

In this section, the content and credibility of the criteria-meeting studies' results are systematically reviewed. This section is broken down into several subsections in order to make the information as easily accessible and understandable as possible.

Outcome Measures. Here, the outcome measures and how they are defined are discussed. This section is particularly important when considering outcome measures that may have some element of variability or when multiple studies use a variety of measures to evaluate the similar outcomes.

Potential Confounders. Potential confounders and the impact they may have on results are described briefly. Further details regarding potential confounders are reported in the adjoining table.

Study Design. The research methodology for the trials is described and the most significant aspects of each are critiqued. Adequacy of follow-up time, the use of masking (blinding patients and physicians to the intervention), and the power given a particular sample size are discussed. In addition, the minimization of bias and confounding through randomization, comparison with a control group, attrition rates, use of an intention to treat analysis, and distinctions between correlation and causation are noted.

Highest Level of Evidence. The results of each trial are described here. When compared groups in high-level trials have significant differences, rate differences and numbers needed to treat are calculated for the reader. The uniformity or nonuniformity of the studies' results are addressed. Also, any limitations imposed by the study designs are addressed.

Applicability. The patient population to which these results apply are described here. This population is defined by the inclusion and exclusion criteria for each study, which are detailed in the adjoining table.

Morbidity/Complications. Any associated perioperative complications and adverse effects of medication are detailed here. If numbers needed to treat could be calculated above, numbers needed to harm are provided when the study data allow.

CLINICAL SIGNIFICANCE AND FUTURE RESEARCH

A brief summary statement begins this section. If a meta-analysis is performed, then this section is moved to follow that later analysis. In this section, the results are placed in their clinical context, both in terms of the particular clinical query and in terms of the chapter subject in general. Expert commentary regarding the evidence and its potential meaning for practice is provided.

Suggestions for future research are also provided. Ways to potentially produce higher-level or more clinically meaningful evidence are proposed. In addition, any study limitations imposed by the disease in question are described.

Layout Part Two: The Tables
The tables highlight key points and facilitate quick comparisons between studies.

The Evidence Condensed: The evidence from each study is described in adjacent tables.

First author, Year of publication	Brief reference information is provided, so that studies may be easily identified in the full bibliography at the end of each review.
Level of evidence (Study design)	The level of evidence and type of study design for each trial is provided to present one quick means of assessment (See chapter 1 for more details regarding leveling of evidence).
Sample size	The number of patients with follow-up is shown (in the context of the original number recruited when relevant) so attrition rates are apparent.
OUTCOMES	
Results of intervention	A numerical summary of the results with the intervention of interest is reported.
Results of control	A numerical summary of the results with a comparison or a control is also noted to place the above results in context.
Measure of statistical significance	The presence or absence of a statistically significant difference between the above results is noted. Since "p-values" are most familiar to the majority of readers, we typically report these values.
Conclusion	The final conclusion of each study is summarized. In other words, **the brief bottom line for each study is here**.
Follow-up time	The results are always presented in the context of the reported follow-up time.
STUDY DESIGN	
Inclusion criteria	The inclusion criteria are described according to the original report so the applicability of results can be determined.
Exclusion criteria	The exclusion criteria are described so it is clear that the results may not apply to all patients.
Patient characteristics	Further relevant details regarding the patient population are provided, such as age or stage of disease.
Study regimens	The regimen for the intervention and control is provided in detail so it may be easily reproduced by a practitioner.
Outcome measure in detail	Details regarding the outcome measure are provided, so that it is clear exactly how investigators tabulated any ambiguities.
Potential confounders	Multiple rows of potential confounders are detailed so as to make clear how well they were addressed by each study.
Further study details	There are also multiple rows of additional relevant study details such as compliance and criteria for withdrawal.
Details of analysis	Any concerns regarding the analysis, such as whether an intention to treat analysis was performed, are also detailed.
Morbidity/complications	The adverse effects of medications and any perioperative complications that are reported are also tabulated.

Layout Part Three: Meta-analyses

In a select group of systematic reviews, numerical meta-analyses are performed.

META-ANALYSIS

In a select group of systematic reviews, the outcome measures are similar enough and the level of evidence is high enough to allow numerical pooling of the data. When this is the case, an additional part is included in the analysis. This part details the meta-analysis of the data, which statistically combines the data from all relevant studies to provide an estimate of the main effect. The data that are pooled and the methods used to pool them are shown. Analyses were performed using the random effects model with inverse variance or Mantel Haenszel weights, using the Comprehensive Meta-Analysis or Stata statistical software packages. In addition, a sensitivity analysis is performed to show how or if results change with various circumstances. Any potential effect of publication bias (a bias that usually favors publication of positive studies, i.e., reports showing a significant difference between an intervention and control) is addressed by determining the hypothetical impact of a number of negative studies.

Each meta-analysis is described with text and tables. Tables show the pooling of data and the relative results of each included study.

Additional Materials

REFERENCES

There is a full bibliography listing all cited references at the conclusion of each review.

HIGHLIGHTS

In certain clinical queries, highlights from the evidence or associated clinical knowledge are featured. Relevant epidemiology, staging systems for disease, and procedure classifications are among the information provided here.

Authors' note: Our goal has been to provide thorough, concise, factual, systematic reviews of the range of clinical queries regarding the management of otolaryngological disease. In order to achieve this goal, we have collectively reviewed over 20,000 articles and *a priori* developed the "Evidence Condensed" format (© Shin, Hartnick, Randolph, 2003) to maximize rapid accessibility of the most relevant and highest quality data. There are, however, several imperfections in this work. First, our systematic reviews have been performed as close to our publication date as possible, but because of the logistics involved in completing, coordinating, and then finally publishing such a large number of reviews, some were performed earlier than others. All reviews are dated, however, so that the reader can easily determine the timing of the search. In addition, the search strategy and inclusion/exclusion criteria are provided so that the interested reader can reproduce it in a future database to see if any further relevant studies have been published since our review. Second, our reviews have been limited to studies available in the English language. It is an admittedly ethnocentric approach, but one that was thought necessary to balance the challenges and limited resources available to produce this initial unique data-rich publication. It is, however, a situation we hope to remedy in future editions where we will have a larger foundation and an even more international authorship. Third, in the vast majority of clinical queries within our field, the number of relevant articles is manageable enough to permit discussion of all relevant studies. In a minority of cases, however, there is an overabundance of evidence, with a plethora of studies addressing the same topic, but few studies reporting very high level data. In these cases, we have focused our reviews on that highest level of evidence, according to the "Best Evidence" approach. Such cases are clearly described in the methods section. In cases where there is an overabundance of evidence with non-uniform consensus, if the study designs and outcomes are similar enough, and if the level of evidence is high enough, a meta-analysis is reported to obtain an estimate of the overall effect.

REFERENCES

1. Juni P, Altman DG, Egger M. Systematic reviews in health care: assessing the quality of controlled clinical trials. BMJ 2001;323(7303):42–46.
2. Sterne JA, Egger M, Smith GD. Systematic reviews in health care: investigating and dealing with publication and other biases in meta-analysis. BMJ 2001;323(7304):101–105.
3. Rosenfeld R. How to systematically review the literature. Otolaryngol Head Neck Surg 1996;115(1):53–63.
4. Sackett D, et al. Evidence Based Medicine: How to Practice and Teach EBM. 2nd ed. New York: Churchill Livingstone; 2000:261.
5. National Comprehensive Cancer Network. Categories of consensus. In: Practice Guidelines in Oncology; 2002. www.nccn.org/professionals/physician_gls/f_guidelines.asp, accessed December 18, 2007.
6. Ball C, Sackett D, Phillips B, Haynes B, Straus S. Levels of Evidence and Grades of Recommendation. National Health Service Center for Evidence Based Medicine; 1999. www.biomedcentral.com, accessed December 18, 2007.
7. Rosenfeld R. Evidence, outcomes, and common sense. Otolaryngol Head Neck Surg 2001;124(2):123–124.

3 English Translations of Statistical Terms, Study Designs, and Methods of Analysis

Jennifer J. Shin, Christopher J. Hartnick, and Sandra S. Stinnett

This chapter contains plain-language summaries of statistical terms, study designs, and methods of analysis. To provide the quickest access to terms, they are arranged in alphabetical order under each of these three headings. In keeping with our goal of trying to present information in a format that is easily accessible for readers, we have broken down each explanation into parts, using the following templates:

Statistical term	Study design	Methods/Analyses
What it is:	What it is:	What it is:
What it means:	What caliber of	In addition, headers
The theoretical	evidence it	specific to the
"best possible"	provides:	terms are
value is:	What can/cannot	provided, such as:
The theoretical	be concluded	Why it's useful;
"worst possible"	from results	How to prevent
value is:	of this study	it; and Statistical
How to calculate it:	design:	summary
For example:	Key elements	
Related terms:	to critique:	

STATISTICAL TERMS

Absolute Risk Increase

What it is: It is the absolute difference in the rate of an undesired outcome with versus without a particular intervention. It answers the question: How much did you increase undesired outcomes by intervening?

What it means: A high absolute risk increase (ARI) suggests that the intervention's undesired effect is strong, whereas a low ARI suggests that the undesired effect is weak.

The theoretical "best possible" value is: 0% or 0.00. This would mean that the intervention resulted in no increase in an undesired effect. Even better, an intervention may result in a decrease in an undesired effect; such a favorable impact, however, is expressed in terms of an absolute risk reduction (ARR).

The theoretical "worst possible" value is: 100% or 1.00. This would mean that with the intervention, all patients had the undesired effect, whereas without it no one had the undesired effect.

How to calculate it: Step 1. Calculate the rate difference = (percent of treated patients with the undesired outcome) − (percent of control patients with the unde-

sired outcome). Step 2. Take the absolute value of Step 1, i.e., if there is a negative sign, delete it.

For example: If 20% of people without intervention turn purple, but 50% of people with intervention turn purple, then the ARI of turning purple with versus without intervention is 50% − 20% = 30%.

Related terms: rate difference, absolute risk reduction, number needed to treat

Absolute Risk Reduction

What it is: It is the absolute difference in the rate of an undesired outcome without versus with a particular intervention. It answers the question: How much did you reduce undesired outcomes by intervening?

What it means: A high ARR suggests that the intervention's desired effect is strong, whereas a low ARR suggests that the effect is weak.

The theoretical "best possible" value is: 100% or 1.00. This would mean that without the intervention, all patients experienced the undesired outcome, but that with the intervention, all of the patients were spared.

The theoretical "worst possible" value is: 0% or 0.00. This would mean that the intervention has no effect on the occurrence of the undesired outcome. Even worse, an intervention may increase the risk of an undesired outcome; such a poor impact, however, is expressed in terms of an ARI.

How to calculate it: Step 1. Calculate the rate difference = (percent of treated patients with the undesired outcome) − (percent of control patients with the undesired outcome). Step 2. Take the absolute value of Step 1 (i.e., if there is a negative sign, delete it).

For example: If 20% of people without intervention turn into pumpkins, but 5% of people with intervention turn into pumpkins, then the ARR of turning into a pumpkin with versus without intervention is 15% (5% − 20% = −15%, the absolute value of which is 15%). Also, in a meta-analysis of the impact of dexamethasone on post-tonsillectomy emesis, the ARR was determined to be 25% (Chapter 4.C.1). This means that the patients who received steroids had 25% fewer episodes of emesis than controls.

Related terms: rate difference, ARI, number needed to treat

Adverse Event

What it is: An adverse event is defined by the Food and Drug Administration as any incident in which the use of a medication, medical device, or nutritional product is suspected to have resulted in an adverse outcome in a patient. It is defined by the National Cancer Institute as any unfavorable experience associated with the use of a medical treatment or procedure, regardless of attribution.

Alpha Level

What it is: It is a way of referring to a type 1 error. It is the level of "significance" of a statistical test that is specified before conducting an analysis. See also "Type 1 Error."

Attrition Bias

What it is: A type of bias that occurs because too many patients do not complete the study.

Why it is bad: If only 1% of the patients complete follow-up, the results from the other 99% patients could have easily outweighed the results from the returning 1%, so the real result remains unknown.

How to check for it: Compare the number of patients who completed the trial with the number of patients who started the trial. If the number completing the trial is <80% of the number who started, then the study may be subject to attrition bias.

Beta Level

What it is: It is a way of referring to a type 2 error. See also "Type 2 Error."

Bias

What it is: An error in the technique of selecting subjects, performing procedures, measuring a characteristic, or analyzing and reporting data.

What it isn't: Bias does not imply stubbornness or willful deceit as in colloquial speech.

Why it is bad: These types of errors can create misleading results.

How to prevent it: Preventative measures depend on the specific type of bias that needs to be controlled. Please see related terms: attrition bias, selection bias, performance bias, detection bias, expectation bias.

Binary Variable

What it is: Another term for dichotomous variable. See also "Dichotomous Variable."

Blinding

What it is: It is a way of preventing the participants and investigators in a trial from knowing whether they are assigned to treatment or control. In a **double-blind** study, neither the subjects nor the clinicians know whether they are receiving treatment or placebo. If only the subjects or only the clinicians are unaware of their study group assignment, then it is a **single-blind** study.

Why it is useful: It helps to eliminate expectation bias, whereby expecting a certain result influences the result itself. Trials that are double-blinded are less likely than nonblinded studies to demonstrate a false treatment effect.

Bottle Method

What it is: A method to assess compliance with a study medication.

How it is done: Look in the bottle and see if the number of pills that are left is more than the number that should be left.

Calendar Method

What it is: A method to assess compliance with a study medication.

How it is done: Compare the number of doses prescribed with the number of doses of medication that the patient said they took.

Case-Control Study

What it is: In this study design, groups who have and do not have a particular outcome are compared. The subjects who have the outcome of interest constitute the "case" group. The subjects who do not have the outcome of interest constitute the "control" group. The "cases" and the "controls" are compared to see if one had different exposure(s) than the other.

For example: Charts of patients who are alive ("cases") or dead ("controls") with T2N0 oral tongue carcinoma who underwent primary surgical treatment (otherwise similar in most respects) were reviewed to determine whether supraomohyoid or modified radical neck dissections (different exposures) were performed more frequently in either group.

What caliber of evidence it provides: Level 3—retrospective studies with an internal control.

What can be concluded from results of this study design: It can be used to show relationships (correlations, if numerical data allow) and generate hypotheses for higher-level study. This method may prove especially useful when rare diseases or conditions requiring prolonged follow-up preclude the use of prospective trials.

What cannot be concluded from results of this study design: It usually cannot prove that the exposure caused or preceded the outcome.

Key elements to critique: Ideally, when the study is set up, the "controls" should match the "cases" in every respect except for the outcome of interest. If the groups are similar in most respects, then any differences in exposure are more likely to be associated with the difference in outcome. Also important is how specifically the exposure is defined, the length of follow-up, the sample size.

Don't get fooled by: A case-control study is different from a comparison of historical cohorts. With historical cohorts, subjects are grouped based on whether or not they had a particular *exposure* (versus a case-control study where they are grouped based on whether or not they had an *outcome*) and followed forward in time to see what outcomes develop.

Case Series

What it is: It is an observational, descriptive account of characteristics observed in a group of patients. There is no control group.

For example: Seventy patients with ectodermal dysplasia were evaluated to determine what proportion had various otologic manifestations.

What caliber of evidence it provides: Level 4.

What can be concluded from results of this study design: Case series can be used to show relationships (correlations, if numerical data allow) and generate hypotheses for higher-level study.

What cannot be concluded from results of this study design: They cannot prove cause and effect.

Key elements to critique: Ideally: 1) consecutive patients are reported; 2) strict inclusion/exclusion and diagnostic criteria are used to identify and evaluate the patients included in the study; 3) the assessment of outcomes was consistent among patients; 4) follow-up was long enough for the outcome of interest; a dose-response gradient can be demonstrated for certain treatments; 5) results are similar to other case series regarding the same topic.

Cohort

What it is: A group of persons with similar characteristics who are observed together from a certain time point and afterward. A cohort in a prospective study is followed from the initiation of the study and afterward. A cohort in a retrospective study is followed from the initiation of a particular intervention and afterward in the chart.

Cohort Study

What it is: A study that identifies groups ("cohorts") with and without an exposure. These cohorts are then followed forward in time to see what outcomes develop.

For example: Patients with T2N0 floor-of-mouth carcinoma who underwent surgical treatment including either supraomohyoid or modified radical neck dissection (exposures compared) were followed to see whether 5-year survival rates (outcomes) were different.

What caliber of evidence it provides: Level 2 (usually). A cohort study is typically a prospective study. However, it can be performed retrospectively by defining exposure groups and examining medical records to follow patients forward in time to determine outcomes (level 3 data if a control group is also followed).

What can be concluded from results of this study design: A single exposure's effect on multiple outcomes can be determined. In addition, the sequence of events can usually be established. This study may yield information about incidence and relative risk (RR).

What cannot be concluded from results of this study design: Usually, a nonrandomized study cannot control for all confounders.

Key elements to critique: First, it is important to determine how well potential confounders were balanced between the exposed group and unexposed group; if the

groups being compared were radically different beyond whether they had or did not have the exposure of interest, then they may be biased toward a certain outcome that could falsely be attributed to the exposure or lack thereof. Second, the methods of data collection and steps taken to minimize expectation bias are key. The use of blinding during outcome measurement, for example, can be very useful. Third, ideally all patients are accounted for at the conclusion of the study. If only cherry-picked patient data are presented, the results are not as compelling as they would be if consecutive patients are presented. Fourth, the length and quality of time after the exposure must also be considered. Fifth, the sample size must be large enough to provide adequate power to detect any difference that may truly exist.

Don't get confused by: A retrospective study can still contain a cohort. A cohort in a prospective study is followed from the initiation of the study and afterward in time. A cohort in a retrospective study is followed from the initiation of a particular intervention and afterward in the chart. A retrospective cohort is also referred to as a "historical cohort."

Compliance

What it is: It is a measure of how much of the study treatment the subjects actually received.

Confidence Interval

What it is: It is a description of the amount of uncertainty in a measurement. In more specific but technical terms, it is a range of values (computed from sample observations) that would contain the true population value with a specified probability on repeated sampling.

What it means: A wide confidence interval means that the uncertainty is high and the precision is low. A narrow confidence interval implies the converse. A 95% confidence interval implies that if the calculation was performed again and again, then 95% of the confidence intervals would be expected to contain the true population value.

What it does not mean: A 95% confidence interval does *not* mean that there is a 95% chance that the true value lies within that interval.

The theoretical "best possible" value is: A range of 0.

The theoretical "worst possible" value is: A range of infinity.

How to calculate it: There are several computer programs available (even simple spreadsheets such as Microsoft Excel) that can help you. A confidence interval is computed as the sample estimate (such as a mean or proportion) plus or minus a critical value times the standard error. The critical value is the value of the theoretical distribution the parameter is assumed to follow that implies the percentage desired (such as 95%).

Application: A confidence interval gives all the estimates that would be "accepted" if a hypothesis test was

21

UHB TRUST LIBRARY
QEH

performed. Values outside the interval would be rejected. One of the most useful features of confidence intervals is that if 95% confidence intervals are shown for two compared values, then by convention, any overlap in the intervals suggests that there is no significant difference between the compared values.

For example: A 95% confidence interval of 2.4% to 10.4% means that one of such intervals would contain the population value 95% of the time upon repeated sampling.

Related terms: null hypothesis, p value

Confounder

What it is: A potential confounder is a factor that can cause the same outcome as the intervention of interest. A factor is said to be confounded with another factor if it is impossible to discern which of the two is responsible for the observed effect.

For example: Consider studying the impact of antibiotics on postoperative pain. Other factors besides antibiotics—such as surgical technique, anesthetic regimen, and use of steroids—may also influence postoperative pain, and could confound the results.

Why it is bad: When confounders are present, a singular cause and effect cannot be demonstrated. With confounding, a measure of the effect of the intervention under investigation is distorted because of the presence of other potential causes of the same effect.

How to prevent it: A high-quality study will try to eliminate confounders or at least carefully account for them. Randomization is one way of carefully accounting for confounders, by ensuring that they are at least balanced in the two groups being compared. Confounders can also be addressed in the data analysis.

Continuous Variable

What it is: Values defined by continuous variables are numeric with an inherent order and the incremental differences between numbers are equal.

For example: Weight, oxygen saturation.

Statistical summarization: Means with standard deviations or medians with ranges.

Statistical analysis: Pearson correlation coefficients, paired or independent *t* tests, and analyses of variance.

Control Group

What it is: A control group is used to provide a measure of what happens without the intervention. This control measure allows comparison of the intervention group to a group that is ideally similar in every other way.

Why it is useful: The use of a control group can be an effective way to thwart many biases.

Correlation Bias

What it is: It is a type of bias that may occur when correlation is equated with causation.

Example: In a retrospective study of survival rates in patients treated with or without chemotherapy, it may be that chemotherapy is correlated with worse survival rates. This does not, however, mean that chemotherapy causes death. It may simply be that chemotherapy was recommended in more advanced cases.

Correlation Coefficient

What it is: It is a measure of the linear relationship between two numerical measurements made on the same set of subjects. It answers the question: Is a change in one variable associated with a change in another variable?

What it means: A value of more than +0.75 suggests a strong positive relationship between the two variables; as one increases, so does the other. A value of less than −0.75 suggests a strong negative relationship between the two variables; as one increases, the other decreases. Remember, however, that correlation does not imply causation.

The theoretical "strongest possible" value is: −1 or +1. A value of −1 indicates a perfect negative linear relationship; as one variable increases, another decreases. A value of +1 indicates a perfect positive relationship; as one variable increases, another increases.

The theoretical "weakest possible" value is: 0. A value of 0 means there is no linear relationship between the two variables.

How to calculate it: Use a computer program or call a statistician. The Pearson product-moment correlation coefficient is dependent on the means and standard deviations of the two variables; it is used for continuous variables. Spearman's rank correlation uses the means and standard deviations of the ranks of the values and is used for ordinal variables or for numerical values with outliers.

For example: A correlation coefficient of 0–0.25 suggests little or no relationship, 0.25–0.50 suggests a fair relationship, 0.50–0.75 suggests a moderate relationship, and >0.75 suggests a good relationship.

Related terms: linear regression

Crossover Study

What it is: In this study design, treatments are swapped halfway through the study. At the beginning, one group receives a treatment medication whereas the other group receives placebo (or alternative treatment) and results are determined. Then, the placebo group (or alternative treatment) begins medication and vice versa and results are determined again.

For example: To determine the impact of erythromycin on recurrent acute otitis media, children in group A received erythromycin, whereas group B received placebo for 2 months. Then, after a "washout" period of 2 weeks during which both groups received no treatment, group A received placebo whereas group B received erythromycin.

What caliber of evidence it provides: Level 1 or 2. In a level 1 crossover study, patients are randomized to treatment medication or placebo/alternative treatment and then crossed over to the opposite treatment midway through the trial. If patients are not initially randomized to their treatment groups, then a crossover study provides level 2 data.

What can/cannot be concluded from results of this study design: This study design allows for direct comparison of treatment and no treatment (or alternative treatment) in the same individuals.

Key elements to critique: A "washout" period when both groups receive neither medication nor placebo is sandwiched between the two treatment periods may prevent lingering effects of medication from altering the results of the post-crossover portion of the trial. The follow-up time in each arm, masking of the patients and caregivers to which treatment is received, and the attrition rate may all affect the strength of the study.

Cross-Sectional Study

What it is: This observational, descriptive study looks at a population at a single point in time. The exposures and outcomes of interest are measured at this one point.

What caliber of evidence it provides: Level 4. It can only show the burden of disease at that given point in time.

What can be concluded from results of this study design: It can be used to generate hypotheses for further study.

What cannot be concluded from results of this study design: No temporal relationship between an exposure and outcome can be determined.

Key elements to critique: Because this study design only looks at a single point in time and no temporal relationship can be determined, the key element to consider is that conclusions from the study should be limited to generating hypotheses for additional study.

Descriptive Study

What it is: It is an observational, nonanalytic study.

For example: Examples of descriptive studies include case series, case reports, and cross-sectional studies.

What caliber of evidence it provides: Usually descriptive studies provide level 4 evidence.

What can be concluded from results of this study design: These studies describe patterns of disease, defining who is affected, and when and where the incidence is highest. These studies are useful for generating hypotheses for higher-level study.

What cannot be concluded from results of this study design: These studies cannot prove cause and effect or a temporal relationship between an exposure and the disease.

Key elements to critique: Ideally, consecutive patients are reported and strict inclusion/exclusion and diagnostic criteria are used to identify and evaluate the patients included in the study.

Detection Bias

What it is: It is a type of bias that occurs if there is a partiality when assessing the outcomes.

Example: See "Expectation Bias."

How to prevent it: Blind subjects and investigators to treatment groups.

Dichotomous Variable

What it is: A dichotomous or binary variable is a particular type of nominal variable that has only two possible categories.

For example: Gender, yes/no.

Statistical summarization: Odds ratio, RR, or rate difference (RD). An RD, also referred to as an absolute risk reduction, is a particularly useful measure, because it can also be used to calculate the number needed to treat (NNT). See also "Rate Difference," "Odds Ratio," "Relative Risk," "Number Needed to Treat."

Efficacy

What it is: The efficacy of an intervention refers to whether it works in a defined population under ideal controlled circumstances.

How it is established: Efficacy is established in a controlled clinical trial.

Effectiveness

What it is: The effectiveness of an intervention refers to whether it works in regular clinical practice.

How it is established: Effectiveness is often demonstrated in prospective, nonrandomized studies.

Expectation Bias

What it is: It is a type of bias that occurs when expecting that a certain result can influence the result itself.

Example: Patients receiving treatment for postoperative pain might expect to have less pain than the control group. This expectation alone can actually result in less pain.

How to prevent it: This expectation bias can be eliminated by administering a placebo to the control group and blinding both patients and physicians.

Floor Effect

What it is: It occurs when the amount of potential recovery is dependent on the severity of the initial presentation. When this is the case, a simple arithmetic change in scale is not a sufficient measure of results.

For example: When measuring audiometric outcomes, the amount of potential recovery is dependent on the amount of initial hearing loss; a 30-decibel (dB) loss can only improve 30 dB, whereas a 120-dB loss has much more room for improvement. Accordingly, a 30-dB improvement in a patient with a 30-dB loss constitutes full recovery, but a 30-dB improvement in a patient with a 120-dB loss still leaves the patient with a profound hearing loss.

How to manage it: Investigators can address this "floor effect" by measuring the percent recovered or by considering patients with more severe initial presentations in a distinct analysis.

Incidence

What it is: The proportion of new cases in the population at risk in a specified period of time.

Related terms: prevalence

Instrument

What it is: It is a rigorously tested survey tool, used to measure patient-reported outcomes.

Why it is useful: A validated instrument has been tested to ensure that the following are true: 1) it measures what it is intended to measure (*convergent validity*, i.e., scores on a valid test of arithmetic skills correlate with scores on other math tests), 2) it does not inadvertently measure irrelevant changes (*discriminant validity*, i.e., scores on a valid test of arithmetic do not correlate with scores on tests of verbal ability), its scores are stable (*reliability*, i.e., a patient with the same disease impact will continue to have the same response), and 4) it is sensitive to change (*responsiveness*, i.e., a patient with a change in disease impact will have a changed score). Overall, this means that the validated instrument does in fact measure what it is meant to measure when it is administered to the intended population.

Intention to Treat Analysis

What it is: In an intention to treat analysis, results are reported in terms of the originally assigned treatment groups regardless of whatever happened to subjects subsequent to their enrollment in the trial.

Why it is useful: An intention to treat analysis minimizes bias in the analysis of results because it preserves the benefits of randomization. It prevents the exclusion of treatment failures and ensures that all patients who had follow-up are included in the analysis.

For example: In a trial in which patients undergo radiation therapy versus surgical resection for laryngeal carcinoma, the survival outcome for a patient who was originally treated with radiation should be included with the data for the radiation therapy group, even if that patient subsequently required surgical salvage.

Level of Evidence

What they are: Evidence levels provide a quick way to rate the caliber of evidence, based on study designs.

Level 1 Randomized controlled trial (RCT) or a meta-analysis of RCTs

Level 2 Prospective (cohort or outcomes) study with an internal control group or a meta-analysis of prospective controlled studies

Level 3 Retrospective (case-control) study with an internal control group or a meta-analysis of retrospective controlled studies

Level 4 Case series (retrospective reviews, uncontrolled cohort) without an internal control group

Level 5 Expert opinion without explicit critical appraisal or on the basis of physiology or bench research alone

Please also see the individual study designs.

Masking

What it is: Masking is a term used to refer to the use of blinding. Also see "Blinding."

Meta-Analysis

What it is: It is a method of quantitatively combining the results from several independent studies of the same outcome. All of the data are statistically pooled in order to provide an estimate of the overall effect of the intervention under review.

What caliber of evidence it provides: It depends on the level of evidence of included studies. Meta-analyses usually incorporate the results of RCTs, yielding level 1 evidence. Meta-analyses may also be performed on levels 2 or 3 data as well, which can yield level 2 or 3 results.

What can be concluded from results of this study design: Meta-analysis can provide a summary effect estimate, which is essentially an average effect that is weighted by the size of each study, and sometimes by the quality of each study. The strength of the meta-analysis, however, is only as good as the strength of the individual study designs.

What cannot be concluded from results of this study design: Meta-analysis cannot provide a meaningful result with data from studies with major clinical differences in design. Again, the strength of the meta-analysis is only as much as the strength of the individual study designs, and meta-analyses of observational studies (i.e., case series, case-control studies, cohort studies, and cross-sectional studies) must be viewed with caution because of the high potential for confounding influences. As noted by one of our chapter authors, misconceptions can be magnified when poor data are added to poor data.

Key elements to critique: The appropriateness of combining the studies and the individual quality of the included studies are key. It is appropriate to combine results if the studies have similar interventions, outcome measurements, and controls (i.e., homogeneous studies). It is inappropriate to combine results of studies with major clinical differences (i.e., heterogeneous studies), which may result in fundamentally different results.

Negative Predictive Value

What it is: This value defines how often a negative test result is correct. Of values that test negative, the negative predictive value (NPV) defines the proportion of values that is actually negative.

What it means: It is a measure of how much you can trust a negative test result.

The theoretical "best possible" value is: 1.00 or 100%. This means that a negative result is always correct.

The theoretical "worst possible" value is: 0.00 or 0%. This means that a negative result is never correct.

How to calculate it: An estimate is provided by NPV = true negatives/(false negatives + true negatives).

	Positive for disease	*Negative for disease*
Positive test result	True positives	False positives
Negative test result	False negatives	True negatives

Many statisticians will further modify this number based on the prevalence of the disease (Bayes theorem).

For example: The NPV of preoperative coagulation testing for post-tonsillectomy bleeding is 0.92 or 92% (see Chapter 4.D). This means that 92% of children who have a negative (normal) test will not bleed postoperatively.

Related terms: positive predictive value, sensitivity, specificity

Nominal Variable

What it is: These variables describe discrete categories with no order.

For example: Color or shape. A triangle, circle, and pentagon are clearly defined, but do not have an inherent order as no shape has more inherent value than the other.

Statistical summarization: Proportions, percentages, and ratios.

Statistical analysis: McNemar's, kappa, Fisher's exact, and chi-square.

Null Hypothesis

What it is: The null hypothesis states that there is no difference between the groups being compared.

Why it is important: Most studies are set up to test the null hypothesis against an alternative hypothesis that postulates a nonzero difference between groups.

Number Needed to Harm

What it is: It measures the number of patients who need to undergo a particular intervention in order for one patient to see an undesired effect. It answers the question: How many people can I treat so that only one patient has a harmful side effect?

What it means: A high number needed to harm (NNH) suggests that the intervention's undesired effect is weak, whereas a low NNH suggests that the undesired effect is strong. A high NNH means your patients have less risk of adverse effects of treatment. It is often helpful to consider NNH in the context of the NNT; if the NNT is far greater than the NNH, then it suggests that the potential for benefit from the intervention outweighs the potential for adverse effects.

The theoretical "best possible" value is: Infinity. This would mean that an infinite number of patients could be treated and only a single patient would experience an adverse effect.

The theoretical "worst possible" value is: One. This would mean that every patient who had a particular intervention would experience an adverse effect.

How to calculate it: NNH = 1/ARI

For example: According to one study, 3.9% of children have persistent tympanic membrane perforations after tympanostomy tube placement (see Chapter 6.D). This reported ARI allows us to calculate that 1/0.039 = 26 children is the NNH. This means that 1 child in 26 experienced a persistent perforation.

Related terms: absolute risk increase, rate difference, number needed to treat

Number Needed to Treat

What it is: It measures the number of patients who need to undergo a particular intervention in order for one patient to see a desired effect. It answers the question: How many people do I need to treat so that one of them will benefit?

What it means: A high NNT suggests that the intervention's desired effect is weak, whereas a low NNT suggests that the effect is strong. A low NNT means you and your patients get more bang for your buck. It is often helpful to consider NNT in the context of the NNH; if the NNT is far greater than the NNH, then it suggests that the potential for benefit from the intervention outweighs the potential for adverse effects.

The theoretical "best possible" value is: One. This would mean that every patient who had a particular intervention would experience the desired benefit.

The theoretical "worst possible" value is: Infinity. This would mean that an infinite number of patients would have to be treated before a single patient would experience a benefit.

How to calculate it: NNT = 1/ARR

For example: To prevent one child from having post-tonsillectomy emesis, four children must receive dexamethasone (Chapter 4.C.1). This means that 3 of 4 children will receive dexamethasone but have no decrease in emesis.

Related terms: absolute risk reduction, rate difference, number needed to harm

Odds

What it is: It is the probability that an event will occur divided by the probability that it will not occur.

What it means: It answers the question: How much more likely is it that the event will happen, rather than not happen?

The theoretical "best possible" value: Depends on whether the event is desired or undesired. If the event is desired, then the theoretical best possible value is infinity. If the event is undesired, then the theoretical best possible value is 0.

The theoretical "worst possible" value: Depends on whether the event is desired or undesired. If the event is desired, then the theoretical worst possible value is 0. If the event is undesired, then the theoretical worst possible value is infinity.

How to calculate it: Odds = (probability that an event will occur)/(the probability that an event will not occur). Stated differently, odds = (proportion with an event)/[1 − (proportion with an event)].

For example: The probability that evidence-based medicine will become a permanent part of medical education and practice is 99%. The probability that it will not become permanently integrated is 1%. Therefore, the odds are 99:1 that evidence-based medicine is here to stay.

Related terms: odds ratio

Odds compared to proportion:

Proportion	Odds
0.01	0.01
0.02	0.02
0.03	0.03
0.04	0.04
0.05	0.05
0.10	0.11
0.20	0.25
0.30	0.43
0.40	0.67
0.50	1.00
0.60	1.50
0.70	2.33
0.80	4.00
0.90	9.00
0.95	19.00
0.96	24.00
0.97	32.33
0.98	49.00
0.99	99.00

Odds Ratio.

What it is: At the risk of being redundant, we'll define this as the ratio of two odds: it is the odds that one group had an outcome divided by the odds that another group had the same outcome. In a case-control study, it is the odds that the cases had an exposure divided by the odds that the controls had the same exposure.

What it means: It is a way of comparing whether the probability of a certain event is the same for two groups. It answers the question: How much more likely was the outcome in one group compared with another? In a case-control study, it answers the question: How much more likely was the exposure in cases than in controls?

The theoretical "best possible" value: Depends on whether it is desirable to have the risk factor associated with the outcome of interest. If an association is desirable, then the theoretical best possible value is infinity. If an association is undesired, then the theoretical best possible value is 1.

The theoretical "worst possible" value: Depends on whether it is desirable to have the risk factor associated with the outcome of interest. If an association is desirable, then the theoretical worst possible value is 1. If an association is undesired, then the theoretical worst possible value is infinity.

How to calculate it: Odds ratio = odds for cases/odds for controls = $[A/N_{cases}/C/N_{cases}]/[B/N_{controls}/D/N_{controls}]$ = $[A/C]/[B/D]$

	Cases	Controls
Had exposure	A	B
Did not have exposure	C	D
	N_{cases}	$N_{controls}$

For example: Suppose that cases are patients with throat cancer and controls are patients with other throat disorders, but not cancer. Suppose that exposure is use of smokeless tobacco in the past. The odds of having used smokeless tobacco in the cases is A/C. The odds of having used smokeless tobacco in the controls is B/D. The ratio of the odds gives how much more likely the cases were to have used smokeless tobacco than were the controls.

For other study designs, the exposure groups would be chosen initially and patients would be followed to determine the outcome. In this case, the odds of the outcome in the exposure group is A/B and the odds of the outcome in the nonexposed group is C/D. Then the odds ratio is $[A/B]/[C/D]$. This gives how much more likely the exposed group was to have the outcome than was the unexposed group.

Related terms: odds, relative risk

Ordinal Variable

What it is: Values defined by ordinal variables are categorical with an inherent order, but incremental differences between adjacent categories are not necessarily equal.

For example: To use the tumor staging example, a T2N1M0 parotid tumor is in a well-defined category. Such a tumor is also clearly less worrisome than a T4N3M1 tumor, because there is an inherent order to the staging. The difference between a T2 and a T3 tumor, however, is not the same as the difference between a T3 and T4 tumor, because incremental differences between categories are not necessarily equal. Another example of an ordinal variable is the House-Brackmann classification system for facial paralysis.

Statistical summarization: Medians with ranges or proportions and percentages.

Statistical analysis: Spearman correlation coefficients, kappa statistics, signed rank tests, Wilcoxon rank sum tests, and Kruskal-Wallis tests.

Outcomes Research

What it is: It is research designed specifically to evaluate patient-based outcomes and the effectiveness of treatment in regular clinical practice (i.e., nontrial conditions).

What caliber of evidence it provides: Level 2 or 3, depending on whether it is prospective or retrospective.

What can/cannot be concluded from the results of this research: It depends to a large extent on the individual study design. Ideally, it provides data regarding clinical endpoints, functional status, and/or quality of life (QOL).

Key elements to critique: Given that so many outcomes studies address patients' own assessments of their medical care, the method of assessment is a key element. Ideally, a validated survey tool called an instrument is utilized (see "Instrument"). In addition, each individual study should be evaluated according to its study design.

Outset

What it is: This is just another way to say "at the beginning of the study" or "before the intervention occurred."

When it is used: Typically, it is used when comparing patient characteristics in a control group and in an intervention group. What you want is for both groups to be similar at the outset, so that differences in outcome can be attributed solely to the presence or absence of the intervention.

p Value

What it is: It is a measure of support for a hypothesis being tested. More specifically, it is the probability of obtaining the observed result (value of a test statistic), or a result that is more extreme, when the null hypothesis (i.e., there is no difference between groups) is true.

What it means: It describes how often we would expect the result we got. A lower p value corresponds to lower support for the null hypothesis, with a p value ≤ 0.05 traditionally thought to be so low that it disproves the null hypothesis and shows a "significant" difference. In more technical terms, the p value indicates probability or area under the curve (distribution) being used for the hypothesis test, for distributions such as the normal and t-distributions. Differences in values of the test statistic on the x-axis correspond to differences in areas under the curve of the distribution on the y-axis. A p value is the area in one or both of the tails of the distribution since those areas correspond to "extreme" results.

What theoretical extreme values mean: If you wished to find significance, then a small p value would be "best." If you did not wish to find significance, then a large p value might be considered "best." However, not finding a significant result does not necessarily imply that a "significant difference" does not exist; it may just mean that with your sample and its size, you could not attain significance.

How to calculate it: A p value is the result of a statistical test. Use an appropriate statistical test for the hypothesis you wish to test. p values corresponding to that test may be found via computer output or in statistical tables.

Related terms: alpha-level, hypothesis test

Performance Bias

What it is: It is a type of bias that occurs when there are inconsistencies in the care that is provided or exposure to other factors apart from the intervention of interest.

Example: In a study of the impact of a medicine on general postoperative pain, results would be tainted by performance bias if only patients undergoing myringot-

omy were chosen to receive treatment whereas only patients undergoing composite resection with free flap were used as controls.

How to prevent it: Randomization of subjects to treatment groups, or other means of balancing potential confounders between groups.

Positive Predictive Value

What it is: This value defines how often a positive test result is correct. Of values that test positive, the proportion of values that is actually positive.

What it means: It is a measure of how much you can trust a positive test result.

The theoretical "best possible" value is: 1.00 or 100%. This means that a positive result is always correct.

The theoretical "worst possible" value is: 0.00 or 0%. This means that a positive result is never correct.

How to calculate it: An estimate is provided by positive predictive value (PPV) = true positives/(false positives + true positives).

	Positive for disease	*Negative for disease*
Positive test result	True positives	False positives
Negative test result	False negatives	True negatives

Many statisticians will further modify this number based on the prevalence of the disease, according to Bayes theorem.

For example: The PPV of a coagulation test for post-tonsillectomy bleeding is 0.02 or 2% (see Chapter 4.D). This means that 2% of children who have a positive test result (i.e., abnormal coagulation test) will actually bleed.

Related terms: positive predictive value, sensitivity, specificity

Prevalence

What it is: The proportion of all cases in the population at risk at a given point in time.

Related terms: incidence

Prospective Study

What it is: In a prospective study, patients are followed forward in time to determine a specific outcome. The term "prospective" just refers to the fact that the study starts with the present population of individuals and follows them into the future. Therefore, prospective studies can be RCTs, cohort studies, or even uncontrolled studies, depending on the other details of the study.

What caliber of evidence it provides: It depends on the other details of the study, such as whether subjects were randomized to treatment groups and the presence of a control group. Please also see "Randomized Controlled Trial," "Cohort Study," and "Case Series."

What can/cannot be concluded from the results of this research: It depends on the other details of the study, such as whether subjects were randomized to treatment groups and the presence of a control group. Please also see "Randomized Controlled Trial," "Cohort Study," and "Case Series."

Key elements to critique: It depends on the other details of the study, such as whether subjects were randomized to treatment groups and the presence of a control group. Please also see "Randomized Controlled Trial," "Cohort Study," and "Case Series."

Power

What it is: The probability that a study will find a difference that actually exists is called the power of a study.

What makes it better or worse: The power of a study depends on multiple factors, beginning with the sample size. One thousand coin flips that show tails are more likely to mean that the coin actually has tails on both sides, as compared with three coin flips that show tails. Therefore, a study's susceptibility to error from chance is partially controlled by the investigators. Power is also influenced by a preset alpha level (acceptable probability that a study finds a difference when in reality no difference exists), which is by convention set at 0.05, or a 5% probability of inaccurately rejecting the null hypothesis because of chance alone. In addition, power depends on the magnitude of difference deemed clinically significant (the delta level); as the delta level increases, the power increases. Therefore, the same study may have a high power for finding a large difference in two populations but a low power for detecting a small difference. In addition, power depends on the final outcome measurements and a calculation of their variance. Because some of these measurements will not be apparent until the study is completed, investigators must rely on estimates from preliminary data when attempting to ensure that a planned study is adequately powered.

How high it should be: Ninety percent power is clearly acceptable. Some clinicians will accept 80% power.

Publication Bias

What it is: It is a type of bias that occurs because published literature has favored the acceptance and publication of reports of studies showing a significant difference in outcome in two groups, making it less likely that reports showing no difference between two groups will be published or disseminated.

Why it is bad: It makes it more likely that results showing a difference between treatment and control will be published, whereas results showing no difference between treatment and control are more likely to remain in a file drawer, without circulation.

Quality of Life

What it is: QOL is a broadly defined concept that encompasses how patients feel and function on multiple levels.

What affects it: Overall QOL is affected by economic, emotional, spiritual, physical, mental, and other factors. A person's health status, or his personal condition because of bodily afflictions or lack thereof, is just one of these issues that affects well-being, but this status is the typical focus of medical studies.

Global QOL versus disease-specific QOL: Global QOL refers to overall QOL and may be used to determine the impact of many different diseases. Examples of instruments measuring global QOL include the Short Form 36 (SF-36) and Child Health Questionnaire (CHQ). Disease-specific QOL, in contrast, explicitly describes the impact of one disease only. Examples of instruments measuring disease-specific QOL include the Otitis Media 6 (OM-6) and Sinonasal Outcome Test 20 (SNOT-20). Often, both types of instruments are used in the same study to provide complementary data.

Randomization

What it is: It is a process in which study participants are assigned to treatments using random numbers and with probabilities that are specified in advance. In a 1:1 randomization to two treatments, patients have an equal probability of assignment to each group.

Why it is useful: Randomization is one way of carefully accounting for confounders, by ensuring that they are at least balanced in the two groups being compared. In fact, the first table in the results section of a well-reported RCT usually details potential confounders and demonstrates that they were distributed similarly in all of the groups that were compared. In addition, randomization should balance potential biases or confounders that lie beyond the imagination of study coordinators. Because patients are randomly assigned, both known and unknown confounders are likely to be balanced between the intervention and control group. If such confounders are not managed properly, then no cause and effect can be demonstrated. By using randomization to prevent bias in allocating patients to one group or the other, however, different results in the two groups may be attributed solely to either the intervention or lack thereof in the control group.

Randomized Controlled Trial

What it is: It is an experimental study in which subjects can be assigned to either the treatment group or the control group with known probability. This randomized design removes selection bias, meaning that it prevents any bias in allocating patients to receive either treatment or no treatment. Randomization also aids in producing groups that are comparable before intervention. It is the gold standard in study designs.

What caliber of evidence it provides: Level 1.

What can/cannot be concluded from results of this study design: The RCT provides the strongest evidence for determining causation, and it is the ideal study design to establish the efficacy of a treatment or procedure. Not every RCT is performed well, however, and the strength of the conclusions is contingent on the rigor with which the study was performed.

Key elements to critique: The first key element is the effectiveness of the randomization process; selection bias is minimized only so far as randomization successfully balanced known potential confounders in the treatment and control groups. A second key factor is whether blinding was utilized, both at the time of treatment (not always possible with surgical intervention) and at the time of outcome measurement. Third, ideally all patients who are enrolled are accounted for at the conclusion of the study. If the majority of patients are lost to follow-up, then the results may be suspect. Fourth, ideally all patients are analyzed with the group to which they were originally assigned; even if patients in the control group eventually required treatment, they should still be considered as part of the control group, according to a strict intention-to-treat analysis. Fifth, the length and quality of follow-up time must also be considered. Sixth, the sample size must provide adequate power to detect any difference that may truly exist. In a well-reported RCT, an *a priori* (i.e., made before the trial) power calculation is described.

Rate Difference

What it is: It is the difference in the rate of a successful outcome without versus with a particular intervention.

What it means: If the RD is less than zero, it suggests that the intervention increases successful outcomes. If the RD is greater than zero, it suggests that the intervention decreases successful outcomes.

The theoretical "best possible" value is: −100% or −1.00. This would mean that without the intervention, no patients had a successful outcome, but that with the intervention, all patients had success.

The theoretical "worst possible" value is: +100% or +1.00. This would mean that without the intervention, all patients had success, but that with the intervention, no one had success.

How to calculate it: RD = (percent of control patients with the desired outcome) − (percent of treated patients with the desired outcome).

For example: In one study of the effect of amoxicillin prophylaxis versus placebo, 58% of the amoxicillin group versus 40% of the placebo group had no further episodes of acute otitis media. The RD in this study was 40% − 58% = −18% (see Chapter 6.A).

Related terms: absolute risk reduction, absolute risk increase, number needed to treat, number needed to harm

Regression

What it is: It is a way to try to establish a relationship between independent variables (exposures/potential causes) and a potentially dependent variable (outcome/potential effect).

Different types: *Linear regression* is performed for continuous variables (assumes a linear relationship between independent and dependent variables). *Logistic regression*

is performed for binary outcome variables (relationships rely on logarithms).

Relative Risk, Also Known as Risk Ratio

What it is: It is a ratio of the probability of an event in the treated group to the probability of the event in the untreated group.

What it means: It answers the question: How much more likely is an event in the treated group than it is in the untreated group? It is usually used in RCTs and cohort studies.

The theoretical "best possible" value: Depends on whether it is desirable to have the event associated with the treatment. If an association is desirable, then the theoretical best possible value is infinity. If an associated is undesired, then the theoretical best possible value is 0.

The theoretical "worst possible" value: Depends on whether it is desirable to have the event associated with the treatment. If an association is desirable, then the theoretical worst possible value is 0. If an associated is undesired, then the theoretical worst possible value is infinity.

How to calculate it: RR = (probability of an event with treatment)/(probability of an event without treatment) = (A/[A+B])/(C/[C+D])

	Had event	Did not have event
Had treatment	A	B
Did not have treatment	C	D

For example: According to one study, the RR of post-tonsillectomy emesis was 0.55 with versus without steroid treatment. This means that the probability of emesis with steroids was 55% of the probability of emesis without steroids.

Related terms: odds ratio, relative risk reduction

Relative Risk Reduction

What it is: It is the percent of risk that is decreased with intervention, relative to the control group's risk.

What it means: It is a measure of the likelihood of an event in the intervention versus control groups, based on the proportion with an event in each group.

The theoretical "best possible" value is: 1.00 or 100%. This means that all of the risk of an event in the control group was eliminated by the treatment.

The theoretical "worst possible" value is: 0.00 or 0%. This means that none of the risk of an event in the control group was eliminated by the treatment.

How to calculate it: Relative risk reduction (RRR) = the absolute value of {[(proportion with an event in the intervention group) − (proportion with an event in the control group)]/[proportion with an event in the control group]} × 100%.

For example: The risk of gaining weight after no exercise change is 25%. The risk of gaining weight after exercising daily is 5%. The RRR is therefore equal to |(5% − 25%)|/25% or 80%.

Related terms: relative risk, odds

Retrospective Review

What it is: It is a study that is undertaken after the original observations have been made.

What caliber of evidence it provides: Level 3 or 4, depending on whether a control group was used. If there is a control group (i.e., it is a historical cohort study or a case-control study), it is a level 3 study. If there is no control group (i.e., it is a retrospective case series), then it is level 4.

What can/cannot be concluded from the results of this research: It depends largely on the specifics of the individual study design. Please also see "Cohort Study," "Case-Control Study," and "Case Series."

Key elements to critique: The major weakness of a retrospective cohort study lies in how prone it is to selection bias, meaning that there was no attempt to ensure that the same factors were present in a treatment group and a control group. The major vulnerability of a case-control study lies in how effectively potential confounders were balanced in the "case" group and the "control" group. The major weakness of a case series lies in the absence of a control group. Please see the individual study designs for further details.

Risk Difference

What it is: Risk difference is used by some people as another term for rate difference. Also see "Rate Difference."

Selection Bias

What it is: It is a form of bias that occurs when study subjects are improperly chosen.

Example: In a study of the impact of a medicine on postoperative pain, results would be tainted by selection bias if only stoic patients were chosen to receive treatment and only timid ones were chosen to receive control.

How to prevent it: Randomization of subjects to treatment groups, or other means of balancing potential confounders between groups.

Sensitivity

What it is: It is the proportion of patients who truly have a disease that test positive for that disease. It is one way to measure the performance of a diagnostic test.

What it means: A high sensitivity means that a negative test result rules out the diagnosis. In other words, the false negative rate is low. To better understand this meaning, consider how sensitivity is calculated: sensitivity = true positives/(true positives + false negatives). If the number of false negatives is 0, sensitivity is 100%. Also, because all patients who truly have disease must test

as either a true positive or a false negative, if the number of false negatives is 0, then all patients who have disease must be true positives. Thus, in general, a high sensitivity also means that the screening test is a good predictor of those with disease.

The theoretical "best possible" value is: 1.00 or 100%. This means that all patients who truly have a disease will test positive for that disease.

The theoretical "worst possible" value is: 0.00 or 0%. This means that no patients who truly have a disease will test positive for that disease.

How to calculate it: Sensitivity = true positives/(true positives + false negatives).

	Positive for disease	Negative for disease
Positive test result	True positives	False positives
Negative test result	False negatives	True negatives

For example: The sensitivity of laboratory coagulation screening in identifying children who will develop post-tonsillectomy bleeding is 0.09, according to one study (see Chapter 4.D.2). This means that 9% of patients who will truly develop post-tonsillectomy bleeding will have an abnormal coagulation panel (positive test). The sensitivity is low, which suggests that a positive test is not a good predictor of postoperative bleeding.

Related terms: specificity, positive predictive value, negative predictive value

Specificity

What it is: It is the proportion of patients who truly are disease-free that test negative for that disease. It is one way to measure the performance of a diagnostic test.

What it means: A high specificity means that a positive result rules in the diagnosis. In other words, the false positive rate is low. To better understand this meaning, consider how specificity is calculated: specificity = true negatives/(true negatives + false positives). Thus, if the number of false positives is 0, then specificity is 100%. Also, because all patients who truly do not have disease must test as either true negatives or false positives, then if the number of false positives is 0, then all patients who do not have disease must be true negatives. Thus, in general, a high specificity also means that the screening test is a good predictor of those without disease.

The theoretical "best possible" value is: 1.00 or 100%. This means that all patients who are disease-free will test negative for that disease.

The theoretical "worst possible" value is: 0.00 or 0%. This means that no patients who are disease-free will test negative for that disease.

How to calculate it: Specificity = true negatives/(true negatives + false positives)

	Positive for disease	Negative for disease
Positive test result	True positives	False positives
Negative test result	False negatives	True negatives

For example: The specificity of laboratory coagulation screening in identifying children who will develop post-tonsillectomy bleeding is 0.98 according to one study (see Chapter 4.D.2). This means that 98% of patients who will not develop postoperative hemorrhage will have a normal coagulation panel (negative test). The specificity is high, which suggests that a normal panel is associated with no bleeding.

Related terms: specificity, positive predictive value, negative predictive value

Systematic Review

What it is: It is a methodical means to identify, summarize, and critique the literature related to a focused clinical query regarding a therapeutic intervention.

What it involves: Performing just one systematic review of the literature relevant to a clinical query usually takes days to weeks, or sometimes months, with MEDLINE searches often yielding hundreds or thousands of potentially related articles that must be considered. Briefly, these methods include the following steps: 1) a focused clinical question is addressed, 2) appropriate inclusion/exclusion criteria are unambiguously defined, 3) an exhaustive computerized and manual search is performed, 4) the validity of the included articles is appraised through an exposition of their study design, 5) the assessments of studies are corroborated by two authors on each subject, 6) results of each study and the consensus or lack thereof is addressed, 7) where appropriate, a meta-analysis is performed to pool data with methods and adjuncts that are well described.

What caliber of evidence it provides: The caliber of evidence depends on two factors: 1) the level of evidence in the included individual trials, and 2) the degree of consensus achieved by the included trials.

What can be concluded from the results of this research: According to David Sackett, one of the pioneers of evidence-based medicine, "the systematic review of the effects of health care is the most powerful and useful evidence available." The results of the review, however, are only as strong as the individual studies it includes.

What cannot be concluded from the results of this research: Conclusions vary according to the level of evidence provided by the studies that are included.

Key elements to critique: First, consider the specificity of the question addressed; ideally this question explicitly characterizes the patient population, intervention, and outcome of interest. Second, the inclusion/exclusion criteria used to select studies for the review should be evaluated. They should be clinically relevant and clearly defined. Third, the original raw data should be presented as part of the focused analysis. Fourth, characteristics and critiques of individual studies should be made apparent. Fifth, methods should be described in detail, so that the analysis can be repeated by another researcher.

Type 1 Error

What it is: It is the probability that a study finds a difference when in reality no difference exists (i.e., the probability of rejecting the null hypothesis when in actuality the null hypothesis is true). This term can also be referred to as the alpha level, which by convention is typically considered acceptable at 0.05 or less.

Type 2 Error

What it is: It is the probability that the study finds that there is no difference when in reality a difference exists (i.e., the probability of accepting the null hypothesis as true when in actuality the null hypothesis is false) is called a type 2 error or the beta level.

Urine Method

What it is: It is a method to assess compliance.

How it is done: There is an assessment of a urine specimen for a marker that the treatment was taken.

SECTION II

Systematic Reviews in Pediatric Otolaryngology

Section Editors

Michael Cunningham, MD

Margaret Kenna, MD, MPH

J. Paul Willging, MD

4 Pediatric Tonsillectomy

4.A.

Tonsillectomy versus no surgery: Impact on number of recurrent throat infections or sore throats

Jennifer J. Shin and Christopher J. Hartnick

METHODS

A computerized Ovid search of MEDLINE 1966–July 2003 was performed. The terms "tonsillitis" and "pharyngitis" were exploded and cross-referenced with articles obtained by exploding "tonsillectomy," yielding 1249 articles. These were limited to clinical trials, resulting in 79 articles which we reviewed in detail. For inclusion criteria, we required the following: 1) distinct patient populations defined as those less than 18 years old with recurrent throat infection or sore throats, 2) intervention with tonsillectomy with or without adenoidectomy or no surgery, and 3) outcome measures consisting of the number of episodes of recurrent throat infection or sore throats. The references of these articles were then reviewed and manually cross-checked to ensure all applicable literature was included. This search strategy yielded five publications [1–6] of randomized controlled trials (RCTs), one of which was an abstract only [4] that reported on preliminary data for a later full publication. One publication contained a report of two RCTs [5] which will be discussed separately. One of these publications contained parallel reports of randomized and nonrandomized prospective trials [3]. The five RCTs identified are discussed in detail below.

RESULTS

Outcome Measures. A throat infection can be defined in many ways, such as by pharyngeal pain, fever, tonsillar exudates, cervical lymphadenopathy, positive throat culture, and improvement on antibiotics. The two earliest trials [1, 6] did not specify exactly how they defined tonsillitis, sore throat, or respiratory illness. The latest three trials [3, 5] provided strict definitions for throat infections and these are detailed in the footnote.

Potential Confounders. In addition to the consistency with which throat infections or sore throats are defined, the accuracy of caretakers' reporting and type of medical management may alter results. In accordance with this, what details are known about the method of follow-up and nonsurgical management are tabulated for the reader. Also, concurrent adenoidectomy can reduce mouth breathing and snoring with potential consequences in terms of postoperative sore throats [7]. Concurrent adenoidectomies are also tabulated for the reader for this reason. It is worth noting, however, that two studies reported no significant difference in throat infections in children undergoing concurrent adenotonsillectomy and tonsillectomy alone [3, 5], suggesting that the addition of adenoidectomy may have minimal effect.

Study Designs. All are RCTs, and three [3, 5] reported on the effectiveness of randomization, showing mostly or all similar baseline characteristics before treatment. The exceptions included the socioeconomic status and distribution of preoperative tonsillitis in the original Paradise report. To address the first issue, they did break down the results by socioeconomic group, and within each group, surgical intervention still resulted in lower rates of postoperative throat infection. As for the second issue, there were actually *higher* rates of preoperative pharyngitis in the *surgical* group, which would theoretically make it even harder to prove that this group had a resulting reduction in the number of subsequent throat infections. Tonsillectomy is clearly an intervention in which the use of blinding and placebo would prove problematic, and these could not reasonably be expected.

Highest Level of Evidence. All five RCTs designed to determine the effect of tonsillectomy versus no surgery on number of episodes of recurrent throat infection or sore throat showed fewer episodes with surgical intervention. The three most recently reported trials [3, 5] included rigorous statistical analysis of results. Whereas the 1984 trial pooled data from adenotonsillectomy and tonsillectomy alone, the follow-up 2002 study of less-severely affected children had a larger patient population, allowing the analysis of these groups separately. That report established that in children without recurrent otitis media or obstructive symptoms necessitating adenoidectomy, there was no significant difference in subsequent number of throat infections with adenotonsillectomy versus tonsillectomy alone [5]. The raw number of throat infections or sore throats that are present in a given year is also very important to consider when evaluating the clinical implications of these data. An operation with a primary risk of hemorrhage is more appealing when no surgical treatment will result in a mean of three infections per year than when no surgical treatment results in a mean of fewer than one infection per year. Because of this, Paradise et al. concluded that whereas tonsillectomy is often indicated for those with severe recurrent throat infections (≥7 episodes in previous year, ≥5 in each of 2 preceding years, ≥3 in each of 3 preceding years), it is not necessarily indicated for those with less-frequently occurring throat infections [3, 5]. In addition, all studies demonstrate that over time, the incidence of throat infection decreases in both surgically and nonsurgically treated groups. Knowledge of this natural history allows for decisions to be made on an individual basis, especially if comorbidities are involved.

Applicability. Based on the inclusion/exclusion criteria for these trials, these results can be applied to 3- to 15-year-old children. The Paradise studies' results can more specifically be applied to those with recurrent sore throats without obstructive symptoms, major physical disease, or hypogammaglobulinemia.

Morbidity. The surgical morbidity reported in these studies is also detailed in the adjoining table. Medical morbidity in the control groups included rashes from antibiotic use (4/48 and 3/138 from the Paradise studies).

CLINICAL SIGNIFICANCE AND FUTURE RESEARCH

There is level 1 evidence showing that surgical intervention decreases the subsequent number of throat infections or sore throats in children who present with recurrent disease. Both adenotonsillectomy and tonsillectomy alone decrease subsequent throat infections in moderately affected children, and pooled data from tonsillectomy with or without adenoidectomy show better outcome after surgery in severely affected children. The evidence, however, also shows that throat infections/sore throats will decrease over time with medical intervention alone. Therefore, when children present with recurrent symptoms, the severity of the infection is a key factor in determining whether tonsillectomy should be performed.

These trials demonstrate the importance of clearly specified parameters to define clinical terms such as "throat infection" or "sore throat," and any future studies should follow suit. In addition, as the technique of tonsillectomy evolves, future studies may have to analyze intracapsular tonsillotomies or other procedures that may leave residual tonsillar tissue as a separate group. Finally, future studies may address the impact of tonsillectomy versus no surgery on child behavior and quality of life with validated scales.

Reference	Paradise, 1984	Paradise, 2002	Paradise, 2002
Level (design)	1 (RCT)	1 (RCT)	1 (RCT)
Sample size*	73 y 1, 60 y 2, 42 y 3 (91)	147 y 1, 124 y 2, 104 y 3 (177)	126 y 1, 112 y 2, 99 y 3 (151)

OUTCOMES			
Outcome measure	No. of episodes of throat infections: all combined, criteria-satisfying,‡ strep positive, and moderate or severe§		
	No. of "sore throat days" (defined as sore throat even mild or intermittent ≥1 h)		
Results of surgery (mean episodes per y)	No. of criteria-satisfying‡ throat infections per y Y 1: 0.76 Y 2: 0.74 Y 3: 0.95	No. of criteria-satisfying‡ throat infections per y Y 1: 0.94,‖ 0.76¶ Y 2: 0.78,‖ 0.47¶ Y 3: 0.36,‖ 0.46¶	No. of criteria-satisfying† throat infections per y Y 1: 1.02 Y 2: 0.72 Y 3: 0.39
Results of no surgery (mean episodes per y)	No. of criteria-satisfying‡ throat infections per y Y 1: 2.66 Y 2: 2.24 Y 3: 1.65	No. of criteria-satisfying‡ throat infections per y Y 1: 1.78 Y 2: 1.70 Y 3: 1.33	No. of criteria-satisfying‡ throat infections per y Y 1: 2.22 Y 2: 1.66 Y 3: 1.29
p Value	Y 1: 0.001 Y 2: 0.001 Y 3: NS	Y 1: <0.001, <0.001 Y 2: <0.001, <0.001 Y 3: <0.001, <0.001	Y 1: <0.001 Y 2: 0.001 Y 3: <0.001
Conclusion	Surgical group with significantly fewer throat infections than control, but control group infections also decrease over time	T&A not different from tonsillectomy alone; both with fewer throat infections than control	Surgical group with significantly fewer infections; both groups with fewer infections over time

STUDY DESIGN			
Inclusion criteria	3- to 15-y-olds with recurrent criteria-satisfying‡ tonsillitis/pharyngitis: ≥7 episodes in previous y, ≥5 in each of 2 preceding y, ≥3 in each of 3 preceding y	3- to 15-y-olds with frequency or clinical features of previous episodes below that of 1984 trial requirements, including those in whom only documentation was lacking	
		Without recurrent OM or obstruction requiring adenoidectomy	With recurrent OM or obstruction requiring adenoidectomy
Exclusion criteria	Airway symptoms, prior tonsil/adenoid surgery, major physical disease, structural middle ear disease, hypogammaglobulinemia, sibling enrolled, inability to meet projected trial schedule	Airway symptoms and those who met eligibility criteria of the Paradise, 1984 trial	
Surgical intervention	Tonsillectomy alone and T&A grouped together	Tonsillectomy alone vs T&A	Adenotonsillectomy
Nonsurgical treatment	If positive throat culture or treated presumptively and improved within 48 h, then penicillin V 250 mg 10 d or erythromycin 10 mg/kg q.i.d. 10 d if allergic		
Adequacy of randomization: baseline characteristics	Similar age, sex, race, tonsil size, referral source, allergy, rate of adenoidectomy. Statistical differences in surgical group vs control: 47 vs 23% with ≥7episodes in 1 y, 42 vs 67% with ≥3 episodes in 3 y, no. of siblings, socioeconomics	No statistically significant difference in age, sex, race, clinical or documented history, tonsil size, sibling no., or socioeconomic status	
Follow-up method	Standardized inquiry biweekly, clinical assessment q 6 wk and with acute episodes. Episodes counted only if reported within 18 d		
Surgical morbidity	4/95** hemorrhage 1/95** severe nausea 2/95** fever	3/209 with intraoperative hemorrhage 7/209 with delayed hemorrhage, with 1 of these requiring transfusion	

RCT = randomized controlled trial, T&A = adenotonsillectomy, OM = otitis media, q.i.d. = four times a day.
* Sample sizes are shown for those completing the study at 1 y, 2 y, and 3 y; with (the originally randomized number of subjects).
‡ For the Paradise studies, throat infection was strictly defined: each episode with documentation and ≥1 of: PO temperature >38.3°C, lad >2 cm or tender, tonsil/pharyngeal exudates, group A beta hemolytic streptococcus positive, antibiotics for proved/suspected streptococcal infection.
§ Throat infections were rated mild, moderate, or severe according to predetermined criteria.
‖ Tonsillectomy alone.　　¶ T&A.　　# Extrapolated from chart.
** Ninety-five patients are derived from the RCT detailed here and the nonrandomized prospective study reported in the same publication.

Reference	Mawson, 1967	Roydhouse, 1970
Level (design)	1 (RCT)	1 (RCT)
Sample size*	361 y 1, 312 y 2 (404)	379 at y 1, 279 at y 2 (379)†

	OUTCOMES	
Outcome measure	No. of episodes of any of these: tonsillitis, sore throat, cervical adenitis (none further defined)	No. of sore throats (not further defined) No. of respiratory illnesses (not further defined)
Results of surgery (mean episodes per y)	No. of episodes per y as described above Y 1: 0.74# Y 2: 0.58#	No. of sore throats, respiratory illnesses per y Y 1: 0.56, 1.88 Y 2: 0.25, 1.35
Results of no surgery (mean episodes per y)	No. of episodes as described above Y 1: 2.25# Y 2: 1.69#	No. of sore throats, respiratory illnesses per y Y 1: 2.25, 3.33 Y 2: 1.86, 3.13
p Value	Statistical significance not reported	Statistical significance not reported
Conclusion	Trend toward fewer infections with surgery; both groups with fewer infections over time	Trend toward fewer infections with surgery; both groups with fewer infections over time

	STUDY DESIGN	
Inclusion criteria	3- to 12-y-old children "in whom operation could be postponed for as long in the 2 y follow-up as ethically could be found possible"	<12 y old Otherwise not reported
Exclusion criteria	Children "with very enlarged, obviously unhealthy tonsils and adenoids from whom we could not in good conscience withhold operation under any circumstances," or if "we could not in good conscience advise operation"	Mainly otologic symptoms
Surgical intervention	Adenotonsillectomy	Adenotonsillectomy
Nonsurgical treatment	Not specified	Not specified
Adequacy of randomization: baseline characteristics	Descriptive data only without statistics: surgical group with more males than females vs control group with fewer females. Surgical group with fewer <4-y-old patients	Not reported
Follow-up method	Clinical examination q 2 mo for 2 y	Not reported
Surgical morbidity	Not reported	16/397 hemorrhage

RCT = randomized controlled trial, T&A = adenotonsillectomy, OM = otitis media, q.i.d. = four times a day.
* Sample sizes are shown for those completing the study at 1 y, 2 y, and 3 y; with (the originally randomized number of subjects).
† Calculated from reported tables.
‡ For the Paradise studies, throat infection was strictly defined: each episode with documentation and ≥1 of: PO temperature >38.3ºC, lad >2 cm or tender, tonsil/pharyngeal exudates, group A beta hemolytic streptococcus positive, antibiotics for proved/suspected streptococcal infection.
§ Throat infections were rated mild, moderate, or severe according to predetermined criteria.
‖ Tonsillectomy alone.   ¶ T&A.   # Extrapolated from chart.
** Ninety-five patients are derived from the RCT detailed here and the nonrandomized prospective study reported in the same publication.

REFERENCES

1. Mawson SR, Adlington P, Evans M. A controlled study evaluation of adeno-tonsillectomy in children. J Laryngol Otol 1967;81(7):777–790.
2. Paradise JL, Bluestone CD, Bachman RZ, et al. History of recurrent sore throat as an indication for tonsillectomy. Predictive limitations of histories that are undocumented. N Engl J Med 1978;298(8):409–413.
3. Paradise JL, Bluestone CD, Bachman RZ, et al. Efficacy of tonsillectomy for recurrent throat infection in severely affected children. Results of parallel randomized and non-randomized clinical trials. N Engl J Med 1984;310(11):674–683.
4. Paradise JL, Bluestone CD, Rogers KD, et al. Comparative efficacy of tonsillectomy for recurrent throat infection in more vs less severely affected children [abstract]. Pediatr Res 1992;31:126A.
5. Paradise JL, Bluestone CD, Colborn DK, Bernard BS, Rockette HE, Kurs-Lasky M. Tonsillectomy and adenotonsillectomy for recurrent throat infection in moderately affected children. Pediatrics 2002;110(1 Pt 1):7–15.
6. Roydhouse N. A controlled study of adenotonsillectomy. Arch Otolaryngol 1970;92(6):611–616.
7. Burton MJ, Towler B, Glasziou P. Tonsillectomy versus non-surgical treatment for chronic/recurrent acute tonsillitis. Cochrane Database Syst Rev 2002(3).

4 Pediatric Tonsillectomy

4.B.

Postoperative systemic antibiotics: Impact on postoperative pain

Jennifer J. Shin and Christopher J. Hartnick

METHODS

A computerized Ovid search of MEDLINE 1966–July 2003 was performed. The terms "tonsillectomy" and "tonsil" were exploded and the resulting articles were combined. The term "antibiotics" was entered as a keyword and mapped to the subject headings "antibiotics, combined," "antibiotics, lactam," "antibiotics, macrolide," "antibiotics, tetracycline," "antibiotics, anthracycline," "antibiotics, aminoglycoside," "antibiotics, peptide," and "antibiotics, antitubercular." These headings were in turn exploded, combined, and cross-referenced with the tonsillectomy/tonsil articles. The resulting 601 articles were limited to "human" and "English language," resulting in 375 publications, whose titles and abstracts were then reviewed. Those publications were then reviewed to see which met the following inclusion criteria: 1) studied a distinct patient population less than 18 years old, 2) intervened with the use of systemic antimicrobials in the first 2 weeks after tonsillectomy, and 3) described the outcomes of postoperative pain. The references of these articles were then reviewed and manually cross-checked to ensure all applicable literature was included. Five prospective controlled trials meeting the inclusion criteria were identified in this manner [1–7]. The four of those that were randomized are summarized in the adjoining table and the highest level of evidence is discussed in detail below.

RESULTS

Outcome Measures. Postoperative pain can be measured in a variety of ways. In these studies, the amount of analgesic required, the time in continuous pain, and a numeric rating of pain severity were the methods used.

Potential Confounders. Postoperative pain may be influenced by factors besides antibiotic use. First, steroid administration may alter post-tonsillectomy morbidity [6]. None of these studies directly reports any concurrent steroid use in either antibiotic or control groups, although most were performed before steroid use was definitively studied in the context of tonsillectomy. The latest study [1] does note that "other premedications" were similar in both groups. Second, the surgical technique may influence subsequent pain [7], and the techniques used in these studies are described in the adjoining table. Third, the type, route, dose, and duration of antibiotic administration may influence the results, and we have also catalogued these for the reader.

Study Designs. All studies were prospective controlled trials (level 1–2). Four of these were randomized (level 1) and so constituted the highest level of evidence. Randomization is performed to minimize differences in the groups before treatment. In accordance with this, three reports [1, 2, 5] provide a detailed analysis of the pretreatment subject characteristics, confirming no significant difference between the antibiotic and the placebo group at the outset. Only one study was double blind with placebo control and reported compliance (approximately 75% of trial medications were consumed) [5]. Another study was the only one to use a validated clinical pain scale [1]. A third study laudably tries to address the potentially confounding factor of surgical technique, but in dividing the 80 subjects into 8 groups of 10 each, has a relatively lower study power as reported [4]. This study may therefore inappropriately fail to reject the null hypothesis because of inadequate power in these comparisons. The fourth randomized controlled trial (RCT) differs in that it compares two antibiotic regimens, rather than comparing antibiotic versus control [2]. The subjects withdrawn from the studies were minimal in number and withdrawn for acceptable reasons, although it is unclear how the three patients withdrawn from the Telian study for noncompliance would have affected the overall outcome.

Highest Level of Evidence. Three RCTs designed specifically to determine the impact of antibiotics versus control in children post-tonsillectomy provide the highest level of evidence addressing this clinical query. All three reported decreased pain with various measurements in one or more groups of patients using antibiotics. Telian reports fewer days of continuous pain with antibiotics. Colreavy reports a lower subjective pain score with antibiotics. Linden reports less pain medicine utilized in groups undergoing electrocautery or laser excision with antibiotics. This study also, however, reports no difference in pain with or without antibiotics in groups undergoing cold dissection, in contrast to the Telian report. The Linden study is, however, less powered to address this issue, with 20 patients undergoing cold dissection with electrocautery hemostasis, versus 85 in the Telian article. Although not directly addressing the impact of antibiotics versus control, a fourth randomized study warrants mention here in that it shows no difference in pain with amoxicillin versus cefaclor therapy.

Applicability. Based on the inclusion/exclusion criteria for these papers, the results can be applied to children undergoing tonsillectomy with or without adenoidectomy, with no known penicillin allergy, no medical condition requiring antibiotics, and who have had no antibiotics for at least 1 week before surgery.

Morbidity. The morbidity of antibiotic use seems to be minimal according to the two randomized studies that reported on associated complications. One study had one rash and one episode of thrush in 45 children taking antibiotics. The second study's antibiotic group had one episode of diarrhea and one hemorrhage (versus four in the control group). None of these studies, however, were directly designed to address this issue.

CLINICAL SIGNIFICANCE AND FUTURE RESEARCH

The use of antibiotics to minimize pain after tonsillectomy is supported by level 1 evidence in three RCTs. One of these trials does, however, report no difference in pain in subgroups who underwent cold dissection, although this study has limitations in power. Overall, it seems that the use of antibiotics to decrease pain after cautery tonsillectomy is warranted, and may be warranted after dissection tonsillectomy as well.

As for the specific antibiotic regimen, the data support the use of lactam antimicrobials for 1 week, with successful use of either amoxicillin [5] or amoxicillin/clavulanic acid [1]. In addition, cefaclor use results in pain control equivalent to that seen with amoxicillin [2].

Future research into this topic may address the potential interaction of antibiotics with surgical method or steroid use. In addition, future research in this area may be best performed with standardized, validated means of postoperative pain reporting in order to facilitate the analysis of pooled data.

Reference	Telian, 1986	Colreavy, 1999	
Level (design)	1 (RCT)	1 (RCT)	
Sample size*	85 (100)	75 (78)	
OUTCOMES			
Outcome measure	Scale: time experiencing continuous pain Time: POD 1–7	Scale 1: 0 (little or no) −10 (unbearable) Scale 2: mean use of analgesic in mg/kg/24 h Time: POD 7	
Antibiotics score	3.3 d	Scale 1: 2.8 Scale 2: 200 mg/kg/d	
No antibiotics score	4.4 d	Scale 1: 6.3 Scale 2: 112 mg/kg/d	
p Value	<0.05	Scale 1: $p = 0.006$ Scale 2: $p = 0.038$	
Conclusion	Less pain with antibiotics	Less pain with antibiotics	
Follow-up	7–14 d postoperatively	7 d postoperatively	
STUDY DESIGN			
Inclusion criteria	All tonsillectomies with or without adenoidectomies	All tonsillectomies with or without fewer procedures	
Exclusion criteria	No known penicillin allergy, no medical condition requiring antibiotics, no antibiotics for 1 wk before surgery	No known penicillin allergy, no medical condition requiring antibiotics, no antibiotics for 1 wk before surgery	
Intervention	Ampicillin/amoxicillin (250 mg PO t.i.d. if ≥20kg, 125mg PO t.i.d. if <20 kg) 7d vs saline/placebo	Amoxicillin with clavulanic acid (dose according to 1996 British National Formulary) 7d vs control group without placebo	

RCT = randomized controlled trial, POD = postoperative day.
* Sample size: numbers shown for those completing the trial and those (initially recruited).
† Estimated from bar chart.

THE EVIDENCE CONDENSED: Antibiotics to decrease post-tonsillectomy pain in children

Reference	Linden, 1990	Jones, 1990
Level (design)	1 (RCT)	1 (RCT)
Sample size*	80 (80)	95 (104)
OUTCOMES		
Outcome measure	Scale: analgesic use, weighted score Time: POD 5	Scale: none, mild, moderate, or severe Time: POD 1–7
Antibiotics score	Excisn/hstasis Diss/ecaut: 1.1† Diss/lig: 0.8† Ecaut/ecaut: 1.3† Laser/laser: 0.9†	Days with mild–severe pain: cefaclor: 3.9 d, amoxicillin: 3.8 d
No antibiotics score	Excisn/hstasis Diss/ecaut: 1.0† Diss/lig: 0.7† Ecaut/ecaut: 0.8† Laser/laser: 1.3†	None
p Value	No p values reported	NS
Conclusion	Diss/ecaut: no effect Diss/lig: no effect Ecaut/ecaut, Laser/laser: "statistically significant decrease in pain medicine required with antibiotics"	No difference in pain between cefaclor and amoxicillin groups
Follow-up	5 d postoperatively	7–14 d postoperatively
STUDY DESIGN		
Inclusion criteria	Not reported	All tonsillectomies with or without adenoidectomies
Exclusion criteria	Not reported	No known penicillin allergy, no medical condition requiring antibiotics, no antibiotics for 1 wk before surgery
Intervention	Antibiotic regimen not specified vs control group without placebo	Ampicillin/amoxicillin (250 mg PO t.i.d. if ≥20 kg, 125 mg PO t.i.d. if <20 kg) vs cefazolin/ cefaclor (250 mg PO t.i.d. if ≥20 kg, 125 mg PO t.i.d. if <20 kg) 7d
Method of excisn/hstasis	As described in the four groups above	Not reported
Compliance	Not reported	Amoxicillin group: 88% of medications were taken Cefaclor group: 89% of medications were taken
Randomization effectiveness	Not reported	No significant difference in age, sex, indication for surgery, or tonsil size in the two groups before antibiotic or placebo treatment
Morbidity/complications of antibiotics	Not reported	Not reported

RCT = randomized controlled trial, POD = postoperative day. For the Linden study, methods of excision and hemostasis are reported: excisn = excision, hstasis = hemostasis, ecaut = electrocautery, diss = blunt dissection with snare excision, lig = ligation, t.i.d.= three times a day.
* Sample size: numbers shown for those completing the trial and those (initially recruited).
† Estimated from bar chart.

REFERENCES

1. Colreavy MP, Nanan D, Benamer M, et al. Antibiotic prophylaxis post-tonsillectomy: is it of benefit? Int J Pediatr Otorhinolaryngol 1999;50(1):15–22.
2. Jones J, Handler SD, Guttenplan M, et al. The efficacy of cefaclor vs amoxicillin on recovery after tonsillectomy in children. Arch Otolaryngol Head Neck Surg 1990; 116(5):590–593.
3. Lee WC, Duignan MC, Walsh RM, McRae-Moore JR. An audit of prophylactic antibiotic treatment following tonsillectomy in children. J Laryngol Otol 1996;110(4):357–359.
4. Linden BE, Gross CW, Long TE, Lazar RH. Morbidity in pediatric tonsillectomy. Laryngoscope 1990;100(2 Pt 1): 120–124.
5. Telian SA, Handler SD, Fleisher GR, Baranak CC, Wetmore RF, Potsic WP. The effect of antibiotic therapy on recovery after tonsillectomy in children. A controlled study. Arch Otolaryngol Head Neck Surg 1986;112(6):610–615.
6. Steward DL, Welge JA, Myer CM. Steroids for improving recovery following tonsillectomy in children. Cochrane Database Syst Rev 2003(1):CD003997.
7. Leinbach RF, Markwell SJ, Colliver JA, Lin SY. Hot versus cold tonsillectomy: A systematic review of the literature. Otolaryngol Head Neck Surg 2003;129:360–364.

4 Pediatric Tonsillectomy

4.C.1.

Single-dose systemic dexamethasone: Impact on postoperative emesis and oral intake

Jennifer J. Shin and Christopher J. Hartnick

METHODS

A computerized Ovid search of MEDLINE 1966–October 2003 was performed. The terms "tonsillectomy" and "tonsil" were exploded and the resulting articles were combined. The term "steroids" was exploded and the resulting articles were cross-referenced with the tonsillectomy/tonsil articles. This process yielded 192 articles. These articles were then reviewed to determine which met the following inclusion criteria: 1) distinct patient population of children (≤18 years old) undergoing tonsillectomy, 2) intervention with a single dose of intravenous steroid, and 3) outcome measurement of postoperative emesis and/or oral intake. Studies of the effects of local steroid injection were excluded. In this manner, we identified nine randomized controlled trials (RCTs) [1–9] and three meta-analyses of those RCTs [10–12]. The meta-analyses were rigorously performed and well reported, and we will discuss these as the highest level of evidence.

RESULTS

Outcome Measures. Postoperative emesis was usually reported as the number of patients who experienced at least one episode of emesis after surgery [1, 4, 6–8]. In the Steward analyses, that period was defined as 24 hours postoperatively. Other primary papers reported the number of patients requiring antiemetic medication [3] or included "retching" in with the outcome of emesis [5]. Oral intake was usually reported as the number of patients advancing to a soft or solid diet on postoperative (POD) 1 or 3.

Potential Confounders. A meta-analysis is only as strong as the quality and quantity of source articles that are included, as well as the thoroughness of the literature search that produces them. Each of these meta-analyses included only level 1 studies with clearly and statistically defined outcomes, and reviewed almost 200 articles with manual cross-checks in order to identify all relevant studies. The results of meta-analyses may also be affected by the publication bias that exists in the otolaryngology literature toward accepting reports of positive more so than negative results [13]. Such a bias may result in the inclusion of more articles with positive findings in a meta-analysis, which can skew the final results. A sensitivity analysis can help address this issue, by determining how many negative studies would be needed to cancel out a positive finding.

Study Designs. All three are high-quality meta-analyses with well-defined *a priori* inclusion and exclusion criteria, closely specified outcome measures, and methodical quantitative analyses. Each clearly defined inclusion and exclusion criteria, the search strategy employed, and the outcome measures utilized. Each also addressed the issue of the impact of publication bias, and utilized more than one author to minimize bias. The most recent study included the largest number of subjects from a larger number of published trials [10]. All used the random effects model for data analysis.

Highest Level of Evidence. The relative risk of post-tonsillectomy emesis is 0.54–0.55, meaning that children who were treated with steroids had half the risk of emesis that children who received placebo had [10–12]. This finding was statistically significant. In addition, all three meta-analyses found a significant rate difference (RD) of −24% to −27% in children experiencing postoperative emesis [10–12]. This RD is the absolute difference in the outcome of interest between the study group and the control group. For example, if results show that 29% of the steroid group had emesis versus 55% of the placebo group, these data have an RD of 29% − 55% = −26%. This RD also allows us to determine the number of children who need to be treated with steroids to prevent one child from having post-tonsillectomy emesis. The number needed to treat (NNT) is the reciprocal of the RD. In this case, to prevent one child from experiencing postoperative emesis, four children must be treated with a single dose of intraoperative dexamethasone.

By the same group of measurements, oral intake was also improved on POD 1, with 21%–22% more children advancing to a soft or normal diet in the steroid group as compared with the placebo group [10–12], with a resulting NNT of 5. The relative risk of 1.69 also corroborates the positive impact of steroid treatment at POD 1. At POD 3, however, there were no statistically significant differences between the oral intake of the steroid or control groups.

Applicability. These results apply to children (≤18 years old) receiving a single intraoperative dose of dexamethasone undergoing adenotonsillectomy or tonsillectomy alone.

Morbidity. The most recent Steward analysis addressed this issue, citing that no adverse effects were noted in any of the included trials. In addition, it cites a 10-year experience of approximately 800 tonsillectomies each year in which there were no adverse events attributable to single-dose steroid use.

CLINICAL SIGNIFICANCE AND FUTURE RESEARCH

There are three meta-analyses of RCTs that show that post-tonsillectomy emesis and oral intake on POD 1 are improved with the use of a single intravenous perioperative dose of steroids. The difference in oral intake at POD 3, however, is not significant.

Future research may consider the dose-dependent effects of steroid administration through randomized-dose control trials in pediatric tonsillectomy patients.

THE EVIDENCE CONDENSED: Post-tonsillectomy steroids to decrease emesis and increase oral intake

Reference	Steward, 2003	Steward, 2001	Goldman, 2000
Level (design)	1 (MA of RCTs)	1 (MA of RCTs)	1 (MA of RCTs)
Sample size*	Emesis 640 (8) Oral intake POD 1: 248 (4) POD 3: 152 (3)	Emesis 534 (7) Oral intake POD 1: 248 (4) POD 3: 152 (3)	Emesis 468 (5) Oral intake POD 1: 191 (3) POD 3: 135 (3)
OUTCOMES			
Emesis RD†	RD = −25 (−37 to −13) p = 0.00004, favors steroids NNT = 4	RD = −24 (−38 to −10) p = 0.0006, favors steroids NNT = 4	RD = −27 (−42 to −12) p < 0.0001, favors steroids NNT = 4
Emesis RR‡	RR 0.54 (0.42 to 0.69) p < 0.00001, favors steroids	RR 0.55 (0.41 to 0.74) p = 0.00007, favors steroids	Not reported
Oral intake POD 1 RD†	RD = 21 (6 to 36) p = 0.006, favors steroids NNT = 5	RD = 21 (6 to 36) p = 0.006, favors steroids NNT = 5	RD = 22 (1 to 44) p < 0.001, favors steroids NNT = 5
Oral intake POD 1 RR‡	RR 1.69 (1.02 to 2.79) p = 0.04, favors steroids	RR 1.69 (1.02 to 2.79) p = 0.04, favors steroids	Not reported
Oral intake POD 3 RD†	RD = 17 (−7 to 41) p = 0.15	RD 17 (−7 to 41) p = 0.15	RD 12 (−19 to 43) p = 0.281
Oral intake POD 3 RR‡	RR = 1.22 (0.81 to 1.86) p = 0.3	RR 1.22 (0.81 to 1.86) p = 0.3	Not reported
STUDY DESIGN			
Inclusion criteria for studies	• Randomized double-blinded placebo controlled trials of a single dose of intravenous intraoperative corticosteroid versus placebo • Pediatric patients (aged ≤18 y) who underwent tonsillectomy or adenotonsillectomy • Foreign-language publications were translated for evaluation	• Randomized double-blinded placebo controlled trials of a single dose of intravenous intraoperative corticosteroid versus placebo • Pediatric patients (age ≤18 y) who underwent tonsillectomy or adenotonsillectomy were included	• Randomized prospective controlled trials of perioperative intravenous dexamethasone versus no steroid • Complete data (numerator and denominator) were available for endpoints in the control and treatment groups • Foreign-language publications were translated for evaluation
Exclusion criteria	• Trials involving adult patients	• Trials involving adult patients • Trials not published or translated into the English language	• Trials focusing on anesthetic technique, obstructive sleep apnea, or other pediatric diseases
Intervention	Dexamethasone single intravenous perioperative dose	Dexamethasone single intravenous perioperative dose	Dexamethasone single intravenous perioperative dose
Potential publication bias addressed?	Sensitivity analysis (calculated fail safe N): 15 studies with a null RR would be required to increase the overall RR of emesis to nonsignificance	Sensitivity analysis (calculated fail safe N): 12 studies with a null RR would be required to increase the overall RR of emesis to nonsignificance	"Publication bias (the preferential tendency of authors and journals to publish positive results) is unlikely because the 95% CI of the overall RD does not approach zero"

MA = meta-analysis, RCT = randomized controlled trial, POD = postoperative day, RD = rate difference, RR = relative risk, NNT= number needed to treat (i.e., the total number of children that must be treated in order for one child to obtain benefit from steroid treatment), CI = confidence interval.

* Sample size: numbers shown for total number of subjects in the trials included in the MA and (the number of publications included).

† The absolute RD is defined as the absolute difference in successful outcomes between the study group and the control group. For example, in the Splinter 1996 study (the largest RCT to date), 71% of the placebo vs 40% of the dexamethasone group had emesis. The RD in this study was 40% − 71% = −31%.

‡ RR is the risk of an event in a patient in the experimental group relative to that of a patient in the control group.

REFERENCES

1. Aouad MT, Siddik SS, Rizk LB, Zaytoun GM, Baraka AS. The effect of dexamethasone on postoperative vomiting after tonsillectomy. Anesth Analg 2001;92(3):636–640.

2. April MM, Callan ND, Nowak DM, Hausdorff MA. The effect of intravenous dexamethasone in pediatric adenotonsillectomy. Arch Otolaryngol Head Neck Surg 1996; 122(2):117–120.

3. Catlin FI, Grimes WJ. The effect of steroid therapy on recovery from tonsillectomy in children. Arch Otolaryngol Head Neck Surg 1991;117(6):649–652.

4. Ohlms LA, Wilder RT, Weston B. Use of intraoperative corticosteroids in pediatric tonsillectomy. Arch Otolaryngol Head Neck Surg 1995;121(7):737–742.

5. Pappas AL, Sukhani R, Hotaling AJ, et al. The effect of preoperative dexamethasone on the immediate and delayed postoperative morbidity in children undergoing adenotonsillectomy. Anesth Analg 1998;87(1):57–61.

6. Splinter WM, Roberts DJ. Dexamethasone decreases vomiting by children after tonsillectomy. Anesth Analg 1996;83(5):913–916.

7. Tom LW, Templeton JJ, Thompson ME, Marsh RR. Dexamethasone in adenotonsillectomy. Int J Pediatr Otorhinolaryngol 1996;37(2):115–120.

8. Vosdoganis F, Baines DB. The effect of single dose intravenous dexamethasone in tonsillectomy in children. Anaesth Intensive Care 1999;27(5):489–492.

9. Volk MS, Martin P, Brodsky L, Stanievich JF, Ballou M. The effects of preoperative steroids on tonsillectomy patients. Otolaryngol Head Neck Surg 1993;109(4):726–730.

10. Steward DL, Welge JA, Myer CM. Steroids for improving recovery following tonsillectomy in children. Cochrane Database Syst Rev 2003(1):CD003997.

11. Goldman AC, Govindaraj S, Rosenfeld RM. A meta-analysis of dexamethasone use with tonsillectomy. Otolaryngol Head Neck Surg 2000;123(6):682–686.

12. Steward DL, Welge JA, Myer CM. Do steroids reduce morbidity of tonsillectomy? Meta-analysis of randomized trials. Laryngoscope 2001;111(10):1712–1718.

13. Bentsianov B, Boruk M, Rosenfeld R. Evidence-based medicine in otolaryngology journals. Otolaryngol Head Neck Surg 2002;126:371–376.

4 Pediatric Tonsillectomy

Single-dose systemic dexamethasone: Impact on postoperative pain

Jennifer J. Shin and Christopher J. Hartnick

METHODS

A computerized Ovid search of MEDLINE 1966–October 2003 was performed as described in section 4.C.1. The resulting 192 articles were reviewed to determine which met the following inclusion criteria: 1) distinct patient population of children (≤18 years old) undergoing tonsillectomy, 2) intervention with a single dose of intravenous steroid, and 3) outcome measurement of postoperative pain or analgesic use. Studies of the effects of local steroid injection or oral prednisone were excluded. Eight level 1 studies [1–8] were located and these are discussed in detail below. In addition, for studies reporting no significant difference between steroid and placebo groups, power calculations were performed.

RESULTS

Outcome Measures. Pain can be measured in multiple ways, including visual analog and numeric scales [1, 3, 8]. The quality of pain can be determined (i.e., minimal, worst), as can its timing (i.e., rare, continuous) [7]. It can also be measured in the number of patients with a certain amount of pain (i.e., percent of patients with severe pain) [5]. Likewise, pain can be indirectly measured by showing the amount of analgesic consumed [1–8], or by having a blinded observer record behavior indicative of the amount of pain [6]. Also, one study reported fewer phone calls from parents of children receiving steroids, although those phone calls were not only for difficulty with pain management, but also for difficulty with nausea or other complaints [4]. Another commented on the relative number of smiles but this parameter could also be confounded by factors other than pain [1].

Potential Confounders. Antibiotic use has been shown to alter postoperative pain in three randomized controlled trials (RCTs) in children (see 16.B). In addition, especially in the immediate postoperative period, other analgesics or anesthetics used may also alter pain outcomes. Also, surgical technique has been shown to influence postoperative pain [9]. Finally, the dose and route of steroid administration may cause discrepancies. All of these factors are cataloged for the reader in the adjoining table.

Study Designs. These studies are all double-blind RCTs with placebo control. All except three confirmed no statistical differences in age, sex, or other pretreatment characteristics in the steroid and placebo groups. Validated pain scales were used in four studies [1, 3, 6, 8], with clearly defined measures of pain provided in two others [5, 7]. All studies also utilized the surrogate measure of analgesic consumption. Four ensured that the potential confounder of antibiotics was standardized throughout [1–3, 7] and six attempted to standardize the anesthetic regimen. Two RCTs evaluated the immediate postoperative period only (up to 24 hours after surgery). One RCT evaluated the first 48 hours, and the remaining RCTs evaluated the first postoperative 7–10 days. Representative time points from each trial are shown. Because many studies reported a negative result (i.e., no significant difference in pain measures between the steroid and control group), we have also tabulated whether an *a priori* power calculation was performed.

Highest Level of Evidence. All except one study showed no difference in reported subjective pain measures between the steroid and placebo groups. The lone exception [5] reported a significant decrease in the percent of patients with severe pain on the first postoperative day (POD) with dexamethasone treatment. Other groups did not measure this particular parameter of percent with severe pain. Also, all except one study reported no difference in the analgesic consumed in the steroid and placebo groups. The single exception [3] showed a statistically significant decrease in the number of patients requiring codeine or acetaminophen on the first POD with steroid use. The two studies that showed a difference in pain outcome were not the result of higher dosing, because the amount of dexamethasone used was comparable to that of other studies showing no effect.

Applicability. The results of these studies are applicable to patients undergoing tonsillectomy with or without adenoidectomy who are 18 years at the oldest and 1 year at the youngest. They are not applicable to children with steroid use previous to the preoperative period, or with comorbidities including diabetes and neurologic disease. Further details of the inclusion/exclusion criteria for specific studies are tabulated below.

Morbidity. None of these studies reported any steroid-associated morbidity.

CLINICAL SIGNIFICANCE AND FUTURE RESEARCH

There is level 1 evidence regarding the effect of steroids on postoperative pain, the preponderance of which shows no difference in reported pain or analgesic use in children who have dexamethasone versus placebo. At least two of these studies are adequately powered to find any true difference that exists. Two of the seven studies show a significant difference in pain on the first POD. None show a difference beyond this time frame, and none show worsening of pain with steroids. Some might argue, however, that the first POD is such a critical period—with worse pain potentially resulting in increased hospitalization and heightened patient/family anxiety—that any potential analgesic benefit may make steroid administration worthwhile. Also, the results of these studies are often considered in the context of the multiple studies that show a decrease in emesis and nearly no morbidity with a single perioperative dose of dexamethasone.

If further research on this topic is performed, it may be best focused on the first 48 hours after tonsillectomy, because this seems to be the area of most debate. Also, it would be of interest to have clear reporting of any *a priori* power calculations for studies, especially when the results show no significant difference between groups. In addition, the use of uniform validated pain scales would facilitate the analysis of pooled data.

THE EVIDENCE CONDENSED: Single-dose systemic dexamethasone for post-tonsillectomy pain

Reference	Ohlms, 1995			Giannoni, 2002		
Level (design)	1 (RCT)			1 (RCT)		
Sample size*	69 (69)			47 (50)		
OUTCOMES						
Pain measure	Mean score on faces pain scale 0 (least pain) to 1 (most pain)			Mean score on visual analog scale 0 = no pain, 10 = worst pain ever		
Time	POD 1	POD 2	POD 7	POD 1	POD 2	POD 5
Steroid	0.50†	0.47†	0.29†	4.8†	3.8†	2.5†
Placebo	0.59†	0.49†	0.32†	5.0†	3.0†	2.4†
p Value	NS overall			>0.05 for overall		
Conclusion	No difference overall			No difference overall		
Analgesic consumed	Percent taking codeine or acetaminophen			Mean doses of codeine		
Time	POD 1	POD 2	POD 7	POD 1	POD 2	POD 5
Steroid	44%†	60%†	54%†	3.0†	2.3†	1.4†
Placebo	78%†	57%†	41%†	3.9†	2.9†	1.5†
p Value	<0.05	NS	NS	>0.05 overall		
Conclusion	Steroids better on POD 1			No difference overall		
STUDY DESIGN						
Inclusion criteria	Patients aged 3–18 y scheduled for tonsillectomy with or without adenoidectomy were eligible for the study			Patients aged 3–15 y scheduled for tonsillectomy were offered enrollment		
Exclusion criteria	"Any patient with a known contraindication to steroid use," penicillin allergy			NR		
Dexamethasone regimen	0.5 mg/kg (maximum 12 mg) IV ×1 before surgery			1 mg/kg (maximum 16 mg) IV ×1 intraoperatively		
Antibiotic use	All received ampicillin 50 mg/kg IV ×2, amoxicillin 50 mg/kg PO ×5 d.			NR		
Other analgesic or anesthetic medications	All received standard anesthetic with halothane, nitrous oxide, isoflurane, morphine sulfate			All received tonsil fossa injection of ropivacaine and clonidine, ibuprofen PO, midazolam, "standard inhalational anesthetic"		
Method of tonsillectomy	Sharp dissection snare technique			NR		
Indications for tonsillectomy	52 adenotonsillar hypertrophy, 17 recurrent tonsillitis			NR		
Age	3–18 y			3–15 y		
Randomization Effectiveness	No significant difference in age, sex, race, tonsil size, other procedures, EBL, procedure length, IV fluids in the operating room in the pretreatment groups			No significant difference in age, sex, and rate of concurrent adenoidectomy		
A priori power calculation	0.95 to detect a difference in pain score of at least 0.2, with 25 patients in each group			0.89, calculated around the visual analog scale, with a sample size of 20 subjects per group		

RCT = randomized controlled trial, POD = postoperative day, NS = not significant, NR = not reported, IV = intravenous.
* Sample size: numbers shown for those completing the trial and those (initially recruited).
† Estimated from graph.
‡ History of cardiac arrhythmia, glucose intolerance, gastrointestinal bleeding, tuberculosis, or neurologic, developmental, or other chronic medical diseases.

THE EVIDENCE CONDENSED: Single-dose systemic dexamethasone for post-tonsillectomy pain

Reference	Volk, 1993			Tom, 1996
Level (design)	1 (RCT)			1 (RCT)
Sample size*	49 (50)			58 (71)
OUTCOMES				
Pain measure	Mean score on pain scale 0 absent, 1 rare, 2 intermittent, 3 continuous			% with "severe pain" from diary including pain report: details NR
Time	POD 1	POD 2	POD 7	POD 1 "Delayed pain"
Steroid	2.1	2.0	1.5	0.20† "No large or clear effects"
Placebo	2.4	2.0	1.4	0.57†
p Value	NS overall			<0.01 NS
Conclusion	No difference overall			Steroids better on POD 1
Analgesic consumed	Mean doses of acetaminophen			Use of acetaminophen–codeine, details NR
Time	POD 1	POD 2	POD 7	Lumped data from PODs 1–7
Steroid	3.6	3.3	2.3	"No large or clear effects," not further described
Placebo	3.8	3.9	2.5	
p Value	NS overall			
Conclusion	No difference overall			No difference overall
STUDY DESIGN				
Inclusion criteria	Patients age 4–12 y "fulfilling previously established criteria" for tonsillectomy with or without adenoidectomy			Patients age 1–18 y scheduled for adenotonsillectomy were eligible
Exclusion criteria	Penicillin allergy; condition requiring antibiotic prophylaxis; history of peritonsillar abscess; recent steroid usage; other medical comorbidities‡			Bisulfate allergy; cardiac problems; craniofacial anomalies; bleeding or neuromuscular disorders
Dexamethasone regimen	10 mg IV ×1 just before intubation			1 mg/kg (maximum 10 mg) IV ×1 intraoperatively
Antibiotic use	All received amoxicillin PO ×10 d postoperatively			NR
Other analgesic or anesthetic medications	NR			Standardized anesthesia with halothane and nitrous oxide, morphine
Method of tonsillectomy	Blunt and sharp dissection; Hemostasis with cautery			Excision and hemostasis with electrocautery
Indications for tonsillectomy	"Upper airway obstruction from tonsillar hypertrophy most common reason"; not further described			NR
Age	4–12 y			1–18 y
Randomization effectiveness	No large differences in age, sex, average number of tonsillitis episodes in the previous year, snoring, mouth breathing, dysphagia, average tonsil size			NR
A priori power calculation	NR			NR

RCT = randomized controlled trial, POD = postoperative day, NS = not significant, NR = not reported, IV = intravenous.
* Sample size: numbers shown for those completing the trial and those (initially recruited).
† Estimated from graph.
‡ History of cardiac arrhythmia, glucose intolerance, gastrointestinal bleeding, tuberculosis, or neurologic, developmental, or other chronic medical diseases.

THE EVIDENCE CONDENSED: Single-dose systemic dexamethasone for post-tonsillectomy pain

Reference	Pappas, 1998	Vosdoganis, 1999		
Level (design)	1 (RCT)	1 (RCT)		
Sample size*	128 (130)	41 (42)		

OUTCOMES				
Pain measure	No. of phone calls to M.D. for complaints of pain, inability to maintain analgesic schedule (also included calls for poor PO, nausea, vomiting)	Median value assigned by blinded observer using the Objective Pain Scale in the first 24 h postoperatively		
Time	Within 24 h after discharge	4 h	8 h	24 h
Steroid	8	1.0	0.0	1.0
Placebo	25	1.0	1.0	1.0
p value	<0.05	NS	NS	NS
Conclusion	Steroids better within 24 h after discharge	No difference overall		
Analgesic consumed	Percent of patients who received fentanyl in PACU	Mean intake in mg/kg/d		
		Paracetamol		Codeine
Time	Duration of PACU stay	Within 24 h of surgery		
Steroid	62	60.2		0.77
Placebo	66	61.2		0.71
p value	NS	NS		NS
Conclusion	No difference	No difference		

STUDY DESIGN		
Inclusion criteria	Ambulatory tonsillectomy or adenotonsillectomy	Elective inpatient tonsillectomy; ASA I, II
Exclusion criteria	Children who received antiemetics, antihistamines, steroids, or psychoactive drugs within 24 h of surgery; history of diabetes; indication for IV induction	Known allergy to dexamethasone, ASA ≥3, history of severe postoperative nausea/vomiting
Dexamethasone regimen	1 mg/kg (maximum 25 mg) IV ×1 before surgery	0.4 mg/kg (maximum 8 mg) IV ×1 at induction
Antibiotic use	NR	NR
Other analgesic or anesthetic medications	All received midazolam, halothane and nitrous oxide with isoflurane, fentanyl; also acetaminophen codeine q 4 h while awake after discharge	Standard anesthetic with halothane or sevoflurane, propofol, nitrous oxide or isoflurane; paracetamol
Method of tonsillectomy	Electrodissection	NR
Indications for tonsillectomy	Not specified	NR
Age	2–12 y	2–12 y
Randomization effectiveness	"Comparable with respect to tonsillar size, surgical indication, surgical procedure"	No difference in age, weight, sex, type of operation, induction or maintenance agent
A priori power calculation reported	0.90 (was powered around emesis outcome) to detect an RD of 50%, with 55 patients in each group	NR

RCT = randomized controlled trial, POD = postoperative day, RD = rate difference, NS = not significant, NR = not reported, PACU = postanesthesia care unit, ASA = American Society of Anesthesiologists, IV = intravenous.
* Sample size: numbers shown for those completing the trial and those (initially recruited).

THE EVIDENCE CONDENSED: Single-dose systemic dexamethasone for post-tonsillectomy pain

Reference	Catlin, 1991	April, 1996
Level (design)	1 (RCT)	1 (RCT)
Sample size*	25 (25)	(80)

OUTCOMES

Pain measure	"Symptoms of pain" not further specified	Faces Pain Rating Scale for children age 3–7 y, Oucher scale for children 8–15 y; "nonverbal indications of pain (e.g., tears, irritability, lethargy, increased respirations)
Time	"No difference noted . . . except for 2 of the control patients who returned on day 7 with complaints of severe throat pain"	10 h 24 h
Steroid		No difference noted.
Placebo		
p value		
Conclusion	No difference overall	No difference overall
Analgesic consumed	Use of meperidine; acetaminophen ± codeine	Acetaminophen consumed
Time	Lumped PODs 1–7	10 h 24 h
Steroid	No significant difference, no further details reported	"Dexamethasone group took more . . . but not a statistical significance"
Placebo		
p value		
Conclusion	No difference	No difference

STUDY DESIGN

Inclusion criteria	Tonsillectomy or adenotonsillectomy	Elective adenotonsillectomy
Exclusion criteria	Steroid or immunotherapy in the past year, other investigational drug use, contraindication to steroid use, known allergy to protocol medications, mental retardation, Down syndrome, peritonsillar abscess	History of ulcers, diabetes, steroid-dependent asthma, chronic medical disease, recent corticosteroid therapy
Dexamethasone regimen	8 mg/m2 IV ×1 before induction (maximum NR)	1 mg/kg (maximum 16 mg) IV ×1 before surgery
Antibiotic use	"Penicillins" at induction, continued for 7 d	Cefazolin 25 mg/kg IV ×1; amoxicillin or cefaclor ×10 d
Other analgesic or anesthetic medications	Induction with halothane in nitrous oxide, maintenance with isoflurane in nitrous; meperidine, acetaminophen with codeine	Thiopental or halothane/nitrous oxide; 36% of steroid group and 47% of placebo group received narcotic during anesthesia
Method of tonsillectomy	Dissection snare, electrocautery hemostasis	Needle tip cautery dissection
Indications for tonsillectomy	NR	Chronic tonsillitis Adenotonsillar hypertrophy
Age	4–12 y	3–15 y
Randomization effectiveness	Dexamethasone group with more males and slightly older; no stats reported	Dexamethasone group with more females and slightly younger; no stats reported
A priori power calculation reported	NR	NR

RCT = randomized controlled trial, POD = postoperative day, RD = rate difference, NS = not significant, NR = not reported, PACU = postanesthesia care unit, ASA = American Society of Anesthesiologists, IV = intravenous.
* Sample size: numbers shown for those completing the trial and those (initially recruited).

REFERENCES

1. April MM, Callan ND, Nowak DM, Hausdorff MA. The effect of intravenous dexamethasone in pediatric adenotonsillectomy. Arch Otolaryngol Head Neck Surg 1996;122(2):117–120.

2. Catlin FI, Grimes WJ. The effect of steroid therapy on recovery from tonsillectomy in children. Arch Otolaryngol Head Neck Surg 1991;117(6):649–652.

3. Ohlms LA, Wilder RT, Weston B. Use of intraoperative corticosteroids in pediatric tonsillectomy. Arch Otolaryngol Head Neck Surg 1995;121(7):737–742.

4. Pappas AL, Sukhani R, Hotaling AJ, et al. The effect of preoperative dexamethasone on the immediate and delayed postoperative morbidity in children undergoing adenotonsillectomy. Anesth Analg 1998;87(1):57–61.

5. Tom LW, Templeton JJ, Thompson ME, Marsh RR. Dexamethasone in adenotonsillectomy. Int J Pediatr Otorhinolaryngol 1996;37(2):115–120.

6. Vosdoganis F, Baines DB. The effect of single dose intravenous dexamethasone in tonsillectomy in children. Anaesth Intensive Care 1999;27(5):489–492.

7. Volk MS, Martin P, Brodsky L, Stanievich JF, Ballou M. The effects of preoperative steroids on tonsillectomy patients. Otolaryngol Head Neck Surg 1993;109(4):726–730.

8. Giannoni C, White S, Enneking FK. Does dexamethasone with preemptive analgesia improve pediatric tonsillectomy pain? Otolaryngology Head Neck Surg 2002;126(3):307–315.

9. Leinbach RF, Markwell SJ, Colliver JA, Lin SY. Hot versus cold tonsillectomy: A systematic review of the literature. Otolaryngol Head Neck Surg 2003;129:360–364.

4 Pediatric Tonsillectomy

4.D.1.

Preoperative coagulation screening tests versus no laboratory testing: Impact on rate of intraoperative/postoperative bleed

Jennifer J. Shin and Christopher J. Hartnick

METHODS

A computerized Ovid search of MEDLINE 1966–July 2003 was performed. The terms "tonsillectomy" and "tonsil" were exploded and the resulting articles were combined into a first group. Next, the term "hemorrhage" was exploded and combined with articles containing the keyword "bleeding," forming a second group. Then, the terms "prothrombin time," "partial thromboplastin time," "bleeding time," "blood coagulation tests," "coagulation protein disorders," and "blood coagulation disorders" were exploded and the resulting articles combined into a third group. Finally, the three groups were cross-referenced, yielding 93 articles. The resulting studies were reviewed and their references manually cross-checked for any further relevant articles. For inclusion criteria, we required the following: 1) a distinct patient population of children (≤19 years old) undergoing tonsillectomy or adenotonsillectomy; 2) analysis of a group that underwent preoperative screening with laboratory coagulation studies and one that did not; and 3) outcome measures of either postoperative and/or intraoperative bleeding. Studies that lumped data from children and adults were excluded, as were those that lumped data from adenoidectomy alone with tonsillectomy. This process yielded only one published report [1].

RESULTS

The only study to meet all inclusion criteria was a level 4 publication which reported on a group that underwent coagulation testing and a group that did not, but was not primarily designed to address the difference in the two groups. In this historical cohort of 339 consecutive patients, 261 children had either prothrombin time (PT) with partial thromboplastin time (PTT) or PTT-alone testing before surgery, whereas 78 children had no testing. Neither group had any intraoperative bleeds, defined as >450 cc of blood loss during the case. In the group with coagulation testing, 5.2% had "hemorrhage after surgery"

(not otherwise defined), with 1% requiring return to the operating room for control of bleeding. In the group without testing, there was a 3.3% rate of postoperative bleeding. Because this study is retrospective, however, it cannot overcome the inherent biases caused by the historical factors that prompted clinicians to test or not test. In addition, this is only one study, and it is not designed specifically to address this issue. Also, nonuniform testing with either PT/PTT or PTT alone was performed. Because of this paucity of evidence from controlled trials, we will also analyze the predictive value of coagulation testing in the subsequent section.

CLINICAL SIGNIFICANCE AND FUTURE RESEARCH

There is insufficient evidence to show whether the use of preoperative coagulation testing versus no testing results in a differential rate of intraoperative or postoperative bleeding with tonsillectomy. No randomized or other prospective clinical trial comparing bleeding rates in children with preoperative coagulation testing versus without preoperative coagulation testing exists in the literature at this time.

We may not see a definitive trial in the near future, but decisions still need to be made regarding the use of coagulation screening for tonsillectomy. With this conundrum in mind, we will next present the evidence regarding the predictive value of coagulation testing and comment on the associated costs, in order to provide the reader with the best current tools available for decision making.

REFERENCE

1. Howells RC 2nd, Wax MK, Ramadan HH. Value of preoperative prothrombin time/partial thromboplastin time as a predictor of postoperative hemorrhage in pediatric patients undergoing tonsillectomy. Otolaryngol Head Neck Surg 1997;117(6):628–632.

4 Pediatric Tonsillectomy

Preoperative coagulation screening tests: Predictive value for intraoperative/postoperative bleeding and for identification of occult bleeding disorders

Jennifer J. Shin and Christopher J. Hartnick

METHODS

Because of the dearth of literature comparing the rate of post-tonsillectomy bleeding in those with versus without preoperative coagulation testing, a second search of MEDLINE 1966–July 2003 was performed. The same Ovid search strategy and exclusion criteria described above were used, but we required modified inclusion criteria: 1) a distinct patient population of children (≤19 years old) undergoing tonsillectomy or adenotonsillectomy, 2) screening with laboratory coagulation studies, 3) outcome measures of either postoperative and/or intraoperative bleeding or newly identified bleeding disorders, and 4) outcomes reported for patients with abnormal versus normal coagulation testing. Positive and negative predictive values were calculated using Bayes theorem, using the disease prevalence reported in the individual studies. This process yielded four published reports [1–4].

RESULTS

Diagnostic and Outcome Measures. Multiple coagulation tests can be used for screening, including PT/international normalized ratio (INR), PTT, bleeding time, and platelet count. Abnormal results of these tests can be defined in terms of absolute values, comparison to controls, or standard deviations above the mean. Bleeding outcomes can be reported as intraoperative or postoperative bleeding. Bleeding itself may be defined by patient history, clinician-observed hemorrhage, amount of blood lost, and the need for readmission to the hospital or return to the operating room. Newly identified coagulation disorders include those that require perioperative intervention (i.e., von Willebrand's disease, factor VIII deficiency) and those that do not (i.e., factor XII deficiency). Because identification of disorders requiring preoperative intervention may also change postoperative bleeding results or potentially justify screening with coagulation testing, we have also analyzed this factor as a separate outcome.

Potential Confounders. Younger age may result in a larger population of patients with occult bleeding disorders, because older patients may be more likely to have already had an event that uncovered a congenital defect in the coagulation cascade. We have attempted to control for this potential confounder by excluding data from adult patients (>19 years old). In addition, data from patients undergoing adenoidectomy alone may dilute data from patients undergoing tonsillectomy or adenotonsillectomy, and we have excluded these results as well. Also, the method of and indications for tonsillectomy could potentially act as confounders. These methods, the variety of coagulation tests, and the reported definitions of bleeding are cataloged for the reader in as much detail as each study provides. In addition, postoperative instructions (i.e., whether regular oral intake is allowed, use of nonsteroidal antiinflammatory drugs, antibiotic use) may have an impact on bleeding, although these are not regularly reported in these trials.

Study Designs. All studies are case series of patients who underwent coagulation testing before tonsillectomy or adenotonsillectomy. Two are prospective with predetermined testing protocols, inclusion criteria, and outcome measurements [3, 4]. Two are retrospective and in one study not all patients received preoperative testing [1, 2]. Studies that do not report a calculated sensitivity, specificity, positive predictive value, and negative predictive value still provide enough information to allow the reader to calculate those items. The follow-up period ranged from 24 hours to 1 month. Results are similar across studies.

Highest Level of Evidence. These level 4 studies suggest that the positive predictive value of coagulation testing (0.03–0.14, combined[1] 0.02) is low for identifying children who will have intraoperative or postoperative bleeding. These values mean that as few as 3% of children with an abnormal panel may actually bleed, which is similar to reported overall rates. According to other results, however, as many as 14% of children with an abnormal panel may bleed, which is notably higher than reported overall rates. The combined[1] results suggest that positive predictive value is on the lower side. The negative predictive value of coagulation testing (0.90–0.98, combined[1] 0.92) is comparatively high, suggesting that 90%–98% of those with normal testing will not bleed. Depending on a surgeon's post-tonsillectomy bleeding rate, however, he or she may already know that a similar number will not bleed at baseline. Therefore, the utility of the positive and negative predictive values partially depends on the baseline bleeding rate for each otolaryngologist's patient population.

---

[1] Combined: The number of true positives, true negatives, false positives, and false negatives from each study were pooled and used to calculate the positive and negative predictive values for the four studies combined.

The other potential benefit of coagulation screening is the identification of patients who have a previously unrecognized bleeding disorder and would benefit from perioperative intervention, such as 1-(3-mercaptopropionic acid)-8-D-arginine vasopressin monoacetate trihydrate (DDAVP) for von Willebrand's disease. For this objective, the positive predictive value is also somewhat low (0.06–0.10, combined[1] 0.10). This means that approximately 10% of children with positive results will have an occult coagulation disorder that would benefit from perioperative intervention. The negative predictive value for identification of occult bleeding disorders is very high (1.00), suggesting that a negative result is highly reassuring, at least in the immediate postoperative period for which we have reported follow-up. The rate of new diagnosis of bleeding disorders is low (0.0%–0.7%, combined[1] 0.3%), suggesting that 333 (range 142–1000) children were screened to identify one occult bleeding disorder.

Applicability. These results are applicable to children undergoing tonsillectomy or adenotonsillectomy.

Cost. The charges for coagulation testing at a representative institution are as follows: PTT $28.50, PT/INR $28.50, platelet count $33.70 (CBC $44.85), bleeding time (this test was approximately $25, but has been discontinued at some institutions). With this in mind, the charge for an initial screen for one patient may be less than $30 for a single test and as high as $126.85 for the gamut of testing. In addition, there is another layer of charges associated with retesting and hematologic consultation. On the other side of the issue are the charges associated with postoperative bleeding. At one institution, charges are approximately as follows: one emergency room visit $863, one hospitalization for 23-hour observation $787, one return to the operating room $2928.

Finally, there is the emotional cost associated with needle sticks in young children and concerns over false positive results. This must be balanced with the emotional cost associated with a postoperative bleeding episode and returns to the hospital or operating room, as well as the morbidity and even potential mortality of these events.

CLINICAL SIGNIFICANCE AND FUTURE RESEARCH

A mix of prospective and retrospective level 4 evidence is available to show the predictive value of laboratory testing in children undergoing tonsillectomy with or without adenoidectomy. In the absence of a controlled trial comparing bleeding rates in children with versus without preoperative coagulation testing, we can use the predictive value of coagulation testing as a surrogate for decision making. In making those decisions, the predictive value of the testing must be balanced against its monetary and ethical cost. To determine where that balance lies, we must answer certain questions: How much is preventing one bleed or identifying one occult bleeding disorder that would require preoperative intervention worth? How does that worth translate to financial terms? How high does the positive or negative predictive value of a test need to be to justify its worth? In this circumstance, the evidence provides only parameters to use in decision making, rather than showing the difference in outcome when deciding to use or not use an intervention. In cases like this, when high-level controlled evidence is lacking, the practice of evidence-based medicine must then rely on more than just knowledge of the available clinical data. This expertise is combined with clinical judgment and awareness of patient preference. It is that clinical judgment that must determine whether the predictive value of coagulation screening in the face of its cost warrants its performance in all, some, or no previously healthy children.

THE EVIDENCE CONDENSED: Preoperative coagulation screening tests for children undergoing tonsillectomy

Reference	Gabriel, 2000		Burk, 1992	
Level (design)	4 (PCS)		4 (PCS)	
Sample size*	1479 (1706)		1603	
OUTCOMES				
	For postoperative bleeding	For disease discovery	For postoperative bleeding	For disease discovery
PPV[†]	0.14	0.10	0.07	0.06
NPV[†]	0.90	1.00	0.98	1.00
Coagulation testing defined as abnormal	PTT >46 s, PT >13.5 s, bleeding time >5 min, platelet count <150,000		PTT prolonged >2 s, PT prolonged >1.5 s, bleeding time prolonged >30 s, platelet counts (CBC) were all normal; these values are >3 standard deviations from the mean for each test	
Overall total rate of bleeding (timing of bleed)	10% (7% intraoperative, 3% postoperative)		2.3% (all postoperative)	
Intraoperative bleeding defined	"Abnormal intraoperative bleeding assessed by yes or no response"		NR	
Postoperative bleeding defined	"Immediate and delayed hemorrhage during the first 24 h requiring admission to the hospital and/or a return to the operating room" (no commentary about bleeding after 24 h)		"Postoperative bleeding severe enough to warrant prolonged hospital stay or readmission . . . in an interval from 1 h to 10 d after surgery"	
Total rate of new diagnosis of bleeding disorders	0.5%		0.1%	
STUDY DESIGN				
Inclusion criteria	Tonsillectomy, not otherwise specified		Tonsillectomy or adenotonsillectomy	
Exclusion criteria	NR		NR	
Age	9 mo–15 y		3–16 y	
Indications for surgery	Infection 54% OSA 33% Both 13%		NR	
Method of surgery	Sharp and blunt dissection at superior pole and snare excision of inferior pole with electrocautery 88%; Sluder technique 12%		NR	

MA = meta-analysis, PCS = prospective case series, RCS = retrospective case series, OSA = obstructive sleep apnea, PT = prothrombin time, PTT = partial thromboplastin time, PPV = positive predictive value, NPV = negative predictive value.

* Sample size: numbers shown for those completing the trial and those (initially recruited).

† Sensitivity, specificity, PPV, NPV reported for all abnormal coagulation testing (whether PT, PTT, bleeding time, platelet count) for bleeding/identification of a disease requiring preoperative intervention.

‡ No newly diagnosed conditions requiring perioperative intervention were identified in the study reported by Howells et al., limiting statistical analysis of this variable.

Reference	Kang, 1994		Howells, 1997
Level (design)	4 (RCS)		4 (RCS)
Sample size*	1061		331
OUTCOMES			
	For postoperative bleeding	For disease discovery	For postoperative bleeding
PPV†	0.10	0.06	0.03 ‡
NPV†	0.98	1.00	0.97 ‡
Coagulation testing defined as abnormal	"Prolonged PTT or bleeding time"; platelet count (CBC) and PT was "normal in all patients"		"Abnormal was defined . . . as two standard deviations above the mean" for PT/PTT or PTT
Overall total rate of bleeding (timing of bleed)	6% (only postoperative reported)		2.9% (0% intraoperative, all postoperative)
Intraoperative bleeding defined	NR		>450 cc intraoperative blood loss
Postoperative bleeding defined	"1) active bleeding requiring return to operating room for control, 2) active bleeding controlled by eschar removal by suctioning and application of anesthetic and vasoconstricting agents with gentle pressure, 3) no active bleeding seen, readmission for observation, 4) bleeding reported by parents at first postoperative visit (7–10 d)"		"Hemorrhage after surgery"; not further described
Total rate of new diagnosis of bleeding disorders	0.7%		0%
STUDY DESIGN			
Inclusion criteria	Adenotonsillectomy		Tonsillectomy or adenotonsillectomy
Exclusion criteria	Complete records not available		Less than 1 mo follow-up
Age	1–19 y		6 mo–12 y
Indications for surgery	Infection 36% Obstructive hyperplasia 37% Both 27%		Infection 43% OSA 8% Hypertrophy 39% Other 10%
Method of surgery	Curette adenoidectomy with electrocautery hemostasis; cold knife tonsil dissection with electrocautery hemostasis		Sharp, blunt, electrocautery dissection with excision at inferior pole with tonsil snare

MA = meta-analysis, PCS = prospective case series, RCS = retrospective case series, OSA = obstructive sleep apnea, PT = prothrombin time, PTT = partial thromboplastin time, PPV = positive predictive value, NPV = negative predictive value.

* Sample size: numbers shown for those completing the trial and those (initially recruited).

† Sensitivity, specificity, PPV, NPV reported for all abnormal coagulation testing (whether PT, PTT, bleeding time, platelet count) for bleeding/identification of a disease requiring preoperative intervention.

‡ No newly diagnosed conditions requiring perioperative intervention were identified in the study reported by Howells et al., limiting statistical analysis of this variable.

REFERENCES

1. Howells RC 2nd, Wax MK, Ramadan HH. Value of preoperative prothrombin time/partial thromboplastin time as a predictor of postoperative hemorrhage in pediatric patients undergoing tonsillectomy. Otolaryngol Head Neck Surg 1997;117(6):628–632.

2. Kang J, Brodsky L, Danziger I, Volk M, Stanievich J. Coagulation profile as a predictor for post-tonsillectomy and adenoidectomy (T + A) hemorrhage. Int J Pediatr Otorhinolaryngol 1994;28(2–3):157–165.

3. Gabriel P, Mazoit X, Ecoffey C. Relationship between clinical history, coagulation tests, and perioperative bleeding during tonsillectomies in pediatrics. J Clin Anesth 2000;12(4):288–291.

4. Burk CD, Miller L, Handler SD, Cohen AR. Preoperative history and coagulation screening in children undergoing tonsillectomy [comment]. Pediatrics 1992;89(4 Pt 2):691–695.

5 Pediatric Obstructive Sleep Apnea

5.A.

Tonsillectomy and/or adenoidectomy: Impact on polysomnogram

Mark Boseley and Christopher J. Hartnick

METHODS

A computerized Ovid search of MEDLINE from 1966 to September 2005 was performed. The term "obstructive sleep apnea" was searched and the resulting articles were cross-referenced with those obtained by exploding "tonsillectomy" or "adenoidectomy." The results were cross-referenced with the phrases "sleep study or respiratory distress index," or "polysomnogram" or "sleep study." A manual search of the bibliographies yielded no additional articles. Articles were identified that met the following inclusion criteria: 1) children <18 years old with at least a clinical history of sleep-disordered breathing (SDB), 2) treatment with a tonsillectomy, adenoidectomy, or both, and 3) evaluation with both pre- and posttreatment nocturnal polysomnogram. Exclusion criteria were preexisting craniofacial abnormalities, history of Down syndrome, retrospective studies, and children who had other surgical procedures than adenotonsillectomy. Six studies that met these inclusion/exclusion criteria were included in the subsequent review [1–6].

RESULTS

Outcome Measures. The outcome measured was posttreatment change in apnea-hypopnea index (AHI) or respiratory distress index (RDI). The AHI is defined as the total number of obstructive apneas and hypopneas per hour of total sleep time. The RDI is equivalent to the AHI score. Each study defined obstructive sleep apnea (OSA) differently based on their interpretation of an abnormal polysomnogram. The criteria used for each are listed in the subsequent summary tables. These values were obtained from a standard overnight polysomnogram.

Potential Confounders. Results may potentially be biased by: 1) attrition as a result of several studies losing a large proportion of their study patients to follow-up, 2) there was a selection bias in that only children of caregivers who were concerned about their child's breathing were included, and 3) some studies only included children with an AHI >1 which would fail to include those who could still have significant sleep fragmentation from SDB. Once again, most studies lacked an internal control, and therefore it is difficult to conclude a direct cause and effect relationship.

Study Designs. There was one prospective trial that compared a group who had surgical intervention with a group who had no surgery [3] and five prospective cohort studies that compared preoperative data with postoperative data [1, 2, 4–6]. Nieminen et al. [3] had an OSA group, a primary snorer group, and a group of healthy children as controls. The remaining studies were prospective cohort studies that used preoperative data as control data [1, 2, 4–6].

Highest Level of Evidence. All six of these level 2 studies concluded that children diagnosed with OSA based on overnight polysomnogram typically show improvement on their postoperative study. However, each study had significant limitations. Suen et al. [1] and Tal et al. [5] had the largest groups of patients who completed a postoperative PSG (26 and 36, respectively), but both had a significant patient dropout rate. Interestingly, both studies revealed that nearly half of patients with symptoms suggestive of OSA will have normal PSGs. Shintani et al. [2] had the largest study group overall (134 patients), but they included all patients in their study regardless if they had a preoperative normal PSG. Interestingly, one might conclude that their results would have even been better had they excluded patients with a normal sleep study. Nieminen et al. [3] had the only study with a separate control group, but 16 of 21 patients in their study group had previously had an adenoidectomy. They found that the study group had an improvement in PSG scores and the control group remained unchanged. Furthermore, through regression analysis, they concluded that tonsil size was larger in the study group. Jain and Sahni [4] had 30 patients in their study group; however, 19 had only an adenoidectomy performed. They found that adenoid size (not tonsil size) correlated to grade of OSA. This seems somewhat contrary to the results from Nieminen et al. Finally, Stewart et al. [6] examined quality of life and PSG data for a group of patients. Unfortunately, only 17 of 47 patients completed a postoperative PSG 1 year after surgery.

Applicability. The conclusions from these studies may be applied to healthy children <18 years old. They should not be applied to children with craniofacial abnormalities or Down syndrome.

Morbidity/Complications. There were no reported morbidities or complications in the studies included in this review.

CLINICAL SIGNIFICANCE AND FUTURE RESEARCH

There are six prospective controlled trials that address the impact of tonsillectomy and adenoidectomy on pediatric OSA. The implications of these results are that clinical history alone may not be sufficient to determine if a child has significant OSA. However, once diagnosed with OSA by PSG, most will have significant improvement after tonsillectomy, adenoidectomy, or both.

Although most of these studies were of adequate sample size to obtain a power of 80% and an alpha of 0.05 (based on their *a priori* calculations), the individual studies often had a large attrition rate that could affect their conclusions. Also, several studies included a combination of treatments for their study group, which could confound their stated results. In addition, the definition of what constituted OSA on PSG was varied among the studies.

Future studies should make an effort to standardize what constitutes an "abnormal" PSG result. Children with abnormal results should then be treated in a standard manner (i.e., adenotonsillectomy). Children with "normal" pretreatment PSGs can serve as a comparison group. Nieminen et al. [3] used this method in their study. Future studies may also focus on the impact on quality of life, especially in this group with "normal" PSGs.

Reference	Suen, 1995	Shintani, 1998	Nieminen, 2000
Level	2 (prospective controlled)	2 (prospective controlled)	2 (prospective controlled)
Sample size*	26 (69)	134 (134)	21 (78)
OUTCOMES			
Intervention	T&A	T&A, adenoidectomy, tonsillectomy, adenomonotonsillectomy	T&A
Mean RDI, preop PSG	18.1 ± 11.3	24.7 ± 13.4	Surgery group (21): 6.9 Nonsurgery (37): 0.4 Control (30): 0
Mean RDI, postop PSG	4.5 ± 8.4	8.2 ± 5.5	Surgery: 0.3 Nonsurgery: 0.2
Statistical significance	$p < 0.001$	$p < 0.005$	$p < 0.01$ (preop vs postop)
Conclusion	Significant improvement with surgery	Significant improvement with surgery	Significant improvement with surgery
Follow-up time	At least 6 wk postop	2 mo postop	6 mo postop
STUDY DESIGN			
Inclusion criteria	All children suspected of having OSA on clinical evaluation and an RDI >5	Children with complaints of snoring and apnea; no specific history of witnessed apneas specified	Symptoms suggestive of OSAS, regular snorers, and/or had apneas during sleep based on clinical history and parental questionnaire
Exclusion criteria	History of neurologic or craniofacial abnormalities	History of mental or motor delay, Down syndrome, craniofacial abnormalities, excessive obesity	Upper airway anomalies and abnormal facial morphology
Intervention regimen details	100% T&A	85% T&A 10% adenoidectomy alone 3% adenomonotonsillectomy 2% tonsillectomy alone	100% T&A
Age	1–14 y	1–9 y	2–10 y
Diagnostic criteria for OSA	RDI ≥5	AHI ≥10	AHI ≥1
Criteria for withdrawal from study (if prospective)	Patient fails to complete preop and postop PSG	Patient fails to complete preop and postop PSG	Patient fails to complete preop and postop PSG or does not follow up
Consecutive patients?	Yes	Yes	Yes
Morbidity/complication	None reported	None reported	None reported

T&A = adenotonsillectomy, preop = preoperative, postop = postoperative, OSA = obstructive sleep apnea, OSAS = obstructive sleep apnea syndrome, PSG = polysomnogram, RDI = respiratory distress index, AHI = apnea-hypopnea index.
* Sample size: numbers shown for those not lost to follow-up and those (initially recruited).

Reference	Jain, 2002	Tal, 2003	Stewart, 2005
Level	2 (prospective controlled)	2 (prospective controlled)	2 (prospective controlled)
Sample size*	40 (40)	36 (70)	29 (31)
Intervention	T, A, or T&A	T&A	T&A
OUTCOMES			
Mean RDI, preop PSG	Obstructive group (I)†: 27.57 Inflammatory group (II): 12.39	4.1	14.8
Mean RDI, postop PSG	Group I: 6.007 Group II: 10.89	0.9	3.16
Statistical significance	Group I: $p < 0.01$ Group II: $p < 0.05$	$p < 0.0001$	$p = 0.004$
Conclusion	Significant improvement after surgery	Significant improvement after surgery	Significant improvement after surgery
Follow-up time	6–8 wk postop	Mean of 4.6 mo postop	12 mo postop
STUDY DESIGN			
Inclusion criteria	Age 4–12 y with adenoid or tonsil hypertrophy; no other history specified	Children with history consistent with SDB, had RDI >1; clinical history also included a parental questionnaire	Children enrolled based on suspicion of SDB from a history and/or audiotape or witnessed apneas
Exclusion criteria	Down syndrome, craniofacial abnormalities, mental retardation, excessive obesity	History of chronic medical illness or facial abnormalities	Non–English-speaking parent or child, chronic medical conditions, diagnosis of ADHD, children taking any stimulants, history of neurologic disorders, craniofacial abnormalities
Intervention regimen details	53% adenoidectomy alone, 20% T&A, 27% tonsillectomy alone	100% T&A	100% T&A
Age	4–12 y	1–12 y	6–12 y
Diagnostic criteria for OSA	AHI >5	RDI >5	AHI >1
Criteria for withdrawal from study (if prospective)	Patient fails to complete preop and postop PSG	Patient fails to complete preop and postop PSG or did not have positive first PSG	Patient fails to complete preop and postop PSG or did not have positive first PSG
Consecutive patients?	Yes	Yes	Yes
Morbidity/complication	None reported	None reported	None reported

T&A = adenotonsillectomy, preop = preoperative, postop = postoperative, OSA = obstructive sleep apnea, SDB = sleep-disordered breathing, PSG = polysomnogram, ADHD = attention deficit hyperactivity disorder, RDI = respiratory distress index, AHI = apnea-hypopnea index, AI = apnea index.
* Sample size: numbers shown for those not lost to follow-up and those (initially recruited).
† Group I = obstructive indications for surgery; Group II = inflammatory indications for surgery.

REFERENCES

1. Suen JS, Arnold JE, Brooks LJ. Adenotonsillectomy for treatment of obstructive sleep apnea in children. Arch Otolaryngol Head Neck Surg 1995;121:525–530.
2. Shintani T, Asakura K, Kataura A. The effect of adenotonsillectomy in children with OSA. Int J Pediatr Otorhinolaryngol 1998;44:51–58.
3. Nieminen P, Tolonen U, Lopponen H. Snoring and obstructive sleep apnea in children: a 6-month follow-up study. Arch Otolaryngol Head Neck Surg 2000;126:481–486.
4. Jain A, Sahni JK. Polysomnographic studies in children undergoing adenoidectomy and/or tonsillectomy. J Laryngol Otol 2002;116:711–715.
5. Tal A, Bar A, Leiberman A, Tarasiuk A. Sleep characteristics following adenotonsillectomy in children with obstructive sleep apnea syndrome. Chest 2003;124:948–953.
6. Stewart MG, Glaze DG, Friedman EM, Smith EO, Bautista M. Quality of life and sleep study findings after adenotonsillectomy in children with obstructive sleep apnea. Arch Otolaryngol Head Neck Surg 2005;131:308–314.

5 Pediatric Obstructive Sleep Apnea

5.B.

Tonsillectomy and/or adenoidectomy: Impact on quality of life

Mark Boseley and Christopher J. Hartnick

METHODS

A computerized Ovid search of MEDLINE from 1966 to September 2005 was performed. The term "obstructive sleep apnea" was searched and the resulting articles were cross-referenced with those obtained by exploding "tonsillectomy" or "adenoidectomy." The results from this search were cross-referenced with the term "quality of life." The bibliographies were also manually checked which yielded no further articles. The articles were then reviewed to identify those that met the following inclusion criteria: 1) children younger than 18 years with at least a clinical history of sleep disordered breathing (SDB) or obstructive sleep apnea (OSA), 2) treatment with tonsillectomy, adenoidectomy, or both, and 3) evaluation with a validated disease-specific quality of life instrument before and after surgery. Excluded were studies that focused on children with preexisting craniofacial abnormalities, history of Down syndrome, retrospective studies, and children who had surgical procedures other than adenotonsillectomy. After applying these criteria, there were six studies that remained for review.

RESULTS

Outcome Measures. Two disease-specific validated instruments were used in these studies. The first of these was the Obstructive Sleep Disorders 6 (OSD-6) instrument. This includes six domains: physical suffering, sleep disturbance, speech or swallowing problems, emotional distress, activity limitations, and caregiver concerns.

The second validated OSA instrument was the OSA-18 instrument. The OSA-18 has 18 questions in five domains: sleep disturbance, physical suffering, emotional distress, daytime problems, and caregiver concerns.

In addition, two of the studies implemented other validated health-related instruments. The Children's Health Questionnaire Parent Form 28 (CHQPF-28) was used to evaluate global health in the child [1]. The Child Behavior Checklist (CBCL) was an instrument used to assess child behavior [2]. The results of these two surveys were not emphasized in the summary charts because they were not the outcomes of interest for this review.

Potential Confounders. Results may potentially be biased by: 1) there was attrition as a result of several studies losing a large proportion of their study patients to follow-up, 2) there was a selection bias in that only children of caregivers who were concerned about their child's breathing were included, 3) there was very likely to be expectation bias among caregivers who wanted to believe that their children had improved after surgery, and 4) most studies were observational in nature, lacking an internal control, and therefore it is difficult to conclude a direct cause and effect relationship.

Study Designs. There were six prospective cohort studies of subpopulations with SDB with comparison of preoperative and postoperative data [1, 3–6]. The deSerres et al. [3, 4] studies used a matched-pairs analysis, with each patient serving as his/her own control.

Highest Level of Evidence. All of the studies consistently reported that the scores on disease-specific surveys improved after surgery. The deSerres et al. [3, 4] studies found that nearly all of their study patients had improved OSD-6 scores. However, most of their patients were diagnosed with OSA on history and physical examination alone, with only a small percentage conducting a preoperative sleep study (6% and 8%, respectively) [3, 4]. Likewise, Goldstein et al. [2] conducted preoperative sleep studies on 8% of their patients. They also had a significant attrition rate (64 of 133 completed the study) and 16% of their study group had a tonsillectomy for chronic tonsillitis [2]. The Flanary [5] study found short- and long-term improvement on the OSD-18, but did not find the same improvement on the generic quality of life instrument. None of their patients underwent a preoperative sleep study [1]. Sohn and Rosenfeld [1] compared the results of two disease-specific instruments (OSD-6 and OSD-18) and found that their change scores had a high level of correlation. They also found that OSD-18 change scores correlated with adenoid and tonsil size [5]. Only the Mitchell et al. [6] study utilized a preoperative sleep study to make the diagnosis of OSA in all of their study patients. They documented a statistically significant improvement in change scores on the OSA-18 after surgery, but did not obtain a postoperative sleep study [6].

Applicability. The conclusions from these studies may be applied to healthy children less than 18 years old. They should not be applied to children with craniofacial abnormalities or Down syndrome.

Morbidity/Complications. There were no reported morbidities or complications in the studies included in this review.

There were two prospective controlled trials included in this review that utilized patients as their own control in a matched-pair design. The remaining four studies were prospective cohort studies comparing preoperative with postoperative data. All of these studies demonstrated significant improvement after tonsillectomy, adenoidectomy, or both. The studies that included patients who had a polysomnogram (PSG) seemed to imply that clinical history and examination alone are not sufficient to determine if a child has significant OSA. Therefore, one might call into question the results of those studies that primarily enrolled patients based only on physical examination findings. However, it is clear that children with symptoms consistent with OSA seem to have improved disease-specific quality of life after surgery.

Future research should attempt to correlate disease-specific survey results with preoperative and postoperative PSG. This might allow the use of these instruments to better classify which children should have surgery without the added expense of performing a sleep study on every patient.

Reference	de Serres, 2000	de Serres, 2002	Goldstein, 2002
Level (design)	2 (prospective controlled)	2 (prospective controlled)	2 (prospective controlled)
Sample size*	62 (100)	101 (115)	64 (131)
OUTCOMES			
Instruments used to measure QOL	OSD-6 (range of scores: 0 = no problems, 6 = could not be worse)	OSD-6 (range of scores: 0 = no problems, 6 = could not be worse)	Child behavior checklist (CBCL) and OSA-18
Results of surgery	Surgical group: 88.4% large change† Nonsurgical group: 100% trivial	74.5% large change,† 6.1% moderate, 7.1% small Preop change: 100% trivial Change score = 2.3	OSA-18 mean: change score of 2.3 Abnormal behavior seen in 16 children preop and 5 postop
Postop scores	88.4% large change score† Mean change score = 3.0	Matched-pairs design: 74.5% large change,† 6.1% moderate, 7.1% small Change score = 2.3	OSA-18 mean: change score of 2.3 Abnormal behavior seen in 16 children preop
Preop scores	Median preop score = 4.5	Preop change: 100% trivial	Abnormal behavior seen in 5 children postop
Nonsurgical group scores	100% trivial change score (n = 12)	No nonsurgical group	No nonsurgical group
Statistical significance	Reliability of change score to clinical response: correlation = 0.86 (>0.7 considered good reliability) This is correlation between degree of clinical change (global QOL) and OSD-6 between pre- and postop scores	Differences in preop and postop scores, p < 0.001	OSA-18 differences preop to postop, p < 0.001 OSA-18 change score had fair correlation with change in CBCL score, r = 0.5, p < 0.001
Conclusion	Change scores show excellent reliability (see above)	Significant improvement in scores after surgery	Significant improvement in scores after surgery
Follow-up time	4–5 wk	4–5 wk	12 wk
STUDY DESIGN			
Inclusion criteria	Patients with T&A hypertrophy and obstructive sleep disorder who were scheduled for T&A	Patients with T&A hypertrophy and obstructive sleep disorder who were scheduled for T&A	Patients scheduled for T&A for OSA or recurrent tonsillitis; including parent history of snoring and apneic pauses
Exclusion criteria	Tonsil pathology other than hypertrophy, non–English-speaking caregivers, procedure being done on same day	Tonsil pathology other than hypertrophy, non–English-speaking caregivers, procedure being done on same day	Down syndrome or other syndromes affecting the head and neck, neuromuscular or psychiatric disorders, history of mental retardation, non–English-speaking caregivers
Intervention regimen details	100% T&A	100% T&A	100% T&A
Age	2–12 y	2–12 y	2–18 y
Diagnostic criteria for	Clinical history and exam—see inclusion criteria; not further defined	Clinical history and exam—see inclusion criteria; not further defined	Clinical history and exam—see inclusion criteria
Criteria for withdrawal from study (if prospective)	Patients decided not to participate or failed to complete postop surveys	Patients decided not to participate or failed to complete postop surveys	Patients decided not to participate or failed to complete postop surveys
Consecutive patients?	Yes	Yes	Yes
Morbidity/complications	None	None	None

OSA = obstructive sleep apnea, QOL = quality of life, OSD-6 = Obstructive Sleep Disorder 6 survey, OSA-18 = Obstructive Sleep Apnea 18 survey, CBCL = Child Behavior Checklist, preop = preoperative, postop = postoperative, T&A = adenotonsillectomy.
* Sample size: numbers shown for those not lost to follow-up and those (initially recruited).
† Change score of <0.5 defined as trivial change; 0.5–0.9 small change; 1–1.4 moderate change; ≥1.4 large change.

THE EVIDENCE CONDENSED: Pediatric OSA: Impact of adenotonsillectomy on QOL

Reference	Flanary, 2003	Sohn, 2003	Mitchell, 2004
Level (design)	2 (prospective controlled)	2 (prospective controlled)	2 (prospective controlled)
Sample size*	57 (60)	69 (69)	60 (66)
OUTCOMES			
Instruments used to measure QOL	CHQPF-28 [scores transformed to 100-point scale (0 = worst possible, 100 = best possible score)] and OSA-18 (1 = none of the time, 7 = all of the time)	OSA-18 (1 = none of the time, 7 = all of the time) and OSD-6 (range of scores: 0 = no problems, 6 = couldn't be worse)	OSA-18 (1 = none of the time, 7 = all of the time)
Postop scores	OSA-18 score = 2.3 (mean at 3–6 wk) OSA-18 score = 2.08 (mean at 6–12 mo) Overall change score for OSA-18† = 2.12	Overall change score for OSA-18† = 1.14	35.8 (total score)
Preop scores	Preop OSA-18 score = 4.2 (mean)	Preop OSA-18 score = 3.1 (mean)	Preop 71.4 (total score)
Statistical significance	OSA-18 differences preop to short- and long-term postop (p < 0.001)	OSA-18 change score had good correlation to OSD-6 change score,† r = 0.71, p < 0.0001 Overall change in OSA-18 after surgery significant (p < 0.001)	p < 0.002
Conclusion	Significant changes in OSA-18 after surgery	OSA-18 and OSD-6 have good correlation in detecting postoperative changes	Significant changes in OSA-18 scores after surgery
Follow-up time	3 wk and 6 mo postop	>4 wk postop	Within 6 mo postop
STUDY DESIGN			
Inclusion criteria	Patients with clinical diagnosis of upper airway obstruction or OSA; had to have a history of loud snoring with an audio tape when reliability was questioned; those with witnessed apneas and >3+ tonsils were classified as having OSA	Patients with a history of snoring or disruptive sleep for >3 mo who were scheduled for surgery	Patients with OSA documented on prior nocturnal sleep study; clinical history from family not included
Exclusion criteria	Surgery being done for any reason other than airway obstruction	Down syndrome or other syndromes affecting the head and neck, neuromuscular or psychiatric disorders, history of mental retardation, non–English-speaking caregivers	Children <3 y or >12 y, previous T&A, craniofacial syndromes, neuromuscular or psychiatric disorders, developmental delay, RDI <1
Intervention regimen details	100% T&A	52% T&A, 44% adenoidectomy alone, 4% tonsillectomy alone	100% T&A
Age	2–16 y	6 mo–12 y	3–12 y
Diagnostic criteria for	Clinical history and exam—see inclusion criteria	Clinical history and exam—see inclusion criteria; not further defined	PSG
Criteria for withdrawal from study (if prospective)	Patients decided not to participate or failed to complete postop surveys	Patients decided not to participate or failed to complete postop surveys	Patients decided not to participate or failed to complete postop surveys
Consecutive patients?	Yes	Yes	Yes
Morbidity/ complications	None	None	None

OSA = obstructive sleep apnea, QOL = quality of life, preop = preoperative, postop = postoperative, CHQPF-28 = Children's Health Questionnaire Parent Form 28, OSA-18 = Obstructive Sleep Apnea 18 survey, OSD-6 = Obstructive Sleep Disorder 6 survey, T&A = adenotonsillectomy, RDI = respiratory distress index, PSG = polysomnogram.
* Sample size: numbers shown for those not lost to follow-up and those (initially recruited).
† Change score of <0.5 defined as trivial change; 0.5–0.9 small change; 1–1.4 moderate change; ≥1.5 large change.

REFERENCES

1. Sohn H, Rosenfeld RM. Evaluation of sleep-disordered breathing in children. Otolaryngol Head Neck Surg 2003;128:344–352.
2. Goldstein NA, Fatima M, Campbell TF, Rosenfeld RM. Child behavior and quality of life before and after tonsillectomy and adenoidectomy. Arch Otolaryngol Head Neck Surg 2002;128:770–775.
3. deSerres LM, Derkay C, Astley S, Deyo RA, Rosenfeld RM, Gates GA. Measuring quality of life in children with obstructive sleep disorders. Arch Otolaryngol Head Neck Surg 2000;126:1423–1429.
4. deSerres LM, Derkay C, Sie K, et al. Impact of adenotonsillectomy on quality of life in children with obstructive sleep disorders. Arch Otolaryngol Head Neck Surg 2002;128:489–496.
5. Flanary VA. Long-term effects of adenotonsillectomy on quality of life in pediatric patients. Laryngoscope 2003;113:1639–1644.
6. Mitchell RB, Kelly J, Call E, Yao N. Quality of life after adenotonsillectomy for obstructive sleep apnea in children. Arch Otolaryngol Head Neck Surg 2004;130:190–194.

6 Pediatric Recurrent Acute Otitis Media

6.A.

Amoxicillin or ampicillin prophylaxis versus placebo: Impact on number of subsequent episodes of acute otitis media, chance of no further episodes of acute otitis media

Jennifer J. Shin, Sandra S. Stinnett, and Christopher J. Hartnick

METHODS

A computerized Ovid search of MEDLINE 1966–January 2004 was performed. The terms "otitis media" and "antibiotics" were exploded and the resulting articles were cross-referenced, yielding 1947 trials. Given the known richness of the otitis media literature and the authority of higher levels of evidence, these articles were then limited to randomized controlled trials (RCTs), resulting in 302 articles. These articles were then reviewed to identify those that met the following inclusion criteria: 1) patient population <18 years of age with documented recurrent acute otitis media (RAOM), 2) intervention with continuous amoxicillin or ampicillin prophylaxis versus placebo control, 3) outcome measured in terms of the number of episodes of acute otitis media (AOM). Articles in which noncontinuous antibiotic therapy was administered were excluded, as were articles that included patients on the basis of chronic middle ear effusion (MEE) alone. Also excluded were articles that were not placebo controlled, as well as those that enrolled children with nonrecurrent AOM (i.e., only one previous episode). The bibliographies of the articles that met these inclusion/exclusion criteria were manually checked to ensure no further relevant articles could be identified. This process yielded nine articles, five of which focused on amoxicillin or ampicillin prophylaxis versus placebo [1–5], and these studies are reviewed below. The other articles are discussed in subsequent sections in this chapter.

RESULTS

Outcome Measures. Outcomes in all three studies were measured in terms of the number of episodes of AOM subsequent to treatment. AOM is diagnosed mainly with otoscopy, with adjunctive information from patient history and tympanometry. There are, however, minor variations in diagnostic criteria among practitioners, and each study here diagnosed AOM "episodes" on the basis of somewhat different criteria. Further details are provided in the adjoining table. Reported here is the mean number of episodes of AOM per child year, as well as the percent of children with no further episodes of AOM in the follow-up period.

Potential Confounders. The incidence of otitis media is known to decrease with increased age and vary with season, making both of these variables potential confounders. Also, the severity and frequency of previous AOM episodes, as well as the presence or absence of MEE at the outset of the study may influence outcomes. In addition, the specifics of the dose and timing of the antibiotic regimen for prophylaxis, as well as for treatment of frank AOM flairs, may alter the results. Finally, allergies, breast milk feeding, gender, genetics, daycare attendance, and exposure to tobacco smoke may affect AOM outcomes. All of these potential confounders or the way in which investigators addressed them have been cataloged for the reader in the adjoining table in as much detail as the original reports allow.

Study Designs. Five RCTs address this clinical query. Randomization proved effective in balancing multiple patient characteristics between the antibiotic and placebo study groups at the outset of each trial (see table for details). Attrition rates (i.e., number of patients who were enrolled but were lost to follow-up) ranged from 0% to 43%, with the higher rates potentially skewing results. Some patients were not lost to follow-up, but were withdrawn from the study prematurely for severe AOM or MEE (see table). In all cases, however, an intention to treat analysis was performed to minimize skewing the data toward less-affected children. Follow-up times ranged from 1 month to 2 years, and the study with a follow-up time of less than 3 months still addressed the seasonal impact by comparing the winter and nonwinter incidence of AOM in the antibiotic versus placebo groups. No significant differences were identified in either the winter (p = 0.88) or nonwinter (p = 0.64) analyses [1]. All five RCTs evaluated once-daily dosing, and one also evaluated twice-daily dosing, but no difference in AOM incidence was identified with the two dosing schedules in that study [1].

Highest Level of Evidence. Four level 1 studies found a significant improvement in the incidence of AOM with amoxicillin or ampicillin prophylaxis, as compared with placebo [2, 3]. In addition, they noted that the chance of having no further episodes of AOM was significantly greater with antibiotic prophylaxis; they reported rate differences (RD)[1] of −16% to −36%. These figures imply that three to seven children need to be treated with continuous amoxicillin therapy in order to allow one child to remain otitis-free in a 1-year period, or that the number needed to treat (NNT)[2] is three to seven children. The fifth RCT, however, reported incongruous results, concluding that there was no difference with amoxicillin prophylaxis versus placebo [1]. In fact, their data even showed a trend toward better outcomes with placebo, although this was not statistically significant. No *a priori* sample size estimate to achieve the standard 90% power was reported for this trial, although the sample size was even larger than that of other studies that did demonstrate a statistical difference. This study excluded patients with MEE at the outset of the trial, but two other trials with the same entry criterion still found a significant difference between amoxicillin and placebo groups

[1, 4]. The divergent study's follow-up period was also shorter than the others', which might potentially account for the difference in their results. Given this one incongruous finding, however, we have numerically combined the data in a subsequent meta-analysis.

Applicability. These results are applicable to children up to 6 years old with RAOM but no major comorbidities.

Morbidity. One study reported a 7% incidence of adverse effects in the antibiotic group, all of which were minor [2]. This figure suggests 15 children could be treated without adverse effects before one child developed a problem. In addition, this study also reported the results of nasopharyngeal and oropharyngeal swabs from children in the amoxicillin versus placebo [2]. The amoxicillin group had a higher percentage of subjects from whom beta-lactamase–producing organisms were isolated (22% amoxicillin versus 13% placebo).

---

[1] RD is the absolute difference in successful outcomes between the study group and the control group. For example, in the Casselbrant, 1992 study, 58% of the amoxicillin group versus 40% of the placebo group had no further episodes of AOM. The RD in this study was 40% − 58% = −18%.

[2] NNT is the total number of children that must be treated in order for one child to obtain benefit from the treatment. It is calculated by determining the inverse of the RD. For example, for the Casselbrant study, the RD is −18%, so that the NNT = 1/0.18 = 5.6. In this case, six children would need to be treated so as to obtain benefit for one child.

THE EVIDENCE CONDENSED: Amoxicillin or ampicillin prophylaxis versus placebo for recurrent acute otitis media

Reference	Roark, 1997		Casselbrant, 1992	
Level (design)	1 (RCT)		1 (RCT)	
Sample size*	158 (194)		100 (178)	
OUTCOMES				
	No. of AOM episodes per child years	% of children with no further AOM episodes	No. of AOM episodes per child years	% of children with no further AOM episodes
Amoxicillin	2.79 (q.d.) 3.16 (b.i.d.)	64% (q.d.) 61% (b.i.d.)	0.60	58%
Placebo	2.62	63%	1.08	40%
p Value	p = 0.71	p = 0.89	p < 0.001	p = 0.03
Conclusion	No difference	No difference	Amoxicillin better	Amoxicillin better
Follow-up time	1–3 mo, n = 91; >3 mo, n = 67		2 y	
STUDY DESIGN				
Inclusion criteria	Age 3 mo–6 y with 3 documented episodes of AOM within 6 mo		Age 7–35 mo, most recent episode in <6 mo, ≥3 episodes of AOM in the preceding 6 mo, or ≥4 in 12 mo; *free from MEE at time of entry*	
Exclusion criteria	*Presence of MEE*, ventilating tubes or associated anatomic defects, immunodeficiency disorders, or allergy to penicillin		Asthma, chronic sinusitis, previous tonsillectomy or adenoidectomy	
Randomization effectiveness	No difference in age, sex, passive smoking, family history of RAOM, history of RAD, use of child care, age of initial otitis episode, history of supine feeding, mouth breathing, or snoring		No difference in age, season, previous number of AOM episodes, sex, race, socioeconomic status	
Age	3 mo–6 y		7–35 mo	
Masking	Double-blind		Double-blind	
Amoxicillin/ ampicillin regimen	Amoxicillin 20 mg/kg/d either split into b.i.d. dosing or in 1 dose (with a second dose of placebo)		Amoxicillin 20 mg/kg/d in 1 nightly dose	
Diagnostic criteria for an episode of AOM	Otoscopic findings of diminished TM mobility associated with a red or yellow color		Otoscopic signs (erythema or white opacification not attributable to scarring, fullness or bulging, and decreased mobility of TM) or ≥1 symptom (fever, otalgia, irritability) with MEE	
Management of AOM episode while on study treatment	Trimethoprim/sulfamethoxazole, erythromycin/ sulfisoxazole, cefixime, cefprozil, cefaclor, or cephalexin ×10 d; cessation of study medication until 10-d course was complete		Amoxicillin 40 mg/kg/d in 3 divided doses ×10 d unless tympanocentesis cultures revealed resistant organisms—then erythromycin 50 mg/kg/d and sulfisoxazole 150 mg/kg/d ×10 d	
Compliance	89%–95% as assessed by diary and urine testing		82%–95% for antibiotic and placebo, as assessed by calendar method, bottle method, and urine specimens	
Criteria for withdrawal from study	MEE >8 wk despite two courses of antibiotics; 2 new AOM episodes in <90 d		1) ≥4 tympanocenteses within 6 mo or ≥5 within 12 mo, 2) ≥180 total d MEE in the same ear within 12 mo, 3) ≥3 tube replacements within 12 mo, 4) suppurative complication, 5) cholesteatoma, 6) significant adverse reaction to amoxicillin	
Intention to treat analysis	Yes		Yes	
Morbidity/ complications	NR		Amoxicillin group with 7.0% adverse reactions (all minor) Beta-lactamase producing bacteria isolated from pharyngeal swabs in 22% of the amoxicillin group vs 13% of the placebo group	

AOM = acute otitis media, RAOM = recurrent AOM, RCT = randomized controlled trial, MEE = middle ear effusion, TM = tympanic membrane, q.d. = once a day dosing, b.i.d. = twice a day dosing, RAD = reactive airway disease, NR = not reported.
* Sample size: numbers shown for those not lost to follow-up and those (initially recruited).

THE EVIDENCE CONDENSED: Amoxicillin or ampicillin prophylaxis versus placebo for recurrent acute otitis media

Reference	Maynard, 1972	
Level (design)	1 (RCT)	
Sample size*	364 (364)	

OUTCOMES		
	No. of AOM episodes per child years	% of children with no further AOM episodes
Amoxicillin	0.42	76%
Placebo	0.79	60%
p Value	p < 0.001 if >67% compliance; p = NS if <67%	p < 0.05
Conclusion	Ampicillin better	Ampicillin better
Follow-up time	1 y	

STUDY DESIGN	
Inclusion criteria	Age <7 y, previous enrollment in a longitudinal epidemiologic study of otitis media
Exclusion criteria	Not otherwise specified
Randomization effectiveness	Matched family size, age, history of middle ear disease for study children within the household. Male to female ratio was 1 : 3 in the ampicillin group and 1 : 2 in the placebo group
Age	<1 to 6 y
Masking	Double-blind
Amoxicillin/ ampicillin regimen	Ampicillin anhydrous 125 mg PO q.d. if ≤2.5 y, 250 mg PO q.d. if >2.5 y
Diagnostic criteria for an episode of AOM	Spontaneous occurrence of purulent drainage from one or both ears after an interval of at least 2 wk without such drainage
Management of AOM episode while on study treatment	"No attempt was made to alter the usual antibiotic therapy for acute episodes of illness as prescribed by the hospital physician and administered by the local health aid"
Compliance	Ranged from >1/3 of study medications to >2/3 of medications, as assessed by bottle method
Criteria for withdrawal from study	NR
Intention to treat analysis	Yes
Morbidity/ complications	NR

AOM = acute otitis media, RAOM = recurrent AOM, RCT = randomized controlled trial, MEE = middle ear effusion, TM = tympanic membrane, q.d. = once a day dosing, b.i.d. = twice a day dosing, RAD = reactive airway disease, NR = not reported.
* Sample size: numbers shown for those not lost to follow-up and those (initially recruited).

THE EVIDENCE CONDENSED: Amoxicillin or ampicillin prophylaxis versus placebo for recurrent acute otitis media

Reference	Principi, 1989		Sih, 1993	
Level (design)	1 (RCT)		1 (RCT)	
Sample size*	63 (67)		40 [Not specified, but for the overall trial 60 (82)]	
OUTCOMES				
	No. of AOM episodes per patient per month	% of patients with no further AOM	No. of AOM episodes per patient per month	% of patients with no further AOM
Amoxicillin	0.06	73%	0.05	85%
Placebo	0.14	37%	0.23	50%
p Value	$p < 0.01$	$p < 0.01$	NR	$p < 0.0005$
Conclusion	Amoxicillin better	Amoxicillin better	Amoxicillin better (?trend)	Amoxicillin better
Follow-up time	6 mo		3 mo	
STUDY DESIGN				
Inclusion criteria	Age 9 mo–5 y; ≥3 otoscopically and tympanometrically documented episodes of AOM in the preceding 6 mo, with the last episode between 15 d and 2 mo before enrollment; presence or absence of MEE was acceptable (97% had unilateral or bilateral effusion at the outset)		Children with ≥3 episodes of AOM over the preceding 12 mo; all children at admission into the study had AOM treated by amoxicillin 50 mg/kg/d ×10 d to treat this acute episode at the outset and then were reexamined—all had no further signs or symptoms and a *type A or type C tympanogram*	
Exclusion criteria	Patients with cleft palate, Down syndrome, immunodeficiency, or a history of allergic reactions to any of the drugs tested; also patients who had undergone placement of tympanostomy tubes		Type B tympanogram after the initial amoxicillin therapy	
Randomization effectiveness	No significant differences in sex, age, presence of MEE, interval since onset of most recent AOM, season at entry, daycare attendance, and history of atopy		Similar age, private clinic vs public hospital, mean no. of recurrences in the previous 12 mo, history of atopy	
Age	9 mo–5 y		9 mo–9 y	
Masking	Single blind		Single vs double blind not specified	
Amoxicillin regimen	20 mg/kg/d in one bedtime dose ×6 mo		20 mg/kg/d in one bedtime dose ×3 mo	
Diagnostic criteria for an episode of AOM	Diagnosis was based on any combination of fever, otalgia, irritability, and on the presence of hyperemia or opacity accompanied by fullness, bulging, or immobility of the TM confirmed by a flat, type B curve		Diagnosed by the following criteria: (a) acute symptoms (otalgia, recent onset of irritability, fever, respiratory symptoms); and (b) pneumootoscopic findings (erythema, bulging, or reduced mobility of the TM)	
Management of AOM episodes	Cefaclor 50 mg/kg/d in 3 doses ×10 d; study drug was discontinued and then resumed when this 10 d course was complete		Cefaclor 50 mg/kg/d in 3 doses ×10 d; study drug was discontinued and then resumed when this 10 d course was complete	
Compliance	94%–97% compliance, with "poor compliance" defined as failure to administer ≥3 doses in the 4–6 wk between follow-ups, as assessed by the bottle method		NR	
Criteria for withdrawal from the study	≥2 episodes of AOM within a 2 mo period		NR	
Intention to treat analysis?	Yes		Yes	
Morbidity/ complications	"No laboratory or clinical evidence of toxic side effects due to treatment with amoxicillin or TMP-SMX"		NR	

AOM = acute otitis media, RCT = randomized controlled trial, MEE = middle ear effusion, TM = tympanic membrane, NR = not reported, TMP-SMX = trimethoprim and sulfamethoxazole.
* Sample size: numbers shown for those completing the trial and those (initially recruited).

META-ANALYSIS

Methods of Meta-Analysis. All of the studies included in this meta-analysis are RCTs (level 1) and they represent the highest level of evidence regarding the impact of amoxicillin versus placebo on RAOM. Further details regarding the search and selection process for these RCTs are as noted in the initial methods of this review.

Results of Meta-Analysis. The data from all five RCTs comparing the impact of amoxicillin or ampicillin prophylaxis versus placebo on RAOM were combined. Two main outcome measures were considered: 1) the percentage of children who remained otitis-free, 2) the incidence density of RAOM episodes per child per month. For both measures, there was a significantly better outcome with amoxicillin or ampicillin prophylaxis, such that the percent of children remaining otitis-free was 16.1% more (RD) and an odds ratio of 1.98. (The associated NNT was seven, which implies that for every seven children treated with amoxicillin, one will become otitis-free). The more precise incidence density measure, which also accounted for the follow-up time intervals, was also better with antibiotic, such that there were 0.030 fewer AOM episodes per child per month. These results were associated with an NNT of 30, which suggests that in order to prevent one episode of otitis media, 30 children should be treated for 1 month or one child should be treated for 30 months.

In a sensitivity analysis, when the data from only papers with more than 1 year of follow-up [1, 3] were combined, there was still a significantly greater chance of children remaining otitis-free [69.9% versus 54.2%, odds ratio 2.0 [95% confidence interval (CI) 1.4–2.8], NNT 6 (95% CI 4–14)]. Likewise, when only data from patients who were effusion-free at the outset [Roark, Casselbrant, Sih] were combined, there was still a significantly better outcome with amoxicillin [62.9% versus 49.7%, odds

ratio 1.1 (95% CI 1.1–2.6), NNT 8 (95% CI 4–34)]. In considering the potential for publication bias (i.e., studies showing a significant difference are more likely to be published than those that do not) for the data overall, 24 negative RCTs would be needed to invalidate the finding that amoxicillin gives better results than placebo. It seems unlikely that 24 such negative unpublished trials exist now or that this number of RCTs with negative results will be published in the future.

CLINICAL SIGNIFICANCE AND FUTURE RESEARCH

There are five RCTs that compare the impact of amoxicillin or ampicillin versus placebo on RAOM. Four of the five trials demonstrate a significant improvement in RAOM with this antibiotic regimen. The fifth RCT shows no difference whether antibiotic was given or not. When the data from all five RCTs are combined, amoxicillin/ampicillin granted a significantly better chance of becoming otitis-free and a significant decrease in the rate of AOM per child per month. A significantly better outcome with antibiotic emerged in sensitivity analyses as well, whether only children followed for more than 1 year or only children who were effusion-free at the outset were analyzed. The magnitude of the improvement with amoxicillin, however, was modest (16.1% more were otitis-free, 0.360 fewer AOM episodes per year). These results must be considered in the context of what one study reported as a 7% rate of adverse effects with antibiotic group, as well as a 7% increase in beta-lactamase–producing bacteria.

Future research may focus on the comparison of the improvement seen with amoxicillin to other medical or surgical regimens. In addition, it may focus on defining the minimal doses or duration of amoxicillin necessary to achieve benefit. Finally, it may focus on determining which children are more likely to benefit from amoxicillin prophylaxis than from other potential treatments.

Percent of children remaining otitis-free with amoxicillin/ampicillin versus placebo

	Amoxicillin/ ampicillin	Placebo
Roark, 1997	62.6% (n = 62/99)	58.1% (n = 37/59)
Casselbrant, 1992	58.1%* (n = 50/86)	40.0%* (n = 32/80)
Maynard, 1972	75.7% (n = 131/173)	60.2% (n = 115/191)
Principi, 1989	72.7% (n = 24/33)	36.7% (n = 11/30)
Sih, 1993	85.0% (n = 17/20)	50% (n = 10/20)
Total	69.1% (n = 284/411)	53.9% (n = 205/380)

* Extrapolated from reported percentages.

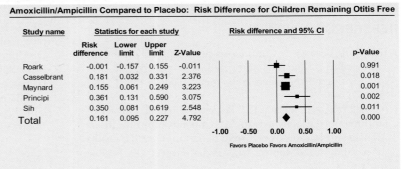

Amoxicillin/Ampicillin Compared to Placebo: Risk Difference for Children Remaining Otitis Free

Study name	Risk difference	Lower limit	Upper limit	Z-Value	p-Value
Roark	-0.001	-0.157	0.155	-0.011	0.991
Casselbrant	0.181	0.032	0.331	2.376	0.018
Maynard	0.155	0.061	0.249	3.223	0.001
Principi	0.361	0.131	0.590	3.075	0.002
Sih	0.350	0.081	0.619	2.548	0.011
Total	0.161	0.095	0.227	4.792	0.000

Favors Placebo / Favors Amoxicillin/Ampicillin

Amoxicillin/Ampicillin Compared to Placebo: Odds Ratio for Children Remaining Otitis Free

Study name	Odds ratio	Lower limit	Upper limit	Z-Value	p-Value
Roark	0.996	0.512	1.940	-0.011	0.991
Casselbrant	2.083	1.121	3.870	2.323	0.020
Maynard	2.061	1.311	3.241	3.133	0.002
Principi	4.606	1.585	13.387	2.806	0.005
Sih	5.667	1.254	25.606	2.254	0.024
Total	1.978	1.464	2.671	4.445	0.000

Favors Placebo / Favors Amoxicillin/Ampicillin

Number of episodes of AOM per child per month (incidence density) with amoxicillin/ampicillin versus placebo

	Amoxicillin/ ampicillin	Placebo
Roark, 1997	0.25 (n = 36/146)	0.22 (n = 20/92)
Casselbrant, 1992	0.05 (n = 103/2064)	0.09 (n = 173/1920)
Maynard, 1972	0.04 (n = 73/2076)	0.06 (n = 141/2292)
Principi, 1989	0.05 (n = 9/198)	0.14 (n = 25/180)
Sih, 1993	0.05 (n = 3/60)	0.23 (n = 14/60)
Total	0.05 (n = 224/4544)	0.08 (n = 373/4544)

Amoxicillin/Ampicillin Compared to Placebo: Risk Difference for Number of Episodes of AOM

Study name	Risk difference	Lower limit	Upper limit	Z-Value	p-Value
Roark	0.029	-0.080	0.139	0.522	0.601
Casselbrant	-0.040	-0.056	-0.024	-4.961	0.000
Maynard	-0.026	-0.039	-0.014	-4.089	0.000
Principi	-0.093	-0.152	-0.035	-3.143	0.002
Sih	-0.183	-0.304	-0.063	-2.985	0.003
Total	-0.034	-0.044	-0.024	-6.871	0.000

Favors Amoxicillin/Ampicillin / Favors Placebo

Amoxicillin/Ampicillin Compared to Placebo: Odds Ratio for Number of Episodes of AOM

Study name	Odds ratio	Lower limit	Upper limit	Z-Value	p-Value
Roark	1.178	0.632	2.195	0.517	0.605
Casselbrant	0.530	0.412	0.683	-4.926	0.000
Maynard	0.556	0.416	0.742	-3.980	0.000
Principi	0.295	0.134	0.651	-3.023	0.003
Sih	0.173	0.047	0.638	-2.633	0.008
Total	0.548	0.459	0.653	-6.724	0.000

Favors Amoxicillin/Ampicillin / Favors Placebo

REFERENCES

1. Roark R, Berman S. Continuous twice daily or once daily amoxicillin prophylaxis compared with placebo for children with recurrent acute otitis media. Pediatr Infect Dis J 1997;16(4):376–381.
2. Casselbrant ML, Kaleida PH, Rockette HE, et al. Efficacy of antimicrobial prophylaxis and of tympanostomy tube insertion for prevention of recurrent acute otitis media: results of a randomized clinical trial. Pediatr Infect Dis J 1992; 11(4):278–286.
3. Maynard JE, Fleshman JK, Tschopp CF. Otitis media in Alaskan Eskimo children. Prospective evaluation of chemoprophylaxis. JAMA 1972;219(5):597–599.
4. Sih T, Moura R, Caldas S, Schwartz B. Prophylaxis for recurrent acute otitis media: a Brazilian study. Int J Pediatr Otorhinolaryngol 1993;25(1–3):19–24.
5. Principi N, Marchisio P, Massironi E, Grasso RM, Filiberti G. Prophylaxis of recurrent acute otitis media and middle-ear effusion. Comparison of Amoxicillin with sulfamethoxazole and trimethoprim. Am J Dis Child 1989; 143(12):1414–1418.

6 Pediatric Recurrent Acute Otitis Media

6.B.

Sulfisoxazole prophylaxis versus placebo: Impact on number of subsequent episodes of acute otitis media, chance of no further episodes of acute otitis media

Jennifer J. Shin, Sandra S. Stinnett, and Christopher J. Hartnick

METHODS

A computerized Ovid search of MEDLINE 1966–January 2004 was performed as described in Section 20.A. The resulting 302 articles were then reviewed to determine which met the following inclusion criteria: 1) patient population <18 years old with documented recurrent acute otitis media (RAOM), 2) intervention with continuous sulfisoxazole prophylaxis versus placebo control, 3) outcome measured in terms of number of episodes of acute otitis media (AOM). Studies in which noncontinuous antibiotic therapy was administered were excluded. Also excluded were studies that enrolled children with nonrecurrent AOM (i.e., only one previous episode). Based on consultation with an infectious disease specialist, studies that considered combination therapy with trimethoprim-sulfamethoxazole were also considered separately, because of differences in antimicrobial activity and spectrum. The bibliographies of the articles that met these inclusion criteria were manually checked to ensure no further relevant articles could be identified. This process yielded nine articles, four of which focused on sulfisoxazole prophylaxis alone [1–4]. The other five articles are discussed in Sections 20.A and 20.C.

RESULTS

Outcome Measures. Outcomes in all three studies were measured in terms of the number of episodes of AOM subsequent to treatment. These "episodes" were, however, diagnosed on the basis of different criteria in each study. One study used a combination of symptoms and signs; the second used otoscopy alone; the third used examination and tympanometry; and the fourth did not use specified diagnostic criteria. Further details are provided in the adjoining table. Reported here is the mean number of episodes of AOM per child year, as well as the percent of children with no further AOM in the follow-up period.

Potential Confounders. Potential confounders are as described in Section 20.A, and are tabulated for the reader here in as much detail as the study reports allow.

Study Designs. Four randomized controlled studies address this issue, three of which are randomized crossover trials (RCOTs). With such a crossover study design, patients are initially assigned to the sulfisoxazole or the placebo group; after a period of 10–12 weeks, patients who initially received sulfisoxazole are switched to placebo, whereas patients who initially received placebo are switched to sulfisoxazole for another 10–12 weeks. This study design has the advantages of increasing power for a given sample size, because each patient provides two data points instead of one. In addition, each patient can serve as his or her own control, having received sulfisoxazole in one period and placebo in another. This study design may also incorporate a "washout period" before the patients cross over, where subjects receive neither drug; this "washout" prevents postcrossover bias from any drug effects that linger even after its discontinuation.

All of these studies were double blinded, and the three crossovers measured compliance, which was >70%. Randomization was shown to be effective in the noncrossover trial, although it was not discussed in detail in the crossover studies, where each patient was used as his own control. It becomes of interest, however, as conflicting results were obtained before and after crossover in two trials. With these inconsistent results, it would have been beneficial to demonstrate that there was no difference between the groups that started with sulfisoxazole and the groups that started with placebo. It would also have been beneficial to have reported if a "washout period" was allowed between the first and second arm of the crossover trials, in order to allow any remaining active sulfisoxazole effect to clear the children's systems before crossover into the placebo group. Attrition rates (i.e., number of patients who were enrolled but were lost to follow-up) were reported in all but one case, and ranged from 19% to 28%. These rates are especially important because the sample sizes for each individual study are somewhat small. A variety of sulfisoxazole doses were prescribed, but these regimens did not seem to correlate with the final results.

Highest Level of Evidence. One RCOT found a considerable decrease in AOM rates with sulfisoxazole in both arms of the trial; both before and after crossover, a significant difference was noted in the number of children who had no further episodes of AOM in the 3-month follow-up period. For the group that received sulfisoxazole before placebo, a rate difference (RD)[1] of 35% was noted, implying that 3 was the number of children that needed to be treated to achieve one otitis-free child (NNT—number needed to treat).[2] For the group that received placebo before sulfisoxazole, there was a lesser RD of 24% which corresponds to an NNT of 5. The other two RCOTs determined that there was a significant difference in AOM outcomes in the group in which placebo was given before sulfisoxazole, but that there was no difference when sulfisoxazole was given first. These results suggested a potential "carryover" effect in which the patients continued to benefit from the agent even after it was discontinued. The fourth study did not use a crossover design, and found no significant difference in the mean number of AOM episodes while taking sulfisoxazole prophylaxis versus placebo. This study had a much longer follow-up time of 6 months. More of the results

[1] Rate difference (RD) is the absolute difference in successful outcomes between the study group and the control group. For example, in the Perrin study before crossover, 89% of the sulfisoxazole group versus 54% of the placebo group had no further episodes of AOM. The RD in this study was 54% − 89% = −35%.

[2] Number needed to treat (NNT) is the total number of children that must be treated in order for one child to obtain benefit from the treatment. It is calculated by determining the inverse of the RD. For example, in the Perrin study, the rate difference is −35%, so that the NNT = 1/0.35 = 2.9. According to this study, 3 children would need to be treated so as to obtain benefit for one child.

from these four trials favor sulfisoxazole therapy, but given the heterogeneity that does exist, a meta-analysis of all of the results is subsequently shown.

Applicability. These results are applicable to children with RAOM with ≥3 episodes in the previous 6–18 months, who also have neither tympanostomy tubes nor a predisposing anatomic deficit such as cleft palate.

Morbidity. Two studies specified that there was a 0% incidence of adverse reactions to sulfisoxazole [1, 4]. Two studies addressed the potential for antimicrobial resistance by following bacterial cultures from either nasopharyngeal swabs or tympanocentesis, and found no difference in microbial pathogens [2, 3]. A third study reported that 2 of 2 patients who experienced spontaneous tympanic membrane perforation after the study had sulfisoxazole-resistant bacteria in cultured otorrhea, although no prestudy or other control data were provided for comparison.

THE EVIDENCE CONDENSED: Sulfisoxazole prophylaxis versus placebo for recurrent acute otitis media

Reference	Perrin, 1974		Liston, 1983	
Level (design)	1 (RCOT)		1 (RCOT)	
Sample size*	54 (75)		35 (43)	
OUTCOMES				
	% of children with no further AOM		Mean AOM episodes per child per month	
	Before crossover	After crossover	Before crossover	After crossover
Sulfisoxazole	89%	96%	0.28†	0.20‡
Placebo	54%	68%	0.56‡	0.30†
p Value	< 0.01	< 0.02	‡< 0.01	†NS
Conclusion	Abx better	Abx better	Abx better	No difference (?carryover)
Follow-up time	3 mo	3 mo	3 mo	3 mo
STUDY DESIGN				
Inclusion criteria	Previous patients of a pediatric practice; ≥3 episodes in the previous 18 mo or ≥5 episodes at any time; "2 children with only 2 previous episodes were entered at the request of group pediatricians"		Age 6 mo–5 y; >3 episodes of AOM occurring at a frequency of at least 1 episode every 2 mo, with at least 2 episodes diagnosed by the study coordinator	
Exclusion criteria	Previous tympanostomy tube placement, predisposing anatomic defects (e.g., cleft palate)		Cleft palate, perforated TM, tympanostomy tubes, prior adenoidectomy, known immunodeficiency	
Randomization effectiveness	Not specified, but crossover design used		Not specified, but crossover design used	
Age	11 mo–8 y		6 mo–5 y	
Sulfisoxazole regimen	500 mg PO b.i.d. (same dose for all children)		75 mg/kg/d in 2 divided doses, rounded to the nearest half teaspoon	
Diagnostic criteria for an episode of AOM	"The diagnosis of AOM was made on exam; no specific criteria for diagnoses were employed . . . any observer bias would apply equally to examinations during both antibiotic and placebo treatment"		Diagnosis required: bulging of an opaque or red pars flaccida with obliteration of the bony landmarks and either a type B tympanogram or purulent drainage from a spontaneous TM perforation	
Management of AOM episode while taking study treatment	"Were treated by the pediatricians in their normal fashion, usually with oral antibiotics for a 10 day period." The study drug was discontinued and resumed when the 10-d course was complete		Amoxicillin 40 mg/kg/d in 3 divided doses ×10 d or if penicillin allergic or culture revealed beta-lactamase–producing organism, then erythromycin 40 mg/kg/d and sulfisoxazole 150 mg/kg/d in 4 divided doses ×10 d. Study drug was discontinued and resumed after the 10 d	
Compliance	71% were considered compliant (>2/3 of drug was taken) as assessed by the bottle method		87.2% overall compliance, as assessed by bottle method	

AOM = acute otitis media, RCT = randomized controlled trial, RCOT = randomized crossover trial, abx = antibiotics, MEE = middle ear effusion, TM = tympanic membrane, b.i.d. = twice a day dosing, NS = not significant, NR = not reported.
* Sample size: numbers shown for those completing the trial and those (initially recruited).

THE EVIDENCE CONDENSED: Sulfisoxazole prophylaxis versus placebo for recurrent acute otitis media

Reference	Varsano, 1985		Gonzalez, 1986	
Level (design)	1 (RCOT)		1 (RCT)	
Sample size*	32 (40)		41 (NR)	

OUTCOMES

	Mean AOM episodes per child per 10 weeks		Mean AOM episodes	% children with no
	Before crossover	After crossover	per child per 6 month	further AOM
Sulfisoxazole	0.4§	0.2‖	1.38	24%
Placebo	1.4‖	0.9§	2.00	15%
p Value	‖<0.01	§NS	NS	NR
Conclusion	Abx better	No difference (?carryover)	No difference	NR
Follow-up time	10 wk	10 wk	6 mo	

STUDY DESIGN

Inclusion criteria	Age 6 mo–5 y, ≥3 separate otoscopically documented episodes of AOM during the preceding 6 mo; free of clinical and otoscopic findings of AOM at the outset; presence or absence of MEE was acceptable		Age 6 mo–10 y, ≥3 episodes of AOM in the preceding 6 mo or ≥4 in 18 mo; presence or absence of MEE was acceptable	
Exclusion criteria	Children who required tympanostomy tube insertion		Cleft palate, Down syndrome, previous tympanostomy tubes, or sulfonamide sensitivity	
Randomization effectiveness	Not specified, but crossover design used		No difference in sex, age, season of entry into the trial	
Age	6 mo–5 y		1–48 mo	
Sulfisoxazole regimen	250 mg PO b.i.d. if <2 y old, 500 mg PO b.i.d. if 2–5 y old		500 mg PO b.i.d. if <5 y old; 1 g PO b.i.d. if >5 y old	
Diagnostic criteria for an episode of AOM	Erythema or white-yellow opacification accompanied by fullness or bulging as well as poor mobility of the TM, or acute spontaneous perforation associated with pus in the ear canal		"Rapid and short onset of signs and symptoms of inflammation in the middle ear. Diagnosis was also based on the following criteria: otalgia (ear tugging in infants), fever, TM erythema or bulging, decreased TM mobility, loss of TM landmarks, otorrhea"	
Management of AOM episode while taking study treatment	Ampicillin or, if penicillin allergic, trimethoprim and sulfamethoxazole ×10 d. Study medication was discontinued and resumed after the 10-d course was completed.		"Antibiotics at standard therapeutic doses for 10 days"	
Compliance	>75% in 27 children, 65%–75% in remaining 5 children, as assessed by counting remaining tablets		"Compliance could not be adequately established in our study"	

AOM = acute otitis media, RCT = randomized controlled trial, RCOT = randomized crossover trial, abx = antibiotics, MEE = middle ear effusion, TM = tympanic membrane, b.i.d. = twice a day dosing, NS = not significant, NR = not reported.
* Sample size: numbers shown for those completing the trial and those (initially recruited).

META-ANALYSIS

Methods of the Meta-Analysis. All of the studies included in this meta-analysis are RCTs (level 1) and they represent the highest level of evidence regarding the impact of sulfisoxazole versus placebo on RAOM. Further details regarding the search and selection process for these RCTs are as noted in the initial methods of this review.

Results of the Meta-Analysis. The data from all four RCTs comparing the impact of amoxicillin or ampicillin prophylaxis versus placebo on RAOM were combined. Two main outcome measures were considered: 1) the percentage of children who remained otitis-free, 2) the incidence density of RAOM episodes per child per month. When all the results from all four studies were numerically combined, 25% more children remained otitis-free with sulfisoxazole. This rate difference corresponded to an overall NNT of 4, suggesting that for every four children treated, one would remain otitis-free. In addition, the combined odds ratio suggested that children treated with sulfisoxazole prophylaxis were 3.35 times as likely to remain otitis-free. To negate this result, there would have to be 19 trials showing no difference between sulfisoxazole and placebo (odds ratio). Even with publication bias (i.e., studies showing a significant difference are more likely to be published than those that do not), it seems unlikely that 19 negative trials exist or will come to exist.

The incidence density measure (number of episodes of AOM per child per month), which also accounted for the follow-up time intervals, was also better with sulfisoxazole, such that there were 0.170 fewer AOM episodes per child per month, or 2.04 fewer AOM episodes per year. These results were associated with an NNT of 6, which suggests that in order to prevent one episode of otitis media, six children should be treated for 1 month

or one child should be treated for 6 months. As for publication bias, 39 negative studies would be needed to negate this combined positive result.

CLINICAL SIGNIFICANCE AND FUTURE RESEARCH

Three level 1 studies conclude that sulfisoxazole prophylaxis results in fewer episodes of AOM, as compared with placebo. The fourth study found no difference between the two groups, but when the results from all four studies were numerically combined in a meta-analysis, a 25% rate difference favored sulfisoxazole prophylaxis. These combined results suggested that sulfisoxazole prophylaxis was more effective than placebo in preventing AOM in certain children, such that for every four children treated, one would remain otitis-free. Meta-analysis data also suggested that sulfisoxazole would result in 2.04 fewer AOM episodes per year, such that six children would need to be treated for 1 month or one child would need to be treated for 6 months in order to prevent one episode of otitis media.

Future research on this subject may further address the interesting question of a potential "carryover" effect by using a noncrossover design or by providing a prolonged follow-up period after patients have discontinued medication. Such an effect could provide multiple advantages, especially in terms of potentially providing the least rigorous dosing schedule for the largest possible benefit. In addition, the impact of experiencing intermittent flairs of AOM versus daily oral medication on quality of life may be explored.

Percent of children remaining otitis-free with sulfisoxazole versus placebo

Study, year	Sulfisoxazole	Placebo
Perrin, 1974	94.3% (n = 50/53)	62.3% (n = 33/53)
Liston, 1983	51.4% (n = 18/35)	41.2% (n = 14/34)
Varsano, 1985	78.1% (n = 25/32)	37.5% (n = 12/32)
Gonzalez, 1986	23.8% (n = 5/21)	15.0% (n = 3/20)
Total	69.5% (n = 98/141)	44.6% (n = 62/139)

Sulfisoxazole vs Placebo: Rate Difference for Children Remaining Otitis-Free

Study name	Risk difference	Lower limit	Upper limit	Z-Value	Risk difference and 95% CI	p-Value
Perrin	0.321	0.176	0.465	4.349		0.000
Liston	0.103	-0.132	0.337	0.858		0.391
Varsano	0.406	0.186	0.627	3.610		0.000
Gonzalez	0.088	-0.152	0.328	0.719		0.472
Total	0.261	0.162	0.359	5.208		0.000

-1.00 -0.50 0.00 0.50 1.00
Favors Placebo   Favors Sulfisoxazole

Sulfisoxazole vs Placebo: Odds Ratio for Children Remaining Otitis-Free

Study name	Odds ratio	Lower limit	Upper limit	Z-Value	Odds ratio and 95% CI	p-Value
Perrin	10.101	2.779	36.719	3.512		0.000
Liston	1.513	0.584	3.918	0.852		0.394
Varsano	5.952	1.977	17.920	3.172		0.002
Gonzalez	1.771	0.363	8.648	0.706		0.480
Total	3.355	1.870	6.021	4.058		0.000

0.01 0.1 1 10 100
Favors Placebo   Favors Sulfisoxazole

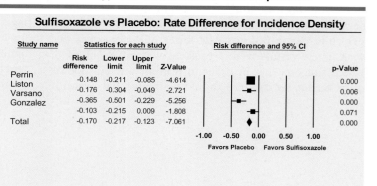

Number of episodes of AOM per child per month (incidence density) with sulfisoxazole versus placebo

Study, year	Sulfisoxazole	Placebo
Perrin, 1974	0.024 (n = 4/162)	0.173 (n = 28/162)
Liston, 1983	0.245 (n = 25/102)	0.421 (n = 43/102)
Varsano, 1985	0.122 (n = 9/74)	0.486 (n = 36/74)
Gonzalez, 1986	0.230 (n = 29/126)	0.333 (n = 40/120)
Total	0.170 (n = 67/394)	0.321 (n = 147/458)

Sulfisoxazole vs Placebo: Rate Difference for Incidence Density

Study name	Risk difference	Lower limit	Upper limit	Z-Value	Risk difference and 95% CI	p-Value
Perrin	-0.148	-0.211	-0.085	-4.614		0.000
Liston	-0.176	-0.304	-0.049	-2.721		0.006
Varsano	-0.365	-0.501	-0.229	-5.256		0.000
Gonzalez	-0.103	-0.215	0.009	-1.808		0.071
Total	-0.170	-0.217	-0.123	-7.061		0.000

-1.00 -0.50 0.00 0.50 1.00
Favors Placebo   Favors Sulfisoxazole

Sulfisoxazole vs Placebo: Odds Ratio for Incidence Density

Study name	Odds ratio	Lower limit	Upper limit	Z-Value	Odds ratio and 95% CI	p-Value
Perrin	0.121	0.041	0.354	-3.857		0.000
Liston	0.445	0.245	0.810	-2.649		0.008
Varsano	0.146	0.064	0.336	-4.525		0.000
Gonzalez	0.598	0.341	1.049	-1.793		0.073
Total	0.358	0.253	0.507	-5.789		0.000

0.01 0.1 1 10 100
Favors Placebo   Favors Sulfisoxazole

REFERENCES

1. Gonzalez C, Arnold JE, Woody EA, et al. Prevention of recurrent acute otitis media: chemoprophylaxis versus tympanostomy tubes. Laryngoscope 1986;96(12):1330–1334.

2. Liston TE, Foshee WS, Pierson WD. Sulfisoxazole chemoprophylaxis for frequent otitis media. Pediatrics 1983;71(4): 524–530.

3. Perrin JM, Charney E, MacWhinney JB Jr, McInerny TK, Miller RL, Nazarian LF. Sulfisoxazole as chemoprophylaxis for recurrent otitis media. A double-blind crossover study in pediatric practice. N Engl J Med 1974;291(13):664–667.

4. Varsano I, Volovitz B, Mimouni F. Sulfisoxazole prophylaxis of middle ear effusion and recurrent acute otitis media. Am J Dis Child 1985;139(6):632–635.

6 Pediatric Recurrent Acute Otitis Media

6.C.

Amoxicillin versus trimethoprim sulfamethoxazole prophylaxis: Impact on number of subsequent episodes of acute otitis media, chance of no further episodes of acute otitis media

Jennifer J. Shin and Christopher J. Hartnick

METHODS

A computerized Ovid search of MEDLINE 1966–January 2004 was performed as described in Section 20.A. The resulting 302 articles were then reviewed to determine which met the following inclusion criteria: 1) patient population <18 years of age with documented recurrent acute otitis media (RAOM), 2) intervention with continuous amoxicillin versus sulfisoxazole prophylaxis, 3) outcome measured in terms of number of episodes of acute otitis media (AOM). Studies in which noncontinuous antibiotic therapy was administered, as well as those that enrolled children with nonrecurrent AOM (i.e., only one previous episode), were excluded. The bibliographies of the articles that met these inclusion criteria were manually checked to ensure no further relevant articles could be identified. This process yielded nine articles, two of which focused on a direct comparison of amoxicillin and trimethoprim-sulfamethoxazole (TMP-SMX) prophylaxis, and these are discussed here [1, 2]. The other seven articles are discussed in detail in other sections in this chapter.

RESULTS

Outcome Measures. Outcomes in both studies were measured in terms of the number of episodes of AOM subsequent to treatment. Both studies used criteria of history and physical examination for diagnosis, with one study requiring tympanogram confirmation of examination findings. Further details are provided in the adjoining table. Reported here is the mean number of episodes of AOM per child year, as well as the percent of children with no further episodes of AOM in the follow-up period.

Potential Confounders. Potential confounders are as described in Section 20.A, and are tabulated here.

Study Designs. Two randomized controlled trials (RCTs) directly compared amoxicillin and TMP-SMX. Randomization provided groups with similar age, history of AOM, and atopy. The Principi study had more stringent entry criteria (three episodes in 6 months) than the Sih study (three episodes in 12 months). Attrition rates were 4% [1] and 47% [2], with the higher rate potentially skewing results. Follow-up times were 6 months [1] and 3 months [2]. The impact of season as a potential con-

founder was addressed in one trial [1]. *A priori* power calculations were not reported in either case, although each demonstrated adequate power to discern a statistically significant rate difference of 32%–36% in their comparison of each antibiotic to placebo.

Highest Level of Evidence. Two level 1 studies found no significant difference in AOM rates with amoxicillin versus TMP-SMX prophylaxis [1, 2]. No *a priori* sample-size estimates for a standard 90% power were reported, although both studies did compare antibiotic groups with a similar-sized placebo group and found statistically significant differences of 32%–36%. As had previously been shown with amoxicillin and sulfisoxazole (see Sections 6.A and 6.B), there was an improvement in outcome with TMP-SMX as compared with placebo.

Applicability. These results are applicable to children at least 9 months of age and up to 5 [1] or 9 years old [2] experiencing RAOM with at least three episodes in the previous 6–12 months.

Morbidity. Neither study reported any adverse effects in the antibiotic groups. Also, neither study addressed the impact of each antibiotic on antimicrobial resistance.

CLINICAL SIGNIFICANCE AND FUTURE RESEARCH

There are two level 1 studies that compared the impact of continuous amoxicillin prophylaxis with continuous TMP-SMX prophylaxis. The number of episodes of AOM and the chance of remaining otitis-free are similar with each choice of daily antibiotic regimen. Therefore, the choice of which antibiotic to use is dependent largely on issues of patient compliance, cost, allergy history, and regional variations in microbial resistance. In addition, these results must again be considered in light of the recommendations from the American Academy of Pediatrics and the American Academy of Otolaryngology regarding concern for antimicrobial resistance.

Given previous results that suggest that the improvement with sulfisoxazole versus placebo is greater than the improvement with amoxicillin versus placebo, future RCTs may directly compare sulfisoxazole versus amoxicillin. Alternatively, studies may focus on determining whether one antibiotic has an increased propensity to promote resistant strains of pathogens.

THE EVIDENCE CONDENSED: Amoxicillin versus trimethoprim sulfamethoxazole prophylaxis for recurrent acute otitis media

Reference	Principi, 1989		Sih, 1993	
Level (design)	1 (RCT)		1 (RCT)	
Sample size*	96 (100)		60 (82)	
OUTCOMES				
	Mean no. of AOM episodes per patient per month	% of patients with no further AOM	Mean no. of AOM episodes per patient per month	% of patients with no further AOM
Amoxicillin	0.06	73%	0.05	80%
TMP-SMX	0.05	73%	0.08	82%
Placebo	0.14	37%	0.23	50%
p Value	NS, amoxicillin vs TMP-SMX	NS, amoxicillin vs TMP-SMX (<0.01, amoxicillin vs placebo) (<0.01, TMP-SMX vs placebo)	NS, amoxicillin vs TMP-SMX	NS, amoxicillin vs TMP-SMX (<0.0005, amoxicillin vs placebo) (<0.0005, TMP-SMX vs placebo)
Conclusion	No difference, amoxicillin vs TMP-SMX	No difference, amoxicillin vs TMP-SMX	No difference, amoxicillin vs TMP-SMX	No difference, amoxicillin vs TMP-SMX
Follow-up time	6 mo		3 mo	
STUDY DESIGN				
Inclusion criteria	Age 9 mo–5 y; ≥3 otoscopically and tympanometrically documented episodes of AOM in the preceding 6 mo, with the last episode between 15 d and 2 mo before enrollment; presence or absence of MEE was acceptable (97% had unilateral or bilateral effusion at the outset)		Children with ≥3 episodes of AOM over the preceding 12 mo; all children at admission into the study had AOM treated by amoxicillin 50 mg/kg/d ×10 d to treat this acute episode at the outset and then were reexamined—all had no further signs or symptoms and a type A or type C tympanogram	
Exclusion criteria	Patients with cleft palate, Down syndrome, immunodeficiency, or a history of allergic reactions to any of the drugs tested; also patients who had undergone placement of tympanostomy tubes		Type B tympanogram after the initial amoxicillin therapy	
Randomization effectiveness	No significant differences in sex, age, presence of MEE, interval since onset of most recent AOM, season at entry, daycare attendance, and history of atopy		Similar age, private clinic vs public hospital, mean number of recurrences in the previous 12 mo, history of atopy	
Age	9 mo–5 y		9 mo–9 y	
Masking	Single blind		Single vs double blind not specified	
Amoxicillin regimen	20 mg/kg/d in 1 bedtime dose ×6 mo		20 mg/kg/d in 1 bedtime dose ×3 mo	
TMP-SMX regimen	12 mg/kg/d in 1 bedtime dose ×6 mo		12 mg/kg/d in 1 bedtime dose ×3 mo	
Diagnostic criteria for an episode of AOM	Diagnosis was based on any combination of fever, otalgia, irritability, and on the presence of hyperemia or opacity accompanied by fullness, bulging, or immobility of the TM confirmed by a flat, type B curve		Diagnosed by the following criteria: (a) acute symptoms (otalgia, recent onset of irritability, fever, respiratory symptoms); and (b) pneumootoscopic findings (erythema, bulging, or reduced mobility of the TM)	
Management of AOM episodes	Cefaclor 50 mg/kg/d in 3 doses ×10 d; study drug was discontinued and then resumed when this 10-d course was complete		Cefaclor 50 mg/kg/d in 3 doses ×10 d; study drug was discontinued and then resumed when this 10-d course was complete	
Compliance	94%–97% compliance, with "poor compliance" defined as failure to administer ≥3 doses in the 4–6 wk between follow-ups, as assessed by the bottle method		NR	
Morbidity/complications	"No laboratory or clinical evidence of toxic side effects attributable to treatment with amoxicillin or TMP-SMX"		NR	

RCT = randomized controlled trial, AOM = acute otitis media, amoxicillin= amoxicillin, MEE = middle ear effusion, TM = tympanic membrane, RAD = reactive airway disease, TMP-SMX = trimethoprim sulfamethoxazole, NR = not reported.
* Sample size: numbers shown for those completing the trial and those (initially recruited).

REFERENCES

1. Principi N, Marchisio P, Massironi E, Grasso RM, Filiberti G. Prophylaxis of recurrent acute otitis media and middle-ear effusion. Comparison of Amoxicillin with sulfamethox-azole and trimethoprim. Am J Dis Child 1989;143(12): 1414–1418.

2. Sih T, Moura R, Caldas S, Schwartz B. Prophylaxis for recurrent acute otitis media: a Brazilian study. Int J Pediatr Otorhinolaryngol 1993;25(1–3):19–24.

6 Pediatric Recurrent Acute Otitis Media

6.D.

Tympanostomy tube placement versus no surgery/no prophylaxis: Impact on subsequent number of episodes of acute otitis media, chance of no further episodes of acute otitis media

Jennifer J. Shin, Sandra S. Stinnett, and Christopher J. Hartnick

METHODS

A computerized Ovid search of MEDLINE 1966–January 2004 was performed. The subject headings "otitis media" and "middle ear ventilation" were exploded and cross-referenced, yielding 807 articles. Given the known richness and high level of the literature on otitis media, these articles were then limited to randomized controlled trials (RCTs), yielding 107 articles. These articles were then reviewed to find those that met the following inclusion criteria: 1) pediatric population of patients <18 years of age with recurrent acute otitis media (RAOM), 2) intervention with tympanostomy tube placement compared with no surgery/no prophylaxis, and 3) outcomes measured in terms of number of episodes of acute otitis media (AOM). Trials that enrolled subjects on the basis of chronic otitis media with effusion (rather than RAOM) were excluded here, although they are analyzed in a subsequent chapter. This search strategy and inclusion/exclusion criteria, along with manual searching of relevant bibliographies, yielded three RCTs [1–3].

RESULTS

Outcome Measures. Outcomes in both studies were measured in terms of the number of episodes of AOM subsequent to treatment. These "episodes" were diagnosed on the basis of physical examination with or without a symptomatic history, with further details provided in the adjoining table. Reported here is the mean number of episodes of AOM, as well as the percent of children with no further episodes of AOM in the follow-up period.

Potential Confounders. Potential confounders include age, tube type and postoperative management, antibiotic regimen for AOM episodes and compliance with it, and presence of middle ear effusion. Also, allergies, breast milk feeding, gender, genetics, daycare attendance, and exposure to tobacco smoke may affect AOM outcomes. Each of these or the way in which each study addressed them are detailed in the adjacent table in as much detail as the studies allow.

Study Designs. Three studies compared AOM outcomes after tympanostomy tube placement versus no surgery/no prophylaxis. Randomization was used to ensure similar age, gender, season of entry, and other characteristics in groups being compared (see table). The proportion of patients lost to follow-up ranged from 9% [3] to 36% [1] in the two cases in which it was reported, with higher numbers associated with increased susceptibility to attrition bias (see Chapter 1 or glossary). Also, in the former study, an additional three of the remaining 98 patients (3%) did not complete the study's half-year follow-up period; in the latter study, an additional 17 of the remaining 111 patients (15%) did not complete the much longer 2-year follow-up period because of treatment failure. In the latter case, these treatment failures were still included in the study's data, so that an intention to treat analysis was performed [1]. Such an intention to treat analysis maximizes the validity of the data. Two studies compared a group receiving tubes to a nonsurgery group that received an oral placebo [1, 2]. The third study had no placebo [3]. No study had a "sham surgery" placebo group. All three studies enrolled children <3–4 years of age [1–3].

Highest Level of Evidence. Three level 1 studies compared AOM outcomes with tympanostomy tubes versus no surgery/no prophylaxis. Two found a statistically significant improvement with tubes in the mean number of AOM episodes and in the chance of remaining otitis-free [2, 3]. There was a 40%–41% difference in the percent of children who had no further AOM in the 6-month follow-up periods. This rate difference suggests that three children need to be treated with tubes to give one child a 6-month otitis-free period. One study, however, found no difference in these same parameters with tube placement versus no surgery/no prophylaxis [1]. This study reported adequate power (90%) to detect a 50% reduction in the average number of episodes of AOM. It did not, however, detect any such reduction, in contrast to the other two studies which showed reductions from 2.00–2.17 to 0.67–0.80 AOM episodes per child per 6 months. It is possible that this one study may have come to a different conclusion than the other two because of differences in its study design, which included: 1) it required children to be free of middle ear effusion at entry; 2) it excluded infants <7 months old; 3) it expanded follow-up time to 2 years (4 times longer). The authors of this report also did note that a secondary outcome measure of "total time with otitis media" (including AOM, otorrhea, or otitis media with effusion) was significantly decreased from 10% in the no-surgery group to 6.6% in the tubes group. In addition, the authors note that because children with tubes were more likely to complete follow-up than those who did not have surgery, and children who were eventually lost to follow-up had more severe disease, the results were biased toward the tympanostomy tube group having a worse outcome. Given that this third study's results did not completely agree with the other two studies, however, a meta-analysis was performed and is shown below.

Applicability. The results of these trials are applicable to children younger than 4 years old with at least three episodes of RAOM in 6 months or less.

Morbidity. Two articles describe tube-associated morbidity over an approximate 2-year period. The incidence of persistent perforation was 0%–3.9% and the incidence of perioperative otorrhea was 9%. Therefore, a number needed to harm (NNH) of at least 26 children must receive tubes to have a persistent perforation at 6 months–2 years. An NNH of 12 children who receive tubes will have otorrhea in the immediate postoperative period.

THE EVIDENCE CONDENSED: Tympanostomy tube insertion versus no surgery or prophylaxis for recurrent acute otitis media

Reference	Casselbrant, 1992		Gebhart, 1981	
Level (design)	1 (RCT)		1 (RCT)	
Sample size*	111(174)		95 (108)	
OUTCOMES				
	No. of AOM episodes per child per year	% of children with no further AOM episodes	No. of AOM episodes per child per 6 months	% of children with no further AOM episodes
Tubes	1.02	35%	0.67	46%
No surgery	1.08	40%	2.17	5%
p Values	=0.25	NR	<0.001	<0.001
Conclusion	No difference	No difference	Tubes better	Tubes better
Follow-up time	2 y		6 mo	
STUDY DESIGN				
Inclusion criteria	7–35 mo of age, most recent episode in <6 mo, ≥3 episodes of AOM in the preceding 6 mo or ≥4 in 12 mo; *free from MEE at time of entry*		<3 y of age, ≥3 episodes of acute purulent otitis media diagnosed and treated by the referring physician in the previous 6 mo; RAOM despite adequate therapy with antibiotics; *presence or absence of MEE was acceptable*	
Exclusion criteria	Asthma, chronic sinusitis, previous tonsillectomy or adenoidectomy		Cleft palate, Down syndrome, recurrent tonsillitis associated with otitis media	
Randomization effectiveness	No difference in age, season of entry, previous no. of AOM episodes, sex, race, socioeconomic status		Similar sex, race, no. of prestudy infections, patient or family history of allergies, season of entry, family history of ear infections, age	
Age	7–35 mo		<3 y	
Diagnostic criteria for an episode of AOM	•Otoscopic signs (erythema or white opacification not attributable to scarring, fullness or bulging and decreased mobility of TM) or ≥1 symptom (fever, otalgia, irritability) in the presence of MEE •If PET in place, then episode of otorrhea was considered equivalent to an episode of AOM		•If tubes not present: hyperemia and thickening of the entire TM, decreased mobility, short process of malleus no longer visible •If tubes in place: drainage through the tympanostomy tubes in the external canal, often with erythema and edema of the TM	
Tube type	Teflon Armstrong tube in the anterosuperior quadrant of TM		Shepard Teflon tubes in the anterosuperior quadrant of the TM	
Response to AOM while tubes in place	Ototopical treatment with neomycin sulfate, polymyxin B sulfate, and hydrocortisone suspension × ≤10 d, amoxicillin 40 mg/kg/d in 3 divided doses ×10 d unless cultures revealed resistant organisms		Ampicillin ×10 d, and if allergic then erythromycin and a sulfonamide ×10 d (doses not specified); Cortisporin otic if otorrhea present; decongestant if nasal congestion or upper respiratory tract infection	
Response to tube obstruction	Ototopical treatment with neomycin sulfate, polymyxin B sulfate, and hydrocortisone; if remained occluded then replaced if <6 mo since insertion, replaced only if AOM/OME developed if 6–12 mo since insertion		If tube obstructed with subsequent AOM, then tube was reinserted	
Response to AOM in group without tubes	Amoxicillin 40 mg/kg/d in 3 divided doses ×10 d unless tympanocentesis cultures revealed resistant organisms—then erythromycin 50 mg/kg/d and sulfisoxazole 150 mg/kg/d ×10 d		Ampicillin ×10 d, and if allergic then erythromycin and a sulfonamide ×10 d (doses not specified); Cortisporin otic if otorrhea present; decongestant if nasal congestion or upper respiratory tract infection	
Morbidity/ complications	Tubes group with 3.9% persistent perforations (3 subjects at 5, 9, and 21 mo; all healed spontaneously at a later date)		9% with persistent drainage beginning <24 h after tube insertion 6% required tube reinsertion 0% persistent perforation 0% cholesteatoma	

RAOM = recurrent acute otitis media, AOM = acute otitis media, RCT = randomized controlled trial, MEE = middle ear effusion, TM = tympanic membrane, NR = not reported, PET = pneumatic equalization tube, OME = otitis media with effusion.
* Sample size: numbers shown for those completing follow-up and (those initially recruited).

THE EVIDENCE CONDENSED: Tympanostomy tube insertion versus no surgery or prophylaxis for recurrent acute otitis media

Reference	Gonzalez, 1986	
Level (design)	1 (RCT)	
Sample size*	42 (NR)	
OUTCOMES		
	No. of AOM episodes per child per 6 months	% of children with no further AOM episodes
Tubes	0.86	55%
No surgery	2.00	15%
p Values	=0.006	=0.01
Conclusion	Tubes better	Tubes better
Follow-up time	6 mo	
STUDY DESIGN		
Inclusion criteria	6 mo–10 y of age, ≥3 episodes of AOM in the preceding 6 mo or ≥4 in 18 mo; *presence or absence of MEE was acceptable*	
Exclusion criteria	Cleft palate, Down syndrome, previous tympanostomy tubes, or sulfonamide sensitivity	
Randomization effectiveness	No difference in sex, age, season of entry into the trial	
Age	1–48 mo	
Diagnostic criteria for an episode of AOM	"Rapid and short onset of signs and symptoms of inflammation in the middle ear." Diagnosis was also based on the following criteria: otalgia (ear tugging in infants), fever, TM erythema or bulging, decreased TM mobility, loss of TM landmarks, otorrhea	
Tube type	Paparella 0.04-mm grommet tubes "in most cases," TM site NR	
Response to AOM while tubes in place	"Antibiotics at standard therapeutic doses for 10 days"	
Response to tube obstruction	NR	
Response to AOM in group without tubes	"Antibiotics at standard therapeutic doses for 10 days"	
Morbidity/ complications	NR	

RAOM = recurrent acute otitis media, AOM = acute otitis media, RCT = randomized controlled trial, MEE = middle ear effusion, TM = tympanic membrane, NR = not reported.
* Sample size: numbers shown for those completing follow-up and (those initially recruited).

Methods of the Meta-Analysis. All of the studies included in this meta-analysis are RCTs (level 1) and they represent the highest level of evidence regarding the impact of tubes versus no surgery/no prophylaxis on patients presenting with RAOM. Further details regarding the search and selection process for these RCTs are as noted in the initial methods of this review.

Results of the Meta-Analysis. The data from all three RCTs comparing the impact of tubes versus no surgery/no prophylaxis on patients with a history of RAOM were combined. Two main outcome measures were considered: 1) the percentage of children who remained otitis-free, and 2) the incidence density of RAOM episodes per child per month. When all the results from all three studies were numerically combined in a meta-analysis, there was an overall 23.5% [95% confidence interval (CI) 13.6–33.4%] improvement in the number of children who remained otitis-free, suggesting that for every four (95% CI 3–8) children treated with tubes, one will remain otitis-free. Children with tubes had a 1.8 times (95% CI 1.05–3.14) greater odds of remaining otitis free. With respect to publication bias, there would need to be seven RCTs with negative findings to neutralize what seems to be an overall beneficial effect of tubes on the chances of remaining otitis-free.

The incidence density of otitis media (number of AOM episodes per child per month) for all of the data combined was 0.025 (95% CI 0.008–0.043) less with tubes than without tubes (or 0.300 per child per year). These incidence densities suggest that 40 (95% CI 23–125) children need to be treated for 1 month or that one child needs to be treated for 40 months to prevent one episode of AOM. To overcome this overall result that tubes cause a lower incidence density of AOM, 28 negative RCTs would be needed; it seems unlikely that even with publication bias, such a large number of negative trials would exist.

CLINICAL SIGNIFICANCE AND FUTURE RESEARCH

Two level 1 studies demonstrated a significant improvement in AOM outcomes with tubes versus no surgery/no prophylaxis, whereas a third found no difference. These conflicting data may result from differences in study design; the study that found no difference between tubes versus no treatment only included patients who were free of middle ear effusion at the outset, whereas the two studies that found better results with tubes included children regardless of their effusion status at the outset. When all of the data are combined in a meta-analysis, there seems to be an overall significant improvement in outcome with tubes versus no surgery/no prophylaxis. Children are 23.5% more likely to remain otitis-free, although the impact on the overall incidence density is modest (0.300 fewer AOM episodes per child per year).

Future research may address whether differences in study design may have impacted some of these results, especially focusing on the impact of middle ear effusion at the outset, age, and follow-up time.

Percent of children remaining otitis-free with tympanostomy tubes versus no surgery/no prophylaxis

Study, year	Tubes	No surgery/no prophylaxis
Casselbrant, 1992	35% (n = 30/77)	40% (n = 32/80)
Gebhart, 1981	46% (n = 25/54)	5% (n = 2/41)
Gonzalez, 1986	55% (n = 12/22)	15% (n = 3/20)
Total	44% (n = 67/153)	26% (n = 37/141)

Tubes vs No Surgery/No Prophylaxis: Rate Difference for Percent Remaining Otitis Free

Study name	Statistics for each study				Risk difference and 95% CI
	Risk difference	Lower limit	Upper limit	p-Value	
Casselbrant	-0.010	-0.163	0.143	0.894	
Gebhart	0.414	0.266	0.563	0.000	
Gonzalez	0.395	0.135	0.656	0.003	
Total	0.235	0.136	0.334	0.000	

-1.00 -0.50 0.00 0.50 1.00

Favors Placebo   Favors Tubes

Tubes vs No Surgery/No Prophylaxis: Odds Ratio for Percent Remaining Otitis Free

Study name	Statistics for each study				Odds ratio and 95% CI
	Odds ratio	Lower limit	Upper limit	p-Value	
Casselbrant	0.957	0.505	1.816	0.894	
Gebhart	16.810	3.683	76.733	0.000	
Gonzalez	6.800	1.537	30.077	0.012	
Total	1.816	1.050	3.143	0.033	

0.01 0.1 1 10 100

Favors Placebo   Favors Tubes

Number of episodes of AOM per child per month (incidence density) with tympanostomy tubes versus no surgery/no prophylaxis

Study, year	Tubes	No surgery/no prophylaxis
Casselbrant, 1992	0.085 (n = 157/1848)	0.090 (n = 173/1920)
Gebhart, 1981	0.111 (n = 36/324)	0.362 (n = 89/246)
Gonzalez, 1986	0.143 (n = 19/132)	0.333 (n = 40/120)
Total	0.092 (n = 212/2304)	0.132 (n = 302/2286)

Tubes vs No Surgery/No Prophylaxis: Rate Difference for Incidence Density

Study name	Statistics for each study				Risk difference and 95% CI
	Risk difference	Lower limit	Upper limit	p-Value	
Casselbrant	-0.005	-0.023	0.013	0.576	
Gebhart	-0.251	-0.320	-0.182	0.000	
Gonzalez	-0.189	-0.293	-0.086	0.000	
Total	-0.025	-0.043	-0.008	0.004	

-0.50 -0.25 0.00 0.25 0.50

Favors Placebo   Favors Tubes

Tubes vs No Surgery/No Prophylaxis: Odds Ratio for Incidence Density

Study name	Statistics for each study				Odds ratio and 95% CI
	Odds ratio	Lower limit	Upper limit	p-Value	
Casselbrant	0.938	0.748	1.175	0.576	
Gebhart	0.221	0.143	0.340	0.000	
Gonzalez	0.336	0.182	0.623	0.001	
Total	0.642	0.531	0.777	0.000	

0.1 0.2 0.5 1 2 5 10

Favors Placebo   Favors Tubes

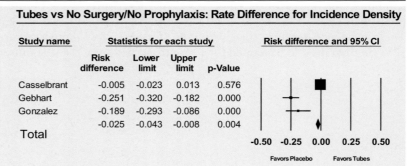

REFERENCES

1. Casselbrant ML, Kaleida PH, Rockette HE, et al. Efficacy of antimicrobial prophylaxis and of tympanostomy tube insertion for prevention of recurrent acute otitis media: results of a randomized clinical trial. [see comment.] Pediatr Infec dis J 1992;11(4):278–286.
2. Gonzalez C, Arnold JE, Woody EA, Erhardt JB, Pratt SR, Getts A, Kueser TJ, Kolmer JW, Sachs M. Prevention of recurrent acute otitis media: chemoprophylaxis versus tympanostomy tubes. Laryngoscope 1986;96(12):1330–1334.
3. Gebhart DE, Tympanostomy tubes in the otitis media prone child. Laryngoscope 1981;91(6):849–866.

6 Pediatric Recurrent Acute Otitis Media

Tympanostomy tube insertion versus antibiotic prophylaxis: Impact on subsequent number of episodes of acute otitis media, chance of no further episodes of acute otitis media

Jennifer J. Shin and Chrisopher J. Hartnick

METHODS

A computerized Ovid search of MEDLINE 1966–January 2004 was performed. The subject headings "otitis media" and "middle ear ventilation" were exploded and cross-referenced, yielding 807 articles. Given the known richness and high level of the literature on otitis media, these articles were then limited to randomized controlled trials (RCTs), yielding 107 articles. These articles were then reviewed to find those that met the following inclusion criteria: 1) pediatric population of patients <18 years of age with recurrent acute otitis media (RAOM), 2) intervention with tympanostomy tube placement compared with continuous antibiotic prophylaxis, and 3) outcomes measured in terms of number of episodes of RAOM. Trials that enrolled subjects on the basis of chronic otitis media with effusion (rather than RAOM) were excluded here, although they are analyzed in a subsequent chapter. Trials in which the antibiotic group received antimicrobial therapy with each episode of acute otitis media (AOM) but did not receive prophylaxis in between flairs were also excluded. These inclusion criteria yielded two RCTs [1, 2], and their bibliographies were also manually searched but no further level 1 trials were uncovered.

RESULTS

Outcome Measures. Outcomes in both studies were measured in terms of the number of episodes of AOM subsequent to treatment. These "episodes" were diagnosed on the basis of history and physical examination, with further details provided in the adjoining table. Reported here is the mean number of episodes of AOM, as well as the percent of children with no further episodes of AOM in the follow-up period.

Potential Confounders. Potential confounders include age, tube type and postoperative management, antibiotic regimen and compliance with it, and presence of middle ear effusion (MEE). First, age may confound the results, because the incidence of AOM decreases with increasing age. The age ranges are fairly tight in these trials, with one study spanning a range of <3 years [1], and the other spanning a range of <4 years [2]. Second, the presence or absence of MEE may also influence the number of AOM events, and one study excluded any patients with MEE at the outset in order to control for this variable

[1]. Third, the tube type, its placement, and the postoperative management of tube occlusions may result in alterations in their longevity and efficacy. Both studies used a standardized tube and one reported in detail their standardized management of tube occlusions. Fourth, the particular antibiotic dose and patient compliance with its administration may affect the outcomes. Both studies clearly reported their prophylaxis regimen, and one study also measured compliance and reported the detailed management of each flair of AOM [1]. Further details are provided in the adjoining table.

Study Designs. Both studies are RCTs with double blinding in the medical arms (i.e., antibiotic prophylaxis and placebo). The rate of noncompletion (i.e., number of patients who were enrolled but did not complete the follow-up) in each trial is a foremost issue when considering the credibility of these results. In one case, more than half of the medical group and 26% of the surgical group did not complete the trial [1], either because they were lost to follow-up or because they were withdrawn from the trial for treatment failure. Subjects who were discharged because of treatment failure, however, were still included in the final data report. In providing this information, the study investigators completed an intention to treat analysis, which ensured that the results were not biased toward patients who responded best to treatment. In the second study, the results for the 65 patients who completed the trial were reported, but the initial number of patients enrolled is unclear [1]. In both cases, therefore, the results may be unintentionally skewed toward a population who was more inclined to complete follow-up, which could reflect either higher satisfaction with care or increased severity of disease. In addition, the length of follow-up is a key factor, because otitis media often has a seasonal component. One study accounted for this factor by following patients for 2 years [1]. The other study followed patients for just 6 months, but accounted for seasonal differences by balancing the number of subjects affected at different seasons through randomization among the three different interventions [2]. One study reported their *a priori* calculation of power: 90% to detect a 50% decrease in episodes of AOM and this power was corroborated by their results which demonstrated a statistically significant difference between groups [1]. The second study did not report their initial power calculation but demonstrated the ability to statistically discern a >57%–72% difference between groups [2].

Highest Level of Evidence. Two RCTs constitute the highest level of evidence comparing tube placements versus antibiotic prophylaxis versus placebo for patients with RAOM. Perhaps because of differences in antibiotic regimens or because of uneven subject withdrawal (please see above), the results of these trials are somewhat conflicting. First, consider the impact of tube placement versus antibiotic prophylaxis. The larger trial showed that in comparison to children undergoing tube placement, children who took antibiotic prophylaxis had a lower mean number of episodes of AOM (p = 0.001), and this was corroborated by the fact that they also were more likely to have no further episodes of AOM in the follow-up period. In contrast, the smaller trial reported the converse: the mean number of episodes of AOM was less in the tubes group and in accordance with this finding, the percent of children with no further episodes of AOM was higher in the tubes group. Statistical significance, however, was not achieved in this case. Second, consider the impact of tympanostomy tubes versus placebo. The larger study found no significant difference, but the smaller study found significantly better outcomes with tubes. Third, consider the effect of antibiotic prophylaxis versus placebo. The larger study found a significant improvement with antibiotics whereas the smaller study found the same trend, although without the statistical significance.

Applicability. The results of both trials are applicable to infants and children 7–35 months of age who have had ≥3 episodes of AOM in the previous 6 months. These results are not necessarily applicable to children with significant comorbidities such as cleft palate, chronic sinusitis, or Down syndrome.

Morbidity. The morbidity of the tubes and antibiotic treatments were described in one study [1] and limited to <7% of the populations studied. Only minor adverse reactions were observed, and all remaining tympanic membrane perforations eventually closed spontaneously.

CLINICAL SIGNIFICANCE AND FUTURE RESEARCH

There are two level 1 studies that directly compared the impact of tubes versus antibiotic prophylaxis, and both studies further placed these results in context through comparison with a third placebo group. Both studies are unfortunately beleaguered by potential biases from subject attrition, and each handled MEE at the outset in different ways, which may account for their diametrically opposed findings regarding the impact of tubes versus antibiotics on the number of episodes of AOM. Likewise, their findings regarding tubes versus placebo and antibiotic prophylaxis versus placebo are not completely similar. Overall, the heterogeneity of the results prevents clean conclusions from being drawn. Future RCTs may attempt to settle this still relatively unresolved issue of the impact of tubes versus antibiotic prophylaxis on the number of episodes of AOM.

THE EVIDENCE CONDENSED: Tympanostomy tube insertion versus antibiotic prophylaxis for recurrent acute otitis media

Reference	Casselbrant, 1992	
Level (design)	1 (RCT)	
Sample size*	264 (74% tubes group, 47% abx, 46% placebo)	
OUTCOMES		
	Mean no. of episodes of AOM, episodes/child/year	% of children with no further episodes in follow-up period
Tubes	1.02	35%
Antibiotics prophylaxis	0.60	58%
Placebo	1.08	40%
p Values	=0.001, tubes vs antibiotics =0.25, tubes vs placebo <0.001, antibiotics vs placebo	NR, tubes vs antibiotics NR, tubes vs placebo =0.03, antibiotics vs placebo
Conclusion	Antibiotics better than tubes	Trend for antibiotics to be better
Follow-up time	2 y (monthly visits and with acute episodes)	
STUDY DESIGN		
Inclusion criteria	7–35 mo of age, most recent episode in <6 mo, ≥3 episodes of AOM in the preceding 6 mo or ≥4 in 12 mo; *free from MEE at time of entry*	
Exclusion criteria	Asthma, chronic sinusitis, previous tonsillectomy or adenoidectomy	
Randomization effectiveness	No difference in age, season, previous number of AOM episodes, sex, race, socioeconomic status	
Age	7–35 mo	
Diagnostic criteria for an episode of AOM	Otoscopic signs (erythema or white opacification not attributable to scarring, fullness or bulging and decreased mobility of TM) or ≥1 symptom (fever, otalgia, irritability) in the presence of MEE If PET in place, then episode of otorrhea was considered equivalent to an episode of AOM	
Tube type	Teflon Armstrong tube in the anterosuperior quadrant of the pars tensa	
Response to AOM while tubes in place	Ototopical treatment with neomycin sulfate, polymyxin B sulfate, and hydrocortisone suspension × ≤10 d, amoxicillin 40 mg/kg/d in 3 divided doses ×10 d unless cultures revealed resistant organisms	
Response to tube obstruction	Ototopical treatment with neomycin sulfate, polymyxin B sulfate, and hydrocortisone; if remained occluded then replaced if <6 mo since insertion, replaced only if AOM/OME developed if 6–12 mo since insertion	
Abx prophylaxis	Amoxicillin 20 mg/kg/d in 1 nightly dose	
Response to AOM in group without tubes	Amoxicillin 40 mg/kg/d in 3 divided doses ×10 d unless tympanocentesis cultures revealed resistant organisms—then erythromycin 50 mg/kg/d and sulfisoxazole 150 mg/kg/d ×10 d	
Compliance	82%–95% for abx and placebo, as assessed by calendar method, bottle method, and urine specimens	
Power	0.90 to detect a 50% reduction in the average number of episodes of AOM	
Morbidity/ complications	Amoxicillin group with 7.0% adverse reactions Tubes group with 3.9% persistent perforations	

RCT = randomized controlled trial, NR = not reported, RAOM = recurrent acute otitis media, AOM = acute otitis media, MEE = middle ear effusion, TM = tympanic membrane, abx = antibiotics, NS = not significant, b.i.d. = twice a day dosing.
* Sample size: numbers shown for those initially recruited and those (completing the trial).

THE EVIDENCE CONDENSED: Tympanostomy tube insertion versus antibiotic prophylaxis for recurrent acute otitis media

Reference	Gonzalez, 1986
Level (design)	1 (RCT)
Sample size*	NR (65)

OUTCOMES		
	Mean no. of episodes of AOM, episodes/child/6 mo	% of children with no further episodes in follow-up period
Tubes	0.86	55%
Abx prophylaxis	1.38	24%
Placebo	2.00	15%
p Values	NR, tubes vs abx =0.006, tubes vs placebo NS, abx vs placebo	=0.08, tubes vs abx =0.01, tubes vs placebo NR, abx vs placebo
Conclusion	Trend for tubes to be better	Trend for tubes to be better
Follow-up time	6 mo (monthly visits and with acute episodes)	

STUDY DESIGN	
Inclusion criteria	6 mo–10 y of age, ≥3 episodes of AOM in the preceding 6 mo or ≥4 in 18 mo; *presence or absence of MEE was acceptable*
Exclusion criteria	Cleft palate, Down syndrome, previous tympanostomy tubes, or sulfonamide sensitivity
Randomization effectiveness	No difference in sex, age, season of entry into the trial
Age	1–48 mo
Diagnostic criteria for an episode of AOM	"Rapid and short onset of signs and symptoms of inflammation in the middle ear." Diagnosis was also based on the following criteria: otalgia (ear tugging in infants), fever, TM erythema or bulging, decreased TM mobility, loss of TM landmarks, otorrhea
Tube type	Paparella 0.04-mm grommet tubes "in most cases," TM site not specified
Response to AOM while tubes in place	"Antibiotics at standard therapeutic doses for 10 days"
Response to tube obstruction	NR
Abx prophylaxis	Sulfisoxazole 500 mg PO b.i.d. if <5 y old; 1 g PO b.i.d. if >5 y old
Response to AOM in group without tubes	"Antibiotics at standard therapeutic doses for 10 days"
Compliance	"Compliance could not be adequately established in our study"
Power	NR
Morbidity/complications	NR

RCT = randomized controlled trial, NR = not reported, RAOM = recurrent acute otitis media, AOM = acute otitis media, MEE = middle ear effusion, TM = tympanic membrane, abx = antibiotics, NS = not significant, b.i.d. = twice a day dosing, PET = pneumatic equalization tube, OME = otitis media with effusion.
* Sample size: numbers shown for those initially recruited and those (completing the trial).

REFERENCES

1. Casselbrant ML, Kaleida PH, Rockette HE, et al. Efficacy of antimicrobial prophylaxis and of tympanostomy tube insertion for prevention of recurrent acute otitis media: results of a randomized clinical trial. [see comment.] Pediatr Infect Dis J 1992;11(4):278–286.

2. Gonzalez C, Arnold JE, Woody EA, et al. Prevention of recurrent acute otitis media: chemoprophylaxis versus tympanostomy tubes. Laryngoscope 1986;96(12):1330–1334.

6 Pediatric Recurrent Acute Otitis Media

6.F.

Adenoidectomy versus no adenoidectomy: Impact on rate of acute otitis media

Jennifer J. Shin and Christopher J. Hartnick

METHODS

A computerized Ovid search of MEDLINE 1966–January 2004 was performed. The terms "otitis media" and "adenoidectomy" were exploded and the resulting articles were cross-referenced, yielding 382 trials. Given the known richness of the otitis media literature and the authority of higher levels of evidence, these articles were then limited to randomized controlled trials (RCTs), resulting in 39 applicable studies. These articles were then reviewed to identify those that met the following inclusion criteria: 1) patient population <18 years of age with documented recurrent acute otitis media (RAOM), 2) intervention with adenoidectomy versus no adenoidectomy, 3) outcome measured in terms of the number of episodes of acute otitis media (AOM). Trials in which persistent middle ear effusion (MEE) was the impetus for surgery or the primary disease process were excluded. Studies focusing on tonsillectomy combined with adenoidectomy are addressed in the next review. The bibliographies of the articles that met these inclusion criteria were manually checked to ensure no further relevant articles could be identified. This process yielded four RCTs and one nonrandomized trial. The four RCTs are discussed in detail below [1–4].

RESULTS

Outcome Measures. Outcomes in all studies except one were measured in terms of the mean rate of AOM episodes per subject over a given period of time [2–4]. The diagnosis of AOM was based on standardized features of the history and physical examination, and the details are tabulated below. The Paradise reports also included the percent of patients with no further AOM episodes in a given year. The Matilla study also included the number of days with otorrhea per person year, which was a reasonable measure because all patients had tympanostomy tubes placed. The most recent study reported a primary outcome of percent of children who failed treatment (two acute episodes in 2 months or three acute episodes in 6 months; or MEE for >2 months as assessed by pneumatic otoscopy) [1].

Potential Confounders. Potential confounders were as described in previous queries in this chapter and are tabulated in the adjoining table in as much detail as the studies allow.

Study Designs. Four RCTs, two of which were reported in one article [3, 4], addressed the impact of adenoidectomy versus no surgery on RAOM. Randomization was effective in controlling cited potential confounders in each study. *These studies differ in key aspects related to the placement of tympanostomy tubes*: 1) the 1999 study and the 2004 study were performed in children who had never been treated with tubes [1, 3]; 2) another study was performed exclusively in children who had previous tube placement but were postextrusion [4]; 3) in the 2003 study, tubes were placed in all subjects as part of the study design [2]. In addition to these differences, two studies focused exclusively on children <2 years of age [1, 2], whereas the others included children up to 15 years old [3, 4]. The reports from 1999 all included an intention to treat analysis [3, 4], whereas the 2003 report used a time-dependent treatment covariate analysis. In this report, control patients who eventually underwent adenoidectomy were analyzed in the control group until the time of their adenoid procedure, after which they were included in the adenoidectomy group [2].

Highest Level of Evidence. The RCTs that evaluated the impact of adenoidectomy alone versus no adenoid surgery on AOM outcomes had variable results. First, in the studies of children with no previous tube placement, adenoidectomy did not improve outcomes [1, 3]. In most parameters measured, there was no difference between the adenoidectomy and control groups. In fact, in the second year of follow-up in the 1999 trial, the control group had a significantly lower rate of AOM episodes per child year than the adenoidectomy group. Second, in the study that focused exclusively on children <2 years of age who had tubes placed either with or without adenoidectomy, there was a trend toward a decreased rate of AOM with adenoidectomy, but no significant difference between groups [2]. Third, in the study regarding children with extruded tubes, adenoidectomy significantly improved outcomes in the first and second years of follow-up [4]. The mean rate of AOM episodes per child year was decreased by 0.58 and 36% more children remained AOM-free; there was a number needed to treat of three children. Likewise, the proportion of days in which otitis was present was significantly decreased. Significant differences were no longer present at the third year of follow-up, but at this point sample size had decreased to 54 patients; with the ensuing decrease in power, it is unclear whether a true difference was obscured or if the effect was simply no longer present after a longer follow-up.

Overall, three studies showed no improvement [1–3] and one showed significant improvement [4] in multiple measures of AOM with adenoidectomy. There is no neat logic that can elucidate exactly why this disparity occurred, although there are several potential explanations. The study that showed improvement differed from the other two in that it focused on a subset of children whose RAOM was so severe that it persisted beyond a period in which they had initially been treated with tubes. This difference alone may have resulted in the observed improvement with adenoidectomy. From a mathematical point of view, when disease is more severe, there is more room for improvement; this fact may make it easier to achieve a demonstrable amount of recovery than when disease is less severe (statistical floor effect). Oddly enough, however, rates of AOM in the control group in this study overall were actually lower than in the control group in a study that enrolled children without previous tympanostomy tube placement. Thus, a purely mathematical explanation may not be complete. In addition, the two studies which found that AOM outcomes were the same regardless of whether adenoidectomy was performed were adequately powered, at least in the initial 1–2 years. In fact, their sample sizes were larger than the study that identified a difference. Also, although one study found no difference when only children under 2 years of age were studied, another study demonstrated adenoidectomy-related improvement that persisted even when adjusting for the impact of age (including an age group of 1- to 2-year-old children). Overall, previous tympanostomy tube placement was the only clear distinction in the one study that identified a significant improvement with adenoidectomy versus no surgery [4].

Applicability. Although all of these studies measured similar interventions and outcomes, each is applicable to a different type of patient. First, the 1999 study (which showed no difference) is applicable to 3- to 15-year-old children who have *not* had previous tympanostomy tubes placement, who present with ≥3 episodes of AOM in the preceding 6 months or ≥4 episodes of AOM in the preceding 12 months *or* MEE in ≥1 ear over ≥180 days in the preceding year. Similarly, the 2004 study is applicable to 10- to 24-month-old children with >3 episodes of AOM in the previous 6 months. Second, the 1990 study

results (which showed improvement with adenoidectomy) are applicable to patients with recurrent and/or persistent otitis media whose previous tympanostomy tubes in one or both ears have extruded. Third, the 2003 study (which showed a nonsignificant trend toward improvement) is applicable to a younger group of patients aged 10 months to 2 years old who present with >3–5 episodes of AOM during the previous 6 months or >4–6 episodes of AOM during the previous 12 months.

Overall, this means that adenoidectomy has demonstrated efficacy only in the treatment of children with RAOM after the extrusion of previously placed tympanostomy tubes. At the same time as the RCT that demonstrated this efficacy, a parallel nonrandomized trial was also conducted in which parents could choose the intervention their child received. In this level 2 trial, results were similar, with more favorable results seen in the adenoidectomy group than in the control group. The presence of this parallel trial allows the statement of efficacy (i.e., adenoidectomy works within a defined population under controlled circumstances) made in the RCT to be expanded to a statement of effectiveness (i.e., adenoidectomy works in regular clinical practice).

Morbidity. Adenoidectomy had a 0%–4.8% complication rate in these trials, suggesting a number needed to harm as low as 21 children. This potential for harm underscores the need to only perform the procedure if more than 1 in 21 children can benefit. (As above, the number needed to treat for children with RAOM after previous tube extrusion was 3, suggesting that 1 in 3 children could benefit from adenoidectomy.)

CLINICAL SIGNIFICANCE AND FUTURE RESEARCH

There are four RCTs that address whether adenoidectomy is a worthwhile endeavor in children with RAOM. The evidence suggests that it is a worthwhile endeavor in the specific population of children who have persistent disease even after the previous placement and extrusion of tympanostomy tubes. Furthermore, it seems that this result can be generalized to a situation in which parental input helps determine whether adenoidectomy is performed. It does not yet seem useful in children who have not previously had tympanostomy tubes placed, regardless of age.

Future research may focus on further defining which characteristics can further identify the subset of children who will benefit from adenoidectomy. In addition, the optimal timing of adenoidectomy relative to other treatments may also be explored.

Reference	Koivunen, 2004		
Level (design)	1 (RCT)		
Sample size*	103 (120)		

	OUTCOMES		
	% of children with treatment failure†		Mean number (SD) of episodes of AOM
Follow-up year	6 mo	2 y	6 mo
Adenoidectomy	42%	76%	1.3 (0.9)
Control	52%	76%	1.3 (0.9)
p Value	NS	NS	NS
Conclusion	No difference	No difference	No difference

	STUDY DESIGN
Inclusion criteria	≥3 AOM during the previous 6 mo, 10–24 mo of age
Exclusion criteria	Previous adenoidectomy or tympanostomy, craniofacial anomalies, documented immunologic disorders, and ongoing antimicrobial chemoprophylaxis
Randomization effectiveness	Similar age, sex, no. of RAOM episodes, daycare, MEE at assignment
Age	10–24 mo
Adenoidectomy details	Adenoidectomy as day care surgery
Additional procedures	12 children in the adenoidectomy group had concurrent tympanostomy tube placement for MEE
Disease details at the outset	55%–62% had >5 previous episodes of RAOM
Diagnostic criteria for AOM	"Acute symptoms together with signs of middle ear inflammation (hyperemic, opaque, or bulging ear drum) and MEE obtained in pneumatic otoscopy or otorrhea"
Management of AOM episode while in study	"Usually amoxicillin for one week"
Management of MEE during study	Amoxicillin and reexamination in 2 wk; if still present then myringotomy; if still present after 2 mo then tympanostomy tube placed
Criteria for withdrawal	"Children who did not get the allocated prophylaxis or whose prophylaxis was changed before defined failure" were defined as "protocol variations"
Intention to treat analysis?	Protocol violations were regarded as dropouts or as treatment failures
Power calculation	A priori calculation of 80% with 57 children in each group
Morbidity/ complications	No complications in the adenoidectomy procedures

RCT = randomized controlled trial, AOM = acute otitis media, RAOM = recurrent AOM, NS = not significant, SD = standard deviation, MEE = middle ear effusion, T&A = adenotonsillectomy, TM = tympanic membrane.

* Sample size: numbers shown for those not lost to follow-up and those (initially recruited).

†Treatment failure in the Koivunen trial was defined as: two acute episodes in 2 mo or three acute episodes in 6 mo; or MEE for >2 mo as assessed by pneumatic otoscopy. The Koivunen trial also compared adenoidectomy with sulfisoxazole prophylaxis and found no significant difference.

Reference	Paradise, 1999
Level (design)	1 (RCT)
Sample size*	140 at y 1, 112 at y 2, 81 at y 3 (177)

OUTCOMES

	Mean rate of AOM episodes per subject			% of patients with no AOM episodes		
Follow-up year	Y 1	Y 2	Y 3	Y 1	Y 2	Y 3
Adenoidectomy	1.8	1.7	1.3	31.1%	26.4%	35.3%
Control	2.1	1.2	1.5	21.5%	37.3%	36.2%
p Value	NS	0.04	NS	NS	NS	NS
Conclusion	No difference	Cnt better	No difference	No difference	No difference	No difference

STUDY DESIGN

Inclusion criteria	3–15 y old; *no previous tympanostomy tube placement*; ≥3 AOM in the preceding 6 mo or ≥4 AOM in the preceding 12 mo, with ≥1 documented episode *or* MEE in ≥1 ear over ≥180 d in the preceding year, documented at least twice at ≥6-mo intervals; free of otitis media at the outset
Exclusion criteria	Indication for tonsillectomy, overt or submucous palatal clefts
Randomization effectiveness	No significant difference in age, sex, race, entry criterion met, MEE, baseline hearing, nasal obstruction, upper respiratory allergy, siblings, parents' socioeconomic status
Age	3–15 y
Adenoidectomy details	Reverse adenotomes, curettes were used under both direct and mirror vision; the fossa of Rosenmüller was curetted routinely
Additional procedures	Myringotomy and aspiration was performed if MEE was present at the time of adenoidectomy or T&A. If in the control group, myringotomy and aspiration was performed if MEE had been present for >90 d without improvement
Disease details at the outset	91.2% RAOM, 5% persistent MEE, 3.4% both
Diagnostic criteria for AOM	MEE with recent otalgia, marked erythema or bulging of the tympanic membrane; otorrhea with otalgia or fever in the presence of tympanostomy tube or TM perforation
Management of AOM episode while in study	"Antimicrobial in the conventional dosage for 10 d to 6 wk, depending on recent clinical course and response to treatment. Amoxicillin was used whenever feasible; second line drugs mainly used were erythromycin-sulfisoxazole and amoxicillin clavulanate"
Management of MEE during study	If MEE ≥90 d without improvement, then myringotomy with aspiration; if recurred within 6 mo and persisted ≥60 d then myringotomy and tube placement
Criteria for withdrawal	Parental wishes, lack of follow-up
Intention to treat analysis?	Yes: patients in the control group who received eventual surgery were analyzed as controls
Power calculation	80% to detect a 25% difference with 57 subjects per treatment group
Morbidity/ complications	Adenoidectomy group with 4.8% postoperative complications

RCT = randomized controlled trial, AOM = acute otitis media, RAOM = recurrent AOM, NS = not significant, SD = standard deviation, MEE = middle ear effusion, T&A = adenotonsillectomy, TM = tympanic membrane, Cnt = control.
* Sample size: numbers shown for those not lost to follow-up and those (initially recruited).

Reference	Paradise, 1990					
Level (design)	1 (RCT)					
Sample size*	86 at y 1, 83 at y 2, 54 at y 3 (99)					

OUTCOMES						
	Mean rate of AOM episodes per subject			% patients with no AOM episodes		
Follow-up year	Y 1	Y 2	Y 3	Y 1	Y 2	Y 3
Adenoidectomy	1.06	1.09	0.89	44%	51%	51%
Control	1.45	1.67	0.87	33%	19%	41%
p Value	NS	0.01	NS	NS	0.01	NS
Conclusion	No difference	Adenoidectomy better	No difference	No difference	Adenoidectomy better	No difference

STUDY DESIGN	
Inclusion criteria	Persistent and/or recurrent otitis media; to therefore *have received tympanostomy tube placement in one or both ears on 1 or more occasions*; and to have developed, *after extrusion of the tube(s)* and within the year that preceded enrollment, ≥1 additional documented episodes of either suppurative (acute) or nonsuppurative (secretory) otitis media; free of MEE at the starting point
Exclusion criteria	Overt or submucous palatal clefts
Randomization effectiveness	No differences in age, sex, race, age at time of onset of otitis media, no. of prior tympanostomy tube procedures, MEE at the time of assignment, tympanostomy tube in place and patent at the start of the trial, baseline hearing sensitivity, degree of nasal obstruction as estimated clinically, degree of nasopharyngeal obstruction as estimated roentgraphically, tonsil-related history, siblings, upper respiratory tract allergy, parents' socioeconomic status
Age	1–15 y
Adenoidectomy details	Reverse adenotomes, curettes were used under both direct and mirror vision; Rosenmüller's fossa was curetted routinely
Additional procedures	Tympanostomy: radial myringotomy and aspiration of middle ear fluid
Disease details at the outset	78% with MEE at the time of assignment, 68% with tubes at the trial start
Diagnostic criteria for AOM	MEE present with at least one of the following: perforation with otorrhea, otalgia, moderate to marked TM erythema, TM bulging; if no MEE, then at least one of the following: otalgia, moderate to marked TM erythema
Management of AOM episode while in study	Antimicrobial drug(s) for 10 d–6 wk, depending on recent clinical course and response to treatment. Ampicillin then amoxicillin was used whenever feasible; the first alternative was erythromycin-sulfisoxazole
Management of MEE during study	If persisted ≥60 d then myringotomy and tube placement
Criteria for withdrawal	Second adenoidectomy
Intention to treat analysis?	Tabulated results are for groups in which control patients were withdrawn if adenoidectomy was subsequently performed; an intention to treat analysis was reported in the text, however, with similar results.
Power calculation	Not specified
Morbidity/complications	No anesthetic complications; 2 patients required nasal packing for 1 d, 10 rashes, 11 persistent TM perforations (1 cholesteatoma, 1 modified radical mastectomy)

RAOM = recurrent acute otitis media, RCT = randomized controlled trial, AOM = acute otitis media, NS = not significant, TM = tympanic membrane, MEE = middle ear effusion, b.i.d.= twice a day dosing.
* Sample size: numbers shown for those not lost to follow-up and those (initially recruited).

Reference	Mattila, 2003	
Level (design)	1 (RCT)	
Sample size*	137 (137)	

OUTCOMES		
	Mean rate of AOM per person year	No. of days with otorrhea per person year
Follow-up year	Up to 2 y old (mean 7 mo)	
Adenoidectomy	2.05	3.62
Control	2.40	3.45
p Value	NS	NS
Conclusion	No difference	No difference

STUDY DESIGN	
Inclusion criteria	Children who had been enrolled at the age of 2 mo in a pneumococcal vaccine study who had >3–5 AOM during the previous 6 mo or 4–6 AOM during the previous 12 mo; 10–23 mo of age
Exclusion criteria	Parental refusal before or after allocation
Randomization effectiveness	No difference in sex, proportion of children with or without siblings, daycare outside home, mean age at operation, no. of AOM episodes before the age of 1 y old, vaccination status
Age	10–23 mo
Adenoidectomy details	Performed with Beckman ring curette, tissue in Rosenmüller's fossa was routinely removed
Additional procedures	*All patients also underwent tympanostomy tube placement* (anterior radial myringotomy)
Disease details at the outset	Mean no. of previous AOMs was 3.4–3.5
Diagnostic criteria for AOM	MEE signs and fever, ear pain, signs of upper respiratory tract infection, irritability, diarrhea, vomiting, or discharge from the ear
Management of AOM episode while in study	Amoxicillin 40 mg/kg PO b.i.d. ×7 d was the first choice antibiotic; if allergic then trimethoprim-sulfadiazine 8 and 25 mg/kg PO b.i.d. ×7 d, cefaclor 40 mg/kg PO b.i.d. ×7 d, or azithromycin 10 mg/kg PO ×1 d then 5 mg/kg PO q.d. ×4 d
Management of MEE during study	All patients had tube placement at the outset
Criteria for withdrawal	Not specified
Intention to treat analysis?	The 5 children in the tympanostomy group who underwent adenoidectomy at a later date were analyzed using a time-dependent treatment covariate (i.e., they were analyzed as part of the adenoidectomy group after the time point where they had this surgery)—may have resulted in underestimation of the effect of adenoidectomy
Power calculation	No *a priori* calculation reported
Morbidity/complications	None reported

RAOM = recurrent acute otitis media, RCT = randomized controlled trial, AOM = acute otitis media, NS = not significant, TM = tympanic membrane, MEE = middle ear effusion, b.i.d.= twice a day dosing.
* Sample size: numbers shown for those not lost to follow-up and those (initially recruited).

REFERENCES

1. Koivunen P, Uhari M, Luotonen J, et al. Adenoidectomy versus chemoprophylaxis and placebo for recurrent acute otitis media in children aged under 2 years: randomised controlled trial. BMJ, 2004;328(7438):487.

2. Mattila PS, Joki-Erkkila VP, Kilpi T, Jokinen J, Herva E, Puhakka H. Prevention of otitis media by adenoidectomy in children younger than 2 years. Arch Otolaryngol Head Neck Surg 2003;129(2):163–168.

3. Paradise JL, Bluestone CD, Colborn DK, et al. Adenoidectomy and adenotonsillectomy for recurrent acute otitis media: parallel randomized clinical trials in children not previously treated with tympanostomy tubes.[see comment]. JAMA 1999;282(10):945–953.

4. Paradise JL, Bluestone CD, Rogers KD, et al. Efficacy of adenoidectomy for recurrent otitis media in children previously treated with tympanostomy-tube placement. Results of parallel randomized and nonrandomized trials. JAMA 1990;263(15):2066–2073.

6 Pediatric Recurrent Acute Otitis Media

6.G.

Adenotonsillectomy versus adenoidectomy alone or no adenotonsillar surgery: Impact on rate of acute otitis media

Jennifer J. Shin and Chrisopher J. Hartnick

METHODS

A computerized Ovid search of MEDLINE 1966–January 2004 was performed as described in 20.F. These articles were then reviewed to identify those that met the following inclusion criteria: 1) patient population <18 years of age with documented recurrent acute otitis media (RAOM), 2) intervention with adenoidtonsillectomy versus no surgery or adenoidectomy alone, 3) outcome measured in terms of the number of episodes of acute otitis media (AOM). Articles in which adenoidectomy alone was the focus are discussed in 20.F. The bibliographies of the articles that met these inclusion criteria were manually checked to ensure no further relevant articles could be identified. This process yielded two randomized controlled trials (RCTs), reported in a single article [1].

RESULTS

Outcome Measures. Outcomes in these studies were measured in terms of the mean rate of AOM episodes per subject over a given period of time, as well as the percent of patients with no further AOM episodes in a given year. The diagnosis of AOM was based on standardized features of the history and physical examination, and the details are tabulated for the reader.

Potential Confounders. Potential confounders were as described in previous queries in this chapter and are detailed in the adjacent table in as much detail as the studies allow.

Study Designs. Two RCTs, both of which were reported in one article [1], addressed the impact of adenotonsillectomy (T&A) on RAOM. In a "three-way" trial, T&A was compared with either adenoidectomy or no surgery, in children without a tonsil-related indication for pharyngeal surgery. In a "two-way" trial, T&A was compared with no surgery in children with a tonsil-related indication for their removal. The three-way and two-way trials were both performed in children who had never been treated with tubes. An intention to treat analysis was reported. Randomization was effective in balancing potential confounders between groups, with the exception of only a single factor (gender) in the two-way trial.

Highest Level of Evidence. The two- and three-way trials that compared T&A with no surgery in children without previous tube placement showed better results with T&A as compared with control. In the three-way trial, there was a significantly lower rate of AOM in the first year and when the data for all 3 years were combined. In the two-way trial, there was no significant difference in individual years but there was again a clear difference in the combined for all years. The amount of improvement (three-way trial, first year) was a decrease of 0.5–0.7 AOM episodes per subject and an increase of 15.1% more children with no further AOM. This absolute risk reduction corresponds to a number needed to treat of seven children; seven children must undergo T&A in order for one of those children to remain otitis-free. Intervention with T&A was also noted to result in a significantly better outcome than adenoidectomy alone in the three-way trial.

Applicability. These studies are applicable to children who have not had previous tympanostomy tubes placement, who present with ≥3 episodes of AOM in the preceding 6 months or ≥4 episodes of AOM in the preceding 12 months *or* MEE in ≥1 ear over ≥180 days in the preceding year.

Morbidity. T&A had a higher rate of complication than adenoidectomy alone (14.6% versus 4.8%) according to the three-way trial. These figures correspond to absolute risk increase of 9.8% from the addition of tonsillectomy. This risk increase means that there is a number needed to harm of 10 children, or that every tenth child undergoing T&A instead of adenoidectomy alone will experience an additional complication. It also means that there is a number needed to harm of seven children undergoing T&A in comparison to no adenotonsillar surgery. This number is unfortunately similar to the number needed to treat noted above. Thus, it seems that a loss must be accepted for every gain if T&A is undertaken.

CLINICAL SIGNIFICANCE AND FUTURE RESEARCH

Two parallel RCTs address the impact of T&A versus no surgery or adenoidectomy alone on RAOM [1]. The evidence in both trials suggests that T&A results in improved AOM outcomes, as compared with no surgery. The extent of that improvement is rather minimal, however, with just a difference of 0.5–0.7 episodes per child at 1 year. Likewise, although T&A results in a significantly different outcome than adenoidectomy alone, the improvement is just 0.4 episodes per child at 1 year. In this case, a statistically significant but clinically minor difference has been demonstrated. Therefore, the intervention's potential for harm becomes especially important, because the demonstrated potential benefit from T&A is small. The T&A-associated morbidity is not negligible (see above); in fact, it is notably higher than the morbidity of adenoidectomy. Therefore, most clinicians believe that the risks of T&A outweigh the potential benefits.

Future research may focus more on the role of adenoidectomy alone, and the preoperative identification of subjects who are likely to benefit from this surgical intervention.

Reference	Paradise, 1990					
Level (design)	1 (randomized controlled trial)					
	"Three-way" trial					
Sample size*	235 at y 1, 201 at y 2, 162 at y 3 (304)					

OUTCOMES						
	Mean rate of AOM episodes per subject			% of patients with no AOM episodes		
Follow-up year	Y 1	Y 2	Y 3	Y 1	Y 2	Y 3
T&A	1.4	1.3	1.2	36.6%	34.3%	36.2%
Adenoidectomy alone	1.8	1.7	1.3	31.1%	26.4%	35.3%
Control	2.1	1.2	1.5	21.5%	37.3%	36.2%
p Value, T&A vs control	<0.001	NS	NS	<0.05	NS	NS
Conclusion, T&A vs control	T&A better	No difference	No difference	T&A better	No difference	No difference
p Value, T&A vs adenoidectomy	0.03	0.04, for all 3 y combined		—	—	—
Conclusion, T&A vs adenoidectomy	T&A better	T&A better in data for all years combined		—	—	—

STUDY DESIGN	
Inclusion criteria	3–15 y old; *no previous tympanostomy tube placement*; ≥3 AOM in the preceding 6 mo or ≥4 AOM in the preceding 12 mo, with ≥1 documented episode *or* MEE in ≥1 ear over ≥180 d in the preceding year, documented at least twice at ≥6-mo intervals; free of otitis media at the outset
	No tonsil-related indication for tonsillectomy
Exclusion criteria	Overt or submucous palatal clefts
Randomization effectiveness	No significant difference in age, sex, race, entry criterion met, MEE, baseline hearing, nasal obstruction, upper respiratory allergy, siblings, parents' socioeconomic status
Age	3–15 y
Intervention regimen details	Reverse adenotomes, curettes were used under both direct and mirror vision; the fossa of Rosenmüller was curetted routinely. Tonsillectomy performed by dissection-snare technique
Additional procedures	Myringotomy and aspiration was performed if MEE was present at the time of adenoidectomy or T&A. If in the control group, myringotomy and aspiration was performed if MEE had been present for >90 d without improvement
Disease details at the outset	91.2% RAOM, 5% persistent MEE, 3.4% both
Diagnostic criteria for AOM	MEE with recent otalgia, marked erythema or bulging of the tympanic membrane; otorrhea with otalgia or fever in the presence of tympanostomy tube or TM perforation
Management of AOM episode while enrolled	"Antimicrobial in the conventional dosage for 10 d to 6 wk, depending on recent clinical course and response to treatment. Amoxicillin was used whenever feasible; second line drugs mainly used were erythromycin-sulfisoxazole and amoxicillin clavulanate"
Management of MEE during study	If MEE ≥90 d without improvement, then myringotomy with aspiration; if recurred within 6 mo and persisted ≥60 d then myringotomy and tube placement
Criteria for withdrawal	Parental wishes, lack of follow-up
Intention to treat analysis?	Yes: Patients in the control group who received eventual surgery were analyzed as controls
Power	80% to detect a 25% difference with 57 subjects per treatment group
Morbidity/complications	Postoperative complications: Adenoidectomy group—4.8% T&A group—14.6%	Postoperative complications included incipient malignant hyperthermia, readmission to hospital, hemorrhage after discharge, pneumonia, and velopharyngeal insufficiency

AOM = acute otitis media, RAOM = recurrent AOM, MEE = middle ear effusion, TM = tympanic membrane, T&A = adenotonsillectomy, NS = not significant.
* Sample size: numbers shown for those not lost to follow-up and those (initially recruited).
p Values and conclusions are listed for adenoidectomy vs control, then adenoidtonsillectomy vs control in the three-way trial.

Reference	Paradise, 1990					
Level (design)	1 (randomized controlled trial)					
	"Two-way" trial					
Sample size*	119 at y 1, 107 at y 2, 88 at y 3 (157)					

	OUTCOMES					
	Mean rate of AOM episodes per subject			% of patients with no AOM episodes		
Follow-up year	Y 1	Y 2	Y 3	Y 1	Y 2	Y 3
T&A	1.7	0.9	0.5	29.5%	50.0%	65.2%
Adenoidectomy alone	—	—	—	—	—	—
Control	2.2	0.9	0.9	22.4%	38.2%	47.7%
p Value, T&A vs control	NS	NS	NS	NS	NS	NS
Conclusion, T&A vs control	No difference in each individual year but T&A better in the data for all 3 y combined			No difference	No difference	No difference

	STUDY DESIGN					
Inclusion criteria	3–15 y old; *no* previous tympanostomy tube placement; ≥3 AOM in the preceding 6 mo or ≥4 AOM in the preceding 12 mo, with ≥1 documented episode *or* MEE in ≥1 ear over ≥180 d in the preceding year, documented at least twice at ≥6-mo intervals; free of otitis media at the outset					
	Tonsil-related indication for tonsillectomy					
Exclusion criteria	Overt or submucous palatal clefts					
Randomization effectiveness	T&A group with significantly more girls than in control. No significant difference in age, sex, race, entry criterion met, MEE, baseline hearing, nasal obstruction, upper respiratory allergy, siblings, parents' socioeconomic status					
Age	3–15 y					
Intervention regimen details	Reverse adenotomes, curettes were used under both direct and mirror vision; the fossa of Rosenmüller was curetted routinely. Tonsillectomy performed by dissection-snare technique					
Additional procedures	Myringotomy and aspiration was performed if MEE was present at the time of adenoidectomy or T&A. If in the control group, myringotomy and aspiration was performed if MEE had been present for >90 d without improvement					
Disease details at the outset	91.2% RAOM, 5% persistent MEE, 3.4% both					
Diagnostic criteria for AOM	MEE with recent otalgia, marked erythema or bulging of the tympanic membrane; otorrhea with otalgia or fever in the presence of tympanostomy tube or TM perforation					
Management of AOM episode while enrolled	"Antimicrobial in the conventional dosage for 10 d to 6 wk, depending on recent clinical course and response to treatment. Amoxicillin was used whenever feasible; second line drugs mainly used were erythromycin-sulfisoxazole and amoxicillin clavulanate"					
Management of MEE during study	If MEE ≥90 d without improvement, then myringotomy with aspiration; if recurred within 6 mo and persisted ≥60 d then myringotomy and tube placement					
Criteria for withdrawal	Parental wishes, lack of follow-up					
Intention to treat analysis?	Yes: Patients in the control group who received eventual surgery were analyzed as controls					
Power	80% to detect a 25% difference with 57 subjects per treatment group					
Morbidity/complications	Postoperative complications included incipient malignant hyperthermia, readmission to hospital, hemorrhage after discharge, pneumonia, and velopharyngeal insufficiency					

AOM = acute otitis media, RAOM = recurrent AOM, MEE = middle ear effusion, TM = tympanic membrane, T&A = adenotonsillectomy, NS = not significant.
* Sample size: numbers shown for those not lost to follow-up and those (initially recruited).

REFERENCE

1. Paradise JL, Bluestone CD, Rogers KD, et al. Efficacy of adenoidectomy for recurrent otitis media in children previously treated with tympanostomy-tube placement. Results of parallel randomized and nonrandomized trials. JAMA 1990;263(15):2066–2073.

7 Pediatric Otitis Media with Effusion

7.A.i.

Amoxicillin versus placebo: Chance of becoming effusion-free

Jennifer J. Shin and Michael J. Cunningham

METHODS

A computerized Ovid search of MEDLINE 1966–January 2004 was performed. The terms "otitis media" and "antibiotics" were exploded and the resulting articles were cross-referenced, yielding 1947 trials. Given the known richness of the otitis media literature and the authority of higher levels of evidence, these articles were then limited to randomized controlled trials (RCTs), resulting in 302 articles. These articles were then reviewed to identify those that met the following inclusion criteria: 1) patient population <18 years of age with documented otitis media with effusion (OME), 2) intervention with amoxicillin therapy alone versus placebo control, 3) outcome measured in terms of presence or absence of middle ear effusion (MEE) with a statistical analysis. Articles comparing intervention with amoxicillin/clavulanate, cephalosporins, trimethoprim-sulfamethoxazole, and erythromycin with placebo were excluded here but are presented separately in this chapter. The bibliographies of articles that met these inclusion criteria were manually examined to determine if any further relevant articles could be identified. This process yielded four RCTs [1–4].

RESULTS

Outcome Measures. All four studies reported the percent of patients with resolution of effusion as the primary outcome measure. In addition, other studies also reported secondary outcomes of percent of patients developing acute otitis media (AOM), percent of time with MEE, percent of patients with recurrent MEE, and episodes of AOM, MEE, and OME per person year.

Potential Confounders. The specificity of the definitions of MEE, OME, and AOM are key, and these are outlined in as much detail as the primary papers allow. In addition, follow-up time, age, history of middle ear disease, duration of effusion at entry, season of the year, history of allergy or nasal obstruction, the status of the adenoid, the specific amoxicillin regimen, including the duration, may also affect results.

Study Designs. All four studies were RCTs. Each study focused on MEE, but there were well-delineated differences regarding the duration of effusions that were studied (ranging from any duration [2, 3] to a minimum of 2–3 months [1, 4]). In addition, there were differences in whether active AOM was present at the outset, with two studies excluding patients with symptoms or signs of AOM [2, 3] whereas one specified that AOM was acceptable in their inclusion criteria [4]. All four reports commented on the effectiveness of randomization in balancing confounders between the amoxicillin and control groups. Also, all were double-blind, placebo-controlled studies. The amoxicillin regimens ranged from 20 to 50 mg/kg/day, for a duration of 2 weeks to 1 year. Compliance was reported in three instances [2–4], as measured by the bottle method, caregiver diary, calendar method, and/or urine specimens. In those three instances, rates of compliance were high. No patients crossed over from one treatment group to another, and additional antimicrobial therapy necessary for the treatment of superimposed AOM were described in detail in three studies. A priori power calculations were noted in two studies [3, 4]; in both instances, the sample sizes were smaller than the estimate required for a 90% power to detect a 20% difference or a 50% reduction in MEE.

Highest Level of Evidence. Of the four RCTs, three showed that after 2 weeks of amoxicillin, there was a significantly higher percentage of effusion-free patients at 2 weeks to 2 months, as compared with placebo. In these three RCTs, rate differences (RD)[1] ranged from 14.7% to 30.0%. These figures suggest numbers needed to treat (NNT)[2] of 4–7, which means that 4–7 children must be treated with 2 weeks of amoxicillin therapy to result in 1 effusion-free child. At 1 year, however, one RCT showed no difference in the percent of patients with MEE after 1 year of amoxicillin or placebo treatment [4]. That same study, however, reported that the amoxicillin group experienced less time with MEE than the control group. In addition, it was reported that the amoxicillin group had a lower rate of new-onset MEE and OME. A

---

[1] RD is the absolute difference in successful outcomes between the study group and the control group. For example, in the Mandel, 1987 study, 28.8% of the amoxicillin group versus 14.1% of the placebo group became effusion-free at 4 weeks. The RD in this study was 14.1% −28.8% = −14.7%.

[2] NNT is the total number of children that must be treated in order for one child to obtain benefit from the treatment. It is calculated by determining the inverse of the RD. For example, for the Mandel, 1987 study, the RD is −14.7%, so that the NNT = 1/0.147 = 6.8. In this case, seven children would need to be treated so to obtain benefit for one child.

second outcome parameter, the percent of children developing subsequent AOM, was reported in three studies [2–4]. In two of these studies, there was no significant difference in the percent of patients developing AOM during the follow-up period [2, 3]. In the third study, however, the rate of AOM per person year was significantly lower in the amoxicillin group [4].

Applicability. These results are applicable to children 7 months to 12 years of age with MEE. Further specifics regarding the applicability of individual trials are tabulated for the reader under "Inclusion Criteria" and "Exclusion Criteria."

Morbidity. Only minor adverse reactions were noted in either the amoxicillin or placebo groups and these are also tabulated for the reader. There is also potential morbidity in regard to development of antibiotic resistance.

CLINICAL SIGNIFICANCE AND FUTURE RESEARCH

There is level 1 evidence that demonstrates improved resolution of OME with amoxicillin, with NNT of 4–7 children. These data, along with those from other trials of antibiotics for OME, are also presented in a meta-analysis in this section. Results regarding the development of superimposed AOM in this patient population are varied.

Additional research may focus specifically on direct comparisons between amoxicillin and newer antibiotic regimens. In addition, the associated risk of sequelae of antibiotic resistance from amoxicillin use may be investigated.

THE EVIDENCE CONDENSED: Amoxicillin versus placebo for pediatric otitis media with effusion

Reference	Mandel, 1987	
Level (design)	1 (randomized controlled trial)	
Sample size*	305 (316)	

OUTCOMES		
	% effusion free	% developing AOM
Amoxicillin	28.8%	10.0%
Placebo	14.1%	14.7%
p Value	= 0.002	NS
Conclusion	Amoxicillin better	No significant difference
Follow-up time	4 wk	

STUDY DESIGN	
Inclusion criteria	7 mo–12 y, OME of any duration (i.e., no evidence of AOM symptoms)
Exclusion criteria	AOM, acute or chronic sinusitis, craniofacial or structural middle ear abnormality, systemic illness, hearing loss not attributable to MEE, history of tonsillectomy/adenoidectomy/tympanostomy tube insertion, severe upper airway obstruction, treatment with sympathomimetics or antihistamines in the past 30 d, hypersensitivity to penicillin
Randomization effectiveness	Similar gender, duration of effusion, previous antimicrobial treatment, race, allergy. Possible difference in laterality, age
Age	7 mo–12 y
Masking	Double blind
Amoxicillin regimen	Amoxicillin 40 mg/kg/d in 3 divided doses ×2 wk
Diagnostic criteria for an AOM episode	Acute symptomatic episode (i.e., fever, otalgia, or both)
Management of AOM during study	Antimicrobial agent other than amoxicillin (i.e., cefaclor or erythromycin-sulfisoxazole)
Diagnostic criteria for OME	Otoscopy, tympanometry, and middle ear muscle reflex testing
Criteria for successful treatment	Effusion-free at 2 or 4 wk
Compliance	85%–91% took at least 75% of medications in amoxicillin group, 77%–84% took at least 75% in placebo group; measured by caregiver records and by bottle method
Criteria for withdrawal from study	Not specified in detail
A priori power calculation	Not specified
Morbidity/ complications	Amoxicillin group: 5% rate of mild sedation or irritability, 3 diarrhea, 3 rash Placebo group: 6% rate of mild sedation or irritability, 1 diarrhea, 0 rash

AOM = acute otitis media, MEE = middle ear effusion, OME = asymptomatic otitis media with effusion, TM = tympanic membrane, % effusion free = % of patients that were without MEE at follow-up, NS = not significant.
* Sample size: numbers shown for those not lost to follow-up and those (initially recruited).

THE EVIDENCE CONDENSED: Amoxicillin versus placebo for pediatric otitis media with effusion

Reference	Mandel, 1991		
Level (design)	1 (randomized controlled trial)		
Sample size*	151 (164)		

OUTCOMES			
	% effusion free	% developing AOM	% MEE recurrence
Amoxicillin	31.6%,† 29.9%‡	8.9%	61.5%
Placebo	14.1%,† 26.7%‡	14.2%	52.5%
p Value	†<0.01, ‡NS	NS	NS
Conclusion	Amoxicillin better at 2 wk No significant difference at 4 wk	No difference	No difference
Follow-up time	†2 wk, ‡4 wk		

STUDY DESIGN			
Inclusion criteria	7 mo–12 y, OME of any duration without symptoms of AOM (e.g., otalgia, fever)		
Exclusion criteria	Symptoms of AOM (otalgia, fever), craniofacial abnormalities, systemic illness, history of tonsillectomy, adenoidectomy, or insertion of a tympanostomy tube, structural middle ear abnormality, hearing loss not attributable to MEE, severe upper airway obstruction, acute or chronic sinusitis, history of hypersensitivity to penicillin		
Randomization effectiveness	Similar characteristics shown in multiple variables, no comment on statistical analysis		
Age	7 mo–12 y		
Masking	Double blind		
Amoxicillin regimen	Amoxicillin 40 mg/kg/d in 3 divided doses ×2 wk		
Diagnostic criteria for an AOM episode	Presence of ≥1 symptom (fever, otalgia, irritability) and 1 sign (bulging or fullness of TM, white fluid level, acute perforation with otorrhea)		
Management of AOM during study	Antimicrobial different in color from assigned medication ×10 d		
Diagnostic criteria for OME	Pneumatic otoscopy, tympanogram, middle ear muscle reflex testing		
Criteria for successful treatment	Effusion-free at 2 or 4 wk		
Compliance	Compliance measured by bottle method (96% in amoxicillin group and 92% in placebo group) and calendar method (93% amoxicillin group and 88% in placebo group)		
Criteria for withdrawal from study	Not specified in detail		
A priori power calculation	250 patients to give a 90% power to detect effusion-free proportions of ≥20% difference with an alpha of 0.05, one-sided; they also reported an interim analysis of stochastic curtailing to evaluate the implications of terminating subject accrual at n = 331; to detect a difference of 0.15 between antimicrobial and placebo, power range was 0.65–0.81		
Morbidity/ complications	1 patient in amoxicillin group with adverse reactions (minor), and 4 patients in the placebo group		

AOM = acute otitis media, MEE = middle ear effusion, OME = asymptomatic otitis media with effusion, TM = tympanic membrane, % effusion free = % of patients that were without MEE at follow-up, NS = not significant.
* Sample size: numbers shown for those not lost to follow-up and those (initially recruited).
†, ‡ Symbols denote which data comparisons correspond to the referenced p-values and follow-up times.

THE EVIDENCE CONDENSED: Amoxicillin versus placebo for pediatric chronic otitis media with effusion

Reference	Mandel, 1996
Level (design)	1 (randomized controlled trial)
Sample size*	79 (111)

OUTCOMES

	% free of new effusions	Rate of new MEE, AOM, OME per person year	% time with MEE
Amoxicillin	21.8%	1.81, 0.28, 1.53	19.7%
Placebo	11.8%	3.18, 1.04, 2.15	33.2%
p Value	NS	<0.001, <0.001, NS	0.002
Conclusion	No difference	MEE: amoxicillin better AOM: amoxicillin better OME: no difference	Amoxicillin better
Follow-up time	1 y		

STUDY DESIGN

Inclusion criteria	7 mo–12 y, effusion free at entry; If had functioning tympanostomy tubes during the previous 12 mo: intact TMs at entry, MEE (either as AOM or OME) documented at least once for ≥2 wk in the previous 3 mo; if no tympanostomy tubes during the previous 12 mo then ≥3 episodes or ≥3 cumulative mo of MEE during the previous 12 mo or both; at least 1 MEE documentation by tympanogram in previous 3 mo
Exclusion criteria	Congenital craniofacial malformation, history of tonsillectomy/adenoidectomy, structural middle ear abnormality, asthma or a seizure disorder, sensorineural hearing loss or conductive hearing loss caused by destructive changes to the middle ear, medical conditions with a predisposition for MEE (i.e., cleft palate, Down syndrome, TM perforation), hypersensitivity to penicillin
Randomization effectiveness	No significant differences in criterion for entry, age group, race, gender, AOM history, parental otologic history, upper respiratory infection at entry, allergy, hearing at entry
Age	7 mo–12 y
Masking	Double blind
Amoxicillin regimen	20 mg/kg PO q.h.s. ×1 y
Diagnostic criteria for AOM episode	Otoscopic diagnosis of MEE and ≥1 symptom (fever >37.2°C orally or >37.8°C rectally, otalgia, irritability) and ≥1 sign of active infection (erythema of TM greater than mild, white opacification of the TM, bulging or fullness of the TM, white fluid level, acute perforation with otorrhea)
Management of AOM during study	Augmentin 40 mg/kg/d (based on the amoxicillin component) or erythromycin-sulfisoxazole 50 mg/kg/d (based on the erythromycin component)
Diagnostic criteria for OME	Based on pneumatic otoscopy, tympanometry, and middle ear muscle reflex
Criteria for successful treatment	Resolution of MEE, AOM, OME
Compliance	Measured by diary (92% compliance in both groups), bottle method (100% vs 103% in amoxicillin vs placebo), and urine specimen (90% vs 92% in amoxicillin vs placebo)
Criteria for withdrawal from study	Treatment failure: 4 consecutive mo of bilateral MEE or 6 consecutive mo of unilateral MEE; 3 episodes of AOM in 6 mo or 4 episodes in 12 mo
A priori power calculation	Sample size of 212 to give a 90% power to detect a 50% reduction in the average number of episodes of MEE in the 1-y period, assuming an alpha = 0.05 two-sided test, 25% dropout rate, and a baseline rate per person year of 0.96 episodes of effusion
Morbidity/ complications	2 treatment failures in the amoxicillin group, 5 treatment failures in the placebo group

MEE = middle ear effusion, AOM = acute otitis media, OME = asymptomatic otitis media with effusion, TM = tympanic membrane, % effusion free = % of patients that were without MEE at follow-up, NS = not significant.
* Sample size: numbers shown for those not lost to follow-up and those (initially recruited).

Reference	Podoshin, 1990
Level (design)	1 (randomized controlled trial)
Sample size*	86 (86)

OUTCOMES	
	% effusion-free
Amoxicillin	30%
Placebo	0%
p Value	"<0.000"
Conclusion	Amoxicillin better
Follow-up time	2 mo

STUDY DESIGN	
Inclusion criteria	OME ≥2 mo duration, no previous treatment for OME, >4 y old, OME as diagnosed by pneumatic otoscopy and flat tympanogram
Exclusion criteria	Recurrent AOM, cleft palate, hypertrophic adenoids (diagnosed by anamnesis history), physical evaluation and lateral skull films with adenoidal-nasopharyngeal ratio ≥0.73, indication of already resolving effusion (fluid lines, air bubbles, or yellow fluid)
Randomization effectiveness	Similar age and gender distributions, statistical analysis not reported, other factors not reported
Age	3 y–8 y
Masking	Double blind
Amoxicillin regimen	50 mg/kg ×14 d
Diagnostic criteria for AOM episode	AOM was not reported as an outcome measure
Management of AOM during study	AOM was not reported as an outcome measure
Diagnostic criteria for OME	Pneumatic otoscopy and tympanometry
Criteria for successful treatment	Normal TM, closure of air-bone gap, and type A tympanogram (partial improvement noted as TM retraction, some conductive hearing loss, or type C tympanogram)
Compliance	Not reported
Criteria for withdrawal from study	Not reported
A priori power calculation	Not reported
Morbidity/ complications	Not reported

MEE = middle ear effusion, AOM = acute otitis media, OME = asymptomatic otitis media with effusion, TM = tympanic membrane, % effusion free = % of patients that were without MEE at follow-up, NS = not significant.
* Sample size: numbers shown for those not lost to follow-up and those (initially recruited).

REFERENCES

1. Podoshin L, Fradis M, Ben-David Y, Faraggi D. The efficacy of oral steroids in the treatment of persistent otitis media with effusion.[see comment.] *Arch Otolaryngol Head Neck Surg*, 1990;16(12):1404–1406.

2. Mandel EM, Rockette HE, Bluestone CD, Paradise JL, Nozza RJ. Efficacy of amoxicillin with and without decongestant-antihistamine for otitis media with effusion in children. Results of a double-blind, randomized trial. N Engl J Med, 1987;316(8):432–437.

3. Mandel EM, Rockette HE, Paradise JL, Bluestone CD, Nozza RJ. Comparative efficacy of erythromycin-sulfisoxazole, cefaclor, amoxicillin or placebo for otitis media with effusion in children. Pediatr Infect Dis J, 1991;10(12): 899–906.

4. Mandel EM, Casselbrant ML, Rockette HE, Bluestone CD, Kurs-Lasky M. Efficacy of antimicrobial prophylaxis for recurrent middle ear effusion. Pediatr Infect Dis J 1996; 15(12):1074–1082.

7 Pediatric Otitis Media with Effusion

7.A.ii.

Amoxicillin/clavulanate versus placebo: Chance of becoming effusion-free

Jennifer J. Shin and Michael J. Cunningham

METHODS

A computerized Ovid search of MEDLINE 1966–January 2004 was performed. The terms "otitis media" and "antibiotics" were exploded and the resulting articles were cross-referenced, yielding 1947 trials. Given the known richness of the otitis media literature and the authority of higher levels of evidence, these articles were then limited to randomized controlled trials (RCTs), resulting in 302 articles. These articles were then reviewed to identify those that met the following inclusion criteria: 1) patient population <18 years of age with documented otitis media with effusion (OME), 2) intervention with combined amoxicillin/clavulanate therapy versus placebo control, 3) outcome measured in terms of presence or absence of middle ear effusion (MEE). Articles which compared intervention with amoxicillin alone (i.e., without clavulanate), trimethoprim-sulfamethoxazole, erythromycin, and cephalosporins to placebo were excluded here but are presented separately in this chapter. The bibliographies of articles that met these inclusion criteria were manually examined to determine if any further relevant articles could be identified. Trials comparing antibiotics to each other were also excluded. This process yielded two RCTs [1, 2].

RESULTS

Outcome Measures. Data were presented in terms of the percentage of children becoming effusion-free (both studies), the amount of time spent with abnormal tympanometry (one study), and the laterality of the effusions (one study).

Potential Confounders. Potential confounders are as noted in Section 21.A.i: The specificity of the definitions of MEE, OME, and acute otitis media are key, and these are outlined in as much detail as the primary papers allow. In addition, follow-up time, age, history of middle ear disease, duration of effusion at entry, seasons, history of allergy or nasal obstruction, the status of the adenoid, the specific amoxicillin/clavulanate regimen may also affect results.

Study Designs. Two RCTs [1, 2] address the impact of amoxicillin with clavulanate versus placebo on MEE. In one trial, potential confounders of age, gender, family distribution, season, and previous otolaryngologic diseases were balanced between the two groups [1]. In the other trial, groups were similar with the exception of gender [2]. Both RCTs were double-blind, placebo-controlled to minimize expectation and detection biases. One study provided 1 month of treatment based on age [1], whereas the other provided 2 weeks of treatment based on weight [2]. Both studies clearly defined their method for diagnosing OME, and these are detailed in the adjoining table. In addition, an attempt to measure compliance was made in each trial. Also, criteria for withdrawal from the study were also clearly delineated. No *a priori* power calculations were performed, but both studies had sufficient enrollment to demonstrate statistically significant differences in the primary outcome.

Highest Level of Evidence. Both studies demonstrated that a higher percentage of children became effusion-free when treated with amoxicillin/clavulanate, as compared with controls, at time periods up to 5 months. Rate differences (RD)[1] of 16%–30% were demonstrated, suggesting that 4–7 children require treatment with amoxicillin/clavulanate so that one child can remain effusion-free [i.e., the number needed to treat (NNT)[2] is 4–7]. These data were corroborated by additional results showing that the mean time with abnormal tympanograms was reduced by 49% with amoxicillin/clavulanate. Likewise, the percent of children with bilateral OME was significantly less with amoxicillin/clavulanate. By 12 months after treatment was initiated, however, any advantage of amoxicillin/clavulanate therapy had dissipated, and no difference between groups could be demonstrated.

---

[1] RD is the absolute difference in successful outcomes between the study group and the control group. For example, in the van Balen study, 23% of the amoxicillin/clavulanate group versus 7% of the placebo group became effusion-free. The RD in this study was 7% − 23% = −16%.

[2] NNT is the total number of children that must be treated in order for one child to obtain benefit from the treatment. It is calculated by determining the inverse of the RD. For example, for the van Balen study, the rate difference is −16%, so that the NNT = 1/0.16 = 6.25. In this case, seven children would need to be treated so as to obtain benefit for one child.

Applicability. These results are applicable to patients aged 6 months to 10 years who present with OME that has been present for at least 3 months.

Morbidity. Overall, there was a trend toward more gastrointestinal symptoms and rash in the patients receiving amoxicillin/clavulanate [1, 2], with a statistical significance demonstrated in one trial [2]. In that one trial, a 5% RD was noted in rash with a 12% RD in gastrointestinal symptoms. These figures correspond to numbers needed to harm of 9–20 children. There were no serious adverse reactions.

CLINICAL SIGNIFICANCE AND FUTURE RESEARCH

There is level 1 evidence that demonstrates benefit with amoxicillin/clavulanate administration, with a resulting increased chance of becoming effusion-free at up to 5 months after the initiation of 2–4 weeks of treatment. This benefit of a 16%–30% increase in effusion-free children must be weighed against the potential risks of adverse reactions (significantly higher with amoxicillin/clavulanate) and potential contribution to antibiotic resistance.

Additional research may focus specifically on direct comparisons between amoxicillin/clavulanate and amoxicillin, which has also demonstrated positive impact on rates of OME (please see Section 21.A.i). This comparison, along with comparisons with other antimicrobial and nonmedical regimens, may help us minimize coverage necessary to achieve benefit, which will ideally help curtail the growing epidemic of antibiotic resistance.

Reference	Thomsen, 1989	
Level (design)	1 (randomized controlled trial)	
Sample size*	221 (264)	

OUTCOMES		
	% effusion-free†	Mean time with abnormal tympanogram
Amoxicillin	61%,✖ 57%,★ 56%ϒ	118 d
Placebo	31%,✖ 32%,★ 45%ϒ	231 d
p Value	✖<0.0001, ★<0.005, ϒNS	<0.002
Conclusion	A/C better at 1 mo, 5 mo. No difference at 12 mo	A/C better
Follow-up time	✖1 mo, ★5 mo, ϒ12 mo	

STUDY DESIGN	
Inclusion criteria	1–10 y old, unilateral and bilateral serous otitis media for ≥3 mo as established by tympanometry at ≥3-mo intervals
Exclusion criteria	Allergy to penicillin
Randomization effectiveness	Comparable with regard to age, gender, family distribution, social background, previous ear-nose-throat–related diseases, season of entry
Age	1–10 y
Masking	Double blind
Amoxicillin/ampicillin regimen	Amoxicillin 125 mg/clavulanate 31.25 mg ×1 mo if aged 1–5 y, amoxicillin 187.5 mg/clavulanate 46.88 mg ×1 mo if aged 6–10 y
Diagnostic criteria for AOM	Not specified in detail
Management of AOM during study	No additional antibiotics while in treatment period; after treatment period, received ampicillin or penicillin V
Diagnostic criteria for OME	Tympanometry only
Criteria for successful treatment	Effusion-free by tympanometry
Compliance	Parental records and bottle method were used actual percentage compliant not reported
Criteria for withdrawal from study	Refusal to take medication, skin reactions, concomitant infection, diarrhea, failure to complete the 4-wk treatment period
A priori power calculation	Not specified
Morbidity/complications	A/C group: 3 withdrawals from skin reactions, 2 withdrawals from diarrhea Placebo group: 1 withdrawal from skin reaction

MEE = middle ear effusion, OME = asymptomatic otitis media with effusion, NS = not significant, TM = tympanic membrane, AOM = acute otitis media, A/C = amoxicillin/clavulanate, t.i.d. = three times a day.
* Sample size: numbers shown for those not lost to follow-up and those (initially recruited).
† Data at the 1-mo and 5-mo follow-up times were interpreted from a chart presented in the orginal report.
✖, ★, ϒ Symbols denote which data comparisons correspond to the referenced p-values and follow-up times.

THE EVIDENCE CONDENSED: Amoxicillin/clavulanate versus placebo for pediatric otitis media with effusion

Reference	van Balen, 1996	
Level (design)	1 (randomized controlled trial)	
Sample size*	153 (162)	

OUTCOMES

	% effusion-free	% with bilateral OME
Amoxicillin	23%	53%
Placebo	7%	84%
p Value	0.03	0.001
Conclusion	A/C better	A/C better
Follow-up time	2 wk	

STUDY DESIGN

Inclusion criteria	6 mo–6 y old, OME of at least 3 mo by the time of randomization, only bilateral OME is treated in the Netherlands
Exclusion criteria	Antimicrobial therapy within 4 wk preceding the trial, penicillin allergy, compromised immunity, craniofacial abnormalities, Down syndrome, cystic fibrosis
Randomization effectiveness	Similar except for gender: placebo group had more boys. Similar age, season at entry, baseline or recurrent upper respiratory tract infection, AOM at baseline or 6 wk before entry, hearing loss, language/speech problems, mouth breathing/snoring, positive family history
Age	6 mo–6 y
Masking	Double blind
Amoxicillin/ampicillin regimen	Amoxicillin 20 mg/kg/d and clavulanate 5 mg/kg/d, each in 3 divided doses ×14 d; both antibiotic and placebo group also received xylometazoline 0.25% nasal drops t.i.d.
Diagnostic criteria for AOM	Not specified in detail
Management of AOM during study	Not specified in detail
Diagnostic criteria for OME	OME = presence of middle ear fluid behind an intact TM without signs or symptoms of acute infection, diagnosed by tympanometry; persistent OME = effusion for ≥3 mo
Criteria for successful treatment	Effusion-free by tympanometry
Compliance	90% of each group took at least 10 d of the study medication
Criteria for withdrawal from study	Side effects precluding compliance with study medication (1 in each group), failure to complete follow-up
A priori power calculation	Not specified
Morbidity/complications	A/C group: 30% gastrointestinal symptoms, 6% pruritus/rash Placebo group: 18% gastrointestinal symptoms, 1% pruritus/rash

MEE = middle ear effusion, OME = asymptomatic otitis media with effusion, NS = not significant, TM = tympanic membrane, AOM = acute otitis media, A/C = amoxicillin/clavulanate, t.i.d. = three times a day.
* Sample size: numbers shown for those not lost to follow-up and those (initially recruited).

Pediatric Otitis Media with Effusion
126

REFERENCES

1. Thomsen J, Sederberg-Olsen J, Balle V, Vejlsgaard R, Stangerup SE, Bondesson G. Antibiotic treatment of children with secretory otitis media. A randomized, double-blind, placebo-controlled study. [see comment]. Arch Otolaryngol Head Neck Surg 1989;115(4):447–451.
2. van Balen FA, de Melker RA, Touw-Otten FW. Double-blind randomised trial of co-amoxiclav versus placebo for persistent otitis media with effusion in general practice. [see comment.] Lancet, 1996;348(9029):713–716.

7 Pediatric Otitis Media with Effusion

Cephalosporin versus placebo: Chance of becoming effusion-free

Jennifer J. Shin and Michael J. Cunningham

METHODS

A computerized Ovid search of MEDLINE 1966–January 2004 was performed. The terms "otitis media" and "antibiotics" were exploded and the resulting articles were cross-referenced, yielding 1947 trials. Given the known richness of the otitis media literature and the authority of higher levels of evidence, these articles were then limited to randomized controlled trials (RCTs), resulting in 302 articles. These articles were then reviewed to identify those that met the following inclusion criteria: 1) patient population <18 years of age with documented otitis media with effusion (OME), 2) intervention with a cephalosporin alone versus placebo control, 3) outcome measured in terms of presence or absence of middle ear effusion (MEE) with a statistical analysis. Articles comparing intervention with amoxicillin alone, amoxicillin/clavulanate, trimethoprim-sulfamethoxazole, and erythromycin with placebo were excluded here but are presented separately in this chapter. Articles comparing one antibiotic to another were also excluded. In addition, papers in which alternate lengths of therapy of cephalosporins were compared were excluded, including one in which the same children were repeatedly randomized into cephalosporin versus control every 2 weeks over 8 weeks after *all* received an initial course of cephalosporin [1]. The bibliographies of articles that met inclusion criteria were manually examined to determine if any further relevant articles could be identified. This process yielded three RCTs [2–4].

RESULTS

Outcome Measures. All three studies focused on the primary outcome measure of the percent of patients who became effusion-free at the designated follow-up times.

Potential Confounders. Potential confounders were as noted in Section 21.A.i: The specificity of the definitions of MEE, OME, and acute otitis media (AOM) are key, and these are outlined in as much detail as the primary papers allow. In addition, follow-up time, age, history of middle ear disease, etiology of the effusion, duration of effusion at entry, season of the year, history of allergy or nasal obstruction, and the status of the adenoid may also affect results. In addition, the specific cephalosporin used is a potentially important factor; cefixime is a third-generation cephalosporin [3] whereas cefaclor is second generation [2, 4]. These generational distinctions translate into differences in the antimicrobial coverage that could impact results.

Study Designs. Three RCTs compared the impact of cephalosporin versus placebo on OME. Follow-up times ranged from 10 days to 6 months. Two focused on effusions of at least 3 months' duration [3, 4], whereas the other studied effusions of any duration [2]. All three studies reported the effectiveness of randomization, although to varying degrees, as further delineated in the adjacent table. Two studies were clearly reported as double blind [2, 3]. Either a 10-day [3, 4] or 14-day course of antibiotic was used [2]. One study allowed no additional antimicrobials during AOM episodes [3], whereas another used a specific protocol for AOM treatment [2]. Compliance was measured in two trials [2, 3], and noted to be high in one [2]. Two studies reported *a priori* power calculations, each reporting a somewhat limited power of about 80% [2, 3]. The third trial reported no power calculations but showed a significant difference between study populations [4].

Highest Level of Evidence. Two RCTs showed no difference between cephalosporin and placebo [2, 3], whereas the third showed a significant improvement with cephalosporin [4]. The two trials that showed no difference, however, were admittedly of limited power, with a ≥20% chance of not detecting a difference that truly exists. The single trial that did demonstrate a significant improvement with cephalosporin demonstrated a 41% rate difference in the chance of becoming effusion-free after 10 days [4]. This rate difference corresponds to a number needed to treat of three, meaning that their results suggest that for every three children treated with cephalosporin, one child will become effusion-free. In this trial, however, no placebo control was used. Therefore, an expectation bias favored a demonstration of improvement with cephalosporin, as subjects who were treated may have expected to improve more than those who did not receive treatment. Overall, the results are mixed, and individual studies are limited by power or by expectation biases.

Applicability. These results are applicable to children 7 months to 12 years old with OME, without craniofacial abnormality or recent active upper respiratory tract infection.

Morbidity. Minor side adverse reactions were noted in both placebo and cephalosporin groups in one study [2], only in the cephalosporin group in another study [3], and not reported in the final study [4].

CLINICAL SIGNIFICANCE AND FUTURE RESEARCH

Three level 1 studies gave mixed results regarding the impact of cephalosporin versus placebo on the resolution of OME. Studies demonstrating no difference were limited by powers of 80% or less (i.e., they had a ≥20% chance of not detecting a difference that truly existed), whereas the study that showed an improvement with cephalosporin lacked a placebo control, biasing results toward such improvement in the cephalosporin group.

Higher-powered, placebo-controlled RCTs may better resolve the impact of cephalosporin versus placebo on OME. In addition, equivalence studies may be performed to determine if cephalosporin achieves the same impact as amoxicillin.

THE EVIDENCE CONDENSED: Cephalosporin versus placebo for pediatric otitis media with effusion

Reference	Mandel, 1991
Level (design)	1 (RCT)
Sample size*	163 (164)

	OUTCOMES
	% effusion-free
Cephalosporin	22.1%, 33.3%
Placebo	14.1, 26.7
p Value	NS, NS
Conclusion	No difference
Follow-up time	2 wk, 4 wk

	STUDY DESIGN
Inclusion criteria	7 mo–12 y old, OME of any duration without symptoms of AOM (e.g., otalgia, fever)
Exclusion criteria	AOM (otalgia, fever), craniofacial abnormality, systemic illness, prior tonsillectomy/adenoidectomy or tympanostomy tube, structural middle ear abnormality, hearing loss not from MEE, severe upper airway obstruction, acute/chronic sinusitis, penicillin hypersensitivity
Randomization effectiveness	Similar characteristics shown in multiple variables, no comment on statistical analysis
Age	7 mo–12 y
Masking	Double blind
Cephalosporin regimen	Cefaclor 40 mg/kg/d in 3 divided doses ×2 wk
Diagnostic criteria for AOM episode	≥1 symptom (fever, otalgia, irritability) and 1 sign (bulging or fullness of TM, white fluid level, acute perforation with otorrhea)
Management of AOM episode while on study treatment	Antimicrobial different in color from assigned medication ×10 d
Diagnostic criteria for OME	Pneumatic otoscopy, tympanogram, middle ear muscle reflex testing
Criteria for successful treatment	Effusion-free at 2 or 4 wk
Compliance	Compliance measured by bottle method (94% in cefaclor group, 92% in placebo group) and calendar method (95% cefaclor group, 88% in placebo group)
Criteria for withdrawal from study	Not specified in detail
A priori power calculation	250 patients for a 90% power to detect ≥20% difference with an alpha of 0.05, one-sided; they also reported an interim analysis of stochastic curtailing to evaluate the implications of terminating subject accrual at n = 331; to detect a 15% difference, power was 65%–81%
Morbidity/ complications	4 patients in cefaclor group with adverse reactions (minor), and 4 patients in the placebo group

RCT = randomized controlled trial, MEE = middle ear effusion, OME = asymptomatic otitis media with effusion, AOM = acute otitis media, TM = tympanic membrane, % effusion-free = % of patients that were without MEE at follow-up, SD = standard deviation.
* Sample size: numbers shown for those not lost to follow-up and those (initially recruited).

Reference	Hemlin, 1997	Ernstson, 1985
Level (design)	1 (RCT)	1 (RCT)
Sample size*	80 (81)	91 (91)

OUTCOMES		
	% effusion-free	% effusion-free
Cephalosporin	19.7%, 13.1%, 11.5%	52%
Placebo	5.0%, 0.0%, 0.0%	11%
p Value	NS, NS, NS	<0.001
Conclusion	No difference	Cefaclor better
Follow-up time	2 wk, 6 wk, 6 mo	10 d

STUDY DESIGN		
Inclusion criteria	Unilateral or bilateral OME for ≥3 mo duration as confirmed by otomicroscopy and tympanometry Jerger type B curve	<12 y old, OME in one or both ears, diagnosed by otomicroscopy and type B tympanometry, persistent at several examinations for >3 mo
Exclusion criteria	Severe underlying disease, immunologic deficiency, cleft palate, known or suspected allergy to penicillins or cephalosporins, history of antibacterial treatment within the preceding 4 wk, or "previous inclusion in the study"	Cleft palate, upper respiratory tract infection during the period of observation, antibiotics within the 4 wk before randomization
Randomization effectiveness	Age, gender, laterality of MEE, season at entry, prior AOM episodes and myringotomies were reported, although a statistical analysis was not reported	Similar age. More girls than boys in the control group. Not further specified
Age	2–12 y	Mean 4.7 y (SD 2.5), range not reported
Masking	Double blind	Not reported
Cephalosporin regimen	Cefixime 8 mg/kg/d in 2 divided doses ×10 d	Cefaclor 20 mg/kg twice daily ×10 d
Diagnostic criteria for AOM episode	AOM not considered as an outcome measure	AOM not considered as an outcome measure
Management of AOM episode while on study treatment	Antimicrobial agents other than the study drugs were not allowed during the study period. "Any other medication considered necessary for the patient's welfare was allowed"	AOM not considered as an outcome measure, nor was management strategy noted
Diagnostic criteria for OME	Immobile and pale TM when examined with otomicroscopy with a flat Jerger type B tympanogram curve	Pneumatic otoscopy and tympanometry
Criteria for successful treatment	OME resolved 2–11 d after treatment: in ≥1 ear if originally had bilateral OME, or in both ears if originally had unilateral OME; normal middle ear status: pale eardrum with normal mobility on otomicroscopy and type A or C tympanogram with a peak of greater than −300 decapascals	Normal otomicroscopy and type A or C1 tympanometry
Compliance	Measured by diary method and bottle method, numerical results not specified	Not reported
Criteria for withdrawal from study	Patients with failure to resolve OME at 2–11 d after treatment completion were not followed further in this study	Not reported
A priori power calculation	80% power to detect a 35% difference with 80 patients, also reported that "the failure to reach a statistically significant difference is most likely due to a type II error," and that their own study "lacks sufficient power to verify the long-term treatment effect of cefixime treatment"	Not reported
Morbidity/ complications	Cefixime group: 6 patients with gastrointestinal symptoms; placebo group with 0 gastrointestinal symptoms	Not reported

RCT = randomized controlled trial, MEE = middle ear effusion, OME = asymptomatic otitis media with effusion, AOM = acute otitis media, TM = tympanic membrane, % effusion-free = % of patients that were without MEE at follow-up, SD = standard deviation.
* Sample size: numbers shown for those not lost to follow-up and those (initially recruited).

REFERENCES

1. Donaldson JD, Martin GF, Maltby CC, Seyward EB. The efficacy of pulse-dosed antibiotic therapy in the management of otitis media with effusion. J Otolaryngol 1990; 19(3):175–178.

2. Mandel EM, Rockette HE, Paradise JL, Bluestone CD, Nozza RJ. Comparative efficacy of erythromycin-sulfisoxazole, cefaclor, amoxicillin or placebo for otitis media with effusion in children. Pediatric Infect Dis J 1991;10(12):899–906.

3. Hemlin C, Carenfelt C, Papatziamos G. Single dose of betamethasone in combined medical treatment of secretory otitis media. Ann Otol Rhinol Laryngol 1997;106(5):359–363.

4. Ernstson S, Anari M. Cefaclor in the treatment of otitis media with effusion. Acta Otolaryngol Suppl 1985;424:17–21.

7 Pediatric Otitis Media with Effusion

Erythromycin versus placebo: Chance of becoming effusion-free

Jennifer J. Shin and Michael J. Cunningham

METHODS

A computerized Ovid search of MEDLINE 1966–January 2004 was performed. The terms "otitis media" and "antibiotics" were exploded and the resulting articles were cross-referenced, yielding 1947 trials. Given the known richness of the otitis media literature and the authority of higher levels of evidence, these articles were then limited to randomized controlled trials (RCTs), resulting in 302 articles. These articles were then reviewed to identify those that met the following inclusion criteria: 1) patient population <18 years of age with documented otitis media with effusion (OME), 2) intervention with erythromycin therapy versus placebo control, 3) outcome measured in terms of presence or absence of middle ear effusion (MEE). Trials comparing erythromycin either with or without concomitant sulfisoxazole were both included, but sulfisoxazole coadministration was considered a potential confounder. Articles that compared intervention with amoxicillin alone, amoxicillin/clavulanate, cephalosporins, or trimethoprim-sulfamethoxazole, were excluded here but are presented separately in this chapter. The bibliographies of articles that met these inclusion criteria were manually examined to determine if any further relevant articles could be identified. This process yielded four RCTs [1–4].

RESULTS

Outcome Measures. Data were presented in terms of the percent of children becoming effusion-free by 2 weeks, 4 weeks, 2 months, or 6 months. In addition, one trial reported the percent of children worsening [3], although the specifics of what was defined as "worsening" were not reported.

Potential Confounders. Potential confounders were as noted in Section 21.A.i: The specificity of the definitions of MEE, OME, and acute otitis media (AOM) are key, and these are outlined in as much detail as the primary papers allow. In addition, follow-up time, age, history of middle ear disease, etiology of the effusion, duration of effusion at entry, season of the year, history of allergy or nasal obstruction, and the status of the adenoid may also affect results. In addition, whether erythromycin was administered alone [1] or in combination with sulfisoxazole [2–4] may affect results.

Study Designs. Four RCTs addressed this issue. Three evaluated a combined regimen of erythromycin-sulfisoxazole [2–4], whereas the third evaluated erythromycin alone [1]. One evaluated OME of any duration [2]; two evaluated OME of 1–3 months' duration [1, 4], and one did not specify [3]. Randomization effectiveness was described in some detail in each report. Three RCTs were double-blind, placebo-controlled studies in an attempt to minimize inadvertent biases [1–3]. One RCT was single blind only, with just the examiner blinded to the intervention [4]. OME was diagnosed based on a combination of pneumatic otoscopy, tympanometry, and audiology. Compliance and power calculations were reported in just one study [2].

Highest Level of Evidence. Three studies reported no difference in the percent of children becoming effusion-free whether erythromycin or placebo was administered at follow-up periods from 2 weeks to 6 months [1–3]. One of these studies reported a significant difference in the percent of children worsening at 2 weeks [3], although how "worsening" was defined was not reported. Interestingly, the study that identified this significant difference had the fewest patients, and thus the lowest relative power. It should be noted that according to the one report that did note its study's power (i.e., probability of detecting a difference that truly exists), these three studies had a <85% chance of detecting a 15% difference between two groups. The fourth study did report a significant difference, with better outcomes with erythromycin intervention [4], but it was the only one to prevent a clear consensus that a 2- to 4-week course of erythromycin, either with or without sulfisoxazole, did not significantly change the chance of becoming effusion-free. In addition, this fourth study was the only study that was not double-blinded, and so may have been subject to expectation bias. This study noted a 17.2% rate difference in the chance of becoming effusion-free, which corresponds to a number needed to treat of six.

Applicability. These results are applicable to children aged 5 months–15 years with OME without symptoms of AOM. Further criteria for individual studies are as tabulated under inclusion and exclusion criteria.

Morbidity. There were no significant differences noted in the minor adverse reactions that occurred in the erythromycin versus placebo groups. In addition, no serious adverse reactions occurred.

CLINICAL SIGNIFICANCE AND FUTURE RESEARCH

There is evidence from three level 1 studies that erythromycin with or without concomitant sulfisoxazole is no better than placebo in its ability to affect the resolution of OME. These results, however, do exist in the context of studies with somewhat limited power. A fourth study contradicts these findings, with a greater chance of becoming effusion-free noted in patients receiving erythromycin. This study, however, was single blind (not double blind) and may be subject to expectation bias. Overall, there is mixed evidence regarding whether erythromycin will result in better resolution of OME, and limited evidence to suggest that it may prevent worsening of disease.

Higher-powered RCTs may better resolve the impact of erythromycin versus placebo on OME, possibly by demonstrating no significant difference despite a >90% chance of doing so. In addition, newer-generation macrolides, such as azithromycin or clarithromycin are proving worthy of study.

THE EVIDENCE CONDENSED: Erythromycin versus placebo for pediatric chronic otitis media with effusion

Reference	Mandel, 1991	Moller, 1990
Level (design)	1 (RCT)	1 (RCT)
Sample size*	158 (165)	141 (147)
OUTCOMES		
	% effusion-free	% effusion-free
Erythromycin	21.3%, 25.0%	17.3%
Placebo	14.1%, 26.7%	26.4%
p Value	NS, NS	NS
Conclusion	No difference	No difference
Follow-up time	2 wk, 4 wk	1 mo
STUDY DESIGN		
Inclusion criteria	7 mo–12 y old, OME of any duration without symptoms of AOM (e.g., otalgia, fever)	Bilateral OME for >3 mo, AOM-free for ≥3 mo, all candidates for tube insertion but entered trial instead
Exclusion criteria	AOM symptoms (otalgia, fever), craniofacial abnormalities, prior tonsillectomy/adenoidectomy or tube insertion, systemic illness, structurally abnormal middle ear, hearing loss not attributable to MEE, acute/chronic sinusitis, severe upper airway obstruction, hypersensitivity to penicillin	Cleft palate or other congenital anomaly, use of antibiotics during the last 3 mo, obstructive adenoid tissue
Randomization effectiveness	Similar characteristics shown in multiple variables, no comment on statistical analysis	Not specified, but no difference in results were noted because of sex or age
Age	7 mo–12 y	1–15 y
Masking	Double blind	Double blind
Erythromycin regimen	Erythromycin-sulfisoxazole 50 mg-150 mg/kg/d in 4 divided doses ×2 wk	Erythromycin 50 mg/kg/d ×2 wk
Diagnostic criteria for AOM	≥1 symptom (fever, otalgia, irritability) and 1 sign (bulging or fullness of TM, white fluid level, acute perforation with otorrhea)	AOM outcomes were not studied
Management of AOM during study	Antimicrobial different in color from assigned medication ×10 d	AOM outcomes were not studied
Diagnostic criteria: OME	Pneumatic otoscopy, tympanogram, middle ear muscle reflex testing	Otomicroscopy by 2 otolaryngologists, tympanometry, and pure tone audiograms
Criteria for successful treatment	Effusion-free at 2 or 4 wk	Air-filled middle ears
Compliance	Compliance measured by bottle method (92% in erythromycin group and 92% in placebo group) and calendar method (90% erythromycin group and 88% in placebo group)	Not reported
Criteria for withdrawal from study	Not specified in detail	"Unable to continue because of intercurrent disease or an unwillingness to participate"
A priori power calculation	250 patients give a 90% power to detect a ≥20% difference with an alpha of 0.05, one-sided‡	Not reported
Morbidity/ complications	Erythromycin group with 3 adverse reactions (gastrointestinal, rash); placebo group with 4 reactions	No adverse effects reported

RCT = randomized control trial, NS = not significant, MEE = middle ear effusion, OME = asymptomatic otitis media with effusion, AOM = acute otitis media, TM = tympanic membrane.
* Sample size: numbers shown for those not lost to follow-up and those (initially recruited).
‡ The authors also reported an interim analysis of stochastic curtailing to evaluate the implications of terminating subject accrual at n = 331; to detect a difference of 0.15 between antimicrobial and placebo, power range was 0.65–0.81.

THE EVIDENCE CONDENSED: Erythromycin versus placebo for pediatric chronic otitis media with effusion

Reference	Corwin, 1986	Schloss, 1987	
Level (design)	1 (RCT)	1 (RCT)	
Sample size*	131 (149)	Not specified (54)	
OUTCOMES			
	% effusion-free	% effusion-free	% worse
Erythromycin	50.0%	24.0%†	0.0%
Placebo	33.8%	29.6%†	22.2%
p Value	=0.031	NS	"Significant"
Conclusion	Erythromycin better	No difference	Erythromycin better
Follow-up time	1 mo	†2 wk, 1 mo, 2 mo, 6 mo	
STUDY DESIGN			
Inclusion criteria	Persistent OME 1 mo after AOM treated with amoxicillin ×10 d, otherwise healthy	Not reported in detail	
Exclusion criteria	>3 episodes of AOM during the previous year, prophylactic antibiotic treatment, chronic MEE	Not reported in detail	
Randomization effectiveness	Similar median age, sex, race, prior AOM rates, bilateral effusion	Not reported	
Age	5 mo–16 y	Not reported	
Masking	Single blind (examiner)	Double blind	
Erythromycin regimen	Erythromycin-sulfisoxazole 50 mg–150 mg/kg/d ×10 d	Erythromycin-sulfisoxazole 50 mg/kg/d in 3 divided doses ×14–28 d	
Diagnostic criteria for AOM	TM bulging, erythema, fullness, or opacification; impaired TM mobility; ≥1 symptom (fever, otalgia)	AOM outcomes were not studied	
Management of AOM during study	"Treated with antibiotics"	AOM outcomes were not studied	
Diagnostic criteria: OME	Minimally mobile gray or opalescent TM in neutral or retracted position, with tympanometry if >2 y old	Pneumatic otoscopy, tympanometry, audiolometry	
Criteria for successful treatment	"Normal ear"	Not reported in detail	
Compliance	Not reported	Not reported	
Criteria for withdrawal from study	Failure to return for follow-up	Not reported	
A priori power calculation	Not reported	Not reported	
Morbidity/ complications	Not reported	"No significant difference"	

RCT = randomized control trial, NS = not significant, MEE = middle ear effusion, OME = asymptomatic otitis media with effusion, AOM = acute otitis media, TM = tympanic membrane, NS = not significant.
* Sample size: numbers shown for those not lost to follow-up and those (initially recruited).
† Symbol denotes that % effusion-free was measured at a follow-up time of 2 weeks.

REFERENCES

1. Moller P, Dingsor G. Otitis media with effusion: can erythromycin reduce the need for ventilating tubes? J Laryngol Otol 1990;104:200–202.

2. Mandel EM, Rockette HE, Paradise JL, Bluestone CD, Nozza RJ. Comparative efficacy of erythromycin-sulfisoxazole, cefaclor, amoxicillin or placebo for otitis media with effusion in children. Pediatr Infect Dis J 1991;10(12):899–906.

3. Schloss MD, Dempsey EE, Rishikof E, Sorger S, Grace M. Double blind study comparing erythromycin-sulfizoxazole to placebo in chronic otitis media with effusion. In Proc 4th Int Symp Recent Adv Otitis Media. New York: BC Decker, 1987.

4. Corwin MJ, Weiner LB, Daniels D. Efficacy of oral antibiotics for the treatment of persistent otitis media with effusion. International J Pediatr Otorhinolaryngol 1986;11(2):109–112.

7 Pediatric Otitis Media with Effusion

7.A.v.

Trimethoprim-sulfamethoxazole versus control: Chance of becoming effusion-free

Jennifer J. Shin and Michael J. Cunningham

METHODS

A computerized Ovid search of MEDLINE 1966–January 2004 was performed. The terms "otitis media" and "antibiotics" were exploded and the resulting articles were cross-referenced, yielding 1947 trials. Given the known richness of the otitis media literature and the authority of higher levels of evidence, these articles were then limited to randomized controlled trials (RCTs), resulting in 302 articles. These articles were then reviewed to identify those that met the following inclusion criteria: 1) patient population <18 years of age with documented otitis media with effusion (OME), 2) intervention with trimethoprim-sulfamethoxazole (TMP-SMX) therapy versus placebo control, 3) outcome measured in terms of middle ear effusion. Trials comparing sulfisoxazole alone to control were not included here but are included in a meta-analysis of the effect of all antibiotics. Articles that compared intervention with amoxicillin alone, amoxicillin/clavulanate, cephalosporins or erythromycin were excluded here but are presented separately in this chapter. The bibliographies of articles that met these inclusion criteria were manually examined to determine if any further relevant articles could be identified. This process yielded five RCTs [1–5].

RESULTS

Outcome Measures. Data were presented in terms of the percent of children becoming effusion-free. In addition, several trials reported the percent of children who developed a new acute otitis media (AOM) within the study's follow-up period [2–5].

Potential Confounders. Potential confounders were as noted in Section 21.A.i: The specificity of the definitions of middle ear effusion, OME, and AOM are key, and these are outlined in as much detail as the primary papers allow. In addition, follow-up time, age, history of middle ear disease, etiology of the effusion, duration of effusion at entry, season of the year, history of allergy or nasal obstruction, and the status of the adenoid may also affect results.

Study Designs. Five RCTs addressed this issue. Two were double blind [1, 2]. One of these blinded trials used Dimetapp as a control [1], whereas the other compared placebo with a stepped regimen of TMP-SMX for up to 6 weeks with prednisone in weeks 3 and 4 [2]. The three remaining trials were not blinded or placebo controlled, exposing them to potential expectation biases [3–5]. Groups were similar after randomization, suggesting that confounders were balanced among groups. Combinations of otoscopy, tympanometry, and audiometry were used to evaluate whether OME was present, with individual trial details provided in the adjoining table. Compliance was evaluated in three instances [2, 3, 5]. No study reported an *a priori* power calculation.

Highest Level of Evidence. TMP-SMX resulted in a higher percentage of effusion-free children at one or more follow-up timepoints in four of the five RCTs. Three of those trials, however, were not blinded, so a placebo effect may have been partially responsible for the favorable results [3, 5]. In addition, one of these trials considered the impact of a regimen which included steroids for part of the treatment [2]. These steroids could also potentially confound results. In the remaining study, in which TMP-SMX was compared with Dimetapp as a control, the rate difference (RD)[1] was 37.1% [1]. This RD suggests that three children must be treated with TMP-SMX in order for one of them to become effusion-free [i.e., the number needed to treat (NNT) is three[2]].

In addition, four trials considered the impact of TMP-SMX on the development of new AOM [2–5], although only three studies included a report of a statistical analysis of that AOM data [2, 4, 5]. In two cases, there was no difference between TMP-SMX or no antibiotic administration, whereas in the third, a smaller percent of the TMP-SMX–treated children developed new AOM.

Applicability. These results are applicable to children aged 6 months–12 years with OME. Further criteria for individual studies are as tabulated under inclusion and exclusion criteria.

---

[1] RD is the absolute difference in successful outcomes between the study group and the control group. For example, in the Marks study, 64% of the TMP-SMX group versus 26.9% of the placebo group became effusion-free. The RD in this study was 26.9% − 64% = −37.1%.

[2] NNT is the total number of children that must be treated in order for one child to obtain benefit from the treatment. It is calculated by determining the inverse of the RD. For example, for the van Balen study, the RD is −16%, so that the NNT = 1/0.371 = 2.7. In this case, three children would need to be treated so to obtain benefit for one child.

Morbidity. In the two trials that reported adverse reactions, they were limited to three cases of neutropenia in the patients receiving TMP-SMX. No other adverse reactions were reported in any of the trials.

CLINICAL SIGNIFICANCE AND FUTURE RESEARCH

Five level 1 studies with limitations from power, expectation bias, and/or confounding concomitant steroid administration addressed the impact of TMP-SMX on OME. Four of the five studies demonstrated a significant improvement in the percent of children who became effusion-free with TMP-SMX. Two of those four studies were somewhat biased toward this TMP-SMX–improved outcome because of a lack of placebo. A potential improvement of 37.1% in effusion rates posttherapy must not only be considered in the face of relevant studies' limitations, but also be balanced against potential risks of TMP-SMX therapy such as neutropenia.

Future research may focus on the impact of TMP-SMX alone in trials utilizing a placebo control with enough subject accrual to achieve 90% power. In addition, direct comparisons between TMP-SMX and other medical therapies may prove useful.

THE EVIDENCE CONDENSED: Trimethoprim-sulfamethoxazole versus control for pediatric otitis media with effusion

Reference	Marks, 1981
Level (design)	1 (randomized controlled trial)
Sample size*	51 (58)

OUTCOMES	
	% improved
TMP-SMX	64.0%
Control	26.9%
p Value	<0.025
Conclusion	TMP-SMX better
Follow-up time	4–6 wk

STUDY DESIGN	
Inclusion criteria	<12 y old, OME
Exclusion criteria	Concurrent respiratory or other otologic disease, cleft palate or stigmata thereof (i.e., bifid uvula), history of sensitivity to sulfonamide/cotrimoxazole
Randomization effectiveness	Similar age, otalgia, AOM, history of tympanostomy tubes or adenoidectomy. Some asymmetry in gender, mouth breathing and snoring, although no statistical analysis reported
Age	2–11 y
Masking	Double blind, Dimetapp controlled
TMP-SMX regimen	"5 mL of cotrimoxazole paediatric suspension" ×4 wk (according to the authors, placebo was 5 cc Dimetapp elixir because it was shown to be equivalent to placebo in previous studies)
Diagnostic criteria for AOM episode	Not specified
Management of AOM during study	Not specified
Diagnostic criteria for OME	"Diagnosis of serous otitis media was made where otoscopic findings suggested this with no other tympanic complications being evident . . . pure tone audiogram with a 15 dB air/bone gap or greater . . . and impedance audiogram flat with negative pressure in excess of −300 mm of water"
Criteria for successful treatment	Change in pure tone average showing a return to normal or >20-dB improvement, impedance audiometry changed so either a flat tracing returned to normal or reverted to one peaked at −300 mm H_2O or better
Compliance	Not reported
Criteria for withdrawal from study	Not reported
A priori power calculation	Not reported
Morbidity/ complications	Not reported in detail

TMP-SMX = trimethoprim-sulfamethoxazole, AOM = acute otitis media, NS = not significant, MEE = middle ear effusion, OME = asymptomatic otitis media with effusion, TM = tympanic membrane, % effusion-free = % of patients that were without MEE at follow-up.
* Sample size: numbers shown for those not lost to follow-up and those (initially recruited).

THE EVIDENCE CONDENSED: Trimethoprim-sulfamethoxazole versus control for pediatric otitis media with effusion

Reference	Daly, 1991
Level (design)	1 (randomized controlled trial)
Sample size*	42 (42)

OUTCOMES		
	% effusion-free	% developing AOM
TMP-SMX	48%	33%
Control	14%	52%
p Value	= 0.02	NS
Conclusion	TMP-SMX better	No difference
Follow-up time	6 wk	

STUDY DESIGN	
Inclusion criteria	6 mo–8 y old, bilateral OME, and ≥1 of the following: daycare attendance for >15 h a week with five or more children, OME ≥4 wk at enrollment as documented in the medical record. Also ≥2 AOM in the preceding 18 mo, last documentation of AOM or OME <4 wk before enrollment; appropriate antibiotic treatment for the most recent AOM episode (≥10 d of ampicillin, amoxicillin, cefaclor, TMP-SMX, or erythromycin/sulfisoxazole), immunizations up to date
Exclusion criteria	Allergy to trimethoprim, sulfonamides, ampicillin, amoxicillin, or oral corticosteroids; significant chronic disease of the kidney, heart, liver, or immune system; hypertension; tympanostomy tubes; concomitant infection; varicella exposure in the preceding 3 wk without a history of varicella
Randomization effectiveness	No significant differences in gender, race, family history of frequent otitis media, status as youngest child in the family, allergy, parental smoking, daycare attendance, bilateral OME, duration of OME, number of prior episodes
Age	6 mo–8 y
Masking	Double blind, placebo controlled
TMP-SMX regimen	8 mg trimethoprim and 40 mg sulfamethoxazole per day in 2 divided doses ×2, 4, or 6 wk (whichever was required for resolution of OME); if there was no resolution of OME by 2 wk, then wk 3 and 4 only were supplemented with prednisone 1 mg/kg/d in 2 divided doses ×7 d then 1 mg/kg on alternate days ×7 d
Diagnostic criteria for AOM episode	Any of the following: 1) OME and erythematous TM, 2) white, yellow, or orange TM in the presence of otalgia, fever, or irritability, 3) TM perforation and otorrhea
Management of AOM during study	Amoxicillin 40 mg/kg/d in 3 divided doses ×10 d
Diagnostic criteria for OME	Findings from otoscopy and tympanometry, with the otoscopist's impression settling any cases of uncertain diagnoses
Criteria for successful treatment	Resolution of OME in both ears, as determined by pneumatic otoscopy and tympanometry according to a previously published algorithm
Compliance	89% in both groups as measured by diary, bottle method, and serum assay for sulfamethoxazole
Criteria for withdrawal from study	Not specified; no patients withdrew
A priori power calculation	Not reported
Morbidity/ complications	TMP-SMX group with 1 patient who reported being "more sleepy and off balance," no adverse reactions in either group

TMP-SMX = trimethoprim-sulfamethoxazole, AOM = acute otitis media, NS = not significant, MEE = middle ear effusion, OME = asymptomatic otitis media with effusion, TM = tympanic membrane, AOM = acute otitis media, % effusion-free = % of patients that were without MEE at follow-up.
* Sample size: numbers shown for those not lost to follow-up and those (initially recruited).

THE EVIDENCE CONDENSED: Trimethoprim-sulfamethoxazole versus control for pediatric chronic otitis media with effusion

Reference	Healy, 1984	
Level (design)	1 (randomized controlled trial)	
Sample size*	196 (200)	

OUTCOMES		
	% effusion-free	% new AOM
TMP-SMX	58%	2/96
Control	6%	5/93
p Value	<0.0001	Not reported
Conclusion	TMP-SMX better	—
Follow-up time	4 wk	

STUDY DESIGN	
Inclusion criteria	2–5 y old, OME of >6 wk duration at the time of enrollment, with persistent OME confirmed again 6 wk after enrollment
Exclusion criteria	Prior tonsillectomy, adenoidectomy, and/or tympanostomy tubes; middle ear abnormality (i.e., TM perforation, cholesteatoma, adhesive otitis media); facial anomalies or congenital syndromes; URI in prior 4 wk; systemic illness such as cystic fibrosis; sinusitis; acute suppurative otitis media; strong family history of allergy; medical therapy for MEE in prior 4 wk
Randomization effectiveness	Patient characteristics of gender, age, season of entry, and laterality of effusions were reported
Age	2–5 y
Masking	Neither double blinded nor placebo controlled
TMP-SMX regimen	TMP-SMX 8 and 40 mg/kg/24 h in 2 divided doses ×4 wk
Diagnostic criteria for AOM episode	Not reported
Management of AOM during study	Not reported
Diagnostic criteria for OME	Pneumatic otoscopy, tympanometry type B, C1, or C2, and middle ear muscle reflex testing in all patients
Criteria for success	Normal pneumatic otoscopic examination and a type A tympanogram
Compliance	Evaluated by calendar and bottle method; 89% of patients received >85% of study medication
Criteria for withdrawal from study	Failure to follow-up
A priori power calculation	Not reported
Morbidity/ complications	Not reported

TMP-SMX = trimethoprim-sulfamethoxazole, NS = not significant, MEE = middle ear effusion, OME = asymptomatic otitis media with effusion, TM = tympanic membrane, URI = upper respiratory tract infection, AOM = acute otitis media.
* Sample size: numbers shown for those not lost to follow-up and those (initially recruited).

THE EVIDENCE CONDENSED: Trimethoprim-sulfamethoxazole versus control for pediatric chronic otitis media with effusion

Reference	Schwartz, 1982	
Level (design)	1 (randomized controlled trial)	
Sample size*	64 (69)	

OUTCOMES		
	% effusion-free	% new AOM
TMP-SMX	58%, 76%	0%
Control	42%, 80%	17%
p Value	NS, NS	<0.05
Conclusion	No difference	TMP-SMX better
Follow-up time	2 wk, 4 wk	

STUDY DESIGN	
Inclusion criteria	AOM within 15 d of entry into study, previous amoxicillin treatment for at least 10 d, persistent OME by otomicroscopy with the "color of the effusion as seen through the eardrum and absence of visible bubbles or fluid lines suggest[ing] a mucoid effusion," and type B tympanometry
Exclusion criteria	Not specified
Randomization effectiveness	Similar age, laterality of OME, percent with OME >6 wk; more boys in the control group although statistical analysis not reported
Age	Mean 41.7–43.9 mo
Masking	Neither double blinded nor placebo controlled
TMP-SMX regimen	TMP-SMX 4 and 20 mg/kg in 1 dose ×14 d then off
Diagnostic criteria for AOM episode	"Bulging of a yellow- or red-appearing TM with obliteration of some or all ossicular landmarks and impaired or absent medial-lateral mobility of the TM to pneumomassage" with coinciding "pain or querulous behavior"
Management of AOM during study	Not specified
Diagnostic criteria for OME	Immobile or minimally mobile TM in the neutral or retracted position with gray or opalescent color on pneumatic otoscopy and flat tympanogram
Criteria for success	"Resolution" of OME by pneumatic otoscopy and tympanometry
Compliance	Not reported
Criteria for withdrawal from study	Failure to follow-up
A priori power calculation	Not reported
Morbidity/ complications	Not reported

TMP-SMX = trimethoprim-sulfamethoxazole, NS = not significant, MEE = middle ear effusion, OME = asymptomatic otitis media with effusion, TM = tympanic membrane, URI = upper respiratory tract infection, AOM = acute otitis media.
* Sample size: numbers shown for those not lost to follow-up and those (initially recruited).

THE EVIDENCE CONDENSED: Trimethoprim-sulfamethoxazole versus control for pediatric chronic otitis media with effusion

Reference	Giebink, 1990	
Level (design)	1 (randomized controlled trial)	
Sample size*	39 (39)	

	OUTCOMES	
	% effusion-free	% new AOM
TMP-SMX	55%, 50%	25%
Control	5%, 30%	45%
p Value	= 0.02, NS	NS
Conclusion	TMP-SMX better at 2 wk, no difference at 4 wk	No difference
Follow-up time	2 wk, 4 wk	8 wk

	STUDY DESIGN	
Inclusion criteria	10–95 mo old, OME for ≥8 wks, ≥3 physician-documented otitis media episodes in the prior 18 mo; AOM or asymptomatic OME diagnosed 10–28 d before entry, completion of >10 d of antibiotics for the most recent AOM, OME documented by otoscopy and tympanometry at entry and at 3 and 6 wk after entry—patients were randomized 6 wk after entry	
Exclusion criteria	History of adverse reactions to sulfonamides; presence of tympanostomy tubes; AOM	
Randomization effectiveness	No significant differences in age, gender, race, OME duration, number of prior OM episodes, hearing loss, speech therapy, prior pneumonia, asthma or "seasonal pollenosis," bottle feeding, family history of otitis media or hearing loss, season of enrollment	
Age	10–95 mo	
Masking	Not blinded	
TMP-SMX regimen	TMP-SMX 8 and 40 mg per day in 2 divided doses for 4 wk	
Diagnostic criteria for AOM episode	OME with erythematous TM; or white, yellow, or orange TM in the presence of fever, otalgia, or irritability; or with tympanic membrane perforation with purulent drainage	
Management of AOM during study	Amoxicillin, cefaclor, or erythromycin ×10 d	
Diagnostic criteria for OME	Pneumatic otoscopy and impedance audiometry algorithm in the absence of symptoms	
Criteria for success	"OME resolution, i.e., no OME in either ear"	
Compliance	97% compliance with TMP-SMX as measured by medication diary, bottle method	
Criteria for withdrawal from study	Refusal to take prednisone, new illness requiring additional treatment,† inadvertent enrollment of a patient with cholesteatoma	
A priori power calculation	Not reported	
Morbidity/ complications	TMP-SMX group: 3 neutropenia Control group: 0 neutropenia	

TMP-SMX = trimethoprim-sulfamethoxazole, NS = not significant, MEE = middle ear effusion, OME = asymptomatic otitis media with effusion, TM = tympanic membrane, URI = upper respiratory tract infection, AOM = acute otitis media.
* Sample size: numbers shown for those not lost to follow-up and those (initially recruited).
† Gastroenteritis, AOM, streptococcal pharyngitis.

REFERENCES

1. Marks NJ, Mills RP, Shaheen OH. A controlled trial of cotrimoxazole therapy in serous otitis media. *J Laryngol Otol* 1981;95(10):1003–1009.
2. Daly K, Giebink GS, Batalden PB, Anderson RS, Lindgren B. Resolution of otitis media with effusion with the use of a stepped treatment regimen of trimoprim sulfamethoxazole and prednisone. *Pediatr Infect Dis J* 1991;10(7):500–506.
3. Healy GB. Antimicrobial therapy of chronic otitis media with effusion. *International J Pediatr Otorhinolaryngol* 1984; 8(1):13–17.
4. Schwartz RH, Rodriguez WJ. Trimethoprim sulfamethoxizole treatment of persistent otitis media with effusion. *Pediatr Infect Dis J* 1982;1(5):333–335.
5. Giebink GS, Batalden PB, Le CT, Lassman FM, Buran DJ, Seltz AE. A controlled trial comparing three treatments for chronic otitis media with effusion. *Pediatr Infect Dis J* 1990; 9(1):33–40.

7 Pediatric Otitis Media with Effusion

7.B.

Tympanostomy tube placement: Impact on quality of life

Jennifer J. Shin and Christopher J. Hartnick

METHODS

A computerized Ovid search of MEDLINE 1966–January 2004 was performed. The term "otitis media" was exploded and the resulting articles were cross-referenced with those obtained by exploding "quality of life." This process yielded 21 articles, and these were reviewed for the following inclusion criteria: 1) children <18 years old with chronic otitis media with effusion (COME) or recurrent acute otitis media (RAOM), 2) treatment with tympanostomy tubes in comparison to a control group, and 3) evaluation with a validated quality of life (QOL) instrument. Reports of evaluations with nonvalidated questionnaires and anecdotal reports were excluded. Pilot reports of noncontrolled evaluations of QOL were also excluded. This process yielded four articles [1–4], which are discussed in detail below.

RESULTS

Outcome Measures. A validated instrument has been tested to ensure that the following are true: 1) it measures what it is intended to measure (convergent validity, i.e., scores on a valid test of arithmetic skills correlate with scores on other math tests), and 2) it does not inadvertently measure irrelevant changes (discriminant validity, i.e., scores on a valid test of arithmetic do not correlate with scores on tests of verbal ability) [5, 6], 3) its scores are stable (reliability, i.e., a patient with the same disease impact will continue to have the same response), and 4) it is sensitive to change (responsiveness, i.e., a patient with a change in disease impact will have a changed score). Overall, this means that the validated instrument does in fact measure what it is meant to measure.

Three validated instruments were used in these studies. Two are disease-specific instruments that are explicitly intended to measure the QOL as a result of otitis media. The first of these is the otitis media 6 (OM-6) instrument, which was validated to measure changes in QOL within an individual over time (Figure 7.B.1). Through the OM-6, caregivers rate the impact of otitis during the previous 4 weeks in six domains: physical suffering, hearing loss, speech impairment, emotional distress, activity limitations, and caregiver concerns. Each domain is scored on a scale of 1 (no problem) to 7 (extreme problem). In addition, a global QOL score from 0 (worst possible) to 10 (best possible) is obtained

using a visual analog scale. The OM-6 is validated for completion by caregivers in children 6 months to 12 years old with chronic otitis media or RAOM.[1]

The second instrument is the OM-22, which is an expanded version of the OM-6 (Figure 7.B.2). In this expanded version of 22 questions regarding the previous year, each domain is broken down into individual variables, to allow for analysis of each of those individual variables. For example, speech problems are dissected into issues of poor pronunciation, difficulty understanding the child, and inability to repeat words clearly. In addition, demographic data are obtained. The OM-22 is validated for children younger than 16 years of age with RAOM or COME.[2]

The third instrument is a global instrument, the TNO-AZL Infant Quality of Life Instrument (TAIQOL). It is not disease-specific and uses mostly 12-point scales to evaluate 13 domains (lungs, stomach, skin, positive emotions, eating problems, appetite, aggressive behavior, emotions of panic, vitality, social behavior, motoric problems, communication problems); the first four of these domains were excluded by the authors of the study detailed below. This instrument is validated for children 1–4 years old.

Potential Confounders. Variations in indications for tube placement, concurrent procedures, tube type, and subject age, gender, and ethnicity could potentially

---

[1] When the OM-6 was validated, specific inclusion criteria were as follows: 1) aged 6 months to 12 years, 2) chronic otitis media (MEE in one or both ears for ≥3 months) or recurrent otitis media (≥3 acute otitis media episodes in the past 12 months), 3) child accompanied by parent or primary caregiver, and 4) child able to complete age-appropriate audiometry with good reliability. Specific exclusion criteria were 1) tympanic membrane perforation, 2) tympanostomy tube(s) at study entry, 3) middle ear pathologic features other than otitis media (e.g., cholesteatoma), 4) known or suspected developmental delay or neurologic disorder, and 5) parent or primary caregiver unable to read and understand the English language.

[2] When the OM-22 was validated, specific inclusion criteria were as follows: 1) age younger than 16 years, 2) a diagnosis of RAOM as defined by five or more episodes of acute otitis media over the past year or a diagnosis of COME defined as the presence of middle ear effusion in one or both ears for 3 months or longer, 3) child's primary caregiver present to complete the survey, and 4) children presenting to the practice of a single pediatric otolaryngologist. Exclusion criteria included 1) presentation to the other physicians within the University of Florida otolaryngology group, 2) previous ear surgery other than myringotomy and/or tympanostomy tube placement, 3) tympanostomy tubes already present at presentation, 4) tympanic membrane perforation, and 5) primary caregiver not present or unable to read and understand English.

Instructions: Please help us understand the impact of ear infections or fluid on your child's quality of life by checking one box [X] for each question below. Thank you.

Physical Suffering: Ear pain, ear discomfort, ear discharge, ruptured ear drum, high fever, or poor balance. How much of a problem for your child during the past 4 weeks?

[ ] Not present/no problem   [ ] Hardly a problem at all   [ ] Quite a bit of a problem
                      [ ] Somewhat of a problem   [ ] Very much a problem
                      [ ] Moderate problem   [ ] Extreme problem

Hearing Loss: Difficulty hearing, questions must be repeated, frequently says "what," or television is excessively loud. How much of a problem for your child during the past 4 weeks?

[ ] Not present/no problem   [ ] Hardly a problem at all   [ ] Quite a bit of a problem
                      [ ] Somewhat of a problem   [ ] Very much a problem
                      [ ] Moderate problem   [ ] Extreme problem

Speech Impairment: Delayed speech, poor pronunciation, difficult to understand, or unable to repeat words clearly. How much of a problem for your child during the past 4 weeks?

[ ] Not present/no problem   [ ] Hardly a problem at all   [ ] Quite a bit of a problem
   (or not applicable)   [ ] Somewhat of a problem   [ ] Very much a problem
                      [ ] Moderate problem   [ ] Extreme problem

Emotional Distress: Irritable, frustrated, sad, restless, or poor appetite. How much of a problem for your child during the past 4 weeks as a result of ear infections or fluid?

[ ] Not present/no problem   [ ] Hardly a problem at all   [ ] Quite a bit of a problem
                      [ ] Somewhat of a problem   [ ] Very much a problem
                      [ ] Moderate problem   [ ] Extreme problem

Activity Limitations: Playing, sleeping, doing things with friends/family, attending school or day care. How limited have your child's activities been during the past 4 weeks because of ear infections or fluid?

[ ] Not limited at all   [ ] Hardly limited at all   [ ] Moderately limited
              [ ] Very slightly limited   [ ] Very limited
              [ ] Slightly limited   [ ] Severely limited

Caregiver Concerns: How often have you, as a caregiver, been worried, concerned, or inconvenienced because of your child's ear infections or fluid over the past 4 weeks?

[ ] None of the time   [ ] Hardly any time at all   [ ] A good part of the time
           [ ] A small part of the time   [ ] Most of the time
           [ ] Some of the time   [ ] All of the time

Overall, how would you rate your child's quality of life as a result of ear infections or fluid? (Circle one number)

0 1 2 3 4 5 6 7 8 9 10
Worse Possible   Halfway Between   Best Possible
Quality-of-Life   Worst and Best   Quality-of-Life

The 6-item health-related quality-of-life survey (OM-6) for chronic and recurrent otitis media.

Figure 7.B.1. OM-6 instrument.
Images reprinted with permission from Arch Otolaryngol 1997 123; 1049-54, copyright 2007 American Medical Association, all rights reserved.

Please try to answer the following questions to the best of your ability and circle the choice that most accurately reflects your experiences.

1. How many ear infections has your child had in the past year?
    None   1-2   3-4   5-6   7-8   9-10   >10

2. How many days had your child missed from school or day care during the last year because of an ear infection?
    None   1-2   3-4   5-6   7-8   9-10   >10

3. How many days have you had to take off from work to care for your child because of an ear infection during the last year?
    None   1-2   3-4   5-6   7-8   9-10   >10

4. How many doctor visits have you made this last year due to your child's ear infections?
    None   1-2   3-4   5-6   7-8   9-10   >10

5. Has your child been in day care during the past year?   yes   no

6. How many other children live in your home?
    None   1   2   3   4   5   6   >6

7. Do you have cat(s) or dog(s) in the home?   yes   no

8. Does anyone smoke cigarettes in the home?   yes   no

9. How often have you, as a caregiver, been worried, concerned, or inconvenienced by your child's ear infections or fluid in the ears over the past year?
    0   1   2   3   4   5
0 = none of the time   1 = hardly any time at all   2 = a small part of the time
3 = good part of the time   4 = most of the time   5 = all of the time

Please help us understand the impact of ear infections on your child by rating your child's symptoms over the past year.

In the last year, how much of a problem have these symptoms been for your child?

Please circle the number that best corresponds to the extent of your child's problem.

0 = not present/no problem   4 = quite a bit of a problem
1 = hardly a problem at all   5 = very much of a problem
2 = somewhat of a problem   6 = extreme problem
3 = moderate problem

1. Ear pain 0 1 2 3 4 5 6
2. Ear discomfort/ear tugging 0 1 2 3 4 5 6
3. Ruptured ear drum/ear drainage 0 1 2 3 4 5 6
4. High fever 0 1 2 3 4 5 6
5. Poor balance 0 1 2 3 4 5 6
6. Difficulty hearing 0 1 2 3 4 5 6
7. Frequently says "what" 0 1 2 3 4 5 6
8. Television played excessively loud ... 0 1 2 3 4 5 6
9. Frequently doesn't respond to verbal commands ... 0 1 2 3 4 5 6
10. Delayed speech 0 1 2 3 4 5 6
11. Poor pronunciation 0 1 2 3 4 5 6
12. Child is difficult to understand 0 1 2 3 4 5 6
13. Child is unable to repeat words clearly 0 1 2 3 4 5 6
14. Irritable 0 1 2 3 4 5 6
15. Frustrated 0 1 2 3 4 5 6
16. Sad 0 1 2 3 4 5 6
17. Restless 0 1 2 3 4 5 6
18. Poor appetite 0 1 2 3 4 5 6

0 = not limited   4 = moderately limited
1 = hardly limited   5 = very limited
2 = very slightly limited   6 = severely limited
3 = slightly limited

19. Playing 0 1 2 3 4 5 6
20. Sleeping 0 1 2 3 4 5 6
21. Doing things with friends/family 0 1 2 3 4 5 6
22. Attending school or day care.......... 0 1 2 3 4 5 6

Figure 7.B.2. OM-22 instrument.

influence results. One study used randomization, whereas the other three used paired data from the same children to manage these issues.

Study Designs. One study was an RCT that compared global QOL in children randomized to undergo tympanostomy tube placement or "watchful waiting" [3]. Despite randomization in this study, there were remaining baseline differences, with older children, more girls, and better hearing in the children in the group allocated for tube placement. QOL scores, however, were not statistically significant. There was minimal attrition, with 90% of patients completing the entire study. In addition, the study was reported as adequately powered, with *post hoc* calculations corroborating this claim. No measure of disease-specific QOL was undertaken in this trial. The other three studies used either the OM-22 [4] or the OM-6 in English [2] or Dutch translation [4] to evaluate disease-specific QOL. In each case, initial scores were compared with scores at the time of surgery and postoperatively. This study design has the benefit of allowing children to serve as their own paired controls, but cannot account for any placebo effect of tube placement itself.

Highest Level of Evidence. Data from the RCT suggests that there is no difference in global QOL in children after 6 months of grommet placement versus 6 months of observation [3]. This result might be attributable to blunted overall sensitivity of such a global instrument to identify more subtle disease-specific changes. No disease-specific QOL evaluation was performed in this study, although other Dutch investigators did later validate and utilize a Dutch translation of the OM-6 instrument in one of the three other prospective studies discussed here [4]. Data from three prospective studies using paired controls suggests that a significant difference in disease-specific QOL exists in children at the time of surgery versus after tube placement. These studies show that subjective improvements parallel the clinically measurable improvements seen in previous level 1 studies (See 6.D.).

Applicability. These results are applicable to 0.5- to 9.9-year-old children who undergo tympanostomy tube placement for bilateral COME or RAOM. These results are not applicable to children who have tympanic membrane perforation or middle ear pathology other than otitis media.

CLINICAL SIGNIFICANCE AND FUTURE DIRECTIONS

There is one level 1 study that shows no difference in global QOL with 6–12 months of tubes or observation, but three level 2 studies that report a significant difference in disease-specific QOL. Differential use of instruments and study designs makes it difficult to directly compare these two sets of results. The latter results are more consistent with previous randomized clinical trials that report the positive impact of tympanostomy tube placement.

Future randomized controlled trials may integrate the use of a disease-specific instrument that is validated for discriminative purposes (meaning that it can distinguish between individuals with different levels of disease, as opposed to an evaluative instrument that evaluates changes within individuals over time). In addition, a global QOL instrument validated for the pediatric population may also simultaneously be administered. Correlations between global and disease-specific QOL could then be drawn and insight may be gained regarding the somewhat conflicting results seen in studies using global versus disease-specific instruments in the trials to date. This information would supplement the clinical outcomes that are traditionally measured (i.e., rates of RAOM or resolution of COME) and directly show whether subjective QOL assessments directly parallel related objective outcomes.

THE EVIDENCE CONDENSED: Quality of life after tympanostomy tubes

Reference	Rovers, 2001	Rosenfeld, 2000
Level (design)	1 (RCT)	2 (POS)†
Sample size*	187 (166)	248 (224, 115)
OUTCOMES		
Instrument	TAIQOL after 6 mo of tubes vs 6 mo of observation	OM-6 survey at surgery vs at least 14 d postoperatively
Quality of life‡ at baseline (before intervention)	Before tubes: Communication: 6.8 (2.3) Social: 3.6 (0.9) Before observation: Communication: 6.4 (2.0) Social: 3.5 (0.8)	Physical suffering: 4.6 (1.8) Hearing loss: 2.7 (1.8) Speech impairment: 2.3 (1.8) Emotional distress: 4.0 (1.8) Activity limitations: 2.4 (1.9) Caregiver concerns: 4.9 (1.7)
Quality of life‡ after tubes	Communication: 6.7 (2.3) Social: 3.5 (0.9)	Change in score: 1.40 (1.3)
Quality of life‡ with no tubes	Communication: 5.8 (2.1) Social: 3.5 (0.9)	Change in score: 0.33 (1.0)
p Value	NS	<0.001
Follow-up time	6 and 12 mo	Mean 34 d (>14 d)
STUDY DESIGN		
Indications for tube placement	100% COME	56% recurrent OM 42% COME 2% retraction
Additional procedures	NR	None
Tube type	Grommet	Grommet
Age	1–2 y	0.5–9.9 y
Inclusion criteria	Infants with persistent (4–6 mo) bilateral OME (confirmed by tympanometry and otoscopy)	6 mo–12 y old with otitis media scheduled for bilateral tympanostomy tube placement as an isolated surgical procedure, accompanied by caregiver
Exclusion criteria	Unwillingness to accept randomization of treatment	Unilateral tympanostomy tube placement, concurrent procedures, middle ear pathology besides otitis media

RCT = randomized controlled trial, POS = prospective outcomes study, TAIQOL = TNO-AZL Infant Quality of Life Instrument, COME = chronic otitis media with effusion, AOM = acute otitis media, RAOM = recurrent AOM, OME = otitis media with effusion, SD = standard deviation, SEM = standard error, CI = confidence interval, NS = not significant, NR = not reported.

* Sample size: numbers shown for those that were initially recruited and those that (completed the trial). In Rosenfeld, 2000, 224 patients had valid change scores (defined by at least a 14-day interval between surveys) after surgery and 115 had valid change scores before and after surgery.

† In POS studies, children were tested at baseline (initial presentation), before or at surgery (without tubes), and after surgery (after tubes). Thus, in this study design, children serve as their own controls.

‡ Quality of life results reported as mean scores (SEM) for Rovers, 2001; change in mean scores (SD) for Rosenfeld, 2000; means scores (95% CI) for Richards, 2002; mean scores (SD) for Timmerman, 2003.

THE EVIDENCE CONDENSED: Quality of life after tympanostomy tubes

Reference	Richards, 2002	Timmerman, 2003
Level (design)	2 (POS)	2 (POS)
Sample size*	123 (68)	77 (69)
OUTCOMES		
Instrument	OM-22 at surgery vs 6 mo postoperatively	OM-6 (translated from English to Dutch) at surgery vs 6–8 wk postoperatively
Quality of life‡ at baseline (before intervention)	Summary score: 49.1 (44.8–53.4)	Summary score: 18 (7)
Quality of life‡ after tubes	Summary score: 15.6 (11.6–19.6)	Summary score: 12 (5)
Quality of life‡ with no tubes	10 patients repeated OM-6 before surgery, with no difference from baseline	Summary score: 19 (7)
p Value	<0.001	<0.001
Follow-up time	1 and 6 mo	6–8 wk
STUDY DESIGN		
Indications for tube placement	38% RAOM 25% COME 37% RAOM and COME	Chronic or recurrent OME
Additional procedures	Adenoidectomy in subset	NR
Tube type	NR	NR
Age	2.42 y (mean)	12–38 mo
Inclusion criteria	<16 y old, RAOM defined by ≥5 episodes of AOM over the past year or a diagnosis of COME defined as the presence of middle ear effusion in 1 or both ears for ≥3 mo, caregiver present, presentation to single otolaryngologist	12–36 mo at entry, bilateral COME or ROME for >3 mo as diagnosed by otoscopy, hearing loss of >20 dB in the better ear, tympanostomy tube insertion scheduled within 2–4 wk after diagnosis, Dutch speaking
Exclusion criteria	Presentation to physicians outside the University of Florida pediatric ORL clinic, previous ear surgery other than M&T, tubes already present, tympanic membrane perforation, non–English speaking	Tympanic membrane perforation, tubes already present, middle ear pathology other than otitis media, neurologic disorder

RCT = randomized controlled trial, POS = prospective outcomes study, TAIQOL = TNO-AZL Infant Quality of Life Instrument, COME = chronic otitis media with effusion, AOM = acute otitis media, RAOM = recurrent AOM, OME = otitis media with effusion, SD = standard deviation, SEM = standard error, CI = confidence interval, NS = not significant, NR = not reported, M&T = myringotomy and tubes, ROME = recurrent otitis media with effusion.

* Sample size: numbers shown for those that were initially recruited and those that (completed the trial). In Rosenfeld, 2000, 224 patients had valid change scores (defined by at least a 14-day interval between surveys) after surgery and 115 had valid change scores before and after surgery.

‡ Quality of life results reported as mean scores (SEM) for Rovers, 2001; change in mean scores (SD) for Rosenfeld, 2000; means scores (95% CI) for Richards, 2002; mean scores (SD) for Timmerman, 2003.

REFERENCES

1. Richards M, Giannoni C. Quality-of-life outcomes after surgical intervention for otitis media. Arch Otolaryngol Head Neck Surg 2002;128(7):776–782.
2. Rosenfeld RM, Bhaya MH, Bower CM, et al. Impact of tympanostomy tubes on child quality of life. Arch Otolaryngol Head Neck Surg 2000;126(5):585–592.
3. Rovers MM, Krabbe PF, Straatman H, Ingels K, van der Wilt GJ, Zielhuis GA. Randomised controlled trial of the effect of ventilation tubes (grommets) on quality of life at age 1–2 years [see comment]. Arch Dis Child 2001;84(1):45–49.
4. Timmerman AA, Anteunis LJ, Meesters CM. Response-shift bias and parent-reported quality of life in children with otitis media. Arch Otolaryngol Head Neck Surg 2003;129(9):987–991.
5. Campbell DT, Fiske DW. Convergent and discriminant validation by the multitrait-multimethod matrix. Psychol Bull 1959;56:81–105.
6. Trochim WM. Research Methods Knowledge Base. Cornell University; 2000.

7 Pediatric Otitis Media with Effusion

7.C.

Adenoidectomy versus no surgery: Impact on resolution, improvement, and audiometry

Grace Chan, Jennifer J. Shin, and Margaret Kenna

METHODS

A computerized PubMed search of MEDLINE 1966–July 2006 was performed. The medical subject headings "adenoidectomy" and "adenoids" were exploded and cross-referenced with those obtained by exploding the medical subject heading "otitis media with effusion." This search strategy yielded 255 trials, of which 30 were randomized controlled trials (RCTs). These articles were reviewed to identify those that met the following inclusion criteria: 1) patient population <18 years old with otitis media with effusion (OME), 2) intervention with adenoidectomy versus no intervention, 3) outcome measured in terms of otoscopic clearance, tympanometry, and audiometry. Articles randomizing children to multiple interventions were included if they reported a separate analysis between adenoidectomy and no-intervention groups. Bilateral myringotomies (with or without ventilation tubes) were considered to be distinct interventions and not included in this analysis. The bibliographies of the articles, which met these inclusion criteria, were manually checked to ensure no further relevant articles could be identified. This process yielded nine articles. The eight articles by Maw followed an open cohort (adding children as the study progressed), and reported results on this same cohort at incremental time points [1–8]. Furthermore, several articles were redundant. Maw (1983) [1] and Maw (1983) [2] were duplicate articles and were considered as a single study in this review. Maw (1985) [3], Maw (1985) [4], and Maw (1985) [5] were also duplicate articles and were considered as a single study. We presented the Maw studies separately at each incremental time point: 1983, 1985, 1988, 1993, 1994.

RESULTS

Outcome Measures. OME is defined as the presence of middle ear effusion in the absence of acute signs of infection. Often, the diagnosis is made with pneumatic otoscopy. Tympanometry and reflectometry are used as adjuncts. Maw (1983) [1,2] and Maw (1985) [3–5] measured an otoscopic clearance rate (the percentage of ears with otoscopic clearance of fluid). In the Maw studies, the terms "otoscopic clearance," "resolution rate," and "improvement rate" were used interchangeably. Maw (1988) [6], Maw (1993) [7], and Maw (1994) [8] were

more comprehensive. In addition to measuring otoscopic clearance, they also measured the mean audiometric hearing threshold [6–8]. Bulman (1984) [9] used only audiometry.

Potential Confounders. Resolution and improvement of OME may be influenced by other factors than the treatments proposed. All studies were RCTs, and thus all theoretically controlled for both measured and unmeasured confounders. Maw (1983) [1,2], Maw (1985) [3–5], Maw (1988) [6], and Maw (1993) [7] discussed effective randomization and found no significant differences between potential confounders such as the time of year, age, sex, and postnasal space airway measured on lateral radiograph. Maw (1994) [8] and Bulman (1984) [9] did not report the distribution of confounders between groups. Maw (1993) [7] reported several variables to have a significant effect on the duration of fluid in the ears and hearing loss: parental smoking, age at onset of hearing loss, duration of preoperative hearing loss. This study controlled these confounders in the regression analysis. It was not discussed whether or not these variables were significantly different between the adenoidectomy and no-surgery groups at the outset. The type of medical management may also influence results. Maw (1983) [1,2] and Maw (1985) [3–5] reported giving an antihistamine-sympathomimetic amine mixture to participants in the study. The Bulman study did not provide any medical treatments during the study [9]. Other studies did not report whether medications were used during the study [3–8]. Unmeasured confounders include the accuracy of caretakers' reporting, which was not discussed in any study. Another potential confounder was the duration of OME before surgery. Long follow-up times made it difficult to measure and standardize the duration of OME before surgery in all studies.

Study Designs. All studies were RCTs yielding the highest level of evidence. Given the surgical intervention, blinding of the patients and surgeons was not feasible. It would have been feasible to blind those who were collecting the outcome measures, such as otoscopic clearance, tympanometry, and audiometry, although none of the papers mentioned the blinding of investigators or data collectors. No report included the sample size needed to achieve adequate power *a priori*, but all studies identified a significant difference between groups in at least one parameter. Follow-up times ranged from 3 months to 10 years. Specifics regarding those lost to follow-up were not detailed in any of the studies. The attrition rate was not reported in Maw (1985) [3–5].

Highest Level of Evidence. All studies found adenoidectomies to have statistically significant benefits compared with no surgery. The absolute difference in the outcome of interest between the study and control group is known as the rate difference (RD). The number needed to treat (NNT) is number needed to treat in order for one child to achieve the outcome of interest. NNT is calculated by taking the reciprocal of RD.

Maw (1983) [1,2] and Maw (1985) [3–5] found significant resolution of OME after adenoidectomy compared with no surgery [1–5]. In the Maw (1983) and Maw (1985) reports, the RD in resolution of OME after 1 year of follow-up was −46% and −45%, respectively. For one child to have resolution of OME, two children need to be treated with adenoidectomy (NNT = 1/0.46). The more recent Maw reports found significant resolution of OME and tympanometric change in the group receiving adenoidectomy [6–8]. RDs in resolution of OME after 1 year of follow-up were similar to the earlier Maw studies. Maw (1993) conducted a survival analysis to examine the time until resolution of OME after adenoidectomy versus no surgery [7]. The log rank test of equality of survival between each pair of treatments was significant (p = 0.0001), indicating a difference between the two groups. Two studies found significant changes in tympanometry with RDs ranging from −25% to −33% [6, 8]. The NNT for one child to achieve tympanometry change is three to four children. Despite improvements in tympanometry, one study did not find a significant improvement in mean hearing [6]. Mean hearing improved significantly among those receiving adenoidectomy in the 1993 and 1994 Maw studies (p < 0.05, p < 0.04, respectively) [7,8]. The Maw articles were from the same cohort followed over time; therefore, their results may be biased toward their particular cohort, data collection methods, and outcome measures [1–8]. The Bulman study (1984) found adenoidectomy to be statistically beneficial only at one timepoint, 3 months postoperation, compared with no surgery. The study measured fewer outcomes and had a relatively smaller sample size compared with the Maw studies. Furthermore, Bulman et al. [9] did not use the same definition of OME. OME was defined as hearing loss secondary to

glue ear; however, their threshold of secondary hearing loss was at 10 dB. Most patients with "glue ear" have at least low-frequency hearing losses in the 30- to 40-dB range, with better hearing in the high frequencies. Otoscopy and tympanometry would be more supportive of actual OME.

Applicability. Based on the inclusion criteria for these trials, the results can be applied to those 2–11 years old with a diagnosis of OME by pneumatic otoscopy, tympanometry, and hearing loss by audiometry, considering that hearing loss was attributable to OME. All studies took place in England and may not be generalizable to other parts of the world where region-specific diagnoses and management of OME may alter the natural course of OME. In many of these studies, the more severe cases of OME were excluded from the analysis, such as those requiring additional surgical treatment. Therefore, the results may not be applicable to those children. Furthermore, there were children who were lost to follow-up or refused to participate in the study. These children may be different than those included in the study. There was a large dropout rate in the 1988 Maw study [6].

Morbidity/Complications. None of the studies reported the incidence of morbidity or complications.

CLINICAL SIGNIFICANCE AND FUTURE RESEARCH

There is level 1 evidence showing that surgical intervention improves the time to otoscopic clearance of OME, tympanometry peak conversions, and audiometric measures of hearing loss. However, the number of studies is limited and one study of small sample size found improvements only to occur at 3 months after surgery [9].

Further research is needed to examine the effect of adenoidectomy versus no surgery. Investigator-blind studies with power calculations to assess adequate sample sizes are needed. Studies should include information on compliance with the treatment protocol, the criteria for withdrawal from study, intention to treat analysis, and a discussion on the morbidity/complication of surgery. Furthermore, more robust statistical analyses are needed. Duration of fluid and hearing loss may be better assessed using Cox-proportional regressions to better account for time to event information. Further studies should research the baseline characteristics between those children who participate in OME clinical trials versus those who do not in order to determine the generalizability of these results.

Reference	Maw, 1983/Maw, 1983
Level (design)	1 (randomized controlled trial)
Sample size*	6 wk: 60 3 mo: 53 6 mo: 53 9 mo: 45 1 y: 60 (69)

	OUTCOMES
Outcome measure	Otoscopic clearance (% of ears in which fluid was no longer present by pneumatic otoscopy)
Adenoidectomy	6 wk: 39% 3 mo: 56% 6 mo: 64% 9 mo: 58% 1 y: 72%
No surgery	6 wk: 16% 3 mo: 22% 6 mo: 26% 9 mo: 19% 1 y: 26%
p Value	6 wk: NR 3 mo: <0.05 6 mo: <0.01 9 mo: <0.01 1 y: <0.001
Conclusion	Significantly more children with resolution of OME after adenoidectomy vs no surgery
Follow-up time	6 wk, 3/6/9 mo, 1 y

	STUDY DESIGN
Inclusion criteria	Bilateral middle ear effusions on 3 occasions during a 3-mo period, audiometric hearing losses in excess of 25 dB at 2 or more frequencies in each ear
Exclusion criteria	Type A tympanogram
Randomization effectiveness	Similar in seasonal time of year, age, sex, and postnasal space airway measured on lateral radiograph
Age	2–11 y
Masking	None
Adenoidectomy details	Curettage
Diagnostic criteria for OME	Pneumatic otoscopy by validated observer with compliance studies, tympanometry, acoustic reflex stimulation, and pure tone audiometry showing a hearing loss in excess of 25 dB
Management of OME/RAOM while in study	Antihistamine-sympathomimetic amine mixture
Compliance	NR
Criteria for withdrawal from study	NR
Intention to treat analysis	NR
Power	NR
Morbidity/complications	NR

OME = otitis media with effusion (vs RAOM = recurrent acute otitis media—do not include if inclusion criteria was just RAOM), NR = not reported.
* Sample size: numbers shown for those not lost to follow-up and those (initially recruited).

Reference	Maw, 1985/Maw, 1985/Maw, 1985
Level (design)	1 (randomized controlled trial)
Sample size*	NR (102)

OUTCOMES	
Outcome measure	Otoscopic clearance
Adenoidectomy	6 wk: 42% 3 mo: 52% 6 mo: 60% 9 mo: 56% 1 y: 72%
No surgery	6 wk: 19% 3 mo: 27% 6 mo: 25% 9 mo: 25% 1 y: 27%
p Value	6 wk: <0.05 3 mo: <0.05 6 mo: <0.01 9 mo: <0.01 1 y: <0.001
Conclusion	Significantly more children with resolution of OME after adenoidectomy vs no surgery
Follow-up time	6 wk, 3/6/9 mo, 1 y

STUDY DESIGN	
Inclusion criteria	Bilateral middle ear effusions on 3 occasions during a 3-mo period, audiometric hearing losses in excess of 25 dB at 2 or more frequencies in each ear
Exclusion criteria	Type A tympanogram
Randomization effectiveness	Similar in seasonal time of year, age, sex, and postnasal space airway measured on lateral radiograph
Age	2–11 y
Masking	None
Adenoidectomy details	Curettage
Diagnostic criteria for OME	Pneumatic otoscopy by validated observer with compliance studies, tympanometry, acoustic reflex stimulation, and pure tone audiometry showing a hearing loss in excess of 25 dB
Management of OME/ RAOM while in study	Antihistamine-sympathomimetic amine mixture
Compliance	NR
Criteria for withdrawal from study	NR
Intention to treat analysis	NR
Power	NR
Morbidity/ complications	NR

OME = otitis media with effusion (vs RAOM = recurrent acute otitis media—do not include if inclusion criteria was just RAOM), NR = not reported.
* Sample size: numbers shown for those not lost to follow-up and those (initially recruited).

THE EVIDENCE CONDENSED: Adenoidectomy versus no intervention for otitis media with effusion

Reference	Maw, 1988		
Level (design)	1 (randomized controlled trial)		
Sample size*	1 y: 120 2 y: 111 3 y: 69 (145)		

	OUTCOMES		
Outcome measure	Otoscopic clearance†	Tympanometry peak conversion (change of type B tympanogram to type A, C1, or C2)†	Mean hearing threshold (average hearing threshold as measured by pure tone audiometry)†
Adenoidectomy	1 y: 62% 2 y: 65% 3 y: 70%	51% 54% 62%	20.9 dB 19.1 dB 18.9 dB
No surgery	1 y: 20% 2 y: 32% 3 y: 59%	26% 26% 50%	28 dB 26.5 dB 22.1 dB
p Value	There are no reported "p values"; however, the results state that with the exception of adenoidectomy at 3 y, the clearance and tympanometry change attributable to adenoidectomy was significant compared with the no-surgery group. At all follow-up times, hearing gain is significantly better in the surgery vs the no-surgery group		
Conclusion	Significantly better otoscopic clearance and tympanometry change with adenoidectomy as compared with no surgery. No difference in audiometry		
Follow-up time	1, 2, 3 y		

	STUDY DESIGN		
Inclusion criteria	Bilateral middle ear effusions on 3 occasions during a 3-mo period, audiometric hearing losses in excess of 25 dB at 2 or more frequencies in each ear		
Exclusion criteria	Type A tympanogram, spontaneous resolution of OME during preoperative period		
Randomization effectiveness	Similar in seasonal time of year, age, sex, and postnasal space airway measured on lateral radiograph		
Age	2–9 y		
Masking	None		
Adenoidectomy details	NR		
Diagnostic criteria for OME	Pneumatic otoscopy by validated observer with compliance studies, tympanometry, acoustic reflex stimulation, and pure tone audiometry showing a hearing loss in excess of 25 dB		
Management of OME/ RAOM while in study	NR		
Compliance	NR		
Criteria for withdrawal from study	NR		
Intention to treat analysis	NR		
Power	NR		
Morbidity/ complications	NR		

OME = otitis media with effusion (vs RAOM = recurrent acute otitis media—do not include if inclusion criteria was just RAOM), NR = not reported.
* Sample size: numbers shown for those not lost to follow-up and those (initially recruited).
† Extrapolated from reported figures.

Reference	Maw, 1993		
Level (design)	1 (randomized controlled trial)		
Sample size*	NR (160) with otoscopy data NR (134) with tympanometry and audiometry data 59 (213)†		
OUTCOMES			
Outcome measure	Otoscopic clearance	Tympanometry peak conversion	Mean hearing threshold
Adenoidectomy	NR	NR	1 y: 12.5 dB 4 y: 16.9 dB 10 y: 18.4 dB
No surgery	NR	NR	1 y: 4.9 dB 4 y: 13.6 dB 10 y: 16.5 dB
p Value	Log rank p = 0.0001	Log rank p = 0.0001	p < 0.05 on at least 4 of 6 follow-ups
Conclusion	Statistically significant improvements in otoscopic clearance and tympanometric change with adenoidectomy alone vs no surgery. Audiometric hearing thresholds improved with fluid resolution		
Follow-up time	10 y		
STUDY DESIGN			
Inclusion criteria	Bilateral middle ear effusions on 3 occasions during a 3-mo period, audiometric hearing losses in excess of 25 dB at 2 or more frequencies in each ear		
Exclusion criteria	Type A tympanogram		
Randomization effectiveness	Similar in seasonal time of year, age, sex, and postnasal space airway measured on lateral radiograph		
Age	2–9 y		
Masking	None		
Adenoidectomy details	NR		
Diagnostic criteria for OME	Pneumatic otoscopy and excess of 25-dB hearing loss at 1 or more frequencies		
Management of OME/RAOM while in study	NR		
Compliance	NR		
Criteria for withdrawal from study	Children whose ears contained fluid at final assessment or at last assessment before lost to follow-up, children who developed severe obstructive symptoms from enlargement of adenoids or tonsils, children who required additional surgery in unoperated ear, severe problems in operated ear, moved or poor attendance		
Intention to treat analysis	Not done		
Power	Not done		
Morbidity/ complications	NR		

NR = not reported, SD = standard deviation, preop = preoperative, postop = postoperative, OME = otitis media with effusion (vs RAOM = recurrent acute otitis media.
* Sample size: numbers shown for those not lost to follow-up and those (initially recruited).
† Assessment of first 150 cases showed that tonsillectomy had no additional benefit compared with adenoidectomy alone. Children were no longer randomized to adenotonsillectomy group. For the analysis, children who received adenotonsillectomy were grouped with those receiving adenoidectomy alone.

Reference	Maw, 1994			Bulman, 1984
Level (design)	1 (randomized controlled trial)			1 (randomized controlled trial)
Sample size*	37 (170)			14 (30)
OUTCOMES				
Outcome measure	Otoscopic clearance	Tympanometry peak conversion	Mean hearing threshold	Pure tone audiometry
Adenoidectomy	1 y: 63.2% 4 y: 85.1% 10 y: 93.8%	54.4% 79.4% 86.7%	21.3 dB 17.4 dB 14.6 dB	Average audiometric value (SD): preop: 10.4 (3.9) postop: 10.1(4.4) 3 mo: 6.6 (3.2) 6 mo: 7.0 (4.8)
No surgery	1 y: 21.5% 4 y: 59.3% 10 y: 95.2%	21.1% 44.1% 79.0%	28.6 dB 20.0 dB 16.6 dB	Average audiometric value (SD): preop: 12.1 (3.8) postop: 8.8 (6.1) 3 mo: 10.0 (5.3) 6 mo: 10.2 (4.8)
p Value	$p < 0.0001$, first 4 y	$p < 0.04$, first 5 y	$p < 0.02$, first 4 y	preop: NS postop: NS 3 mo: $p < 0.05$ 6 mo: NS
Conclusion	Adenoidectomy significantly improved otoscopic clearance and the mean hearing threshold for the first 4 y and tympanometry for the first 5 y after operation compared with no surgery			Adenoidectomy was statistically beneficial compared with no surgery only at 3 mo postop
Follow-up time	Annually for 5 y, 2 further occasions during subsequent 5-y period			3 mo, 6 mo, 2 y
STUDY DESIGN				
Inclusion criteria	Bilateral middle ear effusions on 3 occasions during a 3-mo period, audiometric hearing losses in excess of 25 dB at 2 or more frequencies in each ear			Hearing loss secondary to glue ear
Exclusion criteria	Type A tympanogram			Recurrent earache, recurrent febrile illness, symptoms of nasal obstruction
Randomization effectiveness	NR			NR
Age	3–9 y			4–9 y
Masking	None			None
Adenoidectomy details	NR			NR
Diagnostic criteria for OME	Pneumatic otoscopy and excess of 25-dB hearing loss at 1 or more frequencies			NR
Management of OME/RAOM while in study	NR			No medical management
Compliance	NR			NR
Criteria for withdrawal from study	Further treatment needed such as adenoidectomy, tonsillectomy, myringotomy or grommet insertion in unoperated ear			Further surgical treatment
Intention to treat analysis	NR			NR
Power	NR			NR
Morbidity/ complications	NR			NR

NR = not reported, SD = standard deviation, preop = preoperative, postop = postoperative, OME = otitis media with effusion (vs RAOM = recurrent acute otitis media, NS = not significant.
* Sample size: numbers shown for those not lost to follow-up and those (initially recruited).

REFERENCES

1. Maw AR. Chronic otitis media with effusion and adenotonsillectomy—a prospective randomized controlled study. Int J Pediatr Otorhinolaryngol 1983;6(3):239–246.

2. Maw AR. Chronic otitis media with effusion (glue ear) and adenotonsillectomy: prospective randomised controlled study. Br Med J (Clin Res Ed) 1983;287(6405):1586–1588.

3. Maw AR. Factors affecting adenoidectomy for otitis media with effusion (glue ear). J R Soc Med 1985;78(12):1014–1018.

4. Maw AR. Age and adenoid size in relation to adenoidectomy in otitis media with effusion. Am J Otolaryngol 1985;6(3):245–248.

5. Maw AR. The long-term effect of adenoidectomy on established otitis media with effusion in children. Auris Nasus Larynx 1985;12(Suppl 1):S234–236.

6. Maw AR, Parker A. Surgery of the tonsils and adenoids in relation to secretory otitis media in children. Acta Otolaryngol Suppl 1988;454:202–207.

7. Maw AR, Bawden R, O'Keefe L, Gurr P. Does the type of middle ear aspirate have any prognostic significance in otitis media with effusion in children? Clin Otolaryngol Allied Sci 1993;18(5):396–399.

8. Maw AR, Bawden R. The long-term outcome of secretory otitis media in children and the effects of surgical treatment: a ten year study. Acta Otorhinolaryngol Belg 1994;48(4):317–324.

9. Bulman CH, Brook SJ, Berry MG. A prospective randomized trial of adenoidectomy vs grommet insertion in the treatment of glue ear. Clin Otolaryngol Allied Sci 1984;9(2):67–75.

7 Pediatric Otitis Media with Effusion

7.D.

Adenoidectomy versus tube placement: Impact on resolution, improvement, and audiometry

Grace Chan, Jennifer J. Shin, and Margaret Kenna

METHODS

A computerized PubMed search of MEDLINE 1966–July 2006 was performed. The medical subject headings "adenoidectomy" and "adenoids" were exploded and cross-referenced with those obtained by exploding the medical subject heading "otitis media with effusion." This search strategy yielded 255 trials, of which 30 were randomized controlled trials (RCTs). These articles were reviewed to identify those that met the following inclusion criteria: 1) patient population <18 years old with otitis media with effusion (OME), 2) intervention with adenoidectomy versus tubes, and 3) outcome measured in terms of otoscopic clearance, tympanometry, and audiometry. Articles randomizing children to receive bilateral myringotomies (without ventilation tubes) were excluded. Articles focusing on children with recurrent acute otitis media were also excluded. The bibliographies of the articles that met these inclusion criteria were manually checked to ensure no further relevant articles could be identified. This process yielded two unique RCTs, Maw (1993) [1] and Bulman (1984) [2], which are discussed in detail below.

RESULTS

Outcome Measures. The diagnosis of OME is often made by pneumatic otoscopy (presence of effusion in the absence of signs of acute inflammation), with tympanometry and reflectometry used as adjuncts. Outcome measures for the Maw study [1] included otoscopic clearance rate, or the percentage of ears with otoscopic clearance of fluid, the percentage of ears with tympanometry peak conversion, and the mean audiometric hearing threshold. Bulman [2] used only audiometry.

Potential Confounders. Both studies were randomized, a process that theoretically can distribute potential confounders equally between compared groups. To ensure that the groups receiving adenoidectomy and tubes were similar across other factors, Maw [1] analyzed the effectiveness of randomization and reported no significant differences in the seasonal time of year enrolled, age, sex, and postnasal space airway measured on lateral radiograph. Bulman [2] did not report on any potential pretreatment differences between the two groups. Medical management during the study could also have influenced

the outcome. If, however, medicine was given equitably to both groups and if there was no interaction between the medicine and intervention, the effect of the medication would be nondifferential between the two groups. Maw did not report whether or not medicine was given during the study [1]. Bulman's protocol did not include medical management [2]. There was no report of unmeasured confounders such as the accuracy of caretakers' reporting in either study.

Study Designs. Both studies were RCTs (level 1) which compared adenoidectomy alone to tubes alone. The Maw study [1] had stricter inclusion criteria and a longer follow-up time of 12 years compared with the Bulman study [2], with a follow-up time of 2 years. Neither study could be double blinded because both interventions were surgical. Masking of investigators and examiners during the collection of outcome measures was not done in either study. *A priori* calculations of power were not reported, so it is difficult to put their results and sample sizes in perspective. Such power calculations are especially important when nonsignificant differences are found between groups. The Maw study did not report an attrition rate.

Highest Level of Evidence. The only significant finding was an improvement in average audiometry values immediately postoperatively in the tubes versus the adenoidectomy group in the Bulman study [2]. This audiometric benefit of tubes disappeared over time. Although the Maw study did not yield statistically significantly different results, it suggested a trend toward a benefit with adenoidectomy. More specifically, Maw conducted a survival analysis to look at the time until resolution of OME after adenoidectomy versus tubes [1]. The relative hazard of otoscopic clearance was 1.14 (95% confidence interval 0.8–1.62) suggesting an estimated 14% increase in otoscopic clearance for children receiving adenoidectomy compared with patients receiving tubes. The relative hazard was not significant (p = 0.5). With only two studies of unspecified power using different outcome measures suggesting different results, conclusions must be drawn cautiously.

Applicability. The results of these studies may be applicable to children 4–9 years old with a diagnosis of OME. However, given the exclusion of severe OME cases, and high attrition rates, these two studies may not be representative of the entire span of the general pediatric population with OME.

Morbidity/Complications. Neither study reported the incidence of morbidity or complications.

CLINICAL SIGNIFICANCE AND FUTURE RESEARCH

Based on the available data, there were no clinically significant differences in OME outcomes after adenoidectomy or tubes. More studies with sample sizes based on clear power calculations and with masking of investigators are needed to confirm these results. At this time, it is difficult to definitively conclude that there is equal benefit from adenoidectomies and tubes based on the above studies. Should this conclusion be true, the clinical implications are great.

Further research would be needed to determine differences in morbidity, complications, comfort, and cost between the two interventions. Although there is no difference in the resolution, improvement, and audiometry between adenoidectomy and tubes, differences in other factors may highlight an overall better method. Additional studies should measure cost, quality of life, and morbidity outcomes in addition to clinical outcomes.

THE EVIDENCE CONDENSED: Adenoidectomy versus tubes for otitis media with effusion

Reference	Maw, 1993		
Level (design)	1 (randomized controlled trial)		
Sample size*	NR (167) with otoscopy data NR (164) with tympanometry and audiometry data 59 (213)†		
OUTCOMES			
Outcome measure	Otoscopic clearance	Tympanometry peak conversion	Mean hearing threshold (dBs)
Adenoidectomy	Hazard ratio (adenoidectomy vs no surgery) = 1.14, 95% CI 0.8–1.62	NR	1 y: 12.5 4 y: 16.9 10 y: 18.4
Tube only	Hazard ratio (reference group) = 1	NR	1 y: 13.1 4 y: 14.1 10 y: 16.0
p Value	Log rank test of equality p = 0.25	Log rank p = 0.21	NR
Conclusion	There was no significant difference overall between adenoidectomy only and ventilation tubes alone		
Follow-up time	12 y		
STUDY DESIGN			
Inclusion criteria	Bilateral middle ear effusions on 3 occasions during a 3-mo period, audiometric hearing losses in excess of 25 dB at 2 or more frequencies in each ear		
Exclusion criteria	Type A tympanogram		
Randomization effectiveness	Similar in seasonal time of year, age, sex, and postnasal space airway measured on lateral radiograph		
Age	2–9 y		
Masking	None		
Adenoidectomy details	NR		
Diagnostic criteria for OME	Pneumatic otoscopy and excess of 25-dB hearing loss at one or more frequencies		
Management of OME/ RAOM while in study	NR		
Compliance	NR		
Criteria for withdrawal from study	Children whose ears contained fluid at final assessment or at last assessment before lost to follow-up, children who developed severe obstructive symptoms from enlargement of adenoids or tonsils, children who required additional surgery in unoperated ear, severe problems in operated ear, moved or poor attendance		
Intention to treat analysis	Not done		
Power	Not done		
Morbidity/ complications	NR		

NR = not reported, SD = standard deviation, CI = confidence interval, NS = not significant, preop = preoperative, postop = postoperative, OME = otitis media with effusion (vs RAOM = recurrent acute otitis media—don't include if inclusion criteria was just RAOM).
* Sample size: numbers shown for those not lost to follow-up and those (initially recruited).
† (Assessment of first 150 cases showed that tonsillectomy had no additional benefit compared with adenoidectomy alone. Children were no longer randomized to adenotonsillectomy group. For the analysis, children who received adenotonsillectomy were grouped with those receiving adenoidectomy alone).

Reference	Bulman, 1984
Level (design)	1 (randomized controlled trial)
Sample size*	14 (30)

OUTCOMES	
Outcome measure	Pure tone audiometry
Adenoidectomy	Average audiometric value (SD): preop: 10.4 (3.9) postop: 10.1 (4.4) 3 mo: 6.6 (3.2) 6 mo: 7.0 (4.8)
Tube only	Average audiometric value (SD): preop: 12.1 (3.8) postop: 5.1 (4.0) 3 mo: 6.4 (3.2) 6 mo: 7.9 (4.9)
p Value	preop: NS postop: $p < 0.05$ 3 mo: NS 6 mo: NS
Conclusion	Tubes significantly improved the average audiometric value compared with adenoidectomies immediately postoperation. There was no significant difference between the 2 groups 3 mo postoperation
Follow-up time	2 y

STUDY DESIGN	
Inclusion criteria	Hearing loss secondary to glue ear
Exclusion criteria	Recurrent earache, recurrent febrile illness, symptoms of nasal obstruction
Randomization effectiveness	NR
Age	4–9 y
Masking	None
Adenoidectomy details	NR
Diagnostic criteria for OME	NR
Management of OME/ RAOM while in study	No medical management
Compliance	NR
Criteria for withdrawal from study	Further surgical treatment
Intention to treat analysis	NR
Power	NR
Morbidity/ complications	NR

NR = not reported, SD = standard deviation, CI = confidence interval, NS = not significant, preop = preoperative, postop = postoperative, OME = otitis media with effusion (vs RAOM = recurrent acute otitis media.
* Sample size: numbers shown for those not lost to follow-up and those (initially recruited).

REFERENCES

1. Maw AR, Bawden R, O'Keefe L, Gurr P. Does the type of middle ear aspirate have any prognostic significance in otitis media with effusion in children? Clin Otolaryngol Allied Sci 1993;18(5):396–399.
2. Bulman CH, Brook SJ, Berry MG. A prospective randomized trial of adenoidectomy vs grommet insertion in the treatment of glue ear. Clin Otolaryngol Allied Sci 1984;9(2): 67–75.

7 Pediatric Otitis Media with Effusion

7.E.

Adenoidectomy with tube placement versus tubes alone: Impact on resolution, improvement, and audiometry

Grace Chan, Jennifer J. Shin, and Margaret Kenna

METHODS

A computerized PubMed search of MEDLINE 1966–July 2006 was performed. The medical subject headings "adenoidectomy" and "adenoids" were exploded and cross-referenced with those obtained by exploding the medical subject heading "otitis media with effusion." This search strategy yielded 255 trials, of which 30 were randomized controlled trials (RCTs). These articles were reviewed to identify those that met the following inclusion criteria: 1) patient population <18 years old with otitis media with effusion (OME), 2) intervention with adenoidectomy with tubes versus tubes alone, and 3) outcome measured in terms of otoscopic clearance, tympanometry, and audiometry. Articles randomizing children to receive bilateral myringotomies (without ventilation tubes) were excluded. The bibliographies of the articles meeting the inclusion criteria were manually checked to ensure no further relevant articles could be identified. This process yielded four articles. Gates (1987) [1] and Gates (1989) [2] reported results from the same study. The three unique RCTs, Maw (1993) [3], Gates (1987, 1989) [1, 2], and Black (1986) [4], are discussed in detail below.

RESULTS

Outcome Measures. Each study used different outcome measures to assess the improvement of OME. The study by Maw [3] measured otoscopic clearance, tympanometry changes, and mean audiometric hearing thresholds. The second trial (Gates) [1, 2] measured time with effusion, time with abnormal hearing, time to first recurrence of effusion, and the number of surgical re-treatments needed. The Black [4] study measured mean hearing threshold, tympanometry changes, and parental opinion.

Potential Confounders. Studies were all RCTs which should theoretically distribute confounding variables equally between the two groups. All studies discussed randomization effectiveness and found no significant differences between potential confounders, except the study by Black, which had a disproportionate number of males to females in the nonadenoidectomy group [4]. The study by Gates examined an extensive list of possible confounders, including ethnicity, sex, age, prior treat-

ment with tubes, family income, laterality of effusion at surgery, referral source, and father's education [1, 2]. The study also detailed a course of medical management for patients during the study. The other two studies did not comment on the use of medications [3, 4]. Unmeasured confounders, such as the accuracy of caretakers' reporting, were not discussed in any study.

Study Designs. All three studies were RCTs comparing results after adenoidectomy with tubes versus tubes alone. Two studies attempted to address potential expectation biases through the use of masking. Although the surgeons, patients, and their parents were aware of the intervention received, both Gates and Black blinded the examiners to the type of surgery performed to avoid investigator bias [1, 2, 4]. The Maw study did not report any masking, and so differential results should be considered with more caution. Two studies also attempted to account for any biases that might be introduced by patients who were lost to follow-up. The Black study identified reasons for discontinuation such as missed appointments or the need for further surgery [4]. Gates analyzed differences between those who dropped out and those who continued in the study and found no differences in the demographic characteristics, distribution, and rate of discontinuation between the two treatment groups. The authors concluded that there was no association between treatment group and loss to follow-up [1, 2]. Such an analysis assures the reader that the results have not been skewed because a particularly affected or unaffected group of subjects did not complete the study. The Maw study did not present the attrition rate. The Black study reported a power analysis to determine the sample size needed in order to achieve a significant difference between treatment groups. The study attained statistical significance in three of four outcomes without reaching the predetermined sample size. The other studies did not include an *a priori* power analysis, but they identified a significant difference between groups in at least one parameter. Follow-up times ranged from 1 to 12 years.

Highest Level of Evidence. All three studies found adenoidectomy with tubes to have statistically significant benefits compared with tubes alone with respect to OME. Maw reported improvements in the time to otoscopic clearance and tympanometric change in a survival analysis. There was an estimated 218% increase in oto-scopic clearance (hazard ratio = 2.18, 95% confidence interval 1.53–3.10) for children receiving adenoidectomy with tubes versus children with tubes alone. The two survival curves for tympanometry peak conversion were statistically different (log rank test p = 0.0002) [3]. Gates reported a decrease in the mean number of visits by 26%, decrease in time with abnormal hearing in worse ear by 26%, and a decrease in number of surgical re-treatments by 53%, for children with adenoidectomy with tubes versus tubes alone [1, 2]. Black reported better hearing levels and tympanometry but only at 6 weeks of follow-up; otherwise there was no difference between groups [4].

Applicability. Based on the inclusion and exclusion criteria for these studies, the results can be applied to children with a diagnosis of OME between 4–9 years old, with no history of operations involving their tonsils, adenoids, or ears. Maw [1] included children 2–9 years old, but because the Gates study began at age 4, there was not enough data to include children between the ages of 2–4.

Morbidity/Complications. None of the studies reported the incidence of morbidity or complications.

CLINICAL SIGNIFICANCE AND FUTURE RESEARCH

There is level 1 evidence showing that surgical intervention with both adenoidectomy and tubes improves OME outcomes compared with tubes only. These studies, particularly the Gates and Black studies, were well designed and accounted for those who were lost to follow-up and expectation biases (researchers' and evaluators' knowledge of the randomization groups influencing the interpretation of data). The Black study only found significant beneficial results at 6 weeks follow-up, however the sample size in Black's study was relatively smaller than the other studies, limiting its power.

Future studies should investigate the benefits versus the risks of conducting adenoidectomy with tubes rather than tubes only. Significant improvements in adenoidectomy with tubes would only be valid if its associated morbidity and complications are minimal compared with that of tubes alone. Additional studies are needed to measure morbidity outcomes in addition to outcomes of efficacy.

Reference	Maw, 1993		
Level (design)	1 (randomized controlled trial)		
Sample size*	NR (179) with otoscopy data NR (157) with tympanometry and audiometry data 59 (213)†		
OUTCOMES			
Outcome measure	Otoscopic clearance	Tympanometry peak conversion	Mean hearing threshold (dB)
Adenoidectomy + tubes	Hazard ratio (adenoidectomy + tubes vs tubes alone) = 2.18, 95% CI 1.53–3.10	NR	1 y: 14.12 4 y: 15.53 10 y: 18.10
Tubes alone	Hazard ratio (reference group) = 1	NR	1 y: 13.1 4 y: 14.1 10 y: 16.0
p Value	Log rank test p = 0.0001	Log rank test p = 0.0002	NR
Conclusion	Statistically significant improvements in otoscopic clearance and tympanometric change with adenoidectomy and tubes vs tubes alone		
Follow-up time	12 y		
STUDY DESIGN			
Inclusion criteria	Bilateral middle ear effusions on 3 occasions during a 3-mo period, audiometric hearing losses in excess of 25 dB at 2 or more frequencies in each ear		
Exclusion criteria	Type A tympanogram		
Randomization effectiveness	Similar seasonal time of year, age, sex, and postnasal space airway measured on lateral radiograph		
Age	2–9 y		
Masking	None		
Adenoidectomy details	NR		
Diagnostic criteria for OME	Pneumatic otoscopy and excess of 25-dB hearing loss at one or more frequencies		
Management of OME/RAOM while in study	NR		
Compliance	NR		
Criteria for withdrawal from study	Children whose ears contained fluid at final assessment or at last assessment before lost to follow-up, children who developed severe obstructive symptoms from enlargement of adenoids or tonsils, children who required additional surgery in unoperated ear, severe problems in operated ear, moved or poor attendance		
Intention to treat analysis	NR		
Power	NR		
Morbidity/ complications	NR		

OME = otitis media with effusion (vs RAOM = recurrent acute otitis media—don't include if inclusion criteria was just RAOM), CI = confidence interval, NS = not significant, NR = not reported, preop = preoperative, postop = postoperative.
* Sample size: numbers shown for those not lost to follow-up and those (initially recruited).
† Days to first recurrence (med ± SD).

THE EVIDENCE CONDENSED: Adenoidectomy plus tubes versus tubes alone for otitis media with effusion

Reference	Gates, 1987/Gates, 1989			
Level (design)	1 (randomized controlled trial)			
Sample size*	208 (300)			

OUTCOMES				
Outcome measure	Time with effusion‡	Time with abnormal hearing ≥20 dB‡	Time to first recurrence of effusion†	No. of surgical re-treatments
Adenoidectomy + tubes	0.258 ± 0.212	Better ear 0.065 ± 0.116 Worse ear 0.224 ± 0.221	240 ± 22	17
Tube only	0.349 ± 0.235	Better ear: 0.101 ± 0.141 Worse ear: 0.304 ± 0.227	222 ± 11	36
p Value	$p = 0.0097$	Better ear: $p = 0.1628$ (no difference) Worse ear: $p = 0.0093$ (significant improvement)	$p = 0.2314$	$p = 0.007$
Conclusion	Time spent with chronic effusion, time with hearing loss in worse ear, and number of surgical re-treatments was significantly reduced in those receiving adenoidectomy with tubes versus tubes alone			
Follow-up time	2 y (18 visits)			

STUDY DESIGN				
Inclusion criteria	Presence of chronic effusion based on pneumatoscopic and tympanometric findings. Positive fluid score was given to any ear with "abnormal" pneumatoscopic results (hypomobile, immobile, or air-fluid level) or the combination of "indeterminate" otoscopic results (retracted tympanic membrane with good outward mobility) and tympanogram types 6, 9, 13, 14, 15			
Exclusion criteria	History of tonsil or adenoid operations, tympanostomy tube placement (within 2 y), cleft palate, major chronic illness, those requiring daily medication, other otologic diagnoses or those with advanced or irreversible structural changes of the tympanum, surgical contraindications			
Randomization effectiveness	Comparable across groups of ethnicity, sex, age, prior treatment with tubes, 36 other selected variables			
Age	4–8 y			
Masking	Examiners and investigators blinded			
Adenoidectomy details	Curettage			
Diagnostic criteria for OME	Pneumatoscopic and tympanometric findings			
Management of OME/RAOM while in study	10-d course of fixed combination erythromycin ethyl succinate and sulfisoxazole, 30-d course of decongestant pseudoephedrine hydrochloride			
Compliance	6% refused operation 15% lost to follow-up			
Criteria for withdrawal from study	Cleared effusion before operation			
Intention to treat analysis	Results reported with patient's data ascribed to assigned treatment group, not by treatment received			
Power	NR			
Morbidity/ complications	NR			

OME = otitis media with effusion (vs RAOM = recurrent acute otitis media—don't include if inclusion criteria was just RAOM), CI = confidence interval, NS = not significant, NR = not reported, preop = preoperative, postop = postoperative.
* Sample size: numbers shown for those not lost to follow-up and those (initially recruited).
† Days to first recurrence (med ± SD).
‡ Time = mean no. of visits ± SD.

Reference	Black, 1986		
Level (design)	1 (randomized controlled trial)		
Sample size*	88 (100)		

OUTCOMES			
Outcome Measure	Mean hearing level (SE) (dBs)	Impedance tympanometry % with abnormal tympanometry	Parental opinion % parents with unfavorable opinion
Adenoidectomy + tubes	Preop: 27.9 (1.04) 6 wk: 19.0 (1.01) 6 mo: 19.8 (1.24) 1 y: 21.9 (1.25)	Preop: 89% 6 wk: 54%	Preop: 100% 6 wk: 22% 6 mo: 21%
Tube only	Preop: 29.1 (1.14) 6 wk: 23.0 (1.29) 6 mo: 22.2 (1.23) 1 y: 22.6 (1.38)	Preop: 81% 6 wk: 84%	Preop: 100% 6 wk: 34% 6 mo: 42%
p Value	Preop: NS 6 wk: $p < 0.05$ 6 mo: NS 1 y: NS	Preop: NS 6 wk: $p < 0.05$ 6 mo: NS 1 y: NS	Preop: NS 6 wk: NS 6 mo: $p < 0.05$ 1 y: NS
Conclusion	There were significantly better hearing levels and tympanometry with adenoidectomy with tubes, but only at 6 wk follow-up. Otherwise there was no difference between groups		
Follow-up time	1 y		

STUDY DESIGN			
Inclusion criteria	Children admitted for surgery for bilateral glue ear (serous and secretory otitis media); OME		
Exclusion criteria	Children who previously underwent operations involving either their tonsils, adenoids, or ears; those with sensorineural deafness; and those additional conditions for surgery other than glue ear		
Randomization effectiveness	Similar age, social class, preoperative histories. Different distribution by sex: adenoidectomy equal number of males and females, nonadenoidectomy 2:1 male to female ratio		
Age	4–9 y		
Masking	Examiners blinded		
Adenoidectomy details	NR		
Diagnostic criteria for OME	NR		
Management of OME/RAOM while in study	NR		
Compliance	12% lost to follow-up		
Criteria for withdrawal from study	Children who had or were awaiting further surgery for glue ear		
Intention to treat analysis	NR		
Power	95% power for final study with 200 children. Power for current study not reported		
Morbidity/ Complications	NR		

OME = otitis media with effusion (vs RAOM = recurrent acute otitis media), CI = confidence interval, NS = not significant, NR = not reported, preop = preoperative, postop = postoperative.
* Sample size: numbers shown for those not lost to follow-up and those (initially recruited).

REFERENCES

1. Gates GA, Avery CA, Prihoda TJ, Cooper JC Jr. Effectiveness of adenoidectomy and tympanostomy tubes in the treatment of chronic otitis media with effusion. N Engl J Med 1987;317(23):1444–1451.
2. Gates GA, Avery CA, Cooper JC Jr, Prihoda TJ. Chronic secretory otitis media: effects of surgical management. Ann Otol Rhinol Laryngol Suppl 1989;138:2–32.
3. Maw AR, Bawden R, O'Keefe L, Gurr P. Does the type of middle ear aspirate have any prognostic significance in otitis media with effusion in children? Clin Otolaryngol Allied Sci 1993;18(5):396–399.
4. Black N, Crowther J, Freeland A. The effectiveness of adenoidectomy in the treatment of glue ear: a randomized controlled trial. Clin Otolaryngol Allied Sci 1986;11(3):149–155.

8 Pediatric Sinusitis

8.A.

Antibiotics/conservative treatment versus control for pediatric nonacute sinusitis: Impact on post-treatment clinical examination and imaging results

Manali Amin and Mark Volk

METHODS

A computerized PubMed search of MEDLINE 1966–January 2006 was performed. Articles mapping to the exploded medical subject heading or keyword "sinusitis" were cross-referenced with those mapping to the text words (all fields) "chronic," "recurrent," or "persistent." The resulting articles were then cross-referenced with those mapping to the medical subject headings "antibacterial agents," "clindamycin," "fluoroquinolones," "macrolides," or "lactams," as well as the medical subject headings "child," "infant," "adolescent" or the text word "pediatric." This search process yielded 208 articles. These articles were then reviewed to identify those that met the following inclusion criteria: 1) pediatric patient population between ages 0 and 18 years old with nonacute sinusitis, 2) prospective intervention with antibiotic versus placebo, 3) outcome measured in terms of patient history, examination findings and/or X-ray examination. Articles were excluded if they focused on adults or patients with cystic fibrosis and other systemic diseases. This method yielded four articles. The bibliographies of the articles that met these inclusion criteria were manually checked to ensure no further relevant articles could be identified. This process yielded no additional articles.

RESULTS

Outcome Measures. None of these investigations utilized a reproducible, objective set of diagnostic criteria for evaluating chronic rhinosinusitis. However, no such widely accepted standardized measurement currently exists. All studies measured outcomes using interval history and physical examinations. Plain sinus radiographs were used in three [1–3]. Otten 1994 used cultures and Dohlman used nasal smears to help assess patient outcomes. One study [4] included asthma symptoms and pulmonary function testing before and after treatment.

There were a number of problems with these various measurements. The history and physical examination criteria were not standardized; they were subjective and differed between studies. Additionally, the established reliability of using plain sinus films in diagnosing sinus disease in children is lacking. Similarly, the use of nasal cultures and nasal smears has not been correlated with chronic sinus disease in children.

Potential Confounders. The Otten 1994 study utilized four different otolaryngology practices. There was no control for the multiple examiners involved. The Tsao study was not blinded and therefore subject to potential bias in terms of whether a patient reported improvement. However, as objective measures (FEV_1 and PC_{20}) were also used to study outcome, the potential bias in overall outcome was limited. Although subjects in this study were not randomized, a subject's assignment to a particular group was sequential based on their time of presentation. Therefore, clinical severity of disease would not be expected to be significantly different among the two study groups and the one asthmatic control group.

Study Designs. Three of the studies were randomized, double-blinded, control trials (level 1) [1–3]. Efficacy of randomization was demonstrated in two of the studies with respect to the age, sex, and clinical disease as determined by symptoms [1] or radiographs [3]. The third study did not comment on the effectiveness of randomization. The follow-up time in these three studies was at minimum 3 weeks and up to 26 weeks after initiation of treatment. In each study, the follow-up visit corresponded to the length of treatment and was appropriate for determining whether treatment was effective.

The fourth study [4] to analyze the effectiveness of antibiotics and conservative measures in the treatment of nonacute sinusitis was an open-label study and did not have randomization (level 2). Patients were sequentially assigned to one treatment group or another depending on their time of presentation to the clinic. Follow-up in this study was at 6 and 12 weeks which corresponded to the midpoint and end of the study. Neither patients nor the investigator were blinded to the treatment which could potentially introduce bias as stated in the previous section.

Highest Level of Evidence. The three level 1 studies all demonstrated that antibiotics were no more effective in the treatment of pediatric nonacute rhinosinusitis than placebo. A negative result, however, must be viewed in the context of the power of the study (i.e., the likelihood that it has the statistical strength to demonstrate a difference if a difference truly exists). The first study reported that it had 80% power to determine a 25%–30% difference between groups, whereas the other two randomized controlled trials (RCTs) did not comment on their power. To establish a study with 90% power to determine a 10% difference between groups, more than 300 patients would be required for each group. Thus, the negative results of the three RCTs must be considered in the context of the potential statistical power of these studies. If the results after 6 weeks for the Dohlman and Otten 1994 study are pooled, then there are 171 total patients. Meta-analysis and comparison between studies is also limited because of the different diagnostic criteria used in the studies. The variation in length of total antibiotic therapy in these studies also made direct comparison between them imperfect. Otten 1994 treated subjects for 1 week whereas Otten 1997 used 10 days of therapy and the other two studies treated their rhinosinusitis patients for 6 weeks with antibiotics. One study [3] suggested that patients whose cultures were positive for *Branhamella catarrhalis* may have some improvement from antibiotic therapy, but they were unable to demonstrate this definitively with their sample size.

Finally, the one level 2 study in this group [4] was able to demonstrate improvement of chronic rhinosinusitis symptoms with antibiotic therapy. However, as previously mentioned, because patients were aware of their treatment, the improvement in symptoms must be interpreted with caution. This study was able to objectively demonstrate improvement in bronchial hyperreactivity (PC_{20}) with the use of antibiotic treatment and, therefore, should be considered in the treatment of asthmatic patients with chronic rhinosinusitis.

Applicability. All but one of the studies (Dohlman) included treatment of patients with signs/symptoms of sinusitis for >3 months (chronic). The Dohlman study treated patients who had subacute sinusitis (>3 weeks but <3 months). In addition, patients in all four studies had sinus radiographs consistent with sinus disease. The exact characterization of the radiographs varied from study to study limiting its applicability. The Tsao study is applicable to asthmatic pediatric patients with chronic rhinosinusitis.

Morbidity/Complications. Only one of the studies reported morbidity [1]. One subject of 25 taking amoxicillin developed a rash, two of 26 individuals taking amoxicillin/clavulanic acid had gastrointestinal upset, and one subject of 26 had difficulty with swallowing trimethoprim/sulfamethoxazole.

CLINICAL SIGNIFICANCE AND FUTURE RESEARCH

Of the four studies, only one study [4] was able to demonstrate an objective improvement in treating chronic rhinosinusitis with antimicrobials. Their results showed that asthmatic patients with chronic rhinosinusitis have a decrease in bronchial hyperreactivity with the use of intranasal saline irrigations and antibiotics. The recommended treatment regimen from this open-label crossover trial was intranasal saline irrigations weekly for 6 weeks combined with amoxicillin/clavulanate at 40 mg/kg/day for 6 weeks. There were also three RCTs that demonstrated no difference between antibiotic and placebo groups, but statistical power was limited and differences between study designs and outcome measurements makes pooling of data difficult.

Future research studies focusing on the treatment of chronic rhinosinusitis with conservative therapy (antibiotics, topical decongestants, and saline) would be made more meaningful by first determining objective, reproducible diagnostic and outcome measures. In addition, repeated use of established outcome measures would allow for eventual meta-analysis of large enough sample sizes to either definitively corroborate the negative results seen in the initial three RCTs or to garner enough power to uncover any differences resulting from antibiotic versus placebo therapy that may truly exist.

Reference	Dohlman, 1993
Level (design)	1 (randomized controlled trial)
Sample size*	96 (123)

OUTCOMES

Intervention	Amoxicillin, ACP, or TMP/SMX
Outcome measures	• Nasal discharge, purulent secretions, congestion, mucosal erythema, cough, wheeze, PFT (0: absent, 1: mild, 2: moderate, 3: severe) • Nasal smears (evaluated for eosinophils and polymorphonuclears) • Water's view mucosal thickness <6 mm
Results with abx	After 6 wk of treatment (responders): Amoxicillin 72% (18/25), ACP 73% (19/26), TMP/SMX 69% (18/26), all abx 71% (55/77)
Results of control	Placebo 63% (12/19)
Measure of statistical significance	p = not significant
Additional results	• Of responders (55 abx, 12 placebo), 58 (87%) responded in 3 wk; 9 more improved after 6 wk • No predictor (age, sex, atopy, pretreatment clinical severity) of response • PMNs on nasal smear did not correlate with treatment success in either group
Conclusions	Antimicrobials were no more effective than placebo in treatment of CRS
Follow-up time	Day 5, 10 (phone call); day 5 (nasal smear); 3 wk (visit)
Power	80% to detect a 25–30% difference with alpha = 0.05

STUDY DESIGN

Inclusion criteria	1) Symptoms >3 wk but less than 3 mo 2) Radiographic evidence of sinusitis
Exclusion criteria	Fever; abx in prior 2 wk; systemic disease; adverse reactions to any of the drugs used in the study
Patient characteristics	Ages 2–16 y, 33 female and 63 male
Study regimens	1) All: oral decongestant, nasal spray 2) Randomization to 3 wk of: group A: amox; group B: ACP; group C: TMP/SMX; group D: placebo 3) If sinusitis resolved after 3 wk, study drug was terminated. If partial resolution, study drug was continued for another 3 wk Patients and physicians were blinded to treatment assignment
Compliance	Not measured
Randomization effectiveness	No significant difference by age, sex, atopy, pretreatment clinical severity
Morbidity/ complications	Amox: rash (1), ACP: gastrointestinal upset (2), TMP/SMX: unable to swallow pill (1), placebo: vomiting (1)

Abx = antibiotics, ACP = amoxicillin/clavulanate potassium, *B. catarrhalis* = *Branhamella catarrhalis*, CMS = chronic maxillary sinusitis, PFT = pulmonary function test, TMP/SMX = trimethoprim-sulfamethoxazole, I&D = incision and drainage, CRS = chronic rhinosinusitis.
* Sample size: numbers shown for those not lost to follow-up and those (initially recruited).

Reference	Otten, 1997
Level (design)	1 (randomized controlled trial)
Sample size*	141 (NR)

OUTCOMES

Intervention	Topical xylometazoline, amoxicillin, and/or I&D of maxillary sinus
Outcome measures	Repeat examinations and sinus X-rays
Results with abx	Results not reported separately. The reported percentages were for all patients combined
	• Persistent purulent rhinorrhea: 60% at 2, 6, 12, and 26 wk
Results of control	• Persistent sinusitis: 41% 6 wk; 31% 12 wk
Measure of statistical significance	No p values given. No statistically significant difference between the 4 treatment groups
Additional results	• Of the 42 with persistent symptoms at 12 wk, 26/42 followed up on average 6 y, 3 mo
	• Age at follow-up 9–14 y
	Only 2/26 still had sinusitis; 24/26 asymptomatic, normal examination and X-rays
	No adenoid enlargement in this group
	Chronic Sx resolved—average age 7 y
Conclusions	Medical treatment no more effective than placebo in treatment of CRS; CRS is self-limiting, resolution ~7 y
Follow-up time	Repeat examinations: 2, 6, 12, and 26 wk
	Repeat sinus X-rays: 6 and 26 wk
Power	Not reported

STUDY DESIGN

Inclusion criteria	Diagnosis of CMS: purulent nasal infection ≥3 mo; examination of purulent rhinitis; sinus X-ray with abnormalities
Exclusion criteria	No evidence of adenoid hypertrophy
	No polyposis
Patient characteristics	ages 3–7 y
Study regimens	Randomization to one of four groups:
	1) Placebo (nasal saline)
	2) Xylometazoline nasal drops, amoxicillin
	3) I&D of maxillary sinus
	4) Combination of regimens 2 and 3
Compliance	Not reported
Randomization effectiveness	Not reported
Morbidity/ complications	Not reported

Abx = antibiotics, ACP = amoxicillin/clavulanate potassium, *B. catarrhalis* = *Branhamella catarrhalis*, CMS = chronic maxillary sinusitis, PFT = pulmonary function test, TMP/SMX = trimethoprim-sulfamethoxazole, I&D = incision and drainage, CRS = chronic rhinosinusitis.
* Sample size: numbers shown for those not lost to follow-up and those (initially recruited).

THE EVIDENCE CONDENSED: Antibiotics/conservative treatment versus control for pediatric nonacute sinusitis

Reference	Otten, 1994
Level (design)	1 (randomized controlled trial)
Sample size*	75 (79)
OUTCOMES	
Intervention	Aspiration of sinus contents; cefaclor
Outcome measures	Examination, cultures, and radiograph: Group I: bilateral complete opacity Group II: bilateral mucosal swelling Group III: unilateral mucosal swelling with unilateral sinus opacity Group IV: unilateral opacity
Results with abx	6 wk: 64.8% (24/37) resolved by symptoms/examination; if + for *B. catarrhalis*, 53.8% (7/13) resolved 12 wk: 86% (32/37) resolved
Results of control	6 wk: 52.5% (20/38) resolved by symptoms/examination; if + for *B. catarrhalis*, 35.7% (5/14) resolved 12 wk: 89% (34/38) resolved
Measure of statistical significance	6 wk: $p = 0.28$ (by symptoms/examination) 6 wk: if + for *B. catarrhalis*, $p < 0.3$ 12 wk: p value not reported
Additional results	6 wk: group I and control: 50% (21/42) resolved; groups II–IV: 66.6% (22/33) resolved; $p = 0.08$ 12 wk: of the 9 patients who failed, 8 were originally in group I. In group I, 19% (8/42) failed treatment vs 3% (1/33) in all other groups
Conclusions	No difference between cefaclor and placebo
Follow-up time	6 wk and 12 wk
Power	Not reported
STUDY DESIGN	
Inclusion criteria	• Purulent rhinitis ≥3 mo • Pus in middle meatus on examination • Sinus film with opacity or swelling
Exclusion criteria	Allergy to cephalosporins, anatomical lesion of the ear/nose/throat, abx in prior 3 wk, systemic disease
Patient characteristics	ages 2–12 y, 39 boys and 36 girls
Study regimens	All patients underwent aspiration of sinus contents or antral washout followed by culturing of contents and antroscopy. Randomized to two groups: 1) Cefaclor 20 mg/kg/d divided in 3 equal doses ×1 wk 2) Placebo ×1 wk
Compliance	Not measured
Randomization effectiveness	No significant difference by sex
Morbidity/ complications	Not reported

Abx = antibiotics, ACP = amoxicillin/clavulanate potassium, *B. catarrhalis* = *Branhamella catarrhalis*, CMS = chronic maxillary sinusitis, PFT = pulmonary function test, TMP/SMX = trimethoprim-sulfamethoxazole, I&D = incision and drainage, CRS = chronic rhinosinusitis.
* Sample size: numbers shown for those not lost to follow-up and those (initially recruited).

Reference	Tsao, 2003	
Level (design)	2 (prospective, open-label crossover)	
Sample size*	71 (NR)	

OUTCOMES		
Intervention	NSI, ACP	
Outcome measures	Headache, mucopurulent rhinorrhea, PND, congestion, sore throat, nocturnal cough, PFTs (FEV_1, PC_{20})	
	Group A: ACP/NSI ×6 wk then NSI ×6 wk Group B: NSI ×6 wk then ACP/NSI ×6 wk	
Results: crossover from ACP/NSI to NSI or vice versa	**Group A: ACP/NSI × 6wk then NSI × 6wk**	**Group B: NSI × 6wk then ACP/NSI × 6wk**
	Symptoms (baseline, 6 wk, 12 wk)	
	Headache A: 3, 0, 0;	B: 5, 2, 0
	Rhinorrhea A: 10, 0^1, 0;	B: 8, 4, 0
	PND A: 8, 0^1, 0;	B: 16, 4^1, 0
	Congestion A: 18, 2^1, 0;	B: 18, 12^2, 4^1
	Sore throat A: 8, 0^1, 0;	B: 8, 4, 0
	Noc Cough A: 15, 2^1, 0;	B: 18, 12^2, 4^1
	FEV_1: (baseline, 6 wk, 12 wk) A: 84.1 ± 6.4, 88.3 ± 10.2, 85.3 ± 8.0	B: 84.6 ± 7.2, 83.2 ± 8.1, 84.3 ± 6.2
	PC_{20}: (baseline, after treatment) A: 3.68 ± 0.52, 7.31 ± 0.98^3	B: 3.11 ± 0.45, 7.00 ± 0.90^4 (6 wk, B: unchanged at 3.72 ± 0.83)
Results of nonsinusitis controls	**Group C: NSI × 12wk**	**Group D: NSI × 12wk**
	FEV_1 (baseline, 12 wk): C: 84.3 ± 7.4, N/A, 86.7 ± 6.8	D: 108.9 ± 2.1, 106.0 ± 6.2
	PC_{20} (baseline, 12 wk): C: 2.98 ± 0.43 unchanged	D: unchanged (no value reported)
Measure of statistical significance	Signs/symptoms: $^1 p < 0.01$, $^2 p < 0.05$ FEV_1: No significant difference (no p value) PC_{20}: $^3 p < 0.001$, $^4 p = 0.001$	
Conclusions	Treatment of CRS with antibiotics in asthmatics improves signs/symptoms and decreases bronchial hyperresponsiveness	
Follow-up time	6 and 12 wk	
Power	Not reported	

STUDY DESIGN		
Inclusion criteria	Groups A, B, and C: mild asthma, perennial allergic rhinitis Groups A and B also had CRS: persistent nasal obstruction, headache, and PND for >12 wk, complete opacification or fluid in maxillary and ethmoid on X-ray Group D: healthy children used as controls	
Exclusion criteria	URI ≤1 mo prior (screen for RSV, adenovirus, parainfluenza, influenza) Group D: asthma, allergic rhinitis, chronic sinusitis, medical problems	
Patient characteristics	ages 7–12 y, 47 male, 24 female	
Study regimens	A: NSI weekly and ACP ×6 wk; followed by: 6 wk of weekly NSI B: 6 wk of weekly NSI; followed by: NSI weekly and ACP ×6 wk C and D: weekly NSI ×12 wk	
Compliance	Not reported	
Randomization effectiveness	Not randomized	
Morbidity/complications	Not reported	

ACP = amoxicillin/clavulanate, FEV_1: forced expiration of volume in 1 second (reported as percentage of predicted), NSI = intranasal saline irrigations, PC_{20} = provocative concentration of methacholine causing a 20% decrease in FEV_1- mg/mL, PFT = pulmonary function tests, PND = postnasal discharge, CRS = chronic rhinosinusitis, URI = upper respiratory infection, RSV = respiratory syncytial virus.
* Sample size: numbers shown for those not lost to follow-up and those (initially recruited).

REFERENCES

1. Dohlman AW, Hemstreet MP, Odrezin GT, Bartolucci AA. Subacute sinusitis: are antimicrobials necessary? J Allergy Clin Immunol 1993;91(5):1015–1023.

2. Otten FW. Conservative treatment of chronic maxillary sinusitis in children. Long-term follow-up. Acta Otorhinolaryngol Belg 1997;51(3):173–175.

3. Otten HW, Antvelink JB, Ruyter de Wildt H, Rietema SJ, Siemelink RJ, Hordijk GJ. Is antibiotic treatment of chronic sinusitis effective in children? Clin Otolaryngol Allied Sci 1994;19(3):215–217.

4. Tsao CH, Chen LC, Yeh KW, Huang JL. Concomitant chronic sinusitis treatment in children with mild asthma: the effect on bronchial hyperresponsiveness. Chest 2003; 123(3):757–764.

8 Pediatric Sinusitis

8.B.

Adenoidectomy for pediatric chronic sinusitis refractory to antibiotic therapy: Impact on patient-reported symptoms and clinical evaluation

Manali Amin and Mark Volk

METHODS

A computerized PubMed search of MEDLINE 1966–January 2006 was performed. Articles mapping to the medical subject headings "adenoidectomy" or "adenoids" or the medical subject headings "endoscopy," "surgery," or "surgical procedures, operative" were cross-referenced with those mapping to the medical subject heading or containing the text word "sinusitis." The resulting set of articles were then cross-referenced with those mapping to the text words (all fields) "chronic," "recurrent," or "persistent," as well as the medical subject headings "child," "infant," "adolescent" or the text word "pediatric." This search strategy yielded 408 studies. These articles were then reviewed to identify those that met the following inclusion criteria: 1) patient population with age 0–18 with chronic rhinosinusitis (CRS), refractory to medical (antibiotic) management, 2) surgical intervention with adenoidectomy, 3) outcomes measured by patient-reported symptom resolution or physician evaluations. Articles that were isolated anecdotal case reports were excluded. The bibliographies of the articles that met these inclusion criteria were manually checked to ensure no further relevant articles could be identified. This process yielded two retrospective studies and two prospective studies [1–4].

RESULTS

Outcome Measures. Outcomes were measured in three of the four studies by comparing caregiver responses to preoperative and postoperative questionnaires. Patient symptoms, caregiver expectations, quality of life [1, 2, 4], and any need for additional intervention [1, 2] were evaluated. One study measured visits to the primary care physician's office for upper respiratory tract symptoms as the main parameter [3].

Potential Confounders. One potential confounder is the severity of sinusitis at the outset of treatment. In the Ramadan 2004 study, the adenoidectomy patients had a lower Lund-Mackay score on computed tomography scan than the other groups [2] they analyzed. This implies that the patients in the adenoidectomy group may have shown improvement more readily because they may have had less-severe sinusitis. Ungkanont's study evaluated improvement in sinusitis episodes by recording the number of visits to the pediatrician's office before and after surgery [3]. This methodology did not account for the possibility that parents were seen for problems outside the pediatrician's office.

Study Designs. These four studies attempted to evaluate the impact of adenoidectomy on children with CRS who failed antibiotic therapy. Two of the studies were retrospective, introducing the inherent potential for selection bias which would affect not only the patients who were included in the study, but also which patients received surgical intervention. In both of the Ramadan studies, the decision to have the patient undergo a surgical procedure was made not by any prespecified objective criteria but rather by surgeon/parent preference. Rosenfeld's study analyzed the subjects in a prospective but serial manner. He took 41 consecutive patients and treated all of them with an aggressive antibiotic regimen. Those that failed antibiotic treatment went on to undergo adenoidectomy. In this study design, each patient acted as his/her own control in a realistic clinical situation in which more aggressive therapies were used in the most refractory patients [4].

The Ramadan and Rosenfeld papers went on to treat the patients who failed to improve after adenoidectomy with endoscopic sinus surgery (ESS). Because this section deals only with adenoidectomy, only the adenoidectomy results are shown in the table adjoining this review. The entire data set with additional data and discussion about ESS is presented in the associated review in this chapter.

Highest Level of Evidence. There were two prospective and two retrospective studies addressing the impact of adenoidectomy in children with chronic sinusitis refractory to medical therapy. No study has evaluated the role of adenoidectomy using a concurrent nonsurgical control. Despite the absence of a randomized controlled trial, these studies strongly suggest that adenoidectomy is an appropriate treatment for pediatric patients who fail to improve on antibiotic therapy. Control of symptoms was achieved in 47%–77% of patients in three studies, whereas a significant decrease in the number of sinusitis infections per year was demonstrated in the fourth study.

Applicability. All of the patients who underwent adenoidectomy for their sinusitis had evidence of chronic sinus disease for many months and had failed multiple weeks of broad-spectrum antibiotic therapy. This study largely excluded patients with systemic or syndromic conditions. Adenoidectomy may not be as efficacious in patients with cystic fibrosis, immunodeficiency, ciliary dyskinesia, and craniofacial syndromes.

Morbidity/Complications. No complications of adenoidectomy were reported.

CLINICAL SIGNIFICANCE AND FUTURE RESEARCH

There are two prospective studies and two retrospective studies that suggest that otherwise healthy children with CRS who fail to resolve with aggressive antibiotic therapy will benefit from adenoid removal. For these patients, adenoidectomy provides a safe and at least moderately effective means to treat refractory CRS. Further studies to elucidate the best therapeutic modalities to optimize outcomes for CRS are indicated. The first step in reaching this goal will entail development of objective, standardized criteria for the grading of CRS in children.

THE EVIDENCE CONDENSED: Adenoidectomy for pediatric chronic rhinosinusitis

Reference	Ramadan, 2004	Ramadan, 1999
Level (design)	2 (prospective comparative)	4 (retrospective case series)
Sample size*	183 (202)	61 (69)
OUTCOMES		
Intervention	Success rate	Success rate
Adenoidectomy	52% (n = 33/64)	47% (n = 14/30)
p Value	Not reported	p = 0.01
Conclusion	52% of patients refractory to medical management improved after adenoidectomy	47% of patients refractory to medical management improved after adenoidectomy
Follow-up time	3 and 6 mo after surgery	3, 6, 9, 12 mo after surgery
STUDY DESIGN		
Inclusion criteria	2–13 y old with: 1) sinusitis diagnosed by history, physical exam, and CT scan, 2) chronic sinusitis—no response after 26 wk of antibiotics + topical/oral decongestants, 3) allergy evaluation and management, 4) repeated CT scan documentation of sinusitis after medical therapy	2–14 y old with: 1) sinusitis diagnosed by history, physical exam, and CT scan, 2) no response after 24 wk of antibiotics + topical/oral decongestants, 3) recurrent sinusitis—6 or more episodes of sinusitis at least 3 wk apart, 4) CT evidence of sinusitis after maximum medical treatment, 5) if allergic, treatment for allergy ×6 mo
Exclusion criteria	Cystic fibrosis, immune deficiency, immunosuppression, ciliary dyskinesia, fungal sinusitis, revision ESS/adenoidectomy, craniofacial abnormality, Down syndrome, developmental delay, chronic tonsillitis	Cystic fibrosis, immune deficiency, immunosuppression, ciliary dyskinesia, revision ESS/adenoidectomy
Intervention selection	Selection based on parent/surgeon preference. Adenoidectomy group was noted to have less disease by CT scan (lower Lund-Mackay)	Selection based on parent/surgeon preference
Intervention regimen details	Standard adenoidectomy	Standard adenoidectomy
Outcome measurement	Success was defined as: 1) improvement of symptoms on preoperative and postoperative validated questionnaire, 2) no need for additional surgery	Success was defined as: 1) improvement of symptoms on preoperative and postoperative validated questionnaire, 2) no need for additional surgery
Age	2–13 y, mean age = 6.2 y	2–14 y
Antibiotic use	All patients failed a 26-wk antibiotic regimen before surgery. Antibiotic use after surgical intervention not stated	All patients failed 24-wk antibiotic regimen before surgery. Antibiotic use after surgical intervention not stated
Consecutive patients?	No	No
Morbidity/complications	No complication of adenoidectomy noted	None

CT = computed tomography, ESS = endoscopic sinus surgery, SRS = Sinusitis Response Score.
* Sample size: numbers shown for those not lost to follow-up and those (initially recruited).

Reference	Rosenfeld, 1995	
Level (design)	2 (prospective comparative)	
Sample size*	41 children: 15 treated with antibiotics alone (level 1), 8 treated with antibiotics and adenoidectomy (level 2)	

OUTCOMES		
Intervention	SRS score (early/late)	All major symptoms better or cured (early/late)
Adenoidectomy	86%/82%	50%/75%
p Value	Not reported	Not reported
Conclusion	Adenoidectomy effective in treating patients who fail antibiotics	
Follow-up time	Early/late (2–3 mo/10–12 mo after surgery)	

STUDY DESIGN	
Inclusion criteria	1) Sinusitis documented by plain X-ray or CT scan (80% of patients had a CT; 65% of levels 1 and 2 and 100% of level 3, 2) At least 1 prior 3-wk course of a beta-lactamase stable antibiotic, 3) 3 mo or more of clinical symptoms or 3 or more annual recurrences (sinusitis prone patients)
Exclusion criteria	Obstructive sleep apnea, obstructive adenoid hyperplasia, cystic fibrosis
Intervention selection	Patients with chronic rhinosinusitis were treated with antibiotics. Those failing antibiotics were treated with adenoidectomy
Intervention regimen details	Standard adenoidectomy
Outcome measurement	SRS; this incorporates: 1) caregiver expectations, 2) quality of life issues, 3) response of the 3 most troublesome clinical symptoms to the final intervention The SRS was calculated as a % of points earned relative to points attainable with regard to the above criteria
Age	2–13 y, median 6 y
Antibiotic use	3 wk of therapeutic antibiotics were prescribed if a patient was symptomatic. This was done in addition to a 3-wk course of antibiotics which all patients received Prophylactic antibiotics were prescribed if a patient was asymptomatic. The antibiotic was administered at half the usual daily dosage for ≥2 mo
Consecutive patients?	Yes
Morbidity/ complications	Surgical morbidity was reported only for FESS and simply reported as no postoperative orbital or intracranial complications.

CT = computed tomography, FESS = functional endoscopic sinus surgery, SRS = Sinusitis Response Score.
* Sample size: numbers shown for those not lost to follow-up and those (initially recruited).

Reference	Ungkanont, 2004
Level (design)	3 (retrospective comparative)
Sample size*	37 patients 24 boys, 13 girls

OUTCOMES	
	No. of Infections per year
Pre/post adenoidectomy	13.7/0.76
p Value	<0.001
Conclusion	Statistically significant reduction of episodes/y of rhinosinusitis after surgery that included adenoidectomy
Follow-up time	Mean = 450 d

STUDY DESIGN	

Inclusion criteria	• Pediatric patients
	• Documented recurrent rhinosinusitis within 1 y before surgery (3 or more per y)
	• Diagnosis of sinusitis: upper respiratory tract infection for >10 d with physical findings of mucoid or mucopurulent discharge in the middle meatus and confirmed paranasal sinus X-rays
	• ≥4 mm of mucosal thickening on plain radiographs, air fluid level or total opacification of the sinus
	• Indications for adenoidectomy:
	  1) 3 or more episodes of rhinosinusitis per y with <2- to 3-wk intervals between courses of antibiotics
	  2) Rhinosinusitis with obstructive, infected adenoids resistant to "full" medical management. Full was not defined
	• Rhinosinusitis with OME

Exclusion criteria	• Patients with nasal polyps • Sinusitis from a dental infection or nasal foreign body • Immune deficiency • Immotile cilia syndrome
Intervention selection	1) Recurrent, refractory rhinosinusitis, 2) rhinosinusitis with obstructive adenoid hypertrophy, 3) rhinosinusitis with otitis media
Intervention regimen details	*Adenoidectomy* T&A: 24 M&T and T&A: 7 Adenoidectomy alone: 4 M&T and adenoidectomy: 2
Outcome measurement	No. of doctor visits for a new episode of upper respiratory tract infection symptoms
Age	2.3–12.7 y, mean 6 y
Antibiotic use	Sinus and Allergy Health Partnership Guidelines [5]
Criteria for withdrawal from study	N/A
Consecutive patients?	No
Morbidity/complications	Not reported

OME = otitis media with effusion, M&T = myringotomy and tubes, T&A = tonsillectomy and adenoidectomy.
* Sample size: numbers shown for those not lost to follow-up and those (initially recruited).

REFERENCES

1. Ramadan HH. Adenoidectomy vs endoscopic sinus surgery for the treatment of pediatric sinusitis. Arch Otolaryngol Head Neck Surg 1999;125(11):1208–1211.
2. Ramadan HH. Surgical management of chronic sinusitis in children. Laryngoscope 2004;114(12):2103–2109.
3. Ungkanont K, Damrongsak S. Effect of adenoidectomy in children with complex problems of rhinosinusitis and associated diseases. Int J Pediatr Otorhinolaryngol 2004;68(4): 447–451.
4. Rosenfeld RM. Pilot study of outcomes in pediatric rhinosinusitis. Arch Otolaryngol Head Neck Surg 1995;121(7):729–736.
5. Antimicrobial treatment guidelines for acute bacterial rhinosinusitis. Sinus and Allergy Health Partnership. Otolaryngol Head Neck Surg 2000;123(1 Pt 2):5–31.

8 Pediatric Sinusitis

8.C.

Endoscopic sinus surgery for chronic/recurrent pediatric sinusitis: Chance for subjective and objective improvement

Manali Amin and Mark Volk

METHODS

A computerized PubMed search of MEDLINE 1966–January 2006 was performed. Articles mapping to the text words (all fields) "endoscopic sinus surgery," "maxillary antrostomy," "ethmoidectomy," "sphenoidotomy," "frontal sinusotomy," "frontal recess," or the medical subject heading "endoscopy" were cross-referenced with those mapping to the medical subject heading or text word "sinusitis." The resulting set of publications was then cross-referenced with those containing the text words "chronic," "recurrent," or "persistent," as well as those mapping to the medical subject headings "child," "infant," "adolescent," or the text word "pediatric." This search strategy yielded 316 studies. These articles were then reviewed to identify those that met the following inclusion criteria: 1) patient population with ages 0–18 years old with chronic or recurrent sinusitis, 2) intervention with functional endoscopic surgery (ESS), 3) outcome measured in terms of postoperative subjective or objective improvement. Articles that included adult patients that could not be analyzed for only pediatric outcomes were excluded. Additional articles were excluded if they included patients with systemic disease such as cystic fibrosis who underwent ESS. The bibliographies of the articles that met these inclusion criteria were manually checked to ensure no further relevant articles could be identified. This entire process yielded 14 studies in 13 articles [1–13].

RESULTS

Outcome Measures. Outcome measures varied depending on the study, but were generally a combination of patient/parental questionnaire and chart review of postoperative findings by examination. The outcome measures were a combination of reporting resolution of symptoms, improvement of symptoms, unchanged symptoms, and worsening of symptoms. Additionally, patient satisfaction was queried in many of the studies. Two of the studies used objective measures (pulmonary function tests, number of hospitalizations, use of medications, and number of days missed from routine activities) to increase the validity of their results [1, 2]. The major limitation of most of the studies is that they used patient/parental reporting as their only outcome measure.

Potential Confounders. As with all studies that use patient reporting of improvement and satisfaction, the results must be interpreted with caution. Patient satisfaction is often related to more than the outcome of the procedure. It may be influenced by their overall experience with the surgical procedure and nontechnical factors such as postoperative course or the perioperative environment. This was especially evident in one study in which patient satisfaction was decreased in some patients who underwent ESS with local anesthesia. Patient reporting of symptom improvement is also subjected to the bias of patient expectations and their memory of preoperative disease. Indeed, many of the studies queried parents/patients months after the surgery.

Study Designs. Only two studies were prospective [3, 12]. One of these studies provided a stepwise method to treating pediatric patients with chronic rhinosinusitis (CRS). Patients who underwent a stepwise treatment protocol and were refractory to medical treatment and adenoidectomy were shown to benefit from ESS. The study did not have an untreated control group and did not randomize subjects to different treatment groups. The other prospective study compared results with ESS alone versus adenoidectomy alone versus ESS with adenoidectomy. The remainder of the studies were all retrospective and also lacked an untreated control group [1, 2, 4–11]. All of the studies demonstrated that patients who did not derive benefit from medical treatment of CRS had improvement after ESS. Three of the studies looked at the effect of adenoidectomy after failure of medical therapy but before undertaking ESS. These results were further supported by the only meta-analysis on this topic [5]. Furthermore, this meta-analysis included data from its institution to address the potential of a publication bias of only reporting those studies in which a surgical technique is shown to be beneficial.

Highest Level of Evidence. All of these studies demonstrated an improvement in sinusitis symptoms after ESS. Improvement/cure rates varied from 79% [7] to 100% [3]. In those studies that examined individual symptoms, improvement again varied from only 50% of chronic cough relief in the Lazar study to 97% improvement or resolution of headache in the Chang study. Because all of the studies are level 4, only correlations of symptom improvement with ESS can be made.

Three studies (one retrospective, two prospective) analyzed the results of ESS in combination with or in comparison to adenoidectomy. Two studies showed that success rates were significantly higher with ESS alone than with adenoidectomy alone. One study showed a trend toward better results with adenoidectomy combined with ESS than with ESS alone. Another study suggested that late outcomes were better if ESS was performed on children who failed adenoidectomy.

Applicability. The study subjects are limited to pediatric patients (ages 0–18 y) who have symptoms of CRS (nasal congestion, chronic cough, headache, postnasal drip, and rhinorrhea) and primarily to those children who do not have systemic diseases such as cystic fibrosis. Four of the studies included patients with systemic disease [7, 8, 10, 11]. Lusk noted that all seven of the 31 patients who required revision ESS had some form of systemic disease (immunodeficiency or cystic fibrosis) [8]. Furthermore, in the Wolf study, the only patient (of 124) who had a recurrence of disease had cystic fibrosis [11]. However, two additional cystic fibrosis patients did not require revision or have recurrence. The Lazar study reported that seven of 16 patients who required a revision ESS had a history of systemic disease [7]. However, the study did not report how many of its total 210 patients had systemic disease and whether their response to surgery was different from those individuals without other medical problems. Finally, the Stankiewicz study reported that 47 of its 77 patients had some form of a systemic disease [10]. However, this study combined all patients including those with cystic fibrosis or immunodeficiency with children with allergies or asthma. They also did not analyze their results separately for the different diagnostic groups. Given these discrepancies, the results of these studies are most applicable to those children without systemic medical problems who have CRS refractory to medical management with antibiotics and other conservative measures. Complicating matters is the fact that conservative measures (antibiotics and topical nasal agents) have not been shown to improve outcomes of CRS when testing in level 1 studies (see 8.A.).

Morbidity/Complications. Each of the studies reported morbidity in a different manner. Some reported synechia as a morbidity, regardless of whether it resulted in recurrence of disease or not [2], whereas other studies simply stated that no major complications were encountered [4]. Other studies did not report morbidities [9]. Given all of the papers that reported morbidities [2, 6–8, 10, 11], 176 patients of a total 1197 (14%) who underwent ESS had some form of complication. This is believed to be a conservative measure because it included both minor and major complications. The Hebert meta-analysis reported a 0.6% rate of major complications in 690 subjects.

CLINICAL SIGNIFICANCE AND FUTURE RESEARCH

These studies all demonstrate that ESS is both safe and effective in pediatric patients whose CRS is refractory to medical management. In the right patient, it can result in a significant improvement in quality of life and reduction in symptoms and would be warranted.

Additional research in this area is required to produce further studies with high levels of evidence. A prospective study could analyze patients who are treated with ESS during a particular length of follow-up time (e.g., 6 months) with those patients who receive no surgical treatment over the same time period. The control group could defer surgery until after completion of the study, perhaps in favor of prolonged or intravenous medical therapy. Finally, future studies should focus on better defining those patient characteristics that make a positive outcome more likely.

Reference	Parsons, 1993		Manning, 1994
Level (design)	4 (retrospective)		4 (retrospective)
Sample size*	52		14 (17)
OUTCOMES			
Results of ESS	Symptom	resolved/improved	Sinusitis questionnaire: 93% improved (symptom scores decreased from 9.3 to 5.1)
	Nasal obstruction	81%	Asthma questionnaire: 79% improved (score decreased from 9.2 to 5.8)
	Nasal discharge	88%	
	PND	61%	No significant change in PFTs
	Chronic cough	84%	Average hospital days for asthma: decreased from 21.4 to 6.5
	Halitosis	75%	
	Headache	96%	Elimination or reduction of steroid use: 86%
	Behavior changes	94%	
p Value	N/A		N/A
Conclusion	>80% of parents thought surgery was worthwhile		1) Improved sinusitis symptoms in 13 of 14, 2) improved asthma symptoms in 11 of 14
Follow-up time	12–38 mo (mean 21.8 mo)		12 mo
STUDY DESIGN			
Inclusion criteria	Failure of medical management determined by pediatrician and surgeon		Steroid-dependent asthma and chronic sinusitis patients who failed to resolve with maximum medical management. Included allergic rhinitis and immunodeficient patients
Exclusion criteria	1) Unable to return for follow-up 2) Review of chart <12 mo postoperation		Cystic fibrosis or other disease predisposing to sinusitis
Patient characteristics	7 mo–17 y (mean 7.4 y)		3.5–13 y (mean 8 y)
Intervention regimen details	ESS with/without middle turbinate resection. Middle meatal stents placed. Second look procedure 10–14 d postoperation		ESS (total ethmoidectomies and maxillary antrostomies)
Outcome criteria	Parental perception of improved 7 symptoms: 1) purulent nasal discharge, 2) chronic nasal obstruction, 3) postnasal drainage, 4) cough, 5) halitosis, 6) headaches, 7) behavior changes		Questionnaire: sinusitis questionnaire (cough, congestion, headache, rhinorrhea); asthma questionnaire; change in PFTs; no. of hospitalizations for asthma; steroid use
Main outcome measures	Parental questionnaire and interview		Parental questionnaire
Morbidity/ complications	None reported		None reported

N/A = not applicable, PND = postnasal discharge, CRS = chronic rhinosinusitis, CT = computed tomography, ESS = endoscopic sinus surgery, CSF = cerebrospinal fluid, PFTs = pulmonary function tests.
* Sample size: numbers shown for those not lost to follow-up and those (initially recruited).

Reference	Chang, 2004	
Level (design)	4 (retrospective)	
Sample size*	101 (131)	
OUTCOMES		
Results of ESS	Symptom	Resolved/better
	Congestion	91%
	Rhinorrhea	90%
	PND	90%
	Headache	97%
	Chronic cough	96%
	Overall satisfaction	86%
p Value	N/A	
Conclusion	Most patients were asymptomatic postoperation and had no recurrence	
Follow-up time	27.2 months mean after surgery	
STUDY DESIGN		
Inclusion criteria	1) 12 wk of persistent symptoms and signs of CRS (nasal obstruction, purulent rhinorrhea, postnasal drip, headache, hyposmia, chronic cough) 2) Recurrent episodes of acute rhinosinusitis, 6 times per y, each lasting at least 10 d 3) Failed 2 wk of initial antibiotics; and treated with 4 additional wk of amoxicillin/clavulanate, cefaclor or cefixime 4) CT scan with Levine and May stage 3 or 4 disease	
Exclusion criteria	Asthma, immunodeficiency, antrochoanal polyps	
Patient characteristics	8–18 y (mean 14.5 y)	
Intervention regimen details	ESS (maxillary antrostomies, anterior ethmoidectomy ± posterior ethmoidectomy); 2nd look procedure in selected patients 3–6 wk later	
Outcome criteria	Parental questionnaire administered at least 6 mo after surgery rating whether symptom/signs had changed (nasal obstruction, purulent rhinorrhea, PND, headache, hyposmia, chronic cough) Parental satisfaction rating Chart review	
Main outcome measures	Parental questionnaire	
Morbidity/ complications	No major complications (hemorrhage requiring transfusion, meningitis, CSF leak) were encountered	

N/A = not applicable, PND = postnasal discharge, CRS = chronic rhinosinusitis, CT = computed tomography, ESS = endoscopic sinus surgery, CSF = cerebrospinal fluid.
* Sample size: numbers shown for those not lost to follow-up and those (initially recruited).

THE EVIDENCE CONDENSED: Endoscopic sinus surgery for chronic/recurrent pediatric sinusitis

Reference	Jiang, 2000	Lazar, 1992
Level (design)	4 (retrospective)	4 (retrospective)
Sample size*	104	210
OUTCOMES		
Results of ESS	Overall 84% improved or resolved; 10% unchanged; 6% worse	165 (79%) "successfully treated" score of 4–10: headache (66%), nasal discharge (63%), congestion (50%), cough (55%) Endoscopy findings: adhesions (20%), granulation (10%), persistent polyposis (7%), significant crusting (11%)
p Value	N/A	N/A
Conclusion	Endoscopic sinus surgery is safe and effective for the treatment of CRS	ESS is effective in CRS refractory to medical therapy
Follow-up time	7 mo–9 y 2 mo (mean 3 y 7 mo)	Range: 3–36 mo with a mean of 18 mo
STUDY DESIGN		
Inclusion criteria	Failure of medical treatment after repeated and appropriate • Long-term antibiotics or several courses of antibiotics based on cultures • Mucolytic agents, antihistamines, nasal steroids, and nasal douche CT scan findings (not specified)	CRS refractory to maximal medical therapy >3 mo with primary care physician or allergist Additional therapy (by otolaryngologist) 3 wk of antibiotics, nasal steroids, topical/oral decongestants, and mucolytics Allergy evaluation (196 of 210 had) Positive CT scan
Exclusion criteria	None	None
Patient characteristics	Ages 5–16 y (mean = 12.6) 55 boys, 49 girls Chronic sinusitis without polyps (63); nasal polyps (47); antrochoanal polyps (11) 102 bilateral; 19 unilateral	Ages 14 mo–16 y 145 boys, 65 girls
Intervention regimen details	Maximal medical treatment Extent of surgery dependent on CT scan findings	Bilateral ESS in all patients (maxillary antrostomies, anterior ethmoidectomies ± posterior ethmoidectomies) ± other related procedures; 2nd look 2–3 wk later Postoperation (6 wk): steroid nasal spray, nasal decongestant, saline nasal mist and broad-spectrum oral antibiotic
Outcome criteria	Questionnaire (response rate: 48%) and chart review for: 1) no symptoms (resolved), 2) symptoms improved after surgery, 3) symptoms unchanged, 4) symptoms worse	Postoperative endoscopy findings, patient questionnaire (allergy history, persistent symptoms, results of surgery): parents/caretaker asked to evaluate surgery on a scale of 0–10 with 0 representing no change and 10 representing cure 0–3: no or poor improvement 4–6: moderate improvement 7–10: marked improvement
Main outcome measures	Parental questionnaire, chart review	Parental questionnaire
Morbidity/ complications	4.1% (n = 5): diplopia (1), orbital fat extrusion (2), bleeding requiring blood transfusion (1), bleeding requiring early termination of procedure (1)	Bleeding postoperation that required packing (8), orbital ecchymosis (5), dacrocystorhinitis (3), severe ear pain (3), revision ESS within 1st y (16)

CRS = chronic rhinosinusitis, ESS = endoscopic sinus surgery, N/A = not applicable, CT = computed tomography.

* Sample size: numbers shown for those not lost to follow-up and those (initially recruited).

Reference	Lusk, 1990
Level (design)	4 (retrospective)
Sample size*	31 (168)

OUTCOMES

Results of ESS	1-y parental assessments: essentially normal (score of 8–10): n = 22 (71%) Persistent disease (score of 5–7): n = 7 (23%) Procedure not satisfactory (score of 1–4): n = 2 (8%)
p Value	N/A
Conclusion	ESS is effective in CRS refractory to medical therapy
Follow-up time	Minimum 1 y

STUDY DESIGN

Inclusion criteria	Failed medical therapy ±Failed prior "related" surgical intervention: M&T, adenoidectomy, tonsillectomy, sinus irrigation, nasal antral windows CT scan findings
Exclusion criteria	None
Patient characteristics	Average age 6.6 y Average duration of symptoms: 26 mo (range 4 mo–7.5 y) Asthma (26%), immune deficiency (23%), allergies (23%)
Intervention regimen details	1) 4-wk course of antibiotics, nasal steroid 2) At end of 4 wk: CT assessments of sinuses Depending on severity on CT: ESS (anterior/posterior ethmoidectomies, maxillary antrostomies; 2nd look 7–10 d later
Outcome criteria	Patient/parent symptom reporting at postoperative visits (report of even 1 incidence of a symptom regardless of etiology was considered +) Parent's assessment of surgical success (1–10 with 10 being the highest)
Main outcome measures	Parental questionnaire
Morbidity/ complications	2 cases of synechia with persistent disease Required multiple procedures: 4 had 2 procedures, 3 had 3 procedures

CRS = chronic rhinosinusitis, ESS = endoscopic sinus surgery, N/A = not applicable, CT = computed tomography, M&T = myringotomy and tubes.
* Sample size: numbers shown for those not lost to follow-up and those (initially recruited).

Reference	Stankiewicz, 1995	Wolf, 1995
Level (design)	4 (retrospective)	4 (retrospective)
Sample size*	77	124
OUTCOMES		
Results of ESS	2nd look (34 pts): 50% with evidence of maxillary antrostomy closure; 1/3 with significant granulation and early synechiae 29 (38%) cured 43 (55%) improved subjectively 5 (7%) unchanged or worsened	Complete resolution or improvement: rhinorrhea (93%), nasal obstruction (88%), recurrent infections (91%), headache (85%), pulmonary symptoms (58%), cough (77%) 87% satisfied or very satisfied
p Value	N/A	N/A
Conclusion	ESS is beneficial in CRS refractory to medical therapy	ESS is beneficial in CRS refractory to medical therapy
Follow-up time	2–7 y (average 3.5 y)	Up to 11 y
STUDY DESIGN		
Inclusion criteria	Failed medical therapy: 2 mo anti-beta-lactamase antibiotic and decongestant; ± antihistamines, nasal steroid sprays, and immunotherapy failure CT scan findings of sinusitis	Failed medical management Preoperative radiographical confirmation (X-rays or CT)
Exclusion criteria	None	None
Patient characteristics	Age: 1–18 y 55 female, 28 male 77 pts with sinusitis: chronic sinusitis (36), acute recurrent sinusitis (29), acute/chronic sinusitis (9), polyposis/chronic sinusitis (7), acute complicated sinusitis (3), sphenoid sinusitis (2), fungal sinusitis (2), choanal polyps (1) Of the 77 sinusitis pts, 47 had one or more of the following: cystic fibrosis, immunodeficiency, allergy, or asthma	Ages 3–16 y (mean 12 y) 65 female, 59 male Preoperative adenoidectomy without success (40), adenoids not clinically significantly enlarged (84), diffuse polyposis (53), inhalational allergies (31), bronchial asthma (5), immunodeficiencies (4), cystic fibrosis (3), Kartagener's syndrome (2)
Intervention regimen details	ESS (maxillary antrostomies, ethmoidectomy, sphenoidotomy) ± related procedures. Second look at 3–6 wk	ESS [unilateral in 43 pts (35%), bilateral in 78 pts (63%), only maxillary endoscopy in 2 pts] Postoperative: antibiotics, topical corticosteroids ± packing ×24–48 h
Outcome criteria	Endoscopic examination (Second look) Parental questionnaire	Chart review: symptoms, endoscopy, radiographical findings, anesthetic complications, postoperative course, recurrence
Main outcome measures	Second look results Parental questionnaire	Parental questionnaire
Morbidity/ complications	1.4% temporary nasolacrimal duct injury; nasal/ethmoid growth on CT scan 4 y later (1)	Diffuse bleeding (10.5%), pain (case under local anesthesia) (0.8%), reoperation (16%)

QOL = quality of life, N/A = not applicable, CRS = chronic rhinosinusitis, ESS = endoscopic sinus surgery, CT = computed tomography, pts = patients.
* Sample size: numbers shown for those not lost to follow-up and those (initially recruited).

Reference	Younis, 1996†
Level (design)	4 (retrospective)
Sample size*	500

OUTCOMES

Results of ESS	88% report improvement in QOL Worse prognosis: passive smoke exposure, recurrence of disease, daycare attendance, immune deficiency, and systemic disease
p Value	N/A
Conclusion	ESS outcome is influenced by extent of disease, daycare attendance, exposure to second-hand smoke, postoperative nasal endoscopy findings, and presence of systemic disease
Follow-up time	1–5 y

STUDY DESIGN

Inclusion criteria	Failed medical therapy CT scan findings (stratification based on severity)
Exclusion criteria	None
Patient characteristics	334 boys, 166 girls Ages: 14 mo–16 y Pts with systemic disease (cystic fibrosis, immotile cilia and immunodeficiencies) were included
Intervention regimen details	ESS: all 500—bilateral ethmoidectomies and maxillary antrostomies; 23 pts—sphenoidotomies
Outcome criteria	Physician's assessment Patient's/parent's or caretaker's evaluation of QOL. QOL was assessed by: no. of d/mo that pt was symptomatic, frequency of medications, no. of physician visits each mo, no. of school/work d lost each mo
Main outcome measures	Parental questionnaire Chart review
Morbidity/ complications	Synechiae (74), bleed (16), bleed requiring transfusion (1), meningitis (2), periorbital ecchymosis (1)

QOL = quality of life, N/A = not applicable, CRS = chronic rhinosinusitis, ESS = endoscopic sinus surgery, CT = computed tomography, pts = patients.
* Sample size: numbers shown for those not lost to follow-up and those (initially recruited).
† Note, some of the patients in this case series and those in Lazar, 1992 are likely to be the same because both studies were done at the same institution and the time frame of the two series overlapped.

THE EVIDENCE CONDENSED: Endoscopic sinus surgery for chronic/recurrent pediatric sinusitis

Reference	Hebert, 1998†	Hebert, 1998
Level (design)	4 (retrospective)	4 (MA of retrospective reviews)
Sample size*	50 (83)	882 (832/8 published, 50/1 unpublished)‡
OUTCOMES		
Results of ESS	Positive outcome: 92%	Positive outcome: published reports: 88.4%; unpublished data: 92% Overall positive outcome: 88.7%
p Value	N/A	N/A
Conclusion	ESS is safe and effective in CRS refractory to medical therapy	ESS is safe and effective in CRS refractory to medical therapy
Follow-up time	Not reported	N/A
STUDY DESIGN		
Inclusion criteria	Pts with CRS refractory to medical therapy who underwent ESS	Studies with a score ≥50: —Pts (n): n < 50 (10 pts); n = 50–100 (20 pts); n > 100 (30 pts) —Average follow-up (y): not reported (0 pts); N/A (5 pts); ≤1 (10 pts); >1–≤2 (20 pts); >2 (30 pts) —Study design: retrospective (5 pts); prospective (10 pts) —Status of chronically ill pts: included but % not indicated (0 pt); ≥10% of population (5 pts); <10% of population (10 pts); not mentioned either way (±) (20 pts); excluded/analyzed separately (30 pts)
Exclusion criteria	Pts with significant underlying disease (cystic fibrosis, immunodeficiencies, allergic fungal sinusitis, cleft lip/palate, Down syndrome, Stickler's syndrome) Neoplasm or midface trauma Death (from other causes) before follow-up	Studies of pts with significant underlying disease Studies with a score <50
Patient characteristics	Age ≤18 y	Pediatric pts (≤18 y)
Intervention regimen details	ESS; second look 2–3 wk later	ESS (middle meatal antrostomy, anterior ethmoidectomy, ± complete ethmoidectomy, ± frontal sinusotomy, ± sphenoid sinusotomy)
Outcome criteria	Telephone questionnaire with caregiver Chart review	Follow-up caregiver questionnaires Chart review
Main outcome measures	Parental questionnaire	Follow-up caregiver questionnaires Chart review
Morbidity/complications	No major complications	0.6% (690 reported): meningitis (2), hemorrhage requiring transfusion (2)
Potential publication bias addressed?	N/A	Bias overcome by including unpublished data; unpublished positive outcomes vs published positive outcomes: chi-square: p = 0.38, power = 0.51 Fisher's exact: p = 0.646, power = 0.12

CRS = chronic rhinosinusitis, N/A = not applicable, ESS = endoscopic sinus surgery, pts = patients, MA = meta-analysis.
* Sample size: numbers shown for those not lost to follow-up and those (initially recruited).
† Previously unpublished data from the meta-analysis listed in column 2.
‡ This meta-analysis included eight published papers with a total of 832 subjects and previously unpublished data from the author's institution with 50 subjects.

THE EVIDENCE CONDENSED: Endoscopic sinus surgery for chronic/recurrent pediatric sinusitis

Reference	Ramadan, 2004†	Ramadan, 1999†
Level (design)	2 (prospective comparative)	3 (retrospective comparative)
Sample size*	183 (202)	61 (69)

	OUTCOMES	
Intervention	Success rate	Success rate
Ad	52% (n = 33/64)	47% (n = 14/30)
ESS	75% (n = 30/40)	77% (n = 24/31)
Ad and ESS	87% (n = 69/79)	N/A
p Value	ESS + Ad vs Ad alone, p < 0.001 ESS alone vs Ad alone, p = 0.005	p = 0.01
Conclusion	Ad improved 52% of pts refractory to medical management. ESS + Ad and ESS alone significantly more successful than Ad alone in treating CRS refractory to abx	47% of pts refractory to medical management improved after Ad. ESS significantly more successful than Ad alone in treating CRS refractory to abx
Follow-up time	3 and 6 mo after surgery	3, 6, 9, 12 mo after surgery

	STUDY DESIGN	
Inclusion criteria	1) CRS by history, physical exam, and CT scan, 2) no response after 26 wk of abx + topical/oral decongestants, 3) allergy evaluation and management, 4) repeated CT scan documentation of sinusitis after medical therapy	1) CRS by history, physical exam, and CT, 2) no response after 24 wk of abx + topical/oral decongestants, 3) ≥6 episodes of sinusitis at least 3 wk apart, 4) CT evidence of CRS after maximum medical RX, 5) if allergic—RX for allergy ×6 mo
Exclusion criteria	CF, immune deficiency, immunosuppression, ciliary dyskinesia, fungal sinusitis, revision ESS/Ad, craniofacial abnormality, Down syndrome, develop delay, chronic tonsillitis	CF, immune deficiency, immunosuppression, ciliary dyskinesia, revision ESS/Ad
Intervention selection	Selection based on parent/surgeon preference. Ad group—less disease by CT scan (lower Lund-Mackay)	Selection based on parent/surgeon preference
Intervention regimen details	Nonrandomized assignment to have Ad alone, ESS alone, or both Ad and ESS at the same time	Nonrandomized to either Ad alone or ESS (anterior ethmoidectomy with middle meatal antrostomy) 28% postethmoidectomy, 12% sphenoidotomy
Outcome measurement	Success was defined as: 1) improvement of symptoms on preoperative and postoperative validated questionnaire, 2) no need for additional surgery	Success was defined as: 1) improvement of symptoms on preoperative and postoperative validated questionnaire, 2) no need for additional surgery
Age	2–13 y, mean age = 6.2 y	2–14 y
Antibiotic use	All pts failed a 26-wk abx regimen before surgery. Abx use after surgical intervention not stated	All pts failed 24-wk abx regimen before surgery. Abx use after surgical intervention not stated
Criteria for withdrawal (if prospective)	N/A	N/A
Consecutive patients?	No	No
Morbidity/ complications	4 (2.9%) pts—2 with orbital entry, 2 with ecchymosis	None

Ad = adenoidectomy, abx = antibiotics, CF = cystic fibrosis, CRS = chronic rhinosinusitis, ESS = endoscopic sinus surgery, N/A = not applicable, NS = not significant, pts = patients, CT = computed tomography, SRS = Sinusitis Response Score.
* Sample size: numbers shown for those not lost to follow-up and those (initially recruited).
† Studies used adenoidectomy before ESS.

Reference	Rosenfeld, 1995†		
Level (design)	2 (prospective comparative)		
Sample size*	41 children: 15—abx only (level 1) 8—abx, Ad (level 2) 2—abx, Ad, ESS (level 3) 16—abx, ESS (level 3)		
OUTCOMES			
Intervention	SRS score (early/late)		All major symptoms better or cured (early/late)
Ad	86%/82%		50%/75%
ESS	N/A		N/A
Ad and ESS	88%/88%		44%/100%
p Value	p = NS/p = NS		p = NS/p = 0.02
Conclusion	Ad effective in treating pts who fail abx and ESS is effective in treating pts who fail abx and Ad		
Follow-up time	Early/late (2–3 mo/10–12 mo after surgery)		
STUDY DESIGN			
Inclusion criteria	—Sinusitis by plain film or CT scan —At least 1 prior 3-wk course of a beta-lactamase stable antibiotic —≥3 mo of symptoms or ≥3 annual recurrences		
Exclusion criteria	Obstructive sleep apnea, obstructive adenoid hyperplasia, CF		
Intervention selection	All pts treated with abx were level 1 Abx failures became level 2 and had Ad Pts failing to improve after Ad became level 3 and had ESS		
Intervention regimen details	Level 1 >abx Level 2 >Ad Level 3 >ESS (maxillary antrostomy, ant/postethmoidectomy)		
Outcome measurement	SRS; caregiver expectations, quality of life issues, response of the 3 worst symptoms to the final intervention SRS: % of points earned relative to points attainable		
Age	2–13 y, median 6 y		
Antibiotic use	3 wk of abx. If symptomatic, additional broad-spectrum abx ×3 wk; if asymptomatic, prophylactic abx		
Criteria for withdrawal (if prospective)	None stated		
Consecutive patients?	Yes		
Morbidity/ complications	Surgical morbidity reported only for ESS—no postoperative orbital or intracranial complications		

Ad = adenoidectomy, abx = antibiotics, CF = cystic fibrosis, CRS = chronic rhinosinusitis, ESS = endoscopic sinus surgery, N/A = not applicable, NS = not significant, pts = patients, CT = computed tomography, SRS = Sinusitis Response Score.
* Sample size: numbers shown for those not lost to follow-up and those (initially recruited).
† Studies used adenoidectomy before ESS.

REFERENCES

1. Manning SC, Wasserman RL, Silver R, Phillips DL. Results of endoscopic sinus surgery in pediatric patients with chronic sinusitis and asthma. Arch Otolaryngol Head Neck Surg 1994;120(10):1142–1145.

2. Younis RT, Lazar RH. Criteria for success in pediatric functional endonasal sinus surgery. Laryngoscope 1996; 106(7):869–873.

3. Rosenfeld RM. Pilot study of outcomes in pediatric rhinosinusitis. Arch Otolaryngol Head Neck Surg 1995;121(7): 729–736.

4. Chang PH, Lee LA, Huang CC, Lai CH, Lee TJ. Functional endoscopic sinus surgery in children using a limited approach. Arch Otolaryngol Head Neck Surg 2004;130(9): 1033–1036.

5. Hebert RL 2nd, Bent JP 3rd. Meta-analysis of outcomes of pediatric functional endoscopic sinus surgery. Laryngoscope 1998;108(6):796–799.

6. Jiang RS, Hsu CY. Functional endoscopic sinus surgery in children and adults. Ann Otol Rhinol Laryngol 2000; 109(12 Pt 1):1113–1116.

7. Lazar RH, Younis RT, Gross CW. Pediatric functional endonasal sinus surgery: review of 210 cases. Head Neck 1992;14(2):92–98.

8. Lusk RP, Muntz HR. Endoscopic sinus surgery in children with chronic sinusitis: a pilot study. Laryngoscope 1990; 100(6):654–658.

9. Parsons DS, Phillips SE. Functional endoscopic surgery in children: a retrospective analysis of results. Laryngoscope 1993;103(8):899–903.

10. Stankiewicz JA. Pediatric endoscopic nasal and sinus surgery. Otolaryngol Head Neck Surg 1995;113(3):204–210.

11. Wolf G, Greistorfer K, Jebeles JA. The endoscopic endonasal surgical technique in the treatment of chronic recurring sinusitis in children. Rhinology 1995;33(2):97–103.

12. Ramadan HH. Surgical management of chronic sinusitis in children. Laryngoscope 2004;114(12):2103–2109.

13. Ramadan HH. Adenoidectomy vs endoscopic sinus surgery for the treatment of pediatric sinusitis. Arch Otolaryngol Head Neck Surg 1999;125(11):1208–1211.

9 Pediatric Cochlear Implantation

9.A.

Cochlear implantation in children with or without a history of frequent otitis media: Chance of post-implant acute otitis media and complications

Jennifer J. Shin and Margaret Kenna

METHODS

A computerized PubMed search of MEDLINE 1966–January 2005 was performed. The medical subject headings "otitis media" and "middle ear ventilation" were exploded and the resulting articles were combined. These articles were then cross-referenced with articles mapping to the medical subject headings or text words "cochlear implantation" or "cochlear implants" yielding 61 articles. These articles were then reviewed to identify those that met the following inclusion criteria: 1) pediatric patient population (<18 years old) undergoing cochlear implantation, 2) intervention in children with, ideally versus without, frequent or recent acute otitis media (AOM), 3) outcome measured in terms of episodes of post-implant AOM and its complications. Articles in which serous non-AOM with effusion alone were studied were excluded, as were articles focusing on patients with chronic suppurative otitis media. Also, articles in which data from children were lumped together with data from adults were excluded. The bibliographies of the articles that met these inclusion criteria were manually checked to ensure no further relevant articles could be identified. This process yielded six articles [1–6].

RESULTS

Outcome Measures. AOM after cochlear implantation (post-CI) was measured in terms of the percent of children who developed AOM and the mean number of episodes of AOM. In addition, the trend for AOM episodes to decrease, remain stable, or increase as compared with before implantation (pre-CI) was observed. Discrete definitions of AOM were not reported in each study.

Potential Confounders. The age of children implanted, the type of device used, the state of middle ear mucosa at the time of implant, and the preoperative regimen for AOM control (including ventilation tube placement, adenoidectomy, and time elapsed since the most recent AOM) could all influence results. In addition, the diagnostic criteria for AOM may vary according to geographic region (i.e., Kempf/Germany versus Luntz/Israel versus House/United States). These factors are detailed in the adjoining tables in as much detail as the original reports allow.

Study Designs. There are six studies that addressed the issue of postoperative AOM in children after cochlear implantation. These studies include a prospective observational comparative study which was reported at an early and a late stage of results. These investigators defined an algorithm for control of preoperative AOM, which included a stepwise use of ventilation tubes, topical and systemic antibiotics, and mastoidectomy in severe cases (Figures 9.A.1, 9.A.2). Their results focused on the incidence of postoperative AOM in children with pre-CI OM/tubes versus children with no pre-CI OM/tubes. There is also an earlier retrospective study from the same authors which focused on the same outcomes. Another retrospective controlled study investigated whether there was any correlation between the incidence of pre-CI AOM and post-CI AOM. Finally, there are two case series. One of these case series described postoperative AOM incidence in 366 implanted children. The other case series described the trend toward decreased, stable, or increased incidence of AOM post-CI. In all of these publications, statistical analysis was minimal and *a priori* calculations of statistical power were not reported. Also, masking was not used in any of these studies.

Highest Level of Evidence. There are two reports of prospective comparative observational data (level 2) showing that patients with pre-CI OM/tubes have a trend toward more postoperative AOM than patients with no pre-CI OM/tubes. No further statistical analysis was reported on this topic. Data from these reports, as well as that from level 3 and 4 studies, also suggest that the overall incidence of AOM decreases in children post-CI, as compared with pre-CI [1, 5]. For example, 100% of patients in the OM-prone group had a history of pre-CI OM, but at over 1-year follow-up, just 20% of patients in that OM-prone group had AOM post-CI [1]. The Fayad study showed similar results, even though it only included patients younger than 4 years old.

Complications of AOM were specifically reported in four studies. No cases of meningitis occurred. The incidence of acute mastoiditis ranged from 0% to 3.3% of implanted children. The use of intravenous antibiotics for postoperative infections was reported in 0%–10% of implanted groups. Explantation was reported in three children in one study [4]; two were attributed to implant bed infections and one was attributed to labyrinthitis

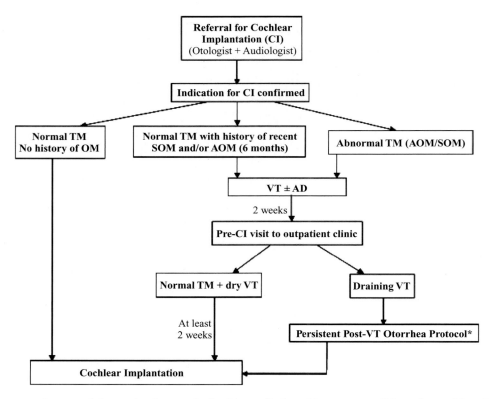

Figure 9.A.1. Structured protocol for optimal control of otitis media in otitis-prone candidates for cochlear implantation. CI: cochlear implantation; TM: tympanic membrane; AOM: acute otitis media; SOM: secretory otitis media; VT: ventilating tube; AD: adenoidectomy. Reprinted from Luntz et al. [6], with permission from Elsevier.

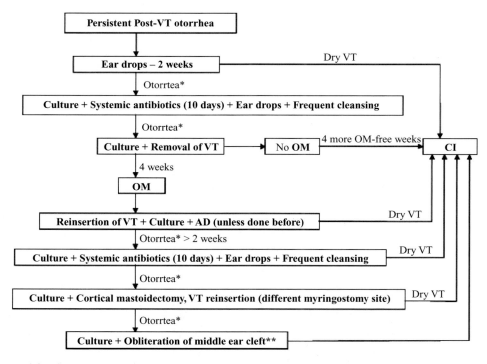

Figure 9.A.2. Protocol for the treatment of persistent drainage through a ventilating tube in candidates for cochlear implantation. * Whenever otorrhea occurs, one or more samples are sent for culture and the antibiotic treatment is changed according to specific growth and susceptibility. ** None of the otitis-prone candidates for cochlear implantation in this study required obliteration of the middle ear cleft. CI: cochlear implantation; VT: ventilating tube; AD: adenoidectomy; OM: otitis media. Reprinted from Luntz et al. [6], with permission from Elsevier.

secondary to rubella. Thus, it is unclear whether these explantations were strictly attributable to AOM or its complications.

Applicability. These data are applicable to children undergoing cochlear implantation. Data from controlled studies can further be specifically applied to patients with or without a history of being prone to OM.

Morbidity/Complications. As noted above, no cases of meningitis were reported. Acute mastoiditis was diagnosed in 0%–3.3% of implanted children. Explantation was reported in two children in one study. One child in the same study developed a cholesteatoma.

CLINICAL SIGNIFICANCE AND FUTURE RESEARCH

There are six studies that addressed the issue of AOM in the pediatric population post-CI. The data contained therein suggests the following: 1) patients with pre-CI OM/tubes have a trend toward more postoperative AOM than patients with no preoperative OM/tubes, 2) OM-prone children tend to develop AOM with decreased frequency post-CI, 3) the incidence of complications of AOM (i.e., acute mastoiditis, meningitis) is low in the overall population of children implanted. These data suggest that children whose preoperative OM is adequately addressed can undergo cochlear implantation with the expectation that AOM will still occur, but with decreased frequency and with low risk of AOM-related complications.

There are many factors that could contribute to the reported decrease in AOM post-CI. In most cases, the pre-CI time period was longer than the post-CI follow-up time, so patients had a longer period to accumulate an AOM-positive history preoperatively. In addition, post-CI children are older, and AOM often decreases in general with age; it is unclear if the decrease in AOM is a global decrease or a phenomenon specific to the implanted ear. In the future, it would be useful to determine the actual incidence of AOM per year within each age group (rather than a general overall average based on records).

A key question that warrants additional research is whether the incidence of AOM-related complications is increased in the children who do develop AOM after implantation. Addressing this issue would also help to more definitively address the question of how aggressive treatment should be for implanted children who develop AOM.

Reference	Luntz, 2004			Luntz, 2001	
Level (design)	2 (prospective observational study)			2 (prospective observational study)	
Sample size*	60 (60)			18 (18)	

OUTCOMES

	AOM within 4 wk postop	AOM after 4 wk postop (isolated, recurrent)	AOM complications	AOM within 1 y postop	AOM after 1 y postop
OM or tubes before implant	14.7%	23.5%, 14.7%	10% required IV antibiotics 3.3% acute mastoiditis 1.7% cholesteatoma	10%	20%
No tubes or recent OM before implant	3.8%	3.8%, 0.0%	0% required IV antibiotics 0% acute mastoiditis 0% cholesteatoma	0%	0%
p Value	Not reported	Not reported		Not reported	Not reported
Conclusion	Group with OM/tubes preimplant with trend toward more postop infections, but overall incidence of OM decreased post-implant			Group with OM/tubes preimplant with trend toward more postop infections, but overall incidence of OM decreased post-implant	
Follow-up time	At least 3 mo (mean 20 mo)			7–19 mo	

STUDY DESIGN

Inclusion criteria	<7 y old, all patients referred to Cochlear Implant Program at the Bnai Zion Medical Center			<7 y old, all patients referred to Cochlear Implant Program at the Bnai Zion Medical Center	
Exclusion criteria	Not specified			Not specified	
Cochlear implant details	n = 9 Nucleus 24, n = 18 Nucleus 24 Contour, n = 5 Clarion preform, n = 2 Clarion with positioner, n = 16 Clarion high focus I with positioner, n = 8 Clarion high focus II with positioner, n = 2 Med-El Combi 40+			n = 9 Nucleus 24, n = 5 Clarion preform, n = 2 Clarion with positioner, n = 2 Clarion high focus with positioner	
Ventilation tubes	There was a history of tubes in 32/34 patients with OM or tubes pre-CI; 28 had tubes at the time of implant			10/10 patients in the "OM/tubes pre-CI" group had tubes present at the time of implant	
Intraoperative findings (CI)	Thick middle ear mucosa in 19/34 of children with pre-CI OM/tubes versus 2/26 control children, obliteration of round window niche by thick mucosa in 16/34 of children with pre-CI OM/tubes versus 0/26 control children			Thick middle ear mucosa in 7/10 of children with pre-CI OM/tubes versus 3/8 control children, obliteration of round window niche by thick mucosa in 7/10 of children with pre-CI OM/tubes versus 0/10 control children	
Age	<7 y (children with pre-CI OM/tubes were 17.3 mo younger at time of first visit and 13.6 mo younger at time of CI)			<7 y	
Masking	None described			None described	
Criteria for preop OM or tubes group	OM diagnosed by otoscopy during the first outpatient examination after referral, at any time between referral and implantation, ventilation tube insertion anytime before referral for AOM, ≥1 AOM or serous otitis media in the previous 6 mo (control group does not meet these criteria)				
Management of OM-prone patients before implantation	Ventilation tube with/without adenoidectomy. If dry/normal TM 2 wk post-tube, then CI after >2 wk. If draining/abnormal TM then stepwise increments of otic drops, systemic antibiotics, reinsertion of tubes, frequent cleansing, and cortical mastoidectomy before CI. Implantation was performed only after middle ear was aerated, TM was thin and transparent, and tube was not draining				
Management of postop AOM	Topical therapy and empirical Augmentin followed by culture-driven therapy if otorrhea was present			Empirical Augmentin	
Criteria for withdrawal	None specified, none withdrew			None specified, none withdrew	
Consecutive patients?	Yes			Not specified	
Morbidity/ complications	No children developed fever or any other fulminant presentation that would have necessitated hospitalization for IV antibiotic or surgical treatment			No children developed complication of OM	

Postop = postoperative, preop = preoperative, IV = intravenous, CI = cochlear implantation, OM = otitis media, AOM = acute otitis media, TM = tympanic membrane.
* Sample size: numbers shown for those not lost to follow-up and those (initially recruited).

Reference	Luntz, 1996				House, 1985
Level (design)	3 (retrospective comparative study)				3 (retrospective comparative study)
Sample size*	50 (60)				20 (26)
OUTCOMES					
	Post-CI mean AOM per year	% with post-CI AOM	Severity of post-CI AOM		% children with post-CI AOM
Multiple AOM requiring tubes pre-CI	0.35 (from 4.0 preop) of AOM	35.7% (from 74% preop)	All post-CI AOM responded to routine abx. No mastoiditis or AOM complications	**AOM pre-CI**	33% (n = 4/12)
No tubes or AOM pre-CI	0 (from 0 preop)	0% (from 0% preop)	No AOM	**No AOM pre-CI**	62.5% (n = 5/8)
p Value	Not reported	Not reported	Not reported		Not reported
Conclusion	Trend toward decreased AOM incidence post-CI				No correlation between pre-CI and post-CI AOM incidence
Follow-up time	Mean 19 mo				1–4 y
STUDY DESIGN					
Inclusion criteria	≤16 y old at time of implant				Children <10 y old who had the implant ≥1 y. Parents and physicians rated the frequency and severity of otitis media
Exclusion criteria	Lack of "complete" information				>10 y old, failure to receive waiver to release medical records
Cochlear implant details	Nucleus mini-22 CI				Fascial plug placed in the round window niche after insertion of the electrode
Ventilation tubes	n = 3 who were implanted with tubes, 1 of these developed post-CI peritubal myringitis which resolved with tube removal				Not reported
Intraoperative findings (CI)	Not described				Not reported
Age	≤16 y				<10 y
Masking	None				None
Extent of preop OM	AOM operationally defined as having occurred when diagnosed by a physician on the basis of fluid in the middle ear, erythema of the tympanic membrane, otalgia, and a systemic symptom such as fever. All children were free of AOM at implantation				60% (n = 7/20) of children whose medical records were available had AOM "over the period in which they had been observed"
Management of OM-prone patients before implantation	Not described in detail				Not reported
Management of postop AOM	"Routine" oral antibiotics				100% of physicians reported they used the same antibiotic management as pre-CI
Consecutive patients?	No				No
Morbidity/ complications	No complications of AOM occurred				Not reported

Postop = postoperative, preop = preoperative, CI = cochlear implantation, OM = otitis media, AOM = acute otitis media, abx = antibiotics.
* Sample size: numbers shown for those not lost to follow-up and those (initially recruited).

THE EVIDENCE CONDENSED: Otitis media in children after cochlear implantation

Reference	Kempf, 2000	Fayad, 2003		
Level (design)	4 (case series)	4 (case series)		
Sample size*	366 (366)	76 (126)		
OUTCOMES				
	All children implanted	Pre-CI ≥1 OM (n = 61)	Pre-CI OM but no M&T (n = 42)	Pre-CI M&T (n = 11)
Post-CI AOM	AOM occurred in 11 children in the implanted side and 9 on the contralateral side for a rate of 5.6%	78% decreased OM, 19% no change, 3% increase	69% decrease, 26% no change, 2% increase	100% decrease
p Value	None	None		
Conclusion	5.6% of patients developed AOM post-CI	Frequency of OM decreased in the majority of patients post-CI		
Follow-up time	"up to 8 y"	5–136 mo (mean 46 mo)		
STUDY DESIGN				
Inclusion criteria	Children who received implants in Hannover 1987–1997	≤4 y old at time of implant		
Exclusion criteria	Not specified	Office charts and medical records not available, phone follow-up incomplete		
CI details	In most cases, a Nucleus 22 mini implant was used; Clarion 1.2 and Nucleus 24M have also been used	Not reported		
Ventilation tubes	Grommets inserted preop for serous OM, no further details	19/76 with history of tubes, 11 had tubes that were left in place beyond the time of cochlear implantation		
Intraoperative findings (CI)	Not reported	Not reported		
Age	1–14 y	Mean 11 mo, range 11–48 mo		
Masking	Not applicable	Not applicable		
Extent of preop OM	Not reported	Of the 76 patients completing the phone survey: 80% had ≥1 OM pre-CI, 36% had >3 pre-CI. Of the 126 patients with complete medical records: 72% had ≥1 OM pre-CI, 31% had >3 pre-CI, and 2% had a history of chronic serous OM		
Management of OM-prone patients before implantation	During the routine pre-implantation investigation, examination of nasopharynx with removal of adenoids was performed, ventilation tubes provided for serous OM	If there was a history of persistent OM within the past 6 mo or active disease at preop evaluation, tubes were placed 6–8 wk pre-CI		
Management of postop AOM	Intravenous antibiotics "a few days longer than normal," if infection is severe then remove the device but leave the electrode in cochlea with reimplantation after 1 y; 7 M&T, 5 postauricular mastoid exploration	1 patient had M&T post-implantation, further details not specified		
Criteria for withdrawal from study (if prospective)	Not applicable	Failure to complete survey or phone survey		
Consecutive patients?	Not reported	Not reported		
Morbidity/complications	0% meningitis, 0.5% explantation, 0.25% cholesteatoma, 0.25% labyrinthitis, 1.25% mastoiditis	Not specified		

CI = cochlear implantation, OM = otitis media, AOM = acute otitis media, preop = preoperative, postop = postoperative, M&T = myringotomy and tubes.
* Sample size: numbers shown for those not lost to follow-up and those (initially recruited).

REFERENCES

1. Luntz M, Teszler CB, Shpak T, Feiglin H, Farah-Sima'an A. Cochlear implantation in healthy and otitis-prone children: a prospective study. Laryngoscope 2001;111(9):1614–1618.

2. Luntz M, Hodges AV, Balkany T, Dolan-Ash S, Schloffman J. Otitis media in children with cochlear implants. Laryngoscope 1996;106(11):1403–1405.

3. House WF, Luxford WM, Courtney B. Otitis media in children following the cochlear implant. Ear Hear 1985; 6(3 Suppl):24S–26S.

4. Kempf HG, Stover T, Lenarz T. Mastoiditis and acute otitis media in children with cochlear implants: recommendations for medical management. Ann Otol Rhinol Laryngol Suppl 2000;185:25–27.

5. Fayad JN, Tabaee A, Micheletto JN, Parisier SC. Cochlear implantation in children with otitis media. Laryngoscope 2003;113(7):1224–1227.

6. Luntz M, Teszler CB, Shpak T. Cochlear implantation in children with otitis media: second stage of a long-term prospective study. Int J Pediatr Otorhinolaryngol 2004;68(3): 273–80.

9 Pediatric Cochlear Implantation

9.B.

Implantation of children with cochleovestibular anomalies versus normal anatomy: Impact on postoperative speech perception and complications

Jennifer J. Shin and Margaret Kenna

METHODS

A computerized PubMed search of MEDLINE 1966–January 2005 was performed. Articles mapping to the medical subject headings "cochlear implantation" and "cochlear implants" were combined with any that had "cochlear implant" as a text word. These articles were cross-referenced with the group that mapped to the medical subject heading "cochlea/*abnormalities" and those containing the text words "common cavity," "cochlear dysplasia," "Mondini," "Scheibe," or "Michel." This search yielded 76 trials. These articles were then reviewed to identify those that met the following inclusion criteria: 1) comparison of patients with cochleovestibular anomalies versus patients with normal anatomy, 2) intervention with cochlear implantation, 3) outcome measured in terms of speech perception and perioperative complications. Isolated case reports and articles without comparative data were excluded, in order to focus on the highest levels of evidence. The bibliographies of the articles that met these inclusion criteria were manually checked to ensure no further relevant articles could be identified. This overall process yielded three articles [1–3].

RESULTS

Outcome Measures. Results were reported in terms of closed- and open-set speech testing. The specific tests used are noted in the adjoining table. In addition, the Eisenman study [2] reported speech category scores, with 0 being the worst and 6 being the best. Again, details are shown in the adjoining table.

Potential Confounders. Age at implantation, duration of deafness, mode of communication, preoperative speech perception, completeness of insertion, number of active electrodes, device encoding strategy, and the extent of cochlear abnormality are all factors that could potentially influence results. These factors are detailed in the adjoining table in as much detail as the individual publications allow.

Study Designs. There are three retrospective controlled studies (level 3) that addressed this topic. The Papsin study [1] compared data from 103 patients with cochleovestibular anomalies to 198 patients with normal anatomy. The larger sample size increases the power of the study, although an a priori power calculation was not reported. The Eisenman and Mylanus studies [2, 3] compared matched pairs in 34 and 20 patients, respectively. Both studies attempted to match pairs for potential confounders (see details in the adjoining table), which can be an effective strategy to minimize the bias of a smaller retrospective analysis. Only the Eisenman study, however, reported a statistical analysis to confirm the adequacy of matching. In that analysis, they found statistically significant, but perhaps clinically insignificant, differences in the age at implantation (difference between means 0.51 years, p = 0.03) and duration of deafness (difference between means 0.68 years, p = 0.04). Follow-up times in the three studies ranged from 6 months to 7.5 years.

Highest Level of Evidence. All three studies showed no noteworthy difference in the range of post-implant speech perception in patients with cochleovestibular anomalies versus normal anatomy. The larger two studies confirmed this finding with statistical analysis. Despite this overall negative finding, all of these articles contained commentary that patients with common cavity deformity, isolated incomplete partition, and narrow internal auditory canal did not perform as well. These patients were relatively few in number compared with the enlarged vestibular aqueduct patients, so did not influence the overall outcome results much (because the range of variability was so wide).

All three studies reported complications of implantation in patients with abnormal inner ear anatomy, including perilymph/cerebrospinal fluid leak, explantation, nonstimulation, facial nerve weakness, and exposed carotid. In addition, the largest study also reported that complicated anatomy resulted in a more challenging surgery in a notable percentage of cases (16% abnormal facial nerve course, 17% abnormal middle ear anatomy), even if there were no associated complications.

Applicability. The results of these studies can be applied to children with common cavity, hypoplastic cochlea, incomplete partition, and enlarged vestibular aqueduct.

Morbidity/Complications. Complications of cochlear implantation in patients with cochleovestibular anomalies are as detailed in the adjoining table and in the above discussion.

There are three retrospective controlled studies showing that post-implant speech perception of children with cochleovestibular anomalies is comparable to that of children with normal inner ear anatomy. Data from the largest of the three studies also suggest that implantation of children with malformed cochleas presents additional intraoperative challenges, and perhaps a more notable incidence of cerebrospinal fluid leaks.

Although these are retrospective level 3 studies, one enrolled nearly 300 patients and the other two utilized matched-pairs analysis in an attempt to minimize bias from confounders. The largest study included nearly all patients with abnormal cochlear anatomy who had been implanted over a 10-year period. The timeframe associated with that larger sample size suggests the logistical difficulty in accruing a reasonable sample size for a prospective study. Thus, retrospective data may remain the highest level of evidence of this topic.

Future research may focus on performing similar studies with magnetic resonance imaging (MRI), as high-quality detailed MRI of the temporal bones becomes more widely available. There may be further radiologic findings that can help explain some of the outcomes in these patients.

Reference	Papsin, 2005
Level (design)	3 (retrospective controlled)
Sample size*	298 : 103 cochleovestibular anomaly, 195 normal anatomy

OUTCOMES

	Open-set speech scores	Closed-set speech scores
Cochleovestibular anomalies	See figure 9.B.1 which shows data from the original publication	See figure 9.B.2 which shows data from the original publication
Normal anatomy	See figure 9.B.1 which shows data from the original publication	See figure 9.B.2 which shows data from the original publication
p Value	>0.05	>0.05
Conclusion	No difference in rate of speech perception improvement	
Follow-up time	Up to 73 mo postoperatively	

STUDY DESIGN

Inclusion criteria	Children implanted 1992–2002
Exclusion criteria	Children who were implanted in a normal ear but had cochleovestibular anomaly in unimplanted ear
Malformation group details	Common cavity n = 8, hypoplastic cochlea n = 16, incomplete partition n = 42, isolated EVA n = 37 (wide notch n = 30, parallel n = 7), concomitant EVA n = 15, posterior labyrinthine dysplasia n = 26, narrowing of IAC or cochlear canal n = 11
Malformation definitions	• Common cavity: cystic cavity representing both cochlea and vestibule, or presence of dilated vestibule and cochlea with marked enlargement of ductus reuniens • Incomplete partition: deficiency in modiolus and incomplete septation within cochlea with <2.5 turns; usually associated with EVA • Cochlear hypoplasia: cochlea smaller than normal but clearly differentiated from vestibular elements • EVA: isolated finding of aqueduct diameter exceeding diameter of posterior SCC; subtypes from less to more severe—wide notch (enlargement caused by endolymphatic sac), parallel (enlarged all the way to the vestibule), funnel
Control group details	Double review of CT scan confirming normal cochleovestibular anatomy
Age	Mean 4.9 y (SD 3.9) for patients with cochleovestibular anomalies; mean 6.0 y (SD 4.4) for patients with normal anatomy
Masking	None specified
CT details	1-mm axial and direct coronal images
Cochlear implant details	Nucleus CI22, CI24, CI24R
Speech testing details	Closed-set tests: test of auditory comprehension, WIPI Open-set tests: Glendonald auditory speech perception test, phonetically balanced kindergarten words and phonemes
Additional malformations studied	Concomitant anomalies studied: • Posterior labyrinthine dysplasia: vestibular anomalies other than EVA • IAC narrowing: <2 mm diameter Findings: children with narrowed IAC performed significantly worse on WIPI speech testing
Consecutive patients?	Not specified
Power	Not reported
Morbidity/ complications	Perilymph/CSF leak n = 9/103, explantation n = 2/103, nonstimulation 2/103, facial nerve weakness 0/103 (abnormal facial nerve course 16%), abnormal middle ear anatomy 18/103; 24% had surgery complicated by CSF/perilymph leak or challenging anatomy

EVA = enlarged vestibular aqueduct, SCC = semicircular canal, IAC = internal auditory canal, GN = Gestel/Nimegen, CI = confidence interval, CT = computed tomography, WIPI = word identification of phoneme index, SD = standard deviation, CSF = cerebrospinal fluid.
* Sample size: numbers shown for those not lost to follow-up and those (initially recruited).

Reference	Eisenman, 2001	
Level (design)	3 (retrospective matched pairs analysis)	
Sample size*	18 : 9 pairs with data at 24 mo 30 : 15 pairs with data at 12 mo 32 : 16 pairs with data at 6 mo (34 : 17 pairs with data initially)	
OUTCOMES		
	Speech group scores at 12 mo	Speech group scores at 24 mo
Cochleovestibular anomalies	Median 3, 25th–75th percentile 2–3	Mean 4.6 (95% CI 3.7–5.8)†
Normal anatomy	Median 4, 25th–75th percentile 3–5	Mean 3.4 (95% CI 2.3–4.7)†
p Value	>0.05 for ESP, GASP-W, GASP-S scores at 6 and 24 mo; <0.04 for RM-ANOVA which demonstrated more rapid rate of improvement in GASP-W testing (F = 6.20)	
Conclusion	Slower rate of improvement with malformation	By 24 mo, no significant difference
Follow-up time	6 mo, 12 mo, 24 mo	
STUDY DESIGN		
Inclusion criteria	All children implanted with osseous cochlear malformations 1991–1998	
Exclusion criteria	Children with isolated vestibular abnormalities	
Malformation group details	Common cavity n = 4, hypoplastic cochlea n = 3, incomplete partition n = 11, concomitant EVA n = 6	
Malformation definitions	Mild malformation: simple incomplete partitioning of the cochlea Severe malformation: hypoplastic cochlea, common cavity	
Control group details	Pairs matched for age at implantation, duration of deafness, preoperative speech perception, primary mode of communication, device type. Small but statistically significant differences in the age at implantation (difference between means 0.51 y, p = 0.03) and duration of deafness (difference between means 0.68 y, p = 0.04)	
Age	1.7–8.9 y	
Masking	None specified	
CT details	Not specified	
Cochlear implant details	Nucleus N22, N24M; Med-El compressed electrode array, Med-El standard electrode array	
Speech testing details	Early speech perception test, Glendonald auditory speech perception test. Speech perception category assignments: 0 no reliable detection of speech, 1 detection of speech signal, 2 pattern perception, 3 beginning word identification, 4 word identification through vowel recognition, 5 word identification through consonant recognition, 6 open-set word recognition	
Additional malformations studied	None specified	
Consecutive patients?	Yes (malformations)	
Power	Not reported	
Morbidity/ complications	CSF outflow from cochleostomy site n = 7 (3 slow, 4 profuse)	

EVA = enlarged vestibular aqueduct, SCC = semicircular canal, IAC = internal auditory canal, GN = Gestel/Nimegen, CI = confidence interval, CT = computed tomography, WIPI = word identification of phoneme index, SD = standard deviation, CSF = cerebrospinal fluid, ESP = Early Speech Perception test, GASP-W = Glendonald Auditory Speech Perception test for Words, GASP-S = Glendonald Auditory Speech Perception test for Sentences.
* Sample size: numbers shown for those not lost to follow-up and those (initially recruited).
† Values extrapolated from graph.

Reference	Mylanus, 2004
Level (design)	3 (retrospective matched pairs analysis)
Sample size*	20 : 10 pairs

OUTCOMES

	GN open-set phenomes	Erber closed set
Cochleovestibular anomalies	40%–95% (n = 8)	54%–75% (n = 2)
Normal anatomy	23%–100% (n = 9)	100% (n = 1)
p Value	Not reported	Not reported
Conclusion	"No great difference in performance between the two groups"	
Follow-up time	Average 4.7 y (range 2.0–7.5)	

STUDY DESIGN

Inclusion criteria	Children undergoing cochlear implantation 1994–2002
Exclusion criteria	Not specified
Malformation group details	Common cavity n = 1, incomplete partition n = 7, EVA n = 3, dysplastic vestibule and canals n = 5
Malformation definitions	As defined by Jackler [4]: total aplasia, severe cochlear aplasia, mild cochlear aplasia (basal turn only), common cavity, severe incomplete partition, mild incomplete partition
Control group details	Pairs matched for age at implantation, duration of deafness, electrode insertion depth
Age	1.0–7.7 y
Masking	None specified
CT details	High-resolution CT scanning interpreted by radiologist specializing in imaging of the temporal bone
Cochlear implant details	Not specified
Speech testing details	Tests consisting of lists of CVC monosyllables; GN test, Bosman test
Additional malformations studied	None specified
Consecutive patients?	Not specified
Power	Not reported
Morbidity/ complications	CSF gusher n = 1/10, aberrant facial nerve n = 1/10, exposed carotid artery n = 1/10

EVA = enlarged vestibular aqueduct, SCC = semicircular canal, IAC = internal auditory canal, GN = Gestel/Nimegen, CI = confidence interval, CT = computed tomography, WIPI = word identification of phoneme index, SD = standard deviation, CSF = cerebrospinal fluid, CVC = consonant-vowel-consonant.
* Sample size: numbers shown for those not lost to follow-up and those (initially recruited).

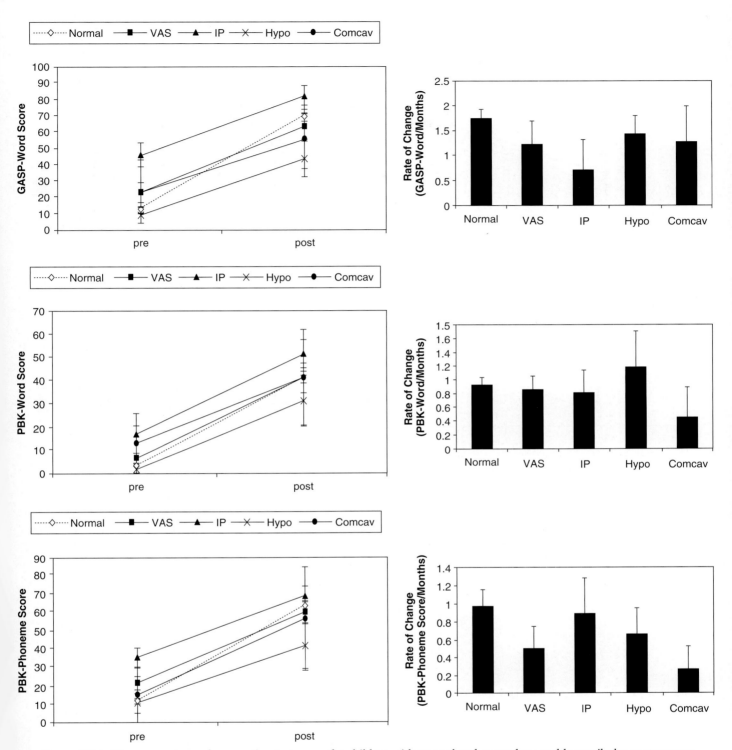

Figure 9.B.1. The open-set speech perception test scores for children with normal and anomalous cochleovestibular anatomy are show in the series of the plots. The score for each test is on the y axis. On the x axis is plotted the preimplant score and the best obtained postoperative score. To the right of each the plot, the rates of progress (best score minus preimplant score/duration of implant use) are shown for each test. Reprinted from Papsin [1] with permission from Lippincott Williams and Wilkins.

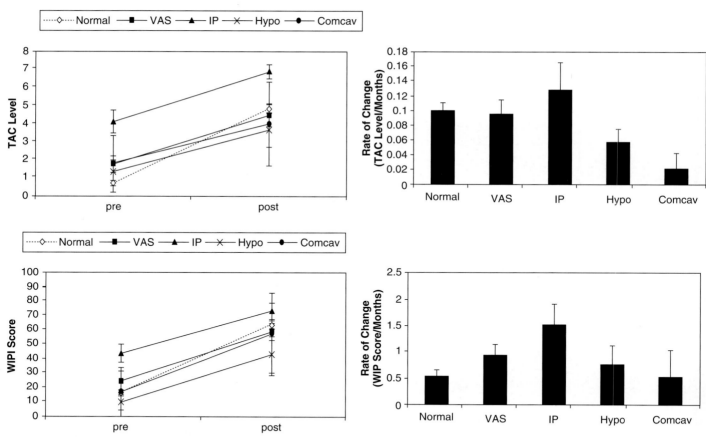

Figure 9.B.2. Results of closed-set speech perception tests. See Figure 9.B.1 legend for details. Reprinted from Papsin [1] with permission from Lippincott Williams and Wilkins.

REFERENCES

1. Papsin BC. Cochlear implantation in children with anomalous cochleovestibular anatomy. Laryngoscope 2005; 115(1 Pt 2 Suppl 106):1–26.
2. Eisenman DJ, Ashbaugh C, Zwolan TA, Arts HA, Telian SA. Implantation of the malformed cochlea. Otol Neurotol 2001;22(6):834–841.
3. Mylanus EA, Rotteveel LJ, Leeuw RL. Congenital malformation of the inner ear and pediatric cochlear implantation. Otol Neurotol 2004;25(3):308–317.
4. Jackler RK, Luxford WM, House WF. Congenital malformations of the inner ear: a classification based on embryogenesis. Laryngoscope 1987;97(suppl 40):1–14.

10 Subglottic Stenosis

10.A.

Single- versus double-stage laryngotracheal reconstruction: Rate of decannulation, need for subsequent procedures

Jennifer J. Shin and Christopher J. Hartnick

METHODS

A computerized Ovid search of MEDLINE 1966–November 2003 was performed. First, the subject heading "laryngostenosis" was exploded and combined with all articles containing the keyword "subglottic stenosis." Second, the terms "treatment outcome," "tracheotomy," and "tracheostomy" were exploded and combined with all articles containing the keywords "outcome" or "decannulation." Third, articles with the keyword "child," "infant," or "pediatric" and those obtained by exploding "pediatrics" were combined. These three groups were then cross-referenced, yielding 338 articles. We then reviewed these reports, as well as the references of any summary articles obtained in order to obtain all relevant references. For inclusion criteria, we required the following: 1) a distinct population of children ≤19 years old with subglottic stenosis, 2) management with single-staged laryngotracheal reconstruction (LTR), preferably in comparison to double-staged LTR, and 3) outcome measures of decannulation and/or need for subsequent salvage procedures. Reports of patients with treatment of purely tracheal or glottic stenosis were excluded. Two articles met these criteria with comparison of single- and double-staged procedures [1, 2]. Five articles met these criteria without such a comparison [3–7]. One 2000 report [4] included patients from a 1995 report [3], and so only the cumulative 2000 report is reported in detail.

RESULTS

Outcome Measures. The major outcome measure is rate of decannulation. This rate can be reported in two ways. The first is to report "operation specific decannulation rates (OSDR)" either at the time of surgery (for single-stage procedures) or at a later date where no other major procedures have been performed in the elapsed time interval (double-stage procedures). The second way of reporting this outcome measure is to report the "overall decannulation rate" regardless of the number of procedures this process necessitated; the total number of salvage procedures required per patient is a second measure of outcome required for this form of reporting.

Potential Confounders. Results may potentially be biased by: 1) the etiology and extent of the stenosis, 2) the presence of tracheomalacia, gastroesophageal reflux disease, concomitant glottic/supraglottic stenosis, 3) surgery as primary or revision procedure, 4) the length of the postoperative follow-up period, and 5) any simultaneous additional procedures. All of these factors are tabulated for the reader in as much detail as the source articles allow.

Study Designs. There are two retrospective controlled studies (level 3) and four retrospective uncontrolled studies (level 4) addressing this topic. The retrospective study design is limited by the inherent biases that prompted surgeons to proceed with single- versus double-stage reconstruction; single-stage reconstruction is preferred with milder stenosis, which bolsters confidence that a tracheotomy will not be replaced. Retrospective studies such as these can attempt to partially address these biases by also reporting potential confounding variables within the two groups and by carefully limiting conclusions drawn from the study. The authors of the controlled studies recognize that patients who are chosen for single-stage reconstruction are more likely to have milder preoperative stenosis (with a more favorable prognosis) and use this knowledge to temper their conclusions. Also, authors of controlled and uncontrolled studies report most of the potential confounders discussed above. Because of the limitations of the retrospective study design, we cannot use these studies to directly compare the effectiveness of the single- and double-staged approach. Instead, we can only conclude that properly selected children with subglottic stenosis can undergo single-stage LTR with acceptable decannulation rates.

Highest Level of Evidence. Both of the level 3 studies show that the rate of decannulation without additional procedures (OSDC) with single-stage LTR was usually equal to or greater than with double-stage LTR. Again, this observation is tempered by the preoperative factors that drove surgeons to opt for the single- versus double-staged approach. One author attempted to account for some of these factors with statistical methods; multiple logistical regression showed that staging was the only preoperative variable that was significantly predictive of decannulation. A higher number of additional procedures, however, was predicted by both a double-staged procedure and a higher grade of stenosis in this report [2]. The other author sorted the data according to the specific procedure and severity of the stenosis. Logistic regression showed no effect of age, in contrast with some previous reports. The grade of initial stenosis again had a significant effect on decannulation rates in double-stage procedures and in single-stage procedures after subsequent salvage reconstructions [1].

Additional evidence is available in the form of retrospective case series, which corroborate that 56%–85% of patients were successfully decannulated after one single-stage LTR, with better rates reported in more recent years. In addition, the 86%–96% decannulation rate after salvage procedures is consistent with the rates seen in controlled studies. In the largest of these series [4], moderate (33%–66% occlusion) or severe (>66% occlusion) tracheomalacia was predictive of the need for postoperative tracheotomy.

Applicability. These results are applicable to further testing of the hypothesis that single-stage LTR can provide acceptable decannulation rates in patients ≤19 years of age, with grade 2–4 subglottic stenosis and no concomitant airway pathology.

Morbidity. Restenosis may occur in the long or short term. Also, short-term postoperative complications of single-stage reconstruction include mucous plugging, wound infection, bleeding, pneumothorax, pneumatocele, and withdrawal from benzodiazepines or narcotics used with long-term sedation for postoperative intubation. These factors were not reported in detail in a distinct population treated for subglottic stenosis in these reports.

CLINICAL SIGNIFICANCE AND FUTURE RESEARCH

There is level 3 evidence to suggest that properly selected children with subglottic stenosis may undergo single-stage LTR with acceptable decannulation rates of 67%–82% (without additional procedures) or 86%–100% (with subsequent salvage surgery). Also, fewer procedures may be required with the single-stage approach, but these results must be tempered by the knowledge that single staging was pursued in patients with less severe preoperative stenosis, in addition to other preoperative factors. Level 4 evidence corroborates the operation-specific and overall decannulation rates reported in these controlled studies. With the inherent biases of the retrospective study design, these studies cannot directly compare outcomes with the single- versus double-staged approach, but they do encourage higher-level testing of the hypothesis that single-staged LTR may be a suitable alternative to the double-staged approach under appropriate circumstances.

Such higher-level testing could either focus on the outcome with single- versus double-staged procedures in patients in standardized circumstances, or it could attempt to identify which variables make patients most suitable for the single-staged approach. For the former, the impact of single- versus double-staged LTR on decannulation and need for subsequent procedures theoretically would ideally be addressed in a randomized controlled trial of grade-specific, operation-specific, and etiology-specific subglottic stenosis. For example, the rate of decannulation with and without subsequent salvage procedures after primary single- versus double-staged LTR in patients ≤18 years of age with grade 2–3 acquired subglottic stenosis and no concomitant airway, pulmonary, cardiac, or neurologic disease would be studied; postoperative steroid usage, intubation duration, and sedation, as well as preoperative screening, incidence, and treatment of gastroesophageal reflux would be standardized in the two groups. Using the single-procedure decannulation rates from one of the controlled studies [2], however, in order to create a study with 90% power to detect a 5% rate difference, a sample size of 320 patients would be necessary. Such a study would require more patients than were included in both controlled studies combined, one of which took 12 years to accumulate 199 patients at one of the busiest airway centers in the United States. Given that we do not expect the results of such a trial soon, future research may otherwise focus on resolving those pivotal preoperative factors that define the most promising candidates for the single-stage approach.

Cotton grading system for subglottic stenosis.* [8]

Grade 1: 0%–70% obstruction
Grade 2: 71%–90% obstruction
Grade 3: 90%–99% obstruction
Grade 4: 100% obstruction

*Based on endoscopic examination

Myer-Cotton grading system for subglottic stenosis.* [9]

Grade 1: 0%–50% obstruction
Grade 2: 51–70% obstruction
Grade 3: 71%–99% obstruction
Grade 4: 100% obstruction

*Based on endotracheal tube outer diameter

Reference	Hartnick, 2001		Saunders, 1999	
Level (design)	3 (HC)		3 (HC)	
Sample size	199 children		69 children	
OUTCOMES				
Intervention	Single stage	Double stage	Single stage	Double stage
Decannulation rate before subsequent procedures*	Grd 2: 82% Grd 3: 79% Grd 4: 67%	Grd 2: 85% Grd 3: 37% Grd 4: 50%	80% (reported 20% of patients required further reconstruction; data from all grades combined)	71% (reported 29% of patients required further reconstruction; data from all grades combined)
Decannulation rate after subsequent procedures	Grd 2: 100% Grd 3: 86% Grd 4: 100%	Grd 2: 95% Grd 3: 74% Grd 4: 86%	91% (reported 9% still with tracheostomy; data from all grades combined)	62% (reported 38% still with tracheostomy; data from all grades combined)
Need for subsequent procedures	1.3 procedures per child (mean)	1.6 procedures per child (mean)	3.2 procedures per child after LTR (mean)	6.2 procedures per child after LTR (mean)
STUDY DESIGN				
Grading	Myer-Cotton system		Cotton system	
Degree of initial stenosis	Grd 2: 49% Grd 3: 47% Grd 4: 3%	Grd 2: 22% Grd 3: 63% Grd 4: 15%	Mean grd 2.14 (includes no grd 4) Pre-LTR tracheostomy: 31%	Mean grd 2.56 Pre-LTR tracheostomy: 100%
Etiology of stenosis	Isolated subglottic stenosis, further details NR		17% congenital 83% acquired	21% congenital 79% acquired
Procedure timing†	Children have "often undergone attempted repair of airway disease before being seen"		3% with previous laryngeal surgery	20% with previous laryngeal surgery
Procedure details	85% costal cartilage	81% costal cartilage	All costal cartilage Postop intubation ×7–10 d	All costal cartilage Postop indwelling stent ×3 mo
Age‡	4.28 y (4.46)	4.62 y (5.67)	2.9 y (0.2–12)	3.4 y (0.5–15)
Concomitant airway pathology	None with concomitant glottic, supraglottic, suprastomal, or tracheal stenosis		"No concomitant airway surgery was undertaken in any of the subject group [*sic*]," further details NR	
Reflux	NR		NR	
Inclusion criteria	<18 y old, preoperative Myer-Cotton grading system available		Patients "for whom sufficient data was available at the time of the study"	
Exclusion criteria	Concomitant glottic, supraglottic disease; concomitant suprastomal collapse or tracheomalacia; anterior cricoid split		Concomitant airway surgery	
Time period	1988–2000		NR	

HC = historical cohort, grd = grade, LTR = laryngotracheal reconstruction, NR = not reported, postop = postoperative.

* In Hartnick, "operation specific" decannulation rates were reported for the procedure without subsequent open surgical repairs; endoscopic procedures did not affect these calculations.

† Primary: no previous open airway procedures; salvage: previous open airway procedure; extended: combined with another procedure (i.e., expansion cartilage grafting or open arytenoid procedure).

‡ Age is reported as the mean, with either (standard deviation or range).

THE EVIDENCE CONDENSED: Laryngotracheal reconstruction for subglottic stenosis

Reference	Gustafson, 2000	Younis, 2003
Level (design)	4 (RCS)	4 (RCS)
Sample size	190 children, 200 cases	35 children
OUTCOMES		
Decannulation rate after SS-LTR alone*	85% (170/200)	83% (29/35)
Decannulation rate after SS-LTR and subsequent procedures†	96% (182/190)	NR
Need for subsequent procedure	9 patients required a 2nd procedure (details NR) for decannulation. 2 patients required a 3rd procedure (details NR) for decannulation. All postop tracheotomy: 30	NR
STUDY DESIGN		
Procedure types	101 ant costal cartilage graft, 39 ant/post costal graft, 29 post costal graft; 15 ant auricular cartilage graft, 7 ant costal graft/post cricoid split, 5 ant/lat costal cartilage graft, 3 ant thyroid ala graft, 1 ant Z-plasty	All 35 received ant and post costal cartilage grafts
Follow-up time	1–11.9 y (mean 5.5 y)	3 mo–6 y
Grading	Myer-Cotton system	Not specified
Degree of initial stenosis	Grd 1: 35%; Grd 2: 35%; Grd 3: 28%; Grd 4: 2%; 64% tracheotomy dependent	Grd 1: 0%; Grd 2: 0%; Grd 3: 60%; Grd 4: 40%
Etiology of stenosis	48% premature, further details NR	35 acquired; 0 congenital
Procedure timing‡	132 primary; 68 salvage	24 primary; 11 salvage
Concomitant airway pathology	18% VCP; 37% BPD; 35% reactive airway disease; 29% tracheomalacia	NR
Reflux	"Most patients" received preop and postop antireflux therapy	All evaluated by gastroenterologist
Age	2 mo–19 y	18 mo–9 y
Inclusion criteria	All children undergoing SS-LTR with at least 1 y follow-up	All children who had SS-LTR
ETT duration	2–17 d	10–24 d
Time period	1987–1998	1992–2000

RCS = retrospective case series, SS-LTR= single-stage laryngotracheal reconstruction, NR = not reported, DS-LTR = double-stage laryngotracheal reconstruction, VCP = vocal cord paralysis, BPD = bronchopulmonary dysplasia, RLN = recurrent laryngeal nerve, ETT = endotracheal tube, ant = anterior, post = posterior, lat = lateral, preop = preoperative, postop = postoperative.
* These rates are not affected by postoperative intubation with an endotracheal tube in children who did not require additional airway modification.
† This includes children who required postoperative tracheotomy who were subsequently decannulated.
‡ Primary: no previous open airway procedures; salvage: previous open airway procedure; extended: combined with another procedure (i.e., expansion cartilage grafting or open arytenoid procedure).

Reference	McQueen, 1999	Lusk, 1991
Level (design)	4 (RCS)	4 (RCS)
Sample size	28 children	9 children
OUTCOMES		
Decannulation rate after SS-LTR alone*	79% (22/28)	56% (5/9)
Decannulation rate after SS-LTR and subsequent procedures†	86% (24/28)	89% (8/9)
Need for subsequent procedure	7 patients required a second procedure for decannulation (3 SS-LTR, 1 DS-LTR, 3 laser excision of granulation at graft site) with 3 of these after postop tracheotomy. All postop tracheotomy: 7	2 patients required a second procedure for decannulation (2 SS-LTR) 1 patient required a 3rd procedure for decannulation (1 DS-LTR then 1 SS-LTR)
STUDY DESIGN		
Procedure types	11% ant and post grafts, 89% ant grafts only	4 ant cricoid split only, 4 auricular cartilage, 1 costal cartilage graft
Follow-up time	2 mo–3 y	1 y–2 y 3mo
Grading	Cotton system	Cotton system
Degree of initial stenosis	Grd 1: 18% Grd 2: 43% Grd 3: 25% Grd 4: 0% Grd unknown: 14% 18% tracheotomy dependent	All stages 2 and 3, further breakdown NR
Etiology of stenosis	23 acquired 5 congenital	5 congenital 9 acquired
Procedure timing‡	All primary	8 primary 1 salvage
Concomitant airway pathology	NR	1 s/p laryngeal cleft repair
Reflux	NR	NR
Age	"Children"	1 mo–12 y
Inclusion criteria	All children undergoing SS-LTR	Single-stage repair of subglottic stenosis
ETT duration	2–14 d	0–13 d
Time period	1993–1996	1987–1990

RCS = retrospective case series, SS-LTR= single-stage laryngotracheal reconstruction, NR = not reported, DS-LTR = double-stage laryngotracheal reconstruction, VCP = vocal cord paralysis, BPD = bronchopulmonary dysplasia, RLN = recurrent laryngeal nerve, ETT = endotracheal tube, ant = anterior, post = posterior, lat = lateral, preop = preoperative, postop = postoperative, S/P = status post.
* These rates are not affected by postoperative intubation with an endotracheal tube in children who did not require additional airway modification.
† This includes children who required postoperative tracheotomy who were subsequently decannulated.
‡ Primary: no previous open airway procedures; salvage: previous open airway procedure; extended: combined with another procedure (i.e., expansion cartilage grafting or open arytenoid procedure).

REFERENCES

1. Hartnick CJ, Hartley BE, Lacy PD, et al. Surgery for pediatric subglottic stenosis: disease-specific outcomes. Ann Otol Rhinol Laryngol 2001;110(12):1109–1113.
2. Saunders MW, Thirlwall A, Jacob A, Albert DM. Single- or two-stage laryngotracheal reconstruction: comparison of outcomes. Int J Pediatr Otorhinolaryngol 1999;50(1):51–54.
3. Cotton RT, Myer CM 3rd, O'Connor DM, Smith ME. Pediatric laryngotracheal reconstruction with cartilage grafts and endotracheal tube stenting: the single-stage approach. Laryngoscope 1995;105(8 Pt 1):818–821.
4. Gustafson LM, Hartley BE, Liu JH, et al. Single-stage laryngotracheal reconstruction in children: a review of 200 cases. Otolaryngol Head Neck Surg 2000;123(4):430–434.
5. Lusk RP, Gray S, Muntz HR. Single-stage laryngotracheal reconstruction. Arch Otolaryngol Head Neck Surg 1991;117(2):171–173.
6. McQueen CT, Shapiro NL, Leighton S, Guo XG, Albert DM. Single-stage laryngotracheal reconstruction: the Great Ormond Street experience and guidelines for patient selection. Arch Otolaryngol Head Neck Surg 1999;125(3):320–322.
7. Younis RT, Lazar RH, Astor F. Posterior cartilage graft in single-stage laryngotracheal reconstruction. Otolaryngol Head Neck Surg 2003;129(3):168–175.
8. Cotton RT. Pediatric laryngotracheal stenosis. J Pediatr Surg 1984;19:699–704.
9. Myer CM 3rd, O'Connor DM, Cotton RT. Proposed grading system for subglottic stenosis based on endotracheal tube sizes. Ann Otol Rhinol Laryngol 1994;103:319–323.

10 Subglottic Stenosis

10.B.

Cricotracheal resection: Chance of decannulation, chance of undergoing subsequent salvage procedure

Jennifer J. Shin and Christopher J. Hartnick

METHODS

A computerized Ovid search of MEDLINE 1966–November 2003 was performed as described in Section 10.A. For inclusion criteria for this clinical query, we required the following: 1) a distinct population of children ≤19 years old, 2) management with cricotracheal resection (CTR) for >50% subglottic stenosis, preferably with comparison to laryngotracheal reconstruction (LTR), and 3) outcome measures of decannulation and/or need for subsequent salvage procedures. Articles were excluded if patients' initial grade was not discernable. For serial reports of case series of a cumulative patient population from the same principal author and institution [1–9], only the most recent update for each institution was included [4, 9]. Just one controlled study [10] and three uncontrolled case series [4, 9, 11] met these criteria.

RESULTS

Outcome Measures. The major outcome measure is rate of decannulation. This rate can be reported either after CTR alone or after CTR *and* subsequent salvage procedures, with the latter being predictably higher. CTR can be performed as a single- or double-stage procedure. Also, the percent of CTR patients that go on to require a subsequent salvage procedure is noted in these reports. Finally, some reports comment on the postoperative voice, and these results are tabulated for the reader, but these outcomes must be viewed with some caution, given the vagaries of nonvalidated subjective descriptions of voice.

Potential Confounders. The stage of stenosis and other potential confounders are as discussed in Section 10.A. In addition, another important possible confounder is the distance of the subglottic stenosis from the true vocal cords themselves. Likewise, gastroesophageal reflux, cardiac, pulmonary, and neurologic disease may alter outcomes.

Study Designs. All studies are retrospective reviews. Two reported data from prospective databases [4, 10]. One study is comparative, reporting outcomes for both CTR and LTR. The results from this comparative historical cohort are summarized below. With the inherent biases of case series and such limited comparative data,

these retrospective study designs can suggest correlations and propose hypotheses, even if they do not establish a direct cause and effect. This means that they can suggest a role of CTR in the treatment of subglottic stenosis, but cannot prove that CTR outcomes are better than or equivalent to LTR outcomes, as higher level prospective controlled studies could.

Highest Level of Evidence. This retrospective evidence suggests that CTR may be an acceptable alternative to LTR in properly selected patients. The one controlled historical cohort reported decannulation rates of 67%–100% after CTR with salvage procedures, and 37%–79% after CTR without subsequent salvage. Likewise, decannulation rates were reported of 83%–88% for LTR without subsequent operations, and 74%–100% for LTR with subsequent salvage. Data from uncontrolled case series are consistent with these results, with 73%–94% decannulation after CTR alone and 86%–100% after CTR and salvage procedures.

Applicability. These results are applicable to patients ≤19 years of age with Myer-Cotton grade 2–4 subglottic stenosis, and suggest that future research on the role of CTR in the management of this disease should focus on this group.

Morbidity. Complications include recurrent laryngeal nerve injury, arytenoid prolapse, dehiscence, and restenosis in a minority of patients, with further details tabulated for the reader.

CLINICAL SIGNIFICANCE AND FUTURE RESEARCH

These retrospective studies suggest that CTR is a reasonable alternative to LTR for >50% subglottic stenosis in carefully chosen patients (Myer-Cotton grade 3–4). Future research will determine whether CTR versus LTR will result in higher, lower, or similar rates of decannulation, additional procedures, and complications. In an ideal world, that future research would be performed as a randomized controlled trial of CTR versus LTR in children ≤19 years old with grade 3–4 subglottic stenosis with ≥3-mm margin 2, 4, 11] of tissue between the stenosis and vocal cords, and no concomitant airway, pulmonary, cardiac, or neurologic disease. Preoperative screening for gastroesophageal reflux would be standardized with prevalence and treatment equal in the two pretreatment groups. Staging, stenting, and timing of the procedures (primary or salvage) would also be standardized or equally distributed between the two groups. The primary outcome measure would be operation-specific

decannulation, with secondary outcome measures of need for subsequent salvage procedure, and validated and/or subjective voice outcome measures [12–15]. To achieve a 90% power to detect a 5% rate difference in decannulation rates of 80% and 85%, a sample size of 492 patients would be necessary. Given that such a study is not immediately forthcoming, future research may focus on identifying the preoperative factors that best predict success with CTR.

THE EVIDENCE CONDENSED (controlled): Cricotracheal resection versus laryngotracheal reconstruction—Decannulation rate

	Cricotracheal resection				Laryngotracheal resection			
	Single stage		Double stage		Single stage		Double stage	
	No salvage	With salvage	No salvage	With salvage	No salvage	With salvage	No salvage	With salvage
Grade 3	75% (6/8)	88% (7/8)	75% (6/8)	88% (7/8)	79% (34/43)	86% (37/43)	37% (23/61)	74% (45/61)
Grade 4	100% (1/1)	—	67% (4/6)	83% (5/6)	67% (2/3)	100% (3/3)	50% (7/14)	86% (12/14)

Source: Adapted with permission from Hartnick CJ, Hartley BE, Lacy PD, et al. Surgery for pediatric subglottic stenosis: disease-specific outcomes. Ann Otol Rhinol Laryngol 2001;110(12):1109–1113 (Annals Publishing Co.).
This is a level 3 study (historical cohort with control) using the Myer-Cotton classification system.

THE EVIDENCE CONDENSED (uncontrolled): Cricotracheal resection for grade 3 or 4 subglottic stenosis

Reference	Monnier, 2003
Level (design)	4 (RCS)
Sample size	60

OUTCOMES	
Decannulation rate: CTR alone	Not reported
Decannulation: CTR and salvage	95%
Need for subsequent procedures	5% (3 revisions for anastomotic dehiscence)
Follow-up period	"≥10 y in 11 children," not otherwise specified

STUDY DESIGN	
Inclusion criteria	All who underwent CTR after 1978
Exclusion criteria	None noted
Procedure timing‡	33 primary 27 salvage
Grading system	Myer-Cotton
Degree of initial stenosis	2 grade 2 41 grade 3 17 grade 4 (46 tracheotomy dependent)
Etiology of stenosis	8 congenital 34 acquired 16 mixed 2 other
Distance from stenosis to cords	11 with stenosis in glottis and subglottis 6 with transglottic stenosis
Concomitant airway disease	12 with bilateral vocal cord fixation 3 with unilateral vocal cord fixation
Reflux	Not reported
Simultaneous procedures	7 Rethi 2 graft of buccal mucosa 7 pedicled graft of membranous trachea 4 vocal cord separation
Age	≤16 y
Stents/staging	38 single stage 22 double stage
Vocal outcome	38 "normal voice or slight dysphonia" 18 "moderate to severe dysphonia"
Morbidity/ complications	1 complete restenosis 1 temporary reintubation 1 death 6 mo after surgery 1 dehiscence 0 RLN injury

RCS = retrospective case series, LTR = laryngotracheal reconstruction, CTR = cricotracheal resection, VCP = vocal cord paralysis, RLN = recurrent laryngeal nerve, BPD = bronchopulmonary dysplasia, PPI = proton pump inhibitor, PRN = as needed, post = posterior, ETT = endotracheal tube.
‡ Primary: no previous open airway procedures; salvage: previous open airway procedure; extended: combined with another procedure (i.e., expansion cartilage grafting or open arytenoid procedure).

THE EVIDENCE CONDENSED (uncontrolled): Cricotracheal resection for grade 3 or 4 subglottic stenosis

Reference	Rutter, 2001*	Triglia, 2001
Level (design)	4 (RCS)	4 (RCS)
Sample size	44	16
OUTCOMES		
Decannulation rate: CTR alone	73%	94%
Decannulation: CTR and salvage	86%	100%
Need for subsequent procedures	16% (4 LTR, 1 laser resection, 2 temporary T tubes)	6% open (1 anastomosis repair) and 37% endoscopic (6 laser resection)
Follow-up period	12–67 mo	Mean 38 mo, >5 y in 5 children
STUDY DESIGN		
Inclusion criteria	All who underwent CTR 1993–1998	All who underwent CTR 1993–2000
Exclusion criteria	None noted	None noted
Procedure timing‡	16 primary 28 salvage	16 primary 0 salvage
Grading system	Myer-Cotton	Myer-Cotton
Degree of initial stenosis	33 (77%) grade 3 10 (23%) grade 4	1 grade 2 12 grade 3 3 grade 4 (10 tracheotomy dependent)
Etiology of stenosis	24 former premature 1 Wegener's granulomatosis Not further specified	2 congenital 13 acquired 1 mixed
Distance from stenosis to cords	Ideally ≥3 mm below the vocal cords, but not limited to these patients	"Minimal residual subglottic space between the stenosis and vocal cords"
Concomitant airway disease	3 laryngotracheoesophageal clefting	All with normal vocal cord function
Reflux	14 taking antireflux therapy 6 post-Nissen fundoplication	Not reported
Simultaneous procedures	2 post-cricoid splits 1 post-cricoid graft 4 arytenoid lateralization 1 arytenoidectomy	None specified
Age	Mean 6 y (range 13 mo–19 y)	Mean 5 y (range 7 mo–17 y)
Stents/staging	22 single stage/ETT 16 T tube 4 suprastomal stent 2 no stent	8 single stage with Portex ETT 8 double stage with reinforced silastic stent
Vocal outcome	Not reported	8 patients demonstrated within-normal-range values for intensity pitch or maximum phonatory time
Morbidity/ complications	"Most" with minor web at the anastomosis 20 arytenoid prolapse (8 required laser arytenoidectomy) 9 restenosis (5 still tracheotomy dependent) 2 RLN injury 1 subglottic collapse 0 dehiscence	1 cervical emphysema 2 dehiscence

RCS = retrospective case series, LTR = laryngotracheal reconstruction, CTR = cricotracheal resection, VCP = vocal cord paralysis, RLN = recurrent laryngeal nerve, BPD = bronchopulmonary dysplasia, PPI = proton pump inhibitor, PRN = as needed, post = posterior, ETT = endotracheal tube.
* Rutter et al. reported that 40 of these children were distinct from the 1997 report by Stern [1].
‡ Primary: no previous open airway procedures; salvage: previous open airway procedure; extended: combined with another procedure (i.e., expansion cartilage grafting or open arytenoid procedure).

REFERENCES

1. Stern Y, Gerber ME, Walner DL, Cotton RT. Partial cricotracheal resection with primary anastomosis in the pediatric age group. Ann Otol Rhinol Laryngol 1997;106(11): 891–896.

2. Walner DL, Stern Y, Cotton RT. Margins of partial cricotracheal resection in children. Laryngoscope 1999;109: 1607–1610.

3. Hartley BE, Cotton RT. Paediatric airway stenosis: laryngotracheal reconstruction or cricotracheal resection? Clini Otolaryngol Allied Sci 2000;25(5):342–349.

4. Rutter MJ, Hartley BE, Cotton RT. Cricotracheal resection in children. Arch Otolaryngol Head Neck Surg 2001; 127(3):289–292.

5. Monnier P, Savary M, Chapuis G. Cricotracheal resection for pediatric subglottic stenosis: update of the Lausanne experience. Acta Oto-Rhino-Laryngol Belg 1995;49(4):373–382.

6. Monnier P, Lang F, Savary M. Partial cricotracheal resection for severe pediatric subglottic stenosis: update of the Lausanne experience. Ann Otol Rhinol Laryngol 1998; 107(11 Pt 1):961–968.

7. Monnier P, Lang F, Savary M. Cricotracheal resection for pediatric subglottic stenosis. Int J Pediatr Otorhinolaryngol 1999;49(Suppl 1):S283–S286.

8. Monnier P, Lang F, SavaryM. [Treatment of subglottis stenosis in children by cricotracheal resection]. Ann Oto-Laryngol Chirug Cervico-Faciale 2001;118(5):299–305.

9. Monnier P, Lang F, Savary M. Partial cricotracheal resection for pediatric subglottic stenosis: a single institution's experience in 60 cases. Eur Arch Oto-Rhino-Laryngol 2003;260(6):295–297.

10. Hartnick CJ, Hartley BE, Lacy PD, Liu J, Willging JP, Myer CM. 3rd, Cotton RT. Surgery for pediatric subglottic stenosis: disease-specific outcomes. Ann Otol Rhinol Laryngol 2001;110(12):1109–1113.

11. Triglia JM, Nicollas R, Roman S. Primary cricotracheal resection in children: indications, technique and outcome. Int J Pediatr Otorhinolaryngol 2001;58(1):17–25.

12. Clary RA, Pengilly A, Bailey M, Jones N, Albert D, Comins J, Appleton J. Analysis of voice outcomes in pediatric patients following surgical procedures for laryngotracheal stenosis. Arch Otolaryngol Head Neck Surg 1996;122(11): 1189–1194.

13. Hartnick CJ, Volk M, Cunningham M. Establishing normative voice-related quality-of-life scores within the pediatric otolaryngology population. Arch Otolaryngol Head Neck Surg 2003;129(10):1090–1093.

14. MacArthur CJ, Kearns GH, Healy GB. Voice quality after laryngotracheal reconstruction. Arch Otolaryngol Head Neck Surg 1994;120(6):641–647.

15. Zalzal GH, Loomis SR, Fischer M. Laryngeal reconstruction in children. Assessment of vocal quality. Arch Otolaryngol Head Neck Surg 1993;119(5):504–507.

SECTION III
Systematic Reviews in Otology

Section Editors

Joseph B. Nadol Jr., MD

Steven D. Rauch, MD

11 Measuring Audiometric Outcomes

Christopher F. Halpin

Audiometry provides evidence to 19 of the topic areas in this book and to much of the otolaryngologic literature. Audiometric evaluations, consisting of pure tone thresholds and word recognition scores are not data points; they are very general evaluations designed to cover all reasonable questions about the peripheral auditory system of the patient. It is clear that audiometric evaluations contain a great deal of useful data, and equally clear that large amounts of the information should be reduced and refocused in order to serve as useful study evidence. This chapter will explore some fine points regarding audiometric data, and attempt to provide support for the process of data reduction and focus. Issues related to pure tones will be addressed first, followed by a discussion of standard word recognition.

PURE TONE THRESHOLDS

Although pure tone thresholds are often used as direct measures of the severity of ear disease, the concept of "hearing loss in dB" contains a pitfall to be considered, particularly in sensorineural cases. Pure tones were originally chosen as clinical stimuli because of their specificity in the frequency domain. The object was to excite the basilar membrane in the most localized manner possible. What is not always clear is that, whereas an electronic analysis of the tone may reflect a single point in the frequency domain, a single hair cell in the cochlea will actually respond to a broad range of frequencies, especially over the very large intensity range of the clinical audiogram. This broad excitation pattern is known as a tuning curve [1] and an example is shown in Figure 11.1. A hair cell tuning curve has a best response, or characteristic frequency (Cf) shown as the sharp peak at 1 kHz. As the stimulus moves away from the Cf, more intensity is required to stimulate the cell, resulting in a steep slope above the best frequency and a characteristic plateau at frequencies below. The complete audiogram in Figure 11.1 is the audiometric threshold pattern expected given a single healthy inner hair cell located at 1 kHz (by "healthy," is also implied all other structures necessary for the normal action of this cell). This means that both the high- and low-frequency slopes of this audiogram show the maximum pure tone "loss" expected adjacent to a healthy cochlear region, because one cell (here at 1 kHz) could be responsible for all these thresholds [2].

Normal audiograms appear flat [near 0 decibel hearing level (dBHL)] because they reflect the sensitivity of the tips of thousands of overlapping tuning curves, each with a different Cf. In the normal cochlear regions,

pure tone thresholds reflect the characteristic frequencies of the healthy hair cells. As hair cells and other structures are damaged by cochlear disease, their sensitivity is reduced or eliminated [3], and the response will arise from cells (with different Cf's) whose tuning curve tail still includes the stimulus region. Even in a region where hair cells are absent, a threshold may be measured because of the responses of these adjacent hair cells in a healthier region of the cochlea. In Figure 11.1, if a cell normally transducing 2 kHz were to die, the patient would continue to raise their hand at 70 dBHL, because the remaining cell at 1 kHz could perceive the 2-kHz tone at that intensity. Thus, the tuning curve concept calls into question the use of hearing thresholds as a continuous scale of severity ("hearing loss in dB"). For example, a patient with an ototoxic reaction and a "steeply sloping high frequency loss" could be modeled as having a flat-topped array of many of these curves (resulting in normal low-frequency thresholds) up to 1 kHz, with the "sloping loss" formed by the high-frequency tail of the tuning curve of the last normal cell. In such a case, pure tone detection arising from the high-frequency response area of that cell (the high-frequency slope in Figure 11.1) would mask the fact that the cochlear transduction elements were completely absent above the 1-kHz region. There are many possible combinations of these relationships, including abnormal tuning curve shapes not discussed here (c.f., Liberman and Dodds [4]). However, investigators using "hearing loss in dB" as a continuous severity variable should be cautious as to whether or not thresholds are likely to reflect graded changes in their location of interest.

If hearing is to be used as an outcome measure, it is critical to remember that elevated audiometric thresholds are a symptom and not a disease. Thus, grouping patients or study subjects on the basis of "hearing loss in dB" is analogous to the formulation: "sickness in degrees of oral temperature." Although it is true that a group of sick people may exhibit a higher average oral temperature than normals, most would agree that they should be parsed into disease-mechanism groups and studied separately. When studying ear disease and treatment outcomes, steps beyond numerical audiometric values are often indicated in order to attempt to study homogeneous groups. This can be done using history items, shared environmental factors, family membership, pilot studies, and more complex use of thresholds and speech audiometry.

With these cautions in mind, the pure tone threshold audiogram remains a critical element in understand-

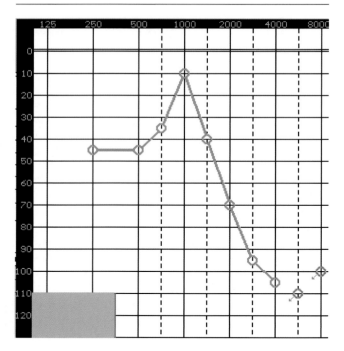

Figure 11.1. The tuning curve. This is the hypothetical audiogram that would be expected to result from a single properly functioning inner hair cell located at 1 kHz. This tuning curve represents the limits of cochlear damping on either side of a cell. Given the very large intensity range of the clinical audiogram, thresholds are expected at nearly all frequencies, even when no other living hair cells are present. This curve places a fundamental limit on the interpretation of pure tone thresholds in sensorineural cases.

ing ear cases. For reasons described above, it is best interpreted in the frequency (or cochlear place) domain where it remains valid and useful. To return to Figure 11.1, the audiogram, with all its limitations, has correctly identified the place of the healthy functioning element, and the regions above and below it which require further investigation are apparent to the clinical eye. Used appropriately, pure tone audiometry is very informative. However, pure tone thresholds were not designed to suffice on their own. They deliver useful place information and are designed to be combined with the more challenging word recognition tests to form useful models of cochlear damage [5]. This approach will be described in the word recognition section of this chapter.

Reliability. Threshold audiometry is occasionally challenged as a "subjective" test in that the patient may choose to respond or not. In addition, audiologists confronted with this assertion seem to have complete confidence in the objectivity of the results without a clearly articulated reason. The underlying misunderstanding all around is that the clinical response in audiometry is not

a handraise, it is control of the handraise by means of the stimulus. In other words, control must clearly shift from the patient to the audiologist such that the response can be automatically elicited under any super-threshold condition, at any time, in any order. For example, after a tentative handraise, as the hand is slowly lowering, the stimulus can be raised 5 dB and re-presented. The patient's hand will shoot back up immediately without conscious thought and this is as "objective" a response as could be desired. During an evaluation, an audiologist can reliably tell if they, or the patient, has control.

The reliability of audiometry is also subject to its physical calibration. The stability of electronic amplifiers and attenuators has improved such that it is rare to find them drifting by as much as 1 dB without a total failure. The transducers (headphones, insert phones, and bone vibrators) are under more physical stress and it remains possible for them to fail in a graded manner (~10 dB) without obviously ceasing to function. Clinical audiometers are calibrated quarterly to specific American National Standards Institute (ANSI) standard physical output values using a sound level meter, an artificial ear (a 6-cc cylinder with a microphone at the bottom), and an artificial mastoid to measure the force output of the bone vibrator. Clinical audiometers are required to have additional testing of attenuator linearity, cross-talk (signal leakage), and other functions annually [6]. These physical calibrations are very reliable and can be backed up by daily listening checks to spot any failures. A good addition to a study archive is a copy of the calibration report for the time period during which the data were taken.

Although a threshold is thought of as the boundary between hearing and not hearing, in functional terms, it is a place on the psychometric function of the rising probability of response with intensity. This place is specified by standardization of the technique for arriving at the value. Audiologists have standardized the Hughson-Westlake bracketing procedure for this purpose [7]. The key point is that the response is defined as two clear responses while ascending from below the threshold. A different (lower) threshold is found when descending, because of the brain's ability to track a known stimulus into physiologic noise a little better than it is able to recognize a signal emerging from it. Even given this amount of specification, some threshold boundary effects vary with ear disease. The sharpest response boundaries are found in cases of cochlear hearing loss. However, at the extremely low intensities where normal listeners' thresholds are found, there is more variability (~5 dB). This amount of variability is also expected in conductive loss cases because the effective energy at the cochlea is the same even though the amount of input sound is higher. Finally, there can be very large inconsistencies (~15 dB) when the disease mechanism is retrocochlear in nature. Because this level of uncertainty can indicate pseudohypoacusis as well, care must be taken to be sure which mechanism is responsible.

Response Limits. Some patients do not hear a tone delivered at the equipment's maximum intensity. The audiometric maxima (for air conduction) reflect not only the output limits of audiometers, but also the likely physiologic range of hearing sensitivity in the majority of cochleas. Output limits, especially from 1 to 6 kHz (i.e., 120–125 dBHL) reflect the boundary between the most severely affected cochleas and the threshold of pain (~130 dBHL). There are exceptions, for example, a very severe mixed loss where a near-maximal conductive component would be applied in addition to a severe (70–90 dB) flat cochlear loss, but these tend to be rare. Except in these cases, the electronics tend to give out in about the range where the cochlea itself gives out.

The inability to elicit a response at the upper limit of the audiometer output should not usually be classified as missing data. Particularly in studies of severe cochlear effects, the out-at-limits symbol clearly indicates a useful magnitude, even though it does not reflect the standard data collection method. Especially when combining these values into pure tone averages (PTAs), out-at-limits must be assigned a numerical value. One approach is to extrapolate data to one step (5dB) above the audiometer output limit. This is the first possible step where a response could have been seen, and is therefore a conservative estimate. Even if a finding of out-at-limits actually represents the complete absence of cochlear function, a number that expresses a high magnitude is often consistent with the goals of a well-constructed study.

There are two special (and common) circumstances in which the magnitude implied by the upper limits of audiometric data must be handled differently. These are the vibrotactile response and the apparent air-bone gap which would result from simply extrapolating the out-at-limits values separately for air and bone conduction. Clearly, vibrotactile responses do not represent auditory events at all. However, they do impose an upper threshold value limit, not by an absent response, but by the presence of a response not related to audition. An audiogram showing the expected thresholds for vibrotactile responses in adults [8] is shown in Figure 11.2 (at 250 and 500 Hz). Vibration is best perceived at low frequencies, high intensities, and also when using the more effective force coupling of the bone vibrator. Also, these responses will not be eliminated by the introduction of masking, so they may appear as either masked or unmasked thresholds. Vibrotactile response areas are well known to audiologists and any combination of transducer, frequency, and intensity approaching these values should elicit further investigation to determine whether the patient perceives the stimulus as sound or vibration. Protocols differ as to whether these levels are plotted on the audiogram (and discussed in the report) or simply excluded. Certainly they must be excluded from any consideration as real values when used in studies of hearing. Bone vibrators require a great deal of force to accelerate the head, and so their output limits are much lower (in dBHL) than those of headphones.

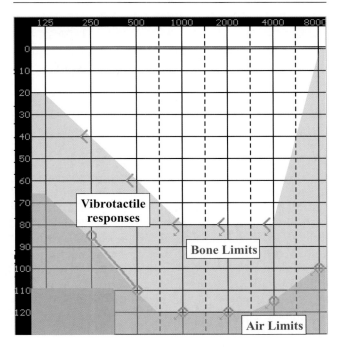

Figure 11.2. Vibrotactile and transducer limits. The 250- and 500-Hz responses by bone and air conduction represent responses expected to arise from vibrotactile rather than auditory perception. Although they are plotted here for reference, they may be omitted from audiograms for clarity and certainly should not be included in study data as pure tone thresholds. The border of the light blue area describes typical bone conduction output limits and the border of the green area, air conduction.

Also, bone vibrators are much more efficient at eliciting vibrotactile sensations and so vibrotactile thresholds occur at lower levels as well. Even though different output limits and vibrotactile responses for air and bone stimuli may be marked on an audiogram, they should never be interpreted as evidence of a real air-bone gap.

The minimum values for audiometric thresholds typically include responses of −10 or −15 dBHL. Both zero and negative values should be discussed with anyone creating data spreadsheets and other such analysis tools. An entry of zero is synonymous with missing values in some data schemes, and care must be taken to allow both audiometric zero and negative threshold values to occur as real magnitudes and to be accommodated in any data set. Conversely, a truly missing point must not act as an audiometric value of zero. There are even instances in which an event that exceeds audiometer limits can occur in the healthy direction. In recent studies of superior semicircular canal dehiscence and other "third cochlear window" disorders, a hypersensitivity to bone-conducted stimuli has been noted [9]. Here, the patient may still be responding to 250 Hz by bone conduction at the lowest possible level. These cases illustrate the need for extrapolated measurements (e.g., addition of one 5-dB step) to appropriately assign a numerical value for what amounts to an out-at-limits response at the opposite end of the stimulus intensity scale.

Conductive Effects. Unlike cochlear pathology, elevated thresholds caused by middle ear disease are more consistent with a model of "hearing loss in dB" as a continuous severity variable. Here, the pure tone thresholds reflect the attenuation of acoustic energy and the relative inefficiency with which it passes through the middle ear system. This inefficiency can indeed be scaled as decibels in the intensity domain. However, it has been shown that different mechanisms such as middle ear fluid volume and viscosity, as well as different sites of lesion, from the tympanic membrane to the stapes footplate, result in different patterns of attenuation as a function of frequency [10]. In general, this means that a fine structure of frequency-specific effects is expected to exist in middle ear cases, even though the mechanism can be modeled as a single load on the system (i.e., the presence of a cholesteatoma). Whether or not it is necessary to report frequency-dependent effects depends on scientific issues specific to each study. It is advisable to first assess all these effects to be sure important frequency-specific findings are not lost before reducing the data set, or combining the thresholds into averages.

There is an assumption in interpretation of conductive hearing loss (as air-bone gap) that the sensitivity of the cochlea is unaffected by the middle ear mechanism. This allows evaluation of the size of the difference between the bone conduction and air conduction thresholds to be used to scale the disease effect. The well-known caveat to point out is the phenomenon known as "Carhart's notch" [11]. In otosclerosis cases, it is clear that the bone conduction threshold at 2 kHz is elevated (by as much as 20 dB) as a consequence of stapes footplate fixation, as opposed to any actual cochlear damage. Carhart's notch may resolve after stapes surgery, and this phenomenon requires some accommodation when studying conductive loss. When subtracting presurgical air versus bone data, the middle ear inefficiency is underestimated. There are several practical ways to address this issue, including ignoring it after having assessed the likely impact on a particular study. Other ways include using the air conduction improvement alone, or concentrating on frequency regions where the effect is not expected. One aspect of this conductive phenomenon which is less well known is that elevated bone conduction thresholds are not necessarily restricted to otosclerosis and are not always narrowly focused on 2 kHz [12]. Here again, knowledge of the disease mechanism under study can guide the investigator in an assessment of whether these effects are likely in their study and how they might be accommodated by using a carefully selected portion of the audiometric evaluation.

Threshold Combinations. A common example of audiometric data reduction and focusing is the combination of 0.5-, 1-, 2-, and 3-kHz thresholds into a standard PTA [13]. The data reduction is achieved by removing 0.25, 4, and 8 kHz and other threshold data, and the focus is achieved because the central frequencies are those found to be most contributory to word recognition. The basic discovery in the area of speech contribution was made by Fletcher, who demonstrated that frequency bands do not add to word recognition in the same manner that they add to loudness. The information content of some bands, especially around 2 kHz, were found to be higher than others [14, 15]. A graph of the speech importance bands is shown in Figure 11.3. Fletcher's predictive model, which he called the Articulation Index (AI) and which is now known as the Speech Intelligibility Index (SII), is a scale of available speech information from 0 to 1. An SII of 1.0 is achieved when all the frequency bands are fully audible. The SII can be thought of as the proportion of speech information in the listening situation given the patient's threshold, the speech level, noise, etc. With this general value derived from the listening conditions, the expected score on any specific speech test can be calculated. For example, an SII of 0.1 (or 1/10th of all possible speech information) will predict a score of 50% of Spondees (i.e., SRT) but only about 18% of standard word recognition monosyllables (i.e., CID W-22) at the same level.

Because the SII predicts the score on the standard monosyllable word recognition tests, this provides a very useful diagnostic tool where cochlear regions can be tested as to whether they are actually contributing the normal amount of information in a specific patient [16]. Figure 11.3 shows that speech information, although best at 2 kHz, is actually fairly evenly distributed throughout frequencies from 310 to 4 kHz. Note that the axis of this graph does not range from 0 to 1.0, but only from 0 to 0.10 because no one band, not even the most important 2-kHz region, contributes as much as one-tenth of the possible speech information. Speech information and word scores actually respond most sensitively to the addition or subtraction of bands. Any set of thresholds that add up to the same SII would result in the same predicted word recognition score. Adding frequencies from 125 up to 750 Hz, or frequencies from 8 down to 2 kHz, or a middle ("most important") set from 1.5 to 3 kHz, each result in an SII value of ~0.4 and a prediction of ~80% correct for clinical word recognition in all three cases.

The red lines in Figure 11.3 are designed to point out a possible alternative to the standard PTA that is based on the behavior of the SII importance values. Most clinicians would argue that 500 Hz should be included in any audiometric model of word recognition. In examining

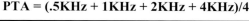

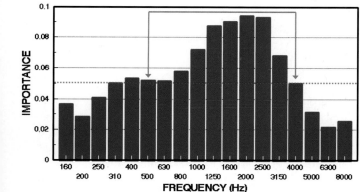

Figure 11.3. Speech importance by frequency. The blue histogram bars represent the contribution of each one-third octave frequency band to speech intelligibility as modeled by the SII. As can be seen in this figure, no one frequency (even those around 2 kHz) contributes more than one-tenth of the possible speech information, and the eventual performance is therefore responsive to the number of available bands. The red lines indicate why 4 kHz might be included in those PTA calculations which also include 500 Hz.

Fletcher's importance values, it can be seen that if the PTA thresholds were restricted to those contributing approximately 0.05 SII (as 500 Hz does), then a case could be made for the inclusion of 4 kHz (also about 0.05 SII). Conversely, if the cut-off was established at 0.07 SII (the 3-kHz importance value) then the 500-Hz band would not qualify.

The SII has been shown over many years to contain sufficient complexity to account for most clinically relevant aspects of the effect of thresholds on word recognition [5]. Conversely, simpler methods (such as PTA) can occasionally fail to accommodate some of these aspects. This is illustrated in Figure 11.4. In the first panel (Case

A), an audiogram is shown with a PTA of 22.5 dB. Because all the frequency bands below 3 kHz contribute their normal weight and sensitivity, the patient's SRT will not be affected (~9 dBHL). Also, the patient will be able to demonstrate the ability to recognize whispered words (94% at 35 dBHL). However, this patient will be very clear that they are experiencing abnormal hearing as a result of a significant dysfunction involving the cochlear base.

The second panel (Case B) shows a case with the same PTA. Here, the different pattern of thresholds does not allow the addition of many central bands until higher levels. The result is very different in the clinic. This patient's SRT will be affected and should rise to more than 25 dBHL. The patient's ability to recognize whispered speech, both at home and in the clinic, will be remarkably worse (~70% at 35 dBHL). The effects in both of these cases are captured using the complexity of the SII calculation, and obscured by attempting to simplify the speech and level effects using PTA. As a practical matter, the calculations required for an "instant" SII calculation were not available during the 1930s when it was discovered by Fletcher and colleagues. Academic institutions can assign a programmer to the creation of small calculation programs (or spreadsheet functions) if the relationship of thresholds to word recognition is an important study consideration. Despite many alternate proposals in this area in academia, clinicians who wish to apply a well-accepted calculation method can use the ANSI standard [17].

A different reason is sometimes given for combining audiometric thresholds in clinical studies. Some investigators would like to use PTA to capture any changes within a wide range of audiometric frequencies. There

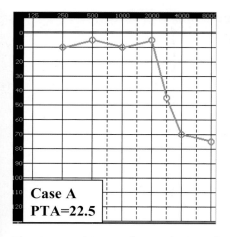

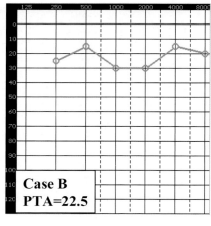

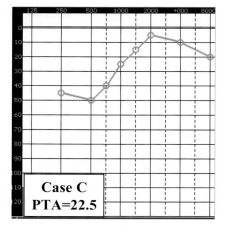

Figure 11.4. PTA can obscure disease effects. These three audiograms have the same PTA (0.5, 1, 2, −4 kHz). If each represented a change from a starting normal ear, most clinicians would suspect that three different disease processes were at work because of clues from the location of affected frequency regions. Clinically, Cases A and B would present with very different impact on whispered speech or SRT. It is important to judge the effect of including all such cases in a proposed study based on the magnitude of PTA alone.

are two important assumptions underlying this approach that must be carefully considered before using such a strategy. One is a qualitative principle suggested by the cases in Figure 11.4. Here, one might imagine a study participant's audiogram changing from normal to one of the audiograms A, B, or C. Many clinicians would interpret these audiograms as evidence of three different disease processes. A report that PTA had decreased by 15 dB in all cases, although true, would tend to obscure this aspect of the study population. Once again, the audiogram, *per se*, is designed to cover all bases rather than to specifically track any one disease effect.

A separate, quantitative effect of attempts to capture changes by combining thresholds into PTA is illustrated in Figure 11.5. The assumption underlying PTA is that the expected effect of the disease will be seen at all PTA frequencies. If this is so, changes across all frequencies will cause sensitive changes in the PTA variable. If, however, changes occur at only one of the PTA frequen-

cies, the inclusion of the other components of the average will act to dilute any change in the apparent outcome. In both cases in Figure 11.5, PTA has decreased by 6.25 dB during the study. In the top case (Case D), a serious noise-induced hearing loss has occurred in the expected 4-kHz frequency region. This localized change of 25 dB is reduced to an apparent change of only 6.25 dB when forced into the PTA combination. However, the case at the bottom (Case E) shows that small changes distributed across a flat hearing loss produce the same quantitative change of 6.25 dB in the PTA with a fairly negligible impact to the clinical observer. Whatever the effects of combining pure tone thresholds into averages, it is important to use the same approach in both the initial and final stages of any study. If, for example, the inclusion criteria specifies loss at only one or two frequencies, a final report using PTA may dilute the impact of changes.

Threshold Data Reduction and Focus. The audiometric effect of the disease or treatment mechanism under study cannot always be known *a priori*. However, the issues

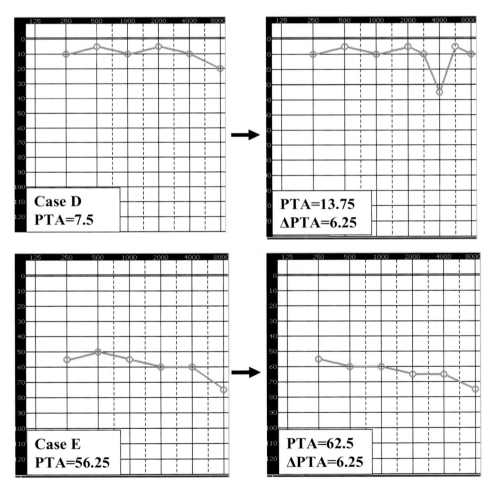

Figure 11.5. Equal change in PTA. These two cases both exhibit a change in PTA of 6.75 dB. In the top case (D), a significant noise-induced hearing loss has developed, but the inclusion of the other PTA frequencies tends to minimize this effect. In Case E, very little of clinical interest has likely occurred, but the fact that the changes are distributed across frequency tends to maximize the resulting change in PTA.

raised above suggest the value of vigorous attempts to apply what is known about the clinical entity in order to reduce and refocus the broad range of information expected from the clinical audiogram. Both quantitative and qualitative features of pure tone audiometry suggest that it is not advantageous to act as if no knowledge exists *a priori*, especially if some expectations can be developed using pilot studies or other means. As is often true in investigations, there is value in removing information from the study construct and keeping a smaller set of variables closely related to the question of interest. One example might include tracking the progression of a sloping loss by reporting only the 2-kHz threshold for each subject [18]. Such an approach does not track all effects, but the reduced variable lends itself to a helpful scatterplot, where variability across subjects can be appreciated by the clinical reader. It is not invalid to produce several such plots for individual frequencies and to decide *post hoc* if choosing one will obscure any significant aspect of the population behavior. The mechanistic approach can, and should be, extended further into expectations of specific changes within the site of lesion. Audiometric variables may be focused on changes at the base of the cochlea in certain ototoxicity studies, on low frequencies when studying the onset of Ménière syndrome, etc.

To keep a data set properly focused on one question, it is often necessary to use different thresholds from the audiograms collected for a study. The obvious example is the evaluation of unmasked and masked thresholds in different cases to arrive at what, in both instances, is an estimate of cochlear sensitivity. It is the sensitivity of the cochlea that should remain the target, whereas the means of arriving at it should be allowed to vary. There is no symbol on the audiogram for the inefficiency of the middle ear, the depopulation of the cochlea, or practically any other directly useful data construct. What actually occurs as these results are used is that a clinician evaluates each audiogram and finds the particular results or relationships that answer the question in that patient. This means that it is expected that some amount of flexible, secondary processing should be expected when using audiograms in order to result in directly meaningful and comparable data. The audiologist, for example, could assist by evaluating each audiogram and reporting (as primary variables) the cochlear sensitivity based on whichever test values represent the best data within that case. These are still reported as numbers (in dBHL) but with the flexibility to decide if masked or unmasked, air or bone thresholds best represent the desired construct, and to properly factor equipment limits, vibrotactile responses, pseudo-conductive losses, etc. These secondary steps should be considered when converting audiometric evaluations into data, rather than expecting the useful data to present in the same form in every case.

Reducing the audiometric data to focus on specific disease mechanisms in each study does not mean that standard reporting conventions should be abandoned. Reporting standards reflect valuable efforts to allow good communication of results across sites. They must necessarily be somewhat general and they often include combining thresholds [13]. If the disease process affects most thresholds, the act of combining the data will not obscure the result. If some aspect under study is more highly localized, a clear change at one frequency can be obscured by forcing it into an average with unaffected regions (as in Figure 11.5). One answer is to start by casting the net wide, by finding any single-frequency changes, and end by considering if using a standard reporting method will preserve those changes when presented to the reader. Any important differences in the audiometric fine structure that are obscured by the more general standard reporting convention should be known to the researcher and presented to the reader.

WORD RECOGNITION

A set of pure tone thresholds may result from the presence of only a few functioning cochlear cells (as in Figure 11.1) or an entire array, thus the pure tone audiogram is not sufficient for a comprehensive evaluation of cochlear disease effects. However, accurate word recognition by the patient requires the combined function of many healthy cells across a broad region (*c.f.*, Young and Sachs [19]) and therefore these data do indeed respond to changes in the health, number, and location of the cochlear population [3]. However, word recognition necessarily involves providing a rapidly changing acoustic stimulus across most of the cochlear array and so the place specificity of the effects is not revealed by words alone. This means that both tones and words provide essential, but fundamentally different, data and one must be combined with the other in order to form a useful model of each patient's ear. The original concept of the audiologic evaluation involved combining the pure tone thresholds and the word recognition results to arrive at a working model of the peripheral auditory system [20]. Stated generally, the approach is to evaluate the severity of missing information using word recognition and then to build (and test) a frequency map of the areas responsible, using the pure tones [5].

Although the principles for combining thresholds and speech scores diagnostically were introduced more than 50 years ago, they involved substantial calculation, and real-time methods for accomplishing this using computer software [21] are only beginning to be implemented. An example is provided here to illustrate how this approach may become very useful both clinically and in studies. Figure 11.6 illustrates the completion of the analysis begun in Figure 11.1. Here again, the hypothetical audiogram is drawn which could result from a very limited patch of functioning cells around 1 kHz.

What has been added using software is a word recognition analysis box on the left. The vertical axis of this box is percent correct for monosyllables, and the horizontal axis is speech level in dBHL. The red bars show the patient's actual scores (central tic) and the critical difference at the p < 0.05 level (red bar height). The SII is used to calculate that ear's performance for monosyllables across level (the red "S" curve). Because the SII calculation was developed using normals, the plotted curve represents the percent scores expected if the cochlea is fully populated with useful (but somehow insensitive) receptors (i.e., if the hearing problem was attributable exclusively to a loss of sensitivity from a middle ear pathology). This line, then, represents the opposite of the tuning-curve hypothesis and, if the patient's actual scores match

the line, this can only result from a near-normal population of functioning cells in the region being stimulated by the speech signal [5].

In the top panel of Figure 11.6, when word recognition is tested at 45 dBHL, the speech spectrum presented is shown by the lower-level green "speech banana" (note the shape of the speech spectrum marked in green). For this test condition, only the frequencies near 1 kHz are sufficiently sensitive to receive the speech information and a fairly low percent score is predicted (~50%). In this case, the patient actually gets a score close to that value (score at base of arrows). The interpretation using both tones and word recognition is that a portion of the middle turn of this cochlea is functioning near-normally. When the speech level is then raised to 90 dBHL, there are then two possible outcomes (arrows). In one case (*a*), the score rises to 92% correct. Because this higher level (the louder speech banana) exceeds the thresholds from

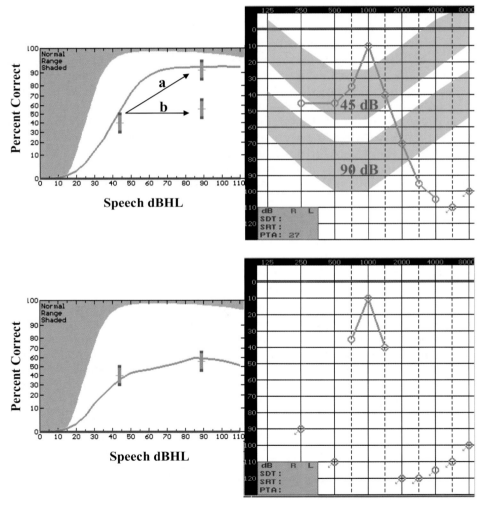

Figure 11.6. Combining pure tones and word recognition. This figure shows the resolution of the diagnostic dilemma posed by Figure 11.1. Here, a speech intelligibility graph is added to the left of the audiogram. The horizontal axis is speech level, and the vertical is percent score of the standard monosyllable word recognition test. The red "S" curve uses the SII to calculate a best-possible performance function based on the audiogram. Two real tests (red bars) were done for comparison (45 and 90 dB, green spectra on top audiogram). Of the two major possibilities (arrows *a* and *b*) the data best support *b*, and the bottom case shows thresholds (regions) hypothetically removed until a narrow region remains which could explain the speech findings.

0.125 to about 2.5 kHz, this high score is evidence that a large amount of the cochlea is healthy enough to contribute to word recognition. The opposite outcome is seen with the lower arrow (*b*). Here, the actual score does not rise with level, even though a broader range of audiometric thresholds are exceeded at 90 dBHL. This second interpretation (*b*) is modeled in the lower panel. Here, both high and low frequencies are removed from the SII equation by placing them out-at-limits. This is acoustically impossible as seen in Figure 11.1, but it is not an impossible model for the actual underlying state of hair cell survival in a real cochlea [22]. Looking to the newly drawn model of expected speech function ("S" curve, lower audiogram) it can be seen that no healthy regions outside of a narrow range from about 0.75 to 1.5 kHz are required to account for the patient's actual word recognition data. The unknown state of the cochlea when examined using thresholds alone in Figure 11.1 can now be resolved into a more useful model by using the audiogram as its own filter and by combining the SII calculation and the actual speech scores.

What is important about this level of analysis is that cases described by the two extreme possibilities (Figure 11.6, *a* versus *b*) may not belong in the same study. Even though they have identical audiograms, one case has a broadly functioning cochlea and the other very narrow. If studies were then performed on a variety of issues, e.g., temporal processing, hearing aid benefit, or general quality of life, the predicted outcomes would be very different. Without adding the word recognition testing, the pure tone audiograms suggest these cases are identical. It is therefore not surprising that when groups are formed using only thresholds in the literature, a widely variable set of results is sometimes found.

Reliability. Unlike pure tones, speech stimuli are not static in frequency and intensity. Rapid changes in level and frequency comprise the speech information itself. However, some relationship to a stable acoustic signal must be made in order to reliably repeat the test and report the results in terms of level. Clinical monosyllables use a steady reference tone (1 kHz) provided along with the materials. The strategy for use of this tone is that the audiologist will play the initial tone track (of a tape or CD) and adjust the sensitivity of the input stage of the audiometer using a V.U. (volume unit) meter. The calibration tone provides a steady input for adjustment of the V.U. meter to "0." This adjustment is generally accurate to within 1 dB. When using the standard CID W-22 monosyllable tests in this manner, each instance of the repeated carrier phrase "You will say . . ." will result in the V.U. meter reaching "0" exactly during the word "say." The remainder of the stimulus is allowed to vary with the "same vocal effort" [23]. Although this may seem to allow a fair amount of internal variation, it is consistent with the nature of speech signals.

The patients' vocal response and the audiologist's "ear" are also factors affecting the reliability and validity of word recognition. Patients as young as 4 years old can and should be tested using the standard materials. The fact that a young patient may not understand the meaning of a word does not invalidate their response. The monosyllable word recognition test is a test of the peripheral end-organ transmission of speech information, and comprehension is not required. If the cochlea picks up the proper sound and the patient repeats it, the item is correct. This also applies to testing patients whose native language is not English. Many patients can at least benefit from a clinical left versus right ear comparison of scores using English word materials even if their familiarity with the language imposes some decrease on those scores. However, considerable care must be taken when switching to the use of speech materials in another language. Very good materials exist for this purpose in many languages but the audiologist must be a fluent speaker of that language such that her/his "ear" is trained to the specific phoneme boundaries, before judgments of correct or incorrect responses can be made. When designing a study, a criterion of "testable in English" may allow better inclusion of local patient populations than a more stringent requirement of "English as a first language." For children, it is also possible to employ pointing tasks for words [i.e., the WIPI (Word Intelligibility by Picture Identification) test] and this can also be adapted to populations with tracheal tubes, etc.

The Effective Range of Word Recognition Scores. The original monosyllable recordings have another quality that makes them remarkably useful for clinical work and research. A well-designed test will not squander any of its operating range on cases outside the range encountered in the clinic. For word recognition, this means that the test will not be so difficult that patients' scores will decrease into the 70% or 80% range before they begin to present in the clinic complaining about communication difficulties. Conversely, a test so easy that people with significant disease can still score 100% will miss the milder disease effects. Over the years, it has become evident that the standard monosyllable tests operate nearly exactly over the range that covers clinical cases most efficiently. A study by Roth et al. [24] has shown that patients begin to come in complaining at about a 94% word recognition score. The standard word recognition test will then track dysfunction down to 0% correct and this range includes the majority of clinical cases and outcomes.

While standard monosyllables track the likely clinical cases, this is precisely because a score of 100% does not reflect a completely healthy cochlea. This relates to the relationship between the underlying speech information available to the cochlea (as calculated by SII) and the prediction of the outcome of a specific test, in this case, monosyllable word recognition. The healthy ear reflects great redundancy in terms of speech information and can absorb significant loss of this ability before standard test scores begin to fall. For example, the 94% score described above is the result of a calculated SII of ~0.5. In other words, patients lose half of their total ability to receive speech information before they begin to be sufficiently challenged to seek care. This level of ability also reflects the upper range of clinical monosyllable scores. The word recognition score then, does not directly scale all cochlear ability, but roughly coincides with the bottom half.

An exception to the useful operating range for standard monosyllables was made apparent as cochlear implants were introduced to the clinic. It was clear that 0% correct for standard monosyllables did not track auditory abilities all the way down to none. This was seen when other tests were given with closed sets of responses, etc. Patients with 0% correct for monosyllables might get a chance-level score (indicating no auditory information) or a score higher than chance, indicating some effect of auditory stimulation on their performance. The problem introduced was that the patients were evaluated before implantation with different speech materials than those that were optimal afterwards. This can be addressed using a special case of monosyllable scoring. In the standard NU#6 monosyllable and similar tests, each word is composed of three phonemes (initial consonant, medial vowel, final consonant). This means that each standard list of 50 items represents 150 chances to guess these phonemes from a limited set, giving rise to an *a priori* probability of about 4% correct. This allows the full-range standard monosyllable test to operate all the way down to scaling no auditory ability (chance level for phonemes), and can then be used after treatment to continue to scale the outcome as high as it might go. Although more complex test strategies are possible, outcome researchers may find it beneficial to maximize the use of standard materials to allow comparisons across treatments and populations. Scaling the test difficulty using sentences, closed set consonants, etc., does not always allow for this valuable cross-comparison in the literature.

Word Recognition Variability and Significant Differences. Standard monosyllable test results are also useful in studies because their within-subject model of variance and significant difference have been carefully specified [25]. Thornton and Raffin noted that word recognition should be viewed as an accumulation of binary responses (correct versus incorrect) and therefore distribute according to a binomial model of variance (rather than the more common normal, or Gaussian distribution). They published a table of significant differences (p = 0.05) from any starting score (reprinted in Halpin and Rauch [26]). This was necessary because, unlike the normal variance model, the binomial critical

differences are narrower at the extremes of the range than they are in the center. For example, comparing a subject's initial score of 50% correct to a post-treatment outcome of 66% (a 16-point change) shows that such a change is not significantly different. However, starting with a score of 2% correct, a post-treatment outcome of 12% (a 10-point change) does exceed the critical difference at the p < 0.05 level. What this means is that no one point-change criterion (i.e., >15%) will serve in all cases given the binomial distribution.

It is reasonable to ask "so what?" when considering factoring this additional complexity into a clinical study. The impact was recently addressed using a large retrospective analysis of the audiometric outcomes using oral steroids for sudden sensorineural hearing loss (n = 318). The result was a constant failure of correct detection in about 9% of cases using any fixed criteria [26]. Higher number criteria (i.e., 15 points change) have few errors of specificity, but allow many misses. Lower numbers (i.e., 10 points change) reduce errors of sensitivity, but allow more false positives. Here again, the *a priori* expectations about the data are important. In studies of conductive loss or normal listeners (where scores near 100% are expected), a narrow significance criteria will reveal all the effects. This is also true when studying cases at the low end of the range (near 0%) because there again, smaller changes are nonetheless significant at the p < 0.05 level. Conversely, a study of late-stage Ménière syndrome, where many scores fall near the middle of the range (50% correct), needs a wide criterion to avoid errors of specificity where significance is claimed when this is not true mathematically. Put simply, there is no single point-change criterion that will accommodate within-subject critical differences properly. Use of the binomial table is not difficult and in many studies, where pre- versus postcomparisons within subjects are made, this level of detail may be indicated.

The critical differences described above assume that the test was given using the standard recorded materials and that full 50-item lists were given. The use of recorded materials is very important, particularly if the results are to be published as data. These materials can be carefully specified where the use of "monitored live voice" cannot. Also, any use of half-lists (25 items) as study data should be discouraged. This practice has emerged from a basic misunderstanding about the performance of monosyllable tests: Although it is true that the central tendency of tests of any length tend to be near the true value, the variability of these lists is very different. The critical difference values for truncated (half) lists are so large that they are not useful for most study applications.

It is possible to introduce more complex tests, as well as simply better-quality recordings of standard tests. The reason to continue to use the standard recordings is not that better-sounding examples are impossible. Every new recording or change in test materials implies a new relationship with the SII. The slope of the "S" curve function in Figure 11.6, for example, is related to the difficulty of the materials including the brightness and quality of the recording and even the accent of the speaker. The original recordings are currently available on compact disc, and staying with these "older" materials allows comparison of performance across many years, thousands of cases, and the full range of disease mechanisms. Many complex psychophysical tasks also exist, but their results are typically translated into speech terms for discussion of clinical impact. What is unique, and valuable, about the standard monosyllable test in quiet is its very well-understood relationship to cochlear regions (as in Figure 11.3), and its specification in both statistical and acoustic terms. In many studies, the primary unknown is the individual health of each patient's ear. When this is the case, a design in which simple but well-understood tests are applied across patients is likely to result in a useful answer.

SUMMARY POINTS

1. The results of audiometry are not expected to act as data points without some additional specification and refocusing given the goals of the study. Focusing audiometric data should include prior knowledge about the expected mechanism of the disease and the expected range of the outcome values.

2. In sensorineural cases, pure tone thresholds have better validity as a map of likely healthy and unhealthy cochlear regions (across frequency) than as a continuous scale of disease severity (in dB). Cochlear "hearing loss in dB" often does not reliably group homogeneous populations, but when combined with word recognition, this can be improved.

3. Audiometry is reliable in terms of both physical calibration and psychophysical technique.

4. It is recommended to collect and observe the fine structure of audiometric data and to determine whether significant findings are obscured using analyses based on recommended reporting standards (i.e., dBPTA). If not, use of the standards is valuable for effective communication.

5. It is possible to integrate audiometric threshold effects in terms of speech performance, but this requires the complexity of the SII calculation in order to be accurate.

6. A monosyllable word recognition test can scale the entire range of auditory ability, from near normal down to none by using phonemic scoring. This approach avoids changing test methods before and after intervention, and allows comparison of familiar tests across populations.

7. It is possible to accurately detect significant differences between a subject's pre- and post-treatment word recognition scores, but this requires the complexity of the use of the binomial difference table, rather than any single percent-difference criterion.

8. The basis of audiometry is to examine the status of each ear using highly specified conditions (simple stimuli in quiet) which have known relationships to the location and nature of peripheral physiologic dysfunction. Each patient's ear, as revealed by simple tests, is often the critical unknown when studying diseases and treatments rather than the general behavior of any group on various complex tasks.

REFERENCES

1. Kiang N, Moxon E. Tails of the tuning curves of auditory nerve fibers. J Acous Soc Am 1974;55:620–630.
2. Halpin C. The tuning curve in clinical audiology. Am J Audiol 2002;11:56–64.
3. Schuknecht H. Pathology of the Ear. 2nd ed. Malvern, PA: Lea & Febiger; 1993.
4. Liberman M, Dodds L. Single neuron labeling and chronic cochlear pathologies. III. Stereocilia damage and alteration of threshold tuning curves. Hear Res 1983;16:55–74.
5. Halpin C, Thornton A, Hou Z. The articulation index in clinical diagnosis and hearing aid fitting. Curr Opin Otolaryngol Head Neck Surg 1996;4:325–334.
6. American National Standards Institute S3.6 Specifications for Audiometers. New York: Author; 2004.
7. Carhart R, Jerger J. Preferred method for determination of pure-tone thresholds. J Speech Hear Dis 1959;24:330.
8. Boothroyd A, Calkwell S. Vibrotactile thresholds in pure-tone audiometry. In: Chaiklin J, Ventry I, Dixon R, eds. Hearing Measurement: A Book of Readings (2nd ed. 1981). New York: Addison-Wesley; 1970:134–139.
9. Rosowski J, Songer J, Nakajima H, Brinsko K, Merchant S. Clinical, experimental, and theoretical investigations of the effect of superior semicircular canal dehiscence on hearing mechanisms. Otol Neurotol 2004;25(3):323–332.
10. Ravicz M, Rosowski J, Merchant S. Mechanisms of hearing loss resulting from middle ear fluid. Hear Res 2004;195:103–130.
11. Tonndorf J. Sensorineural and pseudosensorineural hearing losses. ORL J Ortorhinolaryngol Relat Spec 1988; 50(2):79–83.
12. Ahmad I, Pahor A. Carhart's notch: a finding in otitis media with effusion. Int J Pediatr Otorhinolaryngol 2002; 64(2):165–170.
13. Monsell E. New and revised reporting guidelines from the Committee on Hearing and Equilibrium. Otolaryngol Head Neck Surg 1995;113:176–178.
14. French N, Steinberg J. Factors governing the intelligibility of speech sounds. J Acous Soc Am 1947;19:90–119.
15. Allen J. Harvey Fletcher's role in the creation of communication acoustics. J Acous Soc Am 1996;99: 1825–1839.
16. Fletcher H. A method for calculating the hearing loss for speech from an audiogram. J Acous Soc Am 1950;22:1–5.
17. American National Standards Institute S3.5 Standard Methods for Calculation of the Speech Intelligibility Index. New York: Author; 1997.
18. Halpin C, Khetarpal U, McKenna M. Autosomal-dominant sensorineural hearing loss in a large North American family. Am J Audiol 1996;5(1):105–111.

19. Young E, Sachs M. Representation of steady-state vowels in the temporal aspects of the discharge patterns of populations of auditory nerve fibers. J Acous Soc Am 1979;66: 1381–1403.

20. Carhart R. Individual differences in hearing for speech. Ann Otol Rhinol Laryng 1946;55:233–266.

21. Thornton A, Halpin C, Han Y, Hou Z. The Harvard Audiometer Operating System [software]. Palo Alto, CA: Applitech; 1994.

22. Halpin C, Thornton A, Hasso M. Low frequency sensorineural hearing loss: clinical evaluation and implications for hearing aid fitting. Ear Hear 1994;15:71–81.

23. Hirsh I, Davis H, Silverman E, Reynolds E, Eldert E, Benson R. Development of materials for speech audiometry. In: Chaiklin J, Ventry I, Dixon R, eds. Hearing Measurement: A Book of Readings (2nd ed. 1981). Reading, MA: Addison-Wesley; 1952:183–196.

24. Roth A, Lankford J, Meinke D, Long G. Using the AI to manage patient decisions. Adv Audiol 2001;Nov–Dec: 22–23.

25. Thornton A, Raffin M. Speech discrimination scores modeled as a binomial variable. J Speech Hear Res 1978;21: 507–518.

26. Halpin C, Rauch S. Using audiometric thresholds and word recognition in a treatment study. Otol Neurotol 2006;27(1):110–116.

12 Chronic Otitis Media

12.A.

Topical antibiotic versus placebo or antiseptic alone for chronic active otitis media without cholesteatoma: Impact on resolution of otorrhea

Jennifer J. Shin and J. Gail Neely

METHODS

A computerized PubMed search of MEDLINE 1966–December 2005 was performed. The medical subject heading "otitis media, suppurative" was exploded and the resulting articles were cross-referenced with those mapping to the subject headings "anti-bacterial agents," "macrolides," "fluoroquinolones," "clindamycin," or "lactams," yielding 227 publications. These articles were then reviewed to identify those that met the following inclusion criteria: 1) patient population without cholesteatoma with discharging ears through a chronic perforation, 2) intervention with topical antibiotic drops versus placebo or antiseptic drops, 3) outcome measured in terms of cessation of otorrhea. Because of the richness of the literature, randomized controlled trials (RCTs) were specifically extracted as the best evidence available. Articles in which random allocation could not be confirmed or in which other interventions were allowed were excluded. The bibliographies of the articles that met these inclusion criteria and relevant reviews were manually checked to ensure no further relevant articles could be identified. This process yielded eight articles. It was unknown whether data from one of these articles were included in the reported 1988 Browning article; therefore, the Browning article was preferentially reviewed [1].

RESULTS

We describe herein the results of individual studies. In the subsequent pages are results for the related meta-analysis.

Outcome Measures. Successful treatment in four RCTs was defined in terms of a dry otomicroscopic examination. The other three RCTs defined outcomes in terms of the percent with dry ears (unspecified whether by history or examination) and the percent with cure or improvement (not further specified).

Potential Confounders. The antibiotic regimen used (medication, dose, and duration), compliance, addition of steroids, additional local care, previous surgery, eustachian tube function, and time of follow-up are among variables that could affect results. These potential confounders are provided in as much detail in the adjoining tables as the original reports allow.

Study Designs. All seven of these studies were RCTs (level 1), but only four of them confirmed that basic demographic and risk factors (i.e., potential confounders) were balanced between the groups at the outset. Six different topical antibiotic regimens were compared with either a placebo or antiseptic control: gentamicin, neomycin/polymyxin, ofloxacin, ciprofloxacin, tobramycin, and chloramphenicol. Within five studies, all patients in all groups were also treated with aural toilet. Follow-up times ranged from 1 to 6 weeks. Five of the RCTs were double-blinded to reduce bias. Only one study reported a power calculation, suggesting that with approximately 400 patients they had 80% power to detect a 10% difference between groups. The largest sample size in the remaining trials was 165 patients. One of the studies also examined a subgroup of patients with open mastoid cavities. Based on their data for this subset (38%, n = 9/24 success with treatment versus 22%, n = 4/18 success with placebo), a minimum of 366 subjects would be required to achieve a 90% power to detect a 10% difference between groups with such cavities. Therefore, no definitive conclusions can be inferred about cavity case responses from the currently available subset data.

Highest Level of Evidence. Two RCTs demonstrated significantly more cessation of otorrhea with topical antibiotics in comparison to topical placebo (saline). The remaining five RCTs compared topical antibiotic to topical antiseptic. Two of these five RCTs showed that topical antibiotic resulted in significantly more dry ears than topical antiseptic. These two RCTs studied ciprofloxacin drops compared with boric acid in alcohol or Burow aluminum acetate drops; these two RCTs were also the largest of the studies, with the greatest power to detect any potential true differences between treatment regimens. The remaining data showed no significant difference between topical antibiotic and antiseptic, although the majority did show a trend toward better outcome with antibiotic. The disparate results of these remaining data may be attributable to the following: 1) antibiotics other than ciprofloxacin were tested, 2) different antiseptic agents were used (i.e., povidone iodine), 3) sample sizes were smaller, resulting in less power to find a significant difference between groups. To better understand these results, a detailed meta-analysis has been performed (see the following section) to determine the results of all of the data combined.

Only three RCTs contained data for follow-up periods extending beyond the treatment course. The Macfadyen trial [4] showed better results with antibiotic even 18 days after treatment cessation, but the Jaya RCT [6] showed no difference at the same follow-up time. Browning et al. [1] performed an unofficial substudy in which they followed 14 medication "success" subjects, without cavities, for an average of an additional 6 weeks to determine the rate of activity recurrence and found 43% became active again during that period.

One paper suggested that there was no difference in outcome with antibiotics versus placebo in patients with cavities, but as noted above, in order to achieve adequate power (i.e., ability to find any difference that truly exists), the study would have needed to accrue a much larger number of cavity patients.

Applicability. These results are applicable to patients with suppurative otorrhea in the setting of chronic otitis media with tympanic membrane perforation.

Morbidity/Complications. No complications were reported. However, the data are not sufficiently rigorous to confirm or refute any ototoxicity related to either treatment regimen.

Reference	Browning, 1988			
Level (design)	1 (RCT)			
Sample size*	165 (187)			

OUTCOMES

	% success (no pooling of discharge; noninflamed middle ear mucosa)			
	All patients	**Compliant**	**No cavity**	**Cavity**
Topical abx	45.5% (n = 40/88)	45.8% (n = 38/83)	48.4% (n = 31/64)	37.5% (n = 9/24)
Control	25.3% (n = 19/75)	26.5% (n = 18/68)	25.4% (n = 15/59)	22.2% (n = 4/18)
p Value	=0.009 (χ^2)	Not reported	<0.05	NS
Conclusion	Abx sig. better	Trend toward abx better	Abx sig. better	No difference
Follow-up time	4–6 wk			

STUDY DESIGN

Inclusion criteria	>16 y of age; permanent defect in pars tensa; inflamed middle ear mucosa; mucopurulent discharge after 1 wk of aural toilet and no treatment for 4 wk
Exclusion criteria	Cholesteatoma; aural polyps
Randomization effectiveness	Effective. Comparable groups. Intact canal wall cases (123) and those also associated with open mastoid cavities (42) were stratified before randomization
Age	20–79 y
Masking	Outcome assessment blinded
Antibiotic ear drop regimen	Gentamicin with hydrocortisone ear drops, 4 drops 4× a day, tragal pumping for 4 wk, with an additional 2 wk if not successful at 4 wk
Control regimen	Sterile saline, 1 drop 3× a day or oral placebo tablets for 4 wk, with an additional 2 wk if not successful at 4 wk
Additional local care	Dry mopping with cotton buds before drops in all patients. Aural toilet q wk
Definition of successful treatment	Otoscopically inactive (no pooling of discharge; noninflamed middle ear mucosa)
Management while in study	Weekly follow-up visits during 4 wk, with aural toilet each visit. If dry (see "success" above), considered successful. If still active, treated for another 2 wk and reassessed
Compliance	Compliance was assessed by measuring amount of used medication against amount available for use. Noncompliance = <50%. Compliance was recorded in bins of 10% (i.e., 51%–60%, 61%–70%, 71%–80%, etc.)
Criteria for withdrawal	Failure to attend visits
Intention to treat analysis	All data were reported in 1 table, by cavity/no cavity, treatment/placebo by levels of compliance. The authors did not use intention to treat, but took compliance of ≥70% as "cut-of-point" for analysis and found treatment was significantly better than placebo, except in cavities The analysis (reported above) used all of the data in an intention-to-treat analysis and also found treatment significantly better overall; however, there was not significant difference found in subjects with cavities (42 of 165 total cases) (p = 0.470; power 0.104)
Power	Power = 0.754
Morbidity/complications	Analysis of hearing showed no ototoxicity

RCT = randomized controlled trial, NS = not significant, abx = antibiotics, sig. = significantly, t.i.d. = three times a day.
*Sample size: numbers shown for those not lost to follow-up and those (initially recruited).

THE EVIDENCE CONDENSED: Topical antibiotics versus control for cessation of otorrhea

Reference	van Hasselt, 2002	Kasemsuwan, 1997	
Level (design)	1 (RCT)	1 (RCT)	
Sample size*	88 (88)	35 (50)	

OUTCOMES			
	% dry ears	**% cure**	**% improved**
Topical abx	83% neomycin (n = 29/35) 79% ofloxacin (n = 11/14)	84% (n = 16/19)	5.3% (n = 1/19)
Control	10% (n = 4/39)	12.5% (n = 2/16)	31.3% (n = 5/16)
p Value	Not reported	<0.005	<0.005
Conclusion	Trend toward abx better	Abx sig. better	Abx sig. better
Follow-up time	2 wk	7 d	

STUDY DESIGN		
Inclusion criteria	Chronic suppurative otitis media	Mucopurulent otorrhea, perforated tympanic membrane >3 mo
Exclusion criteria	Not specified	Cholesteatoma, pregnancy, "underlying disease, antibiotics in the previous 2 wk and during the study"
Randomization effectiveness	Not specified	Not specified
Age	Not specified	21–66 y
Masking	Not specified	Double blind
Antibiotic ear drop regimen	0.5% neomycin/0.1% polymyxin B 0.3% ofloxacin t.i.d. ×2 wk	Ciprofloxacin in saline (250 µg/mL) 5 drops t.i.d. for at least 7 d
Control regimen	Antiseptic ear drops: 2% acetic acid/25% spirit	Placebo: saline solution 5 drops t.i.d. for at least 7 d
Additional local care	Suction cleaning for all patients over 2 wk	Ear cleaning on day 1, 4, 7 of treatment
Definition of successful treatment	Not specified	Not specified
Management while in study	Regular visits over 2 wk	Follow-up day 1, 4, 7 over 1 wk of treatment
Compliance	Not specified	Not specified
Criteria for withdrawal	Not specified	Lack of attendance
Intention to treat analysis	Not specified	Not specified
Power	Not specified	Not specified
Morbidity/complications	Not specified	Not specified

RCT = randomized controlled trial, NS = not significant, abx = antibiotics, sig. = significantly, t.i.d. = three times a day.
* Sample size: numbers shown for those not lost to follow-up and those (initially recruited).

THE EVIDENCE CONDENSED: Topical antibiotics versus control for cessation of otorrhea

Reference	Macfadyen, 2005		Fradis, 1997	
Level (design)	1 (RCT)		1 (RCT)	
Sample size*	413 (427)		45, 54 ears (51, 60 ears)	

OUTCOMES

	Both ears resolved	Either or both ears resolved	% cured	% improved
Topical abx	59.4%,† 66.3%§	63.8%,† 72.6%§	Cipro 47.4% Tobra 55.6%	Cipro 31.6% Tobra 16.7%
Control	31.9%,† 45.5%§	38.1%,† 53.0%§	23.5%	17.6%
p Value	†<0.001 §<0.001	†<0.001 §<0.001	Cipro vs control, p = 0.02 Tobra vs control, p = 0.06	
Conclusion	Abx better	Abx better	Cipro sig. better than control Trend to tobra better than control No difference Cipro vs tobra	
Follow-up time	†2 wk, §4 wk		3 wk	

STUDY DESIGN

Inclusion criteria	Kenyan children aged ≥5 y with purulent aural discharge for ≥14 d, pus in the external canal on otoscopy, perforation of the tympanic membrane	Chronic suppurative otitis media
Exclusion criteria	Children treated for ear infection or who received abx for any other disorder in the previous 2 wk, other ear problems (preexisting disease, complicated otitis media, anatomic abnormalities), allergy to study drugs	Aged <18 y, prior middle ear operation, suspicion of cholesteatoma, general health problems, allergy to aminoglycosides or fluoroquinolones
Randomization effectiveness	Similar age, sex, presence of bilateral disease, duration of episode, audiometry, degree of perforation	More males in the tobra group. Otherwise, age and sex similar among groups
Age	4.1–19.3 y	18–73 y
Masking	Participants, caregivers, and outcome assessors blinded	Double blind
Antibiotic ear drop regimen	Cipro 0.3% b.i.d. after dry mopping for 10 consecutive school days (no treatment on weekends)	Cipro or tobra 5 drops t.i.d. ×3 wk
Control regimen	Boric acid 2% in alcohol 45% after dry mopping for 10 consecutive school days (none on weekends)	Burow aluminum acetate 1% solution 5 drops t.i.d. ×3 wk
Additional local care	Dry mopping and cleaning by older children	Not specified
Definition of successful treatment	Resolution of aural discharge	Cessation of otorrhea and eradication of organisms in post-treatment cultures
Management while in study	Follow-up visits at 2 and 4 wk	Otomicroscopy, cultures 24 h after treatment end, cultures before treatment
Compliance	7 children switched treatment bottles with others, resulting in 5 children who received both treatments	Not specified
Criteria for withdrawal	Lost to follow-up at 2 or 4 wk	Lost to follow-up at 3 wk
Intention to treat analysis	Yes, even 7 children who switched their treatment bottles with others were analyzed in their original group	Not specified
Power	80% to detect absolute difference in resolution rates of 10%, at a 2-sided significance level of 5%	Not reported
Morbidity/ complications	Significantly higher rates of ear pain, irritation, bleeding with boric acid	Complications "are minor," not otherwise specified

RCT = randomized controlled trial, NS = not significant, b.i.d. = twice daily, t.i.d. = three times daily, Abx = antibiotics, cipro = ciprofloxacin, tobra = tobramycin, sig. = significantly.
* Sample size: numbers shown for those not lost to follow-up and those (initially recruited).
†, § Symbols denote which data comparisons correspond to the referenced p-values and follow-up times.

THE EVIDENCE CONDENSED: Topical antibiotics versus control for cessation of otorrhea

Reference	Jaya, 2003	Browning, 1983
Level (design)	1 (RCT)	1 (RCT)
Sample size*	36 (40)	38 (NR)
OUTCOMES		
	% inactive	**% inactive**
Topical abx	90%‡	16.7%
Control	88%‡	35.0%
p Value	=0.81	=NS
Conclusion	No difference	No difference Trend toward control better
Follow-up time	1, 2, 3, ‡4 wk	4 wk
STUDY DESIGN		
Inclusion criteria	Aged >10 y, actively discharging chronic suppurative otitis media with moderate to large central perforation	Aged >16 y with active chronic otitis media
Exclusion criteria	Cholesteatoma, aural polyp, impending complications, diabetes mellitus, renal failure, tuberculosis, AIDS, iodine/fluoroquinolone allergy, systemic or topical abx within 10 d	Cholesteatoma, aural polyp
Randomization effectiveness	More males in cipro group. Similar age, disease/discharge duration, otorrhea severity, perforation, middle ear mucosa	Not reported
Age	10 to >40 y	Not specified
Masking	Double blind	Control group not blinded
Antibiotic ear drop regimen	Cipro 0.3% 3 drops t.i.d. by tragal displacement after dry mopping ×10 d	Gentamicin or chloramphenicol t.i.d. ×4 wk
Control regimen	Povidone iodine 5% 3 drops t.i.d. by tragal displacement after dry mopping ×10 d	Aural toilet, boric acid/iodine powder weekly ×4 wk
Additional local care	Dry mopping, weekly aural toilet	Aural toilet weekly in control group
Definition of successful treatment	No active discharge on otomicroscopy	Inactive otorrhea
Management while in study	Otomicroscopy and aural toilet weekly for 4 wk after commencing therapy	Not specified
Compliance	Not specified	Noncompliers if <75% of regimen used
Criteria for withdrawal	Lost to follow-up at time interval examined	Not specified
Intention to treat analysis	Not specified	Not specified
Power	Not reported	Not reported
Morbidity/complications	No patient developed allergic manifestations or ototoxicity	Not reported

RCT = randomized controlled trial, NS = not significant, b.i.d. = twice daily, t.i.d. = three times daily, Abx = antibiotics, cipro = ciprofloxacin, tobra = tobramycin, sig. = significantly.
* Sample size: numbers shown for those not lost to follow-up and those (initially recruited).
‡ Symbol denotes that the % inactive was measured at a follow-up time of 4 weeks.

Methods of Meta-Analysis. A meta-analysis may be useful in considering the data comparing topical antibiotic to antiseptic, because there are multiple relevant trials with negative results and individual sample sizes smaller than that required to provide 90% power. A meta-analysis is a way in which data from multiple studies are pooled together; the pooling creates an increased sample size, which in turn creates more statistical power to uncover any difference that could truly exist. Therefore, to further understand the impact of topical antibiotic versus topical antiseptic on chronic active otitis media, the data from the five RCTs that compared these two regimens have been analyzed. All of the studies included in this meta-analysis provide level 1 data, and they represent the highest level of evidence comparing these two regimens. Data have been combined according to follow-up time, antibiotic class, and antiseptic type. Further details regarding the search and selection process are as noted in the initial methods of this review.

Results of Meta-Analysis. First, results were examined by time of follow-up. At 2 and 4 weeks after treatment, when all of the data were combined, there was a significantly better outcome with topical antibiotic as compared with topical antiseptic. At 2 weeks, odds were 3.7 times better for a dry ear with antibiotic, with a number needed to treat of three (i.e., for every three patients treated, one will benefit). At 4 weeks, odds were 2.7 times better for a dry ear with antibiotic, with a number needed to treat of four. At 3 weeks, there was no significant difference between groups, although there was a trend toward more dry ears with antibiotic. At this 3-week timepoint, there were fewer data for comparison (90 patients, as compared with 538 and 469 at 2 and 4 weeks, respectively). The smaller sample size resulted in less power to detect any difference that may potentially exist.

Second, results were examined according to the class of antibiotic. Data from studies comparing topical quinolone antibiotics and topical antiseptics were combined at the latest follow-up times reported (2–4 weeks). With quinolone drops, there was a 28% greater rate of cessation of otorrhea than with antiseptic, with a number needed to treat of three. Odds for a dry ear with quinolone were 3.5 times better. Likewise, data from studies comparing non-quinolone antibiotics were combined at the latest follow-up times reported (2–4 weeks). Data from neomycin/polymyxin, tobramycin, gentamicin, and chloramphenicol drops were pooled, resulting in nearly 60% resolution of otorrhea. In comparison, the resolution rate with antiseptic was significantly worse (46.8% rate difference). The odds for a dry ear were 4.8 times better with non-quinolone antibiotic with a number needed to treat of three.

Third, we sought to determine if the type of antiseptic could impact results. When the data for studies testing iodine were combined, there were similar rates of dry ears, as compared with the antibiotic group. Even with combined data, however, the total sample size was only 74, so there is still limited power. Therefore, there is no evidence to suggest that iodine antiseptic results in a different outcome than topical antibiotic, but the limited sample sizes leave the issue still open to question.

CLINICAL SIGNIFICANCE AND FUTURE RESEARCH

There are two level 1 studies which agree that topical antibiotic is more effective than topical placebo (saline) in controlling otorrhea from chronically infected ears without cholesteatoma during application. However, the duration of the effect following treatment, recurrence rates, and efficacy for cavity granulations cannot be inferred from these two studies.

There are five level 1 studies that compared the impact of topical antiseptic versus topical antibiotic in controlling drainage from chronic active otitis media. Results are mixed, with two studies showing superior results with antibiotic and the remaining data showing no difference between treatment groups. The discrepancy between the results of these five RCTs may be attributable to differences in antibiotic and antiseptic regimen tests, or to the decreased sample size in studies with negative results; smaller sample sizes may result in decreased ability to detect any difference that may exist.

In a meta-analysis of the data comparing topical antibiotic to topical antiseptic, antibiotic results in a superior outcome at 2 and 4 weeks, and regardless of whether quinolone or non-quinolone antibiotics are analyzed. No difference is demonstrated at 3 weeks and when iodine antiseptic is considered separately. In both of these negative instances, however, the sample sizes are small, providing low power to detect any potential difference between groups.

Future research on this topic may be partially guided by the concern for ototoxicity in a potentially therapeutic regimen. For example, some clinicians may hesitate to use ethanol or iodine containing topical solutions in the presence of a tympanic membrane perforation unless they are presented with evidence to assure them of minimal associated labyrinthine toxicity. Also, in the future, time-to-event rates and intensity-or-event scales of resolution, as well as recurrences over at least 1 year, could be studied to understand more long-lasting effects. Finally, using known non-ototoxic medications with specified standard treatment durations and specific endpoints designed to identify the necessity and timing of surgical intervention would be helpful.

Meta-analysis: Topical antibiotics versus antiseptic control, resolution of otorrhea after 2 weeks

	Topical antibiotics	Antiseptic
Van Hasselt, 2002	29/35 11/14	4/39
Macfadyen, 2005	123/207	65/204
Jaya, 2003	19/21	16/18
Total	**182/277**	**85/261**

Analysis for Publication bias: 29 negative studies (i.e., no difference between groups) would be required to reverse the positive finding (i.e., a significant difference between groups) in this analysis.

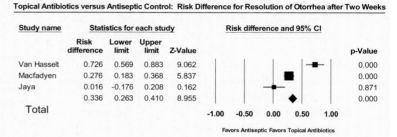

Topical Antibiotics versus Antiseptic Control: Risk Difference for Resolution of Otorrhea after Two Weeks

Study name	Risk difference	Lower limit	Upper limit	Z-Value	Risk difference and 95% CI	p-Value
Van Hasselt	0.726	0.569	0.883	9.062		0.000
Macfadyen	0.276	0.183	0.368	5.837		0.000
Jaya	0.016	-0.176	0.208	0.162		0.871
Total	0.336	0.263	0.410	8.955		0.000

Favors Antiseptic   Favors Topical Antibiotics

Topical Antibiotics versus Antiseptic Control: Odds Ratio for Resolution of Otorrhea After Two Weeks

Study name	Odds ratio	Lower limit	Upper limit	Z-Value	Odds ratio and 95% CI	p-Value
Van Hasselt	42.292	10.882	164.366	5.406		0.000
Macfadyen	3.131	2.089	4.693	5.529		0.000
Jaya	1.188	0.150	9.408	0.163		0.871
Total	3.720	2.541	5.446	6.756		0.000

Favors Antiseptic   Favors Topical Antibiotics

Meta-analysis: Topical antibiotics versus antiseptic control, resolution of otorrhea after 3 weeks

	Topical antibiotics	Antiseptic
Fradis, 1997	9/19 10/18	4/17
Jaya, 2003	18/20	14/16
Total	**37/57**	**n = 18/33**

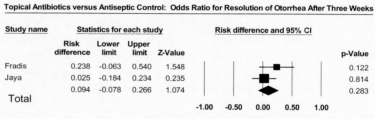

Topical Antibiotics versus Antiseptic Control: Odds Ratio for Resolution of Otorrhea After Three Weeks

Study name	Risk difference	Lower limit	Upper limit	Z-Value	Risk difference and 95% CI	p-Value
Fradis	0.238	-0.063	0.540	1.548		0.122
Jaya	0.025	-0.184	0.234	0.235		0.814
Total	0.094	-0.078	0.266	1.074		0.283

Favors Antiseptic   Favors Topical Antibiotics

Topical Antibiotics versus Antiseptic Control: Odds Ratio for Resolution of Otorrhea After Three Weeks

Study name	Odds ratio	Lower limit	Upper limit	Z-Value	Odds ratio and 95% CI	p-Value
Fradis	2.925	0.695	12.317	1.463		0.143
Jaya	1.286	0.161	10.299	0.237		0.813
Total	2.243	0.687	7.319	1.338		0.181

Favors Antiseptic   Favors Topical Antibiotics

Meta-analysis: Topical antibiotics versus antiseptic control, resolution of otorrhea after 4 weeks

	Topical antibiotics	Antiseptic
Macfadyen, 2005	143/197	90/198
Jaya, 2003	18/20	14/16
Browning, 1983	3/18	7/20
Total	**164/235**	**111/234**

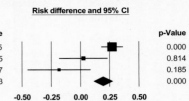

Topical Antibiotics versus Antiseptic Control: Risk Difference for Resolution of Otorrhea After Four Weeks

Study name	Statistics for each study				Risk difference and 95% CI	p-Value
	Risk difference	Lower limit	Upper limit	Z-Value		
Macfadyen	0.271	0.178	0.365	5.705		0.000
Jaya	0.025	-0.184	0.234	0.235		0.814
Browning	-0.183	-0.454	0.087	-1.327		0.185
Total	0.193	0.112	0.274	4.663		0.000

-0.50 -0.25 0.00 0.25 0.50

Favors Antiseptic Favors Topical Antibiotics

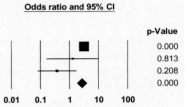

Topical Antibiotics versus Antiseptic Control: Odds Ratio for Resolution of Otorrhea After Four Weeks

Study name	Statistics for each study				Odds ratio and 95% CI	p-Value
	Odds ratio	Lower limit	Upper limit	Z-Value		
Macfadyen	3.178	2.088	4.836	5.398		0.000
Jaya	1.286	0.161	10.299	0.237		0.813
Browning	0.371	0.079	1.738	-1.258		0.208
Total	2.666	1.791	3.968	4.833		0.000

0.01 0.1 1 10 100

Favors Antiseptic Favors Topical Antibiotics

Meta-analysis: Topical quinolone versus antiseptic control, resolution of otorrhea at last follow-up (2–4 weeks)

	Topical antibiotics	Antiseptic
Van Hasselt, 2002	11/14	4/39
Macfadyen, 2005	143/197	90/198
Fradis, 1997	9/19	4/17
Jaya, 2003	18/20	14/16
Total	**181/250**	**112/270**

Analysis for Publication bias: 31 negative studies (i.e., no difference between groups) would be required to reverse the positive finding (i.e., a significant difference between groups) in this analysis.

Study name	Statistics for each study				Risk difference and 95% CI
	Risk difference	Lower limit	Upper limit	p-Value	
Van Hasselt, 2002	0.683	0.448	0.918	0.000	
Macfadyen, 2005	0.271	0.178	0.365	0.000	
Fradis, 1997	0.238	-0.063	0.540	0.122	
Jaya, 2003	0.025	-0.184	0.234	0.814	
Total	0.280	0.203	0.357	0.000	

-1.00 -0.50 0.00 0.50 1.00

Favors Antiseptic Favors Topical

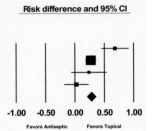

Study name	Statistics for each study				Odds ratio and 95% CI
	Odds ratio	Lower limit	Upper limit	p-Value	
Van Hasselt, 2002	32.083	6.204	165.911	0.000	
Macfadyen, 2005	3.178	2.088	4.836	0.000	
Fradis, 1997	2.925	0.695	12.317	0.143	
Jaya, 2003	1.286	0.161	10.299	0.813	
Total	3.477	2.366	5.107	0.000	

0.01 0.1 1 10 100

Favors Antiseptic Favors Topical

Meta-analysis: Topical non-quinolone versus antiseptic control, resolution of otorrhea at last follow-up (2–4 weeks)

	Topical antibiotics	Antiseptic	Follow-up time
Van Hasselt, 2002	29/35	4/39	2 wk
Fradis, 1997	10/18	4/17	3 wk
Browning, 1983	3/18	7/20	4 wk
Total	**42/71**	**15/76**	

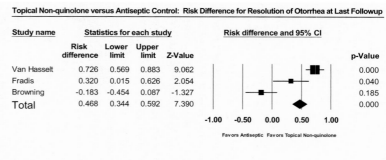

Topical Non-quinolone versus Antiseptic Control: Risk Difference for Resolution of Otorrhea at Last Followup

Study name	Risk difference	Lower limit	Upper limit	Z-Value	p-Value
Van Hasselt	0.726	0.569	0.883	9.062	0.000
Fradis	0.320	0.015	0.626	2.054	0.040
Browning	-0.183	-0.454	0.087	-1.327	0.185
Total	0.468	0.344	0.592	7.390	0.000

Topical Non-quinolone versus Antiseptic Control: Odds Ratio for Resolution of Otorrhea at Last Followup

Study name	Odds ratio	Lower limit	Upper limit	Z-Value	p-Value
Van Hasselt	42.292	10.882	164.366	5.406	0.000
Fradis	4.063	0.947	17.425	1.887	0.059
Browning	0.371	0.079	1.738	-1.258	0.208
Total	4.892	2.123	11.275	3.727	0.000

Meta-analysis: Topical antibiotics versus iodine antiseptic control, resolution of otorrhea at 4 weeks

	Topical antibiotics	Iodine antiseptic
Jaya, 2003	18/20	14/16
Browning, 1983	3/18	7/20
Total	**21/38**	**21/36**

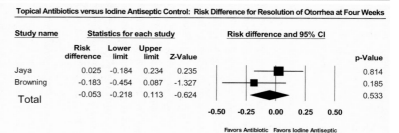

Topical Antibiotics versus Iodine Antiseptic Control: Risk Difference for Resolution of Otorrhea at Four Weeks

Study name	Risk difference	Lower limit	Upper limit	Z-Value	p-Value
Jaya	0.025	-0.184	0.234	0.235	0.814
Browning	-0.183	-0.454	0.087	-1.327	0.185
Total	-0.053	-0.218	0.113	-0.624	0.533

Topical Antibiotics versus Iodine Antiseptic Control: Odds Ratio for Resolution of Otorrhea at Four Weeks

Study name	Odds ratio	Lower limit	Upper limit	Z-Value	p-Value
Jaya	1.286	0.161	10.299	0.237	0.813
Browning	0.371	0.079	1.738	-1.258	0.208
Total	0.577	0.167	1.993	-0.869	0.385

REFERENCES

1. Browning GG, Gatehouse S, Calder IT. Medical management of active chronic otitis media: a controlled study. J Laryngol Otol 1988;102(6):491.

2. van Hasselt P, van Kregten E. Treatment of chronic suppurative otitis media with ofloxacin in hydroxypropyl methylcellulose ear drops: a clinical/bacteriological study in a rural area of Malawi. Int J Pediatr Otorhinolaryngol 2002;63(1):49–56.

3. Kasemsuwan L, Clongsuesuek P. A double blind, prospective trial of topical ciprofloxacin versus normal saline solution in the treatment of otorrhoea. Clin Otolaryngol Allied Sci 1997;22(1):44–46.

4. Macfadyen C, Gamble C, Garner P, et al. Topical quinolone vs. antiseptic for treating chronic suppurative otitis media: a randomized controlled trial. Trop Med Int Health 2005; 10(2):190.

5. Fradis M, Brodsky A, Ben-David J, Srugo I, Larboni J, Podoshin L. Chronic otitis media treated topically with ciprooxacin or tobramycin. Arch Otolaryngol Head Neck Surg 1997;123(10):1057.

6. Jaya C, Job A, Mathai E, Antonisamy B. Evaluation of topical povidone-iodine in chronic suppurative otitis media. Arch Otolaryngol Head Neck Surg 2003;129(10):1098.

7. Browning GG, Picozzi GL, Calder IT, Sweeney G. Controlled trial of medical treatment of active chronic otitis media. Br Med J Clin Res Ed 1983;287(6398):1024.

12 Chronic Otitis Media

12.B.

Topical versus systemic antibiotic therapy for chronic active otitis media without cholesteatoma: Impact on resolution of otorrhea

Jennifer J. Shin and J. Gail Neely

METHODS

A computerized PubMed search of MEDLINE 1966–December 2005 was performed. The medical subject heading "otitis media, suppurative" was exploded and the resulting articles were cross-referenced with those mapping to the subject headings "anti-bacterial agents," "macrolides," "fluoroquinolones," "clindamycin," or "lactams," yielding 227 publications. These articles were then reviewed to identify those that met the following inclusion criteria: 1) patients with chronic suppurative otitis media with chronic perforation and active otorrhea, 2) intervention with topical antibiotics versus systemic antibiotics, 3) outcome measured in terms of cessation of otorrhea. Because of the richness of the literature, randomized controlled trials (RCTs) were specifically extracted as the best evidence available. Trials in which simultaneous topical and systemic antibiotics were administered were excluded. Likewise, articles about patients with cholesteatoma or that compared topical and systemic treatment in patients with inactive chronic otitis media were also excluded. The bibliographies of the articles that met these inclusion criteria were manually checked to ensure no further relevant articles could be identified. This process yielded four RCTs [1–4].

RESULTS

Outcome Measures. Successful outcomes were measured as the percent of patients who experienced "clinical and bacteriological cure" (not otherwise specified), completely dry ear on otomicroscopy, and resolution of otorrhea.

Potential Confounders. The topical and systemic antibiotic regimen used (medication, dose, and duration), compliance, additional local care, previous surgery, eustachian tube function, age, immune status, and time of follow-up are among variables that could affect results. These potential confounders are detailed in the adjoining table in as much detail as the original reports allow.

Study Designs. Four RCTs compared topical to systemic antibiotic administration. Only one compared different delivery routes of the same antimicrobial agent (ciprofloxacin). Topical fluoroquinolones were used in three of the studies, with the fourth testing topical gentamicin or chloramphenicol. Systemic antibiotic regimens included intramuscular gentamicin, as well as oral fluoroquinolones and lactams. Two RCTs demonstrated that age and gender were balanced among groups pretreatment. A third RCT additionally showed that the size of perforation, degree of middle ear mucosal inflammation, and severity of aural discharge were comparable among the groups at the outset. In addition, these three RCTs had no or minimal patient attrition during follow-up. The fourth RCT did not report its randomization effectiveness or its attrition rate. No study used placebo drops or pills to mask patients and providers to their treatment group. Sample sizes were somewhat small, but still managed to demonstrate a statistically significant difference in three trials.

Highest Level of Evidence. Three of the four RCTs showed significantly increased rates of dry ears with topical rather than systemic antibiotic therapy. For otorrhea cessation, topical ciprofloxacin was superior to both intramuscular gentamicin and to oral ciprofloxacin. Likewise, topical ofloxin was superior to oral Augmentin. The fourth RCT demonstrated no difference in the percent of dry ears with topical gentamicin or chloramphenicol versus oral lactams. In fact, it suggested a trend toward a better outcome with systemic antibiotics. The differing result in this trial may be attributable to several factors: 1) a different topical regimen was used (i.e., non-fluoroquinolone therapy), 2) a different oral regimen was used (four different lactams), 3) a smaller sample size was tested, resulting in less statistical power to identify any difference that might truly exist, 4) pretreatment groups may not have been balanced at the outset of the trial (randomization effectiveness was not demonstrated). Overall, although the results were not completely homogeneous, the majority of this level 1 evidence shows more cessation of otorrhea with topical, rather than systemic antibiotics.

When the results from all four studies are combined in a meta-analysis, the overall rate of successful treatment with topical antibiotics is 34.4% better than with systemic antibiotics. These numbers suggest a number needed to treat of three [95% confidence interval (CI) 2–5], which means that if three patients receive topical antibiotics rather than systemic antibiotics, one will receive clear benefit. The comparative numbers also suggest an odds ratio of 4.6 (95% CI 2.3–9.1); this means that patients are nearly 5 times as likely to improve with topical, rather than systemic therapy.

Applicability. These results are applicable to patients with chronic suppurative otitis media that is actively draining at the time of treatment initiation. It does not apply to patients with cholesteatoma.

Morbidity/Complications. No side effects, hypersensitivity reactions, or evidence of ototoxicity was reported in any of these trials.

CLINICAL SIGNIFICANCE AND FUTURE RESEARCH

There were four RCTs that compared topical versus systemic antibiotic therapy for chronic active suppurative otitis media. Three of the four RCTs showed significantly more cessation of otorrhea with topical therapy, whereas one showed no difference between the two delivery vehicles. The negative study may have had an alternate result because it tested different antibiotic regimens and had a smaller sample size, making it less powered to detect any difference that might have truly existed. When all of the data from all four RCTs are combined in a meta-analysis, it suggests that patients receiving topical antibiotics are more than 4 times as likely to develop a dry ear than those receiving systemic therapy.

Additional research may focus on comparing topical therapy alone to topical and systemic therapy combined. In addition, specific antibiotic regimens—particular classes with and without potential associated ototoxicity—are also worthy of comparative study.

THE EVIDENCE CONDENSED: Topical versus systemic antibiotics for otorrhea cessation in chronic suppurative otitis media

Reference	Esposito, 1992		Esposito, 1990	
Level (design)	1 (RCT)		1 (RCT)	
Sample size*	60 (60)		40 (40)	
OUTCOMES				
	% cured	% improved	% cured	% improved
Topical antibiotics	83% (n = 25/30)	4% (n = 1/30)	85% (n = 17/20)	15% (n = 3/20)
Systemic abx	43% (n = 13/30)	24% (n = 7/30)	40% (n = 8/20)	25% (n = 5/20)
p Value	<0.005		<0.05	
Conclusion	Topical better than systemic		Topical better than systemic	
Follow-up time	2–3 wk		14 d after treatment end	
STUDY DESIGN				
Inclusion criteria	Chronic suppurative otitis media—otitis media >3 y, purulent otorrhea at least once annually, recurrent episodes of purulent otorrhea constant for at least 15 d; culture positive for pseudomonas sensitive to cipro and gentamicin		Mild or moderate chronic otitis media in the acute stage	
Exclusion criteria	Cholesteatoma, pregnancy, allergy to quinolones or aminoglycosides, <18 y old, underlying diseases such as diabetes		Cholesteatoma or mastoiditis, pregnancy, allergy to quinolone, <18 y old, underlying disease such as diabetes	
Randomization effectiveness	Similar age, gender		Similar age, gender	
Age	18–65 y		38 y, mean	
Masking	NR		NR	
Antibiotic ear drop regimen	Cipro 250 µg/mL 4 drops b.i.d. ×5–10 d		Cipro 250 µg/mL 3 drops b.i.d. ×5–10 d	
Systemic antibiotic regimen	Gentamicin sulfate 80 mg IM b.i.d. ×5–10 d		Cipro 250 mg PO b.i.d. ×5–10 d	
Definition of successful treatment	Bacteriologic and clinical cure, not otherwise specified		Bacteriologic and clinical cure, not otherwise specified	
Management while in study	Examined before, after, and every 2–3 d during treatment		Examined before, after, and every 2–3 d with treatment	
Compliance	Not specified		Not specified	
Criteria for withdrawal	All completed study		All completed study	
Intention to treat analysis	Not specified		Not specified	
Power	NR		NR	
Morbidity/complications	No side effect or worsened audiometry		No side effect or worsened audiometry	

RCT = randomized controlled trial, NR = not reported, b.i.d. = twice daily, t.i.d. = three times daily, abx = antibiotics, cipro = ciprofloxacin, IM = intramuscularly.

* Sample size: numbers shown for those not lost to follow-up and those (initially recruited).

THE EVIDENCE CONDENSED: Topical versus systemic antibiotics for otorrhea cessation in chronic suppurative otitis media

Reference	Yuen, 1994	Browning, 1983
Level (design)	1 (RCT)	1 (RCT)
Sample size*	56 (60)	31 (NR)
OUTCOMES		
	% dry ear	**% inactive**
Topical antibiotics	76% (n = 22/29)	16.7% (n = 3/18)
Systemic abx	26% (n = 7/27)	38.5% (n = 5/13)
p Value	<0.001	NS
Conclusion	Topical better than systemic	No difference
Follow-up time	2 wk	4 wk
STUDY DESIGN		
Inclusion criteria	Active chronic suppurative otitis media with central perforation	>16 y old with active chronic otitis media
Exclusion criteria	Cholesteatoma, discharging mastoid cavity, aural polyp, acute traumatic perforation, acute otitis media, temporal bone radiation, grommets, otomycosis, prior abx within 1 wk	Cholesteatoma, aural polyp
Randomization effectiveness	Comparable perforation size, mucosal inflammation, nature of aural discharge	NR
Age	18–70 y	Not specified
Masking	NR	NR
Antibiotic ear drop regimen	Ofloxin 0.3% t.i.d. ×1 wk	Gentamicin or chloramphenicol t.i.d. ×4 wk
Systemic antibiotic regimen	Augmentin 375 mg PO t.i.d. ×1 wk	Cephalexin, flucloxicillin, cloxicillin, or amoxicillin 1–2 g/d
Definition of successful treatment	Completely dry ear	Inactive otorrhea
Management while in study	Not specified	Not specified
Compliance	Not specified	Noncompliers: <75% regimen used
Criteria for withdrawal	Failure to follow up or intolerance of medication	Not specified
Intention to treat analysis	Not specified	Not specified
Power	NR	NR
Morbidity/complications	No adverse effects or hypersensitivity reactions	NR

RCT = randomized controlled trial, NR = not reported, b.i.d. = twice daily, t.i.d. = three times daily, abx = antibiotics, cipro = ciprofloxacin, IM = intramuscularly.
*Sample size: numbers shown for those not lost to follow-up and those (initially recruited).

Meta-analysis: Percent (number) of patients with chronic active suppurative otitis media with dry ears post-treatment

	Topical antibiotics	Systemic antibiotic
Esposito, 1992	25/30	13/30
Esposito, 1990	17/20	8/20
Yuen, 1994	22/29	7/27
Browning, 1983	3/18	5/13
Total	**67/97**	**33/90**

Topical Antibiotic versus Systemic Antibiotic: Risk Difference for Cessation of Otorrhea

Study name	Statistics for each study				Risk difference and 95% CI	
	Risk difference	Lower limit	Upper limit	Z-Value		p-Value
Esposito, 1992	0.400	0.178	0.622	3.533		0.000
Esposito, 1990	0.450	0.184	0.716	3.320		0.001
Yuen	0.499	0.272	0.726	4.309		0.000
Browning	-0.218	-0.534	0.098	-1.354		0.176
Total	0.344	0.219	0.469	5.392		0.000

-1.00 -0.50 0.00 0.50 1.00

Favors Systemic   Favors Topical

Topical Antibiotic versus Systemic Antibiotic: Odds Ratio for Cessation of Otorrhea

Study name	Statistics for each study				Odds ratio and 95% CI	
	Odds ratio	Lower limit	Upper limit	Z-Value		p-Value
Esposito, 1992	6.538	1.967	21.739	3.063		0.002
Esposito, 1990	8.500	1.861	38.817	2.762		0.006
Yuen	8.980	2.678	30.115	3.555		0.000
Browning	0.320	0.060	1.698	-1.338		0.181
Total	4.620	2.343	9.112	4.417		0.000

0.01 0.1 1 10 100

Favors Systemic   Favors Topical

REFERENCES

1. Esposito S, Noviello S, D'Errico G, Montanaro C. Topical ciprofloxacin versus intramuscular gentamicin for chronic otitis media. Arch Otolaryngol Head Neck Surg 1992; 118(8):842.
2. Esposito S, D'Errico G, Montanaro C. Topical and oral treatment of chronic otitis media with ciprofloxacin. Arch Otolaryngol Head Neck Surg 1990;116(5):557.
3. Yuen PW, Lau SK, Chau P, et al. Ofloxacin eardrop treatment for active chronic suppurative otitis media: prospective randomized study. Am J Otol 1994;15(5):670.
4. Browning GG, Picozzi GL, Calder IT, Sweeney G. Controlled trial of medical treatment of active chronic otitis media. Br Med J Clin Res Ed 1983;287(6398):1024.

12 Chronic Otitis Media

12.C.

Topical versus combined topical and systemic antibiotic therapy for chronic active otitis media without cholesteatoma: Impact on resolution of otorrhea

Jennifer J. Shin and J. Gail Neely

METHODS

A computerized PubMed search of MEDLINE 1966–December 2005 was performed. The medical subject heading "otitis media, suppurative" was exploded and the resulting articles were cross-referenced with those mapping to the subject headings "anti-bacterial agents," "macrolides," "fluoroquinolones," "clindamycin," or "lactams," yielding 227 publications. These articles were then reviewed to identify those that met the following inclusion criteria: 1) patients with chronic suppurative otitis media with chronic perforation and active otorrhea, 2) intervention with topical antibiotics versus combined topical and systemic antibiotics, 3) outcome measured in terms of cessation of otorrhea. Articles about patients with cholesteatoma or which compared topical and systemic treatment in patients with inactive chronic otitis media were excluded. The bibliographies of the articles that met these inclusion criteria were manually checked to ensure no further relevant articles could be identified. This process yielded two randomized controlled trials (RCTs) [1, 2].

RESULTS

Outcome Measures. Successful outcomes were measured as the percent of patients who experienced "cure," defined as either "a completely dry ear with disappearance of middle ear inflammation and otalgia" or as "clinical and bacteriological cure" (not otherwise specified).

Potential Confounders. The topical and systemic antibiotic regimen used (medication, dose, and duration), compliance, additional local care, previous surgery, eustachian tube function, age, immune status, and time of follow-up are among variables that could affect results. In addition, the sensitivity of pathogens to the specific antibiotics used could affect results: Supiyaphun [1] reported that 96% of all bacterial isolates were sensitive to ofloxacin, but only 57% were sensitive to amoxicillin and chloramphenicol, which would bias results toward a better outcome with ofloxacin.

Study Designs. There were two RCTs that compared topical antibiotics with a combination of topical and systemic antibiotics for chronic active otitis media. The first [1] compared 2-week courses of topical ofloxacin to topical chloramphenicol with oral amoxicillin. Randomization was effective in balancing demographic qualities and multiple potential confounders between groups. Investigators were blinded, with a use of an oral placebo to supplement ofloxacin drops. Patients were followed for 14 days, with good compliance with study medications in >90%. An *a priori* power calculation was not provided.

In the second RCT, topical ciprofloxacin was compared with that same drug given both topically and orally. Randomization was effective in balancing demographics of the two groups. No *a priori* power calculation was provided. Patients were followed until 14 days after treatment end.

Highest Level of Evidence. There were two RCTs that addressed this topic. The larger one [1] suggests that with the goal of cure, topical ofloxacin is superior to topical chloramphenicol and amoxicillin in patients. Cultures from these patients, however, suggest that of all bacterial isolates, 96% were sensitive to ofloxacin, but only 57% were sensitive to amoxicillin and chloramphenicol, so the results may have been caused by the antibiotic sensitivity, rather than the route of medication delivery. The smaller study [2] showed a trend toward more cure with topical ciprofloxacin alone but a trend toward more improvement with topical and oral ciprofloxacin; no significant difference between these two groups was reported.

Applicability. These results are applicable to adult or late-teenage patients with chronic otitis media with active otorrhea. They are not applicable to patients with cholesteatoma or with underlying systemic disease.

Morbidity/Complications. Deterioration in bone conduction was noted after topical chloramphenicol amoxicillin therapy, although the mean loss was small.

CLINICAL SIGNIFICANCE AND FUTURE RESEARCH

There were two RCTs that compared topical with concomitant topical and systemic antibiotics. The larger one suggests that topical ofloxacin alone is better than topical chloramphenicol with oral amoxicillin, but pathogens' differential sensitivity to these two antibiotic classes may have biased the results in this direction. The smaller RCT suggests that there is no difference between topical versus topical and systemic ciprofloxacin. The sample size for this comparison, however, was 40 patients. To obtain a 90% power to detect a 15% difference in rates of cure between groups (using an 80% estimated cure with topical alone, based on these published data), a sample size of more than 200 patients would be required. Therefore, a larger sample size is needed to provide convincing negative data.

Future research on this topic would be beneficial, as the combination of topical and oral therapy is a regularly employed regimen when it seems that topical therapy alone may not suffice for chronic otitis media with active otorrhea. The data, however, do not strictly support this practice. In fact, without the knowledge of the predisposing pathogen sensitivity spectrum, it might even be that combining systemic with topical therapy results in a worse outcome. Current data suggest that when ciprofloxacin is given systemically in addition to topically, there is no further benefit, but the associated study's power is quite limited.

This and the previous two systematic reviews have suggested that 1) topical antibiotics are superior to topical placebo or antiseptic, 2) topical antibiotics are superior to systemic antibiotics, and 3) it is unclear whether the addition of oral antibiotics provides an advantage over topical antibiotics alone. Therefore, these overall data support the strength of topical antibiotic therapy in chronic active otitis media.

THE EVIDENCE CONDENSED: Topical versus topical and systemic antibiotics for otorrhea cessation in chronic suppurative otitis media

Reference	Supiyaphun, 2000		Esposito, 1990	
Level (design)	1 (RCT)		1 (RCT)	
Sample size*	79 (80)		40 (40)	
OUTCOMES				
	% cured	% improved	% cured	% improved
Topical abx	76.9% (n = NR)	92.3% (n = NR)	85% (n = 17/20)	15% (n = 3/20)
Topical and systemic abx	37.0% (n = NR)	86% (n = NR)	75% (n = 15/20)	20% (n = 4/20)
p Value	<0.001	NS	Not specified	Not specified
Conclusion	Topical better	No difference	No large difference	
Follow-up time	14 d		14 d after treatment end	
STUDY DESIGN				
Inclusion criteria	Age >15 y, purulent or mucopurulent otorrhea, and central perforations of the tympanic membrane of >21 d duration		Mild or moderate chronic otitis media in the acute stage	
Exclusion criteria	Cholesteatoma or large aural polyp in the middle ear or mastoid, history of ear surgery within the previous year, therapy with systemic abx or ototopical agents of any kind within 2 wk, pregnant or lactating, allergy to penicillin, chloramphenicol quinolone		Cholesteatoma or mastoiditis, pregnancy, allergy to quinolone, <18 y old, underlying disease such as diabetes	
Randomization effectiveness	Similar age, gender, laterality of infection, size, duration and cause of tympanic membrane perforation, or pathogenic organisms were noted between treatment groups at enrollment		Similar age, gender	
Age	15–78 y old		38 y old, mean	
Masking	Investigator-blind		Not reported	
Topical antibiotic regimen	Ofloxacin solution 0.3% 6 drops b.i.d. and oral placebo t.i.d. ×2 wk		Cipro 250 μg/mL 3 drops b.i.d. ×5–10 d	
Topical and systemic antibiotic regimen	Chloramphenicol 1% 3 drops t.i.d., amoxicillin 500 mg PO t.i.d. ×2 wk		Cipro 250 mg PO b.i.d., topical cipro 250 μg/mL 3 drops b.i.d. ×5–10 d	
Definition of successful treatment	Cure = middle ear inflammation and otalgia disappeared and ear became dry. Improved = symptom/sign scores decreased at least 1 level		Bacteriologic and clinical cure, not otherwise specified	
Management while in study	Examined on day 0, 7, 14 with otalgia, otorrhea, and middle ear inflammation rated 0 (none) to 3 (severe/marked)		Examined before, after, and every 2–3 d with treatment	
Compliance	Compliance was good in >90%, as defined by the number of times the patient forgot to use the drug within 7 d: good (0–3), moderate (4–7), poor (>7)		Not specified	
Criteria for withdrawal	Missed follow-up visits		All completed study	
Intention to treat analysis	Not specified		Not specified	
Power	NR		NR	
Morbidity/complications	Deterioration in bone conduction from 22.8 ± 10.4 to 24.8 ± 10.4 (p < 0.007) after amoxicillin/topical chloramphenicol; no deterioration after topical ofloxacin. Fungal superinfection (n = 1 ofloxacin, n = 2 amoxicillin/chloramphenicol)		No side effect or worsened audiometry	

RCT = randomized controlled trial, NR = not reported, NS = not significant, b.i.d. = twice daily, t.i.d. = three times daily, abx = antibiotics, cipro = ciprofloxacin.
* Sample size: numbers shown for those not lost to follow-up and those (initially recruited).

REFERENCES

1. Supiyaphun P, Kerekhanjanarong V, Koranasophonepun J, Sastarasadhit V. Comparison of ofloxacin otic solution with oral amoxicillin plus chloramphenicol ear drop in treatment of chronic suppurative otitis media with acute exacerbation. J Med Assoc Thai 2000;83(1):61.

2. Esposito S, D'Errico G, Montanaro C. Topical and oral treatment of chronic otitis media with ciprofloxacin. Arch Otolaryngol Head Neck Surg 1990;116(5):557.

12 Chronic Otitis Media

12.D.

Ototopical neomycin: Impact on post-treatment hearing

Jennifer J. Shin, Ming-Yee Lin, and Steven D. Rauch

METHODS

A computerized PubMed search of MEDLINE 1970–December 2004 was performed. The medical subject headings "neomycin" and "otitis media" were exploded and the resulting articles were cross-referenced, yielding 33 publications. These articles were then reviewed to identify those that met the following inclusion criteria: 1) patient population with tympanic membrane perforation or tympanostomy tube, 2) intervention with ototopical neomycin, ideally versus control, 3) outcome measured in terms of sensorineural hearing loss. Articles in which gentamicin or framycetin drops were the primary focus of the study were excluded, as were articles in which the exact ototopical regimen was unclear. Likewise, case reports in which neomycin was used concomitant with an additional aminoglycoside were also excluded. The bibliographies of the articles that met these inclusion criteria, as well as several reviews on this topic, were manually checked to ensure no further relevant English articles could be identified. This process yielded the six articles that are reviewed below [1–6].

RESULTS

Outcome Measures. Outcomes were specifically described in terms of bone conduction pure tone audiometry in four studies. Pediatric audiometry was further described in the Merifield study as shown in the adjacent table. Speech reception thresholds were described in the Welling randomized controlled trial (RCT).

Potential Confounders. There were many potential confounders: neomycin regimen and duration, carrier substances, concomitant ototopical medications, the extent and activity of middle ear disease, and patient age and comorbidities. These factors are detailed in the adjacent tables.

Study Designs. There was one RCT, three retrospective controlled studies, one retrospective case series, and one physician survey that addressed this issue. In the single level 1 study [1], children were randomized to have a single intraoperative Cortisporin dose placed in either the right or left middle ear space after tympanostomy tube insertion. The contralateral ear served as a control, and follow-up time was 4 weeks. Preoperative audiometry was similar in both groups. Based on their sample size, they reported a 99% power to detect a ≥5-dB hearing loss, and a 99.9% power to detect a ≥10-dB hearing loss.

The remaining data were retrospective. In the largest retrospective controlled trial [2], 2 weeks of dexamethasone/polymyxin/neomycin drops were compared with no treatment after 1–3 months follow-up in children with tympanostomy tubes. Pretreatment sensorineural thresholds were ≤5 dB in all patients. This study's design was not immediately apparent in reading the original report, and it was described as a level 1 study in a review on this topic, but direct correspondence with the first author confirmed that it was a retrospective study. In the Podoshin retrospective controlled trial, several durations of dexamethasone/polymyxin/neomycin drops were compared with dexamethasone alone in patients with chronic active otitis media over a 1- to 2-year period. As a second control, hearing in 23 untreated ears with chronic otitis media was compared to contralateral healthy ears over a 7-year period. In the third retrospective controlled study, bone conduction thresholds pre-neomycin and post-neomycin were analyzed in 44 children with tubes. In the retrospective review, evaluation of 134 charts revealed 12 cases with tympanic membrane perforations which were evaluated for ototoxicity. The remaining study was a survey study of 7463 physicians with a 30% response rate [6].

Highest Level of Evidence. A single dose of dexamethasone/neomycin/polymyxin resulted in the same hearing as no treatment in children with tympanostomy tubes in the lone RCT.

Two retrospective studies analyzed the impact of a 2- to 14-day course (level 3–4 data), and showed no difference in audiometry after topical neomycin use in children with tympanostomy tubes. The Rakover retrospective controlled trial (n = 446) showed no difference in sensorineural hearing loss in children with tubes who received dexamethasone/neomycin/polymyxin 3 gtts t.i.d. for 2 weeks versus no treatment. The Merifield retrospective review showed no difference in pretreatment versus post-treatment bone conduction thresholds in children who received neomycin containing ototopicals for 2 days to 2 weeks.

There were also two retrospective evaluations of a more prolonged course (level 3–4 data); they demonstrated worse hearing after topical neomycin. The Podoshin retrospective controlled trial showed that sensorineural hearing was 7.0 dB worse (p < 0.025) with dexamethasone/neomycin/polymyxin use versus dexamethasone alone over 1–2 years. This study, however, also reported that hearing was worse in *untreated* chronically inflamed ears (versus contralateral healthy ears, 11.2-dB difference in bone conduction, p < 0.001). The second report [5] of longer term use showed ototoxicity in 1 patient of 12 with tympanic membrane perforations. This 69-year-old patient used 70 mL of polymyxin/neomycin over 2 months in one ear (average 23 gtts/day) then 70 mL in the contralateral ear over 3 months (average 16 drops per day).

Thus, the three retrospective studies that included only children with tympanostomy tubes and short courses of treatment revealed no hearing loss with ototopical neomycin versus control or with pre- versus post-neomycin treatment. The other two reports of a decrease in sensorineural hearing all occurred in populations in which adults were also studied. The most detailed report of neomycin-attributed sensorineural loss occurred in a patient who was nearly 70 years old.

There was also a report of a physician survey (n = 2235 responses to 7463 questionnaires): 3.4% of respondents believed that they had witnessed ototoxicity from ototopical agents, of which 31.6% believed that Cortisporin was the offending agent (1.1% of all respondents). Cortisporin suspension was used by 94.5% of respondents. There was no response to 70% of questionnaires, so data from that 70% of polled physicians remained unknown. No details regarding the extent of hearing loss or the duration of treatments associated with ototoxicity were reported. Eighty percent of responders agreed with the statement, "The risk of ototoxicity of otitis media is as great as or greater than the risk for ototoxicity of an ototopical preparation."

Applicability. The results from the Welling, Rakover, and Merifield trials can be applied to children with tympanostomy tube placement. The results from the Podoshin and Linder trials can be applied to older patients with chronic suppurative otitis media.

Morbidity/Complications. Discussion of associated morbidity was limited to hearing loss and occasional vertigo in these reports.

CLINICAL SIGNIFICANCE AND FUTURE RESEARCH

There were six publications focused on the impact of ototopical neomycin on sensorineural hearing in the presence of an intubated or perforated tympanic membrane. Overall, the data levels and results were mixed (with some seemingly conflicting results), but suggested

that short courses in children with tympanostomy tubes may be safe, whereas longer, relatively high-dose courses in patients with chronic otitis media with tympanic membrane perforations may result in hearing loss.

The single RCT demonstrated no significant difference with versus without a single dose of neomycin/polymyxin/hydrocortisone in children with tympanostomy tubes. The power of the study was 99% to detect a 5-dB difference, suggesting that the administration of a single dose in this intubated pediatric population should indeed have no notable adverse effects on hearing.

There were two retrospective studies that addressed neomycin use for 2–14 days. They showed no difference in sensorineural hearing with neomycin versus no treatment and with pre- versus post-neomycin use in children with tympanostomy tubes, suggesting that <14-day courses of neomycin may be safe in children with tympanostomy tubes.

Two retrospective studies evaluated longer-term use of neomycin. To place their results into context, the authors of one of these studies also reported that the presence of chronic otitis media alone could correlate with sensorineural hearing loss. The same authors noted that bone conduction thresholds were significantly worse with longer courses of topical neomycin in patients with tympanic membrane perforation and chronic active otitis media. However, the mean hearing loss over 1–2 years was 7 dB, suggesting that the magnitude of impact may be small. The second study, a retrospective review of 12 patients with tympanic membrane perforations, showed a severe sensorineural hearing loss in a 69-year-old patient who used an average of 23 gtts/day of polymyxin/neomycin for 2 months. This study suggested that relatively high doses may result in severe sensorineural hearing loss. It is, however, unclear how frequently such sensorineural loss occurs, whether it occurs with standard dosing, and whether it is limited to this patient's demographic group.

With the exception of a single RCT evaluating single-dose therapy, all of the data regarding this topic are level 3–5. Further high-level study on this topic would potentially be useful, although it must be undertaken with caution. First, the impact of short courses of neomycin-containing drops on patients with tympanic membrane perforation and chronic active otitis media could be further elucidated with prospective studies that control for the important confounder of the otic inflammation itself. The chronically infected ear may already be prone to sensorineural loss (as suggested by Podoshin). Also, exudative, thickened mucosa may alter round window permeability to neomycin. Second, the suggested impact of age and whether the middle ear space is exposed by a tube or a chronic perforation is of interest. Third, the magnitude of any associated hearing loss over time could be studied. Whereas larger studies suggest a small degree of hearing loss with long-term use, case reports suggest that severe, devastating hearing loss may occur. This magnitude is key in clinical decision making, as some practitioners and patients may be willing to accept the risk of a mean 7-dB decrement over a mean 1.5 years (as suggested by the Podoshin study) in order to gain treatment benefits from neomycin-containing drops. Fourth, the comparative efficacy and potential adverse effects of topical nonaminoglycoside therapy are topics for further consideration.

Reference	Welling, 1995		Rakover,1989
Level (design)	1 (randomized controlled trial)		3 (retrospective controlled study)
Sample size*	50 (60)		446 (446)
OUTCOMES			
Audiometry			
	Preop mean	**Postop mean**	**Audiometry**
Neomycin drops	BC PTA: 4.6 dB SRT: 22.6 dB	BC PTA: 3.1 dB SRT: 8.6 dB	"There was no sensorineural hearing loss." Specifics not reported
Control	BC PTA: 5.4 dB SRT: 21.4 dB	BC PTA: 3.9 dB SRT: 13.5 dB	"There was no sensorineural hearing loss." Specifics not reported
p Value	NS	NS	Not reported
Conclusion	No difference	No difference	No hearing loss
Follow-up time	4 wk postop		1–3 mo postop
STUDY DESIGN			
Inclusion criteria	Recurrent acute otitis media or chronic serous otitis media necessitating tympanostomy tube insertion, 4–17 y old		Children undergoing anteroinferior quadrant myringotomy and tympanostomy tube insertion for serous otitis media
Exclusion criteria	<4 y old, >17 y old		SNHL, <3 y old, doubt about cooperation in study
Pretreatment group comparison	The contralateral ear of the same patient was used as a control		0- to 5-dB sensorineural hearing threshold throughout, not further specified
Age	4–17 y		3–8 y
Masking	NR		Not applicable
Neomycin regimen details	Intraoperative 0.5 mL Cortisporin via tube to middle ear: hydrocortisone (10 mg /mL), neo (3.5 mg /mL), polymyxin B (10,000 U/mL), propylene glycol (10%)		Dexamethasone (1 mg /mL), neo (5 mg /mL), polymyxin B (20,000 U/mL) 3 gtts t.i.d. ×2 wk
Control details	The contralateral ear of the same patient was used as a control		No treatment
Hearing change caused by infection	NR		NR
Audiometry measures	Pure tone audiometry, if possible with extended high-frequency audiogram (8, 20 kHz). Speech reception thresholds, within 1 mo before surgery		Pure tone audiograms (250–8 kHz) 2 d before and 1–3 mo postop
Preop audiometry	Mean 4.8 dB§ (SD 4§) in patients receiving Cortisporin, 5.1 dB§ (SD 9§) in control patients		0- to 5-dB sensorineural hearing threshold
Compliance	Not specified		NR
Criteria for withdrawal from study	Oral or other topical antibiotic use during study period, sensitivity to Cortisporin, inability to complete audiogram, lost to follow-up		NR
Intention to treat analysis	NR		Not applicable
Power	99% to detect difference of ≥5 dB, 99.99% to detect a difference of ≥10 dB		NR
Morbidity/complications	Postop otorrhea, 8/100 ears (8%), 1 with 45-dB conductive hearing loss		None reported

Preop = preoperative, postop = postoperative, NR = not reported, PTA = pure tone average, t.i.d. = three times a day, BC = bone conduction, SRT = speech reception threshold, COM = chronic otitis media, neo = neomycin, SNHL = sensorineural hearing loss.
* Sample size for randomized controlled trials: numbers shown for those not lost to follow-up and those (initially recruited).
§ Numbers extrapolated from bar graph.

Reference	Podoshin, 1989			
Level (design)	3 (retrospective controlled study)			
Sample size*	173 (124 treated, 26 cnt, 23 not treated)			
OUTCOMES				
Mean sensorineural hearing				
	Continuous	**Off <3 mo**	**Off 3–6 mo**	**All use**
Neomycin drops	10.9-dB loss†	3.6-dB loss†	1.8-dB loss†	6.1-dB loss†
Control	0.9-dB gain† (treatment duration NR). Additional control: unilateral ears with COM with no treatment (17.8 dB) were compared with the contralateral healthy ears (6.6 dB)‡			
p Value	†<0.025, all neo vs all control		‡<0.001	
Conclusion	Significantly more SNHL with continuous neo use. COM significantly more SNHL than healthy ear			
Follow-up time	†1–2 y, mean 1.5 y ‡7.1 y			
STUDY DESIGN				
Inclusion criteria	COM, as defined by otorrhea, tympanic membrane perforation, and active middle ear cleft disease such as cholesteatoma or granulation tissue			
Exclusion criteria	SNHL from previous ear operation, head trauma, noise exposure, presbycusis, or congenital; <6 or >65 y old; previous therapy with known ototoxic drug (e.g., gentamicin); chronic disease (e.g., diabetes, arteriosclerosis)			
Pretreatment group comparison	Similar age, gender, as well as rates of central perforation, discharge, hearing threshold. Control group with more tinnitus			
Age	39.5% neo treated, 46.5% control group 10–19 y old; others not specified			
Masking	Not applicable			
Neomycin regimen details	Dexamethasone (1 mg), neo (5 mg), polymyxin B (20,000 U/mL) 3 drops t.i.d.—regimen a) continuous, b) with intermissions of <3 mo, c) with intermissions from 3 to 6 mo			
Control details	A) Control group received dexamethasone (1 mg) 3 drops t.i.d. B). No treatment group compared hearing loss in unilateral COM diseased and contralateral healthy ear			
Hearing change caused by infection	Unilateral ears with COM with no treatment (17.8 dB) were compared with the contralateral healthy ears (6.6 dB), p < 0.001			
Audiometry measures	All patients were tested by the same audiometer and by the same audiologist at the beginning of treatment and every 2 mo during the period of follow-up			
Preop audiometry	Mean BC threshold 9.3 dB in group before neo treatment, 8.7 dB in dexamethasone control group			
Compliance	Not specified			
Criteria for withdrawal from study	Not applicable			
Intention to treat analysis	Not applicable			
Power	NR			
Morbidity/complications	None reported			

Preop = preoperative, postop = postoperative, NR = not reported, PTA = pure tone average, t.i.d. = three times a day, BC = bone conduction, SRT = speech reception threshold, COM = chronic otitis media, neo = neomycin, SNHL = sensorineural hearing loss.
* Sample size for randomized controlled trials: numbers shown for those not lost to follow-up and those (initially recruited).
†, ‡ Symbols denote which data comparisons correspond to the referenced p-values and follow-up times.

Reference	Merifield, 1993		
Level (design)	3 (retrospective controlled study)		
Sample size	44 (70 ears)		

OUTCOMES			
Mean BC thresholds*			
	3 kHz	**4 kHz**	**6 kHz**
Post-neomycin drops	9.8 dB	9.6 dB	8.8 dB
Pre-treatment	10.1 dB	10.0 dB	7.6 dB
p Value	NS	NS	NS
Conclusion	No difference	No difference	No difference

Follow-up time	Not specified for all, ≥6 mo of follow-up noted in 1 case		

STUDY DESIGN			
Inclusion criteria	Treatment with ototopical medications for persistent otorrhea unresponsive to oral antibiotics: 1) after intubation with previously dry ears, 2) no evidence of preexisting sensorineural hearing loss, 3) one or both ears with chronic suppurative otitis media characterized by persistent purulent otorrhea		
Exclusion criteria	Not specified		
Definition of ototoxicity	≥10 dB deterioration in one ear at ≥1 frequency		
Age	8 mo–10 y, 9 mo		
Neomycin regimen details	Polymyxin B sulfate–neomycin sulfate–hydrocortisone (Pediotic, Cortisporin suspension and solution); colistin sulfate–neomycin sulfate–hydrocortisone acetate, gentamicin sulfate. Duration of drops: 2 d–2 wk		
Consideration of hearing change caused by middle ear disease	Not addressed		
Audiometry measures	Pre- and post-treatment bone conduction thresholds at 3, 4, 6 kHz with masking when necessary: a) eye shift observation and behavioral responses for age 8 mo–2 y, b) visually reinforced play audiometry for age 2–4 y, traditional ascending thresholds with button response for ≥5 y old		
Preoperative audiometry	As above		
Power	Not reported		
Morbidity/complications	1 patient had a 10-dB change in BC at 1 frequency which resolved by the 6-mo follow-up		

PTA = pure tone average, t.i.d. = three times a day, BC = bone conduction, TM perf. = tympanic membrane perforation, SNHL = sensorineural hearing loss, NS = not significant.
* Data extrapolated from line graph.

Reference	Linder, 1995	Lundy, 1993
Level (design)	4 (retrospective review)	5 (opinion survey)
Sample size	134 charts, 12 with TM perf.	2235 responses (7463 physician questionnaires)
OUTCOMES		
Post-neomycin drops	n = 1 patient diagnosed with neomycin ototoxicity: 69 y old man with slowly progressive AU hearing loss, active chronic otitis media used 70 cc AD over 2 mo, then 70 cc AS over 3 mo. He had rapid loss of hearing AU	3.4% (n = 76/2235) reported inner ear damage from topicals (31.6% believed Cortisporin was responsible), SNHL extent not noted
p Value	No comparative statistics	No comparative statistics
Conclusion	Neomycin high-volume use may result in ototoxicity	Physicians attributed ototoxicity to topicals
Follow-up time	At least 5 mo specified in 1 patient	Not reported
STUDY DESIGN		
Inclusion criteria	From a computerized database (1953–1993), 134 patient charts evaluated by audiology department for possible ototoxicity attributable to local or systemic application of various antibiotics. 12 of the 134 cases assessed antibiotic ear drops in the presence of TM perf	Physician questionnaire
Exclusion criteria	Insufficiently documented cases	Physician questionnaire
Definition of ototoxicity	Accelerated hearing loss	Not specified
Age	69 y (reported single case)	Physician questionnaire
Neomycin regimen details	Otosporin (1 mL containing 10,000 IE polymyxin B sulfate, 238,000 IE neomycin sulfate) 70 cc was used over 2 mo in the right ear only; then 70 cc over 3 mo in the left ear only	94.5% of respondents used Cortisporin suspension, 50.7% used Cortisporin solution. Otherwise, not specified
Consideration of hearing change caused by middle ear disease	Rate of prior sensorineural hearing loss was slow in comparison to post-neomycin; otherwise not specified	Not specified
Audiometry measures	Details not specified	Physician questionnaire
Preoperative audiometry	Potential confounders: previous progressive SNHL	Physician questionnaire
Power	Not applicable	Not reported
Morbidity/complications	As above	As above

PTA = pure tone average, t.i.d. = three times a day, BC = bone conduction, TM perf. = tympanic membrane perforation, SNHL = sensorineural hearing loss, NS = not significant, AD = right ear, AS = left ear, AU = both ears.

REFERENCES

1. Welling DB, Forrest LA, Goll F III. Safety of ototopical antibiotics. Laryngoscope 1995;105:472–474.
2. Rakover Y, Keywan K, Rosen G. Safety of topical ear drops containing ototoxic antibiotics. J Otolaryngol 1989;193(1); 46–50.
3. Podoshin L, Fradis M, Ben David J. Ototoxicity of ear drops in patients suffering from chronic otitis media. J Largyngol Otol 1989;193(1):46–50.
4. Merifield DO, Parker NJ, Nicholson N. Therapeutic management of chronic suppurative otitis media with otic drops. Otolaryngol Head Neck Surg 1993;109:77–82.
5. Linder TE, Zwicky S, Bränle. Ototoxicity of ear drops: a clinical perspective. Am J Otol 1995; 16.
6. Lundy LB, Graham MD. Ototoxicity and ototopical medications: a survey of otolaryngologists. Am J otol 1993;14:141–146.

12 Chronic Otitis Media

12.E.

Staging in tympanoplasty: Impact on audiometric outcomes

Jennifer J. Shin and Saumil Merchant

METHODS

Tympanoplasty may be staged for obtaining either a permanently disease-free ear or for optimal restoration of hearing. Intraoperative findings may prompt a staged approach for several reasons: 1) the discovery of a fixed footplate during surgery for active infection, 2) the anticipation of the need to take a "second look" during the initial cholesteatoma surgery, and 3) the desire to allow mucosal disease to resolve before endeavoring to optimize hearing results. In this third scenario, after granulation and irreversibly diseased mucosa are removed, plastic sheeting is placed over denuded surfaces to prevent adhesions and allow for mucosal healing. This systematic review focused on audiometric outcomes with no staging versus staged tympanoplasty. Our goal was to focus specifically on the impact of staging done for the reason outlined in +3 above (i.e., to allow mucosal disease to resolve so as to optimize the hearing outcome).

A computerized PubMed search of MEDLINE 1966–November 2004 was performed. Articles with the text words "staging," "stage," "staged," "two-stage," "staged," or "unstaged," or "delayed" were identified and cross-referenced with articles obtained by exploding the medical subject heading "tympanoplasty," yielding 121 articles. These articles were then reviewed to identify those that met the following inclusion criteria: 1) patient population with chronic otitis media, 2) comparison of no staging versus staged tympanoplasty, 3) outcome measured in terms of the air-bone gap (ABG) at least 6 months after surgery, ideally at all frequencies (250, 500, 1000, 2000, 4000, and 8000 Hz). Studies reporting results of revision surgeries that occurred >3 years after the original surgery were not included, because they did not seem to be within a reasonable timeframe for planned staging; these data were considered more relevant to unplanned revision surgery, a wholly separate topic. Also excluded were studies in which air conduction without bone conduction was measured. Small case series (n < 10 patients) of new techniques were excluded. The bibliographies of articles meeting these inclusion/exclusion criteria were manually checked to ensure no further relevant articles could be identified. This entire process yielded four controlled studies. The data from these four controlled studies are presented herein as the highest level of relevant evidence [1–4].

RESULTS

Outcome Measures. All four studies reported results in terms of an ABG. Two studies described the mean ABG for each group [2, 4], one with associated standard deviations [4]. All four articles reported the percent of patients achieving an ABG of <10 dB or <20 dB. In the three cases in which the audiometry was detailed [2–4], ABG was measured at 500, 1000, and 2000 Hz, with pure tone averages. Data regarding low frequencies specifically or measurements at 250 Hz were not recorded in any case. Such measurements, however, are often desirable because tympanic membrane perforations predispose to hearing loss at low frequencies.

Potential Confounders. Confounders were clearly present, given the retrospective nature of these studies. The key confounders were those that influenced whether no staging versus staged tympanoplasty was performed: 1) the quality of the mesotympanic mucosa, 2) the presence of active otorrhea, and 3) the extent and/or recurrence of cholesteatoma. In addition, several other factors could have potentially influenced audiometric outcomes, such as surgical technique, patient age, graft material, and condition of the stapes. All of these potential confounders are presented in the adjacent table in as much detail as the original reports allow.

Study Designs. All four studies were retrospective comparative studies, providing level 3 evidence. Thus, these results must be viewed with an understanding of the inherent biases of retrospective data. For example, inherent biases toward performing a staged procedure with more active or extensive disease could have resulted in a group of staged patients that were predisposed to a worse outcome. Potential confounders, however, were mostly well detailed, giving more strength to the studies. By understanding these confounders, readers can identify potential ways in which these retrospective results may have been skewed. One of the three studies specified that consecutive patients were described [4]; in doing so, they conveyed that all available data were presented, not just the results from a selected more favorable population. Also, one study reported the percent of patients that completed follow-up at intervals up to 10 years, which elucidated any potential attrition biases [1]. Follow-up times were at least 6 months after surgery, and were as long as 10 years.

Highest Level of Evidence. The data from these four studies showed either an improved outcome with no staging or no difference between unstaged and staged procedures. These comparative retrospective results, however, were tempered by the fact that patients undergoing staged procedures had worse disease at the outset. In addition, only one statistical comparison of the data regarding no staging versus staged ABG data was reported [1]. Therefore, in most instances, only trends can be noted. Several studies did attempt to identify other potential confounders by subgrouping data according to whether stapes crura were intact or missing [1, 2], or whether ears were dry or draining [3]. These data are presented in the adjacent tables.

Applicability. These studies are applicable to patients undergoing tympanoplasty over a wide age range, from children to elderly patients. They are applicable to patients whose surgeons decide on no staging versus staged tympanoplasty based on intraoperative characteristics of the middle ear.

Morbidity/Complications. Postoperative morbidity was minimally described in these studies. Whereas multiple studies reported the presence of sensorineural hearing loss, only one report specified whether they were postoperative losses (i.e., not present preoperatively). Only one case of sensorineural hearing loss was noted in that report [3]. Sensorineural hearing loss is an important secondary outcome measure, as some otologists believe that each additional otologic surgery places the patient at risk for it, and therefore attempt to avoid staging.

CLINICAL SIGNIFICANCE AND FUTURE RESEARCH

There were four level 3 studies that reported comparative data on no staging versus staged tympanoplasties. Although these data show an improved or equivalent audiometric outcome with unstaged rather than staged tympanoplasty, conclusions must be tempered by the inherent biases of these retrospective results, because patients whose procedures were not staged had preoperative characteristics making them prone to more favorable results.

Therefore, there is no study that directly compared audiometric outcomes after no staging versus staged tympanoplasty, while controlling for potential confounders such as cholesteatoma and mucosal disease. Ideally, a prospective controlled trial of patients undergoing unstaged versus staged tympanoplasty would ensure that these and other potential confounders were either eliminated through exclusion criteria or at least balanced between the two compared groups. For example, patients requiring tympanoplasty in the presence of mucosal disease with active otorrhea but without stapes footplate fixation or cholesteatoma could be selected. Other confounders such as extent and location of the initial perforation and the presence/absence of stapes crura could potentially be accounted for by randomization of subjects to no staging versus a staged procedure. Outcomes of ABGs at all frequencies could be measured, both preoperatively and postoperatively. Using the data from the largest study as "pilot data," the sample size necessary to devise a trial with 90% power to detect a 5% difference between groups can be calculated; 144 patients would need to complete such a trial, which seems to be a realistic goal for subject enrollment. In addition, any impact on sensorineural hearing could also be studied as a secondary outcome measure.

THE EVIDENCE CONDENSED: Audiometric outcome with no staging versus staged tympanoplasty (controlled studies)

Reference	Nomura, 2001
Level (design)	3 (retrospective comparative study)
Sample size*	236 ears (147 no staging, 89 staged)

<table>
<tr><td colspan="3" align="center">OUTCOMES</td></tr>
<tr><td></td><td>% with "success" (see below)</td><td>ABG PTA (mean ± SD)</td></tr>
<tr><td>No staging</td><td>73%</td><td>14 ± 11</td></tr>
<tr><td>Staged</td><td>55%</td><td>18 ± 14</td></tr>
<tr><td>p Value</td><td><0.05</td><td>Not reported</td></tr>
<tr><td>Conclusion</td><td colspan="2">No staging better but with multiple confounders</td></tr>
<tr><td>Follow-up time</td><td colspan="2">1 y</td></tr>
</table>

STUDY DESIGN

Inclusion criteria	New cases undergoing tympanoplasty for middle ear cholesteatoma
Exclusion criteria	Not specified
No staging regimen details	Not specified
Staged regimen details	Indications: cholesteatoma incompletely removed at first operation, TM adherent to promontory caused difficulty in preparing an aerated mesotympanum in 1 stage, or granulation tissue and/or thickened mucosa was present around the stapes. Second stage planned 10–18 mo after first operation
Presence of cholesteatoma	All patients had cholesteatoma
Stapes condition	26% type I tympanoplasty, 59% type III tympanoplasty (minor columella, major columella, stapes columella not specified), 15% type IV tympanoplasty; not broken down by no staging vs staged
Canal wall condition	"All patients underwent the canal wall reconstruction technique in which the canal was widened"; the antrum was opened as necessary to access the attic and mesotympanum
Audiometry	ABG at 500, 1000, 2000 Hz Bone conduction at 4000 Hz
Age	20 to >60 y
Diagnostic criteria for "success"	At least 1 of the following: achievement of postoperative hearing level of ≥30 dB, an ABG closure within 15 dB, hearing gain >20 dB
Graft material	Not specified
Consecutive patients?	Yes
Morbidity/complications	Not specified

ABG = air-bone gap, PTA = pure tone average, TM = tympanic membrane, SD = standard deviation.
*Sample size: numbers shown for those not lost to follow-up and those (initially recruited).

THE EVIDENCE CONDENSED: Audiometric outcome with no staging versus staged tympanoplasty (controlled studies)

Reference	Charachon, 1991			
Level (design)	3 (retrospective comparative study)			
Sample size*	199 patients			

	OUTCOMES			
	Intact stapes (n = 52)		**Missing crura (n = 72)**	
	Mean ABG dB (SD not reported)	**% with ABG <20 dB**	**Mean ABG dB** (SD not reported)	**% with ABG <20 dB**
No staging	14.35,† 12.70‡	83%,† 88%‡	19.44,† 17.66‡	86%,† 80%‡
Staged	27.61,† 28.84‡	50%,† 41%‡	31.72,† 31.27‡	29%,† 28%‡
p Value	Not reported	Not reported	Not reported	Not reported
Conclusion	No staging better but with multiple confounders			
Follow-up time	4 mo, †1 y, 3 y, ‡5 y,10 y			

	STUDY DESIGN			
Inclusion criteria	Patients undergoing reconstructions of "radical mastoidectomy"; "very often, the previous procedures were atticotomy or Bondy operation"			
Exclusion criteria	Not specified			
No staging regimen details	Used only if the mesotympanum was covered by normal mucosa, if a stable ossicular reconstruction was possible, and if there was no risk of residual cholesteatoma recurrence			
Staged regimen details	Used if the above criteria were not met. The second stage was performed 12–18 mo later, or delayed up to 24 mo if the Eustachian tube had been drilled			
Presence of cholesteatoma	94 ears with cholesteatoma			
Stapes condition	Footplate fixed in 4 ears; "usually the ossicular chain was found surrounded and more or less destroyed by cholesteatoma"			
Canal wall condition	"The bony canal was lowered to the level of the floor of the ear canal and to the level of the facial nerve"			
Audiometry	ABG at 500, 1000, 2000 Hz			
Age	<10 to 70 y			
Diagnostic criteria for "success"	Not specified			
Graft material	Head of malleus or incus body homograft placed on the head of the stapes; tragal cartilage autograft or incus homograft positioned on mobile footplate			
Consecutive patients?	Not specified			
Morbidity/complications	Not specified			

ABG = air-bone gap, PTA = pure tone average, TM = tympanic membrane, SD = standard deviation.
*Sample size: numbers shown for those not lost to follow-up and those (initially recruited).
†, ‡ Symbols denote which data comparisons correspond to the referenced p-values and follow-up times.

THE EVIDENCE CONDENSED: Audiometric outcome with no staging versus staged tympanoplasty (controlled studies)

Reference	Charachon, 1989	
Level (design)	3 (retrospective comparative study)	
Sample size*	117 patients (19 no staging, 98 staged)	
OUTCOMES		
	% with ABG <10 dB, <20 dB	
	With intact stapes	**With missing crura**
No staging	31%, 87%	20%, 55%
Staged	22%, 55%	18%, 57%
p Value	Not reported	Not reported
Conclusion	Trend toward no staging better (no statistics reported), multiple confounders	No major difference between groups noted (no statistics reported), multiple confounders
Follow-up time	4 mo (shown), 1 y, 3 y, 5 y (ABG for all patients combined remained 19.5–21 dB throughout all times studied)	
STUDY DESIGN		
Inclusion criteria	Patients undergoing reconstruction of "old radical mastoidectomy cavities" by obliteration tympanoplasty; had previously undergone 2–4 surgical procedures (70% radical mastoidectomy, 30% atticotomy or Bondy operation)	
Exclusion criteria	Not specified	
No staging regimen details	If the mesotympanum was covered by safe mucosa, a single-stage procedure was performed.	
Staged regimen details	If the mucosa in the mesotympanum needed to be dissected, silastic sheeting was placed in the mesotympanum to prevent adhesions and a second stage was performed 12 or 18 mo later	
Presence of cholesteatoma	Cholesteatoma in 41 ears	
Stapes condition	"Destruction of stapes" in 73 ears, footplate luxation in 1 ear	
Canal wall condition	"The bony canal was lowered to the level of the floor of the ear canal and to the level of the facial nerve"	
Audiometry	Details not reported	
Age	<10 to 60 y	
Diagnostic criteria for "success"	Not specified	
Graft material	Fascia graft underlay, malleus head or incus homograft	
Consecutive patients?	Not specified	
Morbidity/complications	Not specified	

ABG = air-bone gap.
* Sample size: numbers shown for those not lost to follow-up and those (initially recruited).

THE EVIDENCE CONDENSED: Audiometric outcome with no staging versus staged tympanoplasty (controlled studies)

Reference	Minatogawa, 1990		
Level (design)	3 (retrospective comparative study)		
Sample size*	32 patients (26 no staging, 6 staged)		
OUTCOMES			
	% success (see below for criteria)		
	Dry ears	**Draining ears**	**All ears**
No staging	82% (n = 17)	33% (n = 6)	65% (n = 26)
Staged	NA (n = 0)	33% (n = 6)	33% (n = 6)
p Value	Not reported	Not reported	Not reported
Conclusion	No comparison possible in this subgroup of patients	No major difference between groups noted (no statistics reported), multiple confounders	Trend toward no staging better (no statistics reported), multiple confounders
Follow-up time	>6 mo		
STUDY DESIGN			
Inclusion criteria	Patients undergoing allograft tympanoplasties		
Exclusion criteria	Not specified		
No staging regimen details	Allograft tympanic membrane with attached malleus and incus columella trimmed to couple allograft manubrium to host stapes		
Staged regimen details	In cases of a draining ear, allograft with attached malleus was implanted at the first stage, then >6 mo later, the incus was trimmed for implantation as the columella		
Presence of cholesteatoma	Not specified		
Stapes condition	Not specified		
Canal wall condition	Not specified		
Audiometry	Audiometry at 500, 1000, 2000 Hz		
Age	Not specified		
Diagnostic criteria for "success"	ABG <20 dB, air conductive hearing gain >15 dB, and mean conductive hearing <40 dB		
Graft material	Allograft tympanic membrane with attached malleus and incus		
Consecutive patients?	Not specified		
Morbidity/complications	1 sensorineural hearing loss in no surgery group		

ABG = air-bone gap.
*Sample size: numbers shown for those not lost to follow-up and those (initially recruited).

REFERENCES

1. Charachon R, Gratacap B, Elbaze D. Anatomical and functional reconstruction of old mastoidectomy cavities by obliteration tympanoplasty. Clin Otolaryngol 1989;14:121–126.
2. Characon R., LeJune JM, Bouchal H. Reconstrutions of radical mastoidectomy by obliteration technique. Ear Nose Throat J 1991;70(12):830–838.
3. Minatogawa T, Jumoi T, Inamori T, Oki K, Machizuka H. Hyogo Ear Bank experience with allograft tympanoplasty: review of tympanoplasty on 68 ears. Am J Otol 1990; 11(3):157–163.
4. Nomura K, Lino Y, Hashimoto H, Suzuki J-I, Kazuoki K. Hearing results after tympanoplasty in elderly patients with middle ear cholesteatoma. Acta Otolaryngol 2001; 121:919–924.

13 Sudden Sensorineural Hearing Loss

13.A.

Systemic steroids versus control: Impact on audiometric outcomes

Jennifer J. Shin and Steven D. Rauch

METHODS

A computerized Ovid search of MEDLINE 1970–March 2004 was performed. The terms "hearing loss," "deafness," "hearing loss, sensorineural," and "hearing loss, sudden" were exploded and the resulting articles were combined. These articles were then cross-referenced with articles obtained by exploding the term "steroids." This process yielded 320 publications. These studies were then reviewed to identify those that met the following inclusion criteria: 1) a discrete set of patients with idiopathic sensorineural hearing loss (SNHL) of "acute" or "sudden" onset or occurring over ≤3 days, 2) intervention with systemic steroids versus placebo or systemic steroids versus no intervention, 3) outcome measured with standard audiometry (i.e., pure tone and speech reception thresholds, speech discrimination scores). Studies with the following characteristics were excluded: a) patients with a known cause of SNHL, non-acute or repetitive SNHL, b) intervention with intratympanic steroids (see Section 13.D), c) comparison of steroids with another therapy, d) amalgamation of patients receiving other treatments with either the steroid or nonsteroid treatment groups. The bibliographies of the articles meeting these inclusion/exclusion criteria were manually checked to ensure no further relevant articles could be identified. This entire process yielded six articles [1–6].

RESULTS

Outcome Measures. Audiometric outcomes can be reported in a variety of ways. Standard pure tone averages (PTAs) of thresholds at 500, 1000, and 2000 Hz [1, 3, 4] or extended averages of pure tone thresholds at frequencies from 250 to 8000 Hz may be used [2]. In addition, speech reception thresholds and speech intelligibility scores may be reported [3, 4]. Furthermore, the magnitude of recovery in any scale may be in decibels (dB) or in the percentage of patients who had a defined minimum improvement. Regardless of the measure used, it is important to realize that the amount of potential recovery is dependent on the amount of initial hearing loss; a 30-dB loss can only improve 30 dB, whereas a 90-dB loss has much more room for improvement. Investigators can address this "floor effect" by measuring the percent of decibels recovered or by con-

sidering patients with more severe SNHL in a distinct analysis.

Potential Confounders. Recovery may be influenced by: 1) the severity of the initial loss, 2) the pattern of SNHL (i.e., high frequency, mid-frequency, low frequency, or otherwise), 3) the time elapsed between onset and treatment, 4) the dosage strength and schedule of the investigated steroid regimen, 5) patient comorbidities (especially vascular, inflammatory, or neurologic), 6) age, 7) presence of vertigo, or 8) the time over which the SNHL evolved. These potential confounders are tabulated for the reader in as much detail as the studies allow.

Study Designs. Two randomized controlled trials (RCTs) addressed this issue [1, 2]. Both strictly defined inclusion/exclusion criteria, used a placebo control, and were double blind. Both attempted to control potential confounders: One reported the degree of effectiveness of randomization at the outset [2], whereas the second reported an analysis of the results in which potential confounders were controlled [1]. The larger [1] of these two RCTs reported data from two centers using nearly equivalent steroid doses (high then tapered) over 10–12 days. The smaller RCT [2] used a constant high steroid dose over 5 days.

In addition to these RCTs, there were several retrospective studies that compared the results in a steroid cohort versus an untreated cohort [3–6], but none of these control groups were rigorously otherwise matched (i.e., they were not strict case control studies—see chapters 1 and 3). In addition, the retrospective nature of these studies prevented the implementation of any uniform strategy for withholding steroids in certain patients. Two of these retrospective studies, however, defined strict inclusion/exclusion criteria and were sizable enough for statistical analysis [3, 4].

Highest Level of Evidence. In the largest level 1 study [1], the steroid group improved significantly more than the placebo group, with 5 : 1 relative odds of >50% recovery of PTA. Furthermore, a "steroid effective zone" was defined, as subjects with 40- to 90-dB losses experienced the most benefit from treatment. In contrast, the smaller RCT [2] demonstrated no difference with or without steroids; at long-term follow-up, "average" thresholds at 250–8000 Hz (80% versus 81%) and speech discrimination scores (93% versus 91.5%) were similar. The difference in the two RCTs' conclusions may be the result of a lower power in the smaller trial (i.e., a lower probability of demonstrating a true difference because of a smaller sample size). In addition, variations within the steroid regimens, inclusion/exclusion criteria, or outcome parameters used could contribute to the seemingly disparate results of these two RCTs. The four retrospective studies also had heterogeneous results, although the two largest and most precisely reported of these studies [3, 4] showed that steroid treatment is correlated with improved outcome.

Applicability. These results apply to patients with idiopathic SNHL of at least 20–30 dB that occurred over ≤3 days. The results of the highest-level trials apply to patients who are seen within 10–14 days of onset.

Morbidity. No adverse effects from steroid use were reported during any of these study periods.

CLINICAL SIGNIFICANCE AND FUTURE RESEARCH

There were two level 1 studies and four level 3 studies that compared outcomes with and without systemic steroids. The larger studies showed significant improvement with steroids, whereas the smaller studies concluded that there was no difference. Smaller sample sizes usually resulted in diminished power, however, or a lesser ability to identify an effect that was truly present.

Future research may focus on those patients who are the least likely to undergo spontaneous recovery and those whose SNHL is so severe that they seem less responsive to this intervention. In addition, dose-dependent effects of steroids on audiometric outcomes may be investigated. Finally, the administration of steroids through local application may also be further explored (see Section 13.D.).

THE EVIDENCE CONDENSED: Systemic steroids versus placebo: Impact on audiometric outcomes

Reference	Wilson, 1980
Level (design)	1 (randomized controlled trial)
Sample size*	67 (67) with 52 additional controls who refused treatment/entry to trial

OUTCOMES	
	% of patients with >50% recovery of speech reception score or PTA
Steroid	61%
Placebo	32%
Untreated	58%
p Value	<0.025, steroid vs placebo
Conclusion	Better recovery with steroids
Follow-up time	4 wk, 3 mo (shown)
Secondary results: recovery according to audiogram type	• Mid-frequency loss: all recovered • Loss at 4 kHz > 8 kHz *or* loss 8 kHz > 4 kHz: 78% recovery in steroid group vs 38% recovery in controls • >90-dB loss in all frequencies: both groups with <20% recovery

STUDY DESIGN	
Inclusion criteria	• ≥30-dB idiopathic SNHL over 3 contiguous frequencies in ≤3 d • <10 d from onset of hearing loss
Exclusion criteria	Prior treatment; "patients for whom steroids would represent a hazard": pregnancy, diabetes
Steroid regimen details	MEEI group: methylprednisolone 16 mg PO t.i.d. ×3 d, then taper to 4 mg PO q.d. over the next 9 d; Kaiser group: dexamethasone 4.5 mg PO b.i.d. ×4 d then taper to 0.75 mg PO q.d. over the next 6 d
Randomization effectiveness	Not specified, although it was reported that results were still significant (p < 0.017) when controlling for MEEI vs Kaiser, age, vertigo
Masking	Double blind
Age	13–89 y, severities evenly distributed across ages
Vertigo	Vertigo did not correlate with worse recovery (relative odds 1.3:1)
Compliance	NR
Criteria for withdrawal	NR
Intention to treat analysis	Not applicable—all patients completed the study
Pre-trial power calculation	NR
Morbidity/complications	"All patients were able to tolerate steroids in the dosages prescribed without adverse effects"; no worsening of hearing on steroids

SNHL = sensorineural hearing loss, PTA = pure tone average (average threshold at 500, 1000, 2000 Hz), NS = not significant, NR = not reported, PO = by mouth, t.i.d. = three times a day, b.i.d. = twice a day, q.d. = one time per day, SD = standard deviation, MEEI = Massachusetts Eye and Ear Infirmary, Kaiser = Kaiser Permanente.
* Sample size: numbers shown for those not lost to follow-up and those (initially recruited) to the randomized controlled trials.

THE EVIDENCE CONDENSED: Systemic steroids versus placebo: Impact on audiometric outcomes

Reference	Cinamon, 2001	Chen, 2003	
Level (design)	1 (randomized controlled trial)	3 (retrospective with control)	
Sample size*	21 (21)	318 total; subset of 161 excluded low-frequency SNHL and PTA loss <60 dB	
OUTCOMES			
	% of patients with >15 dB recovery in "average" pure tone threshold (250–8000 Hz)	Mean dB in PTA recovery (SD)	% patients with improved speech intelligibility
Steroid	60%	16.2 dB (30)	50%
Placebo	63%	None	None
Untreated	None	11.7 dB (18)	35%
p Value	NS	NS	<0.03
Conclusion	No difference with steroids	No difference	Steroids better
Follow-up time	6 d (shown), long-term follow-up at 14–90 d ("average" of 33 d)	Not specified	
Secondary results: recovery according to audiogram type	• "Upsloping": nonsignificant trend toward more recovery for all patients • "Downsloping": nonsignificant trend toward less improvement for all patients	In a subset of patients excluding low-frequency SNHL and PTA loss <60 dB, the mean dB improvement with steroids (28 dB) was significantly better than with no treatment (12.9 dB), p < 0.01	
STUDY DESIGN			
Inclusion criteria	• ≥20-dB idiopathic SNHL compared with the healthy ear, in ≥3 frequencies, of immediate onset • <2 wk from onset	• Idiopathic SNHL of ≥25-dB loss at 3 consecutive frequencies, developed within 72 h • If treated, steroids <1 mo from onset	
Exclusion criteria	Chronic otologic history, prior sudden deafness, pathologic otoscopic findings. "Medical condition that could be a contraindication for treatment (e.g., hypertension, diabetes, active peptic ulcer disease, bronchial asthma)"	Ménière syndrome in either ear, prior ear surgery, blunt or penetrating ear trauma, barotrauma or acoustic trauma just before SNHL, luetic deafness, genetic SNHL with strong family history, craniofacial anomalies, known temporal bone malformations	
Steroid regimen details	Prednisone 1 mg/kg PO q.d. ×5 d	Steroid treatment was given within 1 mo of onset of SNHL	
Randomization effectiveness	At the outset: placebo group (54 dB) with more high-tone loss (4–8 kHz) than steroid group (39 dB); similar "average" thresholds (250–8000 Hz; 41.2 dB steroid, 47.4 dB placebo)	Not applicable	
Masking	Double blind	Not applicable	
Age	12–71 y, no correlation with outcome	13–89 y, severities evenly distributed across all ages	
Vertigo	No statistically significant trend toward worse recovery with vertigo	NR	
Compliance	NR	Not applicable	
Criteria for withdrawal	NR	Not applicable	
Intention to treat analysis	Not applicable—all patients completed the study	Not applicable	
Pre-trial power calculation	NR	Not applicable	
Morbidity/complications	NR	NR	

SNHL = sensorineural hearing loss, PTA = pure tone average (average threshold at 500, 1000, 2000 Hz), NS = not significant, NR = not reported, PO = by mouth, t.i.d. = three times a day, b.i.d. = twice a day, q.d. = one time per day, SD = standard deviation, MEEI = Massachusetts Eye and Ear Infirmary, Kaiser = Kaiser Permanente.
* Sample size: numbers shown for those not lost to follow-up and those (initially recruited) to the randomized controlled trials.

THE EVIDENCE CONDENSED: Systemic steroids versus placebo: Impact on audiometric outcomes

Reference	Moskowitz, 1984	Byl, 1977	Simmons, 1973	
Level (design)	3 (retrospective with control)	3 (retrospective with control)	3 (retrospective with control)	
Sample size	36	25	22	
OUTCOMES				
	% of patients with >50% recovery in SRT or PTA	% of patients with complete or "partial"* recovery	% of patients with recovery to within 10 dB of baseline	% of patients with no recovery
Steroid	89%	89%	55%	9%
No treatment	44%	83%	63%	36%
p Value	<0.01	NR	NR	
Conclusion	Recovery better with steroids	No difference	No difference	
Follow-up time	"Several weeks"	Not specified	Not specified	
STUDY DESIGN				
Inclusion criteria	Idiopathic SNHL, "using the definitions provided by Wilson" (see table, page 275)	Idiopathic SNHL occurring over <12 h; patient seen within 10 d of onset	Idiopathic sudden SNHL, not otherwise specified	
Exclusion criteria	Known cause for hearing loss; bilateral hearing loss	Diagnosis of fluctuant hearing loss, luetic labyrinthitis, Ménière, vestibular Schwannoma, CNS disease	Not specified	
Age	70% >40 y, 30% <40 y; no difference in recovery with age	7–83 y	"Average" 39 y (<9 y to >70 y)	
Steroid regimen details	Decadron® 0.75 mg/kg q.i.d. tapered to 0.5 q.d. over 12 d, route of administration NR	Prednisone 60 mg PO q.d. ×4 d then tapered to 0 mg over 6 more d	NR	
Additional instructions	Rest; salt, alcohol, tobacco restriction	Restrict sodium to <500 mg/d; no stimulants, alcohol, or tobacco	NR	
Reason for no treatment	Not specified	Degree of patient concern and physician preference	Physician preference	
Audiogram "types"	No difference in outcome among mid-frequency, upsloping, or downsloping audiograms	Increased severity of initial loss correlates with worse recovery	NR	
Vertigo	22% (14% in recovering patients, 50% in patients without recovery)	Associated with poor outcome	NR	
Morbidity/ complications	No adverse effects from the use of steroids	NR	NR	

SNHL = sensorineural hearing loss, PTA = pure tone average (average threshold at 500, 1000, 2000 Hz), SRT = speech reception threshold, CNS = central nervous system, PO = by mouth, q.i.d. = four times per day, q.d. = one time per day, NR = not reported.
*"Partial" recovery was not further defined or specified in the Byl, 1974 paper.

REFERENCES

1. Wilson WR, Byl FM, Laird N. The efficacy of steroids in the treatment of idiopathic sudden hearing loss. Arch Otolaryngol Head Neck Surg 1980;106:772–776.
2. Cinamon U, Bendet E, Kronenberg J. Steroids, carbogen, or placebo for sudden hearing loss: a prospective double-blind study. Eur Arch Otorhinolaryngol 2001;258:477–480.
3. Chen CY, Halpin C, Rauch SD. Oral steroid treatment of sudden sensorineural hearing loss: a ten year retrospective analysis. Otol Neurotol 2003;24:728–733.
4. Moskowitz D, Lee KJ, Smith HW. Steroid use in idiopathic sudden sensorineural hearing loss. Laryngoscope 1984;94:664–666.
5. Byl FM. Seventy-six cases of presumed hearing loss occurring in 1973: prognosis and incidence. Laryngoscope 1977;87(5):817–825.
6. Simmons FB. Sudden idiopathic sensorineural hearing loss: some observations. Laryngoscope 1973;83(8):1221–1227.

13 Sudden Sensorineural Hearing Loss

13.B.

Acyclovir adjunct to steroids versus placebo adjunct to steroids: Impact on audiometric outcomes

Jennifer J. Shin and Steven D. Rauch

METHODS

A computerized Ovid search of MEDLINE 1966–February 2004 was performed. The terms "hearing loss, sudden" and "hearing loss, sensorineural" were exploded and the resulting articles were combined. These articles were then cross-referenced with those obtained by exploding the term "antiviral agents," yielding 26 trials. These articles were then reviewed to identify those that met the following inclusion criteria: 1) patient population with idiopathic sensorineural hearing loss (SNHL) of "acute" or "sudden" onset or occurring over ≤3 days, 2) intervention with acyclovir versus placebo, 3) outcome measured by standardized audiometry. Articles evaluating acute hearing loss in the presence of a known etiology (i.e., Ménière syndrome, vestibular Schwannoma) were excluded. Articles reporting the impact of valcyclovir are not discussed here but are discussed in the subsequent clinical query. The bibliographies of the articles meeting these inclusion/exclusion criteria were manually checked to ensure no further relevant articles could be identified. This process yielded three randomized controlled trials (RCTs) [1–3].

RESULTS

Outcome Measures. Outcomes are measured in pure tone averages or in pure tone thresholds at individual frequencies. All three studies reported each group's results relative to the combined results for all patients. Two studies also reported a direct comparison of the acyclovir versus placebo groups [2, 3].

Potential Confounders. Any effect acyclovir may have on recovery of sudden SNHL may obviously be affected by the presence of a virus. In an attempt to account for this fact, two studies tested viral serologies, which were positive in 11% of cases. In addition, multiple other factors may affect the potential for hearing recovery (see this same section in 13.A). Factors that were balanced between the intervention and control groups through randomization and strict inclusion/exclusion criteria are tabulated for the reader.

Study Designs. Three RCTs compared audiometric outcomes with intravenous acyclovir adjunct to steroid therapy versus placebo adjunct to steroid. Randomiza-tion was demonstrated to be effective in one study [2], but in the other two trials, randomization did not balance a potentially key confounder [1, 3]. In both of these cases, the placebo adjunct group had significantly worse hearing at the outset. An initially severe hearing loss has been shown to be predictive of less recovery, which would potentially predispose the placebo group to a worse outcome. This predisposition would not hide a true improvement with acyclovir; it would instead magnify it. It is also conceivable, however, that a "floor effect" (see Section 13.A, Outcome Measures) might be more pronounced in a group with more mild hearing loss, which would make it more difficult to demonstrate improvement in the acyclovir adjunct group. In addition, power may be limited in these trials. As reported in one article, for an 80% power to detect a 25-dB difference with standard deviation of 20 dB, the sample size should be 126. The largest sample size completing the trials described here was 70. All three RCTs have multiple strengths, in that they all defined unambiguous inclusion/exclusion and withdrawal criteria. Also, even with follow-up periods of 1 year, retention rates were near perfect in two trials [2, 3], with a 77% retention rate in the third [1]. These relatively high retention rates minimized attrition bias.

Highest Level of Evidence. All three trials concluded that there is no significant difference with acyclovir versus placebo adjunctive treatment. In addition, when the data are examined in detail, it is apparent that differences between the intervention and control groups are <10 dB or <5% in all of the measured outcome variables. In this regard, there does not even seem to be a trend toward a difference in the two groups. These results, however, must be interpreted with respect to the studies' power and randomization effectiveness (see above, Study Designs). Overall, there is no evidence to support an additional benefit from acyclovir therapy, but the studies may be constrained by limited power to detect a true difference.

Applicability. These results are applicable to patients with idiopathic sudden SNHL of ≥20–30 dB in at least three continuous frequencies who are treated within 7–14 days of the hearing loss, and who are willing to undergo intravenous therapy.

Morbidity. Most, if not all, side effects in these studies were attributed to the concomitant steroid therapy.

CLINICAL SIGNIFICANCE AND FUTURE RESEARCH

There were three RCTs that compared the hearing recovery after treatment with acyclovir and steroid versus placebo and steroid; all concluded that there is no additional benefit from acyclovir therapy. The possibility of a benefit, however, still exists, as power limitations and potential confounders may limit the studies' conclusions. With this conundrum, this topic remains controversial.

Future research may focus on the realization of RCTs with increased power. In addition, it would seem ideal to focus on patients who are the most likely to have a viral etiology for their idiopathic loss. In these studies, viral serologies were positive in 11% of cases. The concentration of patients affected by a virus could potentially be increased through inclusion/exclusion criteria that focused on recent viral symptoms. Alternatively, a larger overall sample could be recruited to a trial, expecting that only a portion of them would have a viral etiology.

Reference	Westerlaken, 2003
Level (design)	1 (randomized controlled trial)
Sample size*	(70) 91

	OUTCOMES
	Difference between the PTA recovery of each group and both groups combined
Acyclovir with steroid	−3.1 dB
Placebo with steroid	+3.5 dB
p Value	NS
Conclusion	No difference
Follow-up time	1 wk, 3 mo, 6 mo, 12 mo after discharge

	STUDY DESIGN
Inclusion criteria	• Idiopathic SNHL of ≥30 dB HL for 3 subsequent 1-octave steps in frequency in the standard pure tone audiogram • Blank otologic history • HL occurring within a period of 24 h
Exclusion criteria	• >14 d since SNHL (though 1 patient with a 16-d lapse was included by clerical error) • Contraindications to use of prednisone or acyclovir
Acyclovir regimen	Acyclovir 10 mg/kg IV t.i.d. ×7 d
Randomization effectiveness	Age, gender equally divided between 2 groups. *Statistically significant difference in the mean SNHL at the outset: 62.9 dB HL acyclovir vs 83.6 dB HL placebo (p = 0.002)*—reported a comparison of hearing recovery for patients with > or < 100-dB HL to address this issue (no difference)
Age	12–80 y
Masking	Double blind
Steroid regimen	Prednisolone—1 mg/kg IV on d 1; diminished in equal steps until 0 mg/kg IV on d 7
Viral serology	8/70 with positive viral serology
Criteria for withdrawal from study	Determination of a nonidiopathic etiology after serology, imaging, and consultant evaluation
Intention to treat analysis	Yes
Pre-trial power calculation	For 80% power to detect a 25-dB difference with SD of 20, the sample size should be 126
Morbidity/complications	All side effects were thought to be steroid related

SNHL = sensorineural hearing loss, HL = hearing loss, PTA = pure tone average (average threshold at 500, 1000, 2000 Hz), NS = not significant, t.i.d. = three times a day, IV = intravenously, URI = upper respiratory infection.
*Sample size: numbers shown for those not lost to follow-up and those (initially recruited).

THE EVIDENCE CONDENSED: Acyclovir versus placebo adjunct to steroids for idiopathic sudden hearing loss

Reference	Uri, 2003	
Level (design)	1 (randomized controlled trial)	
Sample size*	60 (60)	
OUTCOMES		
	Pure tone threshold recovery at each frequency†	% with >15 dB recovery in an impaired frequency
Acyclovir with steroid	250 Hz 14.0 dB 500 Hz 22.0 dB 1 kHz 21.5 dB 2 kHz 17.5 dB 4 kHz 12.0 dB 8 kHz 9.0 dB	78.6%
Placebo with steroid	250 Hz 19.5 dB 500 Hz 21.0 dB 1 kHz 20.5 dB 2 kHz 19.0 dB 4 kHz 19.5 dB 8 kHz 13.0 dB	77.4%
p Value	NS, all frequencies	NS
Conclusion	No difference	No difference
Follow-up time	1 mo, 3 mo, 1 y	
STUDY DESIGN		
Inclusion criteria	• Idiopathic "sudden" SNHL of ≥20 dB in at least 3 frequencies	
Exclusion criteria	• >7 d since SNHL • <18 y old, >60 y old • Hypertension, diabetes, autoimmune, collagen and renal diseases, previous ear disease, or known HL	
Acyclovir regimen	Acyclovir 15 mg/kg/d IV t.i.d. ×7 d	
Randomization effectiveness	No difference in gender, age, day of treatment, presence of tinnitus, presence of dizziness, initial SNHL	
Age	18–60 y	
Masking	Not reported	
Steroid regimen	Hydrocortisone 100 mg IV t.i.d. ×7 d Also all patients were put on bed rest	
Viral serology	Not reported	
Criteria for withdrawal from study	Not reported	
Intention to treat analysis	All patients completed the study	
Pre-trial power calculation	Not reported	
Morbidity/complications	No side effects (renal, hepatic, or nervous system) were observed	

SNHL = sensorineural hearing loss, HL = hearing loss, PTA = pure tone average (average threshold at 500, 1000, 2000 Hz), NS = not significant, t.i.d. = three times a day, IV = intravenously, URI = upper respiratory infection.
* Sample size: numbers shown for those not lost to follow-up and those (initially recruited).
† Estimated from graph.

Reference	Stokroos, 1998	
Level (design)	1 (randomized controlled trial)	
Sample size*	43 (44)	

	OUTCOMES	
	Mean PTA at 12 mo (from the initial PTA)	% with >10 dB recovery in PTA
Acyclovir with steroid	44 dB (from 67 dB)	78%
Placebo with steroid	49 dB (from 91 dB)	82%
p Value	NS	NS
Conclusion	No difference	No difference
Follow-up time	1 wk, 3 mo, 6 mo, 12 mo after discharge	

	STUDY DESIGN	
Inclusion criteria	• Idiopathic SNHL of ≥30 dB for 3 subsequent 1-octave steps in frequency in the standard pure tone audiogram • Blank otologic history • HL occurring within a period of 24 h	
Exclusion criteria	• >14 d since SNHL • Contraindication for use of prednisolone or acyclovir	
Acyclovir regimen	Acyclovir 10 mg/kg IV t.i.d. ×7 d	
Randomization effectiveness	No difference in gender, age, recent URI, history of herpes labialis or herpes zoster, delay to treatment. †Significant difference in initial HL with more profound HL in placebo group—reported a covariate analysis to address this issue (no difference)	
Age	11–71 y	
Masking	Double blind	
Steroid regimen	Prednisolone—1 mg/kg IV on d 1; diminished in equal steps until 0 mg/kg IV on d 7	
Viral serology	5/43 with positive viral serology	
Criteria for withdrawal from study	One patient was diagnosed with a vestibular schwannoma and was excluded	
Intention to treat analysis	The remaining 43 patients completed the study	
Pre-trial power calculation	Not reported	
Morbidity/complications	No. of patients with: headache in 3 placebo, 1 acyclovir; nausea in 1 placebo, 1 acyclovir; abdominal pain in 1 placebo; high glucose in 1 placebo	

SNHL = sensorineural hearing loss, HL = hearing loss, PTA = pure tone average (average threshold at 500, 1000, 2000 Hz), NS = not significant, t.i.d. = three times a day, IV = intravenously, URI = upper respiratory infection.
* Sample size: numbers shown for those not lost to follow-up and those (initially recruited).
† Estimated from graph.

REFERENCES

1. Westerlaken BO, Stokroos RJ, Dhooge IJ, Wit HP, Albers FW. Treatment of idiopathic sudden sensorineural hearing loss with antiviral therapy: a prospective, randomized, double-blind clinical trial. Ann Otol Rhinol Laryngol 2003;112(11):993–1000.

2. Uri N, Doweck I, Cohen-Kerem R, Greenberg E. Acyclovir in the treatment of idiopathic sudden sensorineural hearing loss. Otolaryngol Head Neck Surg 2003;128(4):544–549.

3. Stokroos RJ, Albers FW, Tenvergert EM. Antiviral treatment of idiopathic sudden sensorineural hearing loss: a prospective, randomized, double-blind clinical trial. Acta Otolaryngol 1998;118(4):488–495.

13 Sudden Sensorineural Hearing Loss

13.C.

Valcyclovir adjunct to steroids: Impact on audiometric outcomes

Jennifer J. Shin and Steven D. Rauch

METHODS

A computerized search was performed as described in Section 13.B. These articles were then reviewed to identify those that met the following inclusion criteria: 1) patient population with idiopathic sensorineural hearing loss (SNHL) of "acute" or "sudden" onset or occurring over ≤3 days, 2) intervention with valcyclovir adjunct to steroids, ideally versus placebo adjunct to steroids, 3) outcome measured by standardized audiometry. Exclusion criteria and manual checking was performed as described in Section 13.B. This process yielded just two articles: one randomized controlled trial (RCT) and one retrospective case series [1, 2].

RESULTS

Outcome Measures. In addition to the usual audiometric outcomes (see Sections 13.A and 13.B), the RCT addressing this issue also used validated instruments that assess health status. A validated instrument is a questionnaire that has been tested to ensure that the following are true: 1) it measures what it is intended to measure (*convergent validity*, i.e., scores on a valid test of arithmetic skills correlate with scores on other math tests), and 2) it does not inadvertently measure irrelevant changes (*discriminant validity*, i.e., scores on a valid test of arithmetic do not correlate with scores on tests of verbal ability) [3, 4], 3) its scores are stable (*reliability*, i.e., a patient with the same disease impact will continue to have the same response), and 4) it is sensitive to change (*responsiveness*, i.e., a patient with a change in disease impact will have a changed score). Overall, this means that the validated instrument does in fact measure what it is meant to measure. In this case, the Hearing Screening Inventory was used. It is a disease-specific instrument with 12 questions that evaluate the impact of the patient's hearing ability on common situations.

Potential Confounders. Potential confounders are as described in Sections 13.A and 13.B.

Study Designs. There was one randomized controlled trial that addressed this issue [1]. It had extremely well delineated inclusion/exclusion criteria and outcome measures. According to the authors' pre-trial calculations, there was an 80% power (i.e., probability of detecting a difference that truly exists) on the basis of 84 subjects. Comparative data were reported for the 68 patients with normal contralateral hearing, so power may have been limited in this subset analysis. In the analysis, one patient was excluded because of noncompliance with antiviral medication. Although this precludes the strictest of intention to treat analyses, it is unlikely that the addition of this one patient would have significantly altered the findings. In addition to this RCT, one retrospective case series also addressed this issue [2]. Without the presence of a control group, however, results cannot be definitely directly correlated with the valcyclovir adjunctive therapy. In addition, in this study a steroid course lasting 3 weeks was used; the duration of this regimen was longer than reported in previous trials, also making it difficult to draw direct parallels with other studies.

Highest Level of Evidence. In the RCT, there was no difference with valcyclovir versus placebo adjunct to steroid therapy in the multiple audiometric parameters that were tested [1]. Results for the Hearing Screening Inventory were likewise similar between groups. As noted above, however, these results must be considered in light of potential limitations in the power of their subset analysis. In the retrospective case series, 73% of patients receiving a 1-week course of valcyclovir with a 3-week course of steroids had recovery of at least 50% in pure tone thresholds [2]. This was a higher rate of recovery than noted in other studies, but without an internal control group and with a longer steroid regimen, no direct comparisons can be made.

Applicability. These results are applicable to patients with idiopathic SNHL with ≥30-dB hearing loss in three contiguous frequencies over <3 days who presented within 7–10 days of the onset of symptoms.

Morbidity. Either no or minimal adverse effects from antiviral treatment were reported in these trials.

CLINICAL SIGNIFICANCE AND FUTURE RESEARCH

There was one RCT that compared the hearing recovery after treatment with valcyclovir and steroid versus placebo and steroid, and one retrospective case series of patients who received a combination of valcyclovir and steroid therapy. As with acyclovir, there is evidence to suggest that there is no additional benefit from valcyclovir adjunct to steroid therapy, but this claim could be challenged on the basis of limitations of the study designs. Therefore, the topic of the use of valcyclovir for idiopathic sudden SNHL also remains controversial. Future research may be conducted as described in Section 13.B.

THE EVIDENCE CONDENSED: Valcyclovir adjunct to steroid therapy for idiopathic sudden sensorineural hearing loss

Reference	Tucci, 2002			
Level (design)	1 (randomized controlled trial)			
Sample size*	84 (105), subset of 68 with normal contralateral audiometry was analyzed			

OUTCOMES

	Improvement in HL from initial score			
	PTA mean	4000 Hz mean	Speech discrimination	Hearing Screening Inventory
Antiviral with steroid	30.2 dB	19.4 dB	28.5%	11 d median time to improvement
Placebo with steroid	43.0 dB	15.6 dB	39.0%	8 d median time to improvement
p Value	>0.05	>0.05	>0.05	>0.05
Conclusion	No difference	No difference	No difference	No difference
Follow-up time	2 wk, 6 wk			

STUDY DESIGN

Inclusion criteria	• ≥30 dB HL in 3 contiguous frequencies over <3 d in patients with previous audiometry • "Subjective marked loss of hearing in patients with subjectively normal baseline hearing and no previous record of audiometry" • Seen <10 d from onset of SNHL • No underlying disease that could be associated with sudden SNHL as an etiologic factor (see exclusion criteria) • No contraindications to steroid or antiviral use • Willingness to undergo audiometric, laboratory, and imaging studies
Exclusion criteria	Neoplasms, pregnancy, small vessel disease, insulin-dependent diabetes mellitus requiring treatment for >10 y, autoimmune disorder with +ANA or +RF, recent barotraumas, congenital cochlear malformation, otitis media with abnormal tympanogram, neurologic disorder that may predispose to HL, recent ototoxic medication excluding otic drops, major psychiatric illness, liver or renal dysfunction, <18 y old
Randomization effectiveness	No difference in initial PTA, 4000-Hz thresholds, speech discrimination scores; age; right or left ear; sex; race; days to treatment; tinnitus; vertigo; aural fullness; viral illness within the previous month; days missed from work
Valcyclovir regimen	Valcyclovir 1 g PO t.i.d. ×10 d
Steroid regimen	Prednisone PO Day 1–4: 80 mg Day 5–6: 60 mg Day 7–9: 40 mg Day 10–12: 20 mg
Masking	Double blind
Age	18–82 y (mean 55.8 y)
Compliance	1 patient in valcyclovir group with known noncompliance, not otherwise specified
Criteria for withdrawal from study	Diagnosis of vestibular schwannoma, positive fluorescent treponemal antibody absorption test, realization that inclusion criteria were not met on a second evaluation; adverse events
Intention to treat analysis?	1 patient in valcyclovir group who was compliant only with steroid therapy was excluded; otherwise all patients completed the trial
Pre-trial power calculation	80% power on the basis of 84 subjects (magnitude of the effect that could be detected not specified)
Morbidity/complications	2 adverse events (1 hyperglycemia, 1 gastrointestinal irritability) both attributed to steroid therapy; telephone calls to physician in 60% of valcyclovir group vs 37% of placebo group (p = 0.037)

SNHL = sensorineural hearing loss, HL = hearing loss, PTA = pure tone average (average threshold at 500, 1000, 2000 Hz), ANA = antinuclear antibody, RF = rheumatoid factor, PO = by mouth, t.i.d. = three times a day, q.i.d. = four times per day, q.d. = one time per day.
* Sample size: numbers shown for those not lost to follow-up and those (initially recruited).

THE EVIDENCE CONDENSED: Valcyclovir adjunct to steroid therapy for idiopathic sudden sensorineural hearing loss

Reference	Zadeh, 2003
Level (design)	4 (retrospective case series)
Sample size*	51

OUTCOMES

	% of patients with 50% recovery
Antiviral with steroid	73%
Placebo with steroid	None
p Value	Not applicable
Conclusion	Not applicable
Follow-up time	2 wk after treatment "in the majority of cases"

STUDY DESIGN

Inclusion criteria	• ≥30 dB HL in 3 contiguous frequencies over <3 d • Seen ≤7 d from onset of SNHL
Exclusion criteria	No audiogram available after treatment; "poor candidates for steroid therapy"
Randomization effectiveness	Not applicable
Valcyclovir regimen	Valcyclovir 500 mg PO t.i.d. ×7 d
Steroid regimen	Dexamethasone PO Day 0–14: 4 mg q.i.d. Day 15–16: 1 mg t.i.d. Day 17–18: 0.5 mg t.i.d. Day 19–20: 0.5 mg b.i.d. Day 21: 0.5 mg q.d.
Masking	Not applicable
Age	19–81 y
Compliance	Not applicable
Criteria for withdrawal from study	Not applicable
Intention to treat analysis?	Not applicable
Pre-trial power calculation	Not applicable
Morbidity/complications	"Extremely low incidence of side effects"; otherwise not specified

SNHL = sensorineural hearing loss, HL = hearing loss, PTA = pure tone average (average threshold at 500, 1000, 2000 Hz), ANA = antinuclear antibody, RF = rheumatoid factor, PO = by mouth, t.i.d. = three times a day, q.i.d. = four times per day, q.d. = one time per day.
*Sample size: numbers shown for those not lost to follow-up and those (initially recruited).

REFERENCES

1. Tucci DL, Farmer JC Jr, Kitch RD, Witsell DL. Treatment of sudden sensorineural hearing loss with systemic steroids and valcyclovir. Otol Neurotol 2002;23(3):301–308.

2. Zadeh MH, Storper IS, Spitzer JB. Diagnosis and treatment of sudden-onset sensorineural hearing loss: a study of 51 patients. Otolaryngol Head Neck Surg 2003;128(1):92–98.

3. Campbell DT, Fiske DW. Convergent and discriminant validation by the multitrait-multimethod matrix. Psychol Bull 1959;56:81–105.

4. Trochim WM. Research Methods Knowledge Base. New York: Cornell University; 2000.

13 Sudden Sensorineural Hearing Loss

13.D.

Intratympanic steroids: Impact on audiometric outcomes

Jennifer J. Shin and Steven D. Rauch

METHODS

A computerized and manual search was performed as described in Section 13.A. These articles were reviewed to identify those that met the following inclusion criteria: 1) patients with idiopathic sensorineural hearing loss (SNHL) of "acute" or "sudden" onset or occurring over ≤3 days, 2) intervention with intratympanic steroids, 3) outcome measured in terms of standard audiometry. Studies of patients with a known cause of SNHL, non-acute or repetitive SNHL were excluded, yielding four articles [1–4].

RESULTS

Outcome Measures, Potential Confounders. Outcome measures and potential confounders were as described in Section 13.A.

Study Designs. All four studies were uncontrolled series, with the inherent biases of this study design; these results can suggest correlations and propose hypotheses, even if they do not establish a direct cause and effect. This means that they can suggest a role for intratympanic steroids in the treatment of sudden SNHL, but cannot prove that intratympanic delivery caused any improvement that was observed.

Highest Level of Evidence. Four level 4 studies addressed this issue, each showing potential for improvement in the pure tone average, speech discrimination score, and speech reception threshold in a select group of patients treated with intratympanic methylprednisolone or dexamethasone. Potential for improvement was noted whether steroids were delivered continuously or in discrete boluses.

Applicability. These studies are applicable to patients who had an SNHL of ≥20–30 dB over ≤3 days, with failure to respond to 10–14 days of systemic prednisone therapy, possibly with adjunctive systemic therapies.

Morbidity. Few minor temporary complications were noted. No worsening of hearing during therapy was observed.

CLINICAL SIGNIFICANCE AND FUTURE RESEARCH

Four uncontrolled prospective studies suggest a potential role for treatment of patients with sudden SNHL with intratympanic steroids, especially those patients who are unresponsive to systemic steroids. Future higher-level studies, including a current multicenter randomized controlled trial, will ideally establish whether intratympanic steroids are as effective as oral steroids for the treatment of sudden SNHL.

THE EVIDENCE CONDENSED: Intratympanic steroids for idiopathic sudden sensorineural hearing loss

Reference	Gianoli, 2001	Parnes, 1999	Kopke, 2001	Lefebvre, 2002
Level (design)	4 (prospective uncontrolled cohort)	4 (prospective uncontrolled cohort)	4 (prospective uncontrolled cohort)	4 (prospective uncontrolled cohort)
Sample size	23	13	5	6
OUTCOMES				
Pure tone average	44% of patients with >10 dB recovery; 15.2 dB average improvement in score	Not reported	67.5, 26.5, 55.0, 48.8, 0.0 dB improvements in score	16.3, 17.5, 16.3, 10,* 30* dB improvements in score
Speech discrimination score	35% with improved SDS, 2% average improvement in score	53% of patients had improvements in SDS of ≥40%	96%, 50%, 0%, 96%, 0% improvements in score	80%, 40%, 40%, 75%,* 75%* improvements in score
Speech reception threshold	48% of patients with SRT improved >10%	53% of patients had improvement >20 dB	Not reported	Not reported
Follow-up time	1–2 wk after therapy	Up to 7 y	2–12 mo	11–12 d after therapy
STUDY DESIGN				
Inclusion criteria	• Sudden SNHL of ≥20 dB in ≥3 contiguous audiometric frequencies over ≤3 d • Failure to improve after a course of prednisone 1 mg/kg/d for ≥1 wk (n = 22) *or* inability to tolerate systemic steroids (n = 1)	• Sudden SNHL • <6 wk from onset	• Sudden SNHL over ≤3 d • Failure to respond to 2 wk of oral steroid therapy (prednisone 60 mg/d)	• Idiopathic SNHL >30 dB in 3 consecutive 1-octave frequencies over <24 h • Failure to respond to methylprednisolone ×10 d, carbogen inhalation, nafhydrofuryl, diazepam, and low-molecular-weight heparin
Steroid regimen details	Dexamethasone 0.4–0.6 cc of 25 mg/cc or methylprednisolone 125 mg/2 cc ×30 min 4× over 10–14 d; delivery through a posteroinferior tympanotomy, ventilation tube under local anesthesia	11 patients: methylprednisolone 0.9 cc of 40 mg/cc ×2–29 treatments (combined with 0.1 cc of 1% lidocaine) through a cruciate posterior myringotomy under local anesthesia; 4 patients: dexamethasone ×4–8 treatments	Methylprednisolone (62.5 mg/cc) 10 µL/h ×14 d; delivery through microcatheter insertion into round window niche through tympanomeatal flap	Methylprednisolone (62.5 mg/cc) 10 µL/h ×8–10 d, delivery at the level of the round window with an intraear microcatheter
Age	34–83 y	21–70 y	48–59 y	20–79 y
Time to therapy	0–520 wk	2 d–6 wk	4–6 wk	10 d
Morbidity/complications	1 otitis media	No long-term negative effects	3 small tympanic membrane perforations†	None specified

SDS = speech discrimination score, SRT = speech reception threshold, PTA = pure tone average (average threshold at 500, 1000, 2000 Hz), SNHL = sensorineural hearing loss.
* Estimated from graph.
† One patient who was treated with intratympanic steroids after SNHL secondary to trauma had worsening of hearing.

REFERENCES

1. Lefebvre PP, Staecker H. Steroid perfusion of the inner ear for sudden sensorineural hearing loss after failure of conventional therapy: a pilot study. Acta Otolaryngol 2002; 122:698–702.

2. Parnes LS, Sun AH, Freeman DJ. Corticosteroid pharmacokinetics in the inner ear fluids: an animal study followed by clinical application. Laryngoscope 1999;109(Suppl 91):1–17.

3. Kopke RD, Hoffer ME, Wester D, O'Leary MJ, Jackson RL. Targeted topic steroid therapy in sudden sensorineural hearing loss. Otol Neurotol 2001;22:475–479.

4. Gianoli GJ, Li JC. Transtympanic steroids for treatment of sudden hearing loss. Otolaryngol Head Neck Surg 2001; 125:142–146.

14 Cochlear Implantation

14.A.

Comparative implant performance in postlingually deafened adults: Speech recognition outcomes

Pamela Roehm, Richard S. Tyler, Camille Dunn, and Bruce J. Gantz

METHODS

A computerized search of MEDLINE 1966–March 2004 was performed. The term "cochlear implant" (CI) was exploded and the resulting articles were limited to adults, yielding 1246 studies. These articles were then reviewed to identify those that met the following inclusion criteria: 1) cochlear implantation with multichannel CIs, 2) use of standardized tools to measure speech recognition outcomes, 3) follow-up period ≥6 months. Exclusion criteria used were: 1) patient age <18 years at cochlear implantation, 2) patient age <3 years at onset of severe–profound deafness, 3) study performed before 1985. The bibliographies of the articles that met these inclusion criteria were manually checked to ensure no further relevant articles could be identified. This process yielded four reports of randomized controlled trials (RCTs). Two of these publications reported longer-term results on the same patients in the initial two trials (VA Clinical Trial, Iowa Clinical Trial), so only the longer-term results are presented here.

RESULTS

Outcome Measures. Clinical effectiveness can be measured with many different tools that assess the recognition of phonemes, words, and sentences in noisy or quiet environments. The measurements used in this review consisted of 24 tests that were categorized as measuring: 1) prosodic characteristics, 2) lip-reading enhancement, 3) phonetic level, 4) spondee tests, and 5) open-set speech recognition. These five categories were combined to form one composite score in the Cohen 1991 study [1]. Other measurement tools used in this review consisted of the Northwestern University Auditory Test No. 6 (NU-6) words [2], Minimal Auditory Capabilities Battery (MAC) [3], Iowa Sentence [4], Medial Consonant, and Medial Vowel tests [4]. These tests measured the listener's ability to recognize environmental sounds and to understand words and sentences.

The NU-6 is composed of four lists of 50 phonemically balanced Consonant-Nucleus-Consonant words [2]. The MAC is composed of 13 auditory tests of varying levels of difficulty. The tests evaluate prosody, vowels, consonants, sentences, and word tests [3]. The Iowa Sentence test is composed of 100 sentences with 20 different speakers (10 male and 10 female) [4]. The Iowa Medial

Consonant Test is a 13-alternative forced-choice test in which consonant sounds are presented in an "ee/Consonant/ee" context [4]. The Iowa Medial Vowel test is a 9-alternate forced-choice test in which vowel sounds are presented in an "h/Vowel/d" context [4]. The Iowa Sentence, Medial Consonant, and Medial Vowel tests can be presented in audition only, audiovisual, or vision-only test conditions.

Potential Confounders. In the Cohen 1991 study, 20 patients were randomly assigned to receive a single-channel CI that was later withdrawn by its manufacturer. Additionally, the patients in the Cohen study were predominantly male [1]. Finally, longer follow-up results as reported in VA 1993 may have been affected by the inability of five patients to upgrade to a different sound processor that was used by the remaining 24 patients [5].

Long-term results of the Iowa 1993 study as reported in Tyler, 1997 were affected by some subjects who chose to use different coding strategies. Therefore, scores potentially showed improvements or decrements attributable to strategy changes instead of actual changes in performance [4].

Study Designs. All of the studies reviewed were RCTs measuring the efficacy of different CIs in postlingually deafened adults. In the VA 1991 study, age at implantation, duration of deafness, and gender of subjects in the different cohorts were not mentioned. Only two of the 84 patients were female. Patients were stratified based on participating institution and results of round window electrical stimulation, and subsequently randomized to one of three devices: Nucleus 22, Ineraid 4-channel, or 3M/Vienna single channel [1].

In the Iowa 1993 study, patients were randomized to either Nucleus 21 channel or Ineraid 4-channel CIs. In this study, the duration of deafness in the Nucleus CI cohort was 12.8 years [standard deviation (SD) 9.8]. However, the mean age at implantation was significantly different between the two cohorts, with average age 48 years (SD 15.2) in the Nucleus cohort and 54.9 years (SD 14.5) in the Ineraid group. Gender distribution between the two cohorts was not mentioned in the study, although 23 of the 49 subjects were female [6].

Neither of the studies was masked. Both employed adequate follow-up time, with 12 months' follow-up available in the VA 1991 study and 9 months' follow-up data reported in the Iowa 1993 study.

A priori, the power of the VA 1991 study was set at 0.8 with an $\alpha = 0.05$ for a 50% difference between the three test cohorts. Although not reported in the Iowa 1993 publication, the power was 0.9 for an $\alpha = 0.05$ for a 50% difference between the two test cohorts on a paired t-test.

Highest Level of Evidence. These two level 1 studies showed a significant difference in postoperative word recognition compared with baseline performance with all of the CI models tested. In the VA 1991 study, patients implanted with multichannel implants had significantly better performance on open-set discrimination tests than patients with single-channel implants ($p = 0.001$) [1]. Comparison of the Nucleus versus Ineraid multichannel implants showed significantly better scores for Nucleus users on NU-6 word testing [7] and on composite scores when speech processor upgrades were used [5].

In the Iowa 1993 study, audiologic performance of multichannel CI recipients was correlated with different variables, revealing a few that accounted for $\geq 10\%$ of the variance. The most significant of these was years of profound hearing loss. Other significant factors were the number of frequencies with detectable hearing before implantation and age at implantation. The type of multichannel implant used did not significantly change the variance in this study [6].

Applicability. Results from either of these studies can be applied to postlingually deafened adults with nonsignificant benefits from hearing aids.

Morbidity/Complications. Neither of the initial RCTs mentioned complications. In the continuation of the VA 1991 study, 16 complications out of 80 procedures were reported [5]. Many of those listed in the paper were related to the CI pedestal, which is no longer a component of current CI design. Cohen et al. found in 5/80 patients that the facial nerve was stimulated by the implant. Other complications included 3/80 tympanic membrane perforations, 1/80 with hematoma, 1/80 wound infection, 1/80 device failure, 2/80 changes in sense of taste or increased tinnitus.

CLINICAL SIGNIFICANCE AND FUTURE RESEARCH

There were two RCTs comparing the impact of different CIs on speech recognition. Both studies showed a significant difference in postoperative speech recognition scores compared with preoperative baselines. The VA 1991 study demonstrated a significant increase in speech recognition performance for multichannel CIs versus a single-channel model [1]. Differences between the two types of multichannel CIs were not significant unless speech processing upgrades were included; however, the trend was for improved performance with greater number of channels. Overall, the data showed that implantation of multichannel CIs in the postlingually deafened adult can lead to significant improvement in speech recognition compared with preimplant performance using hearing aids.

Additionally, the Iowa 1993 study showed that the two most powerful predictors of final CI performance are duration of profound deafness and preoperative residual hearing at >4 frequencies. Other factors, such as brand of multichannel CI used, were not predictive of final performance [6]. These findings have an obvious impact on choices of which implant *to use and which ear to implant.*

Future research will focus on new technologies in electrode design and in speech processing. Additionally, studies may focus on bilateral implantation, which can provide patients with advantages of sound localization and improvement in speech understanding in noise [8]. An exciting new application is atraumatic short-electrode implantation in patients with retained low-frequency hearing and severe–profound high-frequency hearing. Initial studies of the short-electrode CI in these patients coupled with a hearing aid in that ear can improve speech recognition to >90% word recognition [9].

Characteristics of implants used in these studies

Implant type	No. of channels	Study using implant type	No. of patients implanted
3M/Vienna	1	VA	n = 21 (30 had been planned; device manufacturing discontinued during study)
Nucleus single-channel	1	VA	n = 1
Ineraid	4	VA, Iowa	n = 30 (VA) n = 24 (Iowa)
Nucleus 22	22	VA, Iowa	n = 30 (VA) n = 24 (Iowa)

THE EVIDENCE CONDENSED: Comparative implant performance in postlingually deafened adults: Speech recognition

Reference	Cohen, 1991 (VA trial)
Level (design)	1 (randomized controlled trial)
Sample size*	82 (82)
OUTCOMES	
Implants tested	Patients randomized to Nucleus-22, Ineraid 4-channel, and 3M/Vienna single-channel CI
Outcome measure	24 tests were grouped into 5 categories: prosodic characteristics, lip-reading enhancement, category phonetic level, spondee tests, and open-set speech recognition. Scores were then calculated and placed into a weighted composite. (Ranges of scores for individuals were not reported)
Preoperative speech recognition	Overall composite indexes were 10–12 for the 3 groups.
Postoperative speech recognition	3 of 6 prosodic characteristics tests showed significant differences between device groups • Lip-reading category: one of three tests showed a significant difference between groups • Phonetic level: five of nine tests showed a significant difference between groups • Spondee and open-set discrimination tests: all showed significant differences between multichannel and single-channel implant groups
p Value	Multichannel implant users scored higher than single-channel CI patients on all test categories ($p = 0.002$–0.0001). Patients with single-channel implants did score significantly higher ($p < 0.05$) on 12 of 26 audiologic tests postoperatively compared with their preoperative scores
Conclusion	Multichannel implants superior to single-channel CIs. Users of single-channel implants had improved scores for more than half of audiologic tests
Follow-up time	3 mo, 12 mo
STUDY DESIGN	
Inclusion criteria	>18 y old, bilateral sensorineural hearing loss, profound hearing loss, postlingually deafened, English speaking and literate
Exclusion criteria	Benefit from appropriate amplification, open-set speech recognition, medical contraindications, psychologic instability
Age	30–80 y
Masking	None
Intervention regimen details	Nucleus-22 (n = 30), Ineraid 4-channel (n = 30), 3M/Vienna single-channel (n = 20), Nucleus single-channel (n = 2)
Predictive measures for implant success	Not reported
Compliance	Not reported
Criteria for withdrawal from study	Not specified
Power	0.8
Morbidity/complications	Not reported

CI = cochlear implant, NU-6 = Northwestern University Auditory Test No. 6, MAC = Minimal Auditory Capabilities Battery, PTA = pure tone average.
* Sample size: numbers shown for those not lost to follow-up and those (initially recruited).

THE EVIDENCE CONDENSED: Comparative implant performance in postlingually deafened adults: Speech recognition

Reference	Gantz, 1993 (Iowa trial)
Level (design)	1 (randomized controlled trial)
Sample size*	48 (48)
OUTCOMES	
Implants tested	Patients randomized to Nucleus-21 vs Ineraid 4-channel CI
Outcome measure	Iowa Sentence test, NU-6, MAC; sound only
Preoperative speech recognition	All patients scored <4% on the CID W-22 or NU-6 word tests
Postoperative speech recognition	Iowa Sentences at 9 mo postoperatively (range 0%–96%): • Ineraid mean: 30% • Nucleus mean: 38% NU-6 words scores at 9 mo (range 0%–46%) • Ineraid mean: 8% • Nucleus mean: 12%
p Value	No statistically significant differences ($p > 0.05$) in speech understanding were reported between Nucleus and Ineraid implant groups after 9 mo of implant use
Conclusion	No significant difference in average scores after implantation with Ineraid vs Nucleus
Follow-up time	9 mo, 12 mo, 24 mo (only data at 9 mo was reported)
STUDY DESIGN	
Inclusion criteria	≥18 y old bilateral PTA >90-dB hearing loss, postlingual deafness, and ≤4% CID, W-22, or NU-6 at 60-dB hearing loss with best-fitted hearing aid
Exclusion criteria	Severe psychiatric illness or personality disorder, score <74 on Wechsler Adult Intelligence Scale–Revised
Age	22–73 y
Masking	None
Intervention regimen details	Nucleus-21 (n = 24), Ineraid 4-channel (n = 24)
Predictive measures for implant success	A focus of this paper was to report on audiologic performance after 9 mo of CI use. Preoperative predictor measures were put into a single predictive index. For subjects with a preoperative index of 20, the median predicted performance was about 12% on Sentence testing at 9 mo. A preoperative predictive index score of 45 achieved ≥40% on the Sentence test. 90% of the recipients with a predictive index score of 60 achieved ≥50% on the Sentence test
Compliance	Not reported
Criteria for withdrawal from study	Not specified
Power	0.9
Morbidity/complications	Not reported

CI = cochlear implant, NU-6 = Northwestern University Auditory Test No. 6, MAC = Minimal Auditory Capabilities Battery, PTA = pure tone average, CID = Central Institute of the Deaf.
* Sample size: numbers shown for those not lost to follow-up and those (initially recruited).

REFERENCES

1. Cohen NL, Waltzman SB, Fisher SG. Prospective randomized clinical trial of advanced cochlear implants. Ann Otol Rhinol Laryngol 1991;100(10):823–829.

2. Tillman TW, Carhart R. An expanded test for speech discrimination utilizing CNC monosyllabic words, in Northwestern University Auditory Test No. 6 Technical Report No. SAM-TR-66-55. 1966, USAF School of Aerospace Medicine: Brooks Air Force Base, Texas.

3. Owens E,Telleen CC. Speech perception with hearing aids and cochlear implants. Arch Otolaryngol 1981;107(3):160–173.

4. Tyler RS, et al. Cochlear Implant Program at the University of Iowa, in Sensorineural Hearing Loss: Mechanisms, Diagnosis, and Treatment, M.J. Collins and L.A. Glattke, Editors. 1986, University of Iowa Press: Iowa City.

5. Cohen NL, Waltzman SB, Fisher SG. A prospective randomized study of cochlear implants. N Eng J Med 1993;328(4):233–237.

6. Gantz BJ, Woodworth GG, Knutson JF, Abbas PJ,Tyler RS. Multivariate predictors of audiologic sucess with multichannel cochlear implants. Ann Otol Rhinol Laryngol 1993;102(12):909–916.

7. Tyler RS, Parkinson AJ, Woodworth GG, Lowder MW, Gantz BJ. Performance over time of adult patients using the Ineraid of Nucleus cochlear implant. J Acoust Soc Am 1997;102(1):508–522.

8. Gantz BJ, Tyler RS, Rubinstein JT, et al. Binaural cochlear implants placed during the same operation. Otol Neurotol 2002;23(2):169-180.

9. Gantz BJ,Turner CW. Combining acoustic and electrical hearing. Laryngoscope 2003;113(10):1726–1730.

14 Cochlear Implantation

14.B.

Cochlear implantation of prelingually deafened adults: Speech recognition outcomes

Pamela Roehm, Richard S. Tyler, Camille Dunn, and Bruce J. Gantz

METHODS

A computerized search of MEDLINE 1966–March 2004 was performed and supplemented with a PubMed search. The subject heading "cochlear implant" was exploded and the resulting articles limited to adults, yielding 199 studies. These articles were then reviewed to identify those that met the following inclusion criteria: 1) cochlear implantation with multichannel cochlear implants, 2) use of standardized tools to measure speech recognition outcomes, 3) follow-up period ≥3 months, 4) English language studies of English-speaking patients. Studies in which patients were age <18 years at cochlear implantation, age >3 at onset of severe–profound deafness, single-channel cochlear implant usage, non-English language studies, and studies performed before 1985 were excluded. Teoh et al. [1] have written a recent review that includes some of the studies excluded by our criteria. The bibliographies of the articles that met these inclusion criteria were manually checked to ensure no further relevant articles could be identified. This process yielded five articles [2–6].

RESULTS

Outcome Measures. Speech perception can be measured with many different standardized tools that record recognition of phonemes, words, and sentences in noisy or quiet environments. Delivery of these tests can be performed with visual cues (lip-reading) to provide additional assistance to the hard-of-hearing patient. The studies referenced in this review used published standardized tools to measure speech recognition.

The measurements used in this review consisted of Consonant-Nucleus-Consonant (CNC) words [7], Northwestern University Auditory Test No. 6 (NU-6) words [7], City University New York (CUNY) sentences [8], Hearing in Noise Test (HINT) sentences [9], and Central Institute of the Deaf (CID) sentences [10]. The CNC words consist of lists of 50 phonemically balanced words. The NU-6 is composed of four lists of 50 phonemically balanced CNC words. CUNY sentences are composed of 72 lists of 12 sentences of various lengths. HINT sentences are made of 25 lists of sentences. The score is based on identification of either key or all of the words

in the sentence. CID sentences include a total of 10 lists with 10 sentences. A total of 50 key words are contained in the sentences and the total percentage of key words correctly identified measures speech recognition.

Some subjects can perform at ceiling levels on sentence tests, especially in quiet. This ceiling effect can be partially controlled for by presenting the sentences in noise. Other subjects can have scores of 0, which also skews the data. Repeated testing can be skewed by learning the sentences, which can be prevented by the use of different sentence sets.

Potential Confounders. The degree of speech recognition after cochlear implantation is dependent on age at onset of deafness, age after implantation, and duration of cochlear implant use and technology (e.g., type of cochlear implant and speech processing used). Motivation is also a key factor in determining whether patients gain sufficient implant usage experience to make optimal benefits from their implants. Frequently these variables are not clearly denoted in these case studies. Possibly the most crucial of these is age at onset of deafness, which is frequently generalized in these reports as "prelingual" without being strictly defined.

Study Designs. All studies were retrospective (level 4 case series) with limited numbers of patients. Follow-up times extended from 4 to 36 months after implantation. The shorter follow-up times may be inadequate to reflect optimal benefits from cochlear implant usage.

Highest Level of Evidence. The highest level of evidence found was level 4. All were nonsequential patients. With the exception of the Waltzman 1992 study [4], all found the potential for some increase in open-set word and sentence understanding. These studies found performance was variable among individual patients, with 5/9 patients in the Schramm study showing no improvement [5]. Because of the type of studies that are available for review, substantial selection bias exists, making it difficult to generalize these results to all prelingually deafened adults.

Applicability. Based on inclusion/exclusion criteria for these series and selection of appropriate patients, these data would be applicable to patients implanted at ages ≥18 years with prelingual or congenital deafness.

Because of the difference in cochlear implants and processing strategy, differences in performance may be observed.

Morbidity/Complications. None reported.

CLINICAL SIGNIFICANCE AND FUTURE RESEARCH

There is limited level 4 evidence that cochlear implantation in prelingually deafened adults may yield limited benefits to open-set word and sentence recognition. However, this benefit is substantially less than that found in prelingually deafened children or postlingually deafened adults following cochlear implantation. Adult prelingually deafened patients undergoing cochlear implantation should be highly motivated and cautioned that their implants will not yield speech recognition equivalent to these other groups of cochlear implant recipients.

Future research on this topic ideally will be performed in a prospective manner and utilize standardized tools for speech recognition measurement. The most current technology for both the cochlear implant as well as speech processing should be used because these factors have shown great influence on speech recognition in other subsets of cochlear implant users. Additionally, a clear definition of what constitutes "prelingual" onset of deafness would be needed in a more rigorous study of this patient population. It would be difficult to design a randomized controlled trial (RCT) to explore this topic, because profoundly deaf patients seeking improved hearing would likely not agree to randomization to surgical intervention versus hearing aids. Additionally, the RCT format may not be the most appropriate for testing hearing benefits from cochlear implants in this setting. Instead, using patients' preoperative scores as their own controls and matching patients by preoperative hearing loss levels may be more appropriate.

THE EVIDENCE CONDENSED: Cochlear implant in prelingually deafened adults: Speech recognition outcomes before and after implantation

Reference	Waltzman, 2002	Waltzman, 1999	Waltzman, 1992
Level (design)	4 (case series)	4 (case series)	4 (case series)
Sample size*	14	2	3
OUTCOMES			
Outcome measure	CNC words, CUNY sentences, HINT sentences	NU-6 words, CID sentences (patient 1), CNC words, HINT sentences (patient 2)	AB phonemes, AB words, CID sentences
Preoperative speech recognition	Means: 4.8% CNC words, 21.8% CNC phonemes, 19.5% CUNY sentences in quiet, 6.5% CUNY in noise, 11.5% HINT	Subject 1: 0% NU-6, 6% CID sentences Subject 2: 6% CNC word test, 16% HINT sentences	9% AB phonemes, AB words and CID sentences not tested preoperatively with sound only; 70% CID sentences lip-reading plus aid
Postoperative speech recognition	At latest follow-up CNC words 12.5%, phonemes 30.2%; CUNY sentences in quiet 32.6%; CUNY sentences in noise 19.9%; HINT sentences 27.5%	Subject 1: 26% NU-6, 64% CID sentences Subject 2: 12% CNC words, 28% HINT sentences	15% AB phonemes, 9% AB words, 2% CID sentences with CI only, 60% CID sentences lip-reading plus CI
p Value	Not reported for adult patients	Statistical significance not reported	Statistical significance not reported
Conclusion	71% with 4%–46% improvement on open-set CNC words; 50% with improvement in CUNY and HINT sentence recognition from 2% to 98%	Some improvement in open-set word and sentence recognition for 2 patients	No statistically significant difference in preoperative testing and postoperative results
Follow-up time	6 mo (all), 12 mo (10 patients), 24 mo (5 patients), 36 mo (2 patients)	3 y (first patient), 3 mo (second patient)	4 mo, 1 y, 2 y
STUDY DESIGN			
Inclusion criteria	Profound congenital hearing loss, ≥18 y old at implantation	Deafness onset <3y old	Profound congenital or prelingual noncongenital hearing loss
Exclusion criteria	Not otherwise specified	Not otherwise specified	Not otherwise specified
Intervention regimen details	Clarion Multi-Strategy CI with CIS processing (3 patients); Nucleus CI24M with ACE (8), SPEAK (3), or CIS (1) processing	Clarion Multi-Strategy CI	Nucleus multichannel CI
Speech processing strategy	Results not stratified by implant type or processing strategy	Speech processing strategy not reported	Speech processing strategy not reported
Age	18–35 y	19 y, 20 y	19–28 y
Masking	None	None	None
Compliance	Not reported	Not reported	Not reported
Consecutive patients?	No	No	No
Morbidity/complications	Not reported	Not reported	Not reported

CNC = Consonant-Nucleus-Consonant, CUNY = City University New York, HINT = Hearing in Noise Test, CID = Central Institute of the Deaf, NU-6 = Northwestern University Auditory Test No. 6, CI = cochlear implant.
* Sample size excludes all patients <18 y old at cochlear implantation or >3 y old at onset of deafness that may have additionally been reported in these series.

THE EVIDENCE CONDENSED: Cochlear implant in prelingually deafened adults: Speech recognition outcomes before and after implantation

Reference	Schramm, 2002	Dawson, 1992
Level (design)	4 (case series)	4 (case series)
Sample size*	9	2
OUTCOMES		
Outcome measure	PBK or NU-6 words, CID sentences, PIPSL Questionnaire	MSTP, Picture Vocabulary test, NU-CHIPS, Segmental Speech Feature Test
Preoperative speech recognition	Words 0%–5%; open-set sentences 1%–23%	Not reported
Postoperative speech recognition	At 6 mo: for open-set words 4 patients improved up to 10%, 5 were unchanged or worse, for open-set words performance improved up to 30% in 4 subjects, 5 patients had no change or decreased scores. At 12 mo: for open-set words 4 patients improved up to 12%, 5 were unchanged or worse, for open-set sentence only 5 patients had scores and only 2/5 improved 5%–20% with 3/5 worse or the same	1 patient scored better on MSTP, Picture Vocabulary test, and vowel place and consonant manner. The other patient scored significantly higher on Segmental Speech Feature in vowel length and consonant place
p Value	Statistical significance not reported	Statistical significance not reported
Conclusion	Although some open-set scores can improve for patients with prelingual deafness, performance is variable	Although some open-set scores can improve, performance is variable
Follow-up time	6 mo, 12 mo	1 time point after 12 mo CI usage
STUDY DESIGN		
Inclusion criteria	≥12 y old at implantation, "prelinguistic deafness," oral English as primary communication mode, auditory-oral or auditory-verbal training during school	>12 mo experience with CI
Exclusion criteria	Not otherwise specified	Not otherwise specified
Intervention regimen details	Nucleus-22 (5 patients), Nucleus-24 (7 patients), Clarion S-series (3 patients)	Nucleus-22 in CG mode
Speech processing strategy	Speech processing program not denoted	
Potential confounders	"Prelinguistic deafness" not clearly defined	One patient only used 15 of 22 electrodes because of short-circuit in the electrode array
Age	20–49 y	19 y, 20 y
Masking	None	None
Compliance	Not reported	Not reported
Consecutive patients?	No	No
Morbidity/complications	Not reported	Not reported

CID = Central Institute of the Deaf, NU-6 = Northwestern University Auditory Test No. 6, CI = cochlear implant.
* Sample size excludes all patients <18 y old at cochlear implantation or >3 y old at onset of deafness that may have additionally been reported in these series.

REFERENCES

1. Teoh SW, Pisoni DB, Miyamoto RT. Cochlear Implantation in adults with prelingual deafness. Laryngoscope 2004;114(9):1536–1540.
2. Waltzman SB, Roland JT, Cohen NL. Delayed implantation in congenitally deaf children and adults. Otol Neurotol 2002;23:333–340.
3. Waltzman SB, Cohen NL. Implantation of patients with prelingual long-term deafness. Ann Otol Rhinol Laryngol 1999;108:84–97.
4. Waltzman SB, Cohen NL, Shapiro WH. Use of a multi-channel cochlear implant in the congenitally and prelingually deaf population. Laryngoscope 1992;102:395–399.
5. Schramm D, Fitzpatrick E, Seguin C. Cochlear implantation for adolescents and adults with prelinguistic deafness. Otol Neurotol 2002;23:698–703.
6. Dawson PW, Balmey PJ, Rowland LC, et al. Cochlear implants in children, adolescents, and prelinguistically deafened adults: speech perception. J Speech Hear Res 1992;35: 401–417.
7. Tillman TW, Carhart R. An expanded test for speech discrimination utilizing CNC monosyllabic words, in Northwestern University Auditory Test No. 6 Technical Report No. SAM-TR-66-55. 1966, USAF School of Aerospace Medicine: Brooks Air Force Base, Texas.
8. Boothroyd A, Hanin L, Hnath T. A sentence test of speech perception: reliability, set equivalence, and short-term learning. 1985, New York: Speech and Hearing Sciences Research Center, City University of New York.
9. Nilsson M, Sullivan JA, et al. Development of the hearing in noise test for the measurement of speech reception thresholds in quiet and in noise. J Acoust Soc Am 1994;95(2):1085–1099.
10. Silverman SRH, et al. Problems related to the use of speech in clinical audiometry. Ann Otol Rhinol Laryngol 1955;64(4):1234–1244.

14 Cochlear Implantation

14.C.

Implantation of adults: Impact on quality of life

Steven Hemmerdinger and Susan Waltzman

METHODS

A computerized PubMed search of MEDLINE 1966–April 2005 was performed. The terms "cochlear implant" and "quality of life" were exploded and then combined. Articles were identified that met the following inclusion criteria: 1) patients >18 years old, 2) intervention with cochlear implantation versus no surgery, 3) outcome measured in terms of quality of life (QOL) or health utility. Studies in which there was no control/nonimplanted group and those prior to 1995 were excluded. The bibliographies of the articles that met these inclusion criteria were manually checked to ensure no further relevant articles could be identified. This process yielded five articles [1–5].

RESULTS

Outcome Measures. Typically, QOL is measured with various questionnaires. Three studies utilized a health utility index (HUI), which is a health-state assessment that includes several domains, including sensation (hearing and vision), mobility, emotion, cognition, self-care, pain, and speech [1–3]. The HUI scale is from 0 (death) to 1.0 (perfect health). The Patient Quality of Life Form, Index Relative Questionnaire Form (IRQF), and Nijmegen Cochlear Implantation Questionnaire are all disease-specific validated instruments regarding an individual's experience as a hearing-impaired person. The IRQF is filled out by the subject's relative [3–5]. The former two are scaled from 1 to 5 (optimal), the latter from 1 to 100 (optimal). The global QOL instrument employed is the Short Form 36, with scores ranging from 1 to 100 (optimal) [4]. Finally, the Hopkins Symptom Check List measures depression and anxiety symptoms ranging from 1 to 4 (most bothered) [4].

Potential Confounders. Overall QOL and how it relates to hearing loss and its treatment can be impacted by many factors such as age, residual hearing, duration of hearing loss, and length of implant or hearing aid (HA) use. These studies uniformly compared the implanted and control groups and, in general, subjects were not significantly different before implantation. In one study, the implant group's mean age was older and they were significantly more likely to be more than 64 years old [1]. Only one study mentioned the duration of HA use in the control group, which was significantly greater than the duration of implant use in the study group [5]. In the same study, 85% of control subjects used bilateral HAs, whereas only 14% of implanted patients used a contralateral HA [5]. This study was also influenced by a high nonresponder rate among controls and lack of HA use in 21%. However, these differences would all seem to underestimate the QOL impact of cochlear implants relative to HAs. One study noted an association between QOL benefit and younger age both at intervention and at study enrollment across both groups [5]. The same study evaluated for associations between duration of deafness or time since intervention and QOL benefit from implantation and found none [5]. Two studies that measured cost per quality-adjusted life-year (QALY) used different values for life expectancy. Because cost per QALY is dependent on length of implant use, both life expectancy and age at implantation are major factors in its calculation [1, 2].

Study Designs. One study was a level 2 prospective controlled study with a follow-up time of 12 months [1]. The other four studies were level 3 retrospective or cross-sectional controlled studies, with the longest mean implant use being 6.3 years. All except one study compared the implant subjects' QOL results to those of the control/nonimplanted group. This exception compared postoperative versus preoperative QOL within implanted subjects [3]. There were no significant differences between the control group QOL scores and the implant subjects' preoperative QOL scores. However, the final results may have been less significant if the implanted subjects' postoperative QOL was compared directly with the control group. The two studies that analyzed preimplant QOL retrospectively are subject to recall bias [3, 5].

Highest Level of Evidence. Although these studies used various instruments to ascertain QOL in persons with a cochlear implant compared with nonimplanted hearing-impaired subjects, each concluded that overall QOL and/or specific domains were significantly improved by cochlear implantation. With the use of HUI, the evidence reveals a significantly better health state among implant recipients and cost-utility analyses suggest that implantation is at least as cost-effective as many common interventions considered to be worthwhile based on their reduction of morbidity and mortality [1, 2].

Applicability. This data can be applied to multichannel cochlear implant recipients 18 years of age and older.

Morbidity/Complications. Only one study addressed complications of cochlear implantation, with six and nine patients reporting one or more minor complications at 6 and 12 months after surgery, respectively [1].

CLINICAL SIGNIFICANCE AND FUTURE RESEARCH

QOL is an important outcome measure in the evaluation of cochlear implantation, because its effect is not produced by preventing disease or mortality as are other common interventions. These studies document the QOL impact provided by implantation. This effect is most pronounced on measures of speech and hearing as well as the more general categories of social functioning, emotion, and mental health. Results such as these, along with the cost-utility analyses presented, show that the impact of cochlear implantation is comparable to hemodialysis, cardiac surgery, and knee replacement surgery (cost/QALY of $86,198, $64,033, and $49,700, respectively) [2].

Numerous studies have documented the audiologic improvements that are seen after cochlear implantation. These are sure to improve with advancements in implants and speech processing strategies. If an association exists between hearing test results and QOL after implantation, future implant recipients could have greater QOL benefits.

A randomized cochlear implant study is unlikely to be undertaken so more prospective studies comparing implant recipients to other hearing-impaired individuals are needed. Ideally, all subjects will have at least 10 years of postimplant follow-up. As the criteria for implantation expand, QOL benefits can be measured according to residual hearing levels. In addition, the impact of bilateral implantation and pediatric implantation on QOL should be studied. Finally, the potential socioeconomic impact of implanted patients entering the workforce and mainstream schools, as well as having an improved lifetime earning potential, should be analyzed.

THE EVIDENCE CONDENSED: Adult cochlear implantation and its impact on quality of life

Reference	Palmer, 1999	Wyatt, 1996	Krabbe, 2000
Level (design)	2 (PCT)	3 (CSCS)	3 (RCS)
Sample size*	Implant 46 (62), control 16 (22)	Implant 229 (301), control 32 (38)	Implant 45 (46), control 46 (53)

OUTCOMES			
QOL measures	HUI at enrollment, 6 mo, 12 mo	Ontario HUI Mark III	NCIQ, SF-36, HUI Mark II
Implanted subjects	Preop 0.58 6 mo: 0.76 12 mo: 0.78	0.793	NCIQ (total) Post-CI: 68.5
Control	Enrollment 0.58 6 mo: 0.57 12 mo: 0.58	0.589	Pre-CI: 36.8 Control: 38.8
p Value	Preop NS 6 mo <0.001 12 mo <0.01	<0.0001	Post- vs pre-CI <0.001
Additional measures/ subdomain analysis	Preop: mobility 6 mo: hearing, sensation 12 mo: hearing, sensation, speech	Hearing: p < 0.001 Speech: p < 0.001 Vision: p = 0.026 Emotion: p = 0.003 Cognition: p = 0.017	HUI post- vs pre-CI Diff. 0.28, p < 0.001 SF-36 post vs pre Vitality, pain NS All others p < 0.01
Audiologic performance and correlation with QOL	Significant improvements in speech recognition at 6 mo, 12 mo (no correlations made)	Not reported	Not reported
Cost-utility analysis	Cost per QALY $14,670	Cost per QALY $15,928	Not reported
Conclusion	Implants significantly improved ratings of health utility within 6 mo of surgery	Implants improved ratings of health utility. Cost compares favorably with other widely accepted interventions	Implants led to a significant improvement in health-related QOL
Follow-up time	12 mo	N/A	N/A

STUDY DESIGN			
Inclusion criteria	>18 y old with postlingual deafness, speech discrim. <30%	Nucleus 22-channel CI	Adult subjects who received a CI from 1989 to 1997
Exclusion criteria	Not implanted with Nucleus 22-channel device	Not reported	Prelingual deafness, single-channel implant
Surgical group	CI	CI	CI
Control	Implant candidates	Candidates awaiting surgery	CI candidates Not used in statistical analysis
Potential confounders	Subjects >65 y, assumed LE 78 y	Assumed LE 80 y	Subjects acted as own controls, recall bias
Age	18 y or older (CI mean 56 y, control mean 49 y)	CI mean 57 y, control mean 55 y	CI mean 50 y, control mean 51 y
Implant use†	6 mo, 12 mo	4.6 y	5 y
Morbidity/complications of surgery	6 mo: 2 wound infection, 5 vertigo, 2 tinnitus 12 mo: 1 facial nerve stimulation, others not reported	Not reported	Not reported

PCT = prospective controlled trial, RCS = retrospective controlled study, CSCS = cross-sectional controlled study, QOL = quality of life, QALY = quality-adjusted life-year, HUI = health utility index, NCIQ = Nijmegen Cochlear Implantation Questionnaire, PQLF = Patient Quality of Life Form, IRQF = Index Relative Questionnaire Form, SF-36 = Short-Form 36, HSCL-25 = Hopkins Symptom Check List, CI = cochlear implant, HA = hearing aid, preop = preoperative, HL = hearing loss, N/A = not applicable, NS = not significant, PIPSL = Performance Inventory for Profound and Severe Loss, LE = life expectancy, discrim = discrimination, Diff. = difference.

Mo et al.: non-CI A subjects met criteria for implantation but awaiting surgery, non-CI B subjects did not meet implant criteria.

HUI domains: vision, mobility, emotion, cognition, self-care, pain, speech, hearing.

NCIQ domains: basic sound perception, advanced sound perception, speech production, self-esteem, activity, social interaction.

SF-36 domains: mental health, vitality, pain, physical functioning, general health, social functioning, role functioning (physical/emotional).

* Sample size: numbers shown for those completing study and (initially recruited).

† Implant use: mean use (range, if reported).

Reference	Mo, 2004	Cohen, 2004
Level (design)	3 (CSCS)	3 (RCS)
Sample size*	Implant 84 (93), control 95 (125)	Implant 24 (27), control 27 (49)

OUTCOMES		
QOL measures	PQLF, IRQF, SF-36, HSCL-25	NCIQ, before HA/CI, and at enrollment
Implanted subjects	PQLF (total) 3.53	QOL benefit score 23.6
Control	A 3.37, B 3.28**, HA 3.57	QOL benefit score 12.0
p Value	A NS (0.11), B 0.05**, HA NS	0.082 (NS)
Additional measures/ subdomain analysis	SF-36 general health CI vs controls: NS HSCL-25 CI vs non-CI A: p = 0.01	Basic sound perception p < 0.001
Audiologic performance and correlation with QOL	PQLF correlates with social hearing ability (PIPSL), p < 0.001, not speech recognition	QOL benefit correlates with speech recognition improvement, p = 0.03
Cost-utility analysis	N/A	N/A
Conclusion	Variable disease-specific QOL benefit with CI. Better QOL associated with younger age, less anxiety/depression, better PIPSL score	Trend of greater overall QOL benefit in CI users vs HA users, significant improvement in basic sound perception
Follow-up time	N/A	N/A

STUDY DESIGN		
Inclusion criteria	Multichannel CI recipients	HA/CI use >12 mo, use began >50 y of age
Exclusion criteria	Psychiatric disease, implant not used	No mailing address
Surgical Group	CI	CI
Control	HA: n = 60, mean 56 y Non-CI (A = 9/B = 16)** Mean 50.7 y	HA users Mean use: 120 mo
Potential confounders	No significant confounders	Length HA/CI used, binaural aid rate, recall bias
Age	18 y or older, mean 54 y (3 were <18 y at implantation)	CI mean 67.2 y, HA mean 77.1 y, difference NS
Implant use†	6.3 y (8 mo–14.5 y)	53 mo (12–156)
Morbidity/complications of surgery	Not reported	Not reported

PCT = prospective controlled trial, RCS = retrospective controlled study, CSCS = cross-sectional controlled study, QOL = quality of life, QALY = quality-adjusted life-year, HUI = health utility index, NCIQ = Nijmegen Cochlear Implantation Questionnaire, PQLF = Patient Quality of Life Form, IRQF = Index Relative Questionnaire Form, SF-36 = Short-Form 36, HSCL-25 = Hopkins Symptom Check List,
CI = cochlear implant, HA = hearing aid, preop = preoperative, HL = hearing loss, N/A = not applicable, NS = not significant, PIPSL = Performance Inventory for Profound and Severe Loss, LE = life expectancy.
**Mo et al.: non-CI A subjects met criteria for implantation but awaiting surgery, non-CI B subjects did not meet implant criteria.
HUI domains: vision, mobility, emotion, cognition, self-care, pain, speech, hearing.
NCIQ domains: basic sound perception, advanced sound perception, speech production, self-esteem, activity, social interaction.
SF-36 domains: mental health, vitality, pain, physical functioning, general health, social functioning, role functioning (physical/emotional).
* Sample size: numbers shown for those completing study and (initially recruited).
† Implant use: mean use (range, if reported).

REFERENCES

1. Palmer CS, Niparko JK, Wyatt JR, Rothman M, de Lissovoy G. A prospective study of the cost-utility of the multichannel cochlear implant. Arch Otolaryngol Head Neck Surg 1999;125:1221–1228.
2. Wyatt JR, Niparko JK, Rothman M, de Lissovoy G. Cost utility of the multichannel cochlear implant in 258 profoundly deaf individuals. Laryngoscope 1996;106(7):816–821.
3. Krabbe PFM, Hinderink JB, van den Broek P. The effect of cochlear implant use in postlingually deaf adults. Int J Technol Assess Health Care 2000;16(3):864–873.
4. Mo B, Harris S, Lindbaek M. Cochlear implants and health status: a comparison with other hearing-impaired patients. Ann Otol Rhinol Laryngol 2004;113:914–921.
5. Cohen SM, Labadie RF, Dietrich MS, Haynes DS. Quality of life in hearing-impaired adults: the role of cochlear implants and hearing aids. Otolaryngol Head Neck Surg 2004;131(4):413–422.

14 Cochlear Implantation

14.D.

Implantation of older adults: Speech recognition outcomes

Rita M. Roure and J. Thomas Roland

METHODS

A computerized PubMed search of MEDLINE 1966–March 2005 was performed. First, articles that mapped to the exploded medical subject headings "cochlear implantation" or "cochlear implants" or the text words "cochlear implantation" or "cochlear implant" were combined to create one group. Second, the keywords "elderly" and "older" were exploded and combined to create a second group. Third, articles mapping to the exploded medical subject headings "audiometry" and "treatment outcome" were combined with those mapping to the textword "speech." These three groups were cross-referenced, and articles mapping to the subject headings "infant" and "child" were excluded, yielding 23 articles. These articles were then reviewed to identify those that met the following inclusion criteria: 1) patient population 65 years and older with postlingual deafness, 2) intervention with cochlear implantation, and 3) outcome measured in terms of preoperative and postoperative audiologic testing. The bibliographies of the articles that met these inclusion/exclusion criteria were manually checked to ensure no further relevant articles could be identified. This process yielded five articles [1–5].

RESULTS

Outcome Measures. Speech recognition was measured with various speech perception measures using monosyllabic words (Northwestern University Test No. 6) or sentence recognition (Center for the Institute of the Deaf Sentences). In addition, the Consonant-Nucleus-Consonant, Word Recognition Scores, and Hearing in Noise Test were used. Elderly patients were defined as >65 years old, with the exception of one study [1] which defined elderly as >70 years old. Although audiologic testing varied from one study to another (see chart), they all compared preoperative aided audiologic testing to results after cochlear implantation. All of the studies except one [5] compared the postoperative audiologic testing results of the elderly group with a control study of adult patients <65 years old.

Potential Confounders. Different audiologic testing techniques and cochlear implants used by each study may alter results and make comparison difficult. Also,

one study [4] noted that patients were divided by their age at the time of the study, which resulted in a lower mean age at time of surgery when compared with other studies. The time period between surgical implantation and audiologic testing (used for comparison) ranged between 6 months and 2 years which could also potentially alter results. Furthermore, the difference in mean duration of deafness between the elderly and control groups could also affect results and was not fully reported by the Chatelin group [1].

Study Designs. All of these studies were retrospective chart reviews. One study [4] matched the control group (<60 years old) based on years of profound sensorineural hearing loss and implant coding strategy to control for the disparity between these two groups. They also defined the age as 65 years at the time of the study, whereas the others defined the age at the time of surgery. All of the other studies, except Waltzman, compared the elderly group to other adults <65 years old who had received cochlear implantation in that same time period.

Highest Level of Evidence. All five studies were designed to determine the benefits of cochlear implants in the elderly population (adults >65 years old). The oldest study [5] demonstrated that there is a statistically significant improvement in hearing after cochlear implantation in the elderly. The other more recent studies went further and compared the postoperative audiologic improvement in the elderly to that of younger adult patients receiving cochlear implantation. Yet, two studies [1, 2] did not perform statistics comparing the preoperative audiologic results to the postoperative audiologic results in the elderly. All four studies except one [1] arrived at the same conclusion: there is no significant difference in the postoperative improvement in hearing for the elderly after cochlear implantation when compared with patients <65 years old. Chatelin, however, noted that even though the elderly received significant auditory improvement postoperatively, they did not perform as well as the younger patients in all three measurements tested in this study (see table).

Applicability. Based on the inclusion/exclusion criteria for these trials, these results can be applied to adults >65 years old with postlingual profound sensorineural hearing loss.

Morbidity/Complications. The reported surgical morbidity was very low in all of these studies, as further detailed in the adjoining table. No adverse vestibular outcomes were reported.

CLINICAL SIGNIFICANCE AND FUTURE RESEARCH

There are multiple retrospective chart reviews demonstrating the benefits of cochlear implantation in the elderly population. Even though they have the inherent biases of retrospective studies, the standardized nature of the audiologic testing contributes to the validity of the results. These studies demonstrate the strong potential for benefit from cochlear implantation in the elderly population with profound sensorineural hearing loss.

As cochlear implantation technology improves, we look forward to further evaluation of evolving techniques for the implantation of patients with the high-frequency hearing loss so commonly seen in older patients. Data regarding hybrid cochlear implants which preserve residual low-frequency hearing in individuals with poor word understanding is currently emerging. Data regarding the resulting audiometric outcomes, quality of life, and associated complications with this newer technology will determine how widespread hybrid implants become.

Reference	Chatelin, 2004		Pasanisi, 2002	
Level (design)	3 (retrospective controlled)		3 (retrospective controlled)	
Sample size*	65 (study) 101 (control) (166)		30 (34)	
OUTCOMES				
	Pre-CI	Post-CI	Pre-CI	Post-CI
Elderly Word and sentence recognition	CNC 9% CID 17% HINT 18%	36% 62% 62%	WRS 0% Sentences 0%	72.5% 72.5%
Younger Word and sentence recognition	CNC 4% CID 17% HINT 11%	45% 78% 79%	WRS 0% Sentences 0%	82% 65.7%
p Value for pre- vs post-CI in elderly patients	Not reported		Not reported	
p Value for elderly vs younger patients post-CI	CNC—p = 0.03 HINT—p = 0.07 CNC—p = 0.07		WRS—p = 0.160 Sentences—p = 0.098	
Conclusion	Marked improvement in auditory performance post-CI in elderly subjects, but less performance enhancement in CNC words when compared with younger patients		Significant open-set speech recognition benefits from cochlear implantation in elderly patients. No significant difference between the elderly and younger adults	
Follow-up time	1 y		1 y	
STUDY DESIGN				
Inclusion criteria	>70 y old who underwent cochlear implantation and random selection of patients <70 y old who underwent cochlear implantation in the same time period, preoperative and postoperative audiologic testing available		>41 y old, full insertion of all active electrodes, a duration of deafness of <36 mo, a nucleus multichannel cochlear implant programmed with speak coding strategy, and at least 1-y follow-up. All were postlingually deaf.	
Exclusion criteria	Not reported		Not reported	
Audiologic testing details	All subjects underwent standardized open-set speech recognition testing before implantation (aided) and at 3, 6, and 12 mo postoperatively		Results of word and everyday sentence recognition tests were obtained preoperatively and at 1 y postoperatively. The speech materials were presented in hearing-only conditions	
Device type	Clarion or Nucleus device		Nucleus CI 22M, CI 24M devices	
Duration of deafness	Mean duration of deafness Elderly—6 y Young—not specified		Mean duration of deafness Elderly—21.4 mo Young—22.7 mo	
Age	70–91 y—study group (mean 76) 24–69 y—control group (mean 48)		65–74 y—study group (mean 66.8) 41–59 y—control group (mean 51.2)	
Morbidity/complications	Study group—6 patients complained of taste alteration Control—1 incomplete placement of electrodes, 1 hematoma/wound infection		None	

CI = cochlear implant, RCR = retrospective chart review, CNC = Consonant-Nucleus-Consonant words, CID = Central Institute for the Deaf sentences, HINT = Hearing in Noise Test, WRS = word recognition scores.
* Sample size: numbers shown for those not lost to follow-up and those (initially recruited).

Reference	Labadie, 2000
Level (design)	3 (retrospective controlled)
Sample size*	16 (study), 20 (control), 36

OUTCOMES

	Pre-CI	Post-CI
Elderly Word and sentence recognition	CNC 6% CID 21%	30% 70%
Younger Word and sentence recognition	CNC 2% CID 22%	36% 70%
p Value for pre- vs post-CI in elderly patients	Elderly patients $p < 0.001$ (Younger patients $p < 0.005$)	
p Value for elderly vs younger patients post-CI	Two age groups—$p > 0.05$ Improvement in both age groups—$p > 0.05$	
Conclusion	Highly significant improvement in audiologic performance in both age groups. No significant differences in post-CI performance between the age groups	
Follow-up time	6 mo	

STUDY DESIGN

Inclusion criteria	>18 y old who underwent cochlear implantation at their institution for postlingual deafness and who underwent both preoperative and postoperative audiologic testing
Exclusion criteria	Prelingual deafness
Audiologic testing details	All subjects underwent standardized open-set speech recognition testing before implantation (aided) and at 3 and 6 mo postoperatively
Device type	Clarion cochlear implant device
Duration of deafness	Mean duration of deafness Elderly—12.5 y Young—9.6 y
Age	>65 y—study group (71.5) 18–64 y—control groups (46.9)
Morbidity/complications	Study group—1 transient facial paralysis Control—none

CI = cochlear implant, RCR = retrospective chart review, CNC = Consonant-Nucleus-Consonant words, CID = Central Institute for the Deaf sentences, HINT = Hearing in Noise Test, WRS = word recognition scores.
* Sample size: numbers shown for those not lost to follow-up and those (initially recruited).

Reference	Kelsall, 1995		Waltzman, 1993	
Level (design)	3 (retrospective controlled)		3 (retrospective controlled)	
Sample size*	28		20	
OUTCOMES				
	Pre-CI	Post-CI	Pre-CI	Post-CI
Elderly Word and sentence recognition	NU-6 Word 0.65% NU-6 Phoneme 4.6% CID 1.5%	15.3% 32.4% 45.6%	4-choice spondee 31.1% NU-6 0% CID 0.25%	66.3% 10.3% 20.8%
Younger Word and sentence recognition	NU-6 Word NU-6 Phoneme CID	19.2% 40.9% 46.5%	None	None–but in the Discussion section they noted that only 45% of the elderly patients received >10% on both the NU-6 and CID sentence test in comparison to 65% of the younger adults that achieve this degree of benefit
p Value for elderly pre- vs post-CI	p = 0.0001		p = 0.001–0.002	
p Value elderly vs younger patients post-CI	p = 0.288–0.896		Not reported	
Conclusion	Elderly recipients of cochlear implants perform comparably on audiologic testing to other adult patients.		The geriatric population with bilateral profound SNHL obtains significant benefit from cochlear implantation.	
Follow-up time	1 y		1 y	
STUDY DESIGN				
Inclusion criteria	>65 y old who underwent cochlear implantation and patients <60 y old who were matched based on years of profound SNHL and implant coding strategy		>65 y old who underwent cochlear implantation with pre/postoperative audiologic testing	
Exclusion criteria	Not reported		Not reported	
Audiologic testing details	Results of pre- and postoperative audiologic testing. They tested using the best aided condition preoperatively and with the cochlear implant postoperatively		All patients underwent audiologic as well as standard pure tone audiometry preoperatively (aided) and postoperatively at 3 mo and 1 y	
Device type	Nucleus 22-channel device		Nucleus 22-channel device	
Duration of deafness	Mean duration of deafness Elderly—13.6 y Control—15.4 y		Mean duration of deafness Elderly—25.3 y	
Age	Study group—65–82 y (mean 68 y at implantation) Control group—23–59 y		65–85 y (mean 70.9 y)	
Morbidity/complications	Study group—1 patient developed flap necrosis and another a wound infection		One patient had partial insertion (15 electrodes)	

RCR = Retrospective chart review, NU-6 = Northwestern University Test No. 6, CID = Central Institute for the Deaf, SNHL = sensorineural hearing loss.
* Sample size: numbers shown for those not lost to follow-up and those (initially recruited).

REFERENCES

1. Chatelin V, Kim EJ, Driscoll C, Larky J, Polite C, Lalwani AK. Cochlear implant outcomes in the elderly. Otol Neurotol 2004;25(3):298–301.
2. Pasanisi E, Bacciu A, Vincenti V, et al. Speech recognition in elderly cochlear implant recipients. Clin Otolaryngol Allied Sci 2003;28(2):154–157.
3. Labadie RF, Carrasco VN, Gilmer CH, Pilsbury HC III. Cochlear implant performance in senior citizens. Otolaryngol Head Neck Surg 2000;123(4):419–423.
4. Kelsall DC, Shallop JK, Burnelli T. Cochlear implantation in the elderly. Am J Otol 1995;16(5):609–615.
5. Waltzman SB, Cohen NL, Shapiro WH. The benefits of cochlear implantation in the geriatric population. Otolaryngol Head Neck Surg 1993;108(4):329–333.

14 Cochlear Implantation

Post-implant surgical-site infection: Management with antibiotics, nonexplant surgery, or explantation

Rita M. Roure and J. Thomas Roland

METHODS

A computerized PubMed search of MEDLINE 1966–March 2005 was performed. Articles mapping to the medical subject headings "cochlear implants" or "cochlear implantation" were exploded and combined. These combined articles were then cross-referenced with those obtained by exploding the medical subject headings "central nervous system infections" or "infection" as well as those mapping to the textword "wound infection." This search strategy resulted in 168 publications. The titles, abstracts, and bibliographies of these publications were then reviewed to identify those that met the following inclusion criteria: 1) children and/or adults undergoing cochlear implantation with postoperative surgical-site infection (minor or major), 2) treatment with conservative (i.e., nonsurgical) and/or with surgical treatment (i.e., local surgery or explantation), and 3) outcomes measured in terms of avoidance of explantation. Publications were excluded if the treatment method for the post-implant infections was not specified. The bibliographies of the articles that met these inclusion criteria were manually checked to ensure no further relevant articles could be identified. This process yielded nine articles regarding localized wound infection, which are reviewed here [1–9]. There were also 9 publications regarding meningitis, and these data are shown in the subsequent review.

RESULTS

Outcome Measures. Post-implant surgical-site infections included local wound infections, complicated otitis media, abscess, and meningitis. Cunningham et al. [3] further characterized infections as major and minor. Major infections were identified as those which resulted in device explantation, surgical wound revision, hospitalization, intravenous antibiotics, or meningitis. Minor complications were identified as those requiring local wound care and/or oral antibiotics.

Potential Confounders. The use of perioperative antibiotics, the time of wound surveillance and follow-up, the threshold for diagnosing local infection, the type of implant (especially the presence of external pedestal), and the immune status of the implanted hosts could all influence the study results. The status of these confounders varied among studies. For example, patients in the Cunningham study [3] did not receive perioperative antibiotics, but those in the Bhatia report [1] received 24 hours of perioperative antibiotics. Yu et al. [2] reported that two of the four patients with a major postoperative infection had an underlying primary immunodeficiency and one of these two patients required the only explantation in this study. The other studies did not specify any potential impact of their patients' immune status.

Study Designs. All nine studies regarding post-implant surgical-site infection were retrospective studies. None of these studies were controlled. Three of the nine studies either entirely or partially focused specifically on post-implant infections, and therefore provided substantial related data on their patients. The remaining six studies focused on post-implant complications in general; because these studies provided little or no infection-related patient characteristics, these six studies are described in the adjacent tables in an abbreviated form. All except one of these studies were retrospective chart reviews (level 4). The exception was a survey of surgeons which, after consultation with the Center for Evidence Based Medicine (the source for levels of evidence), was also rated as a level 4 study. Follow-up times were often not reported, but were >1 year in some instances. The specific timing relative to implantation within these follow-up periods was not clearly specified.

Highest Level of Evidence. Rates of post-implant surgical-site infection ranged from 1% to 12%. Within infected patients, three potential management options were described. First, data from these studies suggested that a wide range (0%–83%) of post-implant infection responded to treatment with oral or intravenous antibiotics alone. Second, the percent of patients requiring surgery without explantation ranged from 0% to 75%. These local surgeries included abscess drainage and local flap and pedestal revisions. Third, explantation rates ranged from 3% to 45%. It was not always entirely clearly specified that patients were explanted only after conservative measures failed (rather than as an initial treatment), but such a stepwise approach was described in several publications. The majority of studies did not elucidate what risk factors increased the chance of post-implant infection and eventual explantation of the implant, but Cunningham et al. [3] noted an increased risk of explantation if the device was exposed.

Applicability. These studies included patients of all ages who underwent cochlear implantation.

Morbidity/Complications. There were no reported adverse effects of antibiotics or surgical interventions performed during these studies. Bhatia et al. [1] noted one episode of facial nerve palsy with a suppurative acute otitis media. Both problems resolved with oral antibiotics.

CLINICAL SIGNIFICANCE AND FUTURE RESULTS

These nine level 4 studies suggest that 55%–97% of patients with post-implant surgical-site infection can avoid explantation. Other successful management options include oral or intravenous antibiotics or more minor surgical intervention. Thus, it seems reasonable to attempt conservative antibiotic treatment and more minor surgery before explantation, despite some infectious disease tenets that would favor removal of any infected foreign-body implants.

This topic would prove difficult to investigate with a higher-level study. Statistically meaningful studies comparing explantation and antibiotic therapy are difficult because of the small percentage of patients with postoperative infections. Retrospective data are therefore likely to continue to be the best evidence available in the near future. Future studies may focus on identifying correlations which may help determine which patients are most likely to respond to antibiotics alone, as well as which situations require intravenous instead of oral antibiotic therapy as an initial treatment.

THE EVIDENCE CONDENSED: Post-implant infection management

Reference	Bhatia, 2004	Yu, 2001	Cunningham, 2004
Level (design)	4 (retrospective review)	4 (retrospective review)	4 (retrospective review)
Sample size	300	241	733
OUTCOMES			
Total % with post-CI infection	4% (n = 12/300)	1.7% (n = 4/241)	4.1% (n = 30/733) 5.9% pediatrics (n = 16/272) 3.0% adults (n = 14/462)
% of total responding to antibiotic alone	83% (n = 10/12)	0 (n = 0/4)	26.7% (n = 8/30) oral antibiotics 13.3% (n = 4/30) intravenous antibiotics
% of total requiring nonexplant surgery	0 (n = 0/12)	75% (n = 3/4) Incision and drainage of abscess	23.3% (n = 7/30) Surgical wound revision
% of total explanted because of infection	17% (n = 2/12)	25% (n = 1/4)	36.7% (n = 11/30)
p Value	Not applicable	Not applicable	Not applicable
Conclusion	The majority of patients responded to antibiotics alone	The majority of patients required surgery but avoided explantation	More than one-third of infections were treated with explantation
Follow-up time	4 y	Not reported	43 mo
STUDY DESIGN			
Inclusion criteria	Children (0–8 y old) that had been implanted by the authors consecutively including reimplantations and referrals	Adults who underwent implantation between 1991–2000 at UCSF and 1997–2000 at University of Iowa	All patients undergoing cochlear implant surgery between January 1993 and October 2002
Exclusion criteria	Reimplantations and referrals from other programs. Age >8 y	None given	Use of perioperative antibiotics (started at this institution in October 2002)
Prophylactic perioperative antibiotics	Cephradine—1 dose at induction and 2 further doses within 24 h	Not reported	No subjects received perioperative antibiotics
Post-implant infection details	Discharging wound infection (n = 2) Acute otitis media with eardrum perforation (n = 2) Suppurative otitis media (n = 1) Flap infection (n = 7)	Mastoid abscess (n = 4)	Wound infections (n = 26) With device exposure (n = 9/26) Complicated acute otitis media (n = 4)
Immunologic status of subjects	None	Two patients with post-implant abscesses were diagnosed with immunodeficiency.	None
Age	5.1 y (0–8 y)	Adult and pediatric patients	271 patients (<18 y) 462 patients (>18 y)
Additional potential confounders	One of the patients that was explanted had a complicated intraoperative course that required a canal wall down procedure	Immunodeficient patients included	Exclusion of patients that received perioperative antibiotics
Morbidity	Facial nerve palsy was associated with infection	Not reported	Not reported

UCSF = University of California at San Francisco, CI = cochlear implant.

THE EVIDENCE CONDENSED: Post-implant infection management

Reference	Hoffman, 1995	Webb, 1991	Cohen, 1988
Level (design)	4 (retrospective review)	4 (retrospective review)	4 (survey of surgeon recollection)
Sample size	3064 adults 1905 children	253	107 questionnaires returned from 108 surgeons [152 questionnaires sent to 115 surgeons (37 were duplicates/non-implant surgeons)]
OUTCOMES			
Total % with post-CI infection	1.2% (n = 37/3064) adults 0.73% (n = 14/1905) children	4.3% (n = 11/253)	5.5% (n = 25/459) flap/scalp problems reported as a broad category, including local infections
% of total responding to nonsurgical treatment	% responding to outpatient treatment: 32.4% (n = 12/37) adults 42.9% (n = 6/14) children % responding to intravenous antibiotics: 8.1% (n = 3/37) adults 28.6% (n = 4/14) children	54.5% (n = 6/11) "uncomplicated" wound infections, not otherwise specified	Not reported
% of total requiring nonexplant surgery	13.5% (n = 5/37) adults 14.3% (n = 2/14) children	27.3% (n = 3/11) "severe but controlled" wound infections, not otherwise specified	64% (n = 16/25) "local treatment of flap problem"
% of total explanted because of infection	45.9% (n = 17/37) adults 14.3% (n = 2/14) children	18.2% (n = 2/11)	3% (n = 9/25) "scalp breakdown, removal of implant"
p Value	Not applicable	Not applicable	Not applicable
Conclusion	The majority of patients did not require explantation	The majority of patients had uncomplicated wound infections	The majority of patients had local treatment of flap problems
Follow-up time	Not specified	Not specified	Not specified
STUDY DESIGN			
Inclusion criteria	Data were provided by implant device manufacturers	The first 153 multiple-channel cochlear implant operations performed at the Medizinische Hochschule in Hannover and the first 100 implantations at the University of Melbourne Clinic	Returned questionnaire. Questionnaires were sent to all surgeons presently implanting the Nucleus 22-channel device, based on the mailing list from Cochlear Corporation

CI = cochlear implant.

Reference	Rubinstein, 1999	Green, 2004	Proops, 1999
Level (design)	4 (retrospective review)	4 (retrospective review)	4 (retrospective review)
Sample size	290	214	100
OUTCOMES			
% with post-CI infection	4.4% (n = 4/90)	4.2% (n = 9/214)	12.0% (n = 12/200)
% of total responding to antibiotics alone	None reported	55.5% (n = 5/9) resolved with intravenous antibiotics alone	91.6% (n = 11/12) wound infection, minor
% of total requiring nonexplant surgery	75% (n = 3/4) responded to local wound (pedestal) revision and systemic antibiotics	11.1% (n = 1/9) persistent infection with intact skin around their implants	
% of total explanted because of infection	25% (n = 1/4) explantation and immediate reimplantation after soaking in antibiotic solution	33.3% (n = 3/9) implant extrusion or explantation from infection	8.3% (n = 1/12) explanted because of cholesteatoma
p Value	Not applicable	Not applicable	Not applicable
Conclusion	The majority of infections responded to local wound revision and antibiotics	The majority of infections responded to intravenous antibiotics alone	The majority of infections were minor wound infections
Follow-up time	Up to 9 y	Not specified	Up to 6 y
STUDY DESIGN			
Inclusion criteria	Implants performed at the University of Iowa Hospitals and Iowa City Veterans Administration	Adult cochlear implants in Manchester between 1988 and 2002—all were available for review	The first 100 adult patients implanted on the Midland Cochlear Implant Program

CI = cochlear implant.

REFERENCES

1. Bhatia K, Gibbin KP, Nikolopoulos TP, O'Donoghue GM. Surgical complications and their management in a series of 300 consecutive pediatric cochlear implantation. Otol Neurotol 2004;25(5):730–739.
2. Yu KC, Hegarty JL, Gantz BJ, Lalwani AK. Conservative management of infections in cochlear implant recipients. Otolaryngol Head Neck Surg 2001;125(1):66–70.
3. Cunningham CD III, Slattery WH III, Luxford WM. Postoperative infection in cochlear implant patients. Otolaryngol Head Neck Surg 2004;131(1):109–112.
4. Hoffman RA, Cohen NL. Complications of cochlear implant surgery. Ann Otol Rhinol Laryngol Suppl 1995;166:420–422.
5. Webb RL, Lehnhardt E, Clark GM, Laszig R, Pyman BC, Franz BK. Surgical complications with the cochlear multiple-channel intracochlear implant: experience at Hannover and Melbourne. Ann Otol Rhinol Laryngol 1991;100(2):131–136.
6. Cohen NL, Hoffman RA, Stroschein M. Medical or surgical complications related to the Nucleus multichannel cochlear implant. Ann Otol Rhinol Laryngol Suppl 1988;135:8–13.
7. Rubinstein JT, Gantz BJ, Parkinson WS. Management of cochlear implant infections. Am J Otol 1999;20(1):46–49.
8. Green KM, Bhatt YM, Saeed SR, Ramsden RT. Complications following adult cochlear implantation: experience in Manchester. J Laryngol Otol 2004;118(6):417–420.
9. Proops DW, Stoddart RL, Donaldson I. Medical, surgical and audiological complications of the first 100 adult cochlear implant patients in Birmingham. J Laryngol Otol Suppl 1999;24:14–17.

14 Cochlear Implantation

Cochlear implantation: Risk of postoperative meningitis

Rita M. Roure and J. Thomas Roland

METHODS

A computerized PubMed search of MEDLINE 1966–March 2005 was performed. The terms "cochlear implants" or "cochlear implantation" were exploded and the resulting articles were cross-referenced with those mapping to the keywords "central nervous system infections," "infection," or "meningitis." This search resulted in 62 publications. These articles were then reviewed to identify those that met the following inclusion criteria: 1) patients undergoing cochlear implantation, 2) articles that included the incidence of postoperative meningitis. Articles focusing on prophylactic measures, such as perioperative antibiotics, were excluded. (Perioperative antibiotics for otologic surgery is reviewed in another chapter in this text.) Editorials without associated data were excluded. The bibliographies of the articles that met these inclusion criteria were manually checked to ensure no further relevant articles could be identified. This overall process yielded 9 publications [1–9].

RESULTS.

Outcome Measures. The primary outcome was the incidence of meningitis. The criteria used to diagnose meningitis were not described in detail by most authors. Reefhuis et al. [1], however, did define symptoms consistent with the presence of bacterial meningitis to include two or more of the following: fever (temperature >38°C), stiff neck or nuchal rigidity, lethargy or altered mental status, and headache. Also, abnormal cerebrospinal fluid was defined by two abnormal findings (protein level >55 mg/dL, white-cell count >10/mm^3, and glucose level of ≤40 mg/dL). The diagnosis of meningitis was further classified as definite, probable, or possible (see table).

Potential Confounders. The quality of these data depended primarily on the accuracy of reporting, either the reporting of adverse events to the manufacturers or the reporting of survey respondents. Such data collection could have been prone to recall bias or underreporting. In addition, the criteria used by respondents for diagnosis of meningitis could have altered results. Such criteria were specified in detail by Reefhuis et al. (see table).

Study Designs. The highest level of evidence was published by Reefhuis et al. [1], and takes the form of a case control study (nested within a larger cohort study). In a case control study, patients who have one outcome are compared with those who do not have that outcome; in the Reefhuis case control study, the authors compared 24 cases with meningitis to 186 controls without meningitis. In an attempt to identify risk factors for meningitis, they assessed a number of factors in the medical history: meningitis before implantation, tympanostomy tube placement, otitis media, ventriculoperitoneal shunt placement, chronic medical conditions that could increase the risk of systemic infections, ossification of the cochlea, vaccination status (pneumococcal, meningococcal, *Haemophilus influenza* type b), radiographic evidence of inner ear malformations, sex, age at implantation, year of implantation, race, and geographic regions. In addition, surgery-related factors were examined: use of a positioner, incomplete insertion of the electrode, presence of a cerebrospinal fluid leak, the use of antibiotics before/during/after the procedure, more than one implant, and signs of middle ear inflammation at the time of surgery. Both a univariate and multivariate analysis were performed.

Reefhuis also provided uncontrolled data regarding the overall incidence of meningitis in young children who received a cochlear implant between 1997 and 2002. They collected data in the following ways: 1) survey of manufacturing companies, 2) questionnaires to all the patients' parents and their primary care providers, and 3) review of available medical records. The incidence of meningitis in the study population was calculated as the number of reported cases of meningitis per person-years from implantation. To place their results in context, Reefhuis also provided previously available historical information about meningitis in the general population.

Uncontrolled data were additionally reported in 2004 by Cohen et al. [2], who surveyed all of the North American cochlear implant centers, as well as manufacturing companies (Advanced Bionics Corporation, Cochlear Corporation, Med-EL Corporation). All three manufacturing companies responded, and of the 401 centers surveyed, 130 replied, for a 32.4% response rate. They estimated that of the 24,000 implants performed, 18,000 were included in this study.

There were four other retrospective reviews [3–6] whose sample sizes were 1–2 orders of magnitude smaller than the two uncontrolled studies already discussed. Because the above studies were designed to be inclusive of these smaller studies' patients, the smaller studies are not discussed in detail, but their numbers are briefly presented in an adjacent table. Likewise, three case reports [7–9] are briefly presented in tabular format.

Highest Level of Evidence. There are level 3–4 data regarding meningitis post-cochlear implantation. Level 3 data from the Reefhuis study includes a multivariate analysis that identified the use of a positioner and the presence of inner ear abnormalities as potential risk factors for meningitis in children. Multiple other potentially related medical and surgical factors were evaluated (see details under "Study Design"), but had no significant correlation with meningitis. The level 4 data describe incidence data from children (Reefhuis) or overall (Cohen) with specific numbers as reported in the adjacent table. To put their data in context, Reefhuis noted that the incidence of streptococcal meningitis in the general population was 1/30 of that in implanted children. Even when only children implanted without a positioner were considered, meningitis was still 16 times more common.

Applicability. These results are applicable to patients undergoing cochlear implantation with devices available

between 1997 and 2002 from the three manufacturers listed.

Mortality. One meningitis-related death was reported in the Cohen and Reefhuis studies.

CLINICAL SIGNIFICANCE AND FUTURE RESEARCH

Level 3–4 data suggest that meningitis is potentially increased after cochlear implantation. These studies also provide correlational data regarding which patients may be at increased risk for meningitis postoperatively, such as those implanted with a positioner or in the presence of inner ear anomalies. Based on these data, the implant with a positioner was removed from the market, serving as an example that evolving evidence changes practice.

Future research may focus further on the identification of risk factors for post-implant meningitis, as well as the impact of vaccination. Ideally, through further research, the risk of meningitis to those receiving implants may someday be indistinguishable from those who have not. The achievement of this goal will become more and more desired as the technology improves and the indications for cochlear implantation expand.

THE EVIDENCE CONDENSED: Post-cochlear implant meningitis

Reference	Reefhuis, 2003		Reefhuis, 2003
Level (design)	3 (case control)		4 (retrospective cohort)
Sample size*	24 (29) cases with bacterial meningitis 186 (200) random controls		4264 implanted subjects
OUTCOMES			
	Factors associated with meningitis		Meningitis details
	Multivariate analysis	Odds ratio (95% confidence interval)	n = 24 definite cases n = 5 possible cases
	Use of a positioner	4.5 (1.3–17.9)	n = 9 ≤30 d postoperatively n = 20 >30 d postoperatively
	Inner ear malformation with CSF leak	6.3 (1.2–94.5)	Incidence 239.3/100,000 (95% confidence interval, 156.4–350.6) person-years for the whole group
Conclusion	These two risk factors significantly correlate with post-CI meningitis		Meningitis post-CI is present at a mean incidence of 239.3/100,000
Follow-up time	3 mo–5 y		3 mo–5 y
STUDY DESIGN			
Inclusion criteria	All children with cases of bacterial meningitis and a random sample of 200 children who did not have post-implantation meningitis (selected with stratified approach so that distributions of year of implantation and of manufacturers were proportionate to those in the total cohort, but controls were not individually matched to children with meningitis)		All children <6 y old who received cochlear implantation between January 1, 1997–August 6, 2002, as identified by warranty lists of the 3 companies marketing CIs (estimated to be 95% complete)
Exclusion criteria	Not further specified		Not further specified
Meningitis case identification	Reports to companies, Food and Drug Administration adverse event reporting system, surveillance systems of Centers for Disease Control as well as state and local health departments, questionnaire to all families of children in the study population (57.3% response rate)		
Meningitis diagnostic criteria	Definite meningitis = isolation of bacteria from CSF or isolation of bacteria from blood with abnormal CSF and symptoms consistent with the presence of bacterial meningitis. Probable meningitis = abnormal CSF, symptoms consistent with bacterial meningitis, and evidence of bacteria in CSF, or histopathologic evidence of bacterial meningitis on autopsy. Possible meningitis = abnormal CSF, symptoms consistent with bacterial meningitis, no evidence suggesting a nonbacterial cause or death after an unexplained illness with compatible symptoms		
Age	<6 y		<6 y
Most common pathogens	*Streptococcus pneumoniae* *Haemophilus influenzae*		
Mortality	1 death from meningitis		

CI = cochlear implant, CSF = cerebrospinal fluid, ABC = Advanced Bionics Corporation, Cochlear = Cochlear Corporation, Med-El = Med-El Corporation.

To provide context: historical data reported by Reefhuis et al.—Centers for Disease Control reported the incidence of streptococcal meningitis in the general population of children <6 y old during the same time period as 4.0/100,000 person-years. Data for that time period for children with severe–profound sensorineural loss was not available.

* Sample size: numbers shown for those not lost to follow-up and those (initially recruited).

Reference	Cohen, 2004		
Level (design)	4 (manufacturer and center survey to obtain their retrospective data)		
Sample size*	3 manufacturers 130 centers (401 centers surveyed) 18,000 estimated (24,488 implants)		

	OUTCOMES		
		ABC	Cochlear	Med-El

		ABC	Cochlear	Med-El
	Manufacturer survey	n = 4	n = 10	n = 0
	Center survey	n = 8	n = 6	n = 0
	Manufacturer + center (accounts for overlap)	n = 8/7271	n = 13/16,517	n = 0/700

Conclusion	Meningitis is a potential problem post-CI		
Follow-up time	Not specified		

	STUDY DESIGN		
Inclusion criteria	1) The 3 manufacturers active in the North American market (ABC, Cochlear, Med-el) 2) Response to survey instrument to query CI centers in North America, using the mailing lists of all 3 manufacturers with follow-up e-mail, fax, or telephone		
Exclusion criteria	Not further specified		
Meningitis case identification	Not specified		
Meningitis diagnostic criteria	Not specified		
Age	Not specified		
Most common pathogens	*Streptococcus pneumoniae* *Haemophilus influenzae*		
Mortality	2 deaths (1 deemed unrelated)		

CI = cochlear implant, CSF = cerebrospinal fluid, ABC = Advanced Bionics Corporation, Cochlear = Cochlear Corporation, Med-El = Med-El Corporation.
To provide context: historical data reported by Reefhuis et al.—Centers for Disease Control reported the incidence of streptococcal meningitis in the general population of children <6 y old during the same time period as 4.0/100,000 person-years. Data for that time period for children with severe–profound sensorineural loss was not available.
* Sample size: numbers shown for those not lost to follow-up and those (initially recruited).

Smaller retrospective reviews	Number with meningitis
Cohen, 1988	n = 1/459
Webb, 1991	n = 0/253
Green, 2004	n = 0/240
Proops, 1999	n = 0/100

Case reports	
Staecker, 1999	Lateral sinus thrombosis and secondary temporal lobe infarction caused by infection of a screw anchoring the percutaneous pedestal of an implant
Daspit, 1991	Meningitis on postoperative day 6 after a profuse perilymph leak was encountered during implantation
Graveriau, 2003	Pneumococcal meningitis in a previously healthy immunocompetent man with a cochlear implant

REFERENCES

1. Reefhuis J, Honein MA, Whitney CG, et al. Risk of bacterial meningitis in children with cochlear implants. N Engl J Med 2003;349(5):435–445.
2. Cohen NL, Roland JT Jr, Marrinan M. Meningitis in cochlear implant recipients: the North American experience. Otol Neurotol 2004;25(3):275–281.
3. Cohen NL, Hoffman RA, Stroschein M. Medical or surgical complications related to the Nucleus multichannel cochlear implant. Ann Otol Rhinol Laryngol Suppl 1988;135:8–13.
4. Webb RL, Lehnhardt E, Clark GM, Laszig R, Pyman BC, Franz BK. Surgical complications with the cochlear multiple-channel intracochlear implant: experience at Hannover and Melbourne. Ann Otol Rhinol Laryngol 1991;100(2):131–136.
5. Green KM, Bhatt YM, Saeed SR, Ramsden RT. Complications following adult cochlear implantation: experience in Manchester. J Laryngol Otol 2004;118(6):417–420.
6. Proops DW, Stoddart RL, Donaldson I. Medical, surgical and audiological complications of the first 100 adult cochlear implant patients in Birmingham. J Laryngol Otol Suppl 1999;24:14–17.
7. Staecker H, Chow H, Nadol JB Jr. Osteomyelitis, lateral sinus thrombosis, and temporal lobe infarction caused by infection of a percutaneous cochlear implant. Am J Otol 1999;20(6):726–728.
8. Daspit CP. Meningitis as a result of a cochlear implant: case report. Otolaryngol Head Neck Surg 1991;105(1):115–116.
9. Graveriau C, Roman S, Garrigues B, Triglia JM, Stein A. Pneumococcal meningitis in an immunocompetent adult with a cochlear implant. J Infect 2003;46(4):248–249.

15 Ménière Disease

Intratympanic gentamicin: Impact on vestibular complaints

Ching Anderson and John P. Carey

METHODS

A computerized PubMed search of MEDLINE 1966–May 2005 was performed. The terms "Meniere disease" and "gentamicin" were exploded, and the resulting articles were combined. The terms "intratympanic" and "transtympanic" were entered as text words as the search term "intratympanic OR transtympanic," and the results were combined with the Ménière disease/gentamicin articles. The resulting 136 articles were limited to the English language, leading to the selection of 115 articles that were reviewed in detail. These articles were reviewed to identify those that met the following inclusion criteria: 1) distinct patient populations defined as those adults with definite Ménière disease, as defined by the 1985 [1] or 1995 [2] guidelines of the Committee on Hearing and Equilibrium of the American Academy of Otolaryngology—Head and Neck Surgery (AAO-HNS), who had failed medical management, 2) intervention with unilateral intratympanic gentamicin therapy, and 3) outcome measures consisting of quantitative or semiquantitative evaluation of vestibular complaints. The bibliographies of the articles that met these inclusion criteria were manually checked to ensure all relevant articles could be identified. This search strategy yielded four publications [3–6]. There was one randomized controlled trial (RCT) report [3] and one prospective study [4] with a control group consisting of patients who refused any surgical treatment. The remaining two reports [5, 6] were meta-analyses that each included several prospective and retrospective case series, but only one prospective controlled trial [4].

RESULTS

Outcome Measures. The impact of intratympanic gentamicin on vestibular complaints was assessed by comparing the frequency of vertigo episodes before and after treatment. Stokroos and Kingma [3] reported the number of vertigo attacks per year for each study subject before and after treatment, for both gentamicin and placebo groups; the time period following treatment for reporting frequency of vertigo episodes was not standardized across all subjects. The remaining three studies [4–6] reported the AAO-HNS–defined class of vertigo control, which compared the number of vertigo episodes during the 6 months before treatment to the number of episodes 18–24 months after treatment [1, 2]. The AAO-HNS classes of vertigo control are as follows: Class A is complete elimination of vertigo, Class B is reduction of episodes to ≤40% of pretreatment frequency, Class C is reduction in number to 41%–80% of pretreatment frequency, Class D is change in number by 81%–120% of pretreatment frequency, Class E is an increase in number by >120%, and Class F is defined by the initiation of secondary treatment because of persistent or recurrent vertigo. Of note, the Chia [6] meta-analysis used the AAO-HNS vertigo control classification scheme but allowed for the inclusion of data that did not meet the AAO-HNS 24-month follow-up period requirement.

Potential Confounders. Given the episodic course of Ménière disease, the frequency of vertigo episodes experienced may fluctuate with time, even in the absence of treatment. This fluctuation may have contributed to the placebo effect seen in the Stokroos and Kingma study [3], in which patients receiving placebo also had a statistically significant decrease in vertigo frequency. Differences in gentamicin dosage, delivery technique, treatment protocols, and follow-up period among the four studies may also have led to variability in results. Accordingly, details about these issues are tabulated for the reader. The two meta-analyses examined each included only one prospective controlled trial, with the remaining trials consisting of prospective and retrospective case series without internal control groups, so the level of evidence of the majority of the data used for these meta-analyses was low. Furthermore, publication bias in the otolaryngology literature [7] may have led to inclusion of more positive studies in these meta-analyses, thus potentially overestimating the success rate of intratympanic gentamicin treatment.

Study Designs. One study [3] was a double-blinded RCT (level 1), one study [4] was a prospective controlled trial (level 2), and the remaining two studies [5, 6] were meta-analyses of mostly prospective and retrospective case series (level 4). In the RCT, one major limitation of the study design was that the groups were not comparable in pretreatment vertigo frequency; the placebo-treated group had significantly fewer vertigo attacks. The study was small (12 subjects received gentamicin, 10 placebo), based on their power calculation to detect a 50% reduction in the frequency of vertigo spells. The follow-up period was relatively short, ranging from 6 to 28 months after treatment. Vertigo frequency before and after treatment was compared within the gentamicin and placebo groups, but no statistical analysis directly comparing gentamicin and placebo groups was presented.

In the prospective controlled trial, the control group was self-selected, not randomized. The gentamicin and control groups were similar in age and disease duration, although the pretreatment mean and standard deviation of vertigo frequency was greater in the gentamicin group (statistical significance was not reported). This potential pretreatment difference in the frequency of vertigo should be considered when interpreting the data from this trial.

Both meta-analyses used well-defined *a priori* inclusion and exclusion criteria, clearly specified outcome measures, and quantitative analyses. The Cohen-Kerem meta-analysis had a smaller sample size, because of the exclusion of studies of <10 subjects or follow-up period of <2 years. No requirement for minimal follow-up period was noted in the Chia meta-analysis. The latter meta-analysis was designed primarily to compare the effectiveness of different gentamicin delivery techniques, but overall effectiveness (taking into account all forms of gentamicin delivery) was calculated as well. The Cohen-Kerem meta-analysis used the random effects model for data analysis. The Chia meta-analysis used the parametric empirical Bayes (PEB) analysis with a β previous and the binomial generalized linear model with backward selection.

Highest Level of Evidence. All four studies suggest that intratympanic gentamicin is >90% effective in achieving complete or substantial control of vertigo. The level 2 Quaranta prospective controlled study was the only one to directly compare gentamicin-treated subjects to a control group, and it found statistically greater control of vertigo after gentamicin treatment. Although the Stokroos RCT does represent level 1 evidence, its limitations included the relatively short follow-up time, lack of a standardized follow-up period for comparison, and lack of statistical analysis on the difference between gentamicin and placebo outcomes. Although not reported by the RCT authors, the response rate (i.e., those who reported at least some effect on vertigo frequency) to gentamicin treatment (100%) was greater than the response rate to placebo (60%) (p = 0.03, Fisher's exact test). Results from the level 1 RCT and the level 2 prospective controlled trial indicate that vertigo control is considerable even with placebo alone or no surgical treatment at all, respectively. These findings are consistent with a previous study from Silverstein et al. [8] which found that 57% of patients with Ménière disease

who declined surgical treatment had control of vertigo at 2 years.

Applicability. Based on the inclusion/exclusion criteria for these studies, the results can be applied to patients with Ménière disease. The Stokroos and Quaranta studies can be more specifically applied to patients with Ménière disease who have failed medical treatment.

Morbidity/Complications. Sensorineural hearing loss as a result of gentamicin ototoxicity is the morbidity most often addressed in studies of intratympanic gentamicin treatment for Ménière disease. The impact of intratympanic gentamicin on audiometry in patients with Ménière disease is examined in the following review. Quaranta et al. [4] also discussed the effects of vestibular hypofunction as a result of intratympanic gentamicin treatment. All treated patients had experienced temporary oscillopsia and dysequilibrium, but these symptoms disappeared within 1–24 months after treatment. In general, the need for vestibular physical therapy/rehabilitation after intratympanic gentamicin treatment was not well addressed in any of the studies reviewed.

CLINICAL SIGNIFICANCE AND FUTURE RESEARCH

There is sparse high-level evidence demonstrating that intratympanic gentamicin treatment is effective in reducing the frequency of vertigo episodes in patients with Ménière disease. The single level 1 study available showed that intratympanic gentamicin significantly reduced the frequency of vertigo attacks. However, placebo also was shown to decrease the frequency of vertigo attacks, again emphasizing the confounding tendency of episodic vertigo to resolve spontaneously in Ménière disease. The single level 2 study available showed a statistically significant improvement in vertigo control with intratympanic gentamicin compared with no surgical treatment. However, one major limitation of that study was the lack of randomization among study subjects. The two meta-analyses presented rely on level 4 evidence (a mixture of prospective and retrospective case series without controls) to demonstrate that intratympanic gentamicin is effective in controlling vertigo. These meta-analyses did not examine vertigo control rates in untreated control subjects for statistical comparison.

Although the current literature does suggest that intratympanic gentamicin is effective in controlling vertigo, the paucity of controlled trials makes it difficult to determine how much more beneficial intratympanic gentamicin treatment is than placebo or medical treatment alone. Ideally, future research would include large multi-institutional double-blind, randomized placebo-controlled trials that are sufficiently powered to determine the true effectiveness of intratympanic gentamicin for vertigo control in Ménière disease.

Intratympanic therapies offer an advantage over endolymphatic sac or destructive surgeries in that injections can be repeated with minimal costs and morbidity, and may be titrated to clinical response. The 1995 AAO-HNS outcomes criteria, requiring 2-year follow-up, were developed with one-time surgical interventions in mind. The advent of intratympanic therapies calls for a rethinking of outcomes criteria. Specifically, does the need for a repeat injection after months or years of symptomatic relief really constitute treatment "failure"? Given the tendency of Ménière attacks to spontaneously decrease in frequency over a few months in any prospective study, future designs should include shorter interval measures of vertigo frequency while still respecting the need for long-term follow-up.

AAO-HNS classes of vertigo control

Class A	Complete elimination of vertigo
Class B	Reduction of episodes to ≤40% of pretreatment frequency
Class C	Reduction in number to 41%–80% of pretreatment frequency
Class D	Change in number by 81%–120% of pretreatment frequency
Class E	Increase in number by >120%
Class F	Initiation of secondary treatment because of persistent or recurrent vertigo

THE EVIDENCE CONDENSED: Intratympanic gentamicin for vestibular complaints in Ménière disease

Reference	Stokroos, 2004		Quaranta, 2001
Level (design)	1 (RCT)		2 (PCT)
Sample size*	22 (22)		30 (30)
OUTCOMES			
Outcome measure	No. of vertigo attacks per year		1995 AAO-HNS vertigo class
Intratympanic gentamicin	Pre-treatment: 74 ± 114 (AAO-HNS Class B-C)	Post-treatment: 0 (AAO-HNS Class A)	Class A: 86% Class B: 7% Class C: 0% Class D: 0% Class E: 7% Class F: 0%
Control	Pre-treatment: 25 ± 31 (AAO-HNS Class B-C)	Post-treatment: 11 ± 10 (AAO-HNS Class B)	Class A: 27% Class B: 20% Class C: 20% Class D: 26% Class E: 0% Class F: 7%
p Value or 95% CI	Gentamicin (pre vs post): 0.002	Placebo (pre vs post): 0.028	<0.05
	Comparison of response rate for gentamicin (100%) vs placebo (60%): 0.03		
Conclusion	Both groups with significantly better vertigo control		Significantly better control of vertigo than control group
Follow-up time	6–28 mo		2 y
STUDY DESIGN			
Inclusion criteria	Active unilateral Ménière disease (1995 AAO-HNS criteria) with no known primary underlying etiology, vertigo attacks at least monthly, failure of at least 6 mo of medical treatment		Recurrent episodic rotational vertigo, aural fullness, tinnitus, and fluctuating sensory hearing loss, absence of vestibular symptoms between vertigo attacks, failure of medical treatment
Exclusion criteria	Contralateral neurotologic pathology, ipsilateral middle ear pathology, allergy to aminoglycosides, cumulative gentamicin dose ≥360 mg for 12 applications, cumulative treatment time >6 mo, hearing loss ≥15 dB for 2 successive frequencies		Evidence of otosyphilis, autoimmune or allergic disorders, and other presumed causes of secondary hydrops
Randomization effectiveness/ confounding factors	Similar age. Gender and side of treated ear for each group not reported. Gentamicin group with greater mean and variation in number of vertigo attacks before intervention, but statistical significance not reported		Self-selected control group consisted of patients who declined surgical treatment. Similar age, disease duration. Difference in mean vertigo frequency, PTA, and SDS, but statistical significance not reported
Intervention regimen details	Intratympanic application of either gentamicin (30 mg/mL in buffer solution, pH 6.4) or buffer solution alone repeated every 6 wk until control of symptoms or one of the exclusion criteria met		Two initial doses of 0.5 mL intratympanic gentamicin (20 mg/mL, pH 7.8) injected once a week, additional doses given if recurrence of vertigo symptoms
No. of treatment doses	Gentamicin: 1.5 ± 0.51 doses Placebo: 2.8 ± 2.7 doses		2.7 ± 0.82 doses
Power	Powered *a priori* (but power value not reported) to detect a 50% decrease in number of vertigo attacks, with sample size of 16–22 patients		Not reported

RCT = randomized controlled trial, PCT = prospective controlled trial, MA = meta-analysis, CI = confidence interval, PTA = pure tone average of threshold (values at 0.5, 1, 2, and 3 kHz), SDS = speech discrimination score.
* Sample size: numbers shown for those not lost to follow-up and those (initially recruited).

Reference	Cohen-Kerem, 2004	Chia, 2004
Level (design)	4 (MA)	4 (MA)
Sample size*	580 (627)	980 (980)
OUTCOMES		
Outcome measure	1985 or 1995 AAO-HNS vertigo class	1995 AAO-HNS vertigo class, with exception of 24-mo follow-up period requirement
Intratympanic gentamicin	Class A: 74.7% Both Class A and B: 92.7%	Complete vertigo control (Class A): 73.6% Effective vertigo control (both Class A and B): 90.2%
Control	Not applicable	Not applicable
p Value or 95% CI	Class A: 67.8%–81.5% Both Class A and B: 89.5%–96.0%	Not reported
Conclusion	Effective in control of vertigo	Effective in control of vertigo
Follow-up time	2 y	Not reported
STUDY DESIGN		
Inclusion criteria	Studies published in years 1985–2003 with ≥10 subjects, Ménière disease definition and results reported in accordance with 1985 or 1995 AAO-HNS guidelines	English language studies published in years 1978–2002, clear description of gentamicin delivery technique, vertigo control results, reports of hearing loss post-treatment
Exclusion criteria	Not reported	Not reported
Randomization effectiveness/ confounding factors	Mixture of prospective and retrospective studies, with different gentamicin dosages and dosing regimens	Mixture of prospective and retrospective studies, with different gentamicin dosages and dosing regimens
Intervention regimen details	2 groups of gentamicin delivery techniques: 1) fixed dose protocol; and 2) titrated dose protocol	5 groups of gentamicin delivery techniques: 1) multiple daily dosing; 2) weekly dosing; 3) low-dose technique; 4) continuous microcatheter technique; and 5) titration technique
No. of treatment doses	Variable; range 1–24 doses	Variable; range not reported
Power	Not applicable	Not applicable

RCT = randomized controlled trial, PCT = prospective controlled trial, MA = meta-analysis, CI = confidence interval, PTA = pure tone average of threshold (values at 0.5, 1, 2, and 3 kHz), SDS = speech discrimination score.
* Sample size: numbers shown for those not lost to follow-up and those (initially recruited).

REFERENCES

1. Pearson BW, Brackmann DE. Committee on Hearing and Equilibrium guidelines for reporting treatment results in Ménière's disease. Otolaryngol Head Neck Surg 1985;93(5): 579–581.
2. Committee on Hearing and Equilibrium guidelines for the diagnosis and evaluation of therapy in Ménière's disease, American Academy of Otolaryngology-Head and Neck Foundation, Inc. Otolaryngol Head Neck Surg 1995;113(3): 181–185.
3. Stokroos R, Kingma H. Selective vestibular ablation by intratympanic gentamicin in patients with unilateral active Ménière's disease: a prospective, double-blind, placebo-controlled, randomized clinical trial. Acta Otolaryngol 2004; 124(2):172–175.
4. Quaranta A, Scaringi A, Aloidi A, Quaranta N, Salonna I. Intratympanic therapy for Ménière's disease: effect of administration of low concentration of gentamicin. Acta Otolaryngol 2001;121(3):387–392.
5. Cohen-Kerem R, Kisilevsky V, Einarson TR, Kozer E, Koren G, Rutka JA. Intratympanic gentamicin for Ménière's disease: a meta-analysis. Laryngoscope 2004;114(12):2085–2091.
6. Chia SH, Gamst AC, Anderson JP, Harris JP. Intratympanic gentamicin therapy for Ménière's disease: a meta-analysis. Otol Neurotol 2004;25(4):544–552.
7. Bentsianov BL, Boruk M, Rosenfeld RM. Evidence-based medicine in otolaryngology journals. Otolaryngol Head Neck Surg 2002;126(4):371–376.
8. Silverstein H, Smouha E, Jones R. Natural history vs. surgery for Meniere's disease. Otolaryngol Head Neck Surg 1989; 100(1):6–16.

15 Ménière Disease

Intratympanic gentamicin: Impact on audiometry

Ching Anderson and John P. Carey

METHODS

A computerized PubMed search of MEDLINE 1966–May 2005 was performed. The terms "Meniere disease" and "gentamicin" were exploded, and the resulting articles were combined. The terms "intratympanic" and "transtympanic" were entered as text words as the search term "intratympanic OR transtympanic," and the results were combined with the Ménière disease/gentamicin articles. The resulting 136 articles were limited to the English language, leading to the selection of 115 articles that were reviewed in detail. These articles were then reviewed to identify those that met the following inclusion criteria: 1) distinct patient populations defined as those adults with definite Ménière disease, as defined by the 1985 [1] or 1995 [2] guidelines of the Committee on Hearing and Equilibrium of the American Academy of Otolaryngology—Head and Neck Surgery (AAO-HNS), who had failed medical management, 2) intervention with unilateral intratympanic gentamicin therapy, and 3) outcome measures consisting of pure tone averages (PTA) and/or speech discrimination scores (SDS) at 1–4 years after intratympanic gentamicin therapy. The bibliographies of the articles that met these inclusion criteria were manually checked to identify any further relevant articles. The search strategy yielded three articles [3–5], which were reviewed in detail: one prospective controlled trial [3], and two meta-analyses [4, 5], each of which included several prospective and retrospective case series.

RESULTS

Outcome Measures. In all three studies, hearing outcomes in subjects after intratympanic gentamicin treatment were based in part on the 1995 AAO-HNS guidelines for determining hearing change, by using 1) PTA of thresholds at 0.5, 1, 2, and 3 kHz; and 2) SDS. Clinically significant hearing change was defined as a change of ≥ 10 dB in PTA or a change of $\geq 15\%$ in SDS at 18–24 months after treatment, with PTA change determining the overall nature of hearing change in situations of change in opposing directions [2]. Both the Quaranta prospective controlled trial [3] and the Cohen-Kerem meta-analysis [4] adhered to the AAO-HNS guidelines for data from the 18- to 24-month follow-up period, whereas the Chia meta-analysis [5] did not. The Quaranta study [3] grouped subjects into one of three categories—"better," "same," or "worse" hearing—based on these guidelines. The Cohen-Kerem meta-analysis [4] compared the mean values of PTA and SDS from pooled data for before and after treatment, but did not analyze the data in terms of clinically significant change. This approach to data analysis unfortunately does not necessarily reflect the intrasubject change in hearing, which is clinically relevant given the fluctuating nature of hearing loss in Ménière disease. The Chia meta-analysis [5] used these same AAO-HNS guidelines, but only reported the percentage of subjects in whom hearing worsened, of which a subset had profound hearing loss, defined by the authors as "anacusis or complete loss of speech discrimination." Validity of the findings presented in this meta-analysis is weakened by the authors' inclusion of data from studies that did not have 24-month follow-up; hearing outcomes data at variable time periods following treatment are pooled together.

Potential Confounders. As addressed in the previous section on the impact of intratympanic gentamicin on vestibular complaints, potential confounding factors in these three studies include differences in gentamicin dosage, delivery technique, treatment protocols, and follow-up period (see Table). The control group in the Quaranta study [3] was not randomized, and this lack of randomization may be a confounding factor when comparing results between the gentamicin-treated and control groups. The level of evidence for data used in the two meta-analyses [4, 5] examined was low; each included only one prospective controlled trial, with the remainder of the data coming from prospective and retrospective case series without internal control groups. Publication bias in the otolaryngology literature [6] may have led these meta-analyses to include more studies that demonstrate gentamicin's effectiveness in vertigo control, perhaps concomitant with higher dosages of gentamicin and thus higher rates of hearing loss. Alternatively, eagerness of authors and journals to demonstrate the low morbidity of intratympanic gentamicin may lead to publication bias in favor of studies showing very little hearing loss, thus underestimating the extent of hearing loss that occurs with the full range of doses used in clinical practice.

Study Designs. Study designs for these three studies have been discussed in the previous section on the impact of intratympanic gentamicin on vestibular complaints, and the relevant points are again presented here. The studies examined included one prospective controlled trial [3] (providing level 2 evidence), and two meta-analyses [4, 5] of mainly prospective and retrospective case series (level 4 evidence). The control group in the prospective trial [3] was self-selected, not randomized. Although gentamicin and control groups were similar in age and disease duration, the gentamicin group seemed to have worse hearing before treatment [higher mean PTA ($p < 0.04$, t-test for difference of means), lower mean SDS ($p < 0.001$)]. As stated earlier, both meta-analyses [4, 5] had well-defined *a priori* inclusion and exclusion criteria, clearly specified outcome measures, and quantitative analyses. The smaller sample size of the Cohen-Kerem meta-analysis was the result of exclusion of studies with <10 subjects or follow-up periods of <2 years. The Chia meta-analysis did not require studies to have a minimal follow-up period for inclusion. Although designed primarily to compare hearing outcomes of different gentamicin delivery techniques, the Chia meta-analysis did report overall hearing outcome for all forms of gentamicin delivery. The Cohen-Kerem meta-analysis used the random effects model for data analysis. The Chia meta-analysis used the parametric empirical Bayes analysis with a β previous and the binomial generalized linear model with backward selection.

Highest Level of Evidence. The level 2 Quaranta study [3] and the level 4 Cohen-Kerem meta-analysis [4] both suggest that intratympanic gentamicin does not affect hearing outcomes in treated patients with Ménière disease. The Quaranta study provides level 2 evidence in that it directly compared gentamicin-treated and control groups with respect to changes in hearing and found no statistical difference between the two groups at 24 months follow-up. The results of the Cohen-Kerem meta-analysis, showing no statistically or clinically significant difference in mean PTA and SDS scores when comparing subjects before and after gentamicin treatment, seem to support the findings of the Quaranta study. The findings of the level 4 Chia meta-analysis [5], when viewed in the context of the natural history of Ménière disease, also suggest that hearing outcome is not much affected by intratympanic gentamicin. The authors found that 25% of gentamicin-treated subjects experienced hearing loss, comparable in percentage to the 22% of medically managed patients with Ménière disease who were found to have hearing loss at 24 months' follow-up in a study by Santos et al. [7]. Statistical power is an issue here, however. The standard deviation of the rate of hearing loss in the Chia meta-anlysis [5] seemed to be approximately 20%. This means that any study attempting to detect a 10% greater rate of hearing loss in gentamicin-treated subjects over that seen in controls with 90% power would require about 70 patients in each group. The number of gentamicin patients observed in individual studies frequently surpassed this number, but no trial has simultaneously examined a similar number of control subjects.

Applicability. These results can be applied to patients with Ménière disease, and the Quaranta study can be more specifically applied to patients with Ménière disease who have failed medical treatment.

Morbidity/Complications. Hearing loss itself is a morbidity associated with intratympanic gentamicin treatment. Other morbidities associated with intratympanic gentamicin have been discussed in the prior section, and are presented again here. Vestibular hypofunction is addressed in the Quaranta study [3]. All treated patients reported temporary oscillopsia and dysequilibrium, but these symptoms resolved within 1–24 months after treatment. As stated earlier, the need for vestibular physical therapy/rehabilitation after intratympanic gentamicin treatment was not well addressed in any of the studies reviewed.

CLINICAL SIGNIFICANCE AND FUTURE RESEARCH

Hearing loss resulting from intratympanic gentamicin treatment seems to be minimal, with the rate of occurrence comparable to that of patients treated with medical management alone. This conclusion is based on limited high-level evidence. The only level 2 study [3] in the literature does not show a statistically significant difference in hearing outcome between gentamicin-treated and control groups, but lack of randomization between treatment groups may be a confounding factor. Furthermore, with 15 subjects in each of the treatment groups, the study had 90% power to detect a 22% or greater difference in hearing loss between the groups. A smaller difference might be clinically significant but still undetected. The two meta-analyses presented used mainly level 4 evidence (a mixture of prospective and retrospective case series without controls) as data sources for evaluating hearing outcome after intratympanic gentamicin; hearing outcomes in untreated control subjects were not analyzed for statistical comparison.

Intratympanic gentamicin seems to be effective in controlling vertigo in patients with Ménière disease, with little proven detriment to hearing beyond what is to be expected from the natural history of the disease. Assuming that intratympanic gentamicin is indeed more effective at controlling vertigo than placebo or medical management alone (see "Clinical Significance" discussion in the prior section regarding the impact of gentamicin on vestibular complaints), the low rate of associated hearing loss makes intratympanic gentamicin an attractive treatment option for patients with Ménière disease. Ideally, the same large multi-institutional double-blind, randomized placebo-controlled trials needed to further establish the effectiveness of intratympanic gentamicin treatment for vertigo control would provide high-quality evidence regarding hearing outcome as well.

THE EVIDENCE CONDENSED: Effects of intratympanic gentamicin for Ménière disease on audiometry after 1–4 years

Reference	Quaranta, 2001	Cohen-Kerem, 2004		Chia, 2004
Level (design)	2 (PCT)	4 (MA)		4 (MA)
Sample size*	30 (30)	PTA: 549 (627) SDS: 395 (627)		980 (980)
OUTCOMES				
Outcome measure	Change in PTA ≥10 dB or SDS ≥15%	PTA	SDS	% overall hearing loss based on PTA ≥10 dB or SDS ≥15% % profound hearing loss (anacusis or complete loss of speech discrimination)
Intratympanic gentamicin	Improved: 40% Unchanged: 53% Worse: 7%	Mean (95% CI) Baseline: 56.6 dB (47.6 to 65.6) Follow-up: 58.2 dB (46.6 to 69.8) Change: 1.5 dB (−12.0 to 9.1)	Mean (95% CI) Baseline: 56.7% (39.1 to 74.3) Follow-up: 55.4% (36.3 to 74.4) Change: 2.0% (−16.5 to 20.4)	Overall loss 25.1% Profound loss 6.6%
Control	Improved: 27% Unchanged: 33% Worse: 40%	Not applicable		Not applicable
p Value or 95% CI	Not reported, but "no significant difference between the two groups"	95% CI includes the value 0; no significant difference in PTA	95% CI includes the value 0; no significant difference in SDS	Not reported
Conclusion	Similar hearing outcomes between gentamicin and control groups	No statistically or clinically significant difference in PTA after gentamicin	No statistically or clinically significant difference in SDS after gentamicin	Overall hearing loss in 25.1% of subjects after gentamicin, with 6.6% profound hearing loss
Follow-up time	2 y	2 y		Not reported
STUDY DESIGN				
Inclusion criteria	Recurrent episodic rotational vertigo, aural fullness, tinnitus, and fluctuating sensory hearing loss, absence of vestibular symptoms between vertigo attacks, failure of medical treatment	Studies published in years 1985–2003 with ≥10 subjects, Ménière disease definition and results reported in accordance with 1985 or 1995 AAO-HNS guidelines		English language studies published in years 1978–2002, clear description of gentamicin delivery technique, vertigo control results, reports of hearing loss after treatments
Exclusion criteria	Evidence of otosyphilis, autoimmune or allergic disorders, and other presumed causes of secondary hydrops	Not reported		Not reported
Randomization effectiveness/ confounding factors	Not randomized: control group consisted of patients who declined surgical treatment. Similar age, disease duration. Difference in mean vertigo frequency, PTA, and SDS, but statistical significance not reported	Mixture of prospective and retrospective studies, with different gentamicin dosages and dosing regimens		Mixture of prospective and retrospective studies, with different gentamicin dosages and dosing regimens
Intervention regimen details	Two initial doses of 0.5 mL intratympanic gentamicin (20 mg/mL, pH 7.8) injected once a week, additional doses given if recurrence of vertigo symptoms	2 groups of gentamicin delivery techniques: 1) fixed dose protocol; and 2) titrated dose protocol		5 groups of gentamicin delivery techniques: 1) multiple daily dosing; 2) weekly dosing; 3) low-dose technique; 4) continuous microcatheter technique; and 5) titration technique
No. of treatment doses	2.7 ± 0.82 doses	Variable; range 1–24 doses		Variable; range not reported
Power	Not reported	Not reported		Not reported

PCT = prospective controlled trial, MA = meta-analysis, CI = confidence interval, PTA = pure tone average (of threshold values at 0.5, 1, 2, and 3 kHz), SDS = speech discrimination score.
* Sample size: numbers shown for those not lost to follow-up and those (initially recruited).

REFERENCES

1. Pearson BW, Brackmann DE. Committee on Hearing and Equilibrium guidelines for reporting treatment results in Ménière's disease. Otolaryngol Head Neck Surg 1985;93(5): 579–581.
2. Committee on Hearing and Equilibrium guidelines for the diagnosis and evaluation of therapy in Ménière's disease, American Academy of Otolaryngology-Head and Neck Foundation, Inc. Otolaryngol Head Neck Surg 1995;113(3): 181–185.
3. Quaranta A, Scaringi A, Aloidi A, Quaranta N, Salonna I. Intratympanic therapy for Ménière's disease: effect of administration of low concentration of gentamicin. Acta Otolaryngol 2001;121(3):387–392.
4. Cohen-Kerem R, Kisilevsky V, Einarson TR, et al. Intratympanic gentamicin for Ménière's disease: a meta-analysis. Laryngoscope 2004;114(12):2085–2091.
5. Chia SH, Gamst AC, Anderson JP, Harris JP. Intratympanic gentamicin therapy for Ménière's disease: a meta-analysis. Otol Neurotol 2004;25(4):544–552.
6. Bentsianov BL, Boruk M, Rosenfeld RM. Evidence-based medicine in otolaryngology journals. Otolaryngol Head Neck Surg 2002;126(4):371–376.
7. Santos PM, Hall RA, Snyder JM, Hughes LF, Dobie RA. Diuretic and diet effect on Meniere's disease evaluated by the 1985 Committee on Hearing and Equilibrium guidelines. Otolaryngol Head Neck Surg 1993;109(4):680–689.

15 Ménière Disease

Endolymphatic shunt surgery versus "sham" surgery or medical therapy:
Impact on control of vertigo

Walter Kutz and William H. Slattery III

METHODS

A computerized PubMed search of MEDLINE 1966–August 2005 was performed. The term "endolymphatic sac/surgery*" was exploded and limited to those in the English language, which revealed 251 articles. These articles were then limited to clinical trials, resulting in 32 articles. The references of the 32 articles were manually cross-checked, and no additional articles were identified. The articles were then reviewed to identify those patients that met the following inclusion criteria: 1) patients with Ménière disease who underwent endolymphatic mastoid or subarachnoid shunt procedure, 2) outcomes measured in terms of vestibular complaints, 3) comparison groups with either "sham" surgery or medical treatment as controls. This search strategy and inclusion criteria resulted in four articles [1–4]. Two of the articles are randomized controlled trials (RCTs) comparing endolymphatic shunt surgery to sham procedures and the other two articles are retrospective controlled studies with medical treatment alone as the comparison group.

RESULTS

Outcome Measures. In an attempt to standardize results after treatment for Ménière disease, the Committee on Hearing and Equilibrium of the American Academy of Ophthalmology and Otolaryngology published guidelines for the diagnosis and evaluation of therapy for Ménière disease in 1972. These guidelines were updated in 1985 and 1995 by the American Academy of Otolaryngology—Head and Neck Surgery (AAO-HNS) Committee on Hearing and Equilibrium. Three of the articles used these guidelines for comparison of outcomes between the patients undergoing endolymphatic shunt placement and control groups [2–4]. The other study by Thomsen [1] compared outcomes using a patient-rated scale evaluating vertigo severity, frequency, and duration recorded daily and averaged monthly. This article did not provide actual numerical data, but rather described the data in graphical format.

Potential Confounders. The definition of Ménière disease is often difficult and tends to be subjective. In response to this, the Committee on Hearing and Equilibrium of the AAO-HNS published more specific criteria for the definition of Ménière disease in 1995. In retrospective trials, however, it is often difficult to accurately establish the criteria for diagnosis. In addition, these guidelines are dependent on patients differentiating definite spells of vertigo from other symptoms and accurately recalling the number of vertiginous episodes. Finally, most controlled trials use patients who refused surgery as the control group. It may be argued these patients may not have as severe symptoms as patients electing surgical intervention.

Study Designs. Two RCTs addressed the issue of vertigo control, comparing endolymphatic shunt surgery versus placebo or sham surgery [1, 2]. In addition, the study comparing endolymphatic mastoid shunt to cortical mastoidectomy was double-blinded, states specific exclusion criteria, and demonstrated effective randomization [1]. The second study by Thomsen [2] was not blinded because of the presence of a postauricular incision in patients who had endolymphatic shunt surgery, did not include exclusion criteria, and had a difference in gender distribution between the two groups.

In addition, two retrospective studies compared endolymphatic shunt procedures with medical therapy alone. The control group was self-selected because patients that declined recommended endolymphatic shunt procedures were used as controls. Patients not willing to undergo surgery may have less severe disease and this is reflected in the study by Silverstein in which reduced vestibular response was lower in the control group compared with patients undergoing endolymphatic shunt, 12.3% compared with 25.7%, respectively [3].

Highest Level of Evidence. The first RCT by Thomsen demonstrated a significant improvement in dizziness and vertigo scores for patients who received endolymphatic mastoid shunt surgery compared with control who underwent mastoidectomy alone. The authors argue that the results would not be significant if the two patients in the placebo group that developed more severe symptoms after treatment were excluded. The second RCT by Thomsen demonstrated complete or substantial control of vertigo in both patients who underwent endolymphatic mastoid shunt surgery and tympanostomy tubes, 53% and 55%, respectively, at 1 year [2]. Both RCTs had small sample sizes and did not include power analysis.

The two retrospective studies that compared endolymphatic shunt surgery to medical treatment alone had conflicting results. The Quaranta study demonstrated a statistical improvement in regard to substantial vertigo control with endolymphatic mastoid shunt compared with medical treatment alone at 2 and 4 years postoperatively, but not 6 years or at last follow-up postoperatively [4]. The Silverstein study showed no statistical difference in vertigo control between patients who received endolymphatic subarachnoid shunt and medical treatment alone [3]. As mentioned previously, the patients who declined surgical intervention in the Silverstein study had less reduced vestibular response and fewer episodes of vertigo per month, making comparison between groups difficult. Overall, the results of endolymphatic shunt surgery compared with other treatments in the management of Ménière vertigo are conflicting, with two studies showing significant results in vertigo control [1, 3].

Applicability. Based on the inclusion/exclusion criteria, these results can be applied to adult patients with a diagnosis of classic Ménière disease.

Morbidity/Complications. Only one study reported an adverse outcome of sensorineural hearing loss after endolymphatic mastoid shunt surgery [2]. There were no deaths or meningitis reported.

CLINICAL SIGNIFICANCE AND FUTURE RESEARCH

The data concerning the efficacy of endolymphatic shunt surgery for the treatment of vertigo in Ménière disease are conflicting. Patients do show improvement of vertigo symptoms after endolymphatic shunt surgery, but some studies demonstrate similar improvements with interventions designed to produce a placebo effect or using medical therapy alone. Currently there is a need for a high-power prospective trial comparing the efficacy of endolymphatic shunt surgery versus other treatment modalities.

Ideally, trials concerning vertigo control after intervention for Ménière disease would have uniform outcome measures to allow comparison between studies. Adhering to the AAO-HNS CHE guidelines could help achieve such uniformity. Future improvements in these guidelines may include a more objective assessment of vertigo severity. In addition, chemical labyrinthectomy is rapidly becoming a popular treatment intervention for patients with Ménière disease refractory to medical therapy. Future studies may compare the outcomes of chemical labyrinthectomy with endolymphatic shunt surgery.

THE EVIDENCE CONDENSED: Endolymphatic shunt surgery versus "sham" or placebo surgery

Reference	Thomsen, 1981
Level (design)	1 (randomized controlled trial)
Sample size*	15 (15) patients underwent endolymphatic shunt surgery compared with 15 (15) who underwent cortical mastoidectomy as a "sham" procedure
OUTCOMES	
	Patient-rated scale (0–3 for vertigo severity, duration, and frequency) recorded daily and averaged monthly
Endolymphatic shunt surgery results	15 of 15 with improved symptoms ($p < 0.01$)
Sham/placebo procedure; results	Cortical mastoidectomy 13 of 15 with improved symptoms ($p < 0.01$)
p Value	<0.05
Conclusion	Slight significant improvement of vertigo with endolymphatic mastoid shunt, although improvement seen in both groups
Follow-up time	12 mo
STUDY DESIGN	
Inclusion criteria	Presence of typical attacks of fluctuating hearing loss, tinnitus, and vertigo (at least 1 attack every 2 wk)
Exclusion criteria	Symptoms <6 mo or >5 y
Randomization effectiveness	Equal gender, comparable age, random assignment
Age	25–69 y
Masking	Double blind
Intervention regimen details	Endolymphatic mastoid shunt with insertion of silastic into the sac, draining out to the mastoid cavity
Diagnostic criteria for vertigo	Patient-rated scale as described in Outcomes section
Management of acute symptoms while in study	Not reported
Additional management while in study	Not reported
Compliance	None reported
Criteria for withdrawal from study	None reported
Intention to treat analysis	Not applicable
Power	Not reported
Morbidity/complications	None reported

AAO-HNS CHE = American Academy of Otolaryngology—Head and Neck Surgery Committee on Hearing and Equilibrium.
* Sample size: numbers shown for those not lost to follow-up and those (initially recruited).

Reference	Thomsen, 1998
Level (design)	1 (randomized controlled trial)
Sample size*	15 (15) patients underwent endolymphatic shunt compared with 14 (14) who underwent placement of a tympanostomy tube

	OUTCOMES
	Vertigo control according to the guidelines of the AAO-HNS CHE (1995) (Results determined after 6 and 12 mo)†

Endolymphatic shunt surgery results	6 mo postoperative (Class): A: 33% B: 27% C: 0% D–F: 40%	12 mo postoperative (Class): A: 33% B: 20% C: 0% D–F: 47%
Sham/placebo procedure; results	Insertion of tympanostomy tube	
	6 mo postoperative (Class): A: 43% B: 36% C: 7% D–F: 14%	12 mo postoperative (Class): A: 36% B: 29% C: 21% D–F: 14%
p Value	>0.05	
Conclusion	No significant benefit in control of vertigo symptoms between the two groups, although both groups demonstrated a significant improvement in dizziness symptoms after treatment	
Follow-up time	12 mo	

	STUDY DESIGN
Inclusion criteria	Typical attacks of vertigo, hearing loss, and tinnitus, and symptoms refractory to medical treatment
Exclusion criteria	None reported
Randomization effectiveness	Higher ratio of males to females in group undergoing endolymphatic mastoid shunt, equal mean age and symptoms' duration, random assignment, significance not reported
Age	27–71 y
Masking	Not blinded (postauricular incision indicated shunt procedure)
Intervention regimen details	Routine endolymphatic mastoid shunt insertion
Diagnostic criteria for vertigo	Outcomes as specified by guidelines of the AAO-HNS CHE (1995)
Management of acute symptoms while in study	None reported
Additional management while in study	None reported
Compliance	None reported
Criteria for withdrawal from study	None reported
Intention to treat analysis	Not applicable
Power	Not reported
Morbidity/complications	1 patient with anacusis after endolymphatic mastoid shunt procedure

AAO-HNS CHE = American Academy of Otolaryngology—Head and Neck Surgery Committee on Hearing and Equilibrium.
*Sample size: numbers shown for those not lost to follow-up and those (initially recruited).
†Vertigo results reported for both 1985 and 1995 criteria by a Numerical Value = $(X/Y) \times 100$ rounded to the nearest whole number, where X is the average number of definitive spells per month for the 6 mo after treatment (18–24 mo) and Y is the average number of definite spells per month for the 6 mo before treatment. 0 = A (complete control of definitive spells), 1–40 = B (substantial control of definitive spells), 41–80 = C (limited control of definitive spells), 81–120 = D (insignificant control of definitive spells), >121 = E (poorer control of definitive spells), F = secondary treatment due to disability per month for the 6 mo before treatment.

Reference	Silverstein, 1989
Level (design)	3 (retrospective with control)
Sample size*	30 (89) underwent endolymphatic shunt surgery compared with 23 (50) who refused recommended endolymphatic shunt surgery and continued medical treatment alone
OUTCOMES	
	Vertigo control according to the AAO-HNS CHE (1985) guidelines†

Results of endolymphatic shunt procedures	2 y follow-up:
	  40% complete control of vertigo (Class A)
	  27% substantial control of vertigo (Class B)
	3 or more y follow-up:
	  77% complete control of vertigo (Class A)
	  10% substantial control of vertigo (Class B)

Results of medical therapy only	2 y follow-up:
	  51% complete control of vertigo (Class A)
	  22% substantial control of vertigo (Class B)
	3 or more y follow-up:
	  74% complete control of vertigo (Class A)
	  13% substantial control of vertigo (Class B)

p Value	Not significant
Conclusion	Endolymphatic shunt procedure offered no benefit over patients declining surgery and continuing medical therapy
Follow-up time	Minimum 2 y, mean 8.7 y
STUDY DESIGN	
Inclusion criteria	Episodic vertigo, tinnitus, and SNHL, failed medical therapy for at least 3 mo
Exclusion criteria	"Vestibular" or bilateral Ménière disease
Intervention regimen details	Endolymphatic subarachnoid shunt
Group assignment	Patients chose whether to have surgery
Data collection	Retrospective questionnaires
Age	49.3 y (all patients undergoing endolymphatic shunt surgery)
Masking	None reported
Diagnostic criteria for vertigo	AAO-HNS CHE (1985) guidelines
Management of episode while receiving study treatment	Not reported
Compliance	Not applicable
Criteria for withdrawal from study (if prospective)	Not applicable
Consecutive patients?	Original cohort was consecutive; however, 38.1% response rate to questionnaires
Morbidity/complications	None reported

AAO-HNS CHE = American Academy of Otolaryngology—Head and Neck Surgery Committee on Hearing and Equilibrium, SD = standard deviation, SNHL = sensorineural hearing loss.

* Sample size: numbers shown for those not lost to follow-up and those (initially recruited).

† Vertigo results reported for both 1985 and 1995 criteria by a Numerical Value = $(X/Y) \times 100$ rounded to the nearest whole number, where X is the average number of definitive spells per month for the 6 mo after treatment (18–24 mo) and Y is the average number of definite spells per month for the 6 mo before treatment. 0 = A (complete control of definitive spells), 1–40 = B (substantial control of definitive spells), 41–80 = C (limited control of definitive spells), 81–120 = D (insignificant control of definitive spells), >121 = E (poorer control of definitive spells), F = secondary treatment due to disability per month for the 6 mo before treatment.

Reference	Quaranta, 1998
Level (design)	3 (retrospective with control)
Sample size*	20 (26) underwent endolymphatic shunt surgery compared with 18 (59) who refused recommended endolymphatic shunt surgery and continued medical treatment alone

	OUTCOMES
	Vertigo control according to the AAO-HNS CHE (1995) guidelines measured in the 6 mo before follow-up evaluation†

Results of endolymphatic shunt procedures	2 y follow-up:
	  65% complete or substantial control of vertigo (Class A or B)
	4 yr follow up:
	  85% complete or substantial control of vertigo (Class A or B)
	Last follow-up:
	  85% complete or substantial control of vertigo (Class A or B)

Results of medical therapy only	2 y follow-up:
	  32% complete or substantial control of vertigo (Class A or B)
	4 y follow-up:
	  50% complete or substantial control of vertigo (Class A or B)
	Last follow-up:
	  72% complete or substantial control of vertigo (Class A or B)

p Value	2 y $p < 0.03$; 4 y $p < 0.04$; last follow-up $p > 0.05$
Conclusion	Endolymphatic shunt surgery decreased the number of definite vertigo episodes in 2 or 4 y follow-up, but did not differ from medical therapy in follow-up >6 y
Follow-up time	Mean 12 y (SD = 3.3 y)

	STUDY DESIGN
Inclusion criteria	Clinical findings consistent with Ménière disease, failed medical therapy
Exclusion criteria	None reported
Intervention regimen details	Endolymphatic mastoid shunt
Group assignment	Patients chose whether to have surgery
Data collection	Retrospective questionnaires
Age	54 y (SD = 9.4 y)
Masking	None reported
Diagnostic criteria for vertigo	AAO-HNS CHE (1995) guidelines
Management of episode while receiving study treatment	None reported
Compliance	Not applicable
Criteria for withdrawal from study (if prospective)	Not applicable
Consecutive patients?	Original cohort was consecutive; however, 46% with adequate follow-up data
Morbidity/complications	Not reported

AAO-HNS CHE = American Academy of Otolaryngology—Head and Neck Surgery Committee on Hearing and Equilibrium, SD = standard deviation, SNHL = sensorineural hearing loss.

* Sample size: numbers shown for those not lost to follow-up and those (initially recruited).

† Vertigo results reported for both 1985 and 1995 criteria by a Numerical Value = $(X/Y) \times 100$ rounded to the nearest whole number, where X is the average number of definitive spells per month for the 6 mo after treatment (18–24 mo) and Y is the average number of definite spells per month for the 6 mo before treatment. 0 = A (complete control of definitive spells), 1–40 = B (substantial control of definitive spells), 41–80 = C (limited control of definitive spells), 81–120 = D (insignificant control of definitive spells), >121 = E (poorer control of definitive spells), F = secondary treatment due to disability per month for the 6 mo before treatment.

REFERENCES

1. Thomsen J, Bonding P, Becker B, Stage J, Tos M. The non-specific effect of endolymphatic sac surgery in treatment of Ménière's disease: a prospective, randomized controlled study comparing "classic" endolymphatic sac surgery with the insertion of a ventilating tube in the tympanic membrane. Acta Otolaryngol 1998;118(6):769–773.
2. Thomsen J, Bretlau P, Tos M, Johnsen NJ. Placebo effect in surgery for Ménière's disease. A double-blind, placebo-controlled study on endolymphatic sac shunt surgery. Arch Otolaryngol 1981;107(5):271–277.
3. Silverstein H, Smouha E, Jones R. Natural history vs. surgery for Ménière's disease. Otolaryngol Head Neck Surg 1989;100(1):6–16.
4. Quaranta A, Marini F, Sallustio V. Long-term outcome of Ménière's disease: endolymphatic mastoid shunt versus natural history. Audiol Neurootol 1998;3(1):54–60.

15 Ménière Disease

Endolymphatic shunt surgery versus "sham" surgery or medical therapy: Impact on audiometry

Walter Kutz and William H. Slattery III

METHODS

A computerized PubMed search of MEDLINE 1966–August 2005 was performed. The term "endolymphatic sac/surgery*" with articles limited to English was exploded, revealing 251 articles. These were then limited to clinical trials, resulting in 32 articles. The references of the 32 articles were then manually cross-checked, and no additional articles were identified. These articles were then reviewed to identify those patients that met the following criteria: 1) patients with Ménière disease who underwent endolymphatic mastoid or subarachnoid shunt procedures, 2) measurement of preoperative and postoperative hearing levels, 3) were compared to either placebo intervention or medical therapy alone. This search strategy yielded four articles [1–4]. Two of these articles are randomized controlled trials (RCTs) comparing endolymphatic mastoid shunt to either "sham" surgery or placebo surgery. The other two articles are retrospective controlled studies with medical treatment alone as a control group.

RESULTS

Outcome Measures. In 1972, the Committee on Hearing and Equilibrium of the American Academy of Ophthalmology and Otolaryngology published guidelines for the diagnosis and evaluation of therapy for Ménière disease in an attempt to standardize findings. These guidelines were updated in 1985 and 1995. Three of the four articles reviewed herein followed these guidelines, although the article by Thomsen [2] did not compare at an 18- to 24-month postoperative interval specified by the 1995 guidelines. Pure tone average (PTA) and speech discrimination scores were used as outcome measures in all four studies.

Potential Confounders. Because fluctuating hearing loss is a distinct finding in patients with Ménière disease, a single audiogram may not be reflective of a patient's overall hearing. The American Academy of Otolaryngology—Head and Neck Surgery Committee on Hearing and Equilibrium (AAO-HNS CHE) guidelines of 1985 and 1995 addressed this by suggesting the comparison of the worst audiogram 6 months before intervention with the worst audiogram in a period between 18 and 24 months after intervention. Of the three articles published after these guidelines, only the article by Goin [4] strictly adhered to this specific time frame and used the worst audiogram. Another potential confounding factor in the articles by Quaranta and Goin [3, 4] is the self-selected control group (patients offered surgery but declining and continuing medical therapy). It is possible these patients did not choose surgery because they had less severe disease. A trend in this direction is demonstrated in the article by Goin in which the control group had a preoperative PTA of 42.94 compared with 47.67 in the operated group (p = 0.09) [4].

Study Designs. Two trials were RCTs that compared endolymphatic shunt procedures versus placebo interventions, mastoidectomy and tympanostomy tubes [1, 2]. The first RCT by Thomsen that compared endolymphatic mastoid shunt with mastoidectomy alone was double blinded, included specific exclusion criteria, and demonstrated effective randomization [1]. The second study by Thomsen was not double blinded because of the presence of a postauricular incision in patients who had endolymphatic shunt surgery, did not include specific exclusion criteria, and had a difference in gender distribution between the two groups.

The other two trials were retrospective controlled trials using a comparison group—medical intervention only in the Goin study [4] and vestibular nerve section and medical therapy in the Quaranta study [3].

Highest Level of Evidence. The first RCT by Thomsen demonstrated significantly better hearing in the endolymphatic mastoid shunt group after 1 year only at 250 Hz [1]. The other frequencies demonstrated no significant change in hearing between endolymphatic mastoid shunt and mastoidectomy. Also, there was no significant change in hearing after intervention in either group. The other RCT by Thomsen showed no statistical difference in hearing after intervention or between endolymphatic mastoid shunt and tympanostomy tube placement.

The remaining two articles used retrospective controls that were self-selected which introduced bias as discussed earlier. The study by Quaranta failed to reveal a significant change in hearing between patients treated with endolymphatic mastoid shunt, vestibular nerve section, or medical therapy [3]. All groups had increased auditory thresholds with time but this is likely reflective of the natural course of Ménière disease. The study by Goin also demonstrated no significant difference in change of hearing between patients undergoing endolymphatic mastoid shunt versus medical therapy using the AAO-HNS CHE 1995 guidelines [4].

Applicability. Based on the inclusion/exclusion criteria, these results can be applied to adult patients with a diagnosis of classic Ménière disease.

Morbidity/Complications. The second article by Thomsen reported one patient with anacusis and one patient with sensorineural hearing loss after surgery. The other three papers did not mention any postoperative complications. There were no reported cases of meningitis or death.

CLINICAL SIGNIFICANCE AND FUTURE RESEARCH

The current evidence does not suggest that endolymphatic shunt surgery alters the long-term deterioration in hearing experienced by many Ménière patients, although data may be limited by the power of the studies. Future research should be directed to new therapies directed at restoring auditory function.

The AAO-HNS CHE guidelines attempt to unify reported data on the diagnosis and treatment results for patients with Ménière disease. Adhering to these guidelines will allow better comparison of data between authors and perhaps more meaningful meta-analysis.

THE EVIDENCE CONDENSED: Endolymphatic shunt surgery versus "sham" surgery: Impact on audiometry

Reference	Thomsen, 1981	Thomsen, 1998
Level (design)	1 (randomized controlled trial)	1 (randomized controlled trial)
Sample size*	30 (30)	29 (29)
OUTCOMES		
	PTA (250 Hz, 500 Hz, 1 kHz)	PTA (500–4000 Hz), SDS using median values following the guidelines of the AAO-HNS CHE (1995) (results determined after 6 and 12 mo)†
Endolymphatic shunt surgery results	8 of 15 with improvement in PTA (p = NS)	Postoperative PTA did not change at 6 or 12 mo. Postoperative SDS did not change at 6 or 12 mo
Sham procedure; results	Cortical mastoidectomy 6 of 15 with improvement in PTA (p = NS)	Insertion of tympanostomy tube Postoperative PTA did not change at 6 or 12 mo Postoperative SDS did not change at 6 or 12 mo
p Value	At 250 Hz, patients undergoing endolymphatic mastoid shunt surgery had better hearing results (p < 0.05), p = NS at 500 Hz, 1 kHz, 2 kHz, 4 kHz	Not significant
Conclusion	Slightly significant improvement in hearing in patients undergoing endolymphatic mastoid shunt at 250 Hz	No significant change in either treatment group and no significant change between the two treatment groups
Follow-up time	12 mo	12 mo
STUDY DESIGN		
Inclusion criteria	Presence of typical attacks of fluctuating hearing loss, tinnitus, and vertigo (at least 1 attack every 2 wk)	Typical attacks of vertigo, hearing loss, and tinnitus, and symptoms refractory to medical treatment
Exclusion criteria	Symptoms <6 mo or >5 y	None reported
Randomization effectiveness	Equal gender, comparable age, random assignment	Higher ratio of males to females in group undergoing endolymphatic mastoid shunt, equal mean age and symptoms' duration, random assignment, significance not reported
Age	25–69 y	27–71 y
Masking	Double blind	Not blinded (postauricular incision indicated shunt procedure)
Intervention regimen details	Endolymphatic mastoid shunt with insertion of silastic into the sac, draining out to the mastoid cavity	Routine endolymphatic mastoid shunt insertion
Diagnostic criteria for hearing loss	PTA	PTA and SDS
Management of acute symptoms while in study	Not reported	Not reported
Additional management while in study	Not reported	None reported
Compliance	None reported	None reported
Criteria for withdrawal from study	None reported	None reported
Intention to treat analysis	Not applicable	Not applicable
Power	Not reported	Not reported
Morbidity/complications	None reported	1 patient with anacusis after endolymphatic mastoid shunt procedure

NS = not significant, PTA = pure tone average, SDS = speech discrimination score, AAO-HNS CHE = American Academy of Otolaryngology—Head and Neck Surgery Committee on Hearing and Equilibrium.

* Sample size: numbers shown for those not lost to follow-up and those (initially recruited).

† Pretreatment hearing level determined by the lowest level in the 6 mo before intervention and post-treatment hearing level is determined by the lowest level in the period between 18 and 24 mo after intervention.

THE EVIDENCE CONDENSED: Endolymphatic shunt surgery versus medical therapy alone: Impact on audiometry

Reference	Quaranta, 1997	Goin, 1992
Level (design)	3 (retrospective with control)	3 (retrospective with control)
Sample size*	17 (17) underwent endolymphatic shunt surgery compared with 29 (29) who underwent vestibular nerve section or 22 (22) who refused surgery and continuing medical therapy alone	30 (101) underwent endolymphatic shunt surgery compared with 30 (178) who were used as a historical control group that continued medical therapy alone
OUTCOMES		
	PTA (500 Hz, 1 kHz, 2 kHz) and SDS according to the AAO-HNS CHE (1985) guidelines†	PTA (250 Hz, 500 Hz, 1 kHz, 2 kHz) and SDS according to the AAO-HNS CHE (1985) guidelines measured in the 6 mo before follow-up evaluation†
Results of endolymphatic shunt procedures	PTA worsened by 13.3 dB and SDS decreased by 25.9%	PTA worsened by 8.81 dB (p < 0.01) and SDS decreased by 16.3% (p < 0.01)
Results of alternative therapy	Medical therapy alone PTA worsened by 18.1 dB and SDS decreased by 19% Vestibular nerve section PTA worsened by 9.3 dB and SDS decreased by 13.2%	Medical therapy alone PTA worsened by 2.8 dB (p = NS) and SDS decreased by 8.37% (p < 0.02)
p Value	Not significant	PTA p = 0.10 SDS p = 0.21
Conclusion	Endolymphatic mastoid shunt does not improve hearing results when compared with vestibular nerve section or medical therapy alone	No significant difference in long-term hearing outcomes in either PTA or SDS between endolymphatic mastoid shunt and medical therapy alone
Follow-up time	≥5 y, mean 12.8 y	Mean 46 mo, minimum 2 y
STUDY DESIGN		
Inclusion criteria	Clinical findings consistent with Ménière disease, failed medical therapy	18–60 y old, ≥20-dB hearing impairment, documented cochlear involvement (fluctuating hearing, EcochG, positive urea test)
Exclusion criteria	Bilateral Ménière disease	Patients >60 y old must not have signs of presbycusis in unaffected ear, >60-dB hearing loss, or normal hearing
Intervention regimen details	Endolymphatic mastoid shunt	Endolymphatic mastoid shunt
Group assignment	Patients chose whether to have surgery	Patients chose whether to have surgery
Data collection	Retrospective study	Retrospective study
Age	23–68 y	18–60 y
Masking	None reported	None reported
Diagnostic criteria for vertigo	PTA and SDS	AAO-HNS CHE (1985) guidelines
Management of episode while receiving study treatment	Not reported	Not reported
Compliance	Not applicable	Not applicable
Criteria for withdrawal from study (if prospective)	Not applicable	Not applicable
Consecutive patients?	Yes	Yes
Morbidity/complications	None reported	None reported

PTA = pure tone average, SDS = speech discrimination score, AAO-HNS CHE = American Academy of Otolaryngology—Head and Neck Surgery Committee on Hearing and Equilibrium, NS = not significant.
* Sample size: numbers shown for those not lost to follow-up and those (initially recruited).
† Pretreatment hearing level determined by the lowest level in the 6 mo before intervention and post-treatment hearing level is determined by the lowest level in the period between 18 and 24 mo after intervention.

REFERENCES

1. Thomsen J, Bonding P, Becker B, Stage J, Tos M. The non-specific effect of endolymphatic sac surgery in treatment of Ménière's disease: a prospective, randomized controlled study comparing "classic" endolymphatic sac surgery with the insertion of a ventilating tube in the tympanic membrane. Acta Otolaryngol 1998;118(6):769–773.

2. Thomsen J, Bretlau P, Tos M, Johnsen NJ. Placebo effect in surgery for Ménière's disease. A double-blind, placebo-controlled study on endolymphatic sac shunt surgery. Arch Otolaryngol 1981;107(5):271–277.

3. Quaranta A, Onofri M, Sallustio V, Iurato S. Comparison of long-term hearing results after vestibular neurectomy, endolymphatic mastoid shunt, and medical therapy. Am J Otol 1997;18(4):444–448.

4. Goin DW, Mischke RE, Esses BA, Young D, Priest EA, Whitmoyer-Goin V. Hearing results from endolymphatic sac surgery. Am J Otol 1992;13(5):393–397.

15 Ménière Disease

15.C.

Surgical labyrinthectomy versus other procedures: Chance of decreased vestibular complaints

Walter Kutz and William H. Slattery III

METHODS

A computerized PubMed search of MEDLINE 1966–August 2005 was performed. The terms "labyrinth/surgery" or "labyrinth disease/surgery" and "Meniere disease" with articles limited to English were exploded revealing 732 articles. These articles were then reviewed to identify those that met the following inclusion criteria: 1) patients with Ménière disease who underwent transmastoid or transcanal labyrinthectomy, 2) controlled study with a comparison procedure included in the data analysis, 3) outcomes measured in terms of vertigo control. Three articles that met these criteria were identified and are described below [1–3]. The references of these articles were manually cross-checked to ensure any additional articles would be included and none were identified.

RESULTS

Outcome Measures. In an attempt to standardize results after treatment for Ménière disease, the Committee on Hearing and Equilibrium of the American Academy of Ophthalmology and Otolaryngology (AAOO) published guidelines for the diagnosis and evaluation of therapy for Ménière disease in 1972. These guidelines were updated in 1985 and 1995 by the American Academy of Otolaryngology—Head and Neck Surgery Committee on Hearing and Equilibrium (AAO-HNS CHE). Two articles used the AAOO (1972) guidelines or the AAO-HNS (1995) CHE [2, 3]. The other study used subjective relief from vertigo as the outcome measure [1].

Potential Confounders. It is difficult to compare labyrinthectomy to other forms of treatment for Ménière disease because this is an ablative procedure. In addition, if labyrinthectomy is offered as a treatment option, patients in general will have significant disability and hearing loss. This makes designing a control group difficult. Also, reporting by the AAOO 1972 classification is difficult because the classification uses hearing and vertigo in the same scale, resulting in either relief of vertigo (Class C) or no relief of vertigo (Class D) in patients after labyrinthectomy. One article used relief from vertigo as the outcome measure but does not give a further definition of this term [1].

Study Designs. Two studies compared labyrinthectomy to middle fossa craniotomy with vestibular nerve section [1, 3]. The study by Kaylie compared labyrinthectomy to either endolymphatic mastoid shunt or suboccipital craniotomy with vestibular nerve section [2]. Only the study by Kaylie used statistical analysis to evaluate for a difference between groups [2]. All three studies were retrospective, with the inherent biases of this type of study.

Highest Level of Evidence. The three studies that met inclusion criteria were level 3 evidence. Control of vertigo after labyrinthectomy was 100% in two studies [1, 2]. The Glasscock study demonstrated a 93% control of vertigo in patients undergoing labyrinthectomy [3]. Two articles compared labyrinthectomy to middle fossa vestibular nerve section and found no statistical difference between the groups [1, 3]. Two articles compared labyrinthectomy to middle fossa vestibular nerve section and found greater than 93% vertigo control in both groups [1, 3]. There was, however, no statistical analysis to allow direct comparison of labyrinthectomy and vestibular nerve section. Level 3 data suggests that labyrinthectomy is more effective in controlling vertigo than endolymphatic shunt procedures (p = 0.047) [2].

Applicability. Based on the inclusion/exclusion criteria, these results can be applied to adult patients with a diagnosis of classic Ménière disease.

Morbidity/Complications. Complications were uncommon with three reported wound infections. There were no reported cases of meningitis or death.

CLINICAL SIGNIFICANCE AND FUTURE RESEARCH

Labyrinthectomy is highly successful in controlling vertigo symptoms in patients with Ménière disease. This procedure is most often used when hearing is poor. Vestibular nerve section offers similar results with the potential of hearing preservation, although this procedure carries more risk, higher cost, and longer recovery.

Future studies will compare surgical labyrinthectomy to chemical ablation procedures. Finally, new treatment options are required for Ménière disease that allow hearing restoration and vertigo control.

THE EVIDENCE CONDENSED: Surgical labyrinthectomy versus other procedures: Chance of decreased vestibular complaints

Reference	Gacek, 1996	Kaylie, 2005
Level (design)	3 (retrospective with control)	3 (retrospective with control)
Sample size*	59 (59) patients underwent surgical labyrinthectomy compared with 30 (30) patients who underwent vestibular nerve section through middle fossa craniotomy	32 (32) patients underwent surgical labyrinthectomy compared with 74 (74) patients who underwent endolymphatic shunt and 83 (83) patients who underwent SOVNS
OUTCOMES		
	Subjective relief of episodic vertigo	Vertigo control according to the guidelines of the AAO-HNS CHE (1995)†
Labyrinthectomy results	100% relief of episodic vertigo in patients with Ménière disease	Class A: 95.2% Class B: 4.8%
Results of comparison group(s)	Middle fossa craniotomy with vestibular nerve section: 96.7% relief from episodic vertigo	Endolymphatic shunt: Class A: 47.3% Class B: 25.5% SOVNS: Class A: 70.6% Class B: 11.8%
p Value	No statistical comparison	Endolymphatic shunt: p = 0.047 SOVNS: p = 0.167
Conclusion	Both labyrinthectomy and vestibular nerve section are successful in relieving vertigo in the vast majority of patients and the choice of procedure depends on preoperative hearing	Patients that underwent labyrinthectomy had better control of vertigo than patients undergoing endolymphatic shunt or vestibular nerve section
Follow-up time	At least 12 mo	Mean 5.1 y, range 2.8–8.5 y
STUDY DESIGN		
Inclusion criteria	Unilateral disease, disabling vertigo that failed medical management, hearing thresholds >50 dB SRT and a <50% SDS	All patients met diagnosis of Ménière disease by AAO-HNS CHE (1995) criteria
Exclusion criteria	None reported	Bilateral Ménière disease
Intervention regimen details	Transcanal labyrinthectomy	Translabyrinthine labyrinthectomy
Design concern #1	Subjective outcome	No predetermined criteria for selection of procedure type
Design concern #2	Retrospective study	Some patients had prior procedures
Age	21–81 y	50.5 y, range 13.3–84.1 y
Masking	None reported	None reported
Diagnostic criteria for vertigo	None reported	AAO-HNS CHE (1995) guidelines
Management of episode while receiving study treatment	Not reported	None reported
Compliance	Not applicable	Not applicable
Criteria for withdrawal from study (if prospective)	Not applicable	Not applicable
Consecutive patients?	No	No
Morbidity/complications	None reported	1 cerebrospinal fluid leak

AAO-HNS CHE = American Academy of Otolaryngology—Head and Neck Surgery Committee on Hearing and Equilibrium, SOVNS = suboccipital vestibular nerve section, SRT = speech reception threshold, SDS = speech discrimination score.

* Sample size: numbers shown for those not lost to follow-up and those (initially recruited).

† Vertigo results reported for both 1985 and 1995 criteria by a Numerical Value = $(X/Y) \times 100$ rounded to the nearest whole number, where X is the average number of definitive spells per month for the 6 mo after treatment (18–24 mo) and Y is the average number of definite spells per month for the 6 mo before treatment. 0 = A (complete control of definitive spells), 1–40 = B (substantial control of definitive spells), 41–80 = C (limited control of definitive spells), 81–120 = D (insignificant control of definitive spells), >121 = E (poorer control of definitive spells), F = secondary treatment as a result of disability per month for the 6 mo before treatment.

THE EVIDENCE CONDENSED: Surgical labyrinthectomy versus other procedures: Chance of decreased vestibular complaints

Reference	Glasscock, 1980
Level (design)	3 (retrospective with control)
Sample size*	71 (71) patients underwent surgical labyrinthectomy compared with 55 (55) patients who underwent middle fossa craniotomy with vestibular nerve section

	OUTCOMES
	Vertigo control according to the AAOO (1972) guidelines. Patients relieved of vertigo Class C and those not relieved are Class D
Labyrinthectomy results	Class C: 93% Class D: 7%
Results of comparison group(s)	Middle fossa craniotomy with vestibular nerve section Class A–C: 96% Class D: 4%
p Value	No statistical comparison
Conclusion	Both labyrinthectomy and vestibular nerve section are successful in relieving vertigo in the vast majority of patients and the choice of procedure depends on preoperative hearing
Follow-up time	15 mo–9 y

	STUDY DESIGN
Inclusion criteria	Classic unilateral Ménière disease, all failed medical management
Exclusion criteria	None reported
Intervention regimen details	Translabyrinthine labyrinthectomy
Design concern #1	Subjective outcome
Design concern #2	Retrospective study
Age	Not reported
Masking	None reported
Diagnostic criteria for vertigo	Not reported
Management of episode while receiving study treatment	Not reported
Compliance	Not applicable
Criteria for withdrawal from study (if prospective)	Not applicable
Consecutive patients?	No
Morbidity/complications	2 wound infections

AAOO = American Academy of Ophthalmology and Otolaryngology.
* Sample size: numbers shown for those not lost to follow-up and those (initially recruited).

REFERENCES

1. Gacek RR, Gacek MR. Comparison of labyrinthectomy and vestibular neurectomy in the control of vertigo. Laryngoscope 1996;106(2 Pt 1):225–230.

2. Kaylie DM, Jackson CG, Gardner EK. Surgical management of Ménière's disease in the era of gentamicin. Otolaryngol Head Neck Surg 2005;132(3):443–450.

3. Glasscock ME 3rd, Hughes GB, Davis WE, Jackson CG. Labyrinthectomy versus middle fossa vestibular nerve section in Ménière's disease. A critical evaluation of relief of vertigo. Ann Otol Rhinol Laryngol 1980;89(4 Pt 1):318–324.

16 Tinnitus

16.A.

Antidepressant agents versus placebo for idiopathic subjective tinnitus: Impact on symptom control

Josh Finnell and Jay F. Piccirillo

METHODS

A computerized PubMed search of MEDLINE 1966–October 2005 was performed. The terms "tinnitus" and "antidepressant-agents" were exploded and the resulting articles were cross-referenced, yielding 26 articles. An additional search of the following subject headings was performed: "tinnitus" was cross-referenced with the textwords and medical subject headings "antidepressive agents," "antidepressive," "antidepressant," "amitriptyline," "clomipramine," "cyclobenzaprine," "desipramine," "desmethyldoxepin," "dothiepin," "doxepin," "imipramine," "iprindole," "lofepramine," "metapramine," "mirtazapine," "nortriptyline," "opipramol," "protriptyline," "tianeptine," "trimipramine." These resulting articles were then reviewed to identify those that met the following inclusion criteria: 1) patients with subjective tinnitus of ≥6-month duration between the ages of 18 and 70, 2) treatment with antidepressant agents versus placebo, 3) outcomes measured in terms of validated scales, and 4) randomized controlled trials. The bibliographies of the articles that met these inclusion criteria were manually checked to ensure no further relevant articles could be identified. This overall process yielded four articles.

RESULTS

Outcome Measures. Tinnitus can be measured in multiple ways, including visual analog and numeric scales [1–4]. The Iowa Tinnitus Handicap Questionnaire (ITHQ) is a 27-item self-assessment scale composed of three subscales or factors: factor 1 (15 items) assesses the patient's physical health and emotional status and the social consequences of tinnitus; factor 2 (8 items) evaluates hearing and communication difficulties relating to tinnitus; and factor 3 (4 items) considers the patient's personal viewpoint of tinnitus. The Multidimensional Pain Inventory scale is a six-point Likert-type scale that assesses disruption of 11 separate daily activities. The Internal Disability Scale is a 0 to 7 visual analog scale that assesses life disruption caused by tinnitus. The Tinnitus Patient Survey [1] and Tinnitus Questionnaire [3] rate tinnitus severity on a scale from 0 to 7 and also provide information concerning the quality, duration, localization, and other attributes of their tinnitus.

The Mini-Mental Status Exam (MMSE) [2] is an important diagnostic tool used to evaluate a patient's orientation, concentration, and memory. The MMSE is scored out of a total of 30 points. A score of 24 or higher is considered within normal range. The frequency and intensity of tinnitus can be determined using auditory brainstem response (ABR) [1–4]. Auditory brainstem response audiometry is a neurologic test of auditory brainstem function in response to auditory stimuli.

Potential Confounders. All four randomized controlled trials (RCTs) introduced a sampling error by checking the response to treatment at variable times. Although the ABR, ITHQ, and visual analog scales may be reliable, they may reflect natural variations in a patient's tinnitus. Moreover, tinnitus reporting may be affected by the natural fluctuations of a patient's mood or attitude toward a patient's symptoms. In addition, only two studies [2, 4] screened for depression and controlled the outcome for an independent measure of depression. Thus, the other studies [1, 3] cannot determine whether the antidepressant directly improved tinnitus or it improved depression which improved tinnitus coping or intrusiveness.

Study Designs. These studies were all double-blind RCTs with placebo control. All four confirmed no statistical differences in age, gender, or other pretreatment characteristics in the antidepressant and placebo groups. Only one study used subjective tinnitus ratings as the primary outcome measure. The other two studies used both a subjective tinnitus rating and either ABR or frequency and intensity matching. Both studies reporting randomization efficacy had more patients in the active drug group than in the placebo group. None of the four RCTs showed *a priori* tabulation of a power calculation.

Highest Level of Evidence. Two of the studies showed no statistical difference in reported subjective tinnitus measures between the antidepressant and placebo groups. The other two studies reported a significant decrease in tinnitus among patients in the active drug group. However, both studies that reported a decrease in subjective tinnitus measures found no statistically significant change in ABR.

Applicability. The results of these studies are applicable to patients with tinnitus of ≥6 months' duration between the ages of 18 years at the youngest and 80 years at the oldest. They are not applicable to children younger than 18 years of age. Further details of the inclusion/exclusion criteria for specific studies are tabulated for the reader below.

Morbidity/Complications. Three studies [1,2,4] reported antidepressant-related morbidity. Amitriptyline was associated with mild sedation and dryness of mouth in all subjects. Nortriptyline was associated with anticholinergic-type side effects as an adverse event. There were no reports of morbidity with trimipramine.

CLINICAL SIGNIFICANCE AND FUTURE RESEARCH

There is level 1 evidence regarding the effects of antidepressants on tinnitus, although limited in scope and with somewhat conflicting results. Two RCTs did report a significant decrease in tinnitus among patients in the active drug group, but no statistically significant change in ABR. Only one of the negative studies was adequately powered to find any true difference that existed; this study found no statistically significant difference in the subjective tinnitus measurement and no clinical significance in the ABR between the two groups.

If further research on this topic is performed, it may be best focused on the development of a standardized measure of tinnitus that accounts for the natural fluctuation in a patient's experience. Moreover, future studies should screen and control the outcome for an independent measure of depression to determine whether antidepressants directly or indirectly improve tinnitus. Also, it would be of interest to have clear reporting of *a priori* power calculations for studies, especially when the results show no significant difference between groups. No study used confidence intervals or reported how much of a difference in tinnitus would be clinically significant.

Overall, assessing the efficacy of drug therapy for tinnitus is difficult as objective measures of tinnitus are problematic and subjective measures are open to wide interpretation. A large simple trial taking in a broad range of tinnitus sufferers, applying one or more treatments, and then performing a factor analysis or discriminant analysis or principal components analysis on the data would potentially define meaningful tinnitus subgroups based on shared clinical features and/or response to therapy. Such objectively defined groups could then become cohorts in subsequent future studies of etiology, mechanism, diagnosis, or treatment.

THE EVIDENCE CONDENSED: Antidepressant agents versus placebo for idiopathic subjective tinnitus

Reference	Bayar, 2001	Sullivan, 1993
Level (design)	1 (RCT)	1 (RCT)
Sample size*	37	92 (117)
OUTCOMES		
Scoring system	*TPS* Range 1–7 1 = very mild 7 = very severe	*MPI* 6-point Likert-type scale *ID VAS* Range 0–7
Intervention	*Amitriptyline* (20 patients) RBT = 4.25 ± 3.08 RAT = 1.30 ± 1.49 LBT = 4.35 ± 3.45 LAT = 1.80 ± 2.40	*Nortriptyline* (49 patients) MPI/BT = 2.8 ± 1.1 MPI/AT = 1.8 ± 1.3 ID/BT = 4.0 ± 1.9 ID/AT = 2.5 ± 2.0
Placebo	*Lactose* (17 patients) RBT = 4.00 ± 3.32 RAT = 4.06 ± 3.44 LBT = 4.53 ± 3.28 LAT = 4.71 ± 3.37	*Lactose* (43 patients) MPI/BT = 2.2 ± 1.3 MPI/AT = 2.4 ± 1.3 ID/BT = 4.0 ± 1.8 ID/AT = 3.4 ± 1.6
p Value	TPS = $p < 0.05$	MPI = $p < 0.01$ ID = $p < 0.05$
Conclusion	Amitriptyline decreases severity of tinnitus	Nortriptyline decreases tinnitus disability
Follow-up time	NR	6 wk
STUDY DESIGN		
Inclusion criteria	≥6-mo duration	50–80 y old ≥6-mo duration Forego other tinnitus treatments
Exclusion criteria	Cardiac pathology	Otologic disorder Drug or alcohol abuse TMJ, CMS Score ≥25 on MMSE
Randomization effectiveness	More patients (20) in the amitriptyline group	More patients (49) in the nortriptyline group. Groups differed on level of depression
Age	18–64 y	50–80 y
Duration of tinnitus	10 patients <1 y 11 patients 1–2 y 12 patients 2–5 y 1 patient 10–20 y	All subjects 13.7 ± 11.5 y
Intervention regimen details	50 mg/night for 1 wk 100 mg/night for 5 wk	25–150 mg for 6 wk
Management of episode while in study	NR	NR
Compliance	NR	Assessed blood levels
Criteria for withdrawal from study	NR	NR
Intention to treat analysis	NR	NR
Power	NR	NR
Morbidity/complications	(NR%) mild sedation (NR%) dry mouth	(NR%) anticholinergic side effects

RCT = randomized controlled trial, ABR = auditory brainstem response, ITHQ = Iowa Tinnitus Handicap Questionnaire, MMSE = Mini-Mental Status Exam, ID = Internal Disability Scale, VAS = visual analog scale, TPS = Tinnitus Patient Survey, MPI = Multidimensional Pain Inventory, RBT = right ear before treatment, LBT = left ear before treatment, RAT = right ear after treatment, LAT = left ear after treatment, BT = before treatment, AT = after treatment, TMJ = temporomandibular joint syndrome, CMS = cervical musculoskeletal problem, NR = not reported.
* Sample size: numbers shown for those not lost to follow-up and those (initially recruited).

THE EVIDENCE CONDENSED: Antidepressant agents versus placebo for idiopathic subjective tinnitus

Reference	Mihail, 1988	Dobie, 1993
Level (design)	1 (RCT)	1 (RCT)
Sample size*	19 (26)	92 (117)
OUTCOMES		
Scoring system	*VAS* Range 1–7 1 = very mild 7 = very severe	*ITHQ* Range 0–100 0 = no difficulty 100 = great difficulty
Intervention	*Trimipramine* (NR) VAS/BT = 4.3 VAS/AT = NR	*Nortriptyline* (49 patients) ITHQ/BT = 64.888 ITHQ/AT = 59.661
Placebo	*Lactose* VAS/ BT = 4.0 VAS/AT = NR	*Lactose* ITHQ/BT = 63.574 ITHQ/AT = 56.335
p Value	NR	ITHQ = $p > 0.05$
Conclusion	No difference	No difference
Follow-up time	NR	6 wk
STUDY DESIGN		
Inclusion criteria	≥6-mo duration	≥6-mo duration Score ≥40 on ITHQ
Exclusion criteria	Hearing aid Drug or alcohol abuse High blood pressure Cardiac problems	Otologic disorder Pregnancy TMJ, CMS Score ≥25 on MMSE
Randomization effectiveness	NR	More patients (49) in the nortriptyline group. Groups differed on level of depression.
Age	29–67 y	50–80 y
Duration of tinnitus	5 patients 6 mo–1 y 7 patients 1–5 y 6 patients 6–10 y 4 patients 11–20 y 4 patients ≥20 y	All Subjects 13.7 ± 11.5 y
Intervention regimen details	150 mg for 6 wk Rest for 4 wk 150 mg for 6 wk	25–150 mg for 6 wk
Management of episode while in study	NR	NR
Compliance	Assessed blood levels	Assessed blood levels
Criteria for withdrawal from study	NR	NR
Intention to treat analysis	NR	NR
Power	NR	NR
Morbidity/complications	(100%) dry mouth	(NR%) anticholinergic side effects

RCT = randomized controlled trial, ABR = auditory brainstem response, ITHQ = Iowa Tinnitus Handicap Questionnaire, MMSE = Mini-Mental Status Exam, ID = Internal Disability Scale, VAS = visual analog scale, TPS = Tinnitus Patient Survey, MPI = Multidimensional Pain Inventory, RBT = right ear before treatment, LBT = left ear before treatment, RAT = right ear after treatment, LAT = left ear after treatment, BT = before treatment, AT = after treatment, TMJ = temporomandibular joint syndrome, CMS = cervical musculoskeletal problem, NR = not reported.
*Sample size: numbers shown for those not lost to follow-up and those (initially recruited).

REFERENCES

1. Bayar N, Boke B, Turan E, Belgin E. Efficacy of amitriptyline in the treatment of subjective tinnitus. J Otolaryngol 2001;30(5):300–303.
2. Sullivan M, Katon W, Russo J, Dobie R, Sakai C. A randomized trial of nortriptyline for severe chronic tinnitus. Arch Intern Med 1993;153(19):2251–2259.
3. Mihail M, Crowley JM, Walden BE, Fishburne J, Reinwall JE, Zajtchuk JT. The tricyclic trimipramine in the treatment of subjective tinnitus. Ann Otol Rhinol Laryngol 1988;97(2 Pt 1):120–123.
4. Dobie RA, Sakai CS, Sullivan MD, Katon WJ, Russo J. Antidepressant treatment of tinnitus patients: report of a randomized clinical trial and clinical prediction of benefit. Am J Otol 1993;14(1):18–23.

16 Tinnitus

16.B.

Anticonvulsant agents versus placebo for idiopathic subjective tinnitus: Impact on symptom control

Josh Finnell and Jay F. Piccirillo

METHODS

A computerized PubMed search of MEDLINE 1966–October 2005 was performed. The terms "tinnitus" and "anticonvulsant-agents" were exploded and the resulting articles were cross-referenced, yielding 61 articles. An additional search of the following subject headings was performed: "carbamazepine," "phenytoin," "valproic acid," "ethosuximide," "clonazepam," "primidone," "felbamate," "gabapentin," "lamotrigine," "levetiracetam," "oxcarbazepine," "tiagabine," "topiramate," "zonisamide." The resulting articles were then reviewed to identify those that met the following inclusion criteria: 1) patients with subjective tinnitus of ≥6 months' duration between the ages of 18 and 70 years, 2) treatment with anticonvulsant agents versus placebo, 3) outcomes measured in terms of validated scales. The bibliographies of the articles that met these inclusion criteria were manually checked to ensure no further relevant articles could be identified. This overall process yielded three articles: a randomized controlled trial (RCT) [1], a retrospective study [2], and a study with no internal control group [3].

RESULTS

Outcome Measures. Tinnitus was measured in multiple ways, including visual analog and patient response. In two studies [1, 2], patients were instructed to mark their experience of tinnitus on a 100-mm line at which 100 represented their worst tinnitus and 0 the absence of tinnitus. The frequency and intensity was determined using audiologic measurements such as pitch matching. The third trial was a review of medical charts in which the primary outcome measure was the patient's opinion of the treatment results.

Potential Confounders. Two of the studies introduced a sampling error by checking the response to treatment at variable times. Although audiologic and visual analog scales may be reliable, they may reflect natural variations in a patient's tinnitus. Moreover, tinnitus reporting may be affected by the natural fluctuations of a patient's mood or attitude toward a patient's symptoms.

Study Designs. The first study was a double-blind RCT with placebo control. There were no statistical differences in age, gender, or other pretreatment characteristics in

the anticonvulsant and placebo groups. This study used a combination of subjective tinnitus ratings and audiologic measurement as the primary outcome measure. This study did not show *a priori* tabulation of a power calculation. The second study was a level 3 retrospective case control study. Records were reviewed to find subjects who had an outcome of tinnitus improvement; these subjects constituted the "case" group. Then records were reviewed to find patients who showed no improvement of tinnitus; these subjects constituted the "control" group. The third study was a level 4–designed study containing no internal control group. The results of intervention were reported in one group of patients without a comparison group.

Highest Level of Evidence. The level 1 study showed no statistically significant difference in reported subjective tinnitus measures or audiologic tests between the anticonvulsant and placebo groups. Moreover, the study revealed fairly poor agreement between the questionnaires and the audiologic test results. Both the level 3 and level 4 studies suggest the potential for anticonvulsant drug therapy to ameliorate tinnitus symptoms.

Applicability. The results of this study are applicable to patients with tinnitus of at least 6 months' duration between the ages of 18 years of age at the youngest and 79 years at the oldest. They are not applicable to children under the age of 18 years or women who are pregnant. Further details of the inclusion/exclusion criteria for specific studies are tabulated for the reader on the adjacent page.

Morbidity/Complications. All three studies reported anticonvulsant-related morbidity. Lamotrigine caused nausea, vomiting, and headache as an adverse event in 3% of the study population. Carbamazepine caused a rash in 3% of the study population. Nausea, mild sedation, and headache were also reported. Clonazepam caused drowsiness, depression, nightmares, and a lower libido in 16.9% of the study population.

CLINICAL SIGNIFICANCE AND FUTURE RESEARCH

There is minimal level 1 evidence regarding the effects of anticonvulsants on tinnitus. The single RCT was not adequately powered to find a difference if one truly existed. Clearly, the response to lamotrigine has not been sufficient to make it a first choice as a treatment for tinnitus. Both carbamazepine and clonazepam show promise as drug therapy treatments for the relief of tinnitus and should be tested under a level 1–designed RCT.

If further research on this topic is performed, it may be best focused on the development of a standardized measure of tinnitus that accounts for the natural fluctuation a patient experiences. Also, it would be of interest to have clear reporting of an *a priori* power calculation for studies, especially when the results show no significant difference between groups. The use of confidence intervals would help the reader interpret the results of the study especially if combined with a statement of how much of a difference would be clinically significant.

Overall, assessing the efficacy of drug therapy for tinnitus is difficult as objective measures of tinnitus are problematic and subjective measures are open to wide interpretation. A large simple trial taking in a broad range of tinnitus sufferers, applying one or more treatments, and then performing a factor analysis or discriminant analysis or principal components analysis on the data would potentially define meaningful tinnitus subgroups based on shared clinical features and/or response to therapy. Such objectively defined groups could then become cohorts in subsequent future studies of etiology, mechanism, diagnosis, or treatment.

THE EVIDENCE CONDENSED: Antiepileptic agents versus placebo for idiopathic subjective tinnitus

Reference	Simpson, 1999	Melding, 1979	Gananca, 2002
Level (design)	1 (randomized controlled trial)	4 (case series)	3 (case control study)
Sample size*	31 (33)	98 (125)	1020
OUTCOMES			
	VAS Range 0–100 0 = no tinnitus 100 = worst tinnitus	*VAS* Range 0–100 0 = no tinnitus 100 = worst tinnitus	*Patient response* Asymptomatic: complete remission Improved: partial remission Unimproved: no change
Intervention	*Baseline* 52.8 (SD ± 4.8) *After placebo* 58.5 (SD ± 4.8) *After lamotrigine* 60.8 (SD ± 4.4)	*Carbamazepine* 56% = good or excellent response 24% = partial response *Diphenylhydantoin* No scores reported	*Clonazepam* 326 (32%) = asymptomatic or improvement of tinnitus
Placebo	Lactose	NR	NR
p Value	NR	NR	NR
Conclusion	No significant difference	Carbamazepine is effective in suppressing tinnitus in some patients	Clonazepam is a very useful and safe drug for the symptomatic treatment of patients with tinnitus
Follow-up time	NR	2–3 wk	NR
STUDY DESIGN			
Inclusion criteria	Patients with tinnitus >6 mo	NR	Patients with vestibular disorder that had been treated with clonazepam as the only antivertigo medication
Exclusion criteria	Age <18 y or >75 y Pregnant women Use of antiepileptic drugs GI, hepatic, or renal insufficiency Score of <5 on VAS Patients with tinnitus <6 mo	NR	Patients treated with antivertigo medication other than clonazepam
Randomization effectiveness	More males than females	NR	NR
Age	Male 53 (SD ± 3) Female 58 (SD ± 3)	22–79 y	18–37 y, mean 49 y
Intervention regimen details	*Lamotrigine* 25 mg 1 PO t.i.d. 2 wk 50 mg 1 PO t.i.d. 2 wk 100 mg 1 PO t.i.d. 4 wk	*Carbamazepine* 100 mg 3 PO t.i.d. for 3 mo *Diphenylhydantoin* if carbamazepine was not tolerated	*Clonazepam* 0.5 or 1.0 mg 60–180 d
Diagnostic criteria	VAS	VAS	Patient response
Management of episode while in study	NR	NR	NR
Duration of tinnitus	NR	2 mo–37 y	Average 1.6 y
Compliance	NR	Assessed with blood levels	NR
Criteria for withdrawal from study	NR	NR	NR
Intention to treat analysis	NR	NR	NR
Power	NR	NR	NR
Morbidity/complications	(3%) *Reported all or some:* Nausea Vomiting Headache	(3%) rash (NR%) mild sedation (NR%) nausea (NR%) headache	(16.9%) *Reported all or some:* Drowsiness Depression Nightmares Lower libido

VAS = visual analog scale, GI = gastrointestinal tract, NR = not reported, t.i.d. = three times a day, SD = standard deviation.
* Sample size: numbers shown for those not lost to follow-up and those (initially recruited).

REFERENCES

1. Simpson JA, Gilbert AM, Weiner GM, Davies WE. The assessment of lamotrigine, an antiepileptic drug, in the treatment of tinnitus. J Laryngol Otol 1999;20:627–631.
2. Melding PS, Goodey RJ. The treatment of tinnitus with oral anticonvulsants. J Laryngol Otol 1979;93:111–122.
3. Gananca MM, Caovilla HH, Gananca FF, et al. Clonazepam in the pharmacological treatment of vertigo and tinnitus. Int Tinnitus J 2002;8(1):50–53.

16 Tinnitus

16.C.

Tinnitus retraining therapy: Impact on loudness, annoyance, and habituation to tinnitus

Carol Bauer and Thomas J. Brozoski

METHODS

A computerized PubMed search of MEDLINE 1966–2004 was performed. The terms "retraining therapy" and "tinnitus" were exploded and the resulting articles were cross-referenced, yielding 12 trials. These articles were then reviewed to identify those that met the following inclusion criteria: 1) patient population with chronic tinnitus present at least 1 year, 2) intervention with tinnitus retraining therapy (TRT) versus placebo or other treatment, 3) objective outcome measures of tinnitus loudness and validated assessment of subjective tinnitus impact. Studies in which there were no measurements of objective or subjective features of tinnitus using validated instruments were excluded. The bibliographies of the articles that met these inclusion criteria were manually checked to ensure no further relevant articles could be identified. This process yielded three articles [1–3].

RESULTS

Outcome Measures. The effect of an intervention on the loudness and annoyance of tinnitus is a challenging outcome to study. Tinnitus is a subjective sensation that is modulated by many factors, which can be difficult to accurately identify and control. Objective outcome measures relevant to tinnitus include audiologic measures of hearing thresholds, tinnitus pitch and loudness matching, and minimal masking levels [1]. Psychologic outcomes of interest are measures of tinnitus impact (the Tinnitus Reaction Questionnaire, the Derogatis Stress Profile, and the Ways of Coping Check List) and self-rated assessment of tinnitus loudness, annoyance, and coping (visual analog scales). The Dineen study appropriately evaluated both objective and subjective features of tinnitus. The outcome measures in the Folmer study were limited to subjective evaluations of tinnitus severity and self-rated emotional distress.

Potential Confounders. Study subjects were randomly allocated to treatment groups in the Dineen study, but the details of the process were not reported. There may have been an unintended systematic bias in the preferred coping style of subjects allocated to the different treatment groups and this may have affected the response to treatment. Neither subjects nor investigators were blinded to the treatment interventions. In the Folmer and Berry studies, there was no control group to compare treat-

ment outcomes. None of the studies monitored compliance with sound therapy, and there was no uniformity in the clinical follow-up between initial treatment and outcome assessment. The Folmer data were based on questionnaire responses and only 190 of 300 questionnaires were returned, posing a possible response bias. The Berry study was a prospective evaluation of patients enrolled in a clinical TRT program, with possible bias related to the cognitive dissonance of subjects who enrolled in a fee-for-service treatment program.

Study Designs. There is only one randomized controlled trial (RCT) available for review and the randomization procedure for allocation was not reported. The follow-up period of 6–12 months is appropriate for studying the effects of TRT. Neither subjects nor investigators were blinded to the treatment group assignments in any of the studies. The *a priori* power analysis was appropriate and the investigators correctly performed a *post hoc* analysis comparing groups [2].

Highest Level of Evidence. There are significant discrepancies in the conclusions regarding TRT among the three studies outlined here. Studying a subjective sensation such as tinnitus, which can have significant associated chronic disability, is easily biased by a number of confounding factors. The level 1 study, whereas not strictly limited to studying TRT, can be used to assess the efficacy of the use of sound therapy in conjunction with counseling in facilitating habituation to tinnitus. Only limited conclusions can be determined from the level 3 and 4 studies described herein. Tinnitus management training does have a significant influence on the level of tinnitus habituation. However, there was no difference in effectiveness of different treatment strategies (counseling alone, sound therapy plus counseling, relaxation therapy plus counseling) in the outcomes of tinnitus habituation and coping ability. There were conflicting outcomes in two studies that examined the effect of sound therapy on the minimal masking level of tinnitus.

Applicability. The efficacy of TRT has been reported to apply to tinnitus of any etiology, although this assertion has never been investigated. It is unknown if the therapeutic efficacy is modulated by tinnitus severity or duration. The Dineen study suggests that an individual's preferred coping strategy impacts the effectiveness of the treatment.

Morbidity/Complications. There were no reported negative effects of treatment from any of the studies.

CLINICAL SIGNIFICANCE AND FUTURE RESEARCH

Tinnitus is a common and potentially debilitating chronic disorder that affects 17% of the general population. Many patients seek treatment for this symptom and consequently are at risk for investing time and money in pursuing interventions that have no evidence for therapeutic efficacy. Clinicians are often frustrated by their inability to offer safe, effective, reliable treatments to their patients who experience tinnitus. Although there has been no evidence of complications resulting from treatment with TRT, it is an expensive and time-consuming therapy that may not be appropriate for all people with tinnitus. The Dineen study demonstrated the positive impact of any form of intervention, without the need for inclusion of sound therapy to achieve improved coping and habituation to tinnitus.

An RCT, with appropriate blinding of participants to the treatment allocation, is necessary to adequately assess the efficacy of TRT. Appropriate assessment would include evaluation of objective measures of tinnitus (loudness match) and auditory function (dynamic range, hyperacusis), combined with validated subjective measures of tinnitus impact (annoyance, sleep disturbance, quality of life).

THE EVIDENCE CONDENSED: Tinnitus retraining therapy versus counseling with or without relaxation training for chronic tinnitus

Reference	Dineen, 1999	
Level (design)	1 (randomized controlled trial)	
Sample size*	65 (96)	
OUTCOMES		
	Changes in subjective ratings of tinnitus loudness, annoyance, and coping ability (VAS), and reaction to tinnitus (TRQ)	
Tinnitus retraining therapy	TRT Loudness: −0.3 Annoyance: −1.9 Coping: +1.4 TRQ: −8.1	
Control	Information alone Loudness: −0.7 Annoyance: −1.4 Coping: +0.3 TRQ: −6.6	
p Value	Loudness: NS Annoyance: 0.0004 Coping: NS TRQ: NS	Loudness: NS Annoyance: 0.0006 Coping: NS TRQ: 0.009
Conclusion	Information and sound therapy significantly decreases the annoyance but not the loudness of tinnitus	Information alone is as effective as information combined with sound therapy in decreasing the annoyance of tinnitus
Follow-up time	12 mo	
STUDY DESIGN		
Inclusion criteria	Age >18 y	
Exclusion criteria	Not reported	
Randomization effectiveness	No significant differences in tinnitus severity, duration, gender between treatment groups	
Age; gender	Range 22–87 y; 43 male, 22 female	
Masking	Not done	
TRT regimen details	Counseling was identical for the TRT, and counseling-alone group	
Compliance	Unknown	
Criteria for withdrawal from study	Unknown	
Intention to treat analysis	NA	
Power	n = 30 for power 0.80 and alpha 0.05	
Morbidity/complications	None reported	

VAS = visual analog scale, TRQ = Tinnitus Reaction Questionnaire, TSI = Tinnitus Severity Index, BDI = Beck Depression Index, THI = Tinnitus Handicap Inventory, LDL = loudness discomfort level, MML = minimal masking level, TRT = tinnitus retraining therapy, NS = not significant, NA = not applicable, RT = relaxation training.
* Sample size: numbers shown for those not lost to follow-up and those (initially recruited).

THE EVIDENCE CONDENSED: Tinnitus retraining therapy versus counseling with or without relaxation training for chronic tinnitus

Reference	Folmer, 2002	Berry, 2002
Level (design)	4 (retrospective case series)	4 (prospective case series)
Sample size*	190 (300)	32
OUTCOMES		
	Changes in subjective ratings of tinnitus loudness, TSI, BDI	THI, pure tone thresholds, LDLs, MMLs, tinnitus awareness
Tinnitus retraining therapy	Comprehensive tinnitus management program including counseling and sound therapy	TRT
Control	No control	No control
p Value	TSI: 0.004 Decrease in the number of subjects reporting depression: 0.02	LDL (n = 9): 0.01 LML (n = 12): 0.38 MML (n = 9): 0.16 THI (n = 32): 0.001
Conclusion	A comprehensive tinnitus management program involving education/counseling and sound therapy significantly reduces the subjective rating of tinnitus severity	TRT is effective in improving the subjective rating of tinnitus disability, and improving the dynamic range of a subset of subjects
Follow-up time	6–36 mo (mean 22 mo)	6 mo
STUDY DESIGN		
Inclusion criteria	Participation in treatment program	Not reported
Exclusion criteria	Not reported	Not reported
Randomization effectiveness	NA	NA
Age; gender	Range 17–87 y; 133 male, 57 female	Range 18–76 y; 25 male, 7 female
Masking	NA	NA
TRT regimen details	Intervention was individualized for each subject, and included education, counseling and sound therapy	Counseling and sound therapy were performed using the Jastreboff protocol [4]
Compliance	Unknown	Unknown
Criteria for withdrawal from study	NA	NA
Intention to treat analysis	NA	NA
Power	NA	Not reported
Morbidity/complications	None reported	None reported

VAS = visual analog scale, TRQ = Tinnitus Reaction Questionnaire, TSI = Tinnitus Severity Index, BDI = Beck Depression Index, THI = Tinnitus Handicap Inventory, LDL = loudness discomfort level, MML = minimal masking level, TRT = tinnitus retraining therapy, NS = not significant, NA = not applicable, RT = relaxation training.
* Sample size: numbers shown for those not lost to follow-up and those (initially recruited).

REFERENCES

1. Berry JA, Gold SL, Frederick EA, Gray WC, Staecker H. Patient-based outcomes in patients with primary tinnitus undergoing tinnitus retraining therapy. Arch Otolaryngol Head Neck Surg 2002;128(10):1153–1157.

2. Dineen R, Doyle J, Bench J, Perry A. The influence of training on tinnitus perception: an evaluation 12 months after tinnitus management training. Br J Audiol 1999;33(1):29–51.

3. Folmer RL. Long-term reductions in tinnitus severity. BMC Ear Nose Throat Disord 2002;2(1):3.

4. Jastreboff PJ, Gray WC, Gold SL. Neurophysiological approach to tinnitus patients. Am J Otol 1996;17(2):236–240.

16 Tinnitus

16.D.

Lidocaine versus placebo: Impact on loudness and annoyance of tinnitus

Carol Bauer and Alison Perring

METHODS

A computerized PubMed search of MEDLINE 1966–2004 was performed. The terms "lidocaine" and "tinnitus" were exploded and the resulting articles were cross-referenced, yielding 63 trials. These articles were then reviewed to identify those that met the following inclusion criteria: 1) evaluation of adult patients with tinnitus, 2) intervention with intravenous lidocaine versus placebo, 3) outcome measured in terms of an objective measurement of tinnitus loudness and/or validated assessment of subjective tinnitus impact, 4) randomized controlled trials. Studies in which there were no measurements of objective or subjective features of tinnitus using validated instruments were excluded. Studies using any route of administration other than intravenous were excluded.

The bibliographies of the articles that met these inclusion criteria were manually checked to ensure no further relevant articles could be identified. This process yielded six articles [1–6].

RESULTS

Outcome Measures. The effect of an intervention on the loudness and annoyance of tinnitus is a challenging outcome to study. Tinnitus is a subjective sensation that is modulated by many internal and external factors, which can be difficult to accurately identify and control. Objective outcome measures included hearing thresholds, tinnitus pitch, and loudness matching. Subjective measures of tinnitus loudness and annoyance were visual analog scales and Likert rating scales. Studies that combine both objective and subjective measures yield important information on the effects of interventions on both the sensory features as well as the emotional and cognitive impact of tinnitus.

Potential Confounders. The primary bias inherent in all the studies relates to the inability to adequately mask subjects to the lidocaine infusion. Most subjects experienced side effects during lidocaine treatment, and therefore were not blinded to the intervention. The duration of tinnitus experienced by subjects before study enrollment was large (4 months to 40 years). Inclusion of acute-onset tinnitus with chronic tinnitus may affect study outcome.

Study Designs. The data were obtained in randomized controlled trials using within-subject comparisons and repeated measures (level 1). The methods used for randomizing the order of intervention (saline versus lidocaine) were not specified in any of the studies, and therefore the possibility of inadequate randomization and blinding of subjects and investigators must be considered. All of the studies examined the acute effects of lidocaine, which is appropriate given the intravenous method of delivery. Some trials were designed to measure bidirectional changes in tinnitus and in fact showed that tinnitus was worsened by lidocaine in some cases [1, 3–6].

Highest Level of Evidence. All the trials utilized within-subject comparisons of change in tinnitus after lidocaine compared with saline infusions. The studies demonstrated a significant temporary reduction in tinnitus loudness, annoyance, and distress after lidocaine in the majority of subjects. Only short-term response to lidocaine was reported in these studies because time periods longer than 30 minutes were not studied.

Applicability. Most of the studies involved subjects with tinnitus from a variety of etiologies. The Baguley study [6] uniquely examined tinnitus in a population of subjects with tinnitus after translabyrinthine excision of acoustic neuroma. Notably, there was only a transitory positive effect, which was not sustained 20 minutes after infusion.

Morbidity/Complications. Although side effects during lidocaine infusion were frequently reported, there were no serious complications or mortality associated with the treatment. Twelve to thirty-two percent of patients experienced a transient worsening of tinnitus loudness and annoyance after lidocaine infusion.

CLINICAL SIGNIFICANCE AND FUTURE RESEARCH

There is a long history of searching for a reliable medical intervention that successfully alleviates tinnitus in the majority of patients. Although many reports documented successful use of lidocaine, even the highest level of evidence available is subject to the criticism of inadequate or incomplete blinding of subjects, which may significantly influence the reported outcomes.

Although lidocaine will not likely be a useful clinical treatment for chronic tinnitus because of the transient nature of the drug's effect, future studies with lidocaine may be useful in investigating tinnitus mechanisms that are unique for different etiologies.

THE EVIDENCE CONDENSED: The effect of intravenous lidocaine versus saline on tinnitus

Reference	Baguley, 2005	Israel, 1982	Majumdar, 1983
Level (design)	1 (RCT)	1 (RCT)	1 (RCT)
Sample size*	16	26	20
OUTCOMES			
	Subjective ratings of tinnitus loudness, pitch, and annoyance or distress		
Lidocaine results	Loudness: −5 Distress: −2	Tinnitus improved in 73%	Tinnitus improved in 65%
Placebo results	Loudness: +3 Distress: +4	Tinnitus improved in 15%	Tinnitus improved in 16%
p Value	5 min: $p < 0.05$ 20 min: NS	0.01 (χ^2)	0.01 (χ^2) for ≥20% change in VAS intensity (0–100)
Conclusion	Improved loudness, pitch, and annoyance of tinnitus after lidocaine infusion		
Follow-up time	5 min and 20 min	30 min	5 min
STUDY DESIGN			
Inclusion criteria	Translabyrinthine surgery	Any etiology and severity	Severe tinnitus
Exclusion criteria	Unknown	Unknown	Unknown
Randomization effectiveness	Injection order randomized	Injection order randomized	Injection order *not* randomized
Lidocaine regimen details	Lidocaine IV, 1.5 mg/kg administered over 5 min		
Placebo regimen details	Saline IV 1-wk separation from lidocaine infusion		Saline IV before lidocaine
Age; gender	50–66 y; 12 male, 4 female	NR; 16 male, 10 female	20–65 y
Masking	Not done	Drug infusion and data collection by separate investigators	NR
Intervention regimen details	Lidocaine and saline were administered 1 wk apart	100% experienced side effects during lidocaine infusion. Lidocaine and saline were administered 1 wk apart	Threshold was a 20% change (13/19 controls)
Diagnostic criteria for improvement	Unknown	Tinnitus improved or absent	Severity scale NS
Criteria for withdrawal from study	Unknown	Unknown	Unknown
Power	NR	NR	NR
Morbidity/complications	Loudness, pitch, and distress were worse in 12.5% after lidocaine. One subject had transient slurred speech and somnolence after lidocaine	Tinnitus worse after lidocaine in 4 of 26 subjects	NR

NR = not reported, NA = not applicable, RCT = randomized controlled trial, VAS = visual analog scale, IV = intravenous.
* Sample size: numbers shown for those not lost to follow-up and those (initially recruited).

THE EVIDENCE CONDENSED: The effect of intravenous lidocaine versus saline on tinnitus

Reference	Duckert, 1983	Martin, 1980	Hulshof, 1984
Level (design)	1 (RCT)	1 (RCT)	1 (RCT)
Sample size*	50	32 (34)	22
OUTCOMES			
	Subjective ratings of tinnitus loudness, and objective measures of tinnitus loudness		Likert scales rating tinnitus disturbance
Lidocaine results	Tinnitus improved in 40% and worsened in 32%	Tinnitus improved in 78%	Tinnitus improved in 82%
Placebo results	Tinnitus improved in 20% and worsened in 0%	Tinnitus improved in 12.5%	Tinnitus improved in 22%
p Value	0.001 (χ^2) for 20% change in VAS intensity (−100 to 0 to +100)	0.05 (χ^2) 0.05 (t-test) 0.001 (McNemar's)	0.002, Fisher's test
Conclusion	Improved loudness, pitch, and annoyance of tinnitus after lidocaine infusion		
Follow-up time	5 min	5 min	5 min
STUDY DESIGN			
Inclusion criteria	Any etiology and severity		
Exclusion criteria	Medical contraindication	Medical contraindication	Unknown
Randomization effectiveness	Injection order randomized		Injection order randomized Method unknown
Lidocaine regimen details	Lidocaine 100 mg administered over 3 min	Lidocaine 2% 1.5 mg/kg	Lidocaine 1.5 mg/kg
Placebo regimen details	Saline IV	Saline IV	Saline IV after lidocaine
Age; gender	Range 19–65 y; 45 male, 5 female	Range 19–70 y; 17 male, 15 female	20–67 y; 11 male, 11 female
Masking	Subjects were masked	Subjects were masked	NR
Intervention regimen details	Equal volumes of saline and lidocaine were administered on the same day	Saline and lidocaine injections were performed on the same day	82% experienced side effects during lidocaine infusion. There was an injection order effect on response
Diagnostic criteria for improvement	Threshold for change was 25%	NR	NR
Criteria for withdrawal from study	NR	NR	NA
Power	NR	NR	NR
Morbidity/complications	32% reported worse tinnitus after lidocaine	Loudness increased in 6% after lidocaine	Loudness increased in 1 of 11 subjects after lidocaine

NR = not reported, NA = not applicable, RCT = randomized controlled trial, VAS = visual analog scale, IV = intravenous.
* Sample size: numbers shown for those not lost to follow-up and those (initially recruited).

REFERENCES

1. Martin FW, Colman BH. Tinnitus: a double-blind crossover controlled trial to evaluate the use of lignocaine. Clin Otolaryngol Allied Sci 1980;5(1):3–11.
2. Majumdar B, Mason SM, Gibbin KP. An electrocochleographic study of the effects of lignocaine on patients with tinnitus. Clin Otolaryngol Allied Sci 1983;8(3):175–180.
3. Israel JM, Connelly JS, McTigue ST, Brumme RE, Brown J. Lidocaine in the treatment of tinnitus aurium. A double-blind study. Arch Otolaryngol 1982;108(8):471–473.
4. Hulshof JH, Vermeij P. The effect of intravenous lidocaine and several different doses of oral tocainide HCl on tinnitus. A dose-finding study. Acta Otolaryngol 1984;98(3–4):231–238.
5. Duckert LG, Rees TS. Treatment of tinnitus with intravenous lidocaine: a double-blind randomized trial. Otolaryngol Head Neck Surg 1983;91(5):550–555.
6. Baguley DM, Jones S, Wilkins I, Axon PR, Moffat DA. The inhibitory effect of intravenous lidocaine infusion on tinnitus after translabyrinthine removal of vestibular schwannoma: a double-blind, placebo-controlled, crossover study. Otol Neurotol 2005;26(2):169–176.

17 Bell's Palsy

17.A.

Systemic steroids alone versus placebo: Impact on recovery to normal or near-normal function

Mark Syms and Mitchell Ramsey

METHODS

A computerized Ovid search of MEDLINE 1966–2005 was performed. The terms "facial paralysis" and "Bell's palsy" were exploded, resulting in 1043 articles. These results were limited to English language and therapy-related subheadings yielding 293 trials, which were reviewed. Trials evaluating steroid treatment were reviewed to identify those that met inclusion criteria consisting of: 1) patients with Bell's palsy (idiopathic facial nerve paralysis), 2) intervention with systemic steroids, 3) treatment within 10 days of onset, 4) outcome measures consisting of normal motor facial recovery [House-Brackmann (HB) or similar scale]. Exclusion criteria included: 1) trials including multiple etiologies of facial paralysis, 2) multiple interventions, 3) treatment initiated after 10 days of onset. The references of these articles were then reviewed and manually cross-checked to ensure all applicable literature was reviewed. This search yielded five randomized controlled trials (RCTs) [1–5] and four systematic reviews [6–9] that met inclusion criteria.

RESULTS

Outcome Measures. The primary outcome measures included: 1) recovery of facial motor function to normal/near normal, and 2) incidence of complications of steroid treatment. The most frequently used assessment tool for facial recovery is the HB system [10]. In this system, a HB grade I–II represents normal or near-normal function, or good recovery. A more detailed analysis of facial recovery was not possible because of trial variations and the lack of stratification. Only one trial [2] stratified recovery based on severity of impairment. Stratification is relevant because recovery is better in incomplete paralysis; 94% of patients with paresis have full recovery compared with 61% of patients with complete paralysis [11]. Other outcome measures including time to recovery, synkinesis, or crocodile tears (gustolacrimal reflex) were not assessed.

Potential Confounders. Three possible confounding factors between studies include diagnostic certainty, steroid dose, and facial assessment. Bell's palsy is a diagnosis of exclusion. It is possible that other etiologies of facial paralysis may have been included in the study population; however, all RCTs have sufficient exclusion criteria that make this unlikely. The dose of steroids administered varied widely among the RCTs. One trial administered a total prednisone equivalent dose of 200 mg [1], another 410 mg [2], and a third 4500 mg [5]. Lastly, the assessment method of facial motor recovery varied among trials. In one trial, the method of motor recovery assessment was based on the clinical examination and considered complete or partial, but not otherwise detailed [1] whereas another divided patients into complete return, fair return, and poor return [2]. Despite these variations, it seems that a "successful" outcome (meaning recovery to normal) for the RCTs was comparable.

Study Designs. All five RCTs reported effective randomization of the study population. Two trials were double blinded [2, 5] and one single blinded [1]. Two trials were of lesser quality [3, 4] because they were not blinded and they did not have a placebo-treated control group. The follow-up period was adequate for four trials (6 months minimum), but only 2–3 months for the last [1]. Trial size was small for the majority of RCTs. No trial calculated *a priori* sample size. Only one of the trials [2] provided outcome stratification based on severity of facial dysfunction. Details of the methods and outcomes of the RCTs are listed in the table "Systemic steroids versus placebo, randomized controlled trials."

The four meta-analyses used typical methods for analyzing data, assessing homogeneity, and pooling results. Review of the meta-analyses demonstrated mild methodology differences, which produced variations in trial inclusion and exclusion. One systematic review [8] included a trial that had unclear methodology [12] and two systematic reviews [6, 8] included an RCT with 71% completion rate [13]. In the fourth review [7], the authors limited the analysis to the treatment effect of steroids on patients with complete paralysis. This review included one RCT with 71% completion rate [13] and one non-randomized prospective trial [14].

Highest Level of Evidence and Study Results. Five trials were evaluated as level 1 trials, but two were considered lesser quality because of potential bias from lack of blinding [3, 4]. No single RCT demonstrated a statistically significant improvement in recovery with steroid treatment compared with the control group; furthermore, none was adequately powered. No trial demonstrated any significant adverse effects resulting from treatment. One trial demonstrated a favorable difference with treatment in the clinical evolution represented by an early worsening of facial strength in the control group [5]. A statistically significant difference in recovery was present at 1 month; however, at 12 months no difference existed. Because the power of individual trials is in question, these studies may fail to uncover any difference that may truly exist.

Four meta-analyses from systematic reviews were assessed. Three of the reviews included all grades of facial impairment in their analysis [6, 8, 9]. One found no benefit [9] and two [6, 8] found evidence of a possible positive treatment effect. The fourth review assessed only patients with complete paralysis and demonstrated a possible benefit with treatment [7]. Each meta-analysis and the trials included in them are listed in the table "Systemic steroids versus placebo, meta-analyses." The variations in their inclusion criteria, as well as the selection of lower quality trials in the three reviews showing possible benefit, limits the collective interpretation of their findings.

Applicability. Based on the inclusion and exclusion criteria of these trials, the population studied likely consisted of patients with Bell's palsy or idiopathic facial nerve paralysis. Bell's palsy has an acute onset of unilateral lower motor neuron facial motor paresis or paralysis not associated with other otologic, neurologic, traumatic, or systemic disease. The results of this review should be applied to patients with Bell's palsy.

Morbidity/Complications. No trial indicated significant complications associated with steroid use. The only quantified side effect of steroids was temporary sleep disturbance noted in 3 of 30 patients [5].

CLINICAL SIGNIFICANCE AND FUTURE RESEARCH

Five RCTs evaluated the effect of steroid treatment for Bell's palsy by comparing systemic steroids against placebo or no treatment. No RCT demonstrated a statistically significant treatment benefit in facial motor recovery. Four systematic reviews with meta-analyses have been performed. Three suggest a possible benefit, and one does not. The four reviews are inconsistent and demonstrate methodologic variation. Although some evidence suggests steroids may be effective, the collective available evidence is moderate and lacks uniformity. A definitive treatment effect remains unproven.

Additional research is necessary to determine the efficacy of steroids. Trial design will require adequate sample size and stratification. Working from the available natural history data, if a 10% difference in the rate of complete recovery is expected, each control and treatment arm will need 310 patients (Fisher's exact test, two-tailed analyses, with significance level of 0.05 and power of 80%). If a larger effect is expected, i.e., 20%, then the numbers in each arm decrease to 71 (Fisher's exact test, two-tailed analyses, with significance level of 0.05 and power of 80%). Future studies need clear stratification based on degree of pretreatment dysfunction, or at the very least stratification into incomplete and complete categories.

THE EVIDENCE CONDENSED: Systemic steroids versus placebo, randomized controlled trials

Reference	Taverner, 1954	May, 1976
Level (design)	1 (randomized controlled trial)	1 (randomized controlled trial)
Sample size*	26 total; 14 in treatment group, and 12 in control group (initial recruitment 26)	51 total; 25 in treatment group and 26 in control group (initial recruitment 51)
OUTCOMES		
Steroid group Complete recovery/total in group	n = 10/14	n = 15/25
Control group Complete recovery/total in group	n = 8/12	n = 17/26
OR (95% CI)†	1.25 (0.25–6.21)	0.79 (0.26–2.43)
RR (95% CI)†	1.07 (0.67–1.73)	0.92 (0.61–1.39)
Chi-square Mantel-Haenszel p value†	$p = 0.797$	$p = 0.69$
Results of treatment on facial motor recovery to HB grade I/II	No difference	No difference
Stratification	No	No
Follow-up time	2–3 mo	3 wk, then monthly until 6 mo
STUDY DESIGN		
Inclusion criteria	Unilateral peripheral facial paralysis, other etiologies ruled out; evaluated within 10 d	Unilateral peripheral facial paralysis; evaluated within 2 d
Exclusion criteria	Evidence of otologic or CNS disease	Otologic, neurologic, neoplastic, or traumatic causes. History of familial or recurrent disease
Randomization effectiveness	Good. Master sheet	Good. Biostatistician designed
Age	12–75 y, mean 40 y	Not reported
Steroid regimen details	Cortisone 200 mg ×3 d, 100 mg ×3 d, 50 mg ×2 d. Total dose 1 g	Prednisone 410 mg in descending dose over 10 d
Control regimen details	Lactose	Vitamin
Diagnostic evaluation	History and physical examination, EMG	History and physical examination
Compliance	100%	100%
Criteria for withdrawal from study	Not reported	Not reported
Intention to treat analysis	Not reported	Not reported
Stratification	No	Partial
Method of facial assessment	Clinical, not otherwise detailed	Recovery was graded as complete, fair, or poor
Power	Not reported	Not reported
Morbidity/complications	Not reported	Not reported

OR = odds ratio, RR = relative risk, CNS = central nervous system, EMG = electromyography.
* Sample size: numbers are those completing trial and (initially recruited).
† These values were generated using the data for the primary outcome measure of normal/near-normal facial motor recovery.

THE EVIDENCE CONDENSED: Systemic steroids versus placebo/control, randomized controlled trials

Reference	Lagalla, 2002
Level (design)	1 (randomized controlled trial)
Sample size*	58 total; 30 in treatment group and 28 in control group (initial recruitment 62)

OUTCOMES	
Steroid group Complete recovery/total in group	n = 25/30
Control group Complete recovery/total in group	n = 21/28
OR (95% CI)†	1.667 (0.48–5.75)
RR (95% CI)†	1.111 (0.86–1.39)
Chi-square Mantel-Haenszel p value†	p = 0.438
Results of treatment on facial motor recovery to HB grade I/II	No long-term difference. An early worsening of motor strength was noted without treatment (p = 0.008) but did not persist over the longer term. Also, time to recovery was better in treatment group (p = 0.005)
Stratification	No
Follow-up time	1 wk, then at 1, 3, 6, and 12 mo

STUDY DESIGN	
Inclusion criteria	Unilateral peripheral facial paralysis; evaluated within 3 d
Exclusion criteria	Otologic or other disease causing facial paralysis. Prior treatment, presentation >3 d, pregnancy, peptic ulcer disease, hypertension, or diabetes
Randomization effectiveness	Potential confounders appear balanced between groups. Performed with random number list
Age	15–84 y, mean 47.5 y
Steroid regimen details	Intravenous prednisone, 1 g daily for 3 d then 0.5 g daily for 3 d with intramuscular polyvitamin therapy over 15 d
Control regimen details	Polyvitaminic therapy
Diagnostic evaluation	History and physical examination, MRI or CT, IgM and IgG antibodies against multiple infectious agents
Compliance	100%
Criteria for withdrawal from study	Positive titers for other infectious causes (4 with herpes zoster excluded)
Intention to treat analysis	Yes
Stratification	No
Method of facial assessment	House-Brackmann system
Power	Not reported
Morbidity/complications	3/32 patients had temporary sleep disturbances.

OR = odds ratio, RR = relative risk, MRI = magnetic resonance imaging, CT = computed tomography, Ig = immunoglobulin.
* Sample size: numbers shown for those not lost to follow-up and those (initially recruited).
† These values were calculated from the data for the primary outcome measure of normal/near normal facial motor recovery.

Reference	Unuvar, 1999	Wolf, 1978
Level (design)	1 (randomized, untreated control group, nonblinded)	1 (randomized, untreated control group, nonblinded)
Sample size*	42 total; 21 in treatment group, and 21 in control group (initial recruitment 42)	239 total; 107 in treatment group, and 132 in control group (initial recruitment 239)
OUTCOMES		
Steroid group Complete recovery/total in group	n = 21/21	n = 94/107
Control group Complete recovery/total in group	n = 21/21	n = 106/132
OR (95% CI)†	1.0 (0.43–2.34)	1.774 (0.87–3.61)
RR (95% CI)†	1.0 (0.65–1.53)	1.094 (0.97–1.20)
Chi-square Mantel-Haenszel p value†	NS	p = 0.117
Results of treatment on facial motor recovery to HB grade I/II	No difference	No difference. A significant difference was noted in the control group for autonomic synkinesis (p < 0.01)
Stratification	No	No
Follow-up time	21 d; 4, 6, and 12 mo	Monthly until full recovery or 1 y
STUDY DESIGN		
Inclusion criteria	Severe unilateral peripheral facial paralysis (HB grade IV–V); evaluated within 3 d	Severe unilateral peripheral facial paralysis; evaluated within 5 d
Exclusion criteria	Otologic, neurologic, or chronic systemic diseases, contraindication to steroid treatment	Otologic, traumatic, neoplasm, disease or evidence of herpes zoster oticus Contraindication to steroid treatment
Randomization effectiveness	Potential confounders appear balanced between groups. Performed with computer randomization	No statistical difference between groups
Age	(Pediatric study) 24–74 mo. Mean age 46.9 mo	5–70 y
Steroid regimen details	Methylprednisolone 1 mg/kg/d ×10 d then 3–5 d taper	Prednisone 60 mg/d ×10 d, then 40 mg/d ×2, then 20 mg/d ×2, then 10 mg/d ×1 d
Control regimen details	No placebo	No placebo
Diagnostic evaluation	History and physical examination	History and physical examination. EMG and nerve latency testing. Blood sugar testing
Compliance	100%	100%
Criteria for withdrawal from study	Not reported	Not reported
Intention to treat analysis	Not reported	Not reported
Stratification	All patients had complete or near-complete paralysis	No
Method of facial assessment	House-Brackmann system	Paralysis was rated as none, mild, moderate, or severe (complete)
Power	Not reported	Not reported
Morbidity/complications	No complications of steroid treatment	No complications of steroid treatment

OR = odds ratio, RR = relative risk, MRI = magnetic resonance imaging, CT = computed tomography, Ig = immunoglobulin, NS = not significant.
* Sample size: numbers shown for those not lost to follow-up and those (initially recruited).
† These values were calculated from the data for the primary outcome measure of normal/near normal facial motor recovery.

THE EVIDENCE CONDENSED: Systemic steroids versus placebo, meta-analyses

Reference	Grogan, 2001	Salinas, 2004	Williamson, 1996	Ramsey, 2000
Level (design)	Meta-analysis	Meta-analysis	Meta-analysis	Meta-analysis
Included trials	1. May 2. Taverner 3. Brown 4. Austin	1. May 2. Lagalla 3. Taverner 4. Unuvar	1. Taverner 2. May 3. Wolf 4. Austin	1. May 2. Austin 3. Shafshak
Pooled OR (95% CI)	1.16 (1.05–1.29)	Not reported	1.63 (Mantel-Haenszel method) (1.01–2.64)	3.27 (0.76–14.10)
Relative Risk (95% CI)	Not reported	0.86 (0.47–1.59)	Not reported	0.17 (rate difference) (0.01–0.32)
Treatment results	Possibly effective	No evidence for effect	Possibly effective	Possibly effective
Methodology highlights	Includes Brown and Austin	None	Includes Wolf and Austin	Includes Shafshak and Austin

OR = odds ratio, CI = confidence interval.

REFERENCES

1. Taverner D. Cortisone treatment of Bell's palsy. Lancet 1954;2:1052–1054.
2. May M, Wette R, Hardin WB Jr, Sullivan J. The use of steroids in Bell's palsy: a prospective controlled study. Laryngoscope 1976;86(8):1111–1122.
3. Wolf SM, Wagner JH, et al. Treatment of Bell palsy with prednisone: a prospective, randomized study. Neurology 1978;28(2):158–161.
4. Unuvar E, Oguz F, et al. Corticosteroid treatment of childhood Bell's palsy. Pediatr Neurol 1999;21(5):814–816.
5. Lagalla G, Logullo F, et al. Influence of early high-dose steroid treatment on Bell's palsy evolution. Neurol Sci 2002;23(3):107–112.
6. Williamson IG, Whelan TR. The clinical problem of Bell's palsy: is treatment with steroids effective? Br J Gen Pract 1996;46(413):743–747.
7. Ramsey MJ, DerSimonian R, et al. Corticosteroid treatment for idiopathic facial nerve paralysis: a meta-analysis. Laryngoscope 2000;110(3 Pt 1):335–341.
8. Grogan PM, Gronseth GS. Practice parameter: steroids, acyclovir, and surgery for Bell's palsy (an evidence-based review): report of the Quality Standards Subcommittee of the American Academy of Neurology. Neurology 2001;56(7):830–836.
9. Salinas R, Alvarez G, et al. Corticosteroids for Bell's palsy (idiopathic facial paralysis). Cochrane Database Syst Rev 2004;(4):CD001942.
10. House JW, Brackmann DE. Facial nerve grading system. Otolaryngol Head Neck Surg 1985;93(2):146–147.
11. Peitersen E. Bell's palsy: the spontaneous course of 2,500 peripheral facial nerve palsies of different etiologies. Acta Otolaryngol Suppl 2002;(549):4–30.
12. Brown JS. Bell's palsy: a 5 year review of 174 consecutive cases—an attempted double blind study. Laryngoscope 1982;92(12):1369–1373.
13. Austin JR, Peskind SP, et al. Idiopathic facial nerve paralysis: a randomized double blind controlled study of placebo versus prednisone. Laryngoscope 1993;103(12):1326–1333.
14. Shafshak TS, Essa AY, et al. The possible contributing factors for the success of steroid therapy in Bell's palsy: a clinical and electrophysiological study. J Laryngol Otol 1994;108(11):940–943.

17 Bell's Palsy

Antiviral therapy versus control: Impact on recovery to normal or near-normal function

Mitchell Ramsey and Mark Syms

METHODS

A computerized Ovid search of MEDLINE 1966–2005 was performed. The terms "facial paralysis" and "Bell's palsy" were exploded, resulting in 1043 articles. This group was then limited to English language and therapy-related subheadings yielding 293 trials, which were reviewed. Trials evaluating antiviral treatment were reviewed to identify inclusion criteria which consisted of: 1) patient's with Bell's palsy (idiopathic facial nerve paralysis), 2) intervention with antiviral medication, 3) treatment initiated within 10 days of onset, 4) outcome measures consisting of normal motor facial recovery [House-Brackmann (HB) or similar scale]. Exclusion criteria included: 1) trials including multiple etiologies of facial paralysis, 2) treatment initiated after 10 days of onset. The references of these articles were then reviewed and manually cross-checked to ensure all applicable literature was reviewed. This search produced two randomized controlled trials (RCTs) [1, 2] and one retrospective review [3].

RESULTS

Outcome Measures. The primary outcome measures were: 1) recovery of facial motor function to normal/near normal, and 2) incidence of complications of antiviral or steroid treatment. Any scale or measure that indicated recovery to normal was accepted. The most frequently used scale is the HB system [4]. An HB grade I–II represents normal or near-normal function, or good recovery. A more detailed analysis of recovery could not be performed because stratified outcomes were not reported. Other outcome measures including time to recovery, synkinesis, or crocodile tears (gustolacrimal reflex) were not evaluated.

Potential Confounders. Both RCTs used acyclovir with similar dose and duration. There was a difference in severity of facial motor dysfunction: one trial had a 20% incidence of complete paralysis whereas the other had a 1% incidence. Neither trial indicated existing comorbidities affecting neural function.

Study Designs. Both RCTs were effectively randomized with similarly matched treatment and control groups. One trial did have a significant randomization difference for hypertension but further analysis showed no differ-

ence in outcomes [2]. One RCT compared steroid and acyclovir versus steroid alone [1]. The other RCT compared acyclovir to prednisone [2]. One RCT is clearly double blinded [1], but the level of masking in the other trial is unclear [2]. Neither trial calculated *a priori* sample size or provided outcome stratification based on severity of facial dysfunction. Both trials used steroid treatment rather than placebo in the control group.

Highest Level of Evidence. Two level 1 RCTs were identified [1, 2]. One RCT compared steroid and acyclovir against steroid with placebo [1], whereas the other compared acyclovir alone to steroid alone [2]. One RCT demonstrated a statistically significant benefit in favor of the acyclovir–prednisone group over the placebo–prednisone group (p = 0.02) [1]. The rate of complete facial recovery (FPRP10) was 92% for the treatment group (acyclovir–prednisone) and 76% for the control group (placebo–prednisone). In contrast, the other RCT demonstrated a beneficial effect for the steroid-only group over the acyclovir-only group [2]. Their data showed that the incidence of complete recovery (graded by HB scale and FPRP) was statistically significant in favor of steroid treatment.

Applicability. Based on the inclusion and exclusion criteria of these trials, the population studied likely consists of patients with Bell's palsy or idiopathic facial nerve paralysis. Bell's palsy is an acute onset of unilateral lower motor neuron facial motor paresis or paralysis not associated with other otologic, neurologic, traumatic, or systemic disease. Bell's palsy, idiopathic facial nerve paralysis, is considered a virally mediated inflammation. If this is the etiology of Bell's palsy, then antiviral medications may have an impact on the recovery of patients.

Morbidity/Complications. Neither RCT reported complications association with treatment. One trial noted that gastrointestinal complaints were the most common, but no data were provided [1]. Both prednisone and acyclovir seemed to be associated with a low incidence of serious side effects in these trials.

CLINICAL SIGNIFICANCE AND FUTURE RESEARCH

Two RCTs evaluating acyclovir for Bell's palsy were reviewed. The first trial demonstrated a statistically significant treatment benefit with acyclovir–prednisone therapy compared with prednisone–placebo [1]. The second trial found a statistically significant treatment benefit with prednisone therapy compared with acyclovir [2]. Methodology variations prevent a meta-analysis. The design differences also limit comparison of the trials to substantiate their outcomes. The data support that steroids combined with acyclovir are more effective than steroids alone, and that steroids are more effective than antivirals alone in improving outcomes in patients with Bell's palsy. However, a direct comparison of acyclovir to placebo was not performed; therefore, no recommendation can be made regarding the use of acyclovir as a sole agent for Bell's palsy.

Considering the prevailing concept that Bell's palsy is a virally mediated condition, further research is warranted to confirm this and determine the treatment effect of antiviral medication. In light of the first section of this chapter, which does not show indisputable evidence for a beneficial treatment effect with steroids, future research should involve a well-designed RCT with at least one arm designed to compare antiviral medication to placebo.

THE EVIDENCE CONDENSED: Antiviral treatment of Bell's palsy

Reference	Adour, 1996		De Diego, 1998	
Level (design)	1 (randomized controlled trial)		1 (randomized controlled trial)	
Sample size	99 total patients; 53 in acyclovir–prednisone group (treatment) and 46 patients in placebo–prednisone group (control). 20 patients lost from trial (Initial recruitment 119)		101 total patients; 54 patients in acyclovir group (treatment) and 47 patients in prednisone group (control) (Initial recruitment 113)	
OUTCOMES				
Antiviral group Complete recovery/total in group	Acyclovir–prednisone	n = 49/53	Acyclovir	n = 42/54
Control group Complete recovery/total in group	Placebo–prednisone	n = 35/46	Prednisone	n = 44/47
Comparative results	92% of patients in steroid group recovered to an FPRP of 10 (HB grade I) compared with 76% in the acyclovir group		93.6% of patients in steroid group recovered to HB grade II or better compared with 77.7% in the acyclovir group	
p Value	Recovery in the acyclovir–prednisone group was significantly better than the placebo–prednisone group ($p = 0.02$)		Recovery in the steroid group was significantly better than the acyclovir group ($p = 0.0016$)	
OR (95% CI)	3.85 (1.18–12.39)		0.239 (0.068–0.852)	
RR (95% CI)	1.22 (1.03–1.36)		0.831 (0.760–0.977)	
Chi-square Mantel-Haenszel p value*	0.02		0.026	
Follow-up time	To recovery or 4 mo		Minimum of 3 mo	
STUDY DESIGN				
Inclusion criteria	Peripheral facial paralysis, ≥18 y, treatment started within 3 d, without contraindications to steroid treatment		Peripheral facial paralysis of acute onset evaluated within 4 d without contraindication to steroid treatment	
Exclusion criteria	Contraindication to steroid treatment, pregnancy, l < 18 y old, evaluation >3 d after onset		Associated middle ear disease, cranial or otologic trauma, known neurologic disorders, autoimmune disease, tumors, and herpes zoster oticus. Contraindication to steroid treatment	
Randomization effectiveness	Potential confounders appear balanced between groups		Incidence of hypertension was found to be statistically different between the 2 groups; however, there was no difference in recovery between groups	
Age	Average 41.9 y (acyclovir–prednisone) 46 y (placebo–prednisone)		Ranged from 14 to 85 y with average of 43 y	
Masking	Double blinded		Unclear if double blinded	
Antiviral regimen details	Acyclovir: 2000 mg ×10 d Prednisone 30 mg (minimum) b.i.d. ×5 d, with taper to 10 mg q.d. over 5 more days		Acyclovir 800 mg t.i.d. for 10 d (2400 mg) vs prednisone 1 mg/kg/d ×10 d with taper over 6 d	
Control regimen details	This group received a placebo with above steroid dose		Prednisone was prescribed as a single daily dose of 1 mg/kg for 10 d, and then tapered over the next 6 d	
Diagnostics	History and physical examination, electrophysiology		History and physical examination	
Compliance	Loss of 20 patients, 17%		Loss of 12 patients, 11%	
Withdrawal criteria	Not reported		Not reported	
Intention to treat analysis	Not reported		Not reported	
Morbidity/complications	GI complaints were most frequently reported. None required treatment		23.4% of prednisone patients, and 24.1% of acyclovir patients had sequelae not otherwise specified	

FPRP = facial paralysis recovery profile (a score of 10 is equivalent to normal facial function [5]), HB = House-Brackmann, OR = odds ratio, CI = confidence interval, b.i.d. = twice a day, t.i.d. = three times a day, q.d. = one time per day, GI = gastrointestinal.

REFERENCES

1. Adour KK, Ruboyianes JM, Von Doersten PG, Byl FM, Trent CS, Quesenberry CP Jr, Hitchcock T. Bell's palsy treatment with acyclovir and prednisone compared with prednisone alone: a double-blind, randomized, controlled trial. Ann Otol Rhinol Laryngol 1996;105(5):371–378.
2. De Diego JI, Prim M P, et al. Idiopathic facial paralysis: a randomized, prospective, and controlled study using single-dose prednisone versus acyclovir three times daily. Laryngoscope 1998;108(4 Pt 1):573–575.
3. Hato N, Matsumoto S, et al. Efficacy of early treatment of Bell's palsy with oral acyclovir and prednisolone. Otol Neurotol 2003;24(6):948–951.
4. House JW, Brackmann DE. Facial nerve grading system. Otolaryngol Head Neck Surg 1985;93(2):146–147.
5. Adour KK, Wingerd J, et al. Prednisone treatment for idiopathic facial paralysis (Bell's palsy). N Engl J Med 1972; 287(25):1268–1272.

17 Bell's Palsy

17.C.

Facial nerve decompression: Impact on recovery to normal or near-normal function

Mitchell Ramsey and Mark Syms

METHODS

A computerized Ovid search of MEDLINE 1966–2004 was performed. The terms "facial paralysis" and "Bell's palsy" were exploded, resulting in 1043 articles. This group was limited to therapy-related subheadings yielding 293 trials that were reviewed to identify trials involving surgical decompression. Articles were reviewed to identify inclusion criteria which consisted of: 1) patients with Bell's palsy (idiopathic facial nerve paralysis), 2) surgical decompression of the meatal foramen, labyrinthine segment, and geniculate ganglion of the facial nerve, 3) treatment initiated within 14 days of onset of paralysis, 4) outcome measures consisting of facial recovery [House-Brackmann (HB) or similar scale]. Exclusion criteria included: 1) trials including multiple etiologies of facial paralysis, 2) treatment initiated after 14 days of onset. The references of these articles were then reviewed and manually cross-checked to ensure all applicable literature was reviewed. This search produced no randomized control trials and one level 2 study.

RESULTS

Outcome Measures. The primary outcome measures included 1) recovery of facial motor function to normal (HB grades I–II), and 2) incidence of surgical complications.

Potential Confounders. The treatment and control groups were well matched. Potential confounding factors include variations in surgical technique and extent of decompression. This trial was conducted at multiple centers and some variation probably existed but it seems to be minimal. Inclusion criteria were stringent and it is unlikely that major variation in severity of facial nerve dysfunction existed within and between the groups. The study was nonblinded and this may be considered a source of bias.

Study Design. Patients were offered surgical decompression if they met inclusion criteria. The treatment was not randomized and patients self-selected surgical decompression or medical treatment. The study was performed at multiple sites. Initially, 14 sites were selected to participate in the study. Only three centers entered patients. The study was initiated in 1982 and the results were published in 1999. Initially, decompression was performed within 3 weeks of onset of paralysis. A few years into the study, the time was changed to 2 weeks. Data are only considered for the patients decompressed within 2 weeks.

Highest Level of Evidence. The best evidence available is a level 2 nonrandomized, prospective cohort study [1]. This study had a control group that self-selected for steroid treatment. Patients were treated with prednisone 80 mg per day for 7 days then rapidly tapered over days 8 through 14 (comparable dose to many other steroid trials). The control and surgical group were matched in terms of severity of facial paralysis and age. None of the control group and only two from the surgical group had diabetes. Follow-up time was a minimum of 7 months. *A priori* calculation of sample size necessary to achieve an adequate power was not performed; however, using the available outcome data from the study, to achieve a power of 90% ($p \leq 0.05$) a sample size of 21 patients in each arm is necessary (see table: "Surgical decompression versus steroid therapy").

Study Results. Individuals with Bell's palsy who have $\geq 90\%$ degeneration demonstrated by electroneuronography (ENoG) within 14 days of onset of total paralysis, who have no motor unit potentials on voluntary electromyogram (EMG), and undergo decompression of the meatal foramen, labyrinthine segments, and the geniculate ganglion, have a 91% chance of recovery to an HB grade I or II 7 months after paralysis. Those patients with the same ENoG and EMG parameters who are treated with steroids only have a 42% chance of an HB grade I or II. This difference was found to be statistically significant ($p = 0.0002$). Refer to table "Surgical decompression compared with steroid treatment" for details.

Applicability. The study applies to patients with Bell's palsy who have therapy initiated within the first 2 weeks of onset. It is important to understand that these results were obtained by very experienced surgeons.

Morbidity/Complications. Of the 19 patients treated at the primary center, one patient had a conductive hearing loss and one patient had a cerebrospinal fluid leak treated with a lumbar drain. There were no dead ears, intracranial complications, or other surgical morbidity in the surgical groups.

CLINICAL SIGNIFICANCE AND FUTURE RESEARCH

The surgical management of Bell's palsy has been a source of controversy for many years. Many confounding factors have limited our understanding of the role of surgery. One prospective trial evaluating decompression of the facial nerve including the labyrinthine segment demonstrated a statistically and clinically significant improvement in the appropriately selected patients [1]. This was a multicentered trial with strict inclusion and exclusion criteria. A steroid control group with similar severity of facial paralysis was analyzed for outcome comparison. The authors found that surgical decompression results in improved facial motor recovery. The rate difference, or absolute risk reduction, demonstrates a 49% improvement in facial recovery with surgical decompression compared with steroid treatment (95% confidence interval 0.29–0.60). The series reported a low complication rate, noting one episode of conductive hearing loss and one episode of cerebrospinal fluid leak. It is also relevant to point out that these results come from very experienced surgeons. Based on these results, surgical decompression probably improves facial recovery in the appropriately selected patients.

The best evidence of surgical efficacy is a prospective nonrandomized, nonblinded trial. Additional research to confirm these results would be ideal. However, higher-quality research is unlikely because of the obvious limitations and difficulty in developing a randomized, placebo-controlled, double-blinded study with a surgical arm. In addition, the proportion of Bell's palsy patients likely benefiting from surgery is small and a prolonged multicenter trial would be necessary to reevaluate the impact of surgical therapy.

THE EVIDENCE CONDENSED: Surgical decompression versus steroid therapy

Reference	Gantz, 1999		
Level (design)	2 (prospective, nonrandomized, controlled, nonblinded)		
Sample size*	70 total, 34 in surgical group, and 36 in steroid group		
Intervention	Surgical decompression vs steroid		
OUTCOMES			
Surgical group HB I–II	HB I, n = 14	HB II, n = 17	HB I–II, n = 31
Surgical group HB III–IV	HB III, n = 2	HB IV, n = 1	HB III–IV, n = 3
Control group HB I–II	HB I, n = 5	HB II, n = 10	HB I–II, n = 15
Control group HB III–IV	HB III, n = 19	HB IV, n = 2	HB III–IV, n = 21
Follow-up time	Minimum of 7 mo		
Conclusion p value	Surgical group had a significantly higher proportion of patients recovering to an HB grade I or II. p = 0.0002		
STUDY DESIGN			
Inclusion criteria	Complete paralysis, >90% degeneration on ENoG, no voluntary motor unit EMG, <14 days after onset		
Exclusion criteria	<90% degeneration on ENoG or voluntary EMG response		
Pretreatment group comparison	Preintervention comparison of treatment and control group not provided		
Age	Treatment group mean age 47 y Control group mean age 32 y		
Masking	No		
Surgical regimen	Middle cranial fossa facial nerve decompression		
Control regimen	Prednisone 80 mg ×7 d then tapered over next 7 d		
Diagnostics	History and physical examination, blood sugar and sedimentation rate, audiogram, ENoG, and EMG. Imaging for surgical group		
Surgical complications	1 episode of conductive hearing loss, 1 cerebrospinal fluid leak		
Intention to treat analysis	Not stated		
Morbidity/complications	No data regarding complications of steroid treatment provided		

HB = House-Brackmann, ENoG = electroneuronography, EMG = electromyogram.
* Sample size: numbers shown for those not lost to follow-up and those (initially recruited).

REFERENCE

1. Gantz BJ, Rubinstein JT, Gidley P, Woodworth GG. Surgical management of Bell's palsy. Laryngoscope 1999;109(8): 1177–1188.

18 Perioperative Antibiotics for Otologic Surgery

18.A.

Perioperative systemic antibiotics versus control for myringoplasty: Impact on surgical site infections, graft success

Jennifer J. Shin and Marlene Durand

METHODS

A computerized PubMed search of MEDLINE 1966–November 2004 was performed. Articles mapping to any of the following medical subject headings were exploded and combined: "antibiotic prophylaxis," "antibacterial agents," "lactams," "fluoroquinolones," "macrolides," "clindamycin." These articles were then cross-referenced with those mapping to either the exploded medical subject heading "myringoplasty" or textword "myringoplasty." This process yielded 21 trials. These articles were then reviewed to identify those that met the following inclusion criteria: 1) a distinct patient population undergoing myringoplasty alone, 2) intervention with perioperative systemic antibiotics versus placebo or other no-antibiotic control, 3) outcome measured in terms of postoperative surgical site infections[1] and/or graft success, 4) randomized controlled trials (RCTs). The outcome of graft success was considered relevant because SSIs have been correlated with graft failure. Articles in which the use of randomization was not clearly specified were excluded. Articles were excluded here if specific data from myringoplasties could not be extracted because it was grouped with data from other procedures, but those articles are discussed in Section 19.D. Studies of patients undergoing tympanoplasty both with or without mastoidectomy were excluded here but are discussed in review 19.B. The bibliographies of the articles that met these inclusion/exclusion criteria were manually checked to ensure no further relevant articles could be identified. This process yielded three RCTs [1–3]. Two of these trials were conducted by the same set of authors, and report data from a subset of overlapping patients [1, 2].

RESULTS

Outcome Measures. Infectious outcomes were reported as the absolute number of patients with SSI [2, 3] or percent with pathogens on postoperative ear swab [1]. In this instance, pathogens were defined as *Staphylococcus* *aureus*, *Pseudomonas*, *Streptococcus pyogenes*, coliforms, and anaerobes. Graft outcomes were reported in terms of the percent of patients with graft success [1, 2]. None of the three articles defined SSI, but it is understood that it is clinically diagnosed (rather than by laboratory data with positive cultures from ear drainage).

Potential Confounders. Many factors besides systemic antibiotics could influence postoperative infections or graft success, and are discussed in further depth in Section 21.D. These factors are detailed in the adjoining tables and include the exact antibiotic regimen, details of any preoperative infection, types of otologic procedures studied, method of preoperative sterilization in the operating room, use of topical antibiotics or antiinflammatory medicines, and compliance with study medications.

Study Designs. Three RCTs addressed the impact of systemic antibiotics on outcomes after myringoplasty. All three studies focused solely on this population. Only one trial commented on the effectiveness of randomization in balancing potential confounders between groups at the outset [2]. All three studies were blinded (double blind [3], observer-blind [1], or unspecified [2]). The same ampicillin and flucloxacillin regimens were tested in two trials [1, 2], with the third trial testing a sulfamethoxazole regimen [3]. None of the studies used anti-Pseudomonal coverage, although it is unclear whether this would have impacted results. Topical antibiotics were used disparately; details are in the adjoining table [1–3].

Highest Level of Evidence. The dearth of SSIs that occurred in both study groups made it impractical to draw meaningful conclusions about this particular outcome in the first RCT [2]. The second RCT reported that there was no significant difference between the two groups, but the statistical power to detect any actual difference was limited in this study because of the relatively small sample size (n = 96 patients completing the study) [3]. Using figures suggested by this article's data at 10 days postoperatively, in order to obtain a 90% power to detect a 5% difference in groups with 95% confidence intervals, data from 2812 patients would be needed. The third RCT did not report data in terms of a clinical SSI. Two studies showed no correlation with preoperative "pathogens" on culture and SSIs or graft take [1, 3].

[1] Surgical site infection (SSI) is the term used by the Centers for Disease Control to specify an infection at the operative site, usually within 30 postoperative days [4]. This term excludes infections at other sites, such as pneumonias.

Graft success was also reported in the two trials with overlapping patient populations. Neither trial reported the comparative statistics, but the differences in the percent of patients with graft success was ≤2% in both reports. Again, however, study power was quite limited.

Applicability. These data are applicable to patients undergoing myringoplasty, with further details regarding inclusion/exclusion criteria provided in the adjacent table. The data regarding graft success are applicable to patients who have not required antibiotic eardrops or oral antibiotics within 1 month of surgery.

Morbidity/Complications. Adverse reactions to systemic antibiotics were reported in one article [3] and were comparable in the two groups, although again sample size may limit these conclusions.

CLINICAL SIGNIFICANCE AND FUTURE RESEARCH

There are three RCTs that addressed the impact of systemic antibiotics on infectious and/or graft outcomes after myringoplasty. The data regarding infectious outcomes are indeterminate, given the limited power of the sample sizes studied and the lack of statistical analysis. The data regarding graft outcomes are highly suggestive of perioperative systemic antibiotics making no impact on graft success, but again study power is limited, so conclusions are not definitive.

Future research into the impact of perioperative systemic antibiotics on SSI and graft success after myringoplasty would ideally be performed with an initial sample size associated with a 90% study power.

Reference	John, 1988	
Level (design)	1 (randomized controlled trial)	
Sample size*	130 (130)	

	OUTCOMES	
	No. with surgical site infections	% graft success
Antibiotic	n = 1/130 wound infection, group not specified	85%
No antibiotics		87%
p Value		Not reported
Conclusion	Indeterminate	No difference

Follow-up time	8 wk	

	STUDY DESIGN	
Inclusion criteria	All patients underwent endaural approach using underlay temporalis fascia graft	
Exclusion criteria	Antibiotic ear drops or oral antibiotics within 1 mo of surgery	
Randomization effectiveness	Lower percentage of wet ears in antibiotic group, not otherwise specified	
Age	14–61 y	
Masking	"Blind," not otherwise specified	
Systemic antibiotic regimen details	Ampicillin 250 mg IM ×1 and flucloxacillin 250 mg IM ×1 1 h preoperatively, then oral continuation of both ×5 d	
Use of topical antibiotics	Not routine: canal packing was impregnated with bismuth, iodoform, and paraffin paste	
Diagnostic criteria	"Successful surgery" not overtly defined, but implied as successful closure of perforation	
Procedural details	Endaural approach taking temporalis fascia, posterior tympanomeatal flap, underlay graft	
Management of infection while in study	Not reported	
Infection sequelae	Not reported	
Timing of first antibiotic dose‡	Appropriate	
Criteria for withdrawal from study	None specified	
Power	Not reported	
Morbidity/complications	Not reported	

NS = not significant, IM = intramuscularly, b.i.d. = twice a day, t.i.d. = three times a day.
* Sample size: numbers shown for those not lost to follow-up and those (initially recruited).
‡ Timing of first antibiotic dose is considered "appropriate" if given within the 2 h preceding the incision.

THE EVIDENCE CONDENSED: Systemic antibiotics versus no antibiotics for myringoplasty

Reference	Donaldson, 1966	Carlin, 1987	
Level (design)	1 (randomized controlled trial)	1 (randomized controlled trial)	
Sample size*	94 (96)	71 (71)	

OUTCOMES

	No. of patients with surgical site infections†	% graft success	% with pathogens on ear swab
Antibiotic	n = 1/47, n = 3/47	82.4%	29.4%, 17.6%, 0%
No antibiotics	n = 3/49, n = 6/49	83.7%	24.3%, 27.0%, 0%
p Value	NS	Statistics not reported	Statistics not reported
Conclusion	No difference	No difference	Trend toward antibiotics better at 3 wk
Follow-up time	10 d, 6 wk	1 wk, 3 wk, 8 wk	

STUDY DESIGN

Inclusion criteria	Myringoplasty	Patients admitted for routine myringoplasty: endaural approach using underlay temporalis fascia graft	
Exclusion criteria	Sulfonamide allergy, rheumatic heart disease requiring prophylactic penicillin	Antibiotic ear drops or oral antibiotics within 1 mo of surgery	
Randomization effectiveness	Not reported	Not reported	
Age	Not reported	Not specified	
Masking	Double blind, placebo controlled	Observer was blinded	
Systemic antibiotic regimen details	Sulfamethoxazole 2 g ×1 the evening before surgery, then 1 g b.i.d. ×10 d if >80 lb.; 75% dose if 60–80 lb., 50% dose if 40–60 lb	Ampicillin 250 mg IM ×1 and flucloxacillin 250 mg IM ×1 1 h preoperatively, then oral continuation of both ×5 d	
Use of topical antibiotics	Postoperative packing was soaked in polymyxin, neomycin, hydrocortisone otic drops	If ear was wet at 3-wk visit, then polymyxin/neomycin/hydrocortisone gets t.i.d. ×2 wk	
Diagnostic criteria	Criteria for diagnosis of postoperative infection not specified	Pathogens: *Staphylococcus aureus, Pseudomonas, Streptococcus pyogenes,* coliforms, anaerobes	
Procedural details	Preparation: auricle and adjacent areas were scrubbed with 3% hexachlorophene liquid soap for 10 min	"The operative procedure was standardized as much as possible . . . an endaural approach was used, taking temporalis fascia. A posterior tympanomeatal flap was elevated and the graft was inserted as an underlay."	
Management of infection while in study	Not specified	Not reported	
Infection sequelae	Not specified	Not reported	
Timing of first antibiotic dose‡	Not appropriate	Appropriate	
Criteria for withdrawal from study	Later determination that 2 patients had transcanal tympanoplasty, 2 had radical mastoidectomy	None specified	
Power	Not reported	Not reported	
Morbidity/complications	"Side effects were no more common in the patient receiving the active medication than the placebo."	Not reported	

NS = not significant, IM = intramuscularly, b.i.d. = twice a day, t.i.d. = three times a day.

* Sample size: numbers shown for those not lost to follow-up and those (initially recruited).

† Figures are extrapolated from reported data: n = 47 in antibiotic group; n = 49 in placebo group; n = 10 patients (in which groups not reported) did not follow up at 10 d; n = 2 patients (in which groups not reported) did not follow up at 10 d.

‡ Timing of first antibiotic dose is considered "appropriate" if given within the 2 h preceding the incision.

REFERENCES

1. Carlin WV, Lesser TH, John DG, Fielder C, Carrick DG, Thomas PL, Hill SS. Systemic antibiotic prophylaxis and reconstructive ear surgery. Clin Otolaryngol Allied Sci 1987;12(6):441–446.

2. John DG, Carlin WV, Lesser TH, Carrick DG, Fielder C. Tympanoplasty surgery and prophylactic antibiotics: surgical results. Clin Otolarngol Allied Scie 1988;13(3):205–207.

3. Donaldson JA, Snyder IS. Prophylactic chemotherapy in myringoplasty surgery. Laryngoscope 1966;76:1201–1214.

4. Managram AJ, Horan TC, Pearson ML, Silver LC, Jarvis WR. Guideline for prevention of surgical site infection. Centers for Disease Control, US Department of Health and Human Services, 1999.

18 Perioperative Antibiotics for Otologic Surgery

18.B.

Perioperative systemic antibiotics versus control for tympanoplasty with or without mastoidectomy: Impact on surgical site infections, graft success

Jennifer J. Shin and Marlene Durand

METHODS

A computerized PubMed search of MEDLINE 1966–November 2004 was performed. Articles mapping to any of the following medical subject headings were exploded and combined: "antibiotic prophylaxis," "antibacterial agents," "lactams," "fluoroquinolones," "macrolides," "clindamycin." These articles were then cross-referenced with those mapping to either the exploded medical subject heading "tympanoplasty" or the textwords "tympanoplasty" or "tympanomastoidectomy." This process yielded 48 trials. These articles were then reviewed to identify those that met the following inclusion criteria: 1) distinct patient population undergoing tympanoplasty with or without mastoidectomy, 2) intervention with perioperative systemic antibiotics versus placebo or other no-antibiotic control, 3) outcome measured in terms of postoperative surgical site infections[1] and/or graft success, 4) randomized controlled trials (RCTs). Articles in which the use of randomization was not clearly specified were excluded. Data for subsets of patients undergoing tympanoplasties that were reported in larger studies of multiple otologic procedures were included. If data specific to tympanoplasties could not be extracted because they were grouped with data from other procedures, they were excluded here, but are discussed in Section 19.D. Articles with data for patients undergoing myringoplasty alone were excluded here but are presented in review 19.A. The bibliographies of articles meeting these inclusion/exclusion criteria were manually checked to ensure no further relevant articles could be identified. This process yielded five RCTs [1–5].

RESULTS

Outcome Measures. Infectious outcomes were measured in terms of the percent of patients with SSI [3] or percent with draining ear [4]. Graft outcomes were reported in terms of the percent of patients with graft success [2, 4], number of patients with graft failure [1], or percent of patients with graft perforation or nonepi-

---

[1] Surgical site infection (SSI) is the term used by the Centers for Disease Control to specify an infection at the operative site within 30 postoperative days [6]. This term excludes infections at other sites, such as pneumonias.

thelialization [5]. Graft and infectious outcomes were grouped together in one trial [5].

Potential Confounders. As noted in Section 21.D, many factors besides systemic antibiotics could influence postoperative infections or graft success. These factors are detailed in the adjoining tables.

Study Designs. Five RCTs addressed the impact of systemic antibiotics on outcomes after tympanoplasty with or without mastoidectomy. Two studies focused solely on this population [4, 5]. Three studies reported a larger patient population undergoing all otologic procedures, but reported a separate analysis for the subset undergoing tympanoplasty with or without mastoidectomy [1–3]. Only one trial characterized the preintervention characteristics in detail [2], however, and none provided clear statistical comparisons of the antibiotic and control groups after randomization. Placebo and masking (i.e., blinding the patient and/or the surgeon to whether subjects were in the antibiotic or control group) were used in three studies. A variety of antibiotic regimens were tested, including cephalothin or cefazolin, cefuroxime, ceftazidime, penicillin, ampicillin, and clindamycin with or without gentamicin. Topical antibiotics were used disparately, with further details in the adjoining table [1–3].

Highest Level of Evidence. Three studies reported the rate of postoperative SSI. One RCT focused on patients with actively draining ears which were culture positive for *Pseudomonas* at the time of surgery; the antibiotic group had a significant improvement in the percent of patients with postoperatively draining ears, but it was not placebo controlled [4]. Therefore, it may be prone to expectation bias, favoring a better outcome with antibiotics. The second RCT reported no difference in SSI [3]. The third study grouped data from infectious and graft outcomes together and found no difference in this combined outcome measure [5]. In these two RCTs with negative results, sample size was small, which translates to a limited statistical power to detect any difference that truly exists.

Graft success was also reported in two trials, both of which found no significant difference in outcome with antibiotics versus none [2, 4]. Sample sizes were 27 and

2186, so one of the studies was well powered to detect a significant difference between the groups. Another trial reported the number of patients with graft failures in the antibiotic versus control groups, but did not note the total number of patients in each study group, so it was not possible to interpret the percent of patients with graft failure in each group [1].

Applicability. These data are applicable to a variety of patients undergoing tympanoplasty with or without mastoidectomy, with further details regarding inclusion/exclusion criteria provided in the adjacent table.

Morbidity/Complications. Adverse reactions to systemic antibiotics were mild and occurred at a rate of ≤1%.

CLINICAL SIGNIFICANCE AND FUTURE RESEARCH

Five RCTs addressed the impact of perioperative antibiotics on patients undergoing tympanoplasty with or without mastoidectomy. Two studies demonstrated no difference in SSIs whether antibiotics were used or not, but small sample sizes limited those studies' power to detect any difference that truly exists. One study demonstrated an improvement in the percent of patients with a draining ear, but this study was not placebo controlled, so may have been biased toward this result. None of the four RCTs that evaluated the graft result with versus without antibiotics demonstrated a significant difference. One of these trials had a sample size of >2000 patients, making it highly likely to have identified any difference that does exist. In this study, the empiric use of first-generation cephalosporins was found to have no impact on the graft outcome.

Future research may focus on identifying any subsets of patients undergoing tympanomastoidectomy who would be more likely to benefit from antibiotic intervention, such as those with preoperatively draining ears (see review 19.C).

THE EVIDENCE CONDENSED: Systemic antibiotics versus no antibiotics for tympanoplasty with/without mastoidectomy

Reference	Jackson, 1988
Level (design)	1 (randomized controlled trial)
Sample size*	2136 [the originally recruited tympanoplasty subgroup size was not reported; for the total sample undergoing all otologic procedures n = 3481 (4000)]

	OUTCOMES	
	% with SSI	% graft success
Antibiotic	No comparative data reported for the subgroup undergoing tympanoplasty	98.8%
No antibiotics		98.5%
p Value		NS
Conclusion	—	No difference
Follow-up time	3 wk (SSI and graft)	

	STUDY DESIGN
Inclusion criteria	Otologic surgery; a subgroup undergoing tympanic membrane grafting in tympanoplasty with or without mastoidectomy was identified
Exclusion criteria	Antibiotic requirement for other conditions within 7 d preoperatively or within postoperative follow-up period
Randomization effectiveness	Overall population very well characterized, not described in terms of antibiotic versus control group
Age	All ages
Masking	Operating surgeon was blinded
Systemic antibiotic regimen details	Cephalothin or cefazolin If immediate and severe penicillin allergy: vancomycin Protocol: 1 g IM preoperatively, then "appropriate dose" IV q 6 h ×24 h postoperatively
Use of topical antibiotics	COM surgery: postoperative pack with Polysporin ointment
Diagnostic criteria	"Clean contaminated": dry COM ears "Contaminated": discharging COM ears
Procedural details	All cases prepared identically: povidone iodine 10% soap and preparation solution ×10 min. Preoperatively draining ears n = 370
Management of infection while in study	Not specified
Infection sequelae	Graft failure vs take with 50% vs 6.6% wound infection rate (n = 2135, p < 0.05)
Timing of first antibiotic dose†	Appropriate
Criteria for withdrawal from study	Unavailable follow-up, requiring antibiotics within this time period for reasons other than surgical infection, incomplete data for the variable under consideration
Power	Not specified
Morbidity/ complications	In the larger group of 3481 enrolled patients: 1 dermatologic reaction to cephalosporin, 1 anaphylaxis to oxacillin

SSI = surgical site infection, NS = not significant, IM = intramuscularly, IV = intravenously, COM = chronic otitis media.
* Sample size: numbers shown for those not lost to follow-up and those (initially recruited).
† Timing of first antibiotic dose is considered "appropriate" if given within the 2 h preceding the incision.

THE EVIDENCE CONDENSED: Systemic antibiotics versus no antibiotics for tympanoplasty with/without mastoidectomy

Reference	Govaerts, 1998
Level (design)	1 (randomized controlled trial)
Sample size*	The size of the tympanoplasty subgroup was not reported; the total sample of all otologic procedures was 750

	OUTCOMES	
	% with SSI†	**No. of graft failures**
Antibiotic	No comparative data	2
No antibiotics	reported for the subgroup	1
p Value	undergoing tympanoplasty	Not reported
Conclusion	—	Indeterminate
Follow-up time	Up to 14 d (SSI)	

	STUDY DESIGN
Inclusion criteria	"All patients undergoing ear surgery"
Exclusion criteria	Otoneurosurgery or cochlear implant surgery, systemic antibiotics during the week preceding the procedure, diabetes or immunodeficiency, requirement for endocarditis prophylaxis
Randomization effectiveness	Not reported
Age	All ages
Masking	Double-blind, placebo controlled
Systemic antibiotic regimen details	Cefuroxime 1.5 g IV at induction (approximately 30 min before the incision), 6 h later, and 12 h later if the procedure was >6 h long
Use of topical antibiotics	Postoperative packing was impregnated with oxytetracycline and polymyxin B ointment
Diagnostic criteria	Wound infection: one of the following: fever, wound inflammation, wound secretion, myringitis, or otitis media
Procedural details	"Surgical procedures were carried out according to the general rules of sterility. Surgery for otosclerosis was performed by means of the stapedotomy technique with a whole Teflon prosthesis interposition. Most tympanoplasties made use of the tympanossicular allograft technique"
Management of infection while in study	"The surgeon was allowed to break the code of the drug and prescribe proper antibiotic therapy"
Infection sequelae	All infections occurred in the tympanoplasty group: 2 graft necroses in cefuroxime group, 1 in placebo group
Timing of first antibiotic dose‡	62% appropriate (received the first dose within 2 h before incision); 38% not appropriate (received the first dose after incision)
Criteria for withdrawal from study	None specified
Power	"Able to detect a reduction in postoperative infection by factor 3 or more"
Morbidity/ complications	0.3% (1 patient) with mild allergic reaction to cefuroxime

SSI = surgical site infection, NS = not significant, IM = intramuscularly, IV = intravenously, COM = chronic otitis media.
* Sample size: numbers shown for those not lost to follow-up and those (initially recruited).
† Numbers obtained from bar graphs presented in the original report.
‡ Timing of first antibiotic dose is considered "appropriate" if given within the 2 h preceding the incision.

THE EVIDENCE CONDENSED: Systemic antibiotics versus no antibiotics for tympanoplasty with/without mastoidectomy

Reference	Eschelman, 1971
Level (design)	1 (randomized controlled trial)
Sample size*	74 (74)

OUTCOMES	
	% SSI
Antibiotic	Penicillin: 11.5%, ampicillin 17.4%
No antibiotics	Placebo 16%
p Value	Not reported
Conclusion	No large difference
Follow-up time	Not specified

STUDY DESIGN	
Inclusion criteria	Tympanomastoidectomy or tympanoplasty was reported as a subset of larger group undergoing all otolaryngologic surgeries
Exclusion criteria	Penicillin allergy, patients receiving surgical treatment for acute infection, patients in whom exposure of the vestibule or labyrinth occurred in the presence of chronic supurative disease, patients having endoscopy, tonsillectomy/adenoidectomy, or myringotomy with or without tubes
Randomization effectiveness	Not specified
Age	Not specified
Masking	Double-blind, placebo controlled
Systemic antibiotic regimen details	Penicillin G 600,000 U IM ×1, then Betapen-VK 250 mg PO q 6 h. Ampicillin 500 mg IM ×1, then 500 mg PO q 6 h Duration of each PO regimen: 5 d or until all packs and drains were removed, for a maximum of 10 d
Use of topical antibiotics	AOM after myringoplasty with perforation of graft was treated with Cortisporin drops
Diagnostic criteria	"Postoperative infections ... were defined on clinical terms"
Procedural details	35 tympanomastoidectomies for cholesteatoma, 39 tympanoplasties and tympanomastoidectomies without cholesteatoma
Management of infection while in study	Not specified
Infection sequelae	3 postoperatively infected TM perforations: 2 TMs closed after treatment with erythromycin/Cortisporin, 1 graft did not take and required reoperation; 2 labyrinthitis "treated with antibiotics, antihistamines, and bedrest," 0 resulting dead ears
Timing of first antibiotic dose†	Not reported
Criteria for withdrawal from study	Not reported
Power	Not reported
Morbidity/ complications	In the larger group of 330 patients undergoing a range of otolaryngologic procedures—penicillin group: 2 rash, 1 hand swelling, 2 vomiting/diarrhea; placebo: 1 nausea

SSI = surgical site infection, NS = not significant, IM = intramuscularly, IV = intravenously, t.i.d. = three times a day, COM = chronic otitis media, AOM = acute otitis media, TM = tympanic membrane.
* Sample size: numbers shown for those not lost to follow-up and those (initially recruited).
† Timing of first antibiotic dose is considered "appropriate" if given within the 2 h preceding the incision.

THE EVIDENCE CONDENSED: Systemic antibiotics versus no antibiotics for tympanoplasty with/without mastoidectomy

Reference	Winerman, 1981	Lindholdt, 1986	
Level (design)	1 (randomized controlled trial)	1 (randomized controlled trial)	
Sample size*	72 (72)	26 (27)	

OUTCOMES			
	% SSI, graft reperforation or nonepithelialization	**% draining ear**	**% graft success**
Antibiotic	11.1%	14.3%, 7.1%	71.4%
No antibiotics	15.6%	83.3%, 58.3%	50.0%
p Value	Not reported	<0.001	NS
Conclusion	No large difference	Antibiotics better	No difference
Follow-up time	3 mo	"Postoperatively," 2 mo	

STUDY DESIGN		
Inclusion criteria	Tympanomastoid surgery (closed cavity) for chronic middle-ear infection	Adult referred for surgical treatment of COM with TM perforation for >3 mo, preoperative draining ear with cultures growing *Pseudomonas*
Exclusion criteria	Not specified	Dry ear preoperatively
Randomization effectiveness	Not specified	Multiple background variables reported, but no mathematical analysis
Age	8–67 y	Mean age 37–44 y
Masking	No placebo	Surgeon not blinded, no placebo
Systemic antibiotic regimen details	Clindamycin 300 mg IV t.i.d. for 3 d preoperatively and 11 d postoperatively Gentamicin 3–6 mg/kg/d divided into 3 doses daily for 3 d preoperatively and 7 d postoperatively; gentamicin was not given to 6 patients who received clindamycin alone because no gram-negative bacilli were identified on preoperative cultures	Ceftazidime 2 g IV ×1 the evening before the procedure, and 2 g q 8 h ×24 h, then 1 g q 8 h ×5 d
Use of topical antibiotics	Not specified	Not specified
Diagnostic criteria	Definitions for "infected operative wound" not specified	Criteria for diagnosis of postoperative infection not specified
Procedural details	Closed cavity procedure, 40 had cholesteatoma, 32 had chronically discharging ear	Not specified
Management of infection while in study	Not specified	Not specified
Infection sequelae	Not specified	Not specified
Timing of first antibiotic dose†	Potentially not appropriate	Not appropriate
Criteria for withdrawal from study	Not specified	Not specified
Power	Not specified	Not reported
Morbidity/ complications	Not specified	"No adverse reactions to ceftazidime were noted."

SSI = surgical site infection, NS = not significant, IM = intramuscularly, IV = intravenously, t.i.d. = three times a day, COM = chronic otitis media, AOM = acute otitis media, TM = tympanic membrane.
* Sample size: numbers shown for those not lost to follow-up and those (initially recruited).
† Timing of first antibiotic dose is considered "appropriate" if given within the 2 h preceding the incision.

REFERENCES

1. Govaerts PJ, Raemaekers J, Verlinden A, Kalai M, Somers T, Offeciers FE. Use of antibiotic prophylaxis in ear surgery. Laryngoscope 1998;108(1):107–110.
2. Jackson CG. Antimicrobial prophylaxis in ear surgery. Laryngoscope 1988;98(10):1116–1123.
3. Eschelman. Prophylactic antibiotics in otolaryngologic surgery: a double blind study. Trans Am Acad Ophthalmol Otolaryngol 1971;75(2):387–394.
4. Lindholdt T, Felding JU, Juul A, Kristensen S, Schouenburg P. Efficacy of perioperative ceftazidime in the surgical treatment of chronic otitis media due to Pseudomonas aeriginosa. Arch Otorhinolaryngol 1986;243(3):167–169.
5. Winerman I, Segal S, Man A. Effectiveness of prophylactic antibiotic treatment in mastoid surgery. Am J Otol 1981; 3(1):65–67.
6. Managram AJ, Horan TC, Pearson ML, Silver LC, Jarvis WR. Guideline for Prevention of Surgical Site Infection. Centers for Disease Control, US Department of Health and Human Services, 1999.

18 Perioperative Antibiotics for Otologic Surgery

18.C.

Perioperative systemic antibiotics in patients with actively draining ears: Impact on postoperative infection, graft success

Jennifer J. Shin and Marlene Durand

METHODS

Because the rate of postoperative infection has been noted to be higher in draining (17%) versus nondraining ears (5%) [1], we reviewed the literature specific to draining ears. A computerized PubMed search of MEDLINE 1966–November 2004 was performed. Articles mapping to any of the following medical subject headings were exploded and combined: "antibiotic prophylaxis," "antibacterial agents," "lactams," "fluoroquinolones," "macrolides," "clindamycin." These articles were then cross-referenced with those mapping to the exploded medical subject heading "otologic surgical procedures." This process yielded 266 trials. These articles were then reviewed to identify those that met the following inclusion criteria: 1) a patient population with actively draining ears that was undergoing otologic surgery, 2) intervention with systemic antibiotics versus placebo or other no-antibiotic control, 3) outcome measured in terms of postoperative surgical site infections[1] and/or graft success, 4) randomized controlled trials (RCTs). Articles in which the use of randomization was not clearly specified were excluded. The bibliographies of the articles that met these inclusion/exclusion criteria were manually checked to ensure no further relevant articles could be identified. This process yielded two RCTs [1, 2].

RESULTS

Outcome Measures. Outcomes were measured in terms of the percent of patients with an SSI (wound or external auditory canal) [1], percent with postoperatively draining ear, and/or the percent of patients with graft success [2]. The outcome of graft success was considered relevant because postoperative infections have been correlated with graft failure, a finding corroborated in one of these trials [1].

Potential Confounders. As discussed in Section 21.D, many factors besides systemic antibiotics could influence postoperative infections or graft success. Such factors are detailed in the adjoining table.

[1] Surgical site infection (SSI) is the term used by the Centers for Disease Control to specify an infection at the operative site, usually within 30 postoperative days [3]. This term excludes infections at other sites, such as pneumonias.

Study Designs. Two RCTs addressed a set of patients with preoperatively draining ears [1, 2], with one focusing on only *Pseudomonas*-infected ears [2]. Although these were randomized trials, the effectiveness of that randomization was not demonstrated; it was not clearly delineated that potential confounders were balanced between the two study groups before treatment with either antibiotic or control. Neither study was placebo controlled, but the surgeon was blinded in one of the studies [1]. The surgical preparation was standardized and reported in one trial [1]. Two first-generation cephalosporins (cephalothin and cefazolin) were tested in one trial, with vancomycin for patients with penicillin allergy [1]. The second RCT examined ceftazidime, a third-generation cephalosporin with anti-Pseudomonal activity, because this organism was found in preoperative cultures of all patients included in this study [2]. The use of topical antibiotics was described in one of the studies [1].

Highest Level of Evidence. The two RCTs that addressed this issue had varying results. One trial showed that antibiotics significantly decreased the percent of patients with a draining ear "postoperatively" (exact time interval not specified) and 2 months after the procedure. There was a rate difference (see Chapter 3 for definition) of 69.0% "postoperatively" and 51.2% at 2 months. These figures translate to numbers needed to treat (see Chapter 3 for definition) of two, which means that two patients with *Pseudomonas*-infected draining ears must be treated with ceftazidime in order to prevent one of them from having a draining ear after surgery. It should be noted, however, that both patients and physicians knew whether antibiotics were administered or not, so a potential placebo effect could create a bias toward a better outcome with antibiotics. This same trial showed a trend toward improved graft success, but with no significant difference whether antibiotics were used or not [2].

The second trial to address this issue found no significant difference whether first-generation cephalosporins were given or not. The antibiotic regimen, however, was empiric, and not based on culture results [1]. The lack of antibiotic impact may therefore be attributed to the use of an antibiotic regimen without activity against potentially relevant organisms such as *Pseudomonas*. Neither study reported an *a priori* power calculation.

Applicability. These data are applicable to patients with actively draining ears who are undergoing otologic surgery. One study is potentially applicable to patients undergoing empiric treatment [1], whereas the other is only applicable to patients with *Pseudomonas* infection treated with an anti-Pseudomonal agent [2].

Morbidity/Complications. Adverse reactions to systemic antibiotics were mild and occurred at a rate of ≤1%.

CLINICAL SIGNIFICANCE AND FUTURE RESEARCH

Two RCTs addressed the impact of systemic antibiotics on outcomes in patients undergoing otologic procedures with actively draining ears. They had disparate results, but measured different outcomes in different populations. One demonstrated a significant improvement in postoperative drainage caused by *Pseudomonas* after treatment with an anti-Pseudomonal antibiotic. The other showed no difference in SSI when a first-generation cephalosporin was used empirically. These varying results may be related to the lack of placebo use in the first trial and lack of culture-driven therapy in the trial showing no difference. In addition, the disparity may be caused by the use of antibiotics for prophylaxis (clean-contaminated surgery) versus for treatment (contaminated or infected surgery).

To address the impact of prophylactic antibiotics on draining ears, a placebo-controlled trial utilizing empiric antibiotics directed at all major pathogens in chronic otitis media (including *Staphylococcus aureus* and *Pseudomonas*) would be necessary. Using the data from the Jackson study, the sample size necessary to achieve a 90% power to detect a 10% difference in infection rate with 95% confidence intervals can be calculated at 622 patients (Jackson study had 370 patients). To detect a 5% difference in infection rates, 3230 patients would be necessary.

Reference	Jackson, 1988	Lindholdt, 1986	
Level (design)	1 (randomized controlled trial)	1 (randomized controlled trial)	
Sample size*	370 [original size of this subset with preoperatively draining ears was not specified, but for the entire group 3481 (4000)]	26 (27)	

OUTCOMES			
	% with surgical site infection (wound, canal, total)	**% with postoperatively draining ear**	**% graft success**
Antibiotic	3.8%, 13.0%, 16.8%	14.3%, 7.1%	71.4%
No antibiotics	6.5%, 11.4%, 17.9%	83.3%, 58.3%	50.0%
p Value	NS, NS, NS	<0.001, <0.01	NS
Conclusion	No difference	Antibiotics better	No difference
Follow-up time	3 wk	"Postoperatively," 2 mo	2 mo

STUDY DESIGN		
Inclusion criteria	Subset of patients with discharging ears undergoing otologic surgery	Adult referred for surgical treatment of COM with a TM perforation observed for >3 mo, preoperative draining ear with cultures containing *Pseudomonas aeruginosa*
Exclusion criteria	Antibiotic requirement for other conditions within 7 d preoperatively or within postoperative follow-up period	Dry ear preoperatively
Randomization effectiveness	Overall population very well characterized, not described in terms of antibiotic vs control group	Multiple background variables reported, but no mathematical analysis
Age	All ages	Mean 37 y (antibiotic group), 44 y (placebo group)
Masking	Operating surgeon was blinded	Surgeon not blinded, no placebo
Systemic antibiotic regimen details	COM: cephalothin or cefazolin Neurotologic cases: oxacillin If immediate and severe penicillin allergy: vancomycin Protocol: 1 g IM preoperatively, then "appropriate dose" IV q 6 h ×24 h postoperatively	Ceftazidime 2 g IV ×1 the evening before the procedure, and 2 g q 8 h ×24 h, then 1 g q 8 h ×5 d
Use of topical antibiotics	COM surgery: postoperative pack with Polysporin ointment	Not specified
Diagnostic criteria	"Clean surgery": neurotologic cases "Clean contaminated": dry COM ears "Contaminated": discharging COM ears	Criteria for diagnosis of postoperative infection not specified. Graft success specified as a graft that was intact and in place (distinction from a perforated or displaced graft)
Procedural details	All cases prepared identically: povidone iodine 10% soap and preparation solution ×10 min; iodophor drapes with neurotologic cases. Tympanoplasty n = 2136; stapedectomy n = 341; CPA tumor n = 431; multiple other otologic surgery types. Preoperatively draining ears n = 370	Not specified
Management of infection while in study	Not specified	Not specified
Infection sequelae	Graft failure vs take with 50% vs 6.6% wound infection rate (in a larger group of patients undergoing tympanoplasty n = 2135, p < 0.05)	Not specified
Timing of first antibiotic dose†	Appropriate	Not appropriate
Criteria for withdrawal from study	Unavailable follow-up, requiring antibiotics within this time period for reasons other than surgical infection, incomplete data for the variable under consideration	Not specified
Power	Not specified	Not reported
Morbidity/complications	In larger group of n = 3481 patients: 1 dermatologic reaction to cephalosporin, 1 anaphylaxis to oxacillin	"No adverse reactions to ceftazidime were noted"

NS = not significant, COM = chronic otitis media, TM = tympanic membrane, IM = intramuscularly, IV = intravenously, CPA = cerebellopontine angle.
* Sample size: numbers shown for those not lost to follow-up and those (initially recruited).
† Timing of first antibiotic dose is considered "appropriate" if given within the 2 h preceding the incision.

REFERENCES

1. Jackson CG. Antimicrobial prophylaxis in ear surgery. Laryngoscope 1988;98(10):1116–1123.
2. Lindholdt T, Felding JU, Juul A, Kristensen S, Schouenburg P. Efficacy of perioperative ceftazidime in the surgical treatment of chronic otitis media due to Pseudomonas aeriginosa. Arch Otorhinolaryngol 1986;243(3):167–169.
3. Managram AJ, Horan TC, Pearson ML, Silver LC, Jarvis WR. Guideline for Prevention of Surgical Site Infection. Centers for Disease Control, US Department of Health and Human Services, 1999.

18 Perioperative Antibiotics for Otologic Surgery

18.D.

Perioperative systemic antibiotic prophylaxis for all types of otologic surgery combined: Impact on postoperative infection, graft success

Jennifer J. Shin and Marlene Durand

METHODS

Although ideally only procedure-specific data would be presented, an analysis of all studies that analyzed data from any type of otologic surgery is also presented. This additional review was undertaken because of the large sample sizes necessary to achieve a study of adequate power on this topic (See reviews 21.A and 21.B); accepting data from trials that included a wider variety of procedures was hoped to provide larger sample sizes. In the spirit of a systematic review, all relevant papers are presented, including those already shown in reviews 21.A–21.C.

A computerized PubMed search of MEDLINE 1966–November 2004 was performed. Articles mapping to any of the following medical subject headings were exploded and combined: "antibiotic prophylaxis," "antibacterial agents," "lactams," "fluoroquinolones," "macrolides," "clindamycin." These articles were then cross-referenced with those mapping to the exploded medical subject heading "otologic surgical procedures." This process yielded 266 trials. These articles were then reviewed to identify those that met the following inclusion criteria: 1) patient population undergoing otologic surgery other than just tympanostomy tube placement, 2) intervention with systemic antibiotics versus placebo or other no-antibiotic control, 3) outcome measured in terms of postoperative surgical site infection[1] and/or graft success, 4) randomized controlled trials (RCTs). Articles in which the use of randomization was not clearly specified were excluded. The bibliographies of the articles that met these inclusion/exclusion criteria were manually checked to ensure no further relevant articles could be identified. This process yielded nine RCTs [1–9].

RESULTS

Outcome Measures. Outcomes usually were measured as the percent of patients with postoperative infections, often localized specifically to the wound or the canal. Only one of these trials, however, detailed the exact specifications for the diagnosis of an SSI [5]. One trial reported the "relative factor of protection from infection"

[1] Surgical site infection (SSI) is the term used by the Centers for Disease Control to specify an infection at the operative site, usually within 30 postoperative days [10]. This term excludes infections at other sites, such as pneumonias.

[5], which was calculated by dividing the percent of placebo-consuming patients with postoperative infections by the percent of antibiotic-consuming patients with postoperative infection. In doing so, they calculated the relative risk of postoperative infection with placebo versus antibiotics. Two RCTs also reported the percent of patients with pathogens in cultures taken from postoperative ear swabs [1, 2]. Several trials also reported the percent of patients with a successful tympanoplasty graft; in fact, one trial reported results as the percent having either SSI or graft complication as one variable [9]. Graft outcome was considered relevant because postoperative infections have been correlated with graft failure, a finding corroborated in one of these trials [6].

Potential Confounders. As detailed in review 19.A, many factors besides systemic antibiotics could influence postoperative infection. These factors are detailed in the adjoining tables and include: the exact antibiotic regimen, details of any preoperative infection, types of otologic procedures studied, method of preoperative sterilization in the operating room, use of topical antibiotics or anti-inflammatory medicines, and timing of administration of study medications.

The timing of the first dose of antibiotics is a key potential confounder. This initial dose should be given within the 2 hours preceding the surgical incision [10, 11]. In the Lindholdt, Winerman, Bagger-Sjoback, and Donaldson studies, antibiotics may not have been given within the appropriate timeframe, which may have influenced their results.

The organisms covered by the antibiotic used is another important potential confounder. Antibiotics that cover *Pseudomonas* [8, 9], *Staphylococcus aureus* [2, 3], but neither *Pseudomonas* nor *Staphylococcus* [1, 4–7] were used. Inadequate coverage of appropriate organisms may clearly affect results. In one study, for example, all graft necroses occurred in the presence of gram-negative rods with a resistance pattern suggestive of *Pseudomonas*, but the antibiotic prophylaxis studied (cefuroxime) did not cover *Pseudomonas* [5].

Study Designs. Nine RCTs addressed the impact of systemic antibiotics on infectious outcomes after otologic surgery. Only one trial characterized the preintervention characteristics in detail [6], however, and none provided clear statistical comparisons of the antibiotic and control groups at the outset. All studies except two [8, 9] were at least single, if not double blinded. The surgical preparation was standardized in two cases. A variety of systemic penicillins and cephalosporins were tested, along with sulfamethoxazole and clindamycin with or without gentamicin. Topical antibiotics were used disparately, with further details in the adjoining table.

Highest Level of Evidence. Two of the nine RCTs showed a significant improvement in the infectious outcome with systemic antibiotics. One of these trials demonstrated that patients with preoperatively draining ears caused by *Pseudomonas* were less likely to have persistent drainage at up to 2 months after surgery if treated with an anti-Pseudomonal antibiotic [8]. This result may not be surprising, as this may represent "contaminated" surgery, and antibiotics would therefore be therapeutic rather than prophylactic. Rate differences were 69.0% and 51.2%, suggesting numbers needed to treat of two. In the second trial, patients who received cefuroxime were 3.1–3.4 times as likely to remain infection-free at 2–7 days [5]. This protective effect, however, dissipated at 14 days.

Six other RCTs showed no noteworthy difference in the rate of postoperative infections, with specified follow-up times between 6 days and 3 months [1–4, 6, 7, 9]. The largest and highest powered trial was among those to demonstrate no difference (at 3 weeks follow-up) [6]. This trial also included an analysis of a smaller subset of patients with preoperatively draining ears in which there was no demonstrated difference between the antibiotic and control groups (see review 19.C). These negative trials had later follow-up periods of ≥1 week; further details are provided in the adjoining chart.

Using figures suggested by one article's data [3], in order to obtain a 90% power to detect a 5% difference in groups with 95% confidence intervals, data from 2812 patients would be needed. Only one of these studies had a sample size of this magnitude [6], and only one other came close [5].

Applicability. These data are applicable to a variety of patients undergoing otologic surgery, with further details regarding inclusion/exclusion criteria provided in the adjacent table.

Morbidity/Complications. Adverse reactions to systemic antibiotics were mild and occurred at a rate of ≤1%.

CLINICAL SIGNIFICANCE AND FUTURE RESEARCH

There were nine RCTs that addressed the impact of systemic antibiotics on otologic surgery outcomes. The majority of data (including data from one study with more than adequate power to identify a difference that truly exists) demonstrated no difference with empiric perioperative antibiotics, with follow-up times typically *exceeding* 1 week. There was, however, one trial that demonstrated a significant improvement in SSI rate with antibiotics that occurred only *within* the first postoperative week. In addition, another trial (whose results are limited by lack of a placebo control) demonstrated efficacy when culture-driven (i.e., *Pseudomonas*-specific) perioperative antibiotics were administered.

Future research may focus more specifically on particular otologic procedures or subsets of patients undergoing a particular procedure, in order to identify those patients that would most benefit from this intervention. Grouping together data from clean and clean/contaminated and contaminated surgery may confound results, so these categories of procedures are best studied separately. Given the larger sample sizes needed to achieve adequate power for clean ear surgery (lower overall rates of infection make it harder to demonstrate a difference that truly exists), it may be necessary to focus on clean-contaminated surgeries with their higher rates of postoperative infection. When planning future research, there are three key outcomes to consider: SSI, graft failure, and persistent otorrhea. Each of these outcomes should be clearly defined, especially SSI, which has the potential for a broader clinical interpretation.

Surgical wound classification [10]

Clean	Uninfected wound with no entry into respiratory or alimentary tract	Primary closure with or without a closed drain	Antibiotic use is prophylaxis
Clean-contaminated	Controlled entry into respiratory or alimentary tract	No unusual contamination	Antibiotic use is prophylaxis
Contaminated	Incision into acute nonpurulent inflammation	Open, fresh, accidental wounds or major break in sterile technique	Antibiotic use is prophylaxis
Dirty	Wound with existing clinical infection or retained devitalized tissue	Organisms causing postoperative infection were present in the operative field prior to surgery	Antibiotic use is therapeutic

THE EVIDENCE CONDENSED: Systemic antibiotics versus no antibiotics for otologic surgery

Reference	Jackson, 1988		
Level (design)	1 (randomized controlled trial)		
Sample size*	3481 (4000)		

	OUTCOMES		
	% infected: wound, canal	**% graft success**	**% preoperative wet ears infected: wound, canal**
Antibiotic	1.4%, 4.6%	98.8%	3.8%, 13.0%
No antibiotics	1.7%, 4.0%	98.5%	6.5%, 11.4%
p Value	NS, NS	NS	NS, NS
Conclusion	No difference	No difference	No difference
Follow-up time	3 wk		

	STUDY DESIGN		
Inclusion criteria	Otologic surgery		
Exclusion criteria	Antibiotic requirement for other conditions within 7 d preoperatively or within postoperative follow-up period		
Randomization effectiveness	Overall population very well characterized, not described in terms of antibiotic versus control group		
Age	All ages		
Masking	Operating surgeon was blinded		
Systemic antibiotic regimen details	COM: cephalothin or cefazolin Neurotologic cases: oxacillin If immediate and severe penicillin allergy: vancomycin Protocol: 1 g IM preoperatively, then "appropriate dose" IV q 6 h ×24 h postoperatively		
Use of topical antibiotics	COM surgery: postoperative pack with Polysporin ointment		
Diagnostic criteria	"Clean surgery": neurotologic cases "Clean contaminated": dry COM ears "Contaminated": discharging COM ears		
Procedural details	All cases prepared identically: povidone iodine 10% soap and preparation solution ×10 min; iodophor drapes with neurotologic cases. Tympanoplasty n = 2136; stapedectomy n = 341; CPA tumor n = 431; multiple other otologic surgery types. Preoperatively draining ears n = 370		
Management of infection while in study	Not specified		
Infection sequelae	Graft failure vs take with 50% vs 6.6% wound infection rate (n = 2135, p < 0.05)		
Timing of first antibiotic dose§	Appropriate		
Criteria for withdrawal from study	Unavailable follow-up, requiring antibiotics within this time period for reasons other than surgical infection, incomplete data for the variable under consideration		
Power	Not specified		
Morbidity/ complications	1 dermatologic reaction to cephalosporin, 1 anaphylaxis to oxacillin		

NS = not significant, IM = intramuscularly, IV = intravenously, COM = chronic otitis media, CPA = cerebellopontine angle.
* Sample size: numbers shown for those not lost to follow-up and those (initially recruited).
§ Timing of first antibiotic dose is considered "appropriate" if given within the 2 h preceding the incision.

THE EVIDENCE CONDENSED: Systemic antibiotics versus no antibiotics for otologic surgery

Reference	Govaerts, 1998	
Level (design)	1 (randomized controlled trial)	
Sample size*	Not specified (750)	

OUTCOMES		
	Relative factor of protection from infection	**Infection rate overall**
Antibiotic	3.1,† 3.4‡	3.1%
No antibiotics	1.0,† 1.0‡	4.7%
p Value	†<0.05, ‡<0.05	NS
Conclusion	Antibiotics better	No difference
Follow-up time	†2 d, ‡7 d,14 d	14 d

STUDY DESIGN	
Inclusion criteria	"All patients undergoing ear surgery"
Exclusion criteria	Otoneurosurgery or cochlear implant surgery, systemic antibiotics during the week preceding the procedure, diabetes or immunodeficiency, requirement for endocarditis prophylaxis
Randomization effectiveness	Not reported
Age	All ages
Masking	Double-blind, placebo controlled
Systemic antibiotic regimen details	Cefuroxime 1.5 g IV at induction (approximately 30 min before the incision), 6 h later, and 12 h later if the procedure was >6 h long
Use of topical antibiotics	Postoperative packing was impregnated with oxytetracycline and polymyxin B ointment
Diagnostic criteria	Wound infection: one of the following: fever, wound inflammation, wound secretion, myringitis, or otitis media
Procedural details	"Surgical procedures were carried out according to the general rules of sterility. Surgery for otosclerosis was performed by means of the stapedotomy technique with a whole Teflon prosthesis interposition. Most tympanoplasties made use of the tympanoossicular allograft technique"
Management of infection while in study	"The surgeon was allowed to break the code of the drug and prescribe proper antibiotic therapy"
Infection sequelae	All infections occurred in the tympanoplasty group: 2 graft necroses in cefuroxime group, 1 in placebo group
Timing of first antibiotic dose§	62% appropriate (received the first dose within 2 h before incision); 38% not appropriate (received the first dose after incision)
Criteria for withdrawal from study	None specified
Power	"Able to detect a reduction in postoperative infection by factor 3 or more"
Morbidity/ complications	0.3% (1 patient) with mild allergic reaction to cefuroxime

NS = not significant, IM = intramuscularly, IV = intravenously, COM = chronic otitis media.
* Sample size: numbers shown for those not lost to follow-up and those (initially recruited).
†, ‡ Symbols denote which data comparisons correspond to the referenced p values and follow-up times.
§ Timing of first antibiotic dose is considered "appropriate" if given within the 2 h preceding the incision.

Reference	John, 1988	
Level (design)	1 (randomized controlled trial)	
Sample size*	130 (130)	

	OUTCOMES	
	Wound infection	**% graft success**
Antibiotic	n = 1/130 wound infection, group not specified	85%
No antibiotics		87%
p Value		Not reported
Conclusion	No conclusion	No difference
Follow-up time	8 wk	

	STUDY DESIGN
Inclusion criteria	All patients underwent endaural approach using underlay temporalis fascia graft
Exclusion criteria	Antibiotic ear drops or oral antibiotics within 1 mo of surgery
Randomization effectiveness	Lower percentage of wet ears in antibiotic group, not otherwise specified
Age	14–61 y
Masking	"Blind," not otherwise specified
Systemic antibiotic regimen details	Ampicillin 250 mg IM ×1 and flucloxacillin 250 mg IM ×1 1 h preoperatively, then oral continuation of both ×5 d
Use of topical antibiotics	Not routine: canal packing was impregnated with bismuth, iodoform, and paraffin paste
Diagnostic criteria	"Successful surgery" not overtly defined, but implied as successful closure of perforation
Procedural details	Endaural approach taking temporalis fascia, posterior tympanomeatal flap, underlay graft
Management of infection while in study	Not reported
Infection sequelae	Not reported
Timing of first antibiotic dose†	Appropriate
Criteria for withdrawal from study	None specified
Power	Not reported
Morbidity/ complications	Not reported

NS = not significant, IM = intramuscularly, b.i.d. = twice a day, t.i.d. = three times a day.
* Sample size: numbers shown for those not lost to follow-up and those (initially recruited).
† Timing of first antibiotic dose is considered "appropriate" if given within the 2 h preceding the incision.

THE EVIDENCE CONDENSED: Systemic antibiotics versus no antibiotics for otologic surgery

Reference	Donaldson, 1966	Carlin, 1987	
Level (design)	1 (randomized controlled trial)	1 (randomized controlled trial)	
Sample size*	94 (96)	71 (71)	

OUTCOMES

	% with infections†	% with pathogens on ear swab	% graft success
Antibiotic	n = 1/47, n = 3/47	29.4%, 17.6%, 0%	82.4%
No antibiotics	n = 3/49, n = 6/49	24.3%, 27.0%, 0%	83.7%
p Value	NS	Statistics not reported	Statistics not reported
Conclusion	No difference	Trend toward antibiotics better at 3 wk	No difference
Follow-up time	10 d, 6 wk	1 wk, 3 wk, 8 wk	

STUDY DESIGN

Inclusion criteria	Myringoplasty	Patients admitted for routine myringoplasty: endaural approach using underlay temporalis fascia graft
Exclusion criteria	Sulfonamide allergy, rheumatic heart disease requiring prophylactic penicillin	Antibiotic ear drops or oral antibiotics within 1 mo of surgery
Randomization effectiveness	Not reported	Not reported
Age	Not reported	Not specified
Masking	Double-blind, placebo controlled	Observer was blinded
Systemic antibiotic regimen details	Sulfamethoxazole 2 g ×1 the evening before surgery, then 1 g b.i.d. ×10 d if >80 lb.; 75% dose if 60–80 lb., 50% dose if 40–60 lb.	Ampicillin 250 mg IM ×1 and flucloxacillin 250 mg IM ×1 1 h preoperatively, then oral continuation of both ×5 d
Use of topical antibiotics	Postoperative packing was soaked in polymyxin, neomycin, hydrocortisone otic drops	If ear was wet at 3-wk visit, then polymyxin/neomycin/hydrocortisone gtts t.i.d. ×2 wk
Diagnostic criteria	Criteria for diagnosis of postoperative infection not specified	Pathogens: *Staphylococcus aureus*, *Pseudomonas*, *Streptococcus* pyogenes, coliforms, anaerobes
Procedural details	Preparation: auricle and adjacent areas were scrubbed with 3% hexachlorophene liquid soap for 10 min	"The operative procedure was standardized as much as possible . . . an endaural approach was used, taking temporalis fascia. A posterior tympanomeatal flap was elevated and the graft was inserted as an underlay"
Management of infection while in study	Not specified	Not reported
Infection sequelae	Not specified	Not reported
Timing of first antibiotic dose‡	Not appropriate	Appropriate
Criteria for withdrawal from study	Later determination that 2 patients had transcanal tympanoplasty, 2 had radical mastoidectomy	None specified
Power	Not reported	Not reported
Morbidity/ complications	"Side effects were no more common in the patient receiving the active medication than the placebo"	Not reported

NS = not significant, IM = intramuscularly, b.i.d. = twice a day, t.i.d. = three times a day.
* Sample size: numbers shown for those not lost to follow-up and those (initially recruited).
† Figures are extrapolated as best possible from reported data: n = 47 in antibiotic group; n = 49 in placebo group; n = 10 patients (in which groups not reported) did not follow up at 10 d; n = 2 patients (in which groups not reported) did not follow up at 10 d.
‡ Timing of first antibiotic dose is considered "appropriate" if given within the 2 h preceding the incision.

THE EVIDENCE CONDENSED: Systemic antibiotics versus no antibiotics for otologic surgery

Reference	Eschelman, 1971
Level (design)	1 (randomized controlled trial)
Sample size*	107 (107)

OUTCOMES	
% infected: wound, middle ear	
Antibiotic	Penicillin 7.9%, ampicillin 16.7%
No antibiotics	12.1%
p Value	NS
Conclusion	No difference
Follow-up time	Not specified

STUDY DESIGN	
Inclusion criteria	All surgical patients undergoing otologic procedures (subset of larger group undergoing all otolaryngologic surgeries)
Exclusion criteria	Penicillin allergy, patients receiving surgical treatment for acute infection, patients in whom exposure of the vestibule or labyrinth occurred in the presence of chronic suppurative disease, patients having endoscopy, tonsillectomy/adenoidectomy, or myringotomy with or without tubes
Randomization effectiveness	Not specified
Age	Not specified
Masking	Double-blind, placebo controlled
Systemic antibiotic regimen details	Penicillin G 600,000 U IM ×1, then Betapen-VK 250 mg PO q 6 h. Ampicillin 500 mg IM ×1, then 500 mg PO q 6 h Duration of each PO regimen: 5 d or until all packs and drains were removed, for a maximum of 10 d
Use of topical antibiotics	AOM after myringoplasty with perforation of graft was treated with Cortisporin drops
Diagnostic criteria	"Postoperative infections ... were defined on clinical terms"
Procedural details	35 tympanomastoidectomies for cholesteatoma, 39 tympanoplasties and tympanomastoidectomies without cholesteatoma, 33 stapedectomy or exploratory tympanotomy
Management of infection while in study	Not specified
Infection sequelae	3 postoperatively infected TM perforations: 2 TMs closed after treatment with erythromycin/Cortisporin, 1 graft did not take and required reoperation. 2 labyrinthitis "treated with antibiotics, antihistamines, and bedrest," 0 resulting dead ears
Timing of first antibiotic dose†	Not reported
Criteria for withdrawal from study	Not reported
Power	Not reported
Morbidity/ complications	Penicillin group: 2 rash, 1 hand swelling, 2 vomiting/diarrhea. Placebo: 1 nausea

NS = not significant, IM = intramuscularly, b.i.d. = twice a day, TM = tympanic membrane, AOM = acute otitis media.
* Sample size: numbers shown for those not lost to follow-up and those (initially recruited).
† Timing of first antibiotic dose is considered "appropriate" if given within the 2 hours preceding the incision.

THE EVIDENCE CONDENSED: Systemic antibiotics versus no antibiotics for otologic surgery

Reference	Bagger-Sjoback, 1987	
Level (design)	1 (randomized controlled trial)	
Sample size*	91 (100)	

OUTCOMES		
	% with clinical infection postoperatively	**% with pathogen microbiologic growth postoperatively**
Antibiotic	19.1%	78.7%
No antibiotics	22.7%	95.5%
p Value	NS	<0.041
Conclusion	No difference	Antibiotics better
Follow-up time	6–8 d	

STUDY DESIGN	
Inclusion criteria	Admitted for middle ear surgical procedure, >15 y old
Exclusion criteria	Allergy to penicillin or cephalosporin, other antibiotics within 7 d before surgery
Randomization effectiveness	Similar rates of preoperative infection, microbiologic growth
Age	>15 y
Masking	Double-blind, placebo controlled
Systemic antibiotic regimen details	Phenoxymethylpenicillin (penicillin V) 1 g administered the evening before a morning case or the morning of an afternoon case, then 1 g PO b.i.d. ×6–8 d postoperatively
Use of topical antibiotics	No topical antibiotics were used
Diagnostic criteria	Criteria for diagnosis of postoperative infection not specified
Procedural details	51 myringoplasty, 30 ossiculoplasty, 15 revision surgery, 7 combined approach tympanoplasty, 6 radical mastoidectomy, 5 stapedectomy. Postoperative packing for radical mastoid surgery was soaked in a 1% hydrocortisone solution ×6–8 d
Management of infection while in study	Patients were withdrawn so known antibiotic regimen could be administered
Infection sequelae	Not specified
Timing of first antibiotic dose†	Not appropriate
Criteria for withdrawal from study	4 patients developed infections and were withdrawn for proper antibiotic treatment; 5 patients were withdrawn because of "nonfulfillment of surgical criteria, incomplete forms, etc."
Power	Not reported
Morbidity/ complications	Not reported

NS = not significant, IM = intramuscularly, b.i.d. = twice a day, TM = tympanic membrane, AOM = acute otitis media.
* Sample size: numbers shown for those not lost to follow-up and those (initially recruited).
† Timing of first antibiotic dose is considered "appropriate" if given within the 2 hours preceding the incision.

THE EVIDENCE CONDENSED: Systemic antibiotics versus no antibiotics for otologic surgery

Reference	Winerman, 1981	Lindholdt, 1986	
Level (design)	1 (randomized controlled trial)	1 (randomized controlled trial)	
Sample size*	72 (72)	26 (27)	
OUTCOMES			
	% SSI, graft reperforation or nonepithelialization	% draining ear	% graft success
Antibiotic	11.1%	14.3%, 7.1%	71.4%
No antibiotics	15.6%	83.3%, 58.3%	50.0%
p Value	Not reported	<0.001	NS
Conclusion	No large difference	Antibiotics better	No difference
Follow-up time	3 mo	"postoperatively," 2 mo	
STUDY DESIGN			
Inclusion criteria	Tympanomastoid surgery (closed cavity) for chronic middle ear infection	Adult referred for surgical treatment of COM with a TM perforation observed for >3 mo, preoperative draining ear with cultures containing *Pseudomonas aeruginosa*	
Exclusion criteria	Not specified	Dry ear preoperatively	
Randomization effectiveness	Not specified	Multiple background variables reported, but no mathematical analysis	
Age	8–67 y	Mean 37–44 y	
Masking	No placebo	Surgeon not blinded, no placebo	
Systemic antibiotic regimen details	Clindamycin 300 mg IV t.i.d. for 3 d preoperatively and 11 d postoperatively. Gentamicin 3–6 mg/kg/d divided into 3 doses daily for 3 d preoperatively and 7 d postoperatively; gentamicin was not given to 6 patients who received clindamycin alone because no gram-negative bacilli were identified on preoperative cultures	Ceftazidime 2 g IV ×1 the evening before the procedure, and 2 g q 8 h ×24 h, then 1 g q 8 h ×5 d	
Use of topical antibiotics	Not specified	Not specified	
Diagnostic criteria	Definitions for "infected operative wound" not specified	Criteria for diagnosis of postoperative infection not specified	
Procedural details	Closed cavity procedure, 40 had cholesteatoma, 32 had chronically discharging ear	Not specified	
Management of infection while in study	Not specified	Not specified	
Infection sequelae	Not specified	Not specified	
Timing of first antibiotic dose†	Potentially not appropriate	Not appropriate	
Criteria for withdrawal from study	Not specified	Not specified	
Power	Not specified	Not reported	
Morbidity/ complications	Not specified	"No adverse reactions to ceftazidime were noted"	

NS = not significant, COM = chronic otitis media, TM = tympanic membrane, SSI = surgical site infection, IV = intravenously, t.i.d. = three times a day.
* Sample size: numbers shown for those not lost to follow-up and those (initially recruited).
† Timing of first antibiotic dose is considered "appropriate" if given within the 2 h preceding the incision.

REFERENCES

1. Bagger-Sjoback D, Mendel L, Nord CE. The role of prophylactic antibiotics in middle ear surgery. A study on phenoxymethylpenecillin prophylaxis. Am J Otol 1987; 8(6):519–523.

2. Carlin WV, Lesser TH, John DG, Fielder C, Carrick DG, Thomas PL, Hill SS. Systemic antibiotic prophylaxis and reconstructive ear surgery. Clin Otololaryng Allied Sci 1987;12(6):441–446.

3. Donaldson JA, Snyder IS. Prophylactic chemotherapy in myringoplasty surgery. Laryngoscope 1966;76:1201–1214.

4. Eschelman. Prophylactic antibiotics in otolaryngologic surgery: a double blind study. Trans Am Acad Ophthalmol Otolaryngol 1971;75(2):387–394.

5. Govaerts PJ, Raemaekers J, Verlinden A, Kalai M, Somers T, Offeciers FE. Use of antibiotic prophylaxis in ear surgery. Laryngoscope 1998;108(1):107–110.

6. Jackson CG. Antimicrobial prophylaxis in ear surgery. Laryngoscope 1988;98(10):1116–1123.

7. John DG, Carlin WV, Lesser TH, Carrick DG, Fielder C. Tympanoplasty surgery and prophylactic antibiotics: surgical results. Clin Otololaryng Allied Sci 1988;13(3): 205–207.

8. Lindholdt T, Felding JU, Juul A, Kristensen S, Schouenburg P. Efficacy of perioperative ceftazidime in the surgical treatment of chronic otitis media due to Pseudomonas aeriginosa. Arch Otorhinolaryngol 1986;243(3):167–169.

9. Winerman I, Segal S, Man A. Effectiveness of Prophylactic Antibiotic Treatment in Mastoid Surgery. Am J Otol 1981; 3(1):65–67.

10. Managram AJ, Horan TC, Pearson ML, Silver LC, Jarvis WR. Guideline for Prevention of Surgical Site Infection. Centers for Disease Control, US Department of Health and Human Services, 1999.

11. Classen DC, Evans RS, Pestotnik SL, Horn SD, Menlove RL, Burke JP. The timing of prophylactic administration of antibiotics and the risk of surgical wound infection. N Engl J Med 1992;326(5):281–286.

SECTION IV
Systematic Reviews in General Otolaryngology

Section Editors

Jay Piccirillo, MD

Gregory W. Randolph, MD

19 Tonsillectomy in Adults

19.A.

Tonsillectomy for recurrent pharyngitis in adults: Impact on clinical improvement

Michael G. Stewart and Christopher Prichard

METHODS

A computerized PubMed search of MEDLINE 1966–February 2005 was performed. The terms "tonsillitis," "tonsil," and "tonsillectomy" were searched, and the resulting articles were cross-referenced, yielding 2020 articles. The search was limited to adult data; this yielded 476 articles. The titles or abstracts of these articles were then reviewed to identify those that met the following entry criteria: 1) adults with recurrent pharyngitis, 2) intervention with tonsillectomy, ideally versus nonsurgical treatment, and 3) comparative outcomes of post-treatment symptoms. One randomized controlled trial (RCT) and two retrospective reviews of outcomes after tonsillectomy met these criteria. The bibliographies of these articles and several narrative review articles were manually checked to ensure no further relevant articles could be identified. This process yielded no additional studies. In addition, we reviewed three published systematic reviews [1–3] on tonsillectomy for recurrent tonsillitis. Those reviews used strict entry criteria and included RCTs only; all reviews reported no appropriate RCTs for adults. Therefore, this overall process yielded three studies [4–6].

RESULTS

Outcome Measures. In the single RCT, a patient questionnaire was the primary and only outcome measure. In the two case series, utilization data and a post-treatment interview were used, and in one study a retrospective quality of life instrument was used, the Glasgow Benefit Inventory (GBI). The GBI is an 18-item postintervention questionnaire designed for retrospective evaluation of improvement in quality of life after otolaryngology intervention. It was not designed for any particular disease, but seems to be sensitive to differences in treatment outcome.

Potential Confounders. In all studies—even the RCT—the questionnaires were completed only after treatment, introducing the possibility of recall bias. In addition, there is a strong possibility of expectation bias from the treatment (placebo) effect. In the two uncontrolled case series, the possibility of regression to the mean also exists. Regression to the mean refers to the tendency in populations for most subjects to cluster near the overall mean. Subjects that are outliers, such as those with multiple infections, tend to move back toward the overall population mean over time, i.e., have fewer infections. Therefore, when only studying patients with more significant disease, it is possible that any reduction in severity or frequency is attributable to regression to the mean. Finally, response rates were suboptimal, introducing potential responder/nonresponder bias.

Study Designs. There was only one RCT, and two retrospective case series. Although the methods seem adequate, the description of randomization protocol in the RCT was quite limited, and it was impossible to use masking in outcome assessment because all patients knew whether or not they had undergone surgery. There was no *a priori* power analysis; because the study was very small, and the final result was "no difference," there is a strong possibility that the study did not have enough subjects to detect a difference that truly exists. Using their data and sample size studied, we calculated that the study had a power of approximately 35% to predict a 20% difference in response/cure rate between the two groups. To detect a larger difference, 30% for example, the study had only 59% power. The methodology and data collection techniques in the retrospective case series were adequate, but they have the inherent underlying biases of the retrospective study design.

Highest Level of Evidence. The single level 1 study found a trend toward improvement after tonsillectomy which was not statistically significant. The sample size, however, was small with a resulting limited power; therefore, a type II error cannot be excluded using their data (i.e., the results may falsely show no difference with versus without tonsillectomy when in reality a true difference exists). The two retrospective case series showed significant improvements with surgery. These retrospective studies are subject to recall bias, treatment bias, and regression to the mean. One study was based on medical records data, which should reduce bias, although patients might voluntarily seek less medical attention after surgical treatment. Even though statistical analysis of a quality of life instrument designed for retrospective use was performed in one study, and statistically significant improvement was noted, the uncontrolled retrospective nature of the study still limits interpretation.

Applicability. The single comparative study is quite small, which limits its potential generalizability. However, there are no other factors that would limit the applicability of these results to other patients.

Morbidity/Complications. No significant morbidity or mortality was reported in any studies.

CLINICAL SIGNIFICANCE AND FUTURE RESEARCH

There were one level 1 study and two level 4 studies that addressed the impact of tonsillectomy in adults with chronic tonsillitis. The RCT showed a trend toward improvement after tonsillectomy which was not statistically significant, but the study's sample size gave it limited power to demonstrate a significant difference that might truly exist. The level 4 evidence showed that tonsillectomy is beneficial in the treatment of recurrent tonsillitis. Retrospective case series are prone to recall bias and treatment placebo bias, but improvements after tonsillectomy in adults are demonstrated in a significant way by these data.

Larger level 1 studies comparing surgery versus observation or antibiotics are clearly needed. Also, the outcome measures in such studies should be carefully considered. Although the frequency of infection is an important outcome measure, infection severity and other symptoms—such as chronic throat pain, and quality-of-life impact—should be assessed as well. In addition, because some adult patients that meet criteria for tonsillectomy will have resolution of infections even without tonsillectomy, identification of factors that could predict which patients are likely to improve without surgery would be a very helpful tool for clinicians.

Reference	Stafford, 1986
Level (design)	1 (randomized controlled trial)
Sample size*	40 (40)

OUTCOMES

Questionnaire: "cured" of symptoms

Tonsillectomy	18 of 20 (90%)
No surgery	14 of 20 (70%)
p Value	= 0.24 (Fisher's exact test)
Conclusion	No significant difference
Follow-up time	18 mo

STUDY DESIGN

Inclusion criteria	4 episodes tonsillitis per year for 2 y; good health between episodes; normal blood count and negative Paul Bunnell test
Exclusion criteria	None specified
Randomization effectiveness	Apparently good; details not specified
Age	≥16 y
Masking	None
Intervention regimen details	Surgery group: tonsillectomy within 6 wk of trial entry. Technique not specified. Observation group: PCN V 250 mg q.i.d. for 8 d after each infectious episode (if PCN allergy, treatment also defined)
Diagnostic criteria for infectious episode	Criteria for infectious episode clearly defined (sore throat, dysphagia, pyrexia, malaise for ≥3 d)
Management of tonsillitis while in study	Each episode of tonsillitis treated with 8 d of antibiotics (PCN, or erythromycin or cotrimoxazole if PCN-allergic). Patients were seen every 3 mo
Data acquisition	Patients seen every 3 mo and questionnaire completed (data not reported). Patients could opt out of observation group and have surgery if desired
Management while in study	Defined above
Compliance	100% follow-up
Criteria for withdrawal from study	Not defined, but no withdrawals
Intention to treat analysis	Yes (no crossover)
Power	Not defined
Other outcome measures	In the tonsillectomy group, the 2 patients not "cured" still rated their outcome as "improved" 6/6 (100%) of patients who failed medical therapy rated themselves "cured" after tonsillectomy No difference between 2 groups in bacteriologic results taken at study entry
Morbidity/complications	None

q.i.d. = four times a day, URI = upper respiratory tract infection, HMO = health maintenance organization, PCN = penicillin, NA = not applicable, SD = standard deviation, QOL = quality of life.
* Sample size: numbers shown for those not lost to follow-up and those (initially recruited).

THE EVIDENCE CONDENSED: Tonsillectomy versus no surgery for recurrent tonsillitis

Reference	Mui, 1998	
Level (design)	4 (retrospective case series)	
Sample size*	147 (254)	

	OUTCOMES	
	Mean number of clinic visits for URI or tonsillitis	**Antibiotic prescriptions**
Tonsillectomy	Before surgery: 3.9 After surgery: 0.4	Before surgery: 2.2 After surgery: 0.1
No surgery	NA	NA
p Value	<0.001	<0.001
Conclusion	Significant improvement after surgery	Significant improvement after surgery
Follow-up time	24 mo	

	STUDY DESIGN	
Inclusion criteria	Underwent tonsillectomy without adenoidectomy in a single HMO health system between 1988–1993 Followed 2 y before and after tonsillectomy	
Exclusion criteria	None specified	
Randomization effectiveness	Not randomized	
Age	≥16 y	
Masking	NA	
Intervention regimen details	Surgical technique not specified Medical management before and after tonsillectomy was not specified	
Diagnostic criteria for infectious episode	Criteria for infectious episodes as preoperative criteria were not clearly defined Final review revealed that 68 patients had surgery for "chronic" tonsillitis, and 65 for "recurrent" tonsillitis; 133 of 147 (90.5%) had surgery for infections (remainder were for sleep apnea, asymmetry, etc.)	
Management of tonsillitis while in study	Not addressed	
Data acquisition	Medical records reviewed for physician visits, infections, and prescriptions. For chart review, infection criteria were standardized somewhat (symptoms or physician diagnosis). Patients that could be reached by telephone (60 of 147) were interviewed with a set of standard questions	
Management while in study	Not addressed	
Compliance	Only patients who completed follow-up were included	
Criteria for withdrawal from study	NA	
Intention to treat analysis	NA	
Power	Not reported	
Other outcome measures	Telephone interview of 60 patients: 88% reported fewer sore throats after surgery, 87% reported fewer severe sore throats, 90% reported fewer sick days, and 88% would recommend tonsillectomy to others. Before surgery 59% reported missing ≥6 d from work or school per year, and after surgery only 10% reported missing ≥6 d per year (Only 39/60 could estimate accurately the number of days missed)	
Morbidity/complications	Not reported	

q.i.d. = four times a day, URI = upper respiratory tract infection, HMO = health maintenance organization, PCN = penicillin, NA = not applicable, SD = standard deviation, QOL = quality of life.
* Sample size: numbers shown for those not lost to follow-up and those (initially recruited).

THE EVIDENCE CONDENSED: Tonsillectomy versus no surgery for recurrent tonsillitis

Reference	Bhattacharyya, 2001	
Level (design)	4 (retrospective case series)	
Sample size*	65 (247)	

OUTCOMES		
	Glasgow Benefit Inventory score	**Patient survey: antibiotic prescriptions**
Tonsillectomy	Total: +27.09 Subscales— General health: +34.68 Social function: +14.36 Physical function: +9.49	Before surgery: mean = 6.9 (SD 7.0) After surgery: 0.6 (0.9)
No Surgery	NA	NA
p Value	<0.001 for all scales	<0.001
Conclusion	Significant improvement after surgery	Significant improvement after surgery
Follow-up time	1 y minimum (mean = 42.6 mo)	

STUDY DESIGN	
Inclusion criteria	Underwent tonsillectomy without adenoidectomy for "chronic infectious tonsillitis." Tonsillectomy between January 1, 1994 and December 31, 1998
Exclusion criteria	Tonsillectomy for suspected neoplasm; simultaneous uvulopalatopharyngoplasty
Randomization effectiveness	Not randomized
Age	>16 y
Masking	NA
Intervention regimen details	Surgical technique not specified Medical management before and after tonsillectomy was not specified
Diagnostic criteria for infectious episode	Criteria for infectious episodes as preoperative criteria were not clearly defined
Management of tonsillitis while in study	Not addressed
Data acquisition	Medical records reviewed for demographic data Patients completed a retrospective survey on time taking antibiotics, workdays missed, and physician visits Patients also completed the Glasgow Benefit Inventory, a validated retrospective QOL instrument, with positive scores for improvement in QOL after treatment, and negative scores if QOL worsened
Management while in study	Not addressed
Compliance	26% response rate. Mean age, gender, and year of surgery were not different between responders and nonresponders
Criteria for withdrawal from study	NA
Intention to treat analysis	NA
Power	Not reported
Other outcome measures	Other patient survey data: Workdays missed, mean = 8.0 (SD 11.3) before surgery, 0.5 (1.4) after surgery Physician visits, 5.8 (5.9) before surgery, 0.3 (0.8) after surgery p < 0.001 for both comparisons
Morbidity/complications	Not reported

URI = upper respiratory tract infection, HMO = health maintenance organization, PCN = penicillin, NA = not applicable, SD = standard deviation, QOL = quality of life.
*Sample size: numbers shown for those not lost to follow-up and those (initially recruited).

REFERENCES

1. McKerrow W. Tonsillitis. Clin Evid 2004;12:808–813.
2. McKerrow W. Tonsillitis. Clin Evid 2003;9:608–612.
3. Burton MJ, Towler B, Glasziou P. Tonsillectomy versus non-surgical treatment for chronic/recurrent acute tonsillitis. Cochrane Database of Systematic Reviews 1999, Issue 3. Art. No.: CD001802. DOI: 10.1002/14651858. CD001802. Accessed 2002.
4. Stafford N, von Haacke N, Sene A, Croft C. The treatment of recurrent tonsillitis in adults. Laryngol Otol 1986;100: 175–177.
5. Mui S, Rasgon BM, Hilsinger RL. Efficacy of tonsillectomy for recurrent throat infection in adults. Laryngoscope 1998;108:1325–1328.
6. Bhattacharyya N, Kepnes LJ, Shapiro J. Efficacy and quality-of-life impact of adult tonsillectomy. Arch Otolaryngol Head Neck Surg 2001;127:1347–1350.

19 Tonsillectomy in Adults

19.B.

Perioperative antibiotics versus placebo: Impact on postoperative symptom control

Michael G. Stewart and Christopher Prichard

METHODS

A computerized PubMed search of MEDLINE 1966–February 2005 was performed. The terms "tonsillectomy" and "tonsil" were exploded and the resulting articles were combined. These articles were then cross-referenced with those obtained by exploding "antibacterial agents," "antibiotic prophylaxis," "lactams," "macrolides," "clindamycin," or "fluoroquinolones." This process yielded 295 trials, of which 33 were randomized controlled trials (RCTs). These articles were then reviewed to identify those that met the following inclusion criteria: 1) a distinct patient population ≥12 years old undergoing tonsillectomy or adenotonsillectomy, 2) intervention with systemic antibiotics versus placebo/no antibiotics, 3) outcome measured in terms of postoperative pain scores, analgesic use, or time with pain. Articles regarding studies of topical or local applications of antibiotics were excluded. Articles in which data from children younger and older than 12 years were pooled together with adult data, were also excluded. The bibliographies of the articles that met these inclusion criteria were manually checked to ensure no further relevant articles could be identified. This process yielded three articles which represent the highest level of evidence [1–3].

RESULTS

Outcome Measures. The Grandis and Cannon studies [1, 2] used logbooks kept by patients for 7 days. The O'Reilly study [3] evaluated daily pain scores for 10 days and conducted interviews at 14 days. Symptom evaluation was fairly standard, with minimal patient burden to complete, but diagnostic criteria were not standardized. There was also no external verification of symptom evaluation, i.e., no validated instrument, culture result, vital signs, or other method used to corroborate findings.

Potential Confounders. Recall bias was a potential problem, particularly for interviews conducted 2 weeks postoperatively. Recall bias would also be amplified if logbooks were not completed each day. Perioperative medications besides antibiotics could also influence postoperative symptoms. Moreover, patients lost to follow-up could have had different outcomes than patients completing the study.

Study Designs. There were three RCTs (level 1 evidence) that compared the impact of antibiotics on postoperative pain. Randomization was well described and effective in balancing potential confounders between groups. All three RCTs were placebo controlled to minimize bias. Follow-up time was adequate and covered the time period of clinical interest. The Grandis report [1] included a power analysis showing that 150 patients were needed to achieve a power of 90% to detect a difference of 1 day). Although more than 150 subjects were enrolled, only 101 patients completed the study. There was no power analysis reported in the Cannon study [2], and the overall sample size was fairly small, raising the possibility it could fail to identify a difference that might truly exist. Likewise, the O'Reilly study [3] also found no difference between treatment groups, but no power analysis was reported. To detect a 20% difference in pain scores, 104 patients would be needed in each group. Using calculations from their data (and an estimated standard deviation, because it was not reported), the Cannon study's sample size provided a 16% power to detect a difference of 20% in pain medication utilization, and a 70% power to detect a 50% reduction. The O'Reilly study seems to have a 75% power to detect a 20% difference in cumulative pain score.

Study Results. None of the three RCTs showed a significant difference in overall pain (measured either as a pain score or analgesic medication use) with antibiotic versus placebo. However, two studies did show some beneficial effects of antibiotic use. The Grandis study showed statistically significant improvements in certain symptoms—mouth odor, time to return of regular diet, and resumption of routine activities—even though pain was not improved. Although the Cannon study showed no statistically significant differences, the study population was small, and there was a trend toward selected improved outcomes in the antibiotic assembly. In particular, fever in the first 48 hours, halitosis, and return to diet trended toward better outcomes in the antibiotic group.

Applicability. These results are applicable to adults undergoing tonsillectomy.

Morbidity/Complications. No unexpected or significant adverse effects of antibiotics were reported. The reported secondary hemorrhage rate in one study was fairly high for all patients, but this included many patients with mild or minimal hemorrhage.

CLINICAL SIGNIFICANCE AND FUTURE RESEARCH

There were three level 1 studies that addressed this issue in adult tonsillectomy. No significant difference was noted in pain scores in any study, but they all had sample sizes/powers that might fail to identify any difference that might truly exist. Other symptoms, however, which seem clinically important—such as time to return of diet, and mouth odor—were improved; in the largest study, the improvements were statistically significant, and in one smaller study there was a trend toward significance. Although the improvements in symptom control after antibiotics were not consistently seen in all three studies, no symptom was worse with antibiotic treatment, and there were no significant complications of antibiotic use.

This topic has been studied more thoroughly in children, and antibiotics are clearly beneficial. Because two adult studies show some benefit, and it is a biologically plausible effect, there does not seem to be a significant demand for further immediate study in adults.

THE EVIDENCE CONDENSED: Antibiotics versus placebo for post-tonsillectomy symptom control

Reference	Grandis, 1992	
Level (design)	1 (randomized controlled trial)	
Sample size*	101 (198)	

	OUTCOMES	
	Mean pain score (1 least severe to 10 most severe)†	**Mouth odor (days with severe odor-scale: 1 none, 2 moderate, 3 severe)**
Antibiotic	4.1	2.5 d
Placebo	4.42	4.2 d
p Value	NS	0.004
Conclusion	No significant difference	Improved on antibiotics
Follow-up time	7 d postoperatively	

	STUDY DESIGN	
Inclusion criteria	≥12 y old, tonsillectomy with or without adenoidectomy	
Exclusion criteria	Medical condition requiring perioperative antibiotics, history of penicillin allergy, antibiotics administered within 1 wk of tonsillectomy	
Randomization effectiveness	Authors reported no significant difference in age, sex, or early discontinuation of medication Male/female: 36%:64%; no p value. Table cited in text (Table I) does not contain age/sex data	
Age	12–48 y	
Masking	Double blind	
Antibiotic regimen details	3.1 g ticarcillin and clavulanic acid IV q 6 h ×3 doses after removal of tonsils, then amoxicillin/clavulanic acid 250 mg PO t.i.d. ×7 d	
Placebo details	Saline IV q 6 h ×3 doses then placebo PO t.i.d. ×7 d	
Diagnostic criteria	Not defined—patient logbooks used	
Indication for tonsillectomy	Not reported	
Analgesic while in study	Acetaminophen with codeine	
Surgical technique	Electrocautery hemostasis for adenoids Hot vs cold tonsillectomy not specified	
Compliance	198 patients recruited; 156 left hospital on study medication (55 did not complete data booklets. 11 patients discontinued study medication for odynophagia (8), nausea (2), rash (1)	
Criteria for withdrawal from study	Failure to receive study medication or complete logbooks: No difference in those completing and not completing the study in age, sex, or treatment group assignment	
Intention to treat analysis	Yes (no crossovers)	
Power	*A priori* calculation: for 90% power to discern a 1-d difference in symptom duration with an alpha value of 0.05, 150 patients would be needed	
Other outcome parameters	Significantly better with antibiotics: time with mouth odor, time to return to regular diet, time to return to work Trend toward improvement with antibiotics but no significant difference in fever >99.9°F, otalgia, headache, number of analgesic doses Trend toward improvement with placebo but no significant difference: nausea, vomiting, diarrhea	
Morbidity/complications	No significant difference in nausea, vomiting, diarrhea, otalgia, postoperative bleeding, rash, headache	

NS = not significant, IV = intravenously, t.i.d. = three times a day.
† Standard deviation not reported.
* Sample size: numbers shown for those not lost to follow-up and those (initially recruited).

THE EVIDENCE CONDENSED: Antibiotics versus placebo for post-tonsillectomy symptom control

Reference	Cannon, 1996	
Level (design)	1 (randomized controlled trial)	
Sample size*	46 (50)	

OUTCOMES		
	Mean number of analgesic doses	**Days to soft diet**
Antibiotic	19.45 (range 6–33)	41.7% on soft diet at d 3
Placebo	19.23 (range 6–41)	27.3% on soft diet at d 3
p Value	NS	NS
Conclusion	No significant difference	No significant difference
Follow-up time	7 d postoperatively	

STUDY DESIGN	
Inclusion criteria	≥12 y old, tonsillectomy
Exclusion criteria	Medical condition requiring perioperative antibiotics, history of allergy to penicillin or cephalosporin, antibiotics within 1 wk of tonsillectomy
Randomization effectiveness	Fewer preoperative infections and more males in the cefonicid group; no comment on whether differences were statistically significant
Age	13–40 y
Masking	Double blind
Antibiotic regimen details	Cefonicid 1 g IV ×1 before initiation of tonsillectomy
Placebo details	Placebo IV ×1 before initiation of tonsillectomy
Diagnostic criteria	Not defined—patient logbooks used
Indication for tonsillectomy	Recurrent episodes of acute tonsillitis "for most of the patients in the group." 27 patients with 4–6 infections in preceding year, 14 with >6 infections
Analgesic while in study	Acetaminophen with codeine
Surgical technique	Blunt dissection with snare and electrocautery hemostasis
Compliance	50 patients enrolled; 46 completed study (4 did not complete their logbook)
Intention to treat analysis	Yes (no crossovers)
Power	Not reported
Other outcome parameters	No significant difference in rates of trismus, postoperative bleeding, eschar, day of highest fever, activity level, or weight loss Trend toward improvement with antibiotics but no significant difference: halitosis, time to resumption of soft diet
Morbidity/complications	No allergic reactions, no phlebitis

NS = not significant, IV = intravenously, t.i.d. = three times a day.
* Sample size: numbers shown for those not lost to follow-up and those (initially recruited).

Reference	O'Reilly, 2003	
Level (design)	1 (randomized controlled trial)	
Sample size*	95 (200)	

OUTCOMES

	Mean sum pain score (1 least severe to 10 most severe summed daily for 10 d)	Request for additional analgesics
Antibiotic	32.59 (range 19–46)	43%
Placebo	31.89 (range 19–50)	46%
p Value	NS	NS
Conclusion	No significant difference	No significant difference
Follow-up time	14 d postoperatively	

STUDY DESIGN

Inclusion criteria	≥16 y old, tonsillectomy
Exclusion criteria	Failure to attend follow-up visit or adequately complete questionnaire
Randomization effectiveness	Authors reported no significant difference in age or sex between treatment/placebo Preoperative antibiotics had been taken by more of the placebo group (stated in text, although data table shows more in active)
Age	16–53 y
Masking	Double blind
Antibiotic regimen details	250 mg IV amoxicillin after anesthesia induction, then amoxicillin 250 mg PO t.i.d. ×7 d
Placebo details	No IV placebo, then placebo PO t.i.d. ×7 d
Diagnostic criteria	Not defined—patient logbooks and interview used
Indication for tonsillectomy	"Elective tonsillectomy for nonmalignant disease"
Analgesic while in study	Acetaminophen with codeine, diclofenac
Surgical technique	"Most used electrodissection"
Compliance	200 patients enrolled; 95 attended follow-up visit and completed data booklet
Criteria for withdrawal from study	Failure to attend follow-up visit or adequately complete questionnaire
Intention to treat analysis	Yes (no crossovers)
Power	Not reported
Other outcome parameters	No significant difference in rates between groups for subsequent consultation to general practitioners for pain, additional antibiotic prescriptions, or secondary hemorrhage
Morbidity/complications	24% secondary hemorrhage rate—mild to major (2 of 95 had major hemorrhage: "requiring transfusion or surgery")

NS = not significant, IV = intravenously, t.i.d. = three times a day.
* Sample size: numbers shown for those not lost to follow-up and those (initially recruited).

REFERENCES

1. Grandis JR, Johnson JT, Vickers RM, et al. The efficacy of perioperative antibiotic therapy on recovery following tonsillectomy in adults: randomized double-blind placebo-controlled trial. Otolaryngol Head Neck Surg 1992;106: 137–142.

2. Cannon CR. The efficacy of a single dose antibiotic regimen in adults undergoing tonsillectomy. J Miss State Med Assoc 1996;37:817–821.

3. O'Reilly BJ, Black S, Fernandes J, Panesar J. Is the routine use of antibiotics justified in adult tonsillectomy? J Laryngol Otol 2003;117:382–385.

19 Tonsillectomy in Adults

Monopolar cautery versus cold dissection tonsillectomy: Impact on operating time, intraoperative blood loss, postoperative pain, return to normal diet, and/or postoperative bleeding

James Denneny and Wade Chien

METHODS

A computerized PubMed search of MEDLINE 1966–May 2006 was performed. Articles mapping to the exploded medical subject heading "tonsillectomy" were obtained, yielding 5497 reports. Given the richness of the literature, these publications were then limited to randomized controlled trials (RCTs), yielding 395 articles. An additional search, which collected articles with the terms "electrocoagulation" or "cautery" or "bovie" or "cautery" or "hot" and "cold" or "dissection snare" or "dissection-snare" or "sluder" or "guillotine" or "sharp" or "knife" and cross-referenced them with those obtained by exploding the medical subject heading "tonsillectomy" was also performed, yielding 41 trials. The 395 and 41 articles were then reviewed to identify those that met the following inclusion criteria: 1) patients undergoing tonsillectomy, 2) intervention with monopolar versus cold dissection for the procedure, 3) outcome measured in terms of operating time, intraoperative blood loss, postoperative pain, return to normal diet, and/or postoperative bleeding. In addition, only RCTs were included. The bibliographies of the articles that met these inclusion criteria were manually checked to ensure no further relevant articles could be identified. This process yielded eight articles [1–8].

RESULTS

Outcome Measures. Outcome measures included: 1) the time required to perform the procedure, 2) intraoperative blood loss, 3) postoperative pain, 4) the time required to return to normal diet, and 5) postoperative hemorrhage. There were different methodologies used to quantify postoperative pain, but within each study the same scale was used. Pain measures ranged from the validated FACES pain scale to simply asking patients who had monopolar tonsillectomy on one side and cold dissection on the other side to pick the more painful side. The remaining parameters were objectively measured.

Potential Confounders. Results after tonsillectomy can be dependent not only on technique, but also on the patient population and perioperative management. Subjects in these studies represent a variety of ages with outliers in terms of bleeding disorders and chronic illness

excluded. Attempts were made to limit the number of operators performing the surgery. Antibiotic and steroid usage were standardized, as were postoperative analgesic choices. Pain could be affected by the use of electrocautery to obtain hemostasis following the tonsillectomy when performed using the "cold" technique. Attempts were made to minimize this factor. In most of the studies, there were several different operators performing the surgery, but all had similar experience.

Study Designs. All eight RCTs compared monopolar cautery to cold dissection tonsillectomy. Monopolar tonsillectomies were performed with the Bovie or suction cautery. Cold tonsillectomies were performed with the knife, the snare, the microdebrider, or blunt dissection. A wide variety of patient ages were represented in the study, ranging from 2 to 42 years old. Most studies included all patients undergoing tonsillectomy, regardless of indication, but one study reported only on patients undergoing surgery for obstructive symptoms. Most studies reported all of the listed outcome measures. Follow-up times ranged from 4 hours to 1 month.

Highest Level of Evidence. Each RCT measured multiple parameters, and results overall were mixed. In the simplest of terms, monopolar cautery was associated with a faster operating time, less intraoperative blood loss, and similar postoperative pain, return to normal diet, and postoperative hemorrhage. The key to data, however, often lies in understanding the subtleties, and so the results are discussed in more detail below.

Operating time was measured in six studies. Monopolar cautery was significantly faster in three studies, but slower in one study, whereas two studies showed no difference. In two of the three studies showing monopolar cautery to be faster, the microdebrider was used for the cold dissection arm. In the third of those studies, cold dissection was performed with the snare. Overall, their average operating time differed by <10 minutes.

Intraoperative blood loss was compared in seven RCTs. Microdebrider usage resulted in significantly more blood loss than monopolar cautery in one trial. Cold knife with snare dissection resulted in significantly more blood loss than monopolar cautery in three trials. In addition, another trial reported an average of 66 cc of blood loss with cold dissection versus 11 cc with monopolar cautery; although there was no statistical comparison reported, this wide discrepancy is again suggestive of more blood loss with cold dissection. The two remaining RCTs suggested no difference in intraoperative bleeding.

Postoperative pain was measured in all eight RCTs, and results were mixed. Pain was significantly less with monopolar cautery in two trials, but significantly worse with monopolar cautery in another two trials. The remaining four trials showed no significant difference between groups.

As a corollary to postoperative pain measurements, the time to return to normal diet was compared in three RCTs. Again, results were heterogeneous, with one trial showing faster normal oral intake with the microdebrider than monopolar cautery, another trial showing faster results with dissection snare than with monopolar dissection, and yet another trial showing no difference.

Finally, postoperative hemorrhage was compared. Of the five RCTs that addressed this issue, none showed a significant difference between groups. None of these studies, however, were powered to address this specific question. When the incidence of an event is low (≤5% in these studies for this parameter), very large sample sizes are required to detect a significant difference between groups. Thus, the postoperative bleeding results are not completely definitive, even though they are uniform.

Applicability. These studies are applicable to patients undergoing tonsillectomy for the range of indications. Each individual study is more specifically applicable to the patient population admitted according to their inclusion/exclusion criteria, as described in the adjacent table.

Morbidity/Complications. The main morbidity of tonsillectomy lies in pain, inability to tolerate a normal diet, and blood loss—both intraoperative and postoperative. These parameters were discussed as the main results of these trials (see above).

CLINICAL SIGNIFICANCE AND FUTURE RESEARCH

There were eight RCTs that compared tonsillectomy using monopolar cautery versus cold techniques. Each RCT measured multiple parameters, and results overall were mixed. In the simplest of terms, monopolar cautery was associated with a faster operating time and less intraoperative blood loss, although results were not completely uniform among all studies. Results regarding postoperative pain and return to normal diet were variable, with balanced numbers of trials showing opposite results or no difference. Postoperative hemorrhage was not significantly different in any of the trials, although these studies were not powered to detect differences in low incidence events such as the <5% rate of bleeding.

Future studies may use uniform outcome measures with clear measures of variance to allow for clean meta-analysis of all reported data. Further studies regarding intracapsular techniques with attention to longer-term regrowth of tonsillar tissue would also be of use. Return to regular activities in addition to diet would be valuable data when considering "total cost" of the various techniques.

THE EVIDENCE CONDENSED: Monopolar electrocautery versus cold dissection tonsillectomy

Reference	Mann, 1984			Sobol, 2006		
Level (design)	1 (randomized controlled trial)			1 (randomized controlled trial)		
Sample size*	92 (95)			74		
OUTCOMES						
Techniques studied	Monopolar cautery (n = 51)	Cold dissection (n = 41)	p Value	Microdebrider intracapsular (n = 38)	Monopolar cautery (n = 36)	p Value
Operating time	10.1 min	12.4 min	NR	20.9 min	16.6 min	0.001
Intraoperative blood loss	11.8 mL	66.3 mL	NR	45.0 mL	30.0 mL	0.01
Postoperative pain	POD 1 n = 22 worse with electrocautery POD 7 n = 3 worse with cold	POD 1 n = 22 worse with cold POD 7 n = 3 worse with cold	NR	4.6 d to little or no pain	3.9 d to little or no pain	>0.05
Time to normal diet	NR	NR	NR	2.7 d	4.4 d	0.04
Postoperative hemorrhage	n = 1/51 <24 h from surgery	n = 1/41 <24 h from surgery	NR	None	n = 1/36, delayed	NS
Conclusion	Electrocautery was faster with less blood loss, but with greater pain (not statistically verified) Postop bleeding was equal			Microdebrider tonsillectomy was slower, higher blood loss, but had a shorter time to resumption of normal diet		
Follow-up time	7–10 d			10 d		
STUDY DESIGN						
Inclusion criteria	All patients meeting criteria for tonsillectomy			All patients not meeting exclusion criteria		
Exclusion criteria	None stated			All patients <3 y or >7 y, history of adenotonsillectomy, nonobstructive indication for tonsillectomy, craniofacial syndrome, developmental delay, mucopolysaccharidoses, expressive language disorders, hematologic and wound-healing disorders, necrotizing dermatoses		
Randomization process	By SS#, each patient was their own control, with electrocautery used on one side and cold dissection on the contralateral side. Not otherwise specified			Sealed envelopes that were to be opened only on the morning of surgery; family was blinded to this process. Children were randomized in blocks of 10 into either group		
Age	NR			3–7 y		
Method of tonsillectomy	Monopolar electrocautery was used on one side. Scissors, snare used on contralateral side			Microdebrider intracapsular tonsillectomy vs monopolar electrocautery		
Indications for tonsillectomy	NR			NR		
Variables studied	OR time, blood loss, postop pain, postop hemorrhage			OR time, blood loss, days to near-normal diet, near-normal activity, little or no pain, little or no medication use		
Pain measurement	Patients were asked to select which side was more painful			FACES pain scale		
Power	NR			For a sample size of 40 control and 40 experimental subjects, there is a 75% power to detect a moderate improvement and 99% power to detect a large improvement ($\alpha = 0.05$)		

NR = not reported, POD = postoperative day, NS = not significant, postop = postoperative, OR = operating room.
*Sample size: numbers shown for those not lost to follow-up and those (initially recruited).

THE EVIDENCE CONDENSED: Monopolar electrocautery versus cold dissection tonsillectomy

Reference	Derkay, 2006		
Level (design)	1 (randomized controlled trial)		
Sample size*	300		

OUTCOMES

Techniques studied	Electrocautery (150)	Microdebrider (150)	p Value
Operating time	8 min	10 min	0.0001
Intraoperative blood loss	99% <25 mL	97% <25 mL	NR
Postoperative pain	3 on FACES pain scale	3 on FACES pain scale	NS
Time to normal diet	3.5 d	3 d	NS
Postoperative hemorrhage	n = 2/150	n = 1/150	NS

Conclusion	Microdebrider was slower, patients returned to normal activity faster, stopped taking pain medications sooner, were more likely to have residual tonsillar tissue
Follow-up time	14 d–1 mo

STUDY DESIGN

Inclusion criteria	Children >2 y of age undergoing tonsillectomy for hyperplasia
Exclusion criteria	History of recurrent tonsillitis, craniofacial syndrome, hematologic disorder, severe developmental disorder, or severe comorbid factors
Randomization process	Random-number generator was used to assign patients into either group. Surgeon was notified of the group status immediately before surgery
Age	Mean 5 y in both groups
Method of tonsillectomy	Pencil electrocautery vs microdebrider tonsillectomy
Indications for tonsillectomy	NR
Variables studied	OR time, blood loss, pain level at discharge, pain medication dosing, time to return to normal diet, postop suffering, complications
Pain measurement	FACES pain scale
Power	Designed to detect difference between groups in time to normal activity in 2 days with a power of 89% ($\alpha = 0.05$)

NR = not reported, POD = postoperative day, NS = not significant, postop = postoperative, OR = operating room.
*Sample size: numbers shown for those not lost to follow-up and those (initially recruited).

Reference	Young, 2001			Nunez, 2000		
Level (design)	1 (randomized controlled trial)			1 (randomized controlled trial)		
Sample size*	50			50 (54)		

OUTCOMES

Techniques studied	Monopolar cautery (27)	Cold dissection (23)	p Value	Monopolar cautery (24)	Cold dissection (26)	p Value
Operating time	7.18 min	16 min	<0.05	Not recorded	Not recorded	
Intraoperative blood loss	4.92 mL	32.17 mL	<0.05	15.1 mL	33.7 mL	<0.001
Postoperative pain	0.869 at 2 h postop; 0.826 at 4 h postop	1.66 at 2 h postop; 1.58 at 4 h postop	0.001	26.7 doses of postop analgesic in 12 d	19.2 doses of postop analgesic in 12 d	<0.05
Time to normal diet	NR	NR		7.5 d	5.0 d	<0.05
Postoperative hemorrhage	NR	NR		n = 2/24	n = 1/26	>0.05
Conclusion	Suction cautery has less operative time, less intraop blood loss, and less postop pain			Cold dissection has a higher EBL, less postop pain (lesser requirement of postop analgesic), shorter time to normal diet, less postop throat pain, and less postop general practitioner consultation		
Follow-up time	4 h postop			2 wk		

STUDY DESIGN

Inclusion criteria	Children between 2–16 y undergoing tonsillectomy, either alone or with adenoidectomy			Children diagnosed with recurrent tonsillitis and/or upper airway obstruction		
Exclusion criteria	Bleeding disorder, craniofacial abnormalities			Patients with allergy, intercurrent disease, bleeding tendencies, using antibiotics, or unable to attend follow-up		
Randomization process	Surgical method determined by a random draw at the time of surgery			NR		
Age	2–15 y, with mean of 7 y			Mean 6.4 y in both groups		
Method of tonsillectomy	Suction cautery vs cold knife dissection with snares			Diathermy dissection tonsillectomy vs cold dissection with a Gwynne-Evans dissector and Eves snare		
Indications for tonsillectomy	NR			NR		
Variables studied	Intraop blood loss, operative time, postop fluid intake and pain			Postop analgesic consumption, time to regain normal diet and activity levels, and complications		
Pain measurement	A simple descriptive word pain scale with levels as none, mild, moderate, severe, or excruciating was used. The descriptives were given a numerical indicator to calculate significance (not shown)			The number of analgesic doses used was recorded		
Power	NR			22 children in each arm could show a difference of 1 SD or greater with α of 0.05 with a power of 0.9		

NR = not reported, POD = postoperative day, NS = not significant, postop = postoperative, intraop = intraoperative, URI = upper respiratory infection, OR = operating room, SD = standard deviation, EBL = estimated blood loss.
* Sample size: numbers shown for those not lost to follow-up and those (initially recruited).

Reference	Tay, 1996		
Level (design)	1 (randomized controlled trial)		
Sample size*	105		

OUTCOMES

Techniques studied	Unipolar diathermy	Ligation	p Value
Operating time	NR	NR	
Intraoperative blood loss	NR	NR	
Postoperative pain	4.76/10 on POD 1	5.23/10 on POD 1	0.028
Time to normal diet	NR	NR	
Postoperative hemorrhage	n = 1/105 (within 24 h)	n = 1/105 (POD 6)	NS
Conclusion	There was less pharyngeal pain on the diathermy side on POD 1, but there was no significant difference in pharyngeal pain and otalgia for the remainder of the postop period		
Follow-up time	2 wk		

STUDY DESIGN

Inclusion criteria	All patients >7 y admitted for elective tonsillectomy were entered into the study		
Exclusion criteria	Patients with URI during the 6 wk before admission, and patients who had adenotonsillectomy or other concurrent operations		
Randomization process	The side of diathermy hemostasis was decided by selecting sealed instructions from a bag in OR		
Age	Mean 17.9 y		
Method of tonsillectomy	Each patient was his/her own control. Tonsillectomy was performed by blunt dissection. Diathermy was used for hemostasis on one side, and suture ligation on the other side		
Indications for tonsillectomy	NR		
Variables studied	Postop pharyngeal pain, otalgia, number of patients on analgesics on PODs 7 and 14, and postop hemorrhage		
Pain measurement	A scale of 0–10 was used, with 0 being no pain, and 10 being very severe pain		
Power	85 patients needed for 80% chance of demonstrating a 50% difference in postop pain response		

NR = not reported, POD = postoperative day, NS = not significant, postop = postoperative, intraop = intraoperative, URI = upper respiratory infection, OR = operating room, SD = standard deviation.
* Sample size: numbers shown for those not lost to follow-up and those (initially recruited).

THE EVIDENCE CONDENSED: Monopolar electrocautery versus cold dissection tonsillectomy

Reference	Leach, 1993			Trent, 1993		
Level (design)	1 (randomized controlled trial)			1 (randomized controlled trial)		
Sample size*	28			29		
OUTCOMES						
Techniques studied	Monopolar cautery	Cold dissection	p Value	Monopolar cautery	Epinephrine injection cold dissection	p Value
Operating time	13.5 min	9.9 min	<0.01	5.4 min	6.1 min	>0.05
Intraoperative blood loss	26.6 mL	78.4 mL	<0.01	6.7 mL	8.2 mL	>0.05
Postoperative pain	7.3/10	4.8/10	<0.05	4/27 patients had more pain on POD 0; 8/25 on POD 1; and 8/24 on PODs 4–7	6/27 patients had more pain on POD 0; 5/25 on POD 1; and 7/24 on PODs 4–7	>0.05
Time to normal diet	NR	NR		NR	NR	
Postoperative hemorrhage	n = 1/28	None	NS	None	n = 1/29	NS
Conclusion	Cautery has a longer operative time, lower blood loss, and greater postop pain			There is no difference between cautery and cold dissection in intraop blood loss, operating time, postop pain, or postop hemorrhage		
Follow-up time	4–7 d			7–10 d		
STUDY DESIGN						
Inclusion criteria	All patients meeting criteria for tonsillectomy for recurrent tonsillitis			All patients meeting criteria for tonsillectomy		
Exclusion criteria	Aspirin use within 2 wk before surgery, OSA, history of bleeding disorder, acute tonsillitis within 6 wk before surgery. Patient <13 y or >50 y			Patients with hypertension, blood dyscrasia, allergy to lidocaine, history of peritonsillar abscess		
Randomization process	NR			Randomization using last digit of patient's medical record number: even—cold dissection, and odd—cautery		
Age	13–32 y, mean 17.9 y			3–42 y, mean 14 y		
Method of tonsillectomy	Each patient was his/her own control. Electrocautery was done on 1 side, and cold dissection with a Fisher knife and snare was done on the other side			Bovie tonsillectomy vs epinephrine-injected cold dissection (injection of epinephrine into tonsillar fossa, and dissection with no. 12 blade)		
Indications for tonsillectomy	≥7 episodes of tonsillitis in 1 y; ≥5 episodes per y for 2 y; or ≥3 episodes per y for 3 y			NR		
Variables studied	Operative time, intraop blood loss, postop pain, and postop hemorrhage			Operative time, intraop blood loss, postop pain, and postop hemorrhage		
Pain measurement	A scale of 0–10 was used, with 0 being no pain, and 10 being severe pain			Pain was assessed by asking patients which side (if either) hurt more on POD 0, 1, and on first postop visit (PODs 4–7)		
Power	NR			NR		

POD = postoperative day, NR = not reported, postop = postoperative, intraop = intraoperative, OSA = obstructive sleep apnea.
* Sample size: numbers shown for those not lost to follow-up and those (initially recruited).

REFERENCES

1. Mann DG, St. George C, Granoff D, Scheiner E, Imber P, Mylnarczyk FA. Tonsillectomy—some like it hot. Laryngoscope 1984;94(5):677–679.

2. Sobol SE, Wetmore RF, Marsh RR, Stow J, Jacobs IN. Postoperative recovery after microdebrider intracapsular or monopolar electrocautery tonsillectomy: a prospective, randomized, single-blinded study. Arch Otolaryngol Head Neck Surg 2006;132(3):270–274.

3. Derkay CS, Darrow DH, Welch C, Sinacori JT. Post-tonsillectomy morbidity and quality of life in pediatric patients with obstructive tonsils and adenoid: microdebrider vs electrocautery. Otolaryngol Head Neck Surg 2006; 134(1):114–120.

4. Young C, MacRae J. Tonsillectomy. A comparative study of dissection/snare vs suction-cautery. Can Oper Room Nurs J 2001;19(3):7–11.

5. Nunez DA, Provan J, Crawford M. Postoperative tonsillectomy pain in pediatric patients: electrocautery (hot) vs cold dissection and snare tonsillectomy—a randomized trial. Arch Otolaryngol Head Neck Surg 2000;126(7):837–841.

6. Tay HL. Post-tonsillectomy pain with selective diathermy haemostasis. J Laryngol Otol 1996;110(5):446–448.

7. Trent CS. Electrocautery versus epinephrine-injection tonsillectomy. Ear Nose Throat J 1993;72(8):520–522, 525.

8. Leach J, Manning S, Schaefer S. Comparison of two methods of tonsillectomy. Laryngoscope 1993;103(6):619–622.

19 Tonsillectomy in Adults

Bipolar cautery versus cold dissection tonsillectomy: Impact on operating time, intraoperative blood loss, postoperative pain, return to normal diet, and/or postoperative bleeding

James Denneny and Wade Chien

METHODS

A computerized PubMed search of MEDLINE 1966–May 2006 was performed. Articles mapping to the exploded medical subject heading "tonsillectomy" were obtained, yielding 5497 reports. Given the richness of the literature, these publications were then limited to randomized controlled trials (RCTs), yielding 395 articles. An additional search, which collected articles with the terms "electrocoagulation" or "cautery" or "bovie" or "cautery" or "hot" and "cold" or "dissection snare" or "dissection-snare" or "sluder" or "guillotine" or "sharp" or "knife" and cross-referenced them with those obtained by exploding the medical subject heading "tonsillectomy" was also performed, yielding 41 trials. The 395 and 41 articles were then reviewed to identify those that met the following inclusion criteria: 1) patient population undergoing tonsillectomy, 2) intervention with bipolar versus cold dissection tonsillectomy, 3) outcome measured in terms of operating time, intraoperative blood loss, postoperative pain, return to normal diet, and/or postoperative bleeding. In addition, only RCTs were included. The bibliographies of the articles that met these inclusion criteria were manually checked to ensure no further relevant articles could be identified. This process yielded six articles [1–6].

RESULTS

Outcome Measures. Outcome measures included: 1) the time required to perform the procedure, 2) intraoperative blood loss, 3) postoperative pain, 4) the time required to return to normal diet, and 5) postoperative hemorrhage. There were different methodologies used to quantify postoperative pain, but within each study the same scale was used. Pain was measured on scales of 1 to 10 or 1 to 4. The remainder of the parameters were able to be objectively measured.

Potential Confounders. Potential confounders are similar to those described in the previous section.

Study Designs. These six RCTs compared bipolar cautery to cold dissection tonsillectomy. Bipolar devices included the microbipolars, the LigaSure Vessel Sealing System, and the bipolar scissors. Cold dissections included knife, dissection ligation, and blunt dissection with snares. A wide age range was studied, spanning patients from 2 to 54 years old. Three studies included patients undergoing tonsillectomy for any reason, whereas two focused only on patients undergoing tonsillectomy for recurrent sore throat. The remaining study did not provide details regarding their tonsillectomy population. All studies were randomized to attempt to balance potential confounders between groups. Follow-up times ranged from 10 to 17 days.

Highest Level of Evidence. These RCTs investigated multiple postoperative parameters after bipolar versus cold tonsillectomy. Overall, results seemed to favor a faster operation and less intraoperative blood loss with the bipolar. Postoperative pain and hemorrhage results were mixed; less pain and postoperative bleeding was seen with the bipolar in some trials, but a similar number of other trials showed no difference. More specific details are as follows: 1) Bipolar cautery was faster than cold dissection in five of the six RCTs. The sixth trial showed a trend toward bipolar cautery being slower, but no statistical analysis specific to this parameter was reported. 2) Intraoperative blood loss was significantly less with bipolar cautery in three RCTs. The other trials did not report a relevant statistical analysis. 3) Postoperative pain was found to be significantly less with bipolar cautery in two of the trials whereas two others found no difference. 4) One trial showed a faster return to normal diet with bipolar cautery, whereas another RCT showed no difference. 5) Two RCTs showed significantly fewer postoperative hemorrhages with bipolar cautery as compared with cold dissection. Three RCTs showed no significant difference in the same parameter.

Applicability. These studies are applicable to patients of a wide age range undergoing tonsillectomy. Each individual study is more specifically applicable to the patient population admitted according to their inclusion/exclusion criteria, as described in the adjacent table.

Morbidity/Complications. The main morbidity of tonsillectomy lies in pain, inability to tolerate a normal diet, and blood loss—both intraoperative and postoperative. These parameters were discussed as the main results of these trials (see above).

CLINICAL SIGNIFICANCE AND FUTURE RESEARCH

There were six RCTs that compared results after bipolar tonsillectomy versus cold dissection tonsillectomy. The majority of results supported a faster operation and less intraoperative blood loss with the bipolar. In addition, postoperative pain and hemorrhage was less with the bipolar in some trials, but a similar number of other trials showed no difference.

Future research may focus on reporting uniform outcome measures of pain so as to facilitate clean meta-analyses of these and future data. Future research may also focus on specific patient populations according to age or indications for tonsillectomy. Studies will evolve further as new techniques are developed for this ubiquitous procedure.

Reference	Lachanas, 2005			Raut, 2002		
Level (design)	1 (randomized controlled trial)			1 (randomized controlled trial)		
Sample size*	200			50		
OUTCOMES						
Techniques studied	**Bipolar cautery** (n = 108)	**Cold dissection** (n = 92)	**p Value**	**Bipolar cautery** (n = 18)	**Cold dissection** (n = 32)	**p Value**
Operating time	15 min	21 min	<0.001	10.5 min	14.5 min	0.001
Intraoperative blood loss	None	125 mL	NR	6 mL	86 mL	<0.001
Postoperative pain	3.63/10	5.09/10	<0.001	Overall score 43.1	Overall score 45.7	>0.05
Time to normal diet	NR	NR	NA	NR	NR	NA
Postoperative hemorrhage	n = 2/108 for secondary	n = 1/92 for primary; 2/92 for secondary	NR	16.6% for secondary bleed	12.5% for secondary bleed	0.253
Conclusion	Bipolar cautery is faster and has less postop pain			Bipolar cautery is faster and has less intraop blood loss		
Follow-up time	14 d			15–17 d		
STUDY DESIGN						
Inclusion criteria	200 consecutive adult patients meeting criteria for tonsillectomy			All children >10 y old with recurrent sore throats (>5 attacks/y)		
Exclusion criteria	Patients undergoing adenoidectomy or other concurrent procedures, history of peritonsillar abscess, bleeding disorders			History of peritonsillar abscess, patients undergoing adenoidectomy or other concurrent procedures, Hx of bleeding disorder, craniofacial anomalies, chronic debilitating diseases		
Randomization process	NR			Block randomization involving balancing the number of patients recruited in both arms after every 20 recruits		
Age	16–46 y, mean 25.3 y			10–16 y, mean 14.3 y		
Method of tonsillectomy	Bipolar tonsillectomy with LigaSure Vessel Sealing System, vs cold knife tonsillectomy			Bipolar scissors vs cold blunt dissection with snares		
Indications for tonsillectomy	Chronic tonsillitis, OSA			Recurrent tonsillitis		
Variables studied	Operative time, intraop blood loss, postop pain, hemorrhage			Operative time, intraop blood loss, postop pain, hemorrhage		
Pain measurement	A scale of 0–10 was used, with 0 being no pain, and 10 being intolerable pain			VAS, with a scale of 0–10		
Power	NR			NR		

NR = not reported, NA = not applicable, postop = postoperative, intraop = intraoperative, VAS = visual analog scale.
*Sample size: numbers shown for those not lost to follow-up and those (initially recruited).

THE EVIDENCE CONDENSED: Bipolar electrocautery versus cold dissection tonsillectomy

Reference	Raut, 2001		
Level (design)	1 (randomized controlled trial)		
Sample size*	183 (200)		

OUTCOMES

Techniques studied	Bipolar cautery (n = 91)	Cold dissection (n = 92)	p Value
Operating time	13 min	20 min	<0.001
Intraoperative blood loss	5 mL	115 mL	<0.001
Postoperative pain	6.9/10	6.9/10	>0.05
Time to normal diet	NR	NR	NA
Postoperative hemorrhage	15% for adults, and 16.6% for children	21.3% for adults, and 12.9% for children	>0.05
Conclusion	Bipolar cautery is faster and has less intraop blood loss		
Follow-up time	15 d		

STUDY DESIGN

Inclusion criteria	All adults and all children >10 y old with recurrent sore throats (>5/y)
Exclusion criteria	History of peritonsillar abscess, patients undergoing adenoidectomy or other concurrent procedures, Hx of bleeding disorder, craniofacial anomalies, chronic debilitating diseases
Randomization process	Block randomization involving balancing the number of patients recruited in both arms after every 20 recruits
Age	10–54 y, mean 22 y
Method of tonsillectomy	Bipolar scissors vs cold blunt dissection with snares
Indications for tonsillectomy	Recurrent tonsillitis
Variables studied	Operative time, intraop blood loss, postop pain, hemorrhage
Pain measurement	VAS, with a scale of 0–10
Power	NR

NR = not reported, NA = not applicable, postop = postoperative, intraop = intraoperative, VAS = visual analog scale.
* Sample size: numbers shown for those not lost to follow-up and those (initially recruited).

Reference	Atallah, 2000			Pizzutto, 2000		
Level (design)	1 (randomized controlled trial)			1 (randomized controlled trial)		
Sample size*	50 (70)			400 (420)		
OUTCOMES						
Techniques studied	**Bipolar cautery**	**Cold dissection**	**p Value**	**Bipolar cautery (n = 200)**	**Cold (n = 100) and hot (n = 100) dissection**	**p Value**
Operating time	4.32 min	10.32 min	<0.0005	24.2 min	18.8 min	NR
Intraoperative blood loss	NR	NR	NR	19.6 mL	26.4 mL	NR
Postoperative pain	1.8/4 in first 2 PODs; but worse than cold dissection after POD 2	2.4/4 in first 2 PODs; but better than cold dissection after POD 2	<0.05 for data in the first 2 PODs; NR for the remainder	NR	NR	
Time to normal diet	NR	NR		7.1 d	7.5 days	NR
Postoperative hemorrhage	None	None		n = 9/188	n = 24/193	<0.001
Conclusion	Cold dissection ligation technique takes longer, but has less postop pain after POD 2			Bipolar cautery has less postop hemorrhage and shorter interval to return to school		
Follow-up time	15 d			10–14 d		
STUDY DESIGN						
Inclusion criteria	All patients meeting criteria for tonsillectomy >10 y of age			Patients 2–16 y of age meeting criteria for tonsillectomy with/without adenoidectomy		
Exclusion criteria	Children <10 y of age			History of bleeding disorder, craniofacial anomalies, diabetes, sickle cell disease, developmental delay, chronic medical problems interfering with expected recovery, patients undergoing other concurrent procedures		
Randomization process	Each patient was his/her own control. The side of cold dissection was determined through a random drawing at the time of surgery			Computerized randomization was used for treatment assignment		
Age	10–37 y, mean 22 y			2–16 y		
Method of tonsillectomy	Bipolar electrodissection vs dissection ligation technique			Microbipolar dissection vs monopolar electrocautery vs cold knife dissection		
Indications for tonsillectomy	NR			NR		
Variables studied	Operative time, postop pain			Intraop blood loss, operative time, postop hemorrhage and other complications, duration of returning to school and normal diet, doses of acetaminophen used		
Pain measurement	A scale of 0–4 was used, with 0 being no pain, and 4 being very severe pain.			NR		
Power	NR			NR		

NR = not reported, POD = postoperative day, postop = postoperative, intraop = intraoperative.
* Sample size: numbers shown for those not lost to follow-up and those (initially recruited).

Reference	Brodsky, 1996		
Level (design)	1 (randomized controlled trial)		
Sample size*	129		

OUTCOMES

Techniques studied	Bipolar cautery	Cold dissection	p Value
Operating time	5 min more than cold dissection	5 min less than bipolar	<0.05
Intraoperative blood loss	15–45 mL greater	14–45 mL less	<0.05
Postoperative pain	NR	NR	
Time to normal diet	Sooner in bipolar cautery	Slower	<0.01
Postoperative hemorrhage	n = 1 (1.5%)	n = 7 (10%)	<0.03
Conclusion	Bipolar cautery takes longer, has greater intraop blood loss, but has a shorter duration to normal diet and less postop hemorrhage		
Follow-up time	10 d		

STUDY DESIGN

Inclusion criteria	Patients undergoing tonsillectomy, not otherwise specified		
Exclusion criteria	Chronic illness, craniofacial anomalies, planned admission to intensive care unit or known coagulopathy		
Randomization process	Standard randomization table stratified for ages 2–6 y and 7–16 y		
Age	2–16 y		
Method of tonsillectomy	Microbipolar dissection vs cold knife tonsillectomy with suction cautery for hemostasis		
Indications for tonsillectomy	NR		
Variables studied	Operative time, intraop blood loss, duration of returning to school and normal diet, postop appearance of tonsillar fossa, and postop hemorrhage		
Pain measurement	NR		
Power	NR		

NR = not reported, POD = postoperative day, postop = postoperative, intraop = intraoperative.
*Sample size: numbers shown for those not lost to follow-up and those (initially recruited).

REFERENCES

1. Lachanas VA, Prokopakis EP, Bourolias CA, et al. Ligasure versus cold knife tonsillectomy. Laryngoscope 2005;115(9): 1591–1594.
2. Raut VV, Bhat N, Sinnathuray AR, Kinsella JB, Stevenson M, Toner JG. Bipolar scissors versus cold dissection for pediatric tonsillectomy—a prospective, randomized pilot study. Int J Pediatr Otorhinolaryngol 2002;64(1):9–15.
3. Raut V, Bhat N, Kinsella J, Toner JG, Sinnathuray AR, Stevenson M. Bipolar scissors versus cold dissection tonsillectomy: a prospective, randomized, multi-unit study. Laryngoscope 2001;111(12):2178–2182.
4. Atallah N, Kumar M, Hilali A, Hickey S. Post-operative pain in tonsillectomy: bipolar electrodissection technique vs dissection ligation technique. A double-blind randomized prospective trial. J Laryngol Otol 2000;114(9):667–670.
5. Pizzuto MP, Brodsky L, Duffy L, Gendler J, Nauenberg E. A comparison of microbipolar cautery dissection to hot knife and cold knife cautery tonsillectomy. Int J Pediatr Otorhinolaryngol 2000;52(3):239–246.
6. Brodsky L, Pizzuto M, Gendler J, Duffy L. Microbipolar dissection vs. cold knife/suction cautery tonsillectomy in children: preliminary results of a prospective study. Acta Otolaryngol Suppl 1996;523:256–258.

19 Tonsillectomy in Adults

19.C.iii.

Monopolar cautery versus ultrasonic/harmonic scalpel tonsillectomy: Impact on operating time, intraoperative blood loss, postoperative pain, return to normal diet, and/or postoperative bleeding

James Denneny and Wade Chien

METHODS

A computerized PubMed search of MEDLINE 1966–May 2006 was performed. Articles mapping to the exploded medical subject heading "tonsillectomy" were obtained, yielding 5497 reports. Given the richness of the literature, these publications were then limited to randomized controlled trials (RCTs), yielding 395 articles. An additional search, which collected articles with the terms "electrocoagulation" or "cautery" or "bovie" or "cautery" or "hot" and "cold" or "dissection snare" or "dissection-snare" or "sluder" or "guillotine" or "sharp" or "knife" and cross-referenced them with those obtained by exploding the medical subject heading "tonsillectomy" was also performed, yielding 41 trials. The 395 and 41 articles were then reviewed to identify those that met the following inclusion criteria: 1) patient population with chronic tonsillitis or tonsillar hypertrophy who met criteria for tonsillectomy, 2) intervention with monopolar cautery versus ultrasound/harmonic scalpel tonsillectomy, 3) outcome measured in terms of operating time, intraoperative blood loss, postoperative pain, return to normal diet, and/or postoperative bleeding. In addition, only RCTs were included. The bibliographies of the articles that met these inclusion criteria were manually checked to ensure no further relevant articles could be identified. This process yielded three articles [1–3].

RESULTS

Outcome Measures. Outcome measures included: 1) the time required to perform the procedure, 2) intraoperative blood loss, 3) postoperative pain, 4) the time required to return to normal diet, and 5) postoperative hemorrhage. There were different methodologies used to quantify postoperative pain, but within each study the same scale was used. Pain was measured on scales of 1 to 10 or in terms of the number of patients requiring narcotics.

Potential Confounders. Potential confounders are similar to those described in Section 19.C.i.

Study Designs. All three RCTs compared monopolar cautery to ultrasound/harmonic scalpel tonsillectomy.

Patients undergoing tonsillectomy for the gamut of indications were included in each study. Patients up to age 19 years were investigated in two studies, with the third study not specifying the age of their subjects. Randomization was shown to balance age, sex, race, and preoperative diagnoses in two RCTs. The randomization effectiveness was not reported in the third trial. None of the studies reported *a priori* power calculations. Follow-up times were up to 15 days.

Highest Level of Evidence. These three RCTs concurred that monopolar operating time was faster and that there were no major differences in postoperative discomfort or intraoperative and postoperative bleeding, but results regarding return to normal oral intake were mixed. Operating time was significantly less with monopolar cautery in the two RCTs that analyzed this parameter. In one case, it took half as much time to do monopolar cautery tonsillectomy. There was no significant difference in intraoperative blood loss or postoperative pain in any of the studies. The time before return to a normal diet was significantly better with ultrasonic/harmonic scalpel tonsillectomy in one of the three studies. There was no difference in this parameter in the other study that analyzed this variable, but it had, as its authors admitted, only a 6% power to detect a difference in the time-to-normal-diet variable. There were no notable differences in postoperative hemorrhage, but again, the studies were not powered to come to a definitive conclusion regarding this particular outcome.

Applicability. These studies are applicable to patients undergoing tonsillectomy with either monopolar cautery or ultrasound/harmonic scalpel. Each individual study is more specifically applicable to the patient population admitted according to their inclusion/exclusion criteria, as described in the adjacent table.

Morbidity/Complications. The main morbidity of tonsillectomy lies in pain, inability to tolerate a normal diet, and blood loss—both intraoperative and postoperative. These parameters were discussed as the main results of these trials (see above).

CLINICAL SIGNIFICANCE AND FUTURE RESEARCH

There were three RCTs that compared the impact of monopolar cautery versus ultrasonic/harmonic scalpel on intraoperative and postoperative parameters. There was consensus among studies, as all three concluded that the procedure was faster with monopolar cautery, but that there were no significant differences in postoperative pain or intraoperative and postoperative hemorrhage. Results regarding return to normal oral intake were mixed, but colored by the lesser power/sample size in the negative study.

Future research may focus on reporting uniform outcomes when comparing these two operative techniques. Reporting uniform outcomes may allow for future meta-analyses that could pool data for increased power to help determine whether certain differences in results (i.e., bleeding, pain) truly exist.

Reference	Walker, 2001			Willging, 2003		
Level (design)	1 (randomized controlled trial)			1 (randomized controlled trial)		
Sample size*	172 (316)			117 (120)		
OUTCOMES						
Techniques studied	**Monopolar cautery (n = 75)**	**Harmonic scalpel (n = 97)**	**p Value**	**Monopolar cautery (n = 59)**	**Harmonic scalpel (n = 61)**	**p Value**
Operating time	NR	NR	NA	4 min 33 s	8 min 45 s	<0.001
Intraoperative blood loss	<25 cc	<25 cc	NS	No significant difference		NS
Postoperative pain	73% took narcotics	68% took narcotics	NS	Trend toward better scores with harmonic scalpel		NS
Time to normal diet	POD 1 22% POD 3 46%	POD 1 44% POD 3 74%	POD 1 <0.003 POD 3 <0.001	NR	NR	NA
Postoperative hemorrhage	5.6%	3.2%	NR	1 primary 5 secondary	3 secondary	NS
Conclusion	Harmonic scalpel offered faster return to normal diet with no increase in operative or postop blood loss			No statistically significant difference in blood loss, postop pain or postop hemorrhage was noted. OR time was greater with harmonic scalpel		
Follow-up time	10–14 d			Days 1–7, 14		
STUDY DESIGN						
Inclusion criteria	All patients meeting criteria for tonsillectomy			Recurrent tonsillitis, adenotonsillar hypertrophy, asymmetry		
Exclusion criteria	None stated			Malignancy, HIV, peritonsillar abscess, mono		
Randomization effectiveness	Not specified			Similar age, sex, race, hypertrophied tonsils		
Age	1–19 y			3–18 y		
Method of tonsillectomy	Monopolar electrocautery Harmonic scalpel			Harmonic scalpel Monopolar electrocautery: 10 W to dissect, 15 W to cauterize		
Indications for tonsillectomy	NR			Recurrent tonsillitis, adenotonsillar hypertrophy, asymmetry		
Variables studied	Blood loss, postop pain, return to normal diet, postop hemorrhage			OR time, blood loss, postop pain, postop hemorrhage		
Pain measurement	Number of patients taking narcotics			Wong-Baker FACES pain rating scale		
Power	NR			NR		

NR = not reported, NA = not applicable, NS = not significant, POD = postoperative day, postop = postoperative, HIV = human immunodeficiency virus, OR = operating room.
* Sample size: numbers shown for those not lost to follow-up and those (initially recruited).

THE EVIDENCE CONDENSED: Monopolar electrocautery versus ultrasound/harmonic scalpel tonsillectomy

Reference	Parsons, 2006		
Level (design)	1 (randomized controlled trial)		
Sample size*	61 (134)		
OUTCOMES			
Techniques studied	**Monopolar cautery (n = 43)**	**Harmonic scalpel (n = 44)**	**p Value**
Operating time	21 min	31.5 min	0.003
Intraoperative blood loss	11.3 cc	18.2 cc	NS
Postoperative pain	3.84	4.20	NS
Time to normal diet	Similar number of days required		0.08
Postoperative hemorrhage	n = 2/41	n = 1/43	NS
Conclusion	Surgical time was less for electrocautery; blood loss, postop bleeding, return to normal diet and activity were not statistically different		
Follow-up time	Days 1–10 postop		
STUDY DESIGN			
Inclusion criteria	Chronic tonsillitis, tonsillar hypertrophy		
Exclusion criteria	Not stated		
Randomization effectiveness	Similar age, sex, preoperative diagnoses before intervention		
Age	Not stated		
Method of tonsillectomy	Monopolar electrocautery Harmonic scalpel Coblation		
Indications for tonsillectomy	Chronic tonsillitis, tonsillar hypertrophy		
Variables studied	OR time, blood loss, postop pain, return to diet and activity, postop hemorrhage		
Pain measurement	Wong-Baker FACES visual analog scale (0 best to 10 worst)		
Power	80% power to detect differences in pain scores, 6% for time to normal food intake		

NR = not reported, NA = not applicable, NS = not significant, POD = postoperative day, postop = postoperative, HIV = human immunodeficiency virus, OR = operating room.
*Sample size: numbers shown for those not lost to follow-up and those (initially recruited).

REFERENCES

1. Walker RA, Syed ZA. Harmonic scalpel tonsillectomy versus electrocautery tonsillectomy: a comparative pilot study. Otolaryngol Head Neck Surg 2001;125(11):449–455.
2. Willging JP, Wiatrak BJ. Harmonic scalpel tonsillectomy in children: a randomized prospective study. Otolaryngol Head Neck Surg 2003;128(3):318–325.
3. Parsons SP, Cordes SR, Comer B. Comparison of posttonsillectomy pain using the ultrasonic scalpel, coblator, and electrocautery. Otolaryngol Head Neck Surg 2006;134(1):106–113.

19 Tonsillectomy in Adults

19.C.iv.

Radiofrequency/plasma (coblation) versus cold dissection tonsillectomy: Impact on operating time, intraoperative blood loss, postoperative pain, return to normal diet, and/or postoperative bleeding

James Denneny and Wade Chien

METHODS

A computerized PubMed search of MEDLINE 1966–May 2006 was performed. Articles mapping to the exploded medical subject heading "tonsillectomy" were obtained, yielding 5497 reports. Given the richness of the literature, these publications were then limited to randomized controlled trials (RCTs), yielding 395 articles. An additional search, which collected articles with the terms "electrocoagulation" or "cautery" or "bovie" or "cautery" or "hot" and "cold" or "dissection snare" or "dissection-snare" or "sluder" or "guillotine" or "sharp" or "knife" and cross-referenced them with those obtained by exploding the medical subject heading "tonsillectomy" was also performed, yielding 41 trials. The 395 and 41 articles were then reviewed to identify those that met the following inclusion criteria: 1) patient population with chronic tonsillitis or tonsillar hypertrophy who met criteria for tonsillectomy, 2) intervention with radiofrequency/plasma/coblation versus cold tonsillectomy, 3) outcome measured in terms of operating time, intraoperative blood loss, postoperative pain, return to normal diet, and/or postoperative bleeding. In addition, only RCTs were included. The bibliographies of the articles that met these inclusion criteria were manually checked to ensure no further relevant articles could be identified. This process yielded four articles [1–4].

RESULTS

Outcome Measures. Outcome measures included: 1) the time required to perform the procedure, 2) intraoperative blood loss, 3) postoperative pain, 4) the time required to return to normal diet, and 5) postoperative hemorrhage. There were different methodologies used to quantify postoperative pain, but within each study the same scale was used. Pain was measured with Likert scales or in terms of analgesics used.

Potential Confounders. Potential confounders are similar to those described in the previous section comparing monopolar cautery to cold dissection.

Study Designs. Four RCTs compared results after radiofrequency/plasma/coblation versus cold tonsillectomy. Sample sizes ranged from 20 to 200 patients. Patients of all ages were studied, ranging from 9 to 51 years of age,

and tonsillectomies were performed for a variety of indications. Follow-up times were up to 3 weeks. Only one study reported an *a priori* power calculation.

Highest Level of Evidence. The four RCTs that compared coblation to cold dissection showed very heterogeneous results, with some contradictory data. First, results regarding operative time were mixed, with one study showing faster results with coblation, whereas the other showed faster results with cold dissection. There were no clear differences in the cold dissection technique used in each study. Ages, however, were very different, with one study (coblation better) focusing on children and the other study (coblation worse) focusing on adults. The other two studies did not consider this parameter. Second, intraoperative blood loss was significantly less with coblation according to one trial, but another RCT showed the exact opposite result. The other two RCTs did not analyze this variable. Third, postoperative pain was significantly better with coblation on postoperative day 1 according to one study, but afterward there was no difference. Also, three other studies showed no difference between coblation and cold dissection. Although it would seem that there was some evidence that coblation resulted in somewhat less pain, analysis of the adjunctive variable of time to return to normal diet suggested the opposite result in another study. Resumption of regular oral intake was shorter with cold dissection according to one RCT. It is difficult to reconcile these two findings. Fourth, there were no major differences in postoperative hemorrhage in any of the studies, although several were too small to be adequately powered to definitively demonstrate no difference in a low-incidence occurrence such as postoperative hemorrhage.

Applicability. These studies are applicable to patients undergoing tonsillectomy with cold dissection versus coblation/radiofrequency/plasma dissection. Each individual study is more specifically applicable to the patient population admitted according to their inclusion/exclusion criteria, as described in the adjacent table.

Morbidity/Complications. The main morbidity of tonsillectomy lies in pain, inability to tolerate a normal diet, and blood loss—both intraoperative and postoperative. These parameters were discussed as the main results of these trials (see above).

CLINICAL SIGNIFICANCE AND FUTURE RESEARCH

There were four RCTs that compared results in patients undergoing coblation tonsillectomy versus cold dissection tonsillectomy. The results of these trials are contradictory, with trials coming to opposite conclusions regarding the comparative impact of the two tonsillectomy techniques on intraoperative bleeding, postoperative pain, time to resumption of normal diet, and intraoperative time. There were no major differences in postoperative hemorrhage in any of the studies, although studies were not powered to provide a definitive answer regarding this parameter.

Future studies should be utilized to clarify the issues of operating times and blood loss. Attempts to clarify these issues would require separating the cohorts both by age groups and indications for tonsillectomy. In addition, it would be useful to ensure that only experienced operators are performing the surgery. These studies should include detailed return to diet and work/school data. In addition, it would be useful to provide uniform outcome measures so as to facilitate future meta-analyses.

Reference	Ragab, 2005			Back, 2001		
Level (design)	1 (randomized controlled trial)			1 (randomized controlled trial)		
Sample size*	184 (200)			37 (40)		
OUTCOMES						
Techniques studied	Bipolar radiofrequency (n = 91)	Cold dissection (n = 93)	p Value	Coblation (n = 18)	Cold dissection (n = 19)	p Value
Operating time	8.5 min	15.5 min	<0.001	27 min	18 min	<0.001
Intraoperative blood loss	13 cc	82 cc	<0.001	80 mL	20 mL	<0.002
Postoperative pain	Median 8, range 6–10	Median 9, range 7–10	<0.05 on POD1, NS after POD1	Median 37, range 16–98	Median 36, range 17–87	NS
Time to normal diet	Not specified	Not specified	NS	NR	NR	NA
Postoperative hemorrhage	Primary 0 Secondary 1	Primary 1 Primary 2	NR	Primary 5 Secondary 9	Primary 3 Secondary 8	NR
Conclusion	Bipolar radiofrequency tonsillectomy offered shorter OR times with less blood loss and similar postop pain and complications as standard cold dissection tonsillectomy			Operating time and blood loss was greater with coblation. Postop pain was similar and postop bleeding was not statistically significant		
Follow-up time	Days 1, 4, 7, 14			3 wk		
STUDY DESIGN						
Inclusion criteria	Chronic tonsillitis, tonsillar hypertrophy			Recurrent or chronic tonsillitis, obstructive hypertrophy, quinsy		
Exclusion criteria	Quinsy, bleeding disorder, craniofacial abnormalities, chronic disease			Pneumonia, unilateral removal, bleeding disorders, chronic disease		
Randomization effectiveness	Double blind randomization, comparative group information not specified			Similar age, weight, sex, history of chronic/recurrent tonsillitis		
Age	9–16 y			18–65 y		
Method of tonsillectomy	Bipolar radiofrequency Cold dissection			Coblation at power level 5–7 (192–160 VRMS) Cold dissection		
Indications for tonsillectomy	Not stated			Chronic infection, hypertrophy, quinsy		
Variables studied	OR time, blood loss, postop pain, return to diet, postop bleeding			OR time, blood loss, postop pain, postop bleeding, protein C, ESR		
Pain measurement	Visual analog scale			Median doses of pain medicine taken		
Power	NR			NR		

NR = not reported, NA = not applicable, POD = postoperative day, NS = not significant, OR = operating room, postop = postoperative, ESR = erythrocyte sedimentation rate.
*Sample size: numbers shown for those not lost to follow-up and those (initially recruited).

Reference	Saengpanich, 2005		
Level (design)	1 (randomized controlled trial)		
Sample size*	20		

OUTCOMES

Techniques studied	Bipolar radiofrequency	Cold dissection	p Value
Operating time	NR	NR	NA
Intraoperative blood loss	NR	NR	NA
Postoperative pain	~0.8 to 3/5 from POD 0–6	~0.3 to 3.2/5 from POD 0–6	>0.05
Time to normal diet	NR	NR	NA
Postoperative hemorrhage	NR	NR	NA
Conclusion	Bipolar radiofrequency tonsillectomy did not show any difference in postop pain compared with cold dissection		
Follow-up time	6 d		

STUDY DESIGN

Inclusion criteria	Patients undergoing tonsillectomy
Exclusion criteria	Asymmetric tonsillar hypertrophy, history of peritonsillar abscess, having other concurrent procedures, abnormal coagulability, hypertension, and diabetes
Randomization effectiveness	Single blind randomization, with each patient serving as his/her own control. The side of radiofrequency tonsillectomy was randomly selected at the time of surgery
Age	13–51 y, mean 29.9 y
Method of tonsillectomy	Radiofrequency bipolar tonsillectomy vs cold blunt dissection with loop ligation
Indications for tonsillectomy	Chronic tonsillitis
Variables studied	Postop pain
Pain measurement	A scale of 0–5, with 0 being no pain, and 5 being intractable pain
Power	NR

NR = not reported, NA = not applicable, POD = postoperative day, NS = not significant, OR = operating room, postop = postoperative.
* Sample size: numbers shown for those not lost to follow-up and those (initially recruited).

Reference	Philpott, 2005		
Level (design)	1 (randomized controlled trial)		
Sample size*	92		

OUTCOMES			
Techniques studied	**Bipolar radiofrequency** (n = 43)	**Cold dissection** (n = 49)	**p Value**
Operating time	NR	NR	NA
Intraoperative blood loss	NR	NR	NA
Postoperative pain	Similar analgesic usage, severity of pain in both groups		NS
Time to normal diet	Longer than cold dissection	Shorter than radiofrequency	0.032
Postoperative hemorrhage	n = 11/43	n = 8/49	NS
Conclusion	Use of radiofrequency tonsillectomy does not confer any symptomatic benefit over cold dissection		
Follow-up time	14 d		

STUDY DESIGN			
Inclusion criteria	Adult patients with recurrent tonsillitis meeting criteria for tonsillectomy		
Exclusion criteria	NR		
Randomization effectiveness	Randomization occurred in the OR by means of a closed-envelope system to allocate patients to radiofrequency or cold dissection group		
Age	18–45 y		
Method of tonsillectomy	Bipolar radiofrequency tonsillectomy vs cold dissection		
Indications for tonsillectomy	Recurrent tonsillitis		
Variables studied	Postop pain, time to normal diet and normal daily activities, postop hemorrhage		
Pain measurement	6-point visual analog scale		
Power	Able to tell a difference between 2 groups of 2 on the visual analog scale with a power of 80% and α of 0.05		

NR = not reported, NA = not applicable, NS = not significant, postop = postoperative, OR = operating room.
* Sample size: numbers shown for those not lost to follow-up and those (initially recruited).

REFERENCES

1. Ragab SM. Bipolar radiofrequency dissection tonsillectomy: a prospective randomized trial. Otolaryngol Head Neck Surg 2005;133(6):961–965.
2. Back L, Paloheimo M, Ylikoski J. Traditional tonsillectomy compared with bipolar radiofrequency thermal ablation tonsillectomy. Arch Otolaryngol Head Neck Surg 2001; 127(9):1106–1112.
3. Saengpanich S, Kerekhanjanarong V, Aramwatanapong P, Supiyaphun P. Comparison of pain after radiofrequency tonsillectomy compared with conventional tonsillectomy: a pilot study. J Med Assoc Thai 2005;88(12):1880–1883.
4. Philpott CM, Wild DC, Mehta D, Daniel M, Banerjee AR. A double-blinded randomized control trial of coblation versus conventional dissection tonsillectomy on post-operative symptoms. Clin Otolaryngol 2005;30(2):143–148.

20 Obstructive Sleep Apnea in Adults

20.A.

Continuous positive airway pressure versus placebo: Impact on sleepiness, quality of life, and driving performance in patients with obstructive sleep apnea

David P. White and Roger S. Smith

METHODS

A computerized PubMed search of MEDLINE 1966–February 2006 was performed. The terms "CPAP" (continuous positive airway pressure) and "randomized clinical trial" were exploded and the resulting articles were cross-referenced, yielding 322 trials. These articles were then reviewed to identify those that met the following inclusion criteria: 1) patient population with obstructive sleep apnea of all severity levels, 2) intervention with CPAP for at least 1 month, and 3) used a realistic placebo methodology (subtherapeutic or sham CPAP [1–3]). All outcomes were examined. Articles in which a pill was used as the placebo were excluded [4–8]. The bibliographies of the articles that met these inclusion criteria were manually checked to ensure no further relevant articles could be identified. This process yielded three articles.

RESULTS

Outcome Measures. In two of the studies, the primary outcomes assessed were measures of sleepiness and quality of life (QOL). In one study [1], these were only assessed with validated questionnaires [Epworth Sleepiness Scale (ESS, range 0 best to 24 worst), Functional Outcomes Sleep Questionnaire (FOSQ, lower mean scores represent worse dysfunction), and Short Form 36 (SF-36, range 0 worst to 100 best)]. In the second study [2], sleepiness was assessed both subjectively (ESS and SF-36) and objectively [modified Maintenance of Wakefulness Test (MWT, minutes to sleep onset)]. In the third study [3], driving ability was assessed on a computer driving simulator.

Potential Confounders. In the first study [1], residual confounding did occur despite randomization. Body mass index (BMI) and current smoking were both higher in the sham CPAP group. There was no residual confounding in the remaining two studies [2, 3] for either demographic variables or baseline values for the outcome measures.

Study Designs. All studies examined were randomized clinical trials with reasonably effective randomization with minimal remaining confounding (see above). The blinding in all three studies was adequate in that the investigator testing the subject was blinded to the form of therapy. Subject blinding with sham CPAP can be diffi-cult. However, in all three studies only CPAP-naïve subjects were included and the machines were identical (appearance, noise) for both real and sham or subtherapeutic CPAP. Thus true masking was accomplished. All three studies were of relatively short duration (1 month–6 weeks) which could have affected outcomes, because longer-duration CPAP may have yielded further improvement in the outcome measures. In the first study [1] the power calculation was determined before initiation of the study whereas in the later two studies [2, 3] final power calculations were reported only after an interim analysis.

Highest Level of Evidence. The two studies that addressed subjective and objective sleepiness found CPAP to be clinically and statistically more effective than sham CPAP. The ESS, FOSQ, and the MWT all improved more with CPAP than sham CPAP and, in most cases, returned to relatively normal values. QOL improved more with CPAP in one study [2], with no difference in this outcome between CPAP and sham CPAP being observed in another [1]. The explanation for this difference between studies is unclear although the smaller sample size, lower compliance rate, and confounding by BMI and smoking status in the negative study [1] may have contributed to the inability of these investigators to find a difference in QOL between groups. The third study [3] demonstrated CPAP to be far superior to sham CPAP in improving driving performance on a simulator. However, even after 1 month of real CPAP, the driving performance did not return to completely normal values based on a control group. Whether performance would have reached truly normal levels had the study been of longer duration is unclear. Thus, all conclusions are limited because of the short duration of the studies. Otherwise the conclusions can likely be generalized to most populations of obstructive sleep apnea patients.

Applicability. All studies included patients with mild to severe obstructive sleep apnea with an apnea-hypopnea index >10. All patients were also subjectively sleepy at the start of the studies. Thus, the findings in these studies may not apply to asymptomatic apnea patients. Exclusion criteria did not otherwise importantly reduce the ability to generalize the findings of these studies to most apnea patients.

Morbidity/Complications. No adverse events were reported in any of the three studies.

CLINICAL SIGNIFICANCE AND FUTURE RESEARCH

These studies reviewed here strongly suggest that obstructive sleep apnea has an important adverse effect on subjective and objective sleepiness, QOL, and driving performance. These effects can be substantially reversed with nasal CPAP which did not occur, or occurred to a significantly lesser extent, in the sham CPAP group. In most cases the outcomes returned to normal or near-normal levels suggesting that the cognitive consequences of sleep apnea are largely reversible. However, driving performance did not fully return to normal. Whether this would have occurred with longer-duration CPAP is unclear.

Although these studies indicate that many of the consequences of sleep apnea are reversible, a number of outcomes were not examined and the studies were of relatively short duration. Tests of neurocognitive function such as attention, memory, learning, and executive function were not examined and need to be. A growing literature suggests that sleep apnea may lead to adverse cardiovascular outcomes (stroke, myocardial infarction, and congestive heart failure). However, there have been no randomized clinical trials assessing whether these adverse outcomes can be prevented with treatment of the apnea. Thus, long-term, randomized trials are needed to address these important questions.

THE EVIDENCE CONDENSED: CPAP versus sham CPAP for the treatment of obstructive sleep apnea

Reference	Montserrat, 2001			Jenkinson, 1999		
Level (design)	1 (randomized controlled trial)			1 (randomized controlled trial)		
Sample size*	45 (48)			101 (107)		
OUTCOMES						
Outcome measures	ESS (range, 0 = best to 24 = worst), FOSQ (lower scores worse), and SF-36 (0 = worst to 100 = best)			ESS (range, 0 = best to 24 = worst), MWT (minutes to sleep), and SF-36		
		Pretreatment	Post-treatment		Pretreatment	Post-treatment
CPAP	ESS	16.1 ± 1.0	6.7 ± 0.7	ESS	15.5 (10–23)	7.0 (0.7–17)
	FOSQ	84.45 ± 4.63	109.43 ± 2.63	MWT	22.5 (7.6–40)	32.9 (11.6–40)
	SF-36	46.5 ± 1.9	50.7 ± 1.6	SF-36 (physical)	43.7 ± 11.6	49.4 ± 10.1
Sham CPAP	ESS	16.9 ± 1.2	14.6 ± 1.1	ESS	15.0 (9–22.5)	13.0 (4–19)
	FOSQ	86.16 ± 5.96	100.66 ± 4.39	MWT	20 (3.5–40)	23.5 (7–40)
	SF-36	45.5 ± 2.2	47.2 ± 1.9	SF-36 (physical)	42.6 ± 10.1	45.5 ± 10.4
p Value	ESS: <0.001 FOSQ: NS to <0.009 SF-36: NS			ESS: <0.0001 MWT: <0.005 SF-36: NS to <0.0001		
Conclusion	CPAP leads to improvement in sleepiness, vigilance, and general productivity, but not global QOL			CPAP leads to improvement in subjective and objective sleepiness plus energy, vitality, and mental summary (SF-36)		
Follow-up time	6 wk			1 mo		
STUDY DESIGN						
Inclusion criteria	1) Symptomatic: excessive daytime sleepiness 2) Sleep apnea: AHI > 10			1) ESS > 10 2) ≥10 falls of ≥4% in SaO_2 per hour during sleep study		
Exclusion criteria	Only not meeting inclusion criteria			Selected other therapy, need urgent CPAP, may lose job because of sleepiness, and mental disability		
Randomization effectiveness	Significant differences remained for BMI and smoking status. No difference in age, AHI, or alcohol use			No significant difference in all primary variables (age, BMI, ESS, MWT, SF-36, and >4% SaO_2 dips/h)		
Age	CPAP: 55.7 ± 9.4 y Sham: 52.6 ± 10.9 y			CPAP: 48 y (36–68 y) Sub-CPAP: 50 y (33–71 y)		
CPAP regimen details	Titrated CPAP versus sham CPAP. All subjects also encouraged to lose weight and given sleep hygiene regimen			Autotitrated CPAP in lab compared with CPAP set at 1 cm H_2O. Managing nurse blinded to treatment type		
Compliance	CPAP: 4.25 ± 2 h Sham: 4.5 ± 2 h			CPAP: 5.4 h (2.2–7.4 h) Sub-CPAP: 4.6 h (0.7–8.5 h) These values are significantly different		
Criteria for withdrawal from study	None			None		
Power	90% at a level of p < 0.05			Interim analysis suggested that 100 subjects was adequate to demonstrate difference of p < 0.01		
Morbidity/ complications	None listed			None listed		

CPAP = continuous positive airway pressure, ESS = Epworth Sleepiness Scale, FOSQ = Functional Outcomes Sleep Questionnaire, SF-36 = Short Form 36, SD = standard deviation, TTC = time prior to crash, OFE = off-road events, QOL = quality of life, NS = not significant, AHI = apnea-hypopnea index, BMI = body mass index, OSA = obstructive sleep apnea, UPPP = uvulopalatopharyngoplasty. Number ± number = mean ± SD. Ranges are reported as number–number).
* Sample size: numbers shown for those not lost to follow-up and those (initially recruited).

Reference	Hack, 2000		
Level (design)	1 (randomized controlled trial)		
Sample size*	59 (69)		
OUTCOMES			
Outcome measures	Steering SD, deterioration of SD, TTC, OFE, reaction time		
		Pretreatment	Post-treatment
CPAP	SD	0.36 (0.15–1.12)	0.21 (0.14–0.63)
	TTC	24.8 (7.6–30)	30 (17.6–30)
	ORE	17.8 (0.4–149)	9.0 (0–76)
Sham CPAP	SD	0.35 (0.15–1.17)	0.30 (0.14–1.19)
	TTC	27.6 (10.9–30)	26.9 (9.1–30)
	ORE	34.8 (0.9–149)	23.0 (0–150)
p Value	Steering SD: $p = 0.03$ Deterioration of SD: $p = 0.04$ Reaction time: $p = 0.04$ Others were NS		
Conclusion	CPAP led to significantly better driving performance compared with both baseline and subtherapeutic CPAP		
Follow-up time	1 mo		
STUDY DESIGN			
Inclusion criteria	1) ESS > 10 2) ≥10 ≥4% falls in SaO_2 per hour during sleep study		
Exclusion criteria	Selected other therapy, need urgent CPAP, may lose job because of sleepiness, and mental disability		
Randomization effectiveness	No significant difference in all primary variables (age, BMI, ESS, MWT, SF-36, and >4% SaO_2 dips/h) nor in baseline driving variables		
Age	CPAP: 50 y (38–68 y) Sub-CPAP: 50 y (35–64 y)		
CPAP regimen details	Autotitrated CPAP in lab compared with CPAP set at 1 cm H_2O. Managing nurse blinded to treatment type		
Compliance	CPAP: 5.6 h (3.0–7.2 h) Sub-CPAP: 5.0 h (1.2–8.5 h) These values are not significantly different		
Criteria for withdrawal from study	None		
Power	Interim analysis suggested that 69 subjects was adequate to test the hypothesis		
Morbidity/ complications	None listed		

CPAP = continuous positive airway pressure, ESS = Epworth Sleepiness Scale, FOSQ = Functional Outcomes Sleep Questionnaire, SF-36 = Short Form 36, SD = standard deviation, TTC = time prior to crash, OFE = off-road events, QOL = quality of life, NS = not significant, AHI = apnea-hypopnea index, BMI = body mass index, OSA = obstructive sleep apnea, UPPP = uvulopalatopharyngoplasty. Number ± number = mean ± SD. Ranges are reported as number–number).
* Sample size: numbers shown for those not lost to follow-up and those (initially recruited).

REFERENCES

1. Montserrat JM, Ferrer M, Hernandex L, et al. Effectiveness of CPAP treatment in daytime function in sleep apnea syndrome. Am J Respir Crit Care Med 2001;164:608–613.
2. Jenkinson C, Davies RJO, Mullins R, Stradling JR. Comparison of therapeutic and subtherapeutic nasal continuous positive airway pressure for obstructive sleep apnoea: a randomised prospective parallel trial. Lancet 1999;353:2100–2105.
3. Hack M, Davies RJO, Mullins R, et al. Randomised prospective parallel trial of therapeutic versus subtherapeutic nasal continuous positive airway pressure on simulated steering performance in patients with obstructive sleep apnoea. Thorax 2000;55:224–231.
4. Barnes M, Houston D, Worsnop CJ, et al. A randomized controlled trial of continuous positive airway pressure in mild obstructive sleep apnea. Am J Respir Crit Care Med 2002;165:773–780.
5. Engleman HM, Kingshott RN, Wraith PK, Mackay TW, Deary IJ, Douglas NJ. Randomized placebo-controlled crossover trial of continuous positive airway pressure for mild sleep apnea/hypopnea syndrome. Am J Respir Crit Care Med 1999;159:461–467.
6. Engleman HM, Martin SE, Deary IJ, Douglas NJ. Effect of CPAP therapy on daytime function in patients with mild sleep apnoea/hypopnoea syndrome. Thorax 1997;52:114–119.
7. Engleman HM, Martin SE, Kingshott RN, Mackay TW, Deary IJ, Douglas NJ. Randomised placebo controlled trial of daytime function after continuous positive airway pressure (CPAP) therapy for the sleep apnoea/hypopnoea syndrome. Thorax 1998;53:341–345.
8. McArdle N, Douglas NJ. Effect of continuous positive airway pressure on sleep architecture in the sleep apnea–hypopnea syndrome: a randomized controlled trial. Am J Respir Crit Care Med 2001;164:1459–1463.

20 Obstructive Sleep Apnea in Adults

20.B.

Continuous positive airway pressure versus uvulopalatopharyngoplasty in the treatment of obstructive sleep apnea

David P. White and Roger S. Smith

METHODS

A computerized PubMed search of MEDLINE 1966–January 2006 was performed. The terms "CPAP" (continuous positive airway pressure) and "UPPP" (uvulopalatopharyngoplasty) were exploded and the resulting articles were cross-referenced, yielding 50 trials. These articles were then reviewed to identify those that met the following inclusion criteria: 1) adult patient population with obstructive sleep apnea, 2) intervention with both CPAP and UPPP in the same study, 3) comparative outcomes including symptom measures, sleep study data, and mortality. Articles in which only CPAP or UPPP was used as intervention were excluded. The bibliographies of the articles that met these inclusion criteria were manually checked to ensure no further relevant articles could be identified. This process yielded six articles, which are discussed below in detail [1–6].

RESULTS

Outcome Measures. Because there were so few studies directly comparing UPPP and CPAP, all such studies were considered regardless of outcome measure. Thus, the outcome measure of death was used in four studies, oxygen desaturation episodes and sleepiness in one study, and respiratory disturbance index, sleep variables, and multiple sleep latency test (MSLT) in one study. Although death would seem to be a definitive outcome, in one study this was only confirmed by relatives [5] and in another only from coded medical records [2]. Both can have errors. In one study [1] sleepiness was quantified subjectively by visual analog scale.

Potential Confounders. Because all of the studies reviewed were either nonrandomized trials or retrospective studies, confounding was an important problem. The greatest such confounder was that in all studies the choice of CPAP versus UPPP was based on multiple nonstandardized variables (likelihood of success, the treatment available at the time in that institution, patient preference) or was not defined. In addition, because of the nature of retrospective or nonrandomized trials, many potentially confounding variables turned out to be poorly matched between groups. This included body mass index [3, 5], gender [3], follow-up time [3, 5], and disease burden [3, 5]. Thus, the groups often could not be fairly compared.

Study Designs. As stated above, all studies addressing this topic were either retrospective or nonrandomized trials. As a result, the baseline characteristics of the groups being compared were often statistically different and the treatment choice was based on subject characteristics. In addition, CPAP compliance was often not monitored or reported. Thus, the conclusions that can be reached from such studies are limited.

Highest Level of Evidence. The trials assessed indicated the following: 1) death occurred more commonly in patients treated with UPPP in one study [5], in patients treated with CPAP in one study [2], with no difference between treatment modalities being reported in two studies [3, 4], and 2) CPAP generally improved sleep disordered breathing, daytime symptoms, objective sleep quality, and MSLT more than UPPP [1, 6]. However, because of the problems with study design and confounding described above, no strong conclusions are possible. That being stated, the cumulative data would suggest that death from all causes is likely similar between patients treated with CPAP and UPPP. However, CPAP seems to reduce apnea severity more effectively than UPPP leading to less subjective and objective sleepiness.

Applicability. All studies assessed included patients with mild to severe obstructive sleep apnea with few exclusion criteria. Several were consecutive series. Thus the results and conclusions described above are likely applicable to the general sleep apnea population and not a more limited segment of patients with this disorder.

Morbidity/Complications. Few complications were reported with CPAP although compliance, when assessed and reported, was often relatively low. One study did report rhinorrhea, dry nose and mouth, mask discomfort, and problems with machine noise in a minority of patients using CPAP. UPPP was associated with velopharyngeal insufficiency, infection, and the need for tracheostomy in a small number of patients. However, complications with either treatment were not often systematically assessed.

These studies suggest that CPAP is probably more successful at reducing apnea severity and improving sleep quality than UPPP. However, CPAP compliance is a problem. Thus, when subsequent death was assessed as the primary outcome measure, no clear differences were obvious between the treatment approaches. This could be a product of similar long-term efficacy of the two treatment modalities or could indicate that sleep apnea does not have an important influence on long-term survival.

For the reasons stated above, there is a real need for randomized clinical trials comparing CPAP and UPPP. It would not likely be possible to blind such trials although outcomes could be assessed in a blinded manner. The outcomes measured should include standard ones such as residual apnea/hypopnea frequency and objective sleep quality. However, these studies should also include more meaningful outcomes such as subjective and objective sleepiness, neurocognitive function, reaction times, and other measures of vigilance. This will provide a more clinically relevant comparison of the two treatment modalities. Such trials should be of a reasonable duration as well, this likely being at least 1 year.

It is not likely possible at this time to compare the two treatment modalities using hard cardiovascular endpoints such as stroke or myocardial infarction in a randomized trial. However, intermediate outcomes such as endothelial function, inflammation (CRP), blood pressure, and insulin regulation could certainly be assessed and would add importantly to our understanding of the relative efficacy of these quite different treatment approaches.

THE EVIDENCE CONDENSED: Nasal continuous positive airway pressure versus uvulopalatopharyngoplasty for all outcomes

Reference	Lojander, 1996	Weaver, 2004
Level (design)	2 (prospective trial)	3 (retrospective study)
Sample size	76 (21 CPAP, 18 surg, 37 conserv therapy)	20,826 (18,754 CPAP and 2072 UPPP)

	OUTCOMES	
Outcome measures	Oxygen desaturation episodes and subjective sleepiness	Death rate
Intervention	UPPP: ODI (4%) 45 (21–72) to 14 (3–54) at 12 mo. CPAP: ODI (4%) 25 (10–92) to 0 (0–2) at 12 mo	UPPP (possibly plus another surgical procedure, number, % dead): 71, 3.4% CPAP (number, % dead): 1339, 7.1%
p Value	Oxygen desaturation: UPPP, p < 0.02 Oxygen desaturation: CPAP, p < 0.001 Sleepiness: UPPP, p < 0.05 Sleepiness: CPAP, p < 0.01 No statistical comparison between UPPP and CPAP groups	p = 0.03 adjusted for confounders in favor of UPPP vs CPAP
Conclusion	CPAP group all improved, but compliance only 62% Surg group only normalized oxygen desaturation in 39%. Symptoms did improve	UPPP had a significantly better survival. There was a 31% greater mortality in CPAP- vs UPPP-treated subjects after controlling for age, gender, race, date of treatment, and comorbidities
Follow-up time	1 y	1–5 y, mean 2.75 ± 1.21 y

	STUDY DESIGN	
Inclusion criteria	ODI > 10, daytime sleepiness, and snoring	Diagnosis of OSA plus either CPAP code or UPPP code. Data from 10/97 to 9/01. Must have 1 y of previous comorbidity data and 1 y follow-up
Exclusion criteria	BMI > 40, asthma, COPD, hypothyroid, other serious illness, sleepiness a risk	Nothing other than not meeting inclusion criteria
Intervention regimen details	CPAP (21) vs conserv therapy (23) randomized. UPPP (12) UPPP + mandib surg (5) vs conserv therapy (14) randomized	All participants either initiated on CPAP or underwent a UPPP (possibly with another surgical procedure). Follow-up per medical records
Confounders	Patients selected for therapy group based on likelihood of success (not randomized)	Only veterans studied and comorbidities only controlled for statistically
Data quality	Sleep apnea diagnosis/therapy results only based on oxygen desaturation episodes	All data acquired from coded medical records (may be subject to error). No sleep data (apnea severity) or CPAP compliance data available
Age	30–65 y	57 ± 12 y
Diagnostic criteria for OSA	Sleep apnea diagnosed based on oxygen desaturation episodes	Coded as OSA from medical records plus CPAP code or UPPP code. No actual sleep data
Compliance	CPAP 62%, surg 100%, conserv 89%	No data on CPAP compliance
Criteria for withdrawal from study	CPAP: noncompliance (n = 8) Symptomatic need for therapy in conservatively managed group (n = 4, 1 CPAP and 3 UPPP)	Retrospective study, thus no withdrawal
Consecutive patients?	Yes, although many refused to participate or met exclusion criteria	All patients coded as above (OSA ± CPAP or UPPP) at all US VA hospitals from 10/97 to 9/01
Morbidity/ complications	Surg: 2 velopharyngeal insufficiency, 1 tracheotomy, 2 infected material needing removal CPAP: 7 rhinorrhea, 2 dry nose or mouth, 2 mask discomfort, 1 machine noise	Death was the primary outcome variable

OSA = obstructive sleep apnea, CPAP = continuous positive airway pressure, UPPP = uvulopalatopharyngoplasty, surg = surgery, conserv = conservative treatment, BMI = body mass index, ODI = oxygen desaturation index, NS = not significant, AHI = apnea-hypopnea index, AI = apnea index, COPD = chronic obstructive pulmonary disease.

THE EVIDENCE CONDENSED: Nasal continuous positive airway pressure versus uvulopalatopharyngoplasty for all outcomes

Reference	Keenan, 1995
Level (design)	3 (retrospective study)
Sample size	362 (154 UPPP, 208 CPAP)

OUTCOMES

Outcome measures	Death rate
Intervention	UPPP: (number, % dead): 6, 4.0% CPAP: (number, % dead): 3, 2.5%
p Value	NS for all patients and only patients with an AI > 20
Conclusion	There was no difference in long-term survival between OSA patients treated with CPAP vs UPPP
Follow-up time	43 ± 13 mo for UPPP 20 ± 14 mo for CPAP

STUDY DESIGN

Inclusion criteria	Diagnosis of OSA (AI > 5 or AHI > 15) Treated with either CPAP or UPPP between 1/84 and 4/90
Exclusion criteria	Subsequent CPAP use for UPPP patients Discontinued CPAP use during follow-up
Intervention regimen details	Either placed on CPAP per titration or underwent UPPP with follow-up polysomnogram
Confounders	Multiple confounders: BMI greater in CPAP group, follow-up longer in UPPP group, more males in UPPP group, AI higher in UPPP group
Data quality	Dead determined by phone calls to patients, families, and physicians plus British Columbia Vital Statistics
Age	UPPP: 50 ± 11 y, CPAP: 52 ± 12 y
Diagnostic criteria for OSA	Sleep apnea defined as AI > 5 or AHI > 15
Compliance	Self-report of using or not using CPAP
Criteria for withdrawal from study	Retrospective study, thus no withdrawal
Consecutive patients?	All patients treated with CPAP or UPPP between 1/84 and 4/90
Morbidity/ complications	Death was primary outcome

OSA = obstructive sleep apnea, CPAP = continuous positive airway pressure, UPPP = uvulopalatopharyngoplasty, surg = surgery, conserv = conservative treatment, BMI = body mass index, ODI = oxygen desaturation index, NS = not significant, AHI = apnea-hypopnea index, AI = apnea index, COPD = chronic obstructive pulmonary disease.

THE EVIDENCE CONDENSED: Nasal continuous positive airway pressure versus uvulopalatopharyngoplasty for all outcomes

Reference	Marti, 2002	He, 1988	Zorick, 1990
Level (design)	3 (retrospective study)	3 (retrospective study)	2 (nonrandomized trial)
Sample size	444 (88 UPPP and 124 CPAP)	385 (60 UPPP and 25 CPAP)	92 (46 UPPP and 46 CPAP)
OUTCOMES			
Outcome measures	Death rate	Death rate	RDI, PSG sleep variables, and MSLT
Intervention	UPPP (number, % dead): 3, 3.4% CPAP (number, % dead): 6, 4.8%	UPPP (number, % dead): 8, 13.3% CPAP (number, % dead): 0, 0%	UPPP: RDI: 71 ± 30 to 43 ± 30 MSLT: 4.1 ± 1 to 5.5 ± 0.9 min CPAP: RDI: 76 ± 23 to 7 ± 9 MSLT: 4.4 ± 0.9 to 10.3 ± 1.1 min
p Value	Not reported, *post hoc* calculation, p = NS	Not reported, *post hoc* calculation, p = 0.06	p < 0.001
Conclusion	No significant difference in survival between CPAP and UPPP	Trend toward better survival with CPAP	CPAP improved sleep, RDI, and MSLT more than UPPP
Follow-up time	UPPP: 7.1 = 2.0 y, CPAP: 5.2 ± 1.9 y	UPPP: 8 y, CPAP: 5 y	6 wk
STUDY DESIGN			
Inclusion criteria	Diagnosis of OSA between 1/82 and 12/92 and could be located in 1996	Diagnosis of OSA between 1978 and 1986 and returned questionnaire	Consecutive patients with a history of loud snoring and daytime sleepiness plus OSA on PSG
Exclusion criteria	<16 y old, trach, hypothyroid, acromegaly, malformation of skull base, not treated after 1988	<15 y old, did not return questionnaire	None other than not meeting inclusion criteria
Intervention regimen details	Either placed on CPAP per titration or underwent UPPP (others treated with diet or not treated)	Either placed on CPAP per titration or underwent UPPP (others treated with trach or not treated)	Either placed on CPAP per titration or underwent UPPP
Study design issues	Retrospective study with no randomization of therapy	Retrospective study with no randomization of therapy	No randomization. Follow-up at only 6 wk
Confounders	Multiple confounders: age, BMI, and coronary disease greater with CPAP, follow-up longer with UPPP	Success of UPPP not known if many patients. Almost 50% did not return questionnaire. Death documented only by relatives	Patients assigned to therapy based on anatomy, patient preference, and medical indications
Age	UPPP: 50 ± 10 y, CPAP: 54 ± 9 y	UPPP: 48.2 ± 11.2 y, CPAP: 50.2 ± 12.2 y	UPPP: 47.2 ± 13.7 y, CPAP: 51.7 ± 10.3 y
Diagnostic criteria for described	Sleep apnea defined as AHI > 10	Sleep apnea defined as AI > 5	Sleep apnea criteria on PSG not defined
Management of episode while on study treatment	Retrospective study, no such management described	Retrospective study, no such management described	None described
Compliance	Subjective: CPAP 6.9 ± 1.7 h/night CPAP compliance only subjective	No information on CPAP compliance	No information on CPAP compliance
Consecutive patients?	All patients with OSA diagnosed from 1/82 to 12/92 who could be located in 1996	All patients diagnosed with OSA between 1978 and 1986 who returned the questionnaire	Yes
Morbidity/ complications	Death was the primary outcome	Death was the primary outcome	None reported

CPAP = continuous positive airway pressure, UPPP = uvulopalatopharyngoplasty, RDI = respiratory disturbance index, MSLT = multiple sleep latency test, OSA = obstructive sleep apnea, BMI = body mass index, NS = not significant, AHI = apnea-hypopnea index, AI = apnea index, trach = tracheotomy, PSG = polysomnogram.

REFERENCES

1. Lojander J, Maasilta P, Partinen M, Brander PE, Salmi T, Lehtonen H. Nasal-CPAP, surgery, and conservative management for treatment of obstructive sleep apnea syndrome. Chest 1996;110:114–119.
2. Weaver ED, Maynard C, Yueh B. Survival of veterans with sleep apnea: continuous positive airway pressure versus surgery. Otolaryngol Head Neck Surg 2004;130(6):659–665.
3. Keenan SP, Burt H, Ryan CF, Fleetham JA. Long-term survival of patients with obstructive sleep apnea treated by uvulopalatopharyngoplasty or nasal CPAP. Chest 1995; 105(1):155–159.
4. Marti S, Sampol G, Munoz X, et al. Mortality in severe sleep apnoea/hypopnoea syndrome patients: impact of treatment. Eur Respir J 2002;20:1511–1518.
5. He J, Kryger MH, Zorick FJ, Conway W, Roth T. Mortality and apnea index in obstructive sleep apnea. Chest 1988; 94(1):9–14.
6. Zorick FJ, Roehrs T, Conway W, Potts G, Roth T. Response to CPAP and UPPP in apnea. Henry Ford Hosp Med J 1990;38(4):223–226.

20 Obstructive Sleep Apnea in Adults

Uvulopalatopharyngoplasty versus oral appliance: Impact on apnea index and quality of life

Mary Beauchamp and Regina P. Walker

METHODS

A computerized PubMed search of MEDLINE 1966–November 2004 was performed. Three groups of articles were identified: 1) articles mapping to the subject headings "sleep apnea, obstructive" or "Pickwickian syndrome" were combined; 2) articles mapping to the medical subject heading "orthodontic appliances, functional" were combined with those mapping to the textwords "mandibular advancement device," "oral appliance," "appliance," "splint," or "device"; 3) articles mapping to the subject heading "otorhinolaryngologic surgical procedures" were combined with those mapping to the textwords "uvulopalatopharyngoplasty" (UPPP) "pharyngoplasty," "palatopharyngoplasty," "surgery," "surgical," or "operative." These three groups were then cross-referenced, yielding 24 studies. These articles were then reviewed to identify those that met the following inclusion criteria: 1) patient population with obstructive sleep apnea (OSA), 2) intervention with oral appliance versus UPPP, and 3) outcome measured in terms of quality of life, treatment success, and long-term compliance and complications. The bibliographies of the articles that met these inclusion criteria were manually checked. This process yielded three articles [1–3]. All three articles refer to overlapping patient groups.

RESULTS

Outcome Measures. In two of the studies, successful treatment was defined as a 50% decrease in or normalization of the apnea index (AI), with the AI defined as the average number of apneas per hour of sleep. Apneas were measured utilizing an in-home portable sleep unit, as these studies were completed in Sweden where the authors had vast experience with these in-home units. (Currently, portable sleep studies are not accepted as the standard of care in the United States for the diagnosis of OSA.) In the third study, subjective success was determined using a validated instrument that was completed in the physician's office [3]. Quality of life was measured using the validated Minor Symptoms Evaluation–Profile. Although not specifically designed to evaluate patients with OSA, it measures vitality, contentment, and sleep.

Potential Confounders. Outcome measures used in these publications included post-treatment sleep studies, subjective questionnaire data, and a quality of life measure. These measures were influenced by other factors; age, weight, and body mass index were evaluated as potential confounders, and no statistically significant differences were identified before intervention. In reporting the outcomes, there was a detection bias. The patients that withdrew from the oral appliance arm of the study were not included in the final comparison between the two treatment arms in all three studies. Also, compliance was not an issue in a surgically treated group whereas it was a major factor in treatment outcome when a patient had to use a device every night. In the end, only the successful oral appliance users were compared with the entire surgical group.

Study Designs. All three studies were randomized controlled studies of patients with OSA. Patients were diagnosed with OSA if they had an AI > 5 or apnea-hypopnea index (AHI) >10 after an in-home sleep evaluation measuring five parameters. As above, the AI was defined as average number of apneas per hour of sleep, whereas the AHI was defined as the average number of apneas plus hypopneas per hour of sleep. After a diagnosis of OSA, patients fulfilling inclusion criteria were randomized using a closed-envelope system in sequential order. All three studies involved the same patient groups undergoing treatment with either oral appliance or UPPP. UPPP was performed using the technique described by Fujita, 1981. The oral appliance that was used advanced the patient's mandible to 50% of the maximum protrusive capacity. Success at 1 year of treatment was evaluated in the first study. The second study looked at the quality of life of these patients after 1 year of treatment. The third study evaluated these patients at 4 years for success of treatment, compliance, and morbidity. The technician evaluating the sleep studies was blinded to treatment group. Before initiation of the studies, it was determined that at least 35 patients in each group were required in order to detect a significant difference (alpha 0.05, beta 0.20). To compensate for potential withdrawals, 45 patients in each group were deemed necessary. Ninety-five patients were recruited, 80 patients completed 1-year follow-up, and 72 patients completed 4-year follow-up. Therefore, these studies were adequately powered in their design.

Highest Level of Evidence. The three studies cited in this review are based on one patient group followed for 4 years. One year into treatment, compliance with the oral appliance was 82%, compared with 100% compliance in the UPPP group. There was a significant difference in favor of the oral appliance at 1 year compared with AI and AHI [3]. There was a significant difference in the normalization rate of the AHI and AI in favor of the oral appliance (63%) compared with the UPPP (33%) at 4 years. However, the compliance rate with the oral appliance at 4 years was 62% [2]. When comparing the quality of life between the two treatments, the UPPP showed a significantly higher level of contentment at 1 year than with the oral appliance [1].

Applicability. These studies are applicable to patients 20–65 years old with mild to moderate OSA (AHI > 10, and/or AI > 5). These results do not apply to patients with AI > 25, mental illness, drug misuse, significant nasal obstruction, insufficient teeth to anchor an oral appliance, periodontal disease, pronounced dental malocclusion, severe cardiovascular disease, neurologic disease, and respiratory disease.

Morbidity/Complications. Perioperative complications associated with UPPP were not reported. Long-term follow-up of the patients undergoing UPPP showed that 8% of these patients had nasopharyngeal regurgitation and 10% of patients reported some difficulty swallowing. Of the patients who were randomized to treatment with the oral appliance, one patient dropped out of the study as a result of recurrent aphthous ulcers. On long-term follow-up including dental evaluations, maximum mouth opening capacity did not change significantly, and there were no changes in protrusive capacity. However, one patient did develop temporomandibular joint syndrome (TMJ), two patients developed TMJ crepitus and/or clicking that were not present before the study, and four patients had minor changes in tooth contacts at intercuspidation.

CLINICAL SIGNIFICANCE AND FUTURE RESEARCH

There is level 1 data comparing oral appliance to UPPP for OSA which suggests that sleep studies are improved or normalized significantly more with oral appliance, but that patient contentment is significantly better with UPPP. Both the sleep study and quality-of-life data are important outcome measures, and so it is somewhat difficult to reconcile these two results. An inherent difficulty in treating OSA lies in striking the balance between contentment/compliance and normalization of sleep study parameters. Patients' quality of life is important in contributing to the success of OSA treatment. Even though oral appliance proved more successful in terms of sleep study outcomes, the efficacy of oral appliance is partially invalidated secondary to issues surrounding compliance and patient contentment. In contrast, a patient undergoing a UPPP is 100% compliant and remains treated during each night of sleep, but has a lower normalization rate of sleep study parameters.

Future research comparing UPPP to oral appliance should address long-term efficacy of clinically relevant outcomes, including nadir oxygen saturation and daytime sleepiness, because this chronic and prevalent disease may have a significant impact on work productivity and driving safety. In addition, it would be beneficial to determine the results of a stratified approach with initial oral appliance use with UPPP for patients who cannot adequately comply.

Reference	Wilhelmsson, 1999			Walker-Engstrom, 2000		
Level (design)	1 (randomized controlled trial)			1 (randomized controlled trial)		
Sample size*	80 (95)			80 (95)		

	OUTCOMES					
	Success rate†		Normalization rate‡	**Quality-of-life scores** (lower scores better)		
	AI	**AHI**	**AI or AHI**	**Vitality**	**Contentment**	**Sleep**
UPPP	70%	60%	51%	26.4	27.4	25.2
Oral appliance	95%	81%	78%	31.6	33.7	29.2
p Value	<0.01	<0.05	<0.05	NS	<0.05	NS
Conclusion	OA with significantly better sleep study results than UPPP at 1 y			UPPP contentment significantly better than OA at 1 y		
Follow-up time	1 y			1 y		

	STUDY DESIGN					
Inclusion criteria	Male patients with AHI > 10, AI > 5 between ages of 20 and 60 y Mild to moderate apnea			Male patients with AHI > 10, AI > 5 between ages of 20 and 60 y Mild to moderate apnea		
Exclusion criteria	AI > 25, mental illness, drug misuse, significant nasal obstruction, insufficient teeth to anchor an appliance, pronounced dental malocclusion, severe cardiovascular disease, neurologic or respiratory disease			AI > 25, mental illness, drug misuse, significant nasal obstruction, insufficient teeth to anchor an appliance, pronounced dental malocclusion, severe cardiovascular disease, neurologic or respiratory disease		
Randomization effectiveness	Patients randomized using closed-envelope system in sequential order, sleep studies' evaluator blinded to study treatment There was not a significant difference between age, weight, and BMI for both groups			Patients randomized using closed-envelope system in sequential order, sleep studies' evaluator blinded to study treatment There was not a significant difference between age, weight, and BMI for both groups		
Age	20–60 y			20–60 y		
Intervention regimen details	Dental appliance—evaluation dentist with fashion of appliance used at pm vs UPPP (Fujita)			Dental appliance—evaluation dentist with fashion of appliance used at pm vs UPPP (Fujita)		
Diagnostic criteria for OSA	Questionnaire/home sleep study Fiberoptic examination/Muller maneuver			Questionnaire/home sleep study		
Management while in study	Repeat evaluation 6 mo/1y			Evaluation after 1y		
Compliance	OA 82%/UPPP 100%			NA		
Criteria for withdrawal from study	Not satisfied with appliance or outcome of appliance No withdrawal after UPPP unless lost to follow-up			NA		
Power	80% (beta = 0.20)			80% (beta = 0.20)		
Morbidity/complications	1 with aphthous ulcers, 1 with TMJ symptoms			Not reported		

OA = oral appliance, UPPP = uvulopalatopharyngoplasty, OSA = obstructive sleep apnea, AI = apnea index, AHI = apnea-hypopnea index, NS = not significant, BMI = body mass index, TMJ = temporomandibular joint syndrome, NA = not applicable.
* Sample size: numbers shown for those not lost to follow-up and those (initially recruited).
† Success rate defined as percentage of patients with at least a 50% reduction in AI.
‡ Normalization defined as AI < 5 or AHI < 10.

THE EVIDENCE CONDENSED: Oral appliance versus uvulopalatopharyngoplasty for obstructive sleep apnea

Reference	Walker-Engstrom, 2002		
Level (design)	1 (randomized controlled trial)		
Sample size*	72 (95)		

OUTCOMES

	Success rate†		Normalization rate‡
	AI	AHI	AI or AHI
UPPP	53%	35%	33%
Oral appliance	81%	72%	63%
p Value	<0.05	<0.01	<0.05

Conclusion	OA with significantly better sleep study results than UPPP at 4 y; significant decrease in compliance with OA
Follow-up time	4 y

STUDY DESIGN

Inclusion criteria	Male patients with AHI > 10, AI > 5 between ages of 20 and 60 y Mild to moderate apnea
Exclusion criteria	AI > 25, mental illness, drug misuse, significant nasal obstruction, insufficient teeth to anchor an appliance, pronounced dental malocclusion, severe cardiovascular disease, neurologic or respiratory disease
Randomization effectiveness	Patients randomized using closed-envelope system in sequential order, sleep studies' evaluator blinded to study treatment There was not a significant difference between age, weight, and BMI between groups
Age	20–60 y
Intervention regimen details	Dental appliance—evaluation by dentist with fashion of appliance used at night vs UPPP (Fujita)
Diagnostic criteria for OSA	Questionnaire/home sleep study
Management while in study	Repeat evaluation 4 y
Compliance	OA 62%/UPPP 100%
Criteria for withdrawal from study	Not satisfied with appliance or outcome of appliance No withdrawal after UPPP unless lost to follow-up
Power	80% (beta = 0.20)
Morbidity/complications	UPPP: 8% nasopharyngeal reflux, 10% difficulty swallowing OA: 1 TMJ, 2 TMJ sounds, 4 minimal

OA = oral appliance, UPPP = uvulopalatopharyngoplasty, OSA = obstructive sleep apnea, AI = apnea index, AHI = apnea-hypopnea index, NS = not significant, BMI = body mass index, TMJ = temporomandibular joint syndrome, NA = not applicable.

* Sample size: numbers shown for those not lost to follow-up and those (initially recruited).
† Success rate defined as percentage of patients with at least a 50% reduction in AI.
‡ Normalization defined as AI < 5 or AHI < 10.

REFERENCES

1. Walker-Engstrom M-L, Wilhelmsson B, Tegelberg A, Dimenas E, Ringqvist I. Quality of life assessment of treatment with dental appliance or UPPP in patients with mild to moderate obstructive sleep apnoea. A prospective randomized 1-year follow-up study. J Sleep Res 2000;9:303–308.
2. Walker-Engstrom M-L, Tegelberg A, Wilhelmsson B, Ringqvist I. Four year follow-up of treatment with dental appliance or uvulopalatopharyngoplasty in patients with obstructive sleep apnea. Chest 2002;121:739–746.
3. Wilhelmsson B, Tegelberg A, Walker-Engstrom M-L, et al. A prospective randomized study of a dental appliance compared with uvulopalatopharyngoplasty in the treatment of obstructive sleep apnea. Acta Otolaryngol (Stockh) 1999; 119:503–509.
4. Fujita S, Conway W, Zorick F, Roth T. Surgical correction of anatomic abnormalities in obstructive sleep apnea syndrome: uvulopalatopharyngoplasty. Otolaryngol Head Neck Surg. 1981 Non–Dec; 89(6): 923–934.

20 Obstructive Sleep Apnea in Adults

20.D.

Tongue suspension: Impact on quality of life, polysomnography, and excessive daytime sleepiness

Kenny Pang and B. Tucker Woodson

METHODS

A computerized PubMed search of MEDLINE 1966–April 2006 was performed. Articles mapping to the exploded medical subject headings "obstructive sleep apnea" and "tongue" were cross-referenced, yielding 122 articles. For inclusion criteria, we required the following: 1) adult patients (>20 years old) with obstructive sleep apnea (OSA), 2) intervention with tongue base suspension (TS), 3) outcome measures in terms of quality of life (QOL), objective polysomnographic data, or a validated daytime sleepiness measure such as the Epworth Sleepiness Scale. The resulting articles were reviewed and their references manually crossed-checked for any relevant articles. Studies that evaluated glossectomy or radiofrequency ablation of the tongue were excluded from this analysis. Articles that compared palatal surgery to oral appliance or continuous positive airway pressure were excluded from this review, but are discussed in the adjacent reviews in this chapter. There were seven articles that met these specific inclusion/exclusion criteria.

RESULTS

Outcome Measures. Results of surgical intervention for OSA can be measured in a number of ways. In general, it is well accepted that successful intervention will reduce the postoperative apnea-hypopnea index (AHI) to half its original preoperative AHI and bring the AHI to <15 (mild levels). Reducing AHI levels to <15 reduces the long-term effects of hypertension, ischemic heart disease, and cerebrovascular accidents. QOL in a patient with OSA is also important. Parameters including daytime alertness, sleepiness, and snore scores do relate to QOL in patients with OSA. The Epworth Sleepiness Scale is frequently used as an outcome measure as well. It is a validated measure of daytime sleepiness in which patients rate their likelihood of falling asleep in eight circumstances. Scores range from 0 (best) to 24 (worst).

Potential Confounders. The pathophysiology of upper airway collapse during sleep is affected by multiple factors. Most authors would concur that OSA is fundamentally a balance between the container (the orofacial) skeleton and the contents (the soft tissues in the oral cavity) [1]. It is the vibration of these soft tissues during sleep that results in snoring, and the collapse, partial or

complete, of these structures that lead to upper airway obstruction during sleep. Patients with retrognathia (small orofacial skeleton) will have less space available, therefore increasing the likelihood of airway compromise during sleep [1]. The level of upper airway collapse is important in patients with OSA; some patients have collapse predominantly in the retropalatal area, whereas others collapse mainly in the retrolingual area [2]. Clinical examination and assessment have a crucial role in the management algorithm; however, these may not be consistent in various clinical studies. Different surgical techniques address different levels of obstruction, making comparison of such techniques difficult unless site-specific diagnoses and surgery are performed. Moreover, different authors used patients with varying body mass index (BMI), age, race, and gender in their series, influencing the overall success rates for surgery and other interventions.

Study Designs. There were seven articles that evaluated results after tongue suspension surgery. One publication was a randomized controlled trial (RCT) which compared results with tongue suspension versus tongue advancement (TA) procedures. This RCT focused on patients with moderate or severe OSA, who had multilevel obstruction and had failed continuous positive airway pressure. Follow-up time was 6 months. The remaining six papers were prospective and retrospective cohort studies that compared preoperative versus postoperative data in patients undergoing tongue suspension. Five of these six papers, however, had a key confounder in that the authors studied patients who not only underwent TS, but also underwent uvulopalatopharyngoplasty (UPPP). Thus, it is difficult to discern whether changes in AHI, QOL, or daytime sleepiness were attributable to TS or UPPP or the combination of the two procedures. Follow-up periods ranged from 2 months to 3 years.

Highest Level of Evidence. The RCT that compared TS to TA showed a small but statistically significant better postoperative daytime sleepiness score with TS [14]. The same study showed a trend toward better AHI as well, although it was not a statistically significant difference. The single cohort study that evaluated patients undergoing TS alone [8] showed significant improvements in QOL, AHI, and daytime sleepiness after 2 months in patients with preoperative AHI 15–60. The five remaining studies, which evaluated TS in conjunction with UPPP, showed either a trend toward, or a statistically significant improvement in most parameters after 3 months to 3 years.

Although one might intuitively expect that AHI improvement would correlate with QOL or excessive daytime sleepiness (EDS) improvement, this correlation was not always seen. Discordance between the sleep-related respiratory events (polysomnographic results) and QOL have been shown by two separate articles [4, 6].

Applicability. These results are applicable to patients with multilevel obstruction.

Morbidity. The morbidity from upper airway surgery was low. These reports did not have any significant mortality.

CLINICAL SIGNIFICANCE AND FUTURE RESEARCH

There are seven studies that focused on the impact of TS on AHI, QOL, and EDS in patients with OSA. Results suggest a somewhat better result than with TA, and suggest that either TS alone or TS with UPPP can result in postoperative improvement in sleep parameters.

Future research in this area should standardize patient parameters (e.g., age, BMI, comorbidities, severity of OSA, clinical examination, and surgical technique). In addition, a study comparing the impact of UPPP alone versus UPPP with TS would be useful.

Reference	Thomas, 2003			Woodson, 2001		
Level (design)	1 (randomized controlled trial)			4 (prospective cohort)		
Sample size	17			28		
OUTCOMES						
Study groups	9 TS, 8 TA			28 pts TS		
	QOL	AHI	EDS	QOL	RDI total	EDS
TS	Preop 9.3 ± 1.0 Postop 3.3 ± 2.1	57% achieved a surgical response	Preop 12.1 ± 7.2 Postop 4.1 ± 3.4	Preop 3.9 ± 0.7 Postop 2.4 ± 1.0	Preop 35.4 ± 13.7 Postop 24.5 ± 14.5	Preop 13.8 ± 3.9 Postop 8.8 ± 2.8
TA	Preop 9.3 ± 1.0 Postop 5.0 ± 0.6	50% achieved a surgical response	Preop 13.3 ± 4.5 Postop 5.0 ± 3.5	Not applicable		
p Value	**TS vs TA** not reported; **TS** preop vs postop, p < 0.02; **TA** preop vs postop, p < 0.04	NS	**TS vs TA** p = 0.007 **TS**, p = 0.007, **TA**, p ≤ 0.002	Preop vs postop, p = 0.04	Preop vs postop, p < 0.009	Preop vs postop, p < 0.02
Conclusion	TS slight advantage over TA in EDS			Improvements in EDS, AHI		
Follow-up time	6 mo			2 mo		
STUDY DESIGN						
Inclusion criteria	Moderate and severe OSA, multilevel obstruction, Fujita 2, failed CPAP			AHI < 15 (snorers), AHI > 15 (OSA)		
Exclusion criteria	Fujita 1, mild OSA			AHI > 60, LSAT < 80%, BMI > 34		
Randomization effectiveness	Similar age, BMI, and ESS scores in both groups at the outset			Nonrandomized		
Age	45 y			47.5 ± 8 y		
Masking	Not reported			Not reported		
Intervention regimen details	Success rate of about 60% noted in the TS group, slight advantage over the TA group			AHI decreased in OSA, p < 0.00, multi-institutional 7 sites, effect size for total FOSQ 0.74–0.79, ESS 1.23–1.00		
QOL measure	Not reported			Functional outcomes of sleep		
EDS measure	ESS			ESS, VAS 10-pt scale		
Criteria for withdrawal from study	Lost to follow-up			Failure to follow-up with PSG. No statistical difference between study group and lost to follow-up group		
Intention to treat analysis	Not reported			Not reported		
Power	Not reported			Not reported		
Morbidity/ complications	Pain, limited tongue protrusion			15% (4 with sialadenitis, 1 dehydration, 1 GI bleed)		

UPPP = uvulopalatopharyngoplasty, pts = patients, EDS = excessive daytime sleepiness, QOL = quality of life, OSA = obstructive sleep apnea, ESS = Epworth Sleepiness Scale, CPAP = continuous positive airway pressure, AHI = apnea hypopnea index, BMI = body mass index, TS = tongue suspension, preop = preoperative, postop = postoperative, NS = not significant, PSG = polysomnogram, TA = tongue advancement, VAS = visual analog scale, GI = gastrointestinal, FOSQ = functional outcomes of sleep questionnaire, RDI = respiratory disturbance index.

Reference	Vicente, 2006		
Level (design)	4 (prospective cohort)		
Sample size	55		
OUTCOMES			
Study groups	55 UPPP TS		
	QOL	**AHI**	**EDS**
TS	Not reported	Preop 52.8 ± 14.9 Postop 14.1 ± 23.5	ESS score: Preop 12.2 ± 3.3 Postop 8.2 ± 6.1
p Value	Not applicable	p < 0.001	p = 0.002
Conclusion	Long-term results show that UPPP TS significantly improve AHI and EDS		
Follow-up time	3 y		
STUDY DESIGN			
Inclusion criteria	AHI > 30, severe OSA, failed CPAP, multilevel obstruction, Fujita 2		
Exclusion criteria	BMI > 40, age > 70 y		
Randomization effectiveness	Nonrandomized		
Age	50 ± 5 y		
Masking	Not reported		
Intervention regimen details	BMI no change, 21 pts also had septoplasty, 78% success rate at 3 y (AHI 50% reduction and <15)		
QOL measure	Not reported		
EDS measure	ESS 12.2 to 8.2		
Criteria for withdrawal from study	Patient moved to another location		
Intention to treat analysis	Not reported		
Power	Not reported		
Morbidity/ complications	Not reported		

UPPP = uvulopalatopharyngoplasty, pts = patients, EDS = excessive daytime sleepiness, QOL = quality of life, OSA = obstructive sleep apnea, ESS = Epworth Sleepiness Scale, CPAP = continuous positive airway pressure, AHI = apnea hypopnea index, BMI = body mass index, NS = not significant, TS = tongue suspension, preop = preoperative, postop = postoperative, NS = not significant, PSG = polysomnogram, TA = tongue advancement, VAS = visual analog scale, GI = gastrointestinal.

THE EVIDENCE CONDENSED: Tongue suspension surgery for adult obstructive sleep apnea

Reference	DeRowe, 2000			Terris, 2002			Kuhnel, 2005		
Level (design)	2 (prospective cohort)			3 (retrospective cohort)			2 (prospective cohort)		
Sample size*	16			19			28		

					OUTCOMES				
Study groups	14 UPPP TS			16 pts UPPP TS			28 UPPP TS		
	QOL	RDI mean	EDS	QOL	AHI	EDS	QOL	AHI	EDS
Preoperative	Snoring as reported by bed partner improved in all cases	35 ± 16.5	Not reported	Not reported	42.8 ± 24.8	11.06 ± .5.4	Not reported	41 ± NR	12 ± 4
Postoperative		17 ± 8			14.4 ± NR	5.4. ± 3.8		28 ± 28	9 ± 4
p Value	Not reported	p = 0.001			p < 0.01	p < 0.005		Not reported	Not reported
Conclusion	TS associated with significant postoperative improvement in RDI			TS associated with significant postoperative improvements in EDS, AHI			TS associated with trend toward improvement in AHI, EDS		
Follow-up time	3 mo			6 mo			1 y		

					STUDY DESIGN				
Inclusion criteria	All OSA with multilevel obstruction, Fujita 2, failed CPAP			AHI > 15 (OSA), moderate and severe OSA, Fujita 2, failed CPAP			Failed CPAP, multilevel obstruction, Fujita 2		
Exclusion criteria	Fujita 1			AHI < 15, BMI > 34			BMI > 40, age > 70 y		
Randomization effectiveness	Nonrandomized phase 1 trial			Nonrandomized			Nonrandomized		
Age	35–74 y			44.9 ± 14.2 y			50 ± 5 y		
Intervention regimen details	Success rate of about 51.4% noted in the TS-treated pts			AHI decreased in OSA, p < 0.01, AHI decreased by 51.7%, AI decreased by 81.4%, success rate 67%			Posterior airway space widened by 2 mm in 60% of pts. 67% improved ESS, 55% improved AHI		
QOL measure	Snoring as reported by bed partners			Not reported			Not reported		
EDS measure	ESS			ESS			ESS 19 to 9		
Criteria for withdrawal from study	Lost to follow-up			Failure to follow up with PSG			Lost to follow-up		
Intention to treat analysis	Not reported			Not reported			Not reported		
Power	Not reported			Not reported			Not reported		
Morbidity/ complications	Pain, limited tongue protrusion, mouth floor cyst			Transient VPI, limited tongue movement			Not reported		

UPPP = uvulopalatopharyngoplasty, pts = patients, EDS = excessive daytime sleepiness, QOL = quality of life, AHI = apnea hypopnea index, CPAP = continuous positive airway pressure, BMI = body mass index, NS = not significant, ESS = Epworth Sleepiness Scale, TS = tongue suspension, PSG = polysomnogram, RDI = respiratory disturbance index.
* Sample size: numbers shown for those not lost to follow-up and those (initially recruited).

Reference	Omur, 2005		
Level (design)	3 (retrospective cohort)		
Sample size*	22 UPPP + TS		
OUTCOMES			
Study groups			
	Snoring score	**RDI mean**	**EDS**
Preoperative	8.72 ± 1.83	47.50 ± 15.74	13.9 ± 2.15
Postoperative	3.04 ± 2.35	17.31 ± 14.17	5.40 ± 4.27
p Value	<0.05	<0.05	<0.05
Conclusion	TS and UPPP reduce RDI and ESS compared with UPPP alone.		
Follow-up time	6 mo		
STUDY DESIGN			
Inclusion criteria	Severe OSA (RDI $\geq$ 30/h)		
Exclusion criteria	Simple snoring, mild and moderate OSA (RDI < 30/h)		
Age	32–60 y		
Intervention regimen results	ESS decreased from 13.9 to 5.4 (61.15%); RDI decreased from 47.5 to 17.31 (63.58%); VAS decreased from 8.72 to 3.04 (72.72%)		
Snoring measure	VAS		
EDS measure	ESS		
Criteria for withdrawal from study	Not reported		
Intention to treat analysis	Not reported		
Power	Not reported		
Morbidity/complications	Bleeding, broken suture, infection		

UPPP = uvulopalatopharyngoplasty, EDS = excessive daytime sleepiness, ESS = Epworth Sleepiness Scale, TS = tongue suspension, VAS = visual analog scale, RDI = respiratory disturbance index.
* Sample size: numbers shown for those not lost to follow-up and those (initially recruited).

REFERENCES

1. Pang KP, Blanchard AR, Terris DJ. Snoring: simple to obstructive apnea. In: Calhoun KH, ed. Geriatric Otolaryngology. London: Taylor & Francis; 2006:429–436.
2. Fujita S. Pharyngeal surgery for OSA and snoring. In: Fairbanks DNF, Fujita S, Ikematsu T, Simmons FB, eds. Snoring and OSA. New York: Raven Press; 1987:101–128.
3. Steward DL, Weaver EM, Woodson BT. Multilevel temperature-controlled radiofrequency for obstructive sleep apnea: extended follow-up. Otolaryngol Head Neck Surg 2005;132(4):630–635.
4. Weaver EM, Woodson BT, Steward DL. Polysomnography indexes are discordant with quality of life, symptoms, and reaction times in sleep apnea patients. Otolaryngol Head Neck Surg 2005;132(2):255–262.
5. Friedman M, Ibrahim H, Lowenthal S, Ramakrishnan V, Joseph NJ. Uvulopalatoplasty (UP2): a modified technique for selected patients. Laryngoscope 2004;114(3):441–449.
6. Li HY, Chen NH, Shu YH, Wang PC. Changes in quality of life and respiratory disturbance after extended uvulopalatal flap surgery in patients with obstructive sleep apnea. Arch Otolaryngol Head Neck Surg 2004;130(2):195–200.
7. Ferguson KA, Heighway K, Ruby RRF. A randomized trial of laser-assisted uvulopalatoplasty in the treatment of mild obstructive sleep apnea. Am J Respir Crit Care Med 2003; 167(1):15–19.
8. Woodson BT. A tongue suspension suture for obstructive sleep apnea and snorers. Otolaryngol Head Neck Surg 2001;124(3):297–303.
9. Cahali MB, Formigoni GGS, Gebrim MMS, Miziara ID. Lateral pharyngoplasty versus uvulopalatopharyngoplasty: a clinical, polysomnographic and computed tomography measurement comparison. Sleep 2004;27(5):942–950.
10. Woodson BT, Robinson S, Lim HJ. Transpalatal advancement pharyngoplasty outcomes compared with uvulopalatopharyngoplasty. Otolaryngol Head Neck Surg 2005; 133(2):211–217.
11. Walker-Engstrom ML, Wilhelmsson B, Tegelberg A, Dimenas E, Ringqvust I. Quality of life assessment of treatment with dental appliance or UPPP in patients with mild to moderate obstructive sleep apnoea. A prospective ran-

domized 1-year follow-up study. J Sleep Res 2000;9(3):303–308.

12. Riley RW, Powell NB, Li KK, Troell RJ, Guilleminault C. Surgery and obstructive sleep apnea: long-term clinical outcomes. Otolaryngol Head Neck Surg 2000;122(3):415–421.

13. Woodson BT, Steward DL, Weaver EM, Javaheri S. A randomized trial of temperature-controlled radiofrequency, continuous positive airway pressure, and placebo for obstructive sleep apnea syndrome. Otolaryngol Head Neck Surg 2003;128(6):848–861.

14. Thomas AJ, Chavoya M, Terris DJ. Preliminary findings from a prospective, randomized trial of two tongue-base surgeries for sleep-disordered breathing. Otolaryngol Head Neck Surg 2003;129(5):539–546.

15. Dixon JB, Schachter LM, O'Brien PE. Polysomnography before and after weight loss in obese patients with severe sleep apnea. Int J Obes (Lond) 2005;29(9):1048–1054.

16. Pang KP, Woodson BT. Expansion sphincter pharyngoplasty: a randomized trial with the traditional UPPP in the treatment of OSA. Presented Sleep, Surgery Breathing II Symposium, Chicago, June 2006. Presented American Academy Otolaryngology Head and Neck Surgery, Toronto, September 2006. Otolaryngol Head Neck Surg. 2007 Jul; 137(1):110–114.

17. Weaver EM, Maynard C, Yueh B. Survival of veterans with sleep apnea: continuous positive airway pressure versus surgery. Otolaryngol Head Neck Surg 2004;130(6):659–665.

18. Marti S, Sampol G, Munoz X, et al. Mortality in severe sleep apnoea/hypopnoea syndrome patients: impact of treatment. Eur Respir J 2002;20(6):1511–1518.

19. Friedman M, Ibrahim H, Bass L. Clinical staging for sleep-disordered breathing. Otolaryngol Head Neck Surg 2002;127:13–21.

20. DeRowe A, Gunther E, Fibbi A, et al. Tongue-base suspension with a soft tissue-to-bone anchor for obstructive sleep apnea: preliminary clinical results of a new minimally invasive technique. Otolaryngol Head Neck Surg 2000;122(1):100–103.

21. Terris DJ, Kunda LD, Gonella MC. Minimally invasive tongue base surgery for obstructive sleep apnoea. J Laryngol Otol 2002;116(9):716–721.

22. Kuhnel TS, Schurr C, Wagner B, et al. Morphological changes of the posterior airway space after tongue base suspension. Laryngoscope 2005;115(3):475–480.

23. Omur M, Ozturan D, Elez F, Unver C, Derman S. Tongue base suspension combined with UPPP in severe OSA patients. Otolaryngol Head Neck Surg 2005;133(2):218–223.

24. Vicente E, Marın JM, Carrizo S, Naya MJ. Tongue-base suspension in conjunction with uvulopalatopharyngoplasty for treatment of severe obstructive sleep apnea: long-term follow-up results. Laryngoscope 2006;116:1223–1227.

21 Allergic Rhinitis

21.A.

Intranasal steroids versus nonsedating antihistamines: Impact on symptoms of seasonal allergic rhinitis

Melissa Pynnonen and Jeffrey Terrell

METHODS

A computerized PubMed search of MEDLINE 1966–March 2005 was performed. The subject headings "histamine H1 antagonists" and "steroids" were exploded and cross-referenced with "intranasal." The resulting 63 articles were limited to "randomized controlled trial," "human," and "English language" resulting in 35 publications. The subject headings "histamine H1 antagonists" and "steroids" were exploded and limited to "humans," "English language," and "meta-analysis" resulting in two publications. These two searches were combined, resulting in 37 publications whose titles and abstracts were reviewed. Bibliographies were also reviewed to identify other relevant publications [1, 2]. These articles were then reviewed to identify those that met the following inclusion criteria: 1) patient population with seasonal allergic rhinitis confirmed by skin testing, 2) intervention with oral antihistamine versus intranasal corticosteroid spray, and 3) outcome measured in terms of relief of rhinitis symptoms or rhinitis quality of life improvement. Articles that contained combination therapy were included if the study design contained treatment arms of intranasal corticosteroid spray and oral antihistamine as monotherapy, and if sufficient data were reported to permit comparison. Articles that contained study drugs no longer available (astemizole or terfenadine), or in which the comparator antihistamine was a traditional, sedating, antihistamine (dexchlorpheniramine) were also excluded.

RESULTS

Outcome Measures. Allergic rhinitis can be measured and reported in terms of an overall rhinitis score, or as individual symptoms of obstruction, rhinorrhea, sneezing, and nasal pruritus. Ocular symptoms may be assessed as well [2, 3]. Symptomatic response to treatment may be reported as the frequency of symptom-free days [3–5] or change in symptom severity [2, 3, 6]. The Rhinoconjunctivitis Quality of Life Questionnaire (RQLQ) is a validated instrument designed to assess rhinoconjunctivitis health status longitudinally and provides a more indirect measure of disease burden [6]. As a global measure of health status, one study [6] utilized the RQLQ whereas two other studies [4, 5] utilized a simple visual analog scale.

Potential Confounders. Each study confirmed the diagnosis of seasonal allergic rhinitis with skin testing and performed the trial during the relevant season. Three studies considered perennial rhinitis an exclusion criterion [2, 3, 5] but only one of them [2] actually tested and attempted to control for perennial allergens. Immunotherapy was a variable exclusion criterion: one study excluded patients who were in the first month of treatment [2], another excluded patients in the dose escalation phase [5], and three others [3, 4, 6] made no mention of this factor. Medications and dosages were similar: four of the five studies utilized fluticasone 220 µg daily and/or loratadine 10 mg daily.

Study Designs. All five studies were randomized controlled trials that compared the relative benefit of relief of allergic rhinitis symptoms of oral antihistamine therapy versus intranasal corticosteroid spray. Four studies were designed to evaluate intranasal steroid (INS) versus oral antihistamine as monotherapy; one study [6] was designed to evaluate these modalities as combined therapy. This latter study also included monotherapy treatment arms and those data were extracted for this review. All studies were double blinded, placebo controlled, parallel group designs. Daily individual symptom measures were obtained from subject diaries [2–6] and periodic global symptom measures were obtained with a visual analog scale [4–6]. Surrogate measures of symptom improvement, such as a clinician's rating of symptomatology [2, 4–6] or measurement of nasal peak inspiratory flow [3] were deemed less meaningful to the patient than the patients' reported symptoms and thus were not considered in this analysis. Each study reported on randomization effectiveness, showing mostly similar baseline characteristics before treatment. One study [3] found a greater prevalence of pre-trial use of antihistamines among subjects randomized to the antihistamine treatment arm. This may have biased the study results and the need for rescue therapy (see below). In the only study that reported compliance rates [6], they were very good: 97%–98% of subjects in each treatment arm achieved at least 80% medication compliance. Three studies [3–5] allowed the use of rescue medications and two of them [3, 5] found greater use of rescue antihistamine among subjects in the antihistamine group than in the nasal steroid group. The one study that found no difference in the use of rescue medication [4] offered only ophthalmic cromolyn drops as rescue therapy. Two studies reported statistical size calculations [3, 6] with 80% and 90% power, respectively, although the latter study did not precisely state the sample-size estimate necessary to reach this power.

Highest Level of Evidence. These level 1 studies demonstrated consistently greater relief of nasal symptoms of seasonal allergic rhinitis with INS spray versus nonsedating, oral antihistamine. This result was consistent across all five studies. Confidence levels were not reported, but were calculated from the data reported in two studies [2, 5]. There were fewer data regarding the relief of ocular symptoms although the data showed a trend toward greater improvement with INS.

Applicability. These data can be applied to patients age 12 years and older with seasonal allergic rhinitis confirmed by skin testing.

Morbidity/Complications. Treatment-related adverse events that resulted in subject withdrawal included: seizure in a patient with a history of seizure disorder (n = 1), dizziness (n = 1), sweating and weakness (n = 1), gastritis (n = 1), eczema (n = 1), and drowsiness (n = 3). Other adverse effects attributed to medication were generally minor, and seemed to be similarly distributed between the two treatment arms, although the details of the data varied substantially among the studies. The overall rate of epistaxis was 4%–8% without definite preponderance with either treatment modality [3, 6]. One study [3] noted a higher incidence of headache in the INS group, but as with epistaxis, the data provided were limited. The similar rate of epistaxis between the two treatment modalities is surprising, as minor epistaxis is anecdotally believed to be a common side effect of INS use. Notably, four of the studies excluded subjects with structural abnormalities. Abnormalities such as severe nasal septal deflection may result in greater medication deposition on the septum and an increased risk of bleeding, as well as poor drug distribution and lower efficacy. Thus, exclusion of patients with such abnormalities may have been a factor in minimizing the rates of epistaxis in these studies.

CLINICAL SIGNIFICANCE AND FUTURE RESEARCH

These data support the use of INS spray as monotherapy for symptomatic treatment of seasonal allergic rhinitis. Nasal steroids consistently show greater benefit versus nonsedating antihistamines for relief of allergic rhinitis, particularly the nasal symptoms. There are fewer data regarding the relief of ocular symptoms, although the data show a trend toward greater improvement with INS. Both medications are generally well tolerated.

Directions for future study include evaluation of the efficacy of intranasal antihistamine versus intranasal corticosteroid as well as evaluation of combined antihistamine and INS use versus either therapy alone.

THE EVIDENCE CONDENSED: Intranasal steroids versus nonsedating antihistamines: Impact on symptoms of seasonal allergic rhinitis

Reference	Jordana, 1996
Level (design)	1 (RCT)
Sample size*	242 (257)
OUTCOMES	
Symptom measure	Symptom-free days (28-d study) Median %
INS	
Blockage PM	14†
Blockage AM	36
Sneezing	50†
Pruritus	56†
Rhinorrhea	56†
Eye	47†
AH	
Blockage PM	0†
Blockage AM	7.7
Sneezing	17†
Pruritus	35
Rhinorrhea	26
Eye	56
Statistical analysis	
Blockage PM	$p < 0.0001$
Blockage AM	$p = 0.0001$
Sneezing	$p = 0.0015$
Pruritus	$p = 0.03$
Rhinnorhea	$p < 0.0001$
Eye	$p = 0.14$
Conclusion	Fluticasone more effective than loratadine for relief of nasal symptoms. No statistical difference in eye symptoms
STUDY DESIGN	
Inclusion criteria	SAR
Exclusion criteria	Perennial rhinitis, sinusitis, structural abnormalities, recent AH, corticosteroids or sodium cromoglycate
Randomization effectiveness	More patients in the AH group reported pre-trial use of AH
Age	12–17 y
Intervention regimen details	Fluticasone 200 µg vs loratadine 10 mg
Management of episode while in study	Rescue AH usage: 21% INS group 39% AH group, $p < 0.0025$ No difference in use of rescue eye drop or bronchodilator
Rescue medications	Terfenadine; naphazoline/pheniramine eye drop; inhaled salbutamol
Compliance	NR
Criteria for withdrawal from study	5 subjects withdrew because of treatment failure (1 INS, 4 AH)
Intention to treat analysis	242 subjects randomized; only 240 included in analysis
Source of funding	Glaxo Canada
Power	0.9 to detect a 20% difference

RCT = randomized controlled trial, INS = intranasal steroid, AH = antihistamine, NR = not reported, SAR = seasonal allergic rhinitis (confirmed by skin testing), URI = upper respiratory infection, NA = not applicable.
*Sample size: numbers shown for those not lost to follow-up and those (initially recruited).
†Estimated from graph.

THE EVIDENCE CONDENSED: Intranasal steroids versus nonsedating antihistamines: Impact on symptoms of seasonal allergic rhinitis

Reference	Schoenwetter, 1995
Level (design)	1 (RCT)
Sample size*	274 (298)
OUTCOME	
Symptom measure	Nasal symptom scores (range 0–3) Mean change
INS	
Blockage PM	NR
Blockage AM	−0.89
Sneezing	−1.13
Pruritus	−1.05
Rhinorrhea	−1.05
Eye	−0.8
AH	
Blockage PM	NR
Blockage AM	−0.43
Sneezing	−0.68
Pruritus	−0.76
Rhinorrhea	−0.52
Eye	−0.69
Statistical analysis	
Blockage PM	NR
Blockage AM	95% CI‡ = −0.61 and −0.28
Sneezing	95% CI‡ = −0.63 and −0.27
Pruritus	95% CI‡ = −0.46 and −0.11
Rhinnorhea	95% CI‡ = −0.70 and −0.36
Eye	95% CI‡ = −0.28 and 0.065
Conclusion	Significantly greater improvement in individual and total rhinitis symptoms with INS; trend for greater improvement in ocular symptoms as well
STUDY DESIGN	
Inclusion criteria	SAR
Exclusion criteria	Recent AH, corticosteroid, or cromolyn. Sinusitis, rhinitis medicamentosa, fungal infection, or structural abnormality. Recent initiation of immunotherapy. Excluded perennial rhinitis by testing
Randomization effectiveness	No differences noted
Age	12–70 y
Intervention regimen details	Triamcinolone acetonide 220 µg vs loratadine 10 mg
Management of episode while in study	None
Rescue medications	NA
Compliance	NR
Criteria for withdrawal from study	16 INS patients withdrew 14 AH patients withdrew
Intention to treat analysis	No
Source of funding	Rhone-Poulenc Rorer Pharmaceuticals
Power	NR

RCT = randomized controlled trial, INS = intranasal steroid, AH = antihistamine, NR = not reported, SAR = seasonal allergic rhinitis (confirmed by skin testing), URI = upper respiratory infection, NA = not applicable.
* Sample size: numbers shown for those not lost to follow-up and those (initially recruited).
‡ Confidence intervals calculated from data provided.

THE EVIDENCE CONDENSED: Intranasal steroids versus nonsedating antihistamines: Impact on symptoms of seasonal allergic rhinitis

Reference	Vervloet, 1997	
Level (design)	1 (RCT)	
Sample size*	237 (238)	
OUTCOMES		
Symptom measure	Symptom-free days (21-d study) Mean %	Global effectiveness
INS		
Blockage PM	57	
Blockage AM	53	
Sneezing	46	
Pruritus	58	88%
Rhinorrhea	58	
Eye	NR	
AH		
Blockage PM	30	
Blockage AM	31	
Sneezing	32	
Pruritus	42	62%
Rhinorrhea	33	
Eye	NR	
Statistical analysis		
Blockage PM	95% CI‡ = 18 and 32	
Blockage AM	95% CI‡ = 13 and 31	
Sneezing	95% CI‡ = 6.2 and 22	
Pruritus	95% CI‡ = 7.0 and 25	$p < 0.001$
Rhinnorhea	95% CI‡ = 8.4 and 26	
Eye	**NR**	
Conclusion	Fluticasone more effective than cetirizine for relief of rhinitis	
STUDY DESIGN		
Inclusion criteria	SAR	
Exclusion criteria	PAR, structure abnormality, sinusitis, URI, recent allergy medication use, current immunotherapy in dose escalation	
Randomization effectiveness	Yes	
Age	≥12 y	
Intervention regimen details	Fluticasone 200 µg vs cetirizine 10 mg	
Management of episode while in study	Rescue AH usage (% of days without rescue medication) 87% INS 80% AH, $p < 0.05$ No difference in use of rescue eye drop	
Rescue medications	Terfenadine; sodium cromoglycate eye drops	
Compliance	NR	
Criteria for withdrawal from study	5 subjects in AH group withdrew because of adverse events	
Intention to treat analysis	238 subjects randomized, only 237 analyzed	
Source of funding	Glaxo Wellcome	
Power	NR	

RCT = randomized controlled trial, INS = intranasal steroid, AH = antihistamine, NR = not reported, SAR = seasonal allergic rhinitis (confirmed by skin testing), URI = upper respiratory infection, NA = not applicable, PAR = perennial allergic rhinitis.
* Sample size: numbers shown for those not lost to follow-up and those (initially recruited).
‡ Confidence intervals calculated from data provided.

THE EVIDENCE CONDENSED: Intranasal steroids versus nonsedating antihistamines: Impact on symptoms of seasonal allergic rhinitis

Reference	Ratner, 1998		Gehanno, 1997	
Level (design)	1 (RCT)		1 (RCT)	
Sample size*	569 (600)		103 (114)	
OUTCOMES				
Symptom measure	Total nasal symptom score (0–400) rated on VAS (mean at end of 14-d study)	RQLQ (mean change from baseline)	Mean symptom-free days for combined symptoms (obstruction, sneezing, itching, rhinorrhea)	Improvement in total nasal symptoms rated on VAS
INS	145†	Global −2.2 Nasal −2.5 Eye −1.9 Activities −2.3 Practical problems −2.5 Sleep −2.1 Emotional −1.9 Other −1.9	21%	72%
AH	208†	Global −1.3 Nasal −1.4 Eye −1.3 Activities −1.5 Practical problems −1.3 Sleep −1.2 Emotional −1.1 Other −1.1	4%	49%
p Value	<0.001	<0.05 for all domains	<0.001	0.009
Conclusion	Fluticasone more effective than loratadine			Fluticasone more effective than loratadine
STUDY DESIGN				
Inclusion criteria	SAR		SAR	
Exclusion criteria	Recent AH, corticosteroid, or cromolyn use; structural abnormality, septal perforation, or prior septoplasty. Did not exclude concurrent immunotherapy		Recent corticosteroid or cromolyn Did not exclude recent antihistamine use or concurrent immunotherapy	
Randomization effectiveness	No differences noted		No differences noted	
Age	≥12 y		≥12 y	
Intervention regimen details	Fluticasone 200 µg vs loratadine 10 mg		Fluticasone 200 µg vs loratadine 10 mg	
Rescue medications	None		Ophthalmic cromolyn	
Management of episode while in study	NA		INS 14% p = 0.89 AH 13%	
Compliance	Fluticasone 97.9% (≥80% compliance) Loratadine 97% (≥80% compliance)		NR	
Criteria for withdrawal from study	28 patients withdrew (8 adverse events, 13 lack of efficacy, 7 other reasons; evenly distributed)		2 INS patients withdrew 9 AH patients withdrew	
Intention to treat analysis	No		Yes	
Source of funding	Glaxo Wellcome		Glaxo Laboratories	
Power	0.80 to detect a 30-point mean change in total nasal symptom scores, with 150 patients in each group		NR	

RCT = randomized controlled trial, VAS = visual analog scale, INS = intranasal steroid, AH = antihistamine, NR = not reported, SAR = seasonal allergic rhinitis, RQLQ = Rhinoconjunctivitis Quality of Life Questionnaire, NA = not applicable.
* Sample size: numbers shown for those not lost to follow-up and those (initially recruited).
† Estimated from graph.

REFERENCES

1. Weiner JM, Abramson MJ, Puy RM. Intranasal corticosteroids versus oral H1 receptor antagonists in allergic rhinitis: systematic review of randomised controlled trials. BMJ 1998;317(7173):1624–1629.

2. Schoenwetter W, Lim J. Comparison of intranasal triamcinolone acetonide with oral loratadine for the treatment of patients with seasonal allergic rhinitis. Clin Ther 1995;17(3): 479–492.

3. Jordana G, Dolovich J, Briscoe MP, et al. Intranasal fluticasone propionate versus loratadine in the treatment of adolescent patients with seasonal allergic rhinitis. J Allergy Clin Immunol 1996;97(2):588–595.

4. Gehanno P, Desfougeres JL. Fluticasone propionate aqueous nasal spray compared with oral loratadine in patients with seasonal allergic rhinitis. Allergy 1997;52(4):445–450.

5. Vervloet D, Charpin D, Desfougeres J-L. Intranasal fluticasone once daily compared with once-daily cetirizine in the treatment of seasonal allergic rhinitis. Clin Drug Invest 1997;13(6):291–298.

6. Ratner PH, van Bavel JH, Martin BG, et al. A comparison of the efficacy of fluticasone propionate aqueous nasal spray and loratadine, alone and in combination, for the treatment of seasonal allergic rhinitis. J Fam Pract 1998;47(2):118–125.

21 Allergic Rhinitis

21.B.

Antihistamines versus montelukast versus antihistamine plus montelukast versus placebo for seasonal allergic rhinitis: Impact on symptoms of seasonal allergic rhinitis, and disease-specific quality of life

Jeffrey Terrell and Melissa Pynnonen

METHODS

A computerized PubMed search of MEDLINE 1966–March 2005 was performed using the subject "leukotriene antagonists" [pharmacological action] and the medical subject headings "rhinitis, allergic, perennial" or "hay fever." The resulting 28 articles and abstracts were reviewed to identify those that met the following inclusion criteria: 1) patient population with seasonal allergic rhinitis confirmed by skin testing, 2) an intervention with an oral second-generation, currently marketed antihistamine versus leukotriene modifier or some combination thereof, and 3) clinical outcomes measured in terms of relief of rhinitis symptoms and/or improvement in a validated rhinitis quality of life (QOL) instrument. Articles that contained other forms of therapies or combination therapies (antihistamine, corticosteroid, or mast cell stabilizer) were included if the study design also contained treatment arms of leukotrienes and oral antihistamine as monotherapy or combined therapy, and if sufficient data were reported to permit comparison. Articles that focused on relief of only a single symptom, such as nasal obstruction, were excluded. The bibliographies of the articles that met these inclusion criteria were manually checked to ensure no further relevant articles could be identified. This process yielded eight articles, which are summarized in the adjoining tables and within the text of this review [1–5, 8–10].

RESULTS

Outcome Measures. Outcome measures for allergic rhinitis are most often reported as individual nasal symptoms scores (congestion, rhinorrhea, sneezing, pruritus most frequently) and eye symptoms (pruritus and lacrimation). Specific details regarding each study are provided in the adjoining tables. As validated rhinitis-related QOL instruments have become available, changes in QOL scores are becoming more common primary or secondary endpoints. The Rhinoconjunctivitis Quality of Life Questionnaire (RQLQ) is a frequently used validated instrument with 28 items in seven domains (sleep, nonrhinoconjunctivitis symptoms, practical problems, nasal symptoms, eye symptoms, activity limitations, and emotional function) [6]. Patients rate each item on a seven-point scale, ranging from 0 (not troubled) to 6

(extremely troubled). Mean changes in RQLQ score of more than approximately 0.5 can be considered clinically important [7].

Potential Confounders. Each study confirmed the diagnosis of seasonal allergic rhinitis with skin prick testing and performed the trial during the relevant season. Block randomization was frequently used to maintain similar treatment group sizes. Groups were similar in demographics and clinical parameters within any particular study. A run-in period, before intervention or placebo, was frequently used. To prevent bias and dropout, all studies excluded patients with asthma that was more severe than mild, intermittent.

Study Designs. All eight studies were randomized controlled trials that compared the relief of allergic rhinitis symptoms from antihistamines versus montelukast or a combination of antihistamine plus montelukast. Five studies also included a placebo control. Two studies compared one antihistamine with a different antihistamine combined with montelukast [1, 4]. All studies were blinded, placebo-controlled, parallel group designs. All except one of the eight studies were double blinded. The one single-blinded study was a crossover study. Daily individual symptom measures were obtained from subject diaries. QOL measures were used in six studies. One study used an objective measure of nasal function (a home peak inspiratory flow meter with nasal attachment), which correlated well with nasal obstruction symptoms [4]. Seven of the eight studies commented on the details of randomization effectiveness and dropout rates, neither of which were concerning. Several studies specified whether an intention to treat analysis was performed. For example, Nayak et al. [2] performed an efficacy analysis for all endpoints in a modified intention-to-treat patient population that included all randomized patients who had a baseline and at least one post-treatment symptom evaluation, as well as no withdrawal from removal of consent, protocol deviations, adverse events, or lack of efficacy. Pullertis analyzed an intent-to-treat population consisting of all subjects who were randomized to treatment and who received at least one dose of study medication. Three studies reported statistical size calculations, each with at least 80% power to detect a clinical change. Several studies were only powered to detect a clinical change compared with placebo, rather than the second active drug [2, 3, 8].

Highest Level of Evidence. Multiple studies demonstrated that montelukast and the second-generation antihistamines, as well as the combination of the two, consistently outperformed placebo control [2, 3, 5, 8, 9].

Six of the eight studies reported no statistical differences between the combination of newer antihistamines (loratadine, fexofenadine) with montelukast versus either agent alone. Two studies, however, suggested that the addition of montelukast to antihistamine may improve results. Kurowski et al. [10] suggested that the addition of montelukast to cetirizine resulted in better relief of rhinorrhea, nasal itching, and eye itching than cetirizine alone. Similarly, Meltzer et al. [8] demonstrated significantly improved nasal symptoms (except nasal congestion) with montelukast and loratadine versus either agent alone or placebo. Results from the RQLQ were not clearly significantly different when comparing combined therapy to unimodality therapy. Several studies had limited power to demonstrate a true significant difference between montelukast with antihistamine versus single-agent therapy, as some studies were designed primarily to test both interventions versus placebo. In fact, only three of the studies reported the associated power calculations.

None of the studies reported statistical differences between these newer antihistamines and montelukast (mostly because of intentional study design/limited power) although three studies showed consistent trends that loratadine was associated with better daytime symptoms, eye symptoms, and QOL scores, but not better nocturnal symptoms [2, 3, 9]. This may be the result of a lesser decongestant effect of antihistamines.

Applicability. These data can be applied to adults with seasonal allergic rhinitis confirmed by skin-prick testing, but may or may not apply to patients with perennial allergic rhinitis or allergic rhinitis with more severe asthma.

Morbidity/Complications. Treatment-related adverse events were infrequent, mild, and self-limited. Headache and upper respiratory infections were most common, but these occurred at similar rates as placebo (or less frequently). Laboratory abnormalities were infrequent and similar among treatment groups in these studies.

CLINICAL SIGNIFICANCE AND FUTURE RESEARCH

These data support the use of montelukast for seasonal allergic rhinitis, either alone or combined with a second-generation antihistamine. Montelukast alone yields consistently improved symptoms when compared with placebo. However, when montelukast was compared with loratadine, loratadine consistently trended toward (although not statistically significantly) giving more daytime and eye symptom relief in three similar studies [2, 3, 9]. As a single agent for seasonal allergic rhinitis, second-generation antihistamines may show more promise, but a future well-powered randomized trial or meta-analysis is needed to definitively answer this question. For patients who experience inadequate relief with antihistamines alone or montelukast alone, the addition of montelukast yields better control of nasal symptoms when compared with antihistamine alone, according to the results of two trials.

It is possible that patients may have comorbidities or preferences that might be strong drivers of physician prescribing behaviors: a deviated septum or nosebleeds may preclude steroid sprays as an option for combined therapy; concomitant persistent asthma may sway a prescriber toward a leukotriene inhibitor as a primary or secondary therapy. This review does not consider the recognized benefit of leukotriene inhibitors for the treatment of persistent asthma [11]. Patients with concurrent persistent asthma and allergic rhinitis may obtain improvement in asthma and allergic rhinitis with montelukast alone. Patients with persistent asthma and allergic rhinitis may also benefit from montelukast plus antihistamine (which demonstrated incremental benefit as noted above) or possibly montelukast plus corticosteroid nasal spray, which was not within the scope of this particular review.

Further studies comparing various combinations of corticosteroid nasal sprays, antihistamines, and leukotriene inhibitors may be beneficial if they are adequately powered. Cost-effectiveness studies would also be beneficial.

THE EVIDENCE CONDENSED: Antihistamines versus montelukast versus antihistamine plus montelukast for allergic rhinitis

Reference	Meltzer, 2000			
Level (design)	1 (randomized controlled trial)			
Sample size	Total n = 458 Placebo (91), ML 10 mg (95), ML 20 mg (90), LRT 10 mg (92), MNT 10 mg + LRT 10 mg (90)			
OUTCOMES				
Measures	**Day symptom scores, night symptom scores, scores on RQLQ instrument**			
Outcome	Change in least square mean from baseline symptom scores			
	Day Sx	Day eye	Noc Sx	Composite
Placebo	−0.25	−0.28	−0.11	−0.24
ML 10 mg	−0.36	−0.28	−0.29	−0.39
Antihistamine	−0.34	−0.25	−0.19	−0.32
ML + antihistamine	−0.61	−0.46	−0.33	−0.54
p Value	<0.05 for ML + AH vs placebo, vs ML alone, vs AH alone			
Conclusion	ML + AH improved each nasal symptom compared with all other treatment groups, except for nasal congestion score, which was not significantly different from ML 10 mg alone.			
Follow-up time	2 wk			
STUDY DESIGN				
Inclusion criteria	Healthy men and women, ages 15–75 y, with seasonal AR, positive skin test to 1 of 8 grass or tree pollens			
Exclusion criteria	Pregnant, unstable asthma, asthma agents other than short-acting inhaled beta-agonists, prolonged QTc interval, recent nasal surgery, recent URI			
Medication restrictions	Recent astemizole, systemic corticosteroids; cetirizine, zileuton, zafirlukast, oral or inhaled beta-agonists, recent antihistamines or decongestants, immunotherapy initiated <6 mo before the entry into the study			
Randomization effectiveness	No clinical differences between groups for demographics, baseline symptoms, secondary diagnoses, concomitant drug therapies			
Age	15–75 y			
Allergy regimen	1 wk placebo run-in, then 2 wk of double-blinded placebo or intervention during allergy season			
Outcome measures	Daytime nasal symptom scores, daytime eye symptoms scores, night-time symptoms, and RQLQ scores			
Compliance	Medication compliance not reported			
Criteria for withdrawal from study	25 patients withdrew from the study, evenly distributed among groups			
Power	Study powered for 80% power to detect (alpha = 0.05, s-sided test) a between-treatment difference of 0.25 in score change from baseline			
Morbidity/complications	No different from placebo group			

ML = montelukast, LRT = loratadine, RQLQ = Rhinoconjunctivitis Quality of Life Questionnaire, AH = antihistamines, URI = upper respiratory infection, NA = not applicable, NSAIDs = nonsteroidal antiinflammatory drugs, Sx = symptoms.

THE EVIDENCE CONDENSED: Antihistamines versus montelukast versus antihistamine plus montelukast for allergic rhinitis

Reference	Kurowski, 2004				
Level (design)	1 (randomized controlled trial)				
Sample size	Total n = 60 in four arm study Placebo (11), ML (11), cetirizine (19), cetirizine + ML (19)				
OUTCOMES					
Measures	**Symptoms of AR and conjunctivitis in daily diaries (congestion, rhinorrhea, itching, sneezing, and eye symptoms)**				
Outcome	Mean in scores in each of symptoms below				
	Congest	Rhin	Itch	Sneeze	Eye Sx
Placebo	1.83	1.72	1.63	2.20	2.01
ML 10 mg		†			
Antihistamine		0.91	1.02		1.16
ML + antihistamine	0.93	0.41	0.53	0.92	0.54
p Value	For bolded comparisons between ML + CT vs cetirizine alone, $p < 0.05$.				
Conclusion	Compared with cetirizine alone, ML + cetirizine gave better relief of rhinorrhea, nasal itching, and eye itching when taken before and during grass allergy season				
Follow-up time	6 wk before season, 6 wk after season				
STUDY DESIGN					
Inclusion criteria	Adults with allergic rhinitis with AR for 2 y, positive skin-prick test to grasses and grass/cereal allergens				
Exclusion criteria	Patients with bronchial asthma, polyvalent pollen allergy, non–pollen-associated rhinitis, on immunotherapy, long QT interval, septal deviation, recent nasal surgery, pregnant				
Medication restrictions	Excluded medications: topical or systemic steroids, cromolyns, NSAIDs, topical or systemic antihistamines, leukotriene modifiers, macrolide antibiotics, imidazole antifungal drugs				
Randomization effectiveness	No differences in age and sex				
Age	18–35 y				
Allergy regimen	Patients randomized to placebo, ML only, cetirizine only, or ML + cetirizine for period of 6 wk before and after the start of grass allergy season (endpoint)				
Outcome measures	Self-reported symptom scores on 6-point Likert scale				
Compliance	Medication compliance not reported				
Criteria for withdrawal from study	48 of the 60 patients completed the study, about evenly distributed among the treatment groups				
Power	Not reported				
Morbidity/complications	Not specified				

ML = montelukast, LRT = loratadine, RQLQ = Rhinoconjunctivitis Quality of Life Questionnaire, AH = antihistamines, URI = upper respiratory infection, NA = not applicable, NSAIDs = nonsteroidal antiinflammatory drugs, Sx = symptoms.
† ML + cetirizine was associated with a significantly better score on rhinorrhea question ($p < 0.05$), but numerical data was not reported.

THE EVIDENCE CONDENSED: Antihistamines versus montelukast versus antihistamine plus montelukast for allergic rhinitis

Reference	Philip, 2002			
Level (design)	Randomized, double-blind, parallel-group trial ML vs LRT vs placebo			
Sample size	Total n = 1302 ML (348), LRT (602), placebo (352)			
OUTCOMES				
Measures	**Day symptom scores, night symptom scores, scores on RQLQ instrument**			
Outcome	Least square mean difference from placebo			
	Day Sx	Noc Sx	Eye Sx	RhCQol
ML 10 mg	−0.13	−0.14	−0.20	−0.89
Antihistamine	−0.24	−0.09	−0.20	−0.99
ML + antihistamine	NA			
p Value	Both different from placebo, no comparisons between active interventions			
Conclusion	Loratadine tended to give more day, and eye symptoms relief and improvements in RQLQ scores, but no statistical comparisons between active interventions			
Follow-up time	2 wk			
STUDY DESIGN				
Inclusion criteria	Adults with allergic rhinitis, spring exacerbations, positive skin-prick test to spring allergen, and mild to moderate symptom severity			
Exclusion criteria	Asthmatics requiring more than short-acting B-2 inhalers, structural nasal disorder, URI, sinusitis, ocular infection, pregnant or lactating women			
Medication restrictions	Other allergy medications stopped but stable dosing of immunotherapy allowed			
Randomization effectiveness	No differences in demographics, sex, race, allergic history, baseline symptoms			
Age	15–81 y			
Allergy regimen	3- to 5-day placebo run-in, followed by 2 wk of study drug or placebo with symptom scores recorded after each daytime			
Outcome measures	Symptom scores recorded after each daytime or night, Likert scale for nasal (congestion, rhinorrhea, pruritus, and sneezing) symptoms, eye symptoms, and sleep. Rhinoconjunctivitis QOL scores using validated instrument			
Compliance	99% compliance by pill counts, all groups			
Criteria for withdrawal from study	Patients discontinued at similar rates for reasons of lack of efficacy, adverse experience, protocol deviation, lost to follow-up, withdrew consent, or other			
Power	Not reported			
Morbidity/complications	No differences between placebo, ML, and LRT in adverse symptoms or labs			

ML = montelukast, LRT = loratadine, RQLQ = Rhinoconjunctivitis Quality of Life Questionnaire, AH = antihistamines, URI = upper respiratory infection, NA = not applicable, NSAIDs = nonsteroidal antiinflammatory drugs, Sx = symptoms.

THE EVIDENCE CONDENSED: Antihistamines versus montelukast versus antihistamine plus montelukast for allergic rhinitis

Reference	van Adelsberg, 2003		
Level (design)	1 (randomized controlled trial)		
Sample size*	Total n = 1191 (1214) ML 10 mg [n = 501 (522)], LRT 10 mg [n = 165 (171)], placebo [n = 492 (521)] × 2 wk		

OUTCOMES

Measures	Mean change from baseline		
Outcome	Composite symptom scores	Patient's global evaluation	Rhinoconjunctivitis QOL
Score ranges	0 best to 3 worst		0 best to 6 worst
Placebo	−0.25	2.49	−0.9
ML	−0.34	2.18	−0.66
AH	−0.39	2.19	−0.98
ML + AH	NA	NA	NA
p Value, ML vs placebo	<0.002	0.001	0.001
p Value, AH vs placebo	<0.001	0.023	<0.001
p Value, other	NR, ML vs AH	NR, ML vs AH	NR, ML vs AH
Conclusion	ML and AH had better symptom scores, global evaluation, and QOL than placebo. Trend toward ML better for eosinophil count, AH better for daytime nasal symptoms		
Follow-up time	2 wk		

STUDY DESIGN

Inclusion criteria	Outpatients, 15–85 y old with seasonal allergic rhinitis with at least 2 y of documented clinical history of allergic rhinitis symptoms during the spring; minimum predefined 3-d cumulative score of 18 on the daily diary, positive skin-prick test to 1 of the allergens active during the study season (wheal diameter ≥3 mm greater than diluent control), nonsmokers, good mental and physical health
Exclusion criteria	URI, sinusitis, infectious rhinitis, ocular infection, perennial rhinitis, clinically significant structural nasal obstruction
Medication restrictions	Nasal, ophthalmic, inhaled, oral and parental corticosteroids; AH; nasal, ophthalmic, and inhaled cromolyn and nedocromil; oral and long-acting inhaled beta-agonists; inhaled anticholinergic agents; theophylline; other antileukotrienes
Randomization effectiveness	No difference in baseline demographics, daytime nasal symptom score, allergic history
Age	15–82 y
Allergy regimen	3- to 5-d placebo run-in period, followed by 2 wk of double-blinded treatment: 1) ML 10 mg, 2) LRT 10 mg, or 3) placebo. Patients received 2 tablets for each day of each treatment period. All medications were taken once daily at bedtime, irrespective of food
Outcome measures	Primary efficacy endpoint was daytime nasal symptoms score, defined by congestion, rhinorrhea, pruritus, and sneezing. Secondary endpoints were night-time symptoms score (defined by difficulty going to sleep, night-time awakenings, nasal congestion on awakening) and daytime eye scores, global evaluations, and rhinoconjunctivitis QOL scores
Masking	Double blind
Compliance	Not specified
Criteria for withdrawal from study	Requirement of medication other than study medication for treating allergic rhinitis
Power	1000 patients (300 + 300 + 100) to have a 93% power to detect a 0.15 difference between ML and placebo
Morbidity/complications	Clinical adverse experiences, n = 89 (17%), 26 (15%), and 83 (16%) patients in the ML, LRT, and placebo treatment groups, respectively

ML = montelukast, LRT = loratadine, SD = standard deviation, SEM = standard error of the mean, QOL = quality of life, AH = antihistamines, RQLQ = Rhinoconjunctivitis Quality of Life Questionnaire, URI = upper respiratory infection, NA = not applicable, NS = not significant, NR = not reported.
*The first sample sizes shown are for those who completed the study and those (initially recruited).

THE EVIDENCE CONDENSED: Antihistamines versus montelukast versus antihistamine plus montelukast for allergic rhinitis

Reference	Nayak, 2002		
Level (design)	1 (randomized controlled trial)		
Sample size*	Total n = 872 (907) ML 10 mg (155), LRT (301), ML and LRT (302), placebo (149)		

OUTCOMES

Measures	Mean difference from placebo		
Outcome	Daytime nasal symptoms	Composite symptom scores	Rhinoconjunctivitis QOL
Score ranges	0 best to 3 worst		0 best to 6 worst
Placebo	NA	NA	−0.80 (−0.98, −0.63)
ML	−0.23 (−0.35, −0.11)	−0.20 (−0.31, −0.10)	−1.09 (−1.26, −0.92)
AH	−0.26 (−0.37, −0.16)	−0.21 (−0.30, −0.12)	−1.06 (−1.19, −0.93)
ML + AH	−0.32 (−0.42, −0.21)	−0.25 (−0.34, −0.16)	−1.16 (−1.29, −1.03)
p Value, ML vs placebo	<0.001	<0.001	0.020
p Value, AH vs placebo	<0.001	<0.001	0.016
p Value, other	<0.001, ML + AH vs placebo	<0.001, ML + AH vs placebo	<0.001, ML + AH vs placebo
Conclusion	ML, AH, and ML + AH had better symptom scores than placebo. No difference between ML vs AH vs ML + AH		
Follow-up time	2 wk		

STUDY DESIGN

Inclusion criteria	Nonsmoking adults, aged 15 to 85 y, symptomatic during the fall allergy season, documented history of seasonal allergic rhinitis of at least 2 y. Eligible patients exhibited a positive skin test (wheal diameter ≥3 mm greater than saline control) to 1 of the regional allergens active during the study season and a predefined level of daytime nasal symptoms that was at least mild to moderate in severity, as rated daily by patients. Patients with mild asthma were allowed to participate, provided they used only inhaled, short-acting beta-agonist bronchodilators to treat their asthma
Exclusion criteria	Perennial rhinitis with little or no seasonal flare-ups; rhinitis medicamentosa; nonallergic rhinitis; substantial, structural nasal obstruction; severe asthma that had required emergency room treatment within 1 mo or hospitalization within 3 mo before the trial; URI; acute or chronic pulmonary disorder; initiation of allergen immunotherapy within the previous 6 mo; pregnant or lactating women; hospitalized patients and patients who had recently undergone a major surgical procedure or who had another clinically significant disorder
Medication restrictions	Other AH; inhaled, oral, parenteral, nasal, and ophthalmic corticosteroids; cromolyn sodium; nedocromil; inhaled anticholinergics; oral or long-acting inhaled beta-agonists; theophylline, and other leukotriene modifiers; decongestants and anti-inflammatory drugs. No allergic rhinitis rescue medications were permitted during the study
Randomization effectiveness	There were no clinically meaningful differences among the treatment groups for any baseline characteristic, including baseline symptom scores, secondary diagnoses, and concomitant drug therapies
Age	15–82 y
Allergy regimen	1) ML 10 mg and LRT 10 mg, 2) LRT 10 mg, 3) ML 10 mg, or 4) placebo. All study medications were taken once daily at bedtime
Outcome measures	Primary endpoint was daytime nasal symptoms score (mean of 4 individual scores: nasal congestion, rhinorrhea, nasal pruritus, and sneezing). Each symptom was scored on a scale: 0, none (symptom not noticeable); 1, mild (symptom noticeable but not bothersome); 2, moderate (symptom noticeable and bothersome some of the time); and 3, severe (symptom bothersome most of the time and/or very bothersome some of the time). Secondary endpoints were: 1) night-time symptoms score, 2) daily composite symptoms score, 3) daytime eye symptoms score, 4) individual daytime nasal symptoms, 5) individual night-time symptoms, 6) global evaluation of allergic rhinitis, 7) RQLQ, 8) peripheral blood eosinophils
Masking	Double blind
Compliance	Study medication compliance rates in the 4 treatment groups, as measured by tablet counts, were similar (approximately 99%)
Criteria for withdrawal from study	Withdrawal of consent, protocol deviations, adverse events, lack of efficacy, lost to follow-up
Power	With 300 patients per group, the study had 80% power to detect a 0.12 difference in change from baseline in daytime nasal symptom score between the combination ML/LRT and ML groups
Morbidity/complications	Overall, 17% of patients in each of the active treatment groups and 20% of patients in the placebo group experienced 1 or more adverse events. The 3 most common adverse events were headache, dry mouth, and asthenia/fatigue. No serious adverse events were recorded in any group

ML = montelukast, LRT = loratadine, SD = standard deviation, SEM = standard error of the mean, QOL = quality of life, AH = antihistamines, RQLQ = Rhinoconjunctivitis Quality of Life Questionnaire, URI = upper respiratory infection, NA = not applicable, NS = not significant, NR = not reported.
* The first sample sizes shown are for those who completed the study and those (initially recruited).

THE EVIDENCE CONDENSED: Antihistamines versus montelukast versus antihistamine plus montelukast for allergic rhinitis

Reference	Pullertis, 2002	
Level (design)	1 (randomized controlled trial)	
Sample size*	Total n = 49 (49) ML 10 mg (16), ML 10 mg and LRT 10 mg (15), placebo (18)	
OUTCOMES		
Measures	Mean score ± SD/SEM	
Outcome	Daytime scores	Night-time scores
Score ranges	0 best to 4 worst	0 best to 4 worst
Placebo	Wk 1–2: 3.5 ± 0.4 Wk 3–5: 5.9 ± 0.6 Wk 6–8: 3.3 ± 0.3	Wk 1–2: 2.1 ± 0.4 Wk 3–5: 3.6 ± 0.5 Wk 6–8: 2.3 ± 0.3
ML	Wk 1–2: 2.6 ± 0.5 Wk 3–4: 4.4 ± 0.6 Wk 6–8: 2.2 ± 0.4†	Wk 1–2: 1.8 ± 0.4 Wk 3–5: 2.8 ± 0.5 Wk 6–8: 1.5 ± 0.3
AH	NA	NA
ML + AH	Wk 1–2: 2.1 ± 0.5† Wk 3–5: 4.0 ± 0.7† Wk 6–8: 1.5 ± 0.4†	Wk 1–2: 1.3 ± 0.4 Wk 3–5: 2.7 ± 0.6 Wk 6–8: 1.2 ± 0.3†
p Value, ML vs placebo	†p <0.05, ML vs placebo. Other scores NS	
p Value, AH vs placebo	NA	NA
p Value, other	†p <0.05, ML + AH vs placebo. Other scores NS	
Conclusion	ML better daytime scores than placebo at 6–8 wk. ML + AH better scores than placebo at 1–8 wk. Other scores no difference	
Follow-up time	up to 8 wk	
STUDY DESIGN		
Inclusion criteria	15–50 y old, known history of allergic rhinitis during the grass pollen season for at least the 2 previous years, allergy to grass pollen confirmed by means of a positive skin-prick test response to the mixture of grass pollen allergens, as well as to 3 locally common grass pollen extracts (*Phleum praténse*, *Lólium perénne*, and *Festúca praténsis*) separately	
Exclusion criteria	A positive skin-prick test response against tree pollens (which pollinate earlier in the year), perennial rhinitis, concurrent purulent nasal infection, use of steroids in any form during the course of the study, or the presence of any serious or unstable concurrent disease	
Medication restrictions	For rescue medication, patients were provided with cromoglycate eyedrops and a limited amount of additional LRT tablets, and patients were instructed to record any use of rescue medication in the daily record cards	
Randomization effectiveness	The patients in the different treatment groups resembled each other regarding age, sex distribution, and duration of allergic rhinitis. No statistically significant differences between treatment groups were observed during the run-in period	
Age	18–50 y	
Allergy regimen	1) Active ML, 10 mg/d + placebo nasal spray + placebo capsules for LRT, 2) active ML, 10 mg/d, + active LRT, 10 mg/d + placebo nasal spray, 3) placebo capsules and nasal spray. Patients were instructed to start treatment on the same predetermined date approximately 2–3 wk before the expected beginning of the grass pollen season. All treatment was administered once a day in the morning and lasted for a total of 50 d, covering the whole pollen season	
Outcome measures	Primary endpoint in the study was the patient's recorded nasal symptom score; for nasal blockage: 0, breathing through the nose freely and easily; 1, slight difficulty breathing through the nose; 2, moderate difficulty breathing through the nose; 3, severe difficulty breathing through the nose; and 4, breathing through the nose is very difficult or impossible; for sneezing, rhinorrhea, and nasal itching, scores of 0–4 indicated no, mild, moderate, severe, and very severe symptoms, respectively	
Masking	Double blind	
Compliance	Not specified	
Criteria for withdrawal from study	Not specified	
Power	Not specified	
Morbidity/complications	Not specified	

ML = montelukast, LRT = loratadine, SD = standard deviation, SEM = standard error of the mean, QOL = quality of life, AH = antihistamines, RQLQ = Rhinoconjunctivitis Quality of Life Questionnaire, URI = upper respiratory infection, NA = not applicable, NS = not significant, NR = not reported.
* The first sample sizes shown are for those who completed the study and those (initially recruited).

THE EVIDENCE CONDENSED: Antihistamines versus montelukast versus antihistamine plus montelukast for allergic rhinitis

Reference	Moinuddin, 2004			
Level (design)	1 (randomized controlled trial)			
Sample size*	Total n = 68 (72) Fexofenadine 60 mg + pseudoephedrine 120 mg twice daily (n = 34), LRT 10 mg + ML 10 mg once daily (n = 34)			
OUTCOMES				
Measures	Median total change from baseline			
Outcome	Sneezing	Runny nose	Stuffy nose	RQLQ
Placebo	NA	NA	NA	
ML	NA	NA	NA	
AH	−7.5	−7.0	−11.5	QOL overall scores were significantly improved after treatment in both groups and were similar between the 2 treatment groups at visit 2
ML + AH	−0.5	0.0	−15.5	
p Value, AH vs placebo	<0.05 at days 1–12			<0.05
p Value, ML + AH vs placebo	<0.05 at days 2–4, 8–12			<0.05
p Value, AH vs ML + AH	NS	NS	NS	NS
Conclusion	Nasal scores: AH better than placebo, ML + AH better than placebo; no difference with AH vs ML + AH			QOL: AH better than placebo, ML + AH better than placebo; no difference with AH vs ML + AH
Follow-up time	12 d			
STUDY DESIGN				
Inclusion criteria	Ragweed seasonal allergic rhinitis, 18–45 y of age, in excellent health, positive puncture skin test result to the ragweed antigen extract and a positive history of allergy symptoms on exposure to ragweed during at least the past 2 y			
Exclusion criteria	Health problems that required daily medications; pregnant or lactating women (urine test to rule out pregnancy was performed on all female participants); use of systemic glucocorticosteroids in the past 30 d, intranasal steroids in the past 2 wk, oral AH or decongestants in the past 7 d, or topical AH or decongestants in the past 24 h			
Medication restrictions	The only additional medications allowed during this investigation were acetaminophen, birth control pills, or medroxyprogesterone acetate			
Randomization effectiveness	The demographic characteristics of age, sex, and race, as well as skin test reactivity as gauged by wheal size, showed no significant differences between the 2 study groups. The QOL questionnaire data analysis showed the 2 treatment groups to be similar at baseline in all domains except for the eye symptom domain, for which the group taking fexofenadine–pseudoephedrine had a higher score (worse QOL) than the LRT–ML group			
Age	18–45 y			
Allergy regimen	2 wk of: 1) fexofenadine hydrochloride, 60 mg, + pseudoephedrine hydrochloride, 120 mg twice daily; or 2) combination of LRT 10 mg + ML 10 mg daily			
Outcome measures	1) Rhinoconjunctivitis QOL instrument; 2) symptom diary card on which patients recorded their symptoms twice a day before taking their medication. Symptoms of sneezing, rhinorrhea, nasal congestion, and itchy eyes were recorded: 0 indicates no symptoms; 1, mild symptoms; 2, moderate symptoms; and 3, severe symptoms;. 3) nasal peak inspiratory flow, measured by flow meter			
Masking	Double blind			
Compliance	Noncompliant patients were excluded			
Criteria for withdrawal from study	2 patients from each treatment group dropped out because of noncompliance with the study protocol			
Power	Not specified			
Morbidity/complications	Not specified			

SAR = seasonal allergic rhinitis, ML = montelukast, LRT = loratadine, QOL = quality of life, AH = antihistamines, RQLQ = Rhinoconjunctivitis Quality of Life Questionnaire, NA = not applicable, NS = not significant.
* The first sample sizes shown are for those who completed the study and those (initially recruited).

THE EVIDENCE CONDENSED: Antihistamines versus montelukast versus antihistamine plus montelukast for allergic rhinitis

Reference	Wilson, 2002		
Level (design)	1 (randomized crossover trial)		
Sample size*	Total n = 37 (46)		
OUTCOMES			
Outcome	Nasal peak flow	Total nasal symptom score	Daily activity
Score ranges	L/min	0 best to 24 worst	0 best to 3 worst
Placebo	102 (98–107)	7.4 (6.7–8.0)	1.3 (1.1–1.5)
ML	NA	NA	NA
AH	111 (107–116)	5.0 (4.3–5.7)	0.7 (0.5–0.9)
ML + AH	113 (109–118)	4.0 (3.3–4.7)	0.5 (0.3–0.8)
p Value, AH vs placebo	<0.05	<0.05	<0.05
p Value, ML + AH vs placebo	<0.05	<0.05	<0.05
p Value, AH vs ML + AH	NS	NS	NS
Conclusion	Nasal peak flow and symptom scores: AH better than placebo, ML + AH better than placebo; no difference with AH vs ML + AH		
Follow-up time	2 wk		
STUDY DESIGN			
Inclusion criteria	Symptomatic SAR, positive skin-prick test to grass pollens, present and past history of SAR requiring treatment		
Exclusion criteria	History of persistent asthma, requirement for inhaled corticosteroids, FEV_1 <90% predicted, history of nasal polyps or aspirin sensitivity, occlusive septal deviation (>50%), requirement for oral prednisolone or antibiotics within the preceding 6 mo		
Medication restrictions	Permitted to use rescue treatment with ocular cromoglycate for eye symptoms up to 4 times per day. Intranasal steroids, nasal decongestants, other AH were stopped before the study		
Randomization effectiveness	No differences were shown before each active treatment		
Age	Mean age 37 y (standard error 2 y)		
Allergy regimen	1) Fexofenadine 120 mg daily, or 2) LRT 10 mg daily + ML 10 mg daily		
Outcome measures	1) Nasal inspiratory flow (main endpoint); 2) nasal symptoms "runny nose," "blocked nose," "itchy nose," and "sneezing:" 0 no symptoms to 3 severe symptoms; 3) eye symptoms; 4) rating of interference of symptoms with daily activity: 0 none to 3 maximal		
Masking	Single blind		
Compliance	>90% compliance with study medications required for completion of study		
Criteria for withdrawal from study	Patients with <90% compliance were excluded; patients chose withdrawal due to social or other commitments, exacerbations of SAR		
Power	Not specified		
Morbidity/complications	1 dry throat, 3 sleepiness, 2 headaches, 1 diarrhea, 1 increased thirst		

SAR = seasonal allergic rhinitis, ML = montelukast, LRT = loratadine, QOL = quality of life, AH = antihistamines, RQLQ = Rhinoconjunctivitis Quality of Life Questionnaire, NA = not applicable, NS = not significant.
* The first sample sizes shown are for those who completed the study and those (initially recruited).

REFERENCES

1. Moinuddin R, et al. Comparison of the combinations of fexofenadine-pseudoephedrine and loratadine-montelukast in the treatment of seasonal allergic rhinitis. Ann Allergy Asthma Immunol 2004;92(1):73–79.

2. Nayak AS, et al. Efficacy and tolerability of montelukast alone or in combination with loratadine in seasonal allergic rhinitis: a multicenter, randomized, double-blind, placebo-controlled trial performed in the fall. Ann Allergy Asthma Immunol 2002;88(6):592–600.

3. van Adelsberg J, et al. Randomized controlled trial evaluating the clinical benefit of montelukast for treating spring seasonal allergic rhinitis. Ann Allergy Asthma Immunol 2003;90(2):214–222.

4. Wilson AM, et al. A comparison of once daily fexofenadine versus the combination of montelukast plus loratadine on domiciliary nasal peak flow and symptoms in seasonal allergic rhinitis. Clin Exp Allergy 2002;32(1):126–132.

5. Pullerits T, et al. Comparison of a nasal glucocorticoid, antileukotriene, and a combination of antileukotriene and antihistamine in the treatment of seasonal allergic rhinitis. J Allergy Clin Immunol 2002;109(6):949–955.

6. Juniper EF, et al. Validation of the standardized version of the Rhinoconjunctivitis Quality of Life Questionnaire. J Allergy Clin Immunol 1999;104(2 Pt 1):364–369.

7. Juniper EF, Guyatt GH, Griffith LE, Ferrie PJ. Interpretation of rhinoconjunctivitis quality of life questionnaire data. J Allergy Clin Immunol 1996;98(4):843–845.

8. Meltzer EO, Malmstrom K, Lu S, et al. Concomitant montelukast and loratadine as treatment for seasonal allergic rhinitis: a randomized, placebo-controlled clinical trial. J Allergy Clin Immunol 2000;105(5):917–922.

9. Philip G, Malmstrom K, Hampel FC, Weinstein SF, LaForce CF, Ratner PH, Malice MP, Reiss TF. Montelukast for treating seasonal allergic rhinitis: a randomized, double-blind, placebo-controlled trial performed in the spring. Clin Exp Allergy 2002;32(7):1020–1028.

10. Kurowski M, Kuna P, Gorski P. Montelukast plus cetirizine in the prophylactic treatment of seasonal allergic rhinitis: influence on clinical symptoms and nasal allergic inflammation. Allergy 2004;59(3):280–288.

11. Ressel GW. NAEPP updates guidelines for the diagnosis and management of asthma. Am Fam Physician 2003;68(1):169–170.

22 Chronic Rhinosinusitis in Adults

22.A.

Comparative oral antibiotic regimens: Impact on rates of cure, failure, relapse

Stacey Gray, Jennifer J. Shin, and Ralph Metson

METHODS

A computerized PubMed search of MEDLINE 1966–April 2006 was performed. Articles mapping to the medical subject heading "sinusitis" and textwords "chronic" or "recurrent" were obtained, yielding 2503 studies. These articles were then cross-referenced with those publications mapping to the medical subject headings "anti-bacterial agents" or "quinolones" or "penicillins" or "macrolides" or "cephalosporins" or "clindamycin" or the textwords "antibiotics" or "antimicrobials." This search strategy yielded 447 articles. These publications were then reviewed to identify those that met the following inclusion criteria: 1) adult patient population (>15 years old) with chronic or recurrent rhinosinusitis, 2) intervention with comparative oral antibiotic regimens, 3) outcome measured in terms of clinical improvement, 4) randomized controlled trials (RCTs). Articles focusing only on patients with acute rhinosinusitis were excluded. Also excluded were articles in which data from patients with chronic rhinosinusitis or acute exacerbations thereof were pooled with data from patients with acute rhinosinusitis alone, such that the data from the chronic population could not be separately analyzed. Articles that included pediatric populations were excluded from this review, but are addressed in Chapter 8. The bibliographies of the articles that met these inclusion criteria were manually checked to ensure no further relevant articles could be identified. This process yielded the three articles that are presented herein [1–3].

RESULTS

Outcome Measures. The primary outcome measure in the Legent study [1] was the disappearance of nasal discharge. In addition, the authors analyzed postnasal drip, intermittent nasal obstruction with or without pain, and/or tenderness in the sinus area. They categorized their patients according to their reported symptoms: 1) cured (nasal discharge had disappeared, together with preexisting pain symptoms) at 10 and 40 days, 2) improved (persistent mucous discharge), or 3) failures (purulent discharge or pain symptoms continued). Huck [3] categorized patients with more emphasis on the overall clinical examination; patients were reported as having had: 1) improvement (signs and symptoms improved during therapy), 2) relapse (signs and symptoms recurred by 2–4 days after treatment ended), or 3) failure (obvious therapeutic failure by clinical examination at any time during therapy). Namyslowski [2] described results similarly, classifying patients as cured (complete resolution of signs and symptoms of infection) or failures (incomplete resolution of signs and symptoms of infection, requiring alternative therapy).

Potential Confounders. One of the key potential confounders in all studies on this topic is which patients are included in a population labeled as having "recurrent or chronic rhinosinusitis." All three RCTs included patients who were required to have sinonasal symptoms but the specific symptoms varied (see adjoining table). All three studies used either endoscopy or radiology as adjunctive diagnostic measures. Legent used either a computed tomography scan from the previous 6 months or nasal endoscopy, whereas the Huck and Namyslowski studies used roentgenograms. Two studies defined chronic rhinosinusitis as disease of more than 3 months' duration, whereas the third study simply defined it as nonresolving disease. Other potential confounders include whether patients had prior sinus surgeries, the number of previous antibiotic courses failed, the duration of symptoms before initiation of treatment. These confounders were not addressed by all studies specifically, although randomization should theoretically balance these factors between the two groups at the outset.

Study Designs. There were three RCTs (level 1 data) that questioned whether one oral antibiotic regimen can provide better symptom improvement and cure rates than another. The Legent study compared 9-day courses of amoxicillin/clavulanic acid (AMX/CA) versus ciprofloxacin in patients with chronic rhinosinusitis. Randomization was shown to be effective in balancing demographic and prior sinus-related treatments in the study groups at the outset. This study was double blind, and thus minimized expectation bias. An intention to treat analysis was not specified, but their attrition rates were low. Although no significant differences were found in their primary endpoints, an *a priori* power calculation was not reported. A reassurance of strong power could help minimize concern that a study might find that there is no difference when in reality a difference exists. Follow-up time was 5–6 weeks.

The Namyslowski RCT compared 14-day courses of AMX/CA versus cefuroxime in patients with chronic rhinosinusitis. Randomization was reported to result in a similar age, severity of infection, and most clinical signs and symptoms in both groups before treatment. This study was not blinded, so expectation bias may have had some role in the final outcomes; if clinicians or patients were more inclined to believe they would improve on AMX/CA, for example, then results could be biased toward a better outcome with AMX/CA. An intention to treat analysis was performed, so other potential biases were removed. Power calculations were also not described in this study. Follow-up time was up to 4 weeks.

The Huck study compared 10-day courses of AMX (no CA) versus cefaclor in patients with chronic or recurrent rhinosinusitis. Randomization balanced demographic factors in both groups. This study benefited from being double blind. There was, however, no power description and this study had the relevant smallest sample size. Follow-up time was up to 3 weeks.

Highest Level of Evidence. Three RCTs compared rates of cure, failure, and relapse of one antibiotic regimen in comparison to another. Overall, three sets of conclusions were drawn: 1) There seemed to be no significant difference when AMX/CA and ciprofloxacin were compared, although there was a trend toward better results with ciprofloxacin. 2) When AMX/CA and cefuroxime were compared, there was significantly less relapse with AMX/CA, and a nearly significant trend toward more cure with AMX/CA. There was no significant difference in failure rates. 3) When AMX and cefaclor were compared, overall no significant differences were reported, although sample sizes were small. Small sample sizes may limit a study's ability to demonstrate a difference that truly exists. Specific results and trends are described in the adjoining table.

Applicability. These results are applicable to adult patients with chronic or recurrent rhinosinusitis.

Morbidity/Complications. Adverse effects were minimal and infrequent, and occurred in all treatment groups in all studies. Further details are shown in the adjoining table.

CLINICAL SIGNIFICANCE AND FUTURE RESEARCH

There were three RCTs that compared the clinical impact of different antibiotic regimens on chronic and recurrent rhinosinusitis. First, cure rates were nearly significantly better with AMX/CA, as compared with cefuroxime. There was no significant difference between cures with AMX/CA versus ciprofloxacin, or with AMX versus cefaclor. Second, failure rates were examined, and no significant differences were found in any of the comparisons. Third, relapse rates were considered. AMX/CA was shown to be superior to cefuroxime in preventing relapse, but no different from ciprofloxacin. There was no difference between AMX and cefaclor.

Interpretation of the results must be tempered by the lack of blinding in the one study that did demonstrate a significant difference, as well as the unreported power of studies with multiple negative results. When considering potential benefits of these antibiotics, the risks must also be considered; adverse reactions were infrequent, and occurred similarly in all antibiotics considered.

Future research may focus on longer durations of antibiotic treatment, as courses longer than 9–14 days are frequently used for chronic rhinosinusitis. In addition, longer follow-up times with outcomes measured in terms of a validated instrument or avoidance of surgery may prove more useful.

THE EVIDENCE CONDENSED: Comparative antibiotic regimens for chronic and recurrent rhinosinusitis

Reference	Legent, 1994		
Level (design)	1 (randomized controlled trial)		
Sample size*	241 (251)		
OUTCOMES			
	Amoxicillin/clavulanate	**Ciprofloxacin**	**p Value**
Cure	50.4%†	57.6%†	NS
Failure	17.1% (n = 21/123)	12.7% (n = 15/118)	NS
Relapse	31.6%§ (n = 39/95)	22.1%§ (n = 21/95)	NR
Conclusion	Trend toward more cure, less failure and relapse with ciprofloxacin, but no significant difference		
Follow-up time	†10 d, §40 d		
STUDY DESIGN			
Inclusion criteria	≥18 y old, unilateral or bilateral chronic sinusitis of more than 3 mo duration (with the exception of nasal polyposis		
Exclusion criteria	Patients with nasal polyposis or fungal sinus infections Patients who had received penicillin or fluoroquinolone within a month of presentation, or other infections requiring antibiotics Patients with hepatic or renal insufficiency, pregnant or lactating patients		
Randomization effectiveness	The 2 groups were equivalent for all characteristics except age; the mean age was higher in the AMX/CA group		
Age	Ciprofloxacin group = 41.7 y AMX/CA group = 47.3 y		
Masking	Double blind		
Intervention regimens	Ciprofloxacin 500 mg b.i.d. or AMX/CA 500 mg t.i.d. for 9 d		
Diagnostic criteria for rhinosinusitis	Chronic sinusitis was defined as symptoms of 3 mo duration Sinusitis was diagnosed by the presence of purulent or mucopurulent nasal discharge or postnasal drip, and intermittent nasal obstruction with or without pain/tenderness in sinus area Sinus endoscopy was performed if computed tomography scan reports were not available from within the preceding 6 mo		
Definition of outcomes	Cured—nasal discharge had disappeared, together with preexisting pain symptoms Improved—persistent mucous discharge Failure—purulent discharge or pain symptoms continued		
Criteria for withdrawal	Completion of <7 d of treatment, absence of initial rhinorrhea, withdrawal of consent		
Intention to treat analysis	Not specified		
Power	NR		
Morbidity/complications	AMX/CA: n = 31/124; most frequently reported were GI related (diarrhea, loose stools, abdominal pain, nausea/vomiting). Ciprofloxacin: n = 15/121; most frequently reported were GI related. One case of allergy to ciprofloxacin occurred (with facial edema) and required short-term steroid treatment		

NS = not significant, NR = not reported, AMX/CA = amoxicillin/clavulanic acid, b.i.d. = twice a day, t.i.d. = three times a day, GI = gastrointestinal.
* Sample size: numbers shown for those not lost to follow-up and those (initially recruited).

Reference	Namyslowski, 2002		
Level (design)	1 (randomized controlled trial)		
Sample size*	(206) 231		

	OUTCOMES		
	Amoxicillin/clavulanate	Cefuroxime	p Value
Cure	95%‡ (n = 99/104)	88%‡ (n = 90/102)	0.07
Failure	3%‡ (n = 3/104)	8%‡ (n = 8/102)	NR
Relapse	0%‖ (n = 0/98)	8%‖ (n = 7/89)	0.0049
Conclusion	Significantly less relapse with AMX/CA. Trend toward higher cure and less failure with AMX/CA, but no significant difference		
Follow-up time	‡15–18 d, ‖2–4 wk		

	STUDY DESIGN		
Inclusion criteria	Hospitalized and nonhospitalized patients, ≥18 y old, presenting with either chronic sinusitis or acute exacerbation of chronic sinusitis, requirement to submit to antral sinus puncture <48 h before treatment, evidence for presence of infection for which AMX/CA or cefuroxime was appropriate		
Exclusion criteria	History of hypersensitivity reaction to beta-lactam antibiotics or receiving antibiotic therapy within 2 wk before inclusion, presence of serious underlying disease or concomitant infection that would preclude evaluation of patient response to study medication, confirmed or suspected allergic rhinitis, intraorbital or intracranial complications that would interfere with interpretation of X-ray investigation of sinuses; scheduled surgery for treatment of sinuses, renal impairment, hepatic impairment, planned or existing pregnancy or lactation		
Randomization effectiveness	Similar age, severity of infection, and most clinical signs and symptoms in both groups. Slightly more females, fever, number of patients with more than 3 episodes in 1 y in the AMX/CA group		
Age	Mean age at enrollment: 37 y (AMX/CA), 41 y (cefuroxime)		
Masking	None (open label)		
Intervention regimens	AMX 875 mg/CA 125 mg PO b.i.d. ×14 d or cefuroxime acetil 500 mg PO b.i.d.		
Diagnostic criteria for rhinosinusitis	Chronic sinusitis: at least 1 symptom (postnasal discharge, rhinorrhea, or cough) together with appropriate constitutional symptoms (headache, facial pain, tooth pain, halitosis, sore throat, earache, increased wheeze, or fever) plus abnormal X-ray assessment (opacification, abnormal air-fluid levels, >5 mm mucosal swelling) lasting for >3 mo		
Definition of outcomes	Cure: complete resolution of signs and symptoms of infection Failure: incomplete resolution of signs and symptoms of infection, requiring alternative therapy		
Criteria for withdrawal	Violation of assessment visit schedule, adverse events, insufficient therapeutic effect, lost to follow-up		
Intention to treat analysis	Yes		
Power	NR		
Morbidity/complications	4 diarrhea, 1 urticaria, 1 eye disorder, 1 cardiovascular disorder		

NS = not significant, NR = not reported, AMX/CA = amoxicillin/clavulanic acid, b.i.d. = twice a day.
* Sample size: numbers shown for those not lost to follow-up and those (initially recruited).

Reference	Huck, 1993		
Level (design)	1 (randomized controlled trial)		
Sample size*	40 (NR)		
OUTCOMES			
	Amoxicillin	**Cefaclor**	**p Value**
Cure	NR	NR	NR
Improvement	RS: 56% (n = 5/9) CS: 40% (n = 4/10)	RS: 56% (n = 9/16) CS: 20% (n = 1/5)	RS: NR CS: NR
Failure	RS: 44% (n = 4/9) CS: 60% (n = 6/10)	RS: 31% (n = 5/16) CS: 80% (n = 4/5)	RS: NR CS: NR
Relapse	RS: 0% CS: 0%	RS: 13% (n = 2/16) CS: 0%	RS: NR CS: NR
Conclusion	Trend toward less failure but more relapse of recurrent sinusitis with cefaclor. Trend toward more improvement, less failure for chronic sinusitis with amoxicillin. Overall, no significant differences reported		
Follow-up time	10–12 d, 16–18 d		
STUDY DESIGN			
Inclusion criteria	>15 years old, symptoms of acute (results of patients with acute sinusitis were excluded in this review), recurrent, and chronic maxillary sinusitis (facial pain and/or purulent discharge), sinus roentgenogram (Waters view) consistent with maxillary sinusitis (air fluid levels, opacity, mucosal thickening at the lateral angle of the sinus)		
Exclusion criteria	Hepatic or renal disease, condition that would preclude evaluation of response to therapy, necessity for other systemic antibiotics between pretherapy and posttherapy evaluation, pregnancy		
Randomization effectiveness	Similar age and gender in both groups, although there were more males in the amoxicillin group		
Age	16–73 y		
Masking	Double blind		
Intervention regimens	Cefaclor 500 mg PO b.i.d. ×10 d, amoxicillin 500 mg PO t.i.d. ×10 d		
Diagnostic criteria for rhinosinusitis	Recurrent sinusitis: sinusitis (facial pain and/or purulent discharge) accompanied by >1 episode per year of acute sinusitis with clinical improvement between episodes Chronic sinusitis: nonresolving sinus disease		
Definition of outcomes	Improvement: end of therapy clinical examination revealing the patient's signs and symptoms had improved during therapy Relapse: signs and symptoms recurred by 2–4 d after treatment ended Failure: obvious therapeutic failure by clinical examination at any time during therapy		
Criteria for withdrawal	No pretreatment or negative pretreatment roentgenogram, no pretherapy culture, assessment of "unable to evaluate" for symptomatic response		
Intention to treat analysis	NR		
Power	NR		
Morbidity/complications	Cefaclor: n = 2/54 adverse events (vaginitis) Amoxicillin: n = 5/54 (vaginitis, epistaxis, diarrhea, edema, herpes simplex)		

NR = not reported, RS = recurrent rhinosinusitis, CS = chronic rhinosinusitis, b.i.d. = twice a day, t.i.d. = three times a day.
* Sample size: numbers shown for those not lost to follow-up and those (initially recruited).

REFERENCES

1. Legent F, Bordure P, Beauvillain C, Berche P. A double-blind comparison of ciprofloxacin and amoxycillin/clavulanic acid in the treatment of chronic sinusitis. Chemotherapy 1994;40(Suppl 1):8–15.
2. Namyslowski G, Misiolek M, Czecior E, et al. Comparison of the efficacy and tolerability of amoxycillin/clavulanic acid 875 mg b.i.d. with cefuroxime 500 mg b.i.d. in the treatment of chronic and acute exacerbation of chronic sinusitis in adults. J Chemother 2002;14(5):508–517.
3. Huck W, Reed BD, Nielsen RW, et al. Cefaclor vs amoxicillin in the treatment of acute, recurrent, and chronic sinusitis. Arch Fam Med 1993;2(5):497–503.

22 Chronic Rhinosinusitis in Adults

22.B.

Oral antibiotic therapy for one month or longer: Impact on sinonasal symptoms, quality of life

Stacey Gray, Jennifer J. Shin, and Ralph Metson

METHODS

A computerized PubMed search of MEDLINE 1966–April 2006 was performed. Articles mapping to the medical subject heading "sinusitis" and textwords "chronic" or "recurrent" were obtained, yielding 2503 studies. These articles were then cross-referenced with those publications mapping to the medical subject headings "anti-bacterial agents" or "quinolones" or "penicillins" or "macrolides" or "cephalosporins" or "clindamycin" or the textwords "antibiotics" or "antimicrobials." This search strategy yielded 447 articles. These publications were then reviewed to identify those that met the following inclusion criteria: 1) adult patient population (>15 years old) with chronic rhinosinusitis, 2) intervention with an oral antibiotic regimen of at least 1 month duration, 3) outcome measured in terms of clinical improvement, 4) comparative data, either as antibiotic versus placebo or pretreatment versus posttreatment. Articles in which the specific numerical results were not reported were excluded. Articles focusing only on patients with acute rhinosinusitis or only on microbiological culture data were excluded. Articles that included pediatric populations or patients treated with intravenous antibiotics were excluded from this review, but are addressed in Chapter 8. Isolated case reports were excluded. The bibliographies of the articles that met these inclusion criteria were manually checked to ensure no further relevant articles could be identified. This process yielded the four articles that are presented herein [1–4].

RESULTS

Outcome Measures. All four papers used numerical scales through which patients rated their sinonasal symptoms. For example, Cervin et al. [2] asked patients to rate symptoms on a visual analog scale of 0 (best) to 100 (worst). Wallwork et al. [1] used symptom scales and the Sinonasal Outcome Test 20 (SNOT-20), which is a validated, rhinosinusitis-specific instrument in which patients are asked to answer 20 questions regarding their nasal symptoms and quality of life. Subramanian et al. [3] reported radiographic outcomes, in addition to symptom scores. They described radiographic disease, using the Lund-Mackay system, in which each sinus is graded as: 0 normal, 1 mild mucosal thickening or opacification, or 2 extensive mucosal thickening or opacifica-

tion; total scores range from 0 (best) to 24 (worst). Hashiba et al. [4] used both symptom scores and clinical examination. They rated observed changes as "excellent," "good," "fair," "no change," or "worse," based on numerical ratings (see adjoining table for further details).

Potential Confounders. Potential confounders include the antibiotic regimen used, the duration of treatment, and the severity of disease before treatment. Other potential confounders include whether patients had prior sinus surgeries, the types of antibiotics to which patients had previously been exposed, the number of previous antibiotic courses failed, and the duration of symptoms before initiation of treatment. These potential confounders are detailed as much as the original publications allow in the adjoining tables.

Another key potential confounder in all studies on this topic is which patients are included in a population that has "chronic rhinosinusitis." Two of the four papers specified that they used diagnostic features based on consensus statements (Rhinosinusitis Task Force, American Academy of Otolaryngology–Head and Neck Surgery). Understanding the specifics of these consensus statements can help readers understand which patients may derive similar results from the interventions described.

Study Designs. There was one randomized controlled trial (RCT), two prospective studies, and one retrospective study that addressed symptom control with at least 1 month of oral antibiotic therapy. The RCT compared symptom scores and SNOT-20 scores in patients receiving 3-month courses of roxithromycin versus placebo. Patients were included if they met the diagnostic criteria defined by the most recent Rhinosinusitis Task Force. The diagnosis was further confirmed with computed tomography (CT), using the Lund-Mackay scoring system. The study was double blinded, minimizing expectation bias. Also, they exceeded the sample size required to achieve power of 80% at the 1% level of significance in their reported *a priori* power analysis.

The remaining three studies compared pretreatment results with posttreatment results. These studies (two prospective, one retrospective) showed improved symptoms after treatment with prolonged antibiotic courses. The regimens studied prospectively were: 1) erythromycin succinate 250 mg PO b.i.d. or clarithromycin 250 mg PO daily for 3–12 months, and 2) clarithromycin 200 mg

PO b.i.d. ×8–12 weeks. The retrospective report analyzed results after multiagent therapy that included antibiotics for 4–8 weeks, oral steroids for 10 days, nasal saline irrigation, and intranasal steroids. The three lower-level studies did not note whether they reported consecutive patients, or whether outcomes were measured by blinded observers. No placebo controls were used in the prospective studies. The Subramanian study has the limitations of the retrospective study design.

Highest Level of Evidence. The highest level of evidence was provided by the RCT, which showed that treatment of chronic rhinosinusitis with 3 months of roxithromycin resulted in better symptom scores and quality of life scores than treatment with 3 months of placebo. This effect was shown to be statistically significant at 3 months (i.e., at the completion of treatment). By 6 months, however, the effect was lessened; although there was still a trend toward a better quality of life with roxithromycin, results were no longer statistically significant.

Two prospective studies evaluated two other macrolides: clarithromycin and erythromycin. The results of these studies showed that sinonasal symptom scores were improved after 2–3 months of treatment. Cervin et al., who focused on the population that had already undergone sinus surgery, showed statistically significant improvements, whereas Hashiba et al. reported no statistical comparisons. Cervin et al. showed that sinonasal symptoms were significantly improved even after 1 year. General well-being, however, was improved, but not significantly so. All of these results may have been influenced by expectation bias, given that no placebo control was used. Overall, these results mimic those of the RCT, except that they continued to show significantly better results at longer follow-up times.

The fourth study was retrospective, and showed better symptom and CT scores in a case series treated with 4–8 weeks of antibiotics in combination with other treatments. Specific antibiotic regimens were not described and it may be difficult to determine whether results were attributable to the antibiotics or to the other medicines administered.

Applicability. These results are applicable to adult patients with chronic rhinosinusitis, based on the diagnostic criteria specified in the reports (see adjoining table). The results of the Cervin study are more specifically relevant to patients who have chronic rhinosinusitis even after previous sinus surgery.

Morbidity/Complications. Only one study reported the details of adverse effects and these were limited to nausea/vomiting with roxithromycin.

CLINICAL SIGNIFICANCE AND FUTURE RESEARCH

There were four studies that investigated the symptom impact of oral antibiotics administered for 1 month or longer in patients with chronic rhinosinusitis. The highest level of evidence was provided by one RCT, which showed significantly better symptoms and quality of life after 3 months of roxithromycin (versus placebo). There was still better quality of life at 6 months, but differences were no longer statistically significant in this study. Level 2 and 4 data echoed these results, also suggesting improvement in symptoms with prolonged antibiotic courses.

Future research may focus on long-term treatments with comparative antibiotics or on comparing other antibiotics (i.e., nonmacrolides) with placebo. Ideally, prospective RCTs will be performed with long follow-up times, given the chronic nature of this disease. Future research may also continue to utilize standardized definitions of chronic rhinosinusitis, as well as validated outcome instruments to measure symptoms and disease-specific quality of life.

Chronic Rhinosinusitis Task Force: Clinical criteria to diagnose chronic rhinosinusitis

- Continuous symptoms for more than 12 consecutive weeks or more than 12 weeks of physical findings.
- One sign of inflammation (i.e., discolored nasal drainage, edema or erythema of the middle meatus or ethmoid bulla, generalized or localized erythema, edema, or granulation tissue, or confirmation from a computed tomography scan or plain sinus radiograph) must be present and identified in association with ongoing symptoms of chronic rhinosinusitis.

This definition has been endorsed by the American Academy of Otolaryngology–Head and Neck Surgery, the American Academy of Otolaryngic Allergy, the American Rhinologic Society, and the Sinus and Allergy Health Partnership.

Reference	Wallwork, 2006			Cervin, 2002		
Level (design)	1 (randomized controlled trial)			2 (prospective with pretreatment control)		
Sample size*	64 (64)			n = 12/17 completed 12 mo n = 5/17 completed 3 mo		
OUTCOMES						
	Roxithromycin	Placebo	p Value	Symptom scale 0 best to 100 worst		
	Patient scale: 3.11 ± 0.17†	Patient scale: 3.84 ± 12*	p < 0.01	Nasal congestion	48, 8, 18	p < 0.01 post- vs pretreatment
	SNOT-20 score: 2.34 ± 0.19† 2.49 ± 0.18‡	SNOT-20 score: 2.88 ± 0.12† 2.84 ± 0.15‡	p < 0.05 p = NS	General well- being	24, 18, 5	p = NS post- vs pretreatment
Conclusion	Roxithromycin with significantly better patient symptoms at 12 wk. No difference in SNOT-20 scores at 24 wk			Significantly better nasal congestion at 3 and 12 mo. Significantly better headache, rhinorrhea at 12 mo. No change in general well-being, sense of smell, cough		
Follow-up time	†12 wk, ‡24 wk			Pretreatment, 3 mo, 12 mo		
STUDY DESIGN						
Inclusion criteria	>18 y old, history consistent with diagnosis of chronic rhinosinusitis as outlined by the Rhinosinusitis Task Force. CT confirmation of diagnosis with Lund-Mackay scoring system			Persistent symptoms of chronic sinusitis after 1 or several functional endoscopic sinus surgeries, previously treated with systemic steroids and long-term antibiotics other than macrolides		
Exclusion criteria	History of cystic fibrosis, primary ciliary dyskinesia, immune deficiency, allergic fungal sinusitis, nasal polyposis, impairment of liver or renal function, pregnant, breast-feeding, taking medication with known adverse interaction with macrolides, history of macrolide sensitivity, use of topical or systemic corticosteroids within 4 wk of entry into the study			Immunodeficiency		
Randomization effectiveness	No significant differences between groups in terms of age, sex, immunoglobulin E, CT scores, baseline values of SNOT-20 scores, peak nasal inspiratory flow, saccharine transit time, nasal endoscopy, olfactory function scores, and lavage data			NA		
Age	>18 y			18–67 y		
Masking	Double blinded			NA		
Intervention regimens	Roxithromycin 150 mg PO daily for 3 mo, or placebo PO daily for 3 mo			Erythromycin succinate 250 mg PO b.i.d. or clarithromycin 250 mg PO daily for 3 mo. If patients responded, treatment was continued and reassessed after 12 mo of treatment. If no response, then treatment was discontinued		
Diagnostic criteria for rhinosinusitis	As outlined by the Rhinosinusitis Task Force			Chronic sinusitis as defined by the American Academy of Otolaryngology–Head and Neck Surgery		
Definition of outcomes	Patient response scale (primary outcome): linear rating scale—1 completely improved, 2 much improved, 3 slightly improved, 4 not improved, 5 slightly worse, 6 much worse			Median visual analog scale at 3 and 12 mo: 0 no discomfort, 100 worst possible discomfort		
Criteria for withdrawal	Adverse effects (2 placebo, 1 roxithromycin), lost to follow-up (1 from each group)			Yes		
Intention to treat analysis	Not specified			Not reported		
Power	A priori power analysis predicted sample sizes of 25 in each group would be required to achieve power of 80% at the 1% level of significance			Not specified		
Morbidity/ complications	Placebo n = 2 (rash, abdominal pain), roxithromycin n = 1 (nausea/vomiting)			Not specified		

NS = not significant, CT = computed tomography, SNOT-20 = Sinonasal Outcome Test 20, NA = not applicable, b.i.d. = twice a day.
* Sample size: numbers shown for those not lost to follow-up and those (initially recruited).

THE EVIDENCE CONDENSED: Prolonged oral antibiotic regimens for chronic and recurrent rhinosinusitis

Reference	Subramanian, 2002				Hashiba, 1996
Level (design)	4 (retrospective case series)				2 (prospective with pretreatment control)
Sample size*	40 (NA)				34 (42)

OUTCOMES

		Pretreatment	Posttreatment	p Value	Symptom scores
	Symptom score	7.8 ± 1.9	3.8 ± 2.3	0.0005	47.7% "good"(n = 21/44) at 4 wk 62.8% "good"(n = 37/43) at 8 wk 70.6% "good" (n = 24/34) at 12 wk
	CT score	10.9 ± 48	5.4 ± 3.7	0.0005	At end of treatment: n = 14 excellent, n = 18 good, n = 11 fair, n = 2 no change
	Relapse	n = 14 patients relapsed symptoms necessitating re-treatment within 8 wk of their initial treatment			Statistical comparisons not reported
Conclusion	Symptoms and CT findings improved significantly after treatment				The majority of patients had better symptom scores after treatment
Follow-up time	6–8 wk				Up to 12 wk

STUDY DESIGN

Inclusion criteria	Newly referred or established patients who were undergoing intensive therapy for chronic sinusitis for the first time		Chronic sinusitis patients, principally comprising intractable cases refractory to surgical and other types of therapy, duration ≥2 y, clearly known therapeutic history during the 3 mo before clarithromycin therapy
Exclusion criteria	Not specified		Not specified
Age	17–78 y		18–78 y
Intervention regimens	Antibiotics for 4–8 wk, "chosen for broad-spectrum coverage" Prednisone 20 mg PO b.i.d. ×5 d, then 20 mg PO daily ×5 d Adjunctive therapy: nasal saline irrigation, intranasal steroids Leukotriene blockers used in 14 patients		Clarithromycin 200 mg PO b.i.d. ×8–12 wk Continuation of already existing nebulizer therapy was permitted
Diagnostic criteria for rhinosinusitis	Not specified, but symptom scores were based on Rhinosinusitis Task Force definitions		Not specified
Definition of outcomes	First relapse: time interval starting at the end of antibiotics treatment at which recurrence of symptoms necessitated reinstitution of antibiotics and/or steroids Radiographic response graded according to Lund-Mackay system 0 best to 24 worst: each sinus graded 0 normal, 1 mild mucosal thickening or opacification, 2 extensive Symptom score: 0 none, 1 mild, 2 moderate, 3 severe		Subjective symptom scale (rhinorrhea, postnasal drip, nasal obstruction): 0 no symptoms to 3 severe or highly pronounced Observed changes: excellent = 4 points (3→0 or 2→0), good = 3 points (3→1 or 1→0), fair = 2 points (3→2, 2→1), no change = 1 point, worse
Criteria for withdrawal	NA		Not reported
Consecutive patients	Not reported		Not reported
Power	Not reported		Not reported
Morbidity/ complications	Not reported		No side effects were observed

NS = not significant, CT = computed tomography, SNOT-20 = Sinonasal Outcome Test 20, NA = not applicable, b.i.d. = twice a day, RS = recurrent rhinosinusitis, CS = chronic rhinosinusitis, CT = computed tomography.
* Sample size: numbers shown for those not lost to follow-up and those (initially recruited).

REFERENCES

1. Wallwork B, Coman W, Mackay-Sim A, Greiff L, Cervin A. A double-blind, randomized, placebo-controlled trial of macrolide in the treatment of chronic rhinosinusitis. Laryngoscope 2006;116(2):189–193.
2. Cervin A, Kalm O, Sandkull P, Lindberg S. One-year low-dose erythromycin treatment of persistent chronic sinusitis after sinus surgery: clinical outcome and effects on mucociliary parameters and nasal nitric oxide. Otolaryngol Head Neck Surg 2002;126(5):481–489.
3. Subramanian HN, Schechtman KB, Hamilos DL. A retrospective analysis of treatment outcomes and time to relapse after intensive medical treatment for chronic sinusitis. Am J Rhinol 2002;16(6):303–312.
4. Hashiba M, Baba S. Efficacy of long-term administration of clarithromycin in the treatment of intractable chronic sinusitis. Acta Otolaryngol Suppl 1996;525:73–78.

22 Chronic Rhinosinusitis in Adults

22.C.

Aerosolized antibiotics: Impact on sinonasal outcomes

Stacey Gray, Jennifer J. Shin, and Ralph Metson

METHODS

A computerized PubMed search was performed as described in the previous two reviews. The 447 resulting publications were then reviewed to identify those that met the following inclusion criteria: 1) adult patient population with chronic rhinosinusitis, 2) intervention with intranasal antibiotic compared with intranasal control, 3) outcome measured in terms of clinical improvement and/or quality of life. Articles in which a combination of topical and oral antibiotics was used without comparative control data were excluded. Articles without sufficient numerical data (i.e., regimen was used in 50 patients but the number of successes/failures not reported) were excluded. Articles reporting noncontrolled data from topical antibiotics used only in combination with other treatments (topical decongestants, steroids) were also excluded. Articles focusing only on acute sinusitis were excluded. The bibliographies of the articles that met these inclusion criteria were manually checked to ensure no further relevant articles could be identified. This process yielded three articles, one of which was a retrospective case series and two of which were the randomized controlled trials (RCTs) that are presented herein.

RESULTS

Outcome Measures. Outcome measures included quality of life and symptom scores. The Juniper Rhinoconjunctivitis Quality of Life Questionnaire and a visual analog symptom scale were used in the Desrosiers et al. study [1]. Sykes et al. [2] measured the percent with symptomatic improvement, radiographic improvement, or overall improvement.

Potential Confounders. One of the key potential confounders in all studies about chronic rhinosinusitis has been defining which patients carry that diagnosis. One study provided their working definition; the diagnosis was made based on a modified version of previously published recommendations. Prior sinus surgeries could have also influenced results, and the smaller RCT focused only on postsurgical patients. Intranasal antibiotics could have theoretically been more readily delivered in patients who had surgically widened sinus ostia. Other potential confounders included the number and type of previous antibiotic courses received (in one RCT, all patients received a recent course of oral antibiotics) and the dura-
tion/severity of symptoms before initiation of treatment. These potential confounders are detailed as much as the original reports allow in the adjacent table.

Study Designs. Two RCTs compared topical antibiotic to topical control in patients with chronic rhinosinusitis. The larger study compared topical neomycin-dexamethasone-tramazoline versus dexamethasone-tramazoline alone versus placebo in patients with chronic mucopurulent nasal discharge. Randomization resulted in similar symptoms and radiographic findings in all three groups before treatment. This study was double blinded, minimizing expectation bias. *A priori* power calculations for the study were not reported, and sample sizes were small for each group (n = 10–20 patients per group), making it difficult to accept a negative result as definitive.

The smaller RCT compared topical tobramycin solution with topical placebo in patients with chronic rhinosinusitis, diagnosed as defined by previously published recommendations from Lanza and Kennedy [3]. Sample size was small, with 18 total patients completing the Juniper Rhinoconjunctivitis Quality of Life Questionnaire and a visual analog symptom scale that were used. Thus, again, negative results were not definitive.

Highest Level of Evidence. There were two RCTs that compared results of topical antibiotic with topical control. The larger study showed that both neomycin-dexamethasone-tramazoline and dexamethasone-tramazoline alone had significantly more symptom and radiographic improvement than placebo, but no difference when compared with each other. Thus, it would seem that dexamethasone-tramazoline alone is enough to improve symptoms in comparison to placebo. The study was small, however, and so a result that shows no difference cannot be accepted as definitive, because power is limited.

The smaller study showed no difference in quality of life with topical tobramycin versus placebo. Pain was improved more with antibiotics at 2 weeks, but this improvement did not last even as long as the 4-week treatment course. Also, nasal congestion was worse than with placebo at 2–8 weeks. Individual symptom scores showed no significant difference in postnasal drip, mucosal edema, or secretions. Again, however, sample size limits the power of this study, so that a negative result is not definitive.

Applicability. These results can be applied to adult patients with chronic rhinosinusitis. More specifically, the results of the Desrosiers paper can be applied to patients whose symptoms persist despite endoscopic sinus surgery and medi-cal management.

Morbidity/Complications. Reported morbidity was minimal. The only adverse event noted occurred in a placebo group; one patient developed pneumonia and was treated with oral antibiotics.

CLINICAL SIGNIFICANCE AND FUTURE RESEARCH

Two RCTs compared intranasal antibiotics to intranasal control for adults with chronic rhinosinusitis. One study showed that the addition of neomycin to a topical steroid-decongestant regimen resulted in no significant additional benefit. The other RCT showed that pain was significantly better with antibiotic, but only transiently. Meanwhile, nasal congestion was worse with antibiotic and quality of life was no different. Neither publication, however, reported the power associated with their sample sizes, leaving a negative result open to question. Using the percent with symptom improvement in the Sykes study for estimates, the sample size necessary to achieve a 90% power to identify a 15% difference between response rates (alpha 0.05) can be calculated; 326 patients would be required in each group to minimize the probability of falsely accepting the null hypothesis to 10%. Further research is therefore needed to definitively confirm or refute the effect of topical antibiotic therapy.

THE EVIDENCE CONDENSED: Topical antibiotics for chronic and recurrent sinusitis

Reference	Desrosiers, 2001		
Level (design)	1 (randomized controlled trial)		
Sample size*	18 (20)		

	OUTCOMES		
	Tobramycin	**Placebo**	**p Value**
QOL‡	2.5, 2.5, 2.3	2.2, 2.1, 1.8	NS
Pain‡	30, 38, 28	35, 28, 35	<0.05 at 2 wk
Congestion‡	39, 50, 49	40, 30, 28	<0.05 at 4, 8 wk

Conclusion	No significant difference in QOL. Pain significantly better with tobramycin at 2 wk. Nasal congestion significantly better with placebo at 4, 8 wk
Follow-up time	2, 4, 8 wk

	STUDY DESIGN
Inclusion criteria	Patients who had undergone successful ESS but who presented with symptoms of rhinosinusitis that persisted beyond the normal 8- to 12-wk healing period after surgery who failed further medical management. An additional 21 d of abx therapy was administered to all patients before their entry into the study
Exclusion criteria	Severe renal insufficiency, allergies to tobramycin or quinine, patients using loop diuretics, patients with preexisting hearing loss, isolated frontal rhinosinusitis
Randomization effectiveness	There was no difference between the placebo and treated groups in distribution of demographic parameters or in organisms cultured
Age	Mean 49 y (range 23–89 y)
Masking	Double blind
Intervention regimens	Abx: 4 mL of a 20 mg/mL solution of tobramycin applied t.i.d. for 4 wk. Aerosols were introduced into the sinus cavities with the RinoFlow Nasal and Sinus Wash System Placebo: 4 mL of 0.9% sodium chloride with quinine (1 mg/mL) to duplicate the bitter taste of tobramycin. This was applied t.i.d. for 4 wk with the RinoFlow Nasal and Sinus Wash System
Diagnostic criteria for sinusitis	Symptoms of persistent rhinosinusitis were adapted from the "consensus group" recommendations for chronic rhinosinusitis
Definition of outcomes	QOL measured with Juniper Rhinoconjunctivitis Quality of Life Questionnaire. Symptom measurement with visual analog scale Sinonasal endoscopy for assessment of sinonasal mucosa
Criteria for withdrawal	Not specified
Power	NR
Morbidity/complications	One patient developed pneumonia and was treated with oral abx (occurred in the placebo group)

Abx = antibiotics, NS = not significant, NR = not reported, q.i.d. = four times a day, t.i.d. = three times a day, dex = dexamethasone, tram = tramazoline, QOL = quality of life.
* Sample size: numbers shown for those not lost to follow-up and those (initially recruited).
† p Values reported for abx-dex.tram vs dex-tram, abx-dex.tram vs placebo, dex-tram vs placebo.
‡ Numbers as extrapolated from reported line graphs.

THE EVIDENCE CONDENSED: Topical antibiotics for chronic and recurrent sinusitis

Reference	Sykes, 1986
Level (design)	1 (randomized controlled trial)
Sample size*	50 (50)

OUTCOMES

	Abx-dex-tram	Dex-tram	Placebo	p Value†
Overall response rate	62%	60%	12%	NR
% Symptom improvement	60%–80%	55%–72%	14%–20%	NS, <0.05, <0.05
% Radiographic improvement	50%	45%	0%	NS, <0.05, <0.05
Conclusion	Both neomycin-dex-tram and dex-tram alone had significantly better symptom and radiographic improvement than placebo, but no difference when compared with each other			
Follow-up time	2 wk, further follow-up not specified			

STUDY DESIGN

Inclusion criteria	Chronic mucopurulent rhinosinusitis: chronic anterior and/or posterior purulent nasal discharge
Exclusion criteria	Nasal polyps
Randomization effectiveness	Similar symptoms and sinus radiograph abnormalities; similar number of atopic patients
Age	20–70 y
Masking	Double blind
Intervention regimens	1) 100 μg neomycin, dex 20 μg, tram 120 μg q.i.d. ×2 wk 2) Dex 20 μg, tram 120 μg q.i.d. ×2 wk 3) Placebo: propellant alone q.i.d. ×2 wk
Diagnostic criteria for sinusitis	100% with mucopurulent nasal discharge, not otherwise specified
Definition of outcomes	Response to treatment was judged to have occurred if symptoms completely cleared or were greatly improved; if nasal airways resistance decreased by ≥50%; if nasal mucociliary clearance was >30 min and improved by >20 min; if a pathogenic microorganism isolated before treatment was eradicated; if mucosal thickening or opacity on sinus radiographs cleared; or if intranasal mucosal inflammation and/or hypertrophy resolved
Criteria for withdrawal	Not specified
Power	NR
Morbidity/complications	NR

Abx = antibiotics, NS = not significant, NR = not reported, q.i.d. = four times a day, t.i.d. = three times a day, dex = dexamethasone, tram = tramazoline, QOL = quality of life.
* Sample size: numbers shown for those not lost to follow-up and those (initially recruited).
† p Values reported for abx-dex.tram vs dex-tram, abx-dex.tram vs placebo, dex-tram vs placebo.
‡ Numbers as extrapolated from reported line graphs.

REFERENCES

1. Desrosiers MY, Salas-Prato M. Treatment of chronic rhinosinusitis refractory to other treatments with topical antibiotic therapy delivered by means of a large-particle nebulizer: results of a controlled trial. Otolaryngol Head Neck Surg 2001;125(3):265–269.

2. Sykes DA, Wilson R, Chan KL, Mackay IS, Cole PJ. Relative importance of antibiotic and improved clearance in topical treatment of chronic mucopurulent rhinosinusitis. A controlled study. Lancet 1986;2(8503):359–360.

3. Lanza DC, Kennedy DM. Adult rhinosinusitis defined. Otolaryngol Head Neck Surg 1997;117:S1–7.

22 Chronic Rhinosinusitis in Adults

22.D.

Intranasal antifungal therapy: Impact on computed tomography, symptoms, quality of life, and endoscopy

Stacey Gray, Jennifer J. Shin, and Ralph Metson

METHODS

A computerized PubMed search of MEDLINE 1966–February 2005 was performed. The terms "sinusitis" and "antifungal agents" were exploded and the resulting articles were cross-referenced, yielding 295 articles. These articles were then reviewed to identify those that met the following inclusion criteria: 1) adult patient population with chronic rhinosinusitis, 2) intervention with intranasal antifungal treatment, 3) outcome measured in terms of change in mucosal thickening on computed tomography (CT) scan, change in endoscopic examination, and/or change in symptom scores. Articles that analyzed the impact of oral antifungal treatments were excluded. Pilot studies from the same authors who published later higher-level studies were likewise excluded. The bibliographies of the articles that met these inclusion criteria were manually checked to ensure no further relevant articles could be identified. Among the resulting articles were two randomized controlled trials (RCTs), which are presented as the highest level of evidence.

RESULTS

Outcome Measures. Multiple outcome measures were used in these two RCTs. Both groups used the CT scan as the main outcome measure. In the Ponikau study [1], a graphics program was used to digitally measure the extent of mucosal thickening before and after treatment. The reproducibility of this method was independently confirmed by three blinded investigators. In the Weschta study [2], a modified Lund and Mackay CT score was applied that classified sinus opacification into five stages: 0 not opacified, 1 less than 1/3 opacified, 2 between 1/3 and 2/3 opacified, 3 more than 2/3 opacified, but still air-containing, 4 complete opacification (no air). Each maxillary, anterior and posterior ethmoidal, sphenoidal and frontal sinus was evaluated to give an overall score.

These studies also scored quality of life, symptom, and endoscopy as secondary outcomes. Ponikau used the Sinonasal Outcome Test 20, a validated, rhinosinusitis-specific instrument with 20 questions regarding nasal symptoms and quality of life. Ponikau also rated endoscopic findings: 0 no evidence of disease, 1 inflammatory mucosal changes confined to the middle meatus superior to the lower edge of the middle turbinate, 2 polypoid

changes between the lower edge of the middle turbinate and the root of the inferior turbinate, 3 polypoid changes between the root of the inferior turbinate and the lower edge of the inferior turbinate, and 4 polypoid changes below the lower edge of the inferior turbinate. The stages of the two sides were added to produce a total score of 0 (best) to 8 (worst).

The Weschta study used the rhinosinusitis quality of life score, based on subjective estimates on a seven-point scale: 0 (not troubled by nose symptoms) to 6 (extremely troubled by nose symptoms). Symptom scores were assessed with a visual analog scale. Patients were asked about nasal blockage, facial pain, smell disturbance, nasal discharge, and sneezing. Endoscopy scores were classified from 0 (no polyps) to 3 (polyps fill whole nasal cavity) for each side.

Potential Confounders. Potential confounders included the antifungal regimen used, the duration of treatment, prior medical and surgical therapies, and the severity of symptoms before initiation of treatment. For this particular topic, there was also the important confounder that not all patients with chronic rhinosinusitis have a fungal etiology for their inflammation, which could blunt the reaction to the intervention that these authors hoped to test.

Study Designs. There were two RCTs that compared the impact of intranasal amphotericin B with intranasal placebo on chronic rhinosinusitis. The Ponikau study evaluated the effect of intranasal amphotericin irrigation versus placebo for 6 months. The Weschta study analyzed results after treatment with amphotericin or placebo nasal spray for 8 weeks. Both studies showed that randomization was mostly effective in creating two similar patient groups before treatment. There were, however, significantly more males in the amphotericin group in the Weschta study. Both studies reported *a priori* power calculations that showed a need to recruit 60–70 patients to achieve an 80% power. One of the studies achieved this recruitment goal, but the other accrued just 30 patients. Negative results in a low-powered study must be viewed with caution.

Highest Level of Evidence. There were two RCTs that compared treatment of chronic sinusitis with intranasal amphotericin versus intranasal placebo. CT scan change was used as the primary outcome measure for these studies, and results were dissimilar. The Ponikau study showed a significantly better CT scan score with antifungal treatment, whereas the Weschta study showed no difference. Some differences between the two study designs may explain this discrepancy; different methods were used to score CT findings, deliver study medications, and to include/exclude patients with previous sinus surgery.

Whereas one study showed that CT scores were better with antifungal, the other found that symptom scores were better with placebo. Weschta demonstrated that symptom scores improved significantly more after placebo. Both studies, however, showed no significant difference in quality of life measures, and there was a trend toward posttreatment improvement with both intranasal antifungal and with placebo. The Ponikau study likewise showed no significant difference in endoscopy scores when antifungal was compared with placebo.

Applicability. These results are applicable to adult patients with chronic rhinosinusitis who are not pregnant or immunocompromised.

Morbidity/Complications. Several patients withdrew from the study because of nasal burning or irritation in the antifungal treatment group. No major morbidity or complications occurred.

CLINICAL SIGNIFICANCE AND FUTURE RESEARCH

There were two RCTs focusing on this topic, one of which showed better CT scores with antifungal treatment, and one of which showed better symptom scores with placebo. There was no significant difference in other scores, including measures of quality of life. The actual impact of intranasal antifungal therapy thus remains elusive, and more study is needed to provide a definitive answer. Future research may ideally include high power RCTs that focus on subpopulations of adult chronic rhinosinusitis patients with eosinophilic disease or proven antifungal allergy.

Reference	Ponikau, 2005			Weschta, 2004		
Level (design)	1 (RCT)			1 (RCT)		
Sample size*	24 (30)			60 (78)		
OUTCOMES						
Outcome measure	Reduction from baseline in percentage of inflammatory mucosal thickening on CT scan; change from baseline of mucosal thickening on endoscopic staging; SNOT-20 to measure disease-specific quality of life			CT scan score, modified after Lund and Mackay (score 0–4); symptom score (0–30) and RQL assessment of quality of life score; endoscopic score (0–6)		
	CT score mean change	Endoscopy score median change	SNOT-20 median change	CT score median pre/posttreatment	Symptom score median pre/posttreatment	RQL score median pre/posttreatment
Intranasal antifungal	−8.8%	−1.3	−0.3	29/26.5	28/26	22.5/20.5
Intranasal placebo	+2.5%	0	−0.3	28.5/26.5	26.5/16.5	20/10
p Value	0.03	NS	NS	NS	<0.005	NS
Conclusions	Antifungal better	No significant difference	No significant difference	No significant difference	Placebo better	No significant difference
Follow-up time	6 mo			8 wk		
STUDY DESIGN						
Inclusion criteria	CRS symptoms for >3 mo Mucosal thickening on coronal CT >5 mm in ≥2 sinuses Patients were recruited regardless of medications or previous ESS			Age >18 y; symptom score >14; endoscopy score >2; CT score >19		
Exclusion criteria	Patients <18 y old, pregnant/lactating, immunocompromised patients, orbital or CNS complications of CRS, antibiotics use in last 7 d, systemic steroid use in last 3 mo, systemic antifungal use in last 7 d			Pregnant/lactating; recent ESS; mental impairment or severe illness; recent start on antiallergic immunotherapy, steroid therapy, antihistamines, ASA desensitization; antimycotic or immunosuppressive therapy; clinical suspicion of AFRS		
Randomization effectiveness	There was similar age, sex, asthma rates, previous sinus surgery in both groups. The amphotericin group was somewhat older with a longer mean duration of sinusitis			Demographic and clinical characteristics were similar in both groups, except sex. There were significantly more males in the amphotericin group		
Age, mean (range)	Placebo: 49.7 y (33–75 y) Antifungal tx: 56.9 y (27–85 y)			Placebo: 48 y (25–77 y) Antifungal tx: 54 y (37–67 y)		
Antifungal regimen details	20 cc amphotericin B solution (250 µg/cc dissolved in sterile water) to each nostril b.i.d. with bulb syringe for 6 mo			2 puffs per nostril q.i.d. (total daily dose of 4.8 mg amphotericin B) for 8 wk Solutions freshly prepared every 2 wk		
Placebo regimen details	20 cc sterile water colored with yellow dye to each nostril b.i.d. with bulb syringe			2 puffs per nostril q.i.d. control spray containing tartrazine, chinin sulfate in 5% glucose solution		
Compliance	5 patients in antifungal group did not complete study; 1 patient in placebo group did not complete study			15 study withdrawals—intolerance to study medication (6 antifungal group, 1 placebo group), discontinuation after acute exacerbation of CRS in 1 patient in antifungal group		
Power	Study was designed to enroll 70 patients (35 per group) for 80% chance of detecting a 20% difference between the group means			80% with sample size of 30 patients per group		
Morbidity/complications	2 patients in antifungal group had a burning sensation on intranasal application			No significant side effects		

RCT = randomized controlled trial, CT = computed tomography, SNOT-20 = Sinonasal Outcome Test 20, RQL = rhinosinusitis quality of life, NS = not significant, b.i.d. = twice a day, q.i.d. = four times a day, CRS = chronic rhinosinusitis, ESS = endoscopic sinus surgery.
* Sample size: numbers shown for those not lost to follow-up and those (initially recruited).

REFERENCES

1. Ponikau JU, Sherris DA, Weaver A, Kita H. Treatment of chronic rhinosinusitis with intranasal amphotericin B: a randomized, placebo-controlled, double-blind pilot trial. J Allergy Clin Immunol 2005;115(1):125–131.

2. Weschta M, Rimek D, Formanek M, Polzehl D, Podbielski A, Riechelmann H. Topical antifungal treatment of chronic rhinosinusitis with nasal polyps: a randomized, double-blind clinical trial. J Allergy Clin Immunol 2004;113(6):1122–1128.

22 Chronic Rhinosinusitis in Adults

22.E.i.

Endoscopic sinus surgery: Impact on disease-specific quality of life

Jennifer J. Shin and Gregory W. Randolph

METHODS

A computerized Ovid search of MEDLINE 1966–March 2004 was performed. The articles that mapped to the terms "quality of life," "outcome and process assessment (health care)," or "treatment outcome" were pooled together. These articles were then cross-referenced with those articles obtained by exploding the terms "sinusitis" and "endoscopy." This process yielded 197 articles. These articles were then reviewed to identify those that met the following inclusion criteria: 1) patient population with chronic or recurrent acute sinusitis, 2) prospective intervention with endoscopic sinus surgery (ESS), ideally versus medical therapy, 3) preoperative and postoperative symptomatic outcome measured by a validated instrument. Studies that used nonvalidated questionnaires, nonvalidated modifications of instruments, or that used validated instruments to assess neurotic tendencies only were excluded. Retrospective studies that reported only postoperative scores were excluded. The bibliographies of the articles that met these inclusion criteria were manually checked to ensure no further relevant articles could be identified. This rigorous process yielded eight articles (two with overlapping study populations) using disease-specific instruments, which are discussed herein [1–8]. This process also yielded four articles using global instruments which are discussed in the next section.

RESULTS

Outcome Measures. A validated instrument has been tested to ensure that the following are true: 1) it measures what it is intended to measure (convergent validity, i.e., scores on a valid test of arithmetic skills correlate with scores on other math tests), and 2) it does not inadvertently measure irrelevant changes (discriminant validity, i.e., scores on a valid test of arithmetic do not correlate with scores on tests of verbal ability) [9, 10], 3) its scores are stable (reliability, i.e., a patient with the same disease impact will continue to have the same response), and 4) it is sensitive to change (responsiveness, i.e., a patient with a change in disease impact will have a changed score). Overall, this means that the validated instrument in fact measures what it is meant to measure.

These studies used five validated instruments to evaluate sinusitis-specific symptoms: Chronic Sinusitis Survey [1–4], Rhinosinusitis Symptom Inventory [5], Quebec French Rhinosinusitis Outcome Measure [6], Sinonasal Outcome Test 20 [7], and Sinonasal Assessment Questionnaire [8]. More than 20 sinusitis-specific instruments have been critiqued and reviewed in the literature [11]. The Chronic Sinusitis Survey is a duration-based (8 weeks), sinus-specific health survey containing a symptom subscale and a medication subscale. The Rhinosinusitis Symptom Inventory catalogs major and minor symptoms of sinusitis, medicine use, physician visits, and missed workdays. The Quebec Measure is based on a validated translation of the Rhinosinusitis Outcome Measure of the American Academy of Otolaryngology–Head and Neck Surgery Foundation (AAO-HNSF). The Sinonasal Outcome Test 20 assesses physical, functional, and emotional problems from sinusitis. The Sinonasal Assessment Questionnaire is an instrument with 11 questions developed to ensure that symptoms of nasal obstruction and hyposmia are specifically assessed.

Potential Confounders. The extent of initial disease, ESS technique and indications, otolaryngologic comorbidities such as nasal allergies or polyps, and the length of follow-up could all influence outcomes. These factors, among others, are cataloged for the reader in the adjacent table.

Study Designs. These prospective outcomes studies that compared disease-specific quality of life before and after ESS provide level 2 evidence. One team additionally compared pre-ESS and post-ESS data with data from a group who underwent medical intervention only [2, 4]. One study specifically examined frontal sinus surgery [3]. Four teams specified the inclusion of consecutive patients, in order to minimize selection bias [1–5]. Most studies specified clinical criteria for ESS, often as described by the AAO-HSNF 1997 Task Force recommendations [12]. Follow-up times ranged from 3 months to more than 1 year. There were no level 1 studies (i.e., randomized controlled trials) that addressed this issue.

Highest Level of Evidence. In all seven studies, post-ESS scores were statistically significantly better than pre-ESS scores. This conclusion did not differ, regardless of changes in the instrument used, the institution/surgeon, nuances in the indications for surgery, or the time of follow-up. Also, one study showed that scores after medical intervention were improved over time, but not as improved as scores after surgery. The medical treatment group, however, was different from the surgical group at the outset; the medical group had significantly more females, fewer comorbidities, and higher baseline scores on the Chronic Sinusitis Survey. Thus, although the medical group improved less, they also had less room for improvement (statistical floor effect).

Applicability. These results are applicable to adult patients undergoing ESS for chronic or recurrent acute sinusitis. These results may not be applicable to patients with severe comorbidities such as cystic fibrosis.

Morbidity. Complications were usually not described.

CLINICAL SIGNIFICANCE AND FUTURE RESEARCH

There were seven level 2 studies that compared disease-specific quality of life scores in patients before and after ESS for chronic or recurrent acute sinusitis. In each case, scores were significantly improved after surgery. One study compared outcomes after medical treatment alone versus after surgery, and found that whereas both groups improved, those in the surgical group improved significantly more. This result suggests that both groups have the potential to improve, so that the severity of the disease at the outset must be carefully considered when deciding on treatment. (Similar conclusions were made from the randomized controlled trials evaluating the role of tonsillectomy in treating pediatric recurrent sore throats; see Section 4.A.) Future research may therefore focus on defining exactly what severity of disease warrants medical versus surgical therapy.

THE EVIDENCE CONDENSED: Disease-specific quality of life before versus after endoscopic sinus surgery

Reference	Wang, 2002	Gliklich, 1997; Metson, 2000
Level (design)	2 (prospective outcomes study)	2 (prospective outcomes study)
Sample size*	230 (230)	160 (160)
OUTCOMES		
Validated instrument	Chronic Sinusitis Survey (Chinese translation)	Chronic Sinusitis Survey
	Total score: mean ± SD	Total score: mean ± SD
Scale	0 (worst) to 100 (best)	0 (worst) to 100 (best)
Pre-ESS score	63 ± 20.3	39.1 ± 19
Post-ESS score	83.9 ± 18.8	61.7 ± 23
p Value	0.0001	<0.0001
Medical therapy only (no ESS) score	None	Medical group also improved (from 30.4 to 43.9) after 3 mo (p < 0.007), but surgical group improved even more (p = 0.001)
Conclusion	Post-ESS better than pre-ESS	Post-ESS better than pre-ESS, post-ESS better than medical management alone
Follow-up time	6 mo	3, 6, 12 mo
STUDY DESIGN		
Inclusion criteria	ESS for chronic sinusitis, as defined by the 1997 AAO-HNSF Rhinosinusitis Task Force†	ESS for chronic sinusitis, defined by symptoms/signs of sinusitis (facial pressure, pain, headache; rhinorrhea or postnasal drainage; nasal congestion or obstruction) for more than 3 mo
Exclusion criteria	Not specified	Previous nasal or sinus surgery
Selection bias minimization	Consecutive patients	Consecutive patients, fewer males and comorbidities in medical (vs surgical) group
Age	Mean 40.1 ± 14.6 y	20–76 y
Preoperative disease details	Lund-Mackay CT staging system [14]: 51.3% 0–4, 23.5% 5–8	Surgical cohort: CT staging‡ [15]: 0 4%, I 19%, II 29%, III 26%, IV 22%; 37% with polyposis Medical cohort: 8% polyps
ORL-related comorbidities	Nasal allergy 47%, asthma triad 0.9%, anatomic variation 62%	Surgical cohort: 36% asthma, 50% allergies, 2% Samter's triad, 74% nasal septal deviation. Medical cohort: 13% asthma, 62% septal deviation
ESS details	"ESS was performed using the standard anterior to posterior approach ... with or without residents"	87% ethmoidectomy with maxillary antrostomy, 43% sphenoidotomy, 9% frontal sinusotomy
Morbidity/complications	8.6% hemorrhage, 0.4% lamina injury, 0% dura or nasolacrimal duct injury	None noted

SD = standard deviation, ESS = endoscopic sinus surgery, AAO-HNSF = American Academy of Otolaryngology–Head and Neck Surgery Foundation, CT = computed tomography.

* Sample size: numbers shown for those not lost to follow-up and those (initially recruited).

† The 1997 AAO-HNSF Task Force on Rhinosinusitis defined the clinical diagnosis of chronic sinusitis: duration >12 wk, strong history as defined by >2 major factors (facial pain/pressure, facial congestion/fullness, nasal obstruction/blockage, nasal discharge/purulence/discolored postnasal drainage, hyposmia/anosmia, purulence in nasal cavity on examination) or 1 major factor and 2 minor factors [headache, fever (nonacute), halitosis, fatigue, dental pain, cough, ear pain/pressure/fullness] or nasal purulence on examination [12].

‡ CT staging system: Stage I anatomic abnormalities, Stage II bilateral ethmoid disease with involvement of 1 dependent sinus, Stage III bilateral ethmoid disease with 2 or more dependent sinuses on each side, Stage IV diffuse sinonasal polyposis [15].

THE EVIDENCE CONDENSED: Disease-specific quality of life before versus after endoscopic sinus surgery

Reference	Bhattacharyya, 2003	Metson, 1998
Level (design)	2 (prospective outcomes study)	2 (prospective outcomes study)
Sample size*	100 (150)	53 (63)
OUTCOMES		
Validated instrument	Rhinosinusitis Symptom Inventory	Chronic Sinusitis Survey
	Total score: mean	Total score: mean ± SD
Scale		0 (worst) to 100 (best)
Pre-ESS score	45.1	46.4 ± 19.5
Post-ESS score	19.4	62.2 ± 18.9
p Value	<0.001	<0.01
Conclusion	Post-ESS better than pre-ESS	Post-ESS better than pre-ESS
Follow-up time	Mean 19 mo (range 6.4–36.6 mo)	3, 6, 12 mo postoperatively
STUDY DESIGN		
Inclusion criteria	ESS for chronic sinusitis, as defined by the 1997 AAO-HNSF Task Force,† radiographic evidence [13], no response to >12 wk of topical nasal steroids and broad-spectrum antibiotics	Frontal sinus ESS for CT evidence of frontal sinusitis or recurrent frontal headaches with radiologic or endoscopic evidence of paranasal disease
Exclusion criteria	Not specified	Frontal sinus drillouts were analyzed in a separate retrospective study (most also had relief with surgery)
Selection bias minimization	Consecutive patients	Consecutive patients
Age	Mean 41 y	24–76 y
Preoperative disease details	As defined in the inclusion criteria	CT stage‡ [15]: III 55.6%, IV 44.4%
ORL-related comorbidities	None specified	None specified
ESS details	"Standard technique in outpatient setting ... extent of surgery determined according to preoperative CT and nasal endoscopy"	Frontal recess was opened and frontal ostium probed or enlarged
Morbidity/complications	None noted	None noted in this group

SD = standard deviation, ESS = endoscopic sinus surgery, AAO-HNSF = American Academy of Otolaryngology–Head and Neck Surgery Foundation, CT = computed tomography.

* Sample size: numbers shown for those not lost to follow-up and those (initially eligible).

† The 1997 AAO-HNSF Task Force on Rhinosinusitis defined the clinical diagnosis of chronic sinusitis: duration >12 wk, strong history as defined by >2 major factors (facial pain/pressure, facial congestion/fullness, nasal obstruction/blockage, nasal discharge/purulence/discolored postnasal drainage, hyposmia/anosmia, purulence in nasal cavity on examination) or 1 major factor and 2 minor factors [headache, fever (nonacute), halitosis, fatigue, dental pain, cough, ear pain/pressure/fullness] or nasal purulence on examination [12].

‡ CT staging system: Stage I anatomic abnormalities, Stage II bilateral ethmoid disease with involvement of 1 dependent sinus, Stage III bilateral ethmoid disease with 2 or more dependent sinuses on each side, Stage IV diffuse sinonasal polyposis.

THE EVIDENCE CONDENSED: Disease-specific quality of life before versus after endoscopic sinus surgery

Reference	Durr, 2003		Jones, 1998	Fahmy, 2002	
Level (design)	2 (prospective outcomes study)		2 (prospective outcomes study)	2 (prospective outcomes study)	
Sample size*	51 (58)		49 (55)	27 (40)	
OUTCOMES					
Validated instrument	Quebec French Rhinosinusitis Outcome Measure		Sinonasal Outcome Test 20	Sino-Nasal Assessment Questionnaire-11	Sinonasal Outcome Test 20
	First set	Second set	Total score	Total score	Total score
Scale	0 (best) to 7.5 (worst)	1 (best) to 4 (worst)	0 (best) to 100 (worst)	0 (best) to 80 (worst)	0 (best) to 100 (worst)
Pre-ESS score	4.7 ± 1.6	2.8 ± 0.5	38.2% mean percent difference between presurgery and postsurgery (± 37.2%)	37.4	31.9
Post-ESS score	2.1 ± 1.7	1.9 ± 0.7		21.4	20.9
p Value	<0.001	<0.001	<0.05 (extrapolated from text)	0.0001	0.005
Conclusion	Post-ESS better than Pre-ESS		Post-ESS better than pre-ESS	Post-ESS better than pre-ESS	Post-ESS better than pre-ESS
Follow-up time	3 mo		6 mo	6 mo postoperatively	
STUDY DESIGN					
Inclusion criteria	Recurrent acute chronic sinusitis, chronic rhinosinusitis, or nasal polyposis "as confirmed by history, endoscopic exam, and computed tomography"; nomenclature based on the Task Force†		Adult patients undergoing sinus surgery	Patients participating in the Royal College of Surgeons Endoscopic Sinus Surgery National Comparative Audit	
Exclusion criteria	Other severe disease (e.g., cystic fibrosis), previous sinus surgery		Lack of follow-up, unavailable CT scans	Not specified	
Consecutive patients?	Not specified		Not specified	Not specified	
Age	Mean 43.7 y		17–71 y	18–68 y	
Preoperative disease details	9.8% recurrent acute rhinosinusitis, 37.3% chronic rhinosinusitis, 52.9% nasal polyposis		55% chronic sinusitis, 45% recurrent acute sinusitis or predisposing conditions, 46.9% had prior surgery, 53% after 28-d antibiotic trial, "a combination of chronic and/or acute sinusitis with predisposing conditions"	Not specified	
ORL-related comorbidities	31% asthma, 59% inhalent allergies confirmed by skin testing		6% asthma, 4% polyps	Not specified	
ESS details	Not reported		Not reported	Not reported	
Morbidity/ complications	None noted		None noted	None noted	

CT = computed tomography, ESS = endoscopic sinus surgery, ORL = otolaryngology.

* Sample size: numbers shown for those not lost to follow-up and those (initially recruited).

† The 1997 AAO-HNSF Task Force on Rhinosinusitis defined the clinical diagnosis of chronic sinusitis: duration >12 wk, strong history as defined by >2 major factors (facial pain/pressure, facial congestion/fullness, nasal obstruction/blockage, nasal discharge/purulence/discolored postnasal drainage, hyposmia/anosmia, purulence in nasal cavity on examination) or 1 major factor and 2 minor factors [headache, fever (nonacute), halitosis, fatigue, dental pain, cough, ear pain/pressure/fullness] or nasal purulence on examination [12].

REFERENCES

1. Wang PC, Chu CC, Liang SC, Tai CJ. Outcome predictors for endoscopic sinus surgery. Otolaryngol Head Neck Surg 2002;126(2):154–159.

2. Metson RB, Gliklich RE. Clinical outcomes in patients with chronic sinusitis. Laryngoscope 2000;110(3 Pt 3):24–28.

3. Metson R, Gliklich RE. Clinical outcome of endoscopic surgery for frontal sinusitis [see comment]. Arch Otolaryngol Head Neck Surg 1998;124(10):1090–1096.

4. Gliklich RE, Metson R. Effect of sinus surgery on quality of life. Otolaryngol Head Neck Surg 1997;117:12–17.

5. Bhattacharyya N. Symptom outcomes after endoscopic sinus surgery for chronic rhinosinusitis. Arch Otolaryngol Head Neck Surg 2004;130:329–333.

6. Durr DG, Desrosiers M. Evidence-based endoscopic sinus surgery. J Otolaryngol 2003;32(2):101–106.

7. Jones ML, Piccirillo JF, Haiduk A, Thawley SE. Functional endoscopic sinus surgery: do ratings of appropriateness predict patient outcomes? Am J Rhinol 1998;12(4):249–255.

8. Fahmy FF, McCombe A, McKiernan DC. Sino nasal assessment questionnaire, a patient focused, rhinosinusitis specific outcome measure. Rhinology 2002;40(4):195–197.

9. Campbell DT, Fiske DW. Convergent and discriminant validation by the multitrait-multimethod matrix. Psychol Bull 1959;56:81–105.

10. Trochim WM. Research Methods Knowledge Base. Cornell University; 2000.

11. Linder JA, Singer DE, van den Ancker M, Atlas SJ. Measures of health-related quality of life for adults with acute sinusitis. J Gen Intern Med 2003;18:390–401.

12. Lanza D, Kennedy DW. Adult rhinosinusitis defined. Otolaryngol Head Neck Surg 1997;117(3 Pt 2):S1–S7.

13. Bhattacharyya N, Fried MP. The accuracy of computed tomography in the diagnosis of chronic sinusitis. Laryngoscope 2003;113:125–129.

14. Lund VJ, Mackay IS. Staging in rhinosinusitis. Rhinology 1993;107:183–184.

15. Gliklich RE, Metson R. A comparison of sinus computed tomography staging systems for outcomes research. Am J Rhinol 1994;8:291–297.

22 Chronic Rhinosinusitis in Adults

22.E.ii.

Endoscopic sinus surgery: Impact on global quality of life

Jennifer J. Shin and Gregory W. Randolph

METHODS

A computerized and manual search of the literature from 1966 to March 2004 was performed as described in Section 4.C.1. This section discusses the articles using instruments assessing global quality of life [1–5].

RESULTS

Outcome Measures. Validated instruments have the advantages described in Section 4.C.1. These four studies used the Short Form 36 (SF-36) instrument, a validated survey that assesses overall health-related quality of life. This instrument does not focus only on rhinosinusitis-related symptoms, as did the disease-specific instruments discussed in 4.C.1. In the SF-36, eight domains are assessed: physical functioning, role functioning–physical, bodily pain, general health, vitality, social functioning, role functioning–emotional, and mental health. Scores are standardized to a scale of 0 (worst) to 100 (best), and population norms are available.

Potential Confounders. The extent of initial disease, endoscopic sinus surgery (ESS) technique and indications, the length of follow-up, and general comorbidities such as hypertension and tobacco use could all influence outcomes. These factors, among others, are cataloged for the reader in the adjacent table.

Study Designs. These studies provide level 2 evidence regarding preoperative and postoperative global health-related quality of life scores. Three of the four studies specified the use of consecutive patients [1–5]. No studies compared SF-36 scores of a parallel group receiving only medical treatment with post-ESS scores. One study specifically examined frontal sinus surgery. Follow-up times ranged from 3 to 12 months.

Highest Level of Evidence. In all four studies, improvement was seen in some or all domains of the SF-36. The study that focused on frontal sinus surgery showed an improvement in only one domain at 12 months, but had demonstrated improvement in domains of general health, vitality, mental health, and social functioning at 6 months, before losing sample size with subject attrition at the 12-month follow-up point. In each study, most or all SF-36 scores reached population norms postoperatively.

Applicability. These results are applicable to adult patients undergoing ESS for chronic or recurrent acute sinusitis. These results may not be applicable to patients with severe comorbidities such as cystic fibrosis.

Morbidity. One study noted that there were no orbital or central nervous system complications. None were reported in other studies.

CLINICAL SIGNIFICANCE AND FUTURE RESEARCH

There were four level 2 studies that compared global quality of life scores in patients before and after ESS for chronic or recurrent acute sinusitis. Scores in some or all domains of the SF-36 instrument were significantly improved after surgery. These results suggest that overall health-related quality of life was improved in patients who qualified for ESS in these studies. Future research may therefore focus on further delineating those clinical criteria that make patients the best candidates for ESS, or on a direct comparison of selected patients who receive medical versus surgical therapy. Results of an ongoing randomized controlled trial comparing medical to surgical intervention are eagerly awaited.

THE EVIDENCE CONDENSED: Global quality of life before versus after endoscopic sinus surgery

Reference		Gliklich, 1997; Metson, 2000		
Level (design)		2 (prospective outcomes study)		
Sample size*		160 (160)		
		Pre-ESS	Post-ESS	p Value
SF-36 domain mean score	**PF**	85.1	89.0	<0.01
	RP	60.4	73.9	<0.01
	BP	64.6	74.2	<0.001
	GH	67.8	69.3	NS
	SF	73.0	83.7	<0.001
	VT	52.5	60.0	<0.001
	RE	81.8	86.6	NS
	MH	72.6	76.7	<0.01
Post-ESS score vs population norm		Mean normative values reached by 6 mo postoperatively in all domains except RP		
Conclusion		Post-ESS improved from pre-ESS		
Follow-up time		3, 6, 12 mo		
Inclusion criteria		Chronic sinusitis, as defined by the presence of symptoms and signs of sinusitis (facial pain, pressure or headache, rhinorrhea or postnasal drainage, nasal congestion or obstruction) for >3 mo		
Exclusion criteria		Previous nasal or sinus surgery		
Selection bias minimization		Consecutive patients		
Preoperative disease details		Surgical cohort: CT staging†: 0 4%, I 19%, II 29%, III 26%, IV 22%; 37% with polyposis		
General health comorbidities		11% smokers, 9% hypertension, 2% congestive heart failure, 4% previous myocardial infarction, 5% depression, 2% diabetes mellitus		
ESS details		87% ethmoidectomy with maxillary antrostomy, 43% sphenoidotomy, 9% frontal sinusotomy		
Morbidity/complications		Not reported		

ESS = endoscopic sinus surgery, SF-36 = Short Form 36, NS = not significant; SF-36 domains: PF = physical functioning, RP = role physical, BP = bodily pain, GH = general health, VT = vitality, SF = social functioning, RE = role emotional, MH = mental health.
† CT staging system: Stage I anatomic abnormalities, Stage II bilateral ethmoid disease with involvement of 1 dependent sinus, Stage III bilateral ethmoid disease with 2 or more dependent sinuses on each side, Stage IV diffuse sinonasal polyposis.

THE EVIDENCE CONDENSED: Global quality of life before versus after endoscopic sinus surgery

Reference		Winstead, 1998			Metson, 1998			Durr, 2003		
Level (design)		2 (prospective outcomes study)			2 (prospective outcomes study)			2 (prospective outcomes study)		
Sample size*		84 at 6 mo, 40 at 12 mo (125)			56 (63)			51 (58)		
OUTCOMES										
		All four studies used the SF-36 Health Survey Scale 0 (worst)–100 (best)								
		Pre-ESS	Post-ESS	p Value	Pre-ESS	Post-ESS	p Value	Pre-ESS	Post-ESS	p Value
SF-36	PF	82.8	91.2	<0.05	90.1	92.3	NS	80.0	82.0	NS
domain	RP	43.5	81.7	<0.05	68.9	79.2	NS	53.1	70.4	0.01
mean	BP	53.9	73.2	<0.05	52.4	55.0	NS	54.9	62.8	NS
score	GH	61.5	70.6	<0.05	70.7	70.3	NS	61.0	61.5	NS
	SF	65.4	79.4	<0.05	81.7	90.8	NS	24.2	60.5	<0.001
	VT	45.4	56.2	<0.05	57.5	63.1	NS	47.9	80.6	<0.001
	RE	65.4	82.4	<0.05	87.3	89.1	NS	63.8	80.4	0.01
	MH	64.2	73.8	<0.05	76.5	79.9	<0.05	62.8	68.1	NS
Post-ESS score vs population norm		Post-ESS scores at 6 and 12 mo without significant variance from population norms			Mean normative scores were reached in all domains except BP, VT			Not reported		
Conclusion		Post-ESS improved from pre-ESS			Post-ESS improved from pre-ESS			Post-ESS improved from pre-ESS		
Follow-up time		6, 12 mo (only 12 mo shown)			3, 6, 12 mo postoperatively			3 mo		
STUDY DESIGN										
Inclusion criteria		All patients scheduled to undergo ESS; all had unresponsive chronic sinusitis, defined as >3 mo of facial pressure, pain, headache, or recurring episodes of acute rhinosinusitis associated with abnormalities on the CT and/or nasal endoscopic examination			Frontal sinus ESS for CT evidence of frontal sinusitis or recurrent frontal headaches with radiologic or endoscopic evidence of paranasal disease			Recurrent acute chronic sinusitis, chronic rhinosinusitis, or nasal polyposis "as confirmed by history, endoscopic exam, and computed tomography"; nomenclature based on the Task Force meeting, Alexandria VA, 1996‡		
Exclusion criteria		Cystic fibrosis, ESS for drainage of subperiosteal orbital abscess, repair of cerebrospinal fluid fistula, or excision of inverted papilloma			Frontal sinus drillouts were analyzed in a separate retrospective study (most also had relief with surgery)			Other severe disease (e.g., cystic fibrosis), previous sinus surgery		
Selection bias minimization		Consecutive patients			Consecutive patients			Use of consecutive patients not specified		
Preoperative disease details		CT staging†: I 23%, II 26%, III 43%, IV 7%			CT stage [6]: III 55.6%, IV 44.4%			9.8% recurrent acute rhinosinusitis, 37.3% chronic rhinosinusitis, 52.9% nasal polyposis		
General health comorbidities		37% tobacco use, 22 depression, 1.5% diabetes mellitus			23.8% with ≥1 comorbidity, hypertension most common			14% smokers, not otherwise specified		
ESS details		"Surgical technique in all patients was uniform with strict adherence to the functional concepts of Stammberger"; 41% with concomitant septal surgery			Frontal recess was opened and frontal ostium probed or enlarged			Not reported		
Morbidity/ complications		No orbital or central nervous system complications			None noted in this group			Not reported		

ESS = endoscopic sinus surgery, SF-36 = Short Form 36, NS = not significant, CT = computed tomography; SF-36 domains: PF = physical functioning, RP = role physical, BP = bodily pain, GH = general health, VT = vitality, SF = social functioning, RE = role emotional, MH = mental health.
* Sample size: numbers shown for those not lost to follow-up and those (initially recruited).
† CT staging system: Stage I anatomic abnormalities, Stage II bilateral ethmoid disease with involvement of 1 dependent sinus, Stage III bilateral ethmoid disease with 2 or more dependent sinuses on each side, Stage IV diffuse sinonasal polyposis.
‡ The 1997 AAO-HNSF Task Force on Rhinosinusitis defined the clinical diagnosis of chronic sinusitis: duration ≥12 wk, strong history as defined by ≥2 major factors (facial pain/pressure, facial congestion/fullness, nasal obstruction/blockage, nasal discharge/purulence/discolored postnasal drainage, hyposmia/anosmia, purulence in nasal cavity on exam) or 1 major factor and 2 minor factors [headache, fever (nonacute), halitosis, fatigue, dental pain, cough, ear pain/pressure/fullness] or nasal purulence on examination [7].

REFERENCES

1. Gliklich RE, Metson R. Effect of sinus surgery on quality of life. Otolaryngol Head Neck Surg 1997;117:12–17.
2. Metson RB, Gliklich RE. Clinical outcomes in patients with chronic sinusitis. Laryngoscope 2000;110(3 Pt 3):24–28.
3. Winstead W, Barnett SN. Impact of endoscopic sinus surgery on global health perception: an outcomes study. Otolaryngol Head Neck Surg 1998;119(5):486–491.
4. Metson R, Gliklich RE. Clinical outcome of endoscopic surgery for frontal sinusitis [see comment]. Arch Otolaryngol Head Neck Surg 1998;124(10):1090–1096.
5. Durr DG, Desrosiers M. Evidence-based endoscopic sinus surgery. J Otolaryngol 2003;32(2):101–106.
6. Gliklich RE, Metson R. A comparison of sinus computed tomography staging systems for outcomes research. Am J Rhinol 1994;8:291–297.
7. Lanza D, Kennedy DW. Adult rhinosinusitis defined. Otolaryngol Head Neck Surg 1997;117(3 Pt 2):S1–S7.

23 Adult Laryngopharyngeal Reflux

23.A.

Proton pump inhibitor therapy versus placebo: Impact on symptom scores and laryngeal signs

James Hartman

METHODS

A computerized PubMed search of MEDLINE 1966–January 2006 was performed using the terms "laryngopharyngeal reflux" (LPR) and "supraesophageal reflux disease." The resulting articles were combined into a first group and cross-referenced with a second group of articles using the keywords "treatment of reflux." This process yielded 91 articles which were reviewed. Their references were manually cross-checked for any further relevant articles which yielded three additional pertinent studies. This search was reverified by cross-referencing studies that mapped to both the medical subject heading "gastroesophageal reflux" and "laryngeal disease." All of these articles were reviewed to determine which met the following inclusion criteria: 1) distinct patient population of adults (≥18 years old) with symptoms and signs suggesting LPR, 2) intervention with a proton pump inhibitor (PPI) versus placebo, 3) outcome measured by patient questionnaire and video laryngoscopy. Studies were excluded if a) medical treatment other than PPIs was used, b) surgical treatment was used, and c) laryngeal diagnoses other than those caused by reflux were studied. This process yielded five level 1 articles [1–5].

RESULTS

Outcome Measures. LPR is typically diagnosed empirically by history of associated symptoms and findings of posterior laryngitis. Questionnaires have been established to score patients' reflux histories and videolaryngoscopy has been used to score laryngopharyngeal findings [1–5]. The presence of LPR can also be established by a 24-hour dual pH probe, as was required for entry into four trials [2–5]. This probe, however, remains an uncomfortable test for patients and therefore can be an arduous diagnostic tool for routine use. In accordance with this realization, Steward et al. [1] modified their protocol to make the probe optional when accrual became threatened. In addition, only two reports [2, 4] had follow-up pH probes in their protocol and these were performed only in some patients. Finally, quality of life measurements (Short Form 36) of the impact a condition has on an individual were utilized in one study [1].

Potential Confounders. Lifestyle choices may result in activities that have a proclivity for causing gastroesopha-geal reflux. Two studies controlled for these lifestyle choices [1, 4] and demonstrated no significant difference between intervention and placebo groups. In addition, compliance with study medication, as well as the dosage and duration of treatment could affect results. Details of treatment regimens are detailed in the adjoining table.

Study Designs. These five studies are all double-blind randomized controlled trials (RCTs) with placebo control. One study is also a crossover study with a 2-week washout in between treatment regimens [2]. All of the studies used reflux symptom questionnaires. Four used videolaryngoscopy grading, whereas a fifth [5] used laryngoscopy grading. Four required pH studies for entry [2–5].

All five studies demonstrated to different degrees that the patients who were to receive either PPI or placebo were similar before receiving the different therapies. Three of the studies confirmed that there were no statistical differences in demographic data [1, 3, 4], whereas one study did not reveal demographic data but did note that there was no significant difference in pH study results at the outset [2]. The remaining study demonstrated only minor demographic differences between its two groups but did not statistically evaluate them [5]. In addition to demographic comparisons, there were also analyses of reflux severity at the outset. In one study [5], the group treated with placebo then a PPI had worse esophageal scores but no difference in laryngeal symptom scores. Pretreatment comparisons of videolaryngoscopy scores were not reported. Two studies concluded that there was no significant difference in baseline laryngeal measures [1, 4], but one study showed some differences in initial symptom scores [3]. When statistically evaluated, however, only the difference in initial hoarseness scores was found to have been significant. The PPI-treated group was initially more hoarse and this group had a significantly greater response than did the placebo-treated group. Such a difference in hoarseness creates concern for a potential floor effect, i.e., the amount of potential recovery is dependent on the severity of initial symptoms.

Follow-up evaluation ended at the conclusion of treatment: 2 months in two studies [1, 3], 3 months in two studies [4, 5], and in 6.5 months in the crossover study [2]. Masking was adequate as each study was double blinded. An *a priori* calculation of the sample size needed to demonstrate a declared power was performed in three studies [1, 2, 4]. An intention to treat analysis was performed in two studies [1, 4], whereas all five studies tabulated their attrition.

Highest Level of Evidence. The five RCTs had disparate results, with two studies showing significantly better results with PPI than with placebo and three studies showing no difference between the two types of therapy. The two studies that demonstrated statistically significant improvement in laryngopharyngeal symptoms did not show a notable difference in the laryngopharyngeal examination for the group treated with a PPI versus placebo [3, 4]. This result suggests that signs may not be rigorously correlated with symptoms of LPR. Of the three studies that showed no statistically significant difference for adults with laryngopharyngeal reflux treated with PPI versus those treated with placebo [1, 2, 5], there was a trend toward a better result with PPI in two of the studies. Although not statistically significant, one study did show greater improvement in nearly all measures for the PPI-treated group [1]. The greatest impact on results in that study, however, was linked to lifestyle modifications; when reported by patients, they were significantly correlated with global symptom improvement in the total population and the control group. All three studies that showed no difference in outcome may have been subject to limitations in power because of small sample size. For example, the authors of one study, which 36 subjects completed, noted a need for 66 patients even while assuming a large difference in response rate of 67% versus 33%. Thus, there may not have been sufficient enrollment to uncover any differences that may truly exist. The wide 95% confidence intervals, because of small sample size, for all the studies suggest that definitive conclusions about clinical effectiveness are difficult to make.

Applicability. The results of these studies are applicable to adult patients presenting with symptoms and signs attributable to laryngopharyngeal reflux in the absence of other identifiable causes for laryngopharyngeal symptoms.

Morbidity/Complications. None of these studies reported any serious morbidity and only one patient withdrew because of drug-related side effects (abdominal complaints) [4].

CLINICAL SIGNIFICANCE AND FUTURE RESEARCH

There is conflicting level 1 evidence regarding the impact of PPIs on symptomatic adults with laryngopharyngeal reflux. Two RCTs showed a significantly better result with PPI, whereas three RCTs showed no benefit compared with placebo. All studies had small sample sizes, with associated wide ranges in confidence intervals around the difference between PPI and placebo. Therefore, it is possible that among the negative studies, based on statistical significance (i.e., p value > 0.05), a clinically significant effect cannot be ruled out. Likewise, a clinically insignificant effect could also be possible among the statistically significant studies. Unfortunately, multiple different scales of measurement were used for measurement of outcomes, making meta-analysis to increase power a less attractive option. One of the RCTs did find significant benefit to the utilization of lifestyle modifications; the authors even suggested that a 2-month trial of these modifications was a reasonable alternative to medical therapy. There were almost no reported adverse effects of PPIs in the trials, suggesting that the risk of PPI therapy may be low. When the positive impact found in two of the studies are considered with the very low adverse reactions rate, an empiric trial of a PPI remains an attractive therapy alternative.

If further research on this topic is performed, the impact of lifestyle modifications should be studied. For example, a prospective trial of modifications versus a medication group could be performed. More accurate power calculations with larger subject accrual would likely serve to address the conflicting results of the currently available studies. All future studies should ideally have a longer treatment period (preferably at least 3 months) and utilize the same validated reflux symptom questionnaire and reflux sign grading system to facilitate the ability to analyze pooled data.

Reference	Steward, 2004
Level (design)	1 (RCT)
Sample size*	36 (42)

OUTCOMES	
Reflux measures	Reflux symptom scores. Sum of scores 0–4 for severity and frequency for 9 symptoms. Maximum 72
	Videolaryngoscopy Reflux grade 0 Sum of scores to 4 for 6 items Maximum 24 Lifestyle questionnaire (SF-36) Mental and physical components
PPI-treated group	Mean change in total reflux score of 9.7, p ≤ 0.002 Mean change in laryngoscopy grade 0.6, p ≤ 0.19 Mean change in SF-36 mental 0.03, p ≤ 0.99 Mean change in SF-36 physical −2.1, p ≤ 0.64
Placebo-treated group	Mean change in total reflux score of 6.6, p ≤ 0.03 Mean change in laryngoscopy grade 0.5, p ≤ 0.44 Mean change in SF-36 mental −0.9, p ≤ 0.64 Mean change in SF-36 physical 1.2 p ≤ 0.51
Difference of mean changes: PPI vs control	**Total reflux score:** −3.06 (95% CI: −10.99 to 4.86) [p = 0.44] **Laryngoscopy Grade:** −0.11 (95% CI: −1.65 to 1.43) [p = 0.69] **SF-36 mental:** −0.92 (95% CI: −7.36 to 5.51) [p = 0.77] **SF-36 physical:** 3.34 (95% CI: −2.71 to 9.40) [p = 0.27] Negative values indicate more improvement from PPI
Conclusion	No statistically significant differences between the 2 groups though greater improvement for most outcome measures was seen in the PPI-treated group
Time of assessment	Entry, 2 mo

STUDY DESIGN	
Inclusion criteria	Patients ≥18 y old with history of hoarseness, throat clearing, dry cough, globus, or sore throat >4 wk. Physical examination consistent with diagnosis of laryngopharyngeal reflux. pH probe optional
Exclusion criteria	Previous reflux surgery or current tracheostomy, gastrostomy, hypersecretory disorder, recent use of a PPI or H2 blocker, allergy to PPIs, current systemic steroid use, history of laryngeal or pharyngeal tumor or neck irradiation, recent intubation, vocal cord paralysis, or granulomatous disease
Randomization effectiveness	No significant difference in reflux symptoms scores, laryngeal reflux grade, or SF-36 summary
Patient characteristics	≥18 y old Mean 52.8 y Male 23.8%
PPI regimen	Rabeprazole 20 mg b.i.d. for 2 mo
Other treatment used for reflux	Lifestyle modifications (reflux precautions) both groups
Masking	Double blind
Pretrial power calculation	33 patients in each group with assumption that PPI to placebo response was 67%–30% (5% alpha error, power = 80% with 10% dropout rate)
Morbidity	No serious adverse events

RCT = randomized controlled trial, SF-36 = Short Form 36, PPI = proton pump inhibitor, ANCOVA = analysis of covariance, CI = confidence interval, b.i.d. = twice a day.
* Sample size: numbers shown for those completing the trial and those initially enrolled.

Reference	Eherer, 2003
Level (design)	1 (RCT crossover)
Sample size*	14 (21)

OUTCOMES

Reflux measures	Reflux symptom scores. Sum of frequency scores 0–4 multiplied by the intensity score 0–3, esophageal 0–48, laryngeal 0–72
	Videolaryngoscopy Scores 1–3 10 items, maximum score of 30
Crossover group results	Mean change for laryngeal symptom scores: PPI/placebo group 8.3 Placebo/PPI group 10.3 Mean change for esophageal scores: PPI/placebo group 2.2 Placebo/PPI group 5.4 Mean change for laryngeal signs scores: PPI/placebo 8.0 Placebo/PPI 5.6
Difference of mean changes: PPI vs contro	**Laryngeal symptom scores:** −2.0 (95% CI: −13.151 to 9.151) [p = 0.7107] **Esophageal scores:** −3.20 (95% CI: −9.777 to 3.377) [p = 0.3202] **Laryngeal signs scores:** 2.40 (95% CI: −3.804 to 8.604) [p = 0.4270]
Conclusion	PPIs may be helpful in reflux laryngitis patients but the long-term advantage over placebo is not clear
Time of assessment	Entry, 3 mo, 6.5 mo

STUDY DESIGN

Inclusion criteria	Patients ≥18 y old with hoarseness, other laryngeal symptoms of 2 mo duration, and laryngitis on examination, and abnormal 24-h dual pH probe
Exclusion criteria	Smokers, other identifiable causes of laryngitis, laryngeal malignancy or history of laryngeal surgery
Randomization effectiveness	Not reported
Patient characteristics	20–70 y old Mean 48 y Male 76.2%
PPI regimen	Pantoprazole 40 mg b.i.d. for 3 mo, followed by a 2-wk washout then a crossover to placebo b.i.d. for 3 mo or vice versa
Other treatment used for reflux	Not reported
Masking	Double blind
Pretrial power calculation	15 total patients with assumption placebo was half as effective as treatment (5% alpha error, power of 0.8)
Morbidity	No adverse events

RCT = randomized controlled trial, SF-36 = Short Form 36, PPI = proton pump inhibitor, ANCOVA = analysis of covariance, CI = confidence interval, b.i.d. = twice a day.
* Sample size: numbers shown for those completing the trial and those initially enrolled.

Reference	Noordzij, 2001
Level (design)	1 (RCT)
Sample size*	30 (30)

OUTCOMES	
Reflux measures	Reflux symptoms questionnaire Laryngeal score sum of 6 items severity 0–100 × frequency in past 14 d Maximum is 1400 for each symptom Videostrobolaryngoscopy Scores 0–3 for 5 items
PPI-treated group	Mean change in laryngeal score 976.4 p = 0.039 from repeated-measures ANCOVA Range of mean changes for 5 signs 0.00–0.08
Placebo-treated group	Mean change in laryngeal score 454.4 p = 0.827 from repeated-measures ANCOVA Range of mean changes for 5 signs −0.13 to 0.21
Difference of mean changes: PPI vs control	**Laryngeal score:** p = 0.098 from repeated-measures ANCOVA (nonsignificant for all 5 signs) Difference of mean changes: 522 (95% CI: −962.35 to 2006.35)
Conclusion	Significant improvement in laryngeal symptom score occurred for the PPI-treated group vs the control group; however, endoscopic signs did not change significantly.
Time of assessment	Entry, 1 mo, 2 mo

STUDY DESIGN	
Inclusion criteria	Adult patients with at least 1 symptom of reflux laryngitis for 3 mo and >4 episodes of laryngopharyngeal reflux on 24-h dual pH probe
Exclusion criteria	Infectious laryngitis, laryngeal cancer, vocal fold lesions, seasonal allergies, occupational laryngitis
Randomization effectiveness	No significant difference in laryngeal reflux scores, laryngeal reflux signs, or LPR episodes on pH probe
Patient characteristics	Adults Mean 48.7 y Male 53.3%
PPI regimen	Omeprazole 40 mg b.i.d. for 2 mo
Other treatment used for reflux	Lifestyle modifications were discouraged.
Masking	Double blind
Pretrial power calculation	Not reported
Morbidity	No adverse reactions

RCT = randomized controlled trial, SF-36 = Short Form 36, PPI = proton pump inhibitor, ANCOVA = analysis of covariance, CI = confidence interval, b.i.d. = twice a day.
* Sample size: numbers shown for those completing the trial and those initially enrolled.

Reference	El-Serag, 2001
Level (design)	1 (RCT)
Sample size*	20 (22)

OUTCOMES

Reflux measures	Reflux symptoms (8) items. Complete resolution of all 8 or not
	Videolaryngoscopy signs (4), complete resolution of all 4 or not
PPI-treated group	6 symptom complete responders and 6 partial responders 2 signs complete responders 5 partial responders
Placebo-treated group	1 symptom complete responder and 9 partial responders 0 signs complete responders and 3 partial responders
Difference of mean changes: PPI vs control	**Symptom resolution:** Difference of proportions: 40% (95% CI: 0.9%54.9%) [p = 0.0449] **Signs resolution:** Difference of proportions: 28.3% (95% CI: −13.2% to 59.7%)
Conclusion	Significant symptomatic benefit to adult patients with reflux laryngitis when treated with a PPI; however, laryngoscopy signs did not change significantly.
Time of assessment	Entry, 6 wk, 3 mo

STUDY DESIGN

Inclusion criteria	Adult patients with idiopathic chronic laryngitis with hoarseness, throat clearing, dry cough, globus, or sore throat for at least 3 wk, and physical findings of posterior laryngitis. Pathologic reflux on 24-h dual pH probe
Exclusion criteria	Infectious or allergic causes of laryngitis, aerodigestive cancers, history of radiation or gastrointestinal surgery
Randomization effectiveness	No significant difference in laryngeal reflux symptoms or signs, or results from 24-h dual pH probe
Patient characteristics	Adults Mean 61.7 y Male 95.5%
PPI regimen	Lansoprazole 30 mg b.i.d. for 3 mo
Other treatment used for reflux	Not reported
Masking	Double blind
Pretrial power calculation	11 patients in each group to detect 70% difference in efficacy (5% alpha error, 20% beta error)
Morbidity	Not reported

RCT = randomized controlled trial, SF-36 = Short Form 36, PPI = proton pump inhibitor, ANCOVA = analysis of covariance, CI = confidence interval, b.i.d. = twice a day.
* Sample size: numbers shown for those completing the trial and those initially enrolled.

Reference	Havas, 1999
Level (design)	1 (RCT)
Sample size*	15 (20)

OUTCOMES

Reflux measures	Reflux cervical symptom scores. Sum of scores 0–3 for severity and 0–4 for frequency for 4 items. Maximum 28
	Laryngoscopy signs staged 0–5
PPI-treated group	Mean change in symptoms score 3.875 Mean change in laryngoscopy grade 1.25
Placebo-treated group	Mean change in symptom score 3.860 Mean change in laryngoscopy grade 1.17
Difference of mean changes: PPI vs control	**Cervical Symptoms:** 0.015 (95% CI: −6.43 to 6.46) [p = 0.9961] **Laryngoscopy grade:** 0.08 (95% CI: −1.52 to 1.68) [p = 0.92]
Conclusion	PPI treatment was no better than placebo in the treatment of patients with posterior pharyngolaryngitis.
Time of assessment	Entry, 6 wk, 12 wk

STUDY DESIGN

Inclusion criteria	Adult patients with posterior laryngitis
Exclusion criteria	Patients with neurologic disorders, chronic airway obstruction, use of current antisecretory medicines, severe erosive esophagitis, and professional voice users
Randomization effectiveness	No significant difference in reflux symptoms or laryngeal grade
Patient characteristics	32–76 y old Mean 53.6 y Male 46.7%
PPI regimen	Lansoprazole 30 mg b.i.d. for 3 mo
Other treatment used for reflux	Not reported
Masking	Double blind
Pretrial power calculation	Not reported
Morbidity	No adverse reactions

RCT = randomized controlled trial, SF-36 = Short Form 36, PPI = proton pump inhibitor, ANCOVA = analysis of covariance, CI = confidence interval, b.i.d. = twice a day.
* Sample size: numbers shown for those completing the trial and those initially enrolled.

REFERENCES

1. Steward DL, Wilson KM, Kelly DH, et al. Proton pump inhibitor therapy for chronic laryngo-pharyngitis: a randomized placebo-control trial. Otolaryngol Head Neck Surg 2004;131(4):342–350.
2. Eherer AJ, Habermann W, Hammer HF, Kiesler K, Friedrich G, Krejs GJ. Effect of pantoprazole on the course of reflux-associated laryngitis: a placebo-controlled double-blind crossover study. Scand J Gastroenterol 2003;(5):462–467.
3. Noordzij JP, Khidr A, Evans BA, et al. Evaluation of omeprazole in the treatment of reflux laryngitis: a prospective, placebo-controlled, randomized, double-blind study. Laryngoscope 2001;111(12):2147–2151.
4. El-Serag HB, Lee P, Buchner A, Inadomi JM, Gavin M, McCarthy DM. Lansoprazole treatment of patients with chronic idiopathic laryngitis: a placebo-controlled trial. Am J Gastroenterol 2001;96(4):979–983.
5. Havas T, Huang S, Levy M, et al. Posterior pharyngolaryngitis double-blind randomised placebo-controlled trial of proton pump inhibitor therapy. Aust J Otolaryngol 1999; 3(3):243–246.

24 Unilateral Vocal Cord Paralysis

24.A.

Unilateral vocal cord paralysis: Introductory overview

Randall C. Paniello

METHODS OVERVIEW

For initial inquiries into this topic, a computerized PubMed search of Medline listings from 1966–2005 was performed in January, 2006, using key words "vocal", "fold" or "cord", "paralysis" or "paresis" or "immobility" or "movement impairment", and "treatment." The search was filtered to include only papers published in English, involving human subjects, and including abstracts. This process yielded 1,930 publications. The search was then further limited by excluding single case reports, papers on the incidence or etiology of vocal fold paralysis, review articles with no new patient data (except meta-analyses), duplicate or follow-up papers, and papers focusing on non-voice outcomes such as swallowing. The remaining papers were reviewed and graded for their level of evidence, and then categorized into the subheadings of this chapter to the extent possible. The bibliographies of the selected papers were reviewed to determine whether any additional studies had been missed in the search, and these were added.

DATA OVERVIEW

The final list included 154 studies. Most studies focused on a single treatment method—a certain injectable agent or operation. A few studies compared two varieties of the same operation, such as two different injectable agents or two different types of medialization surgery; such studies are considered in their respective topic-specific section below. Other studies compared two completely different approaches to treating unilateral vocal fold paralysis (UVFP), such as medialization versus reinnervation; these studies were considered in a separate section to emphasize their importance.

Thus, the set of papers was further organized into the following topics for this chapter on UVFP.

Vocal fold injection methods (24.B)
Laryngeal framework surgery methods
   Medialization laryngoplasty (24.C.i)
   Arytenoid adduction (24.C.ii)
Laryngeal reinnervation (24.D)
Studies comparing methods from above groups (24.E, 24.F)

A number of important topics related to vocal fold paralysis were omitted from this review because of the relative paucity of relevant publications. These include vocal fold paralysis in children; diagnostic studies such as electromyography; intraoperative monitoring of the laryngeal nerves; and the role of primary voice/speech therapy for treatment.

POTENTIAL COMMON CONFOUNDERS AND BIASES

One problem common to every paper reviewed was that the criteria for the diagnosis of vocal fold paralysis were not specifically defined. Many otolaryngologists believe that the range of possible vocal fold mobility follows a continuum from normal, to mild–moderate–severe weakness (paresis), to complete adductor paralysis. Thus, it is never entirely clear where an author draws the distinction among normal, paresis, and paralysis. For this review, the authors' diagnoses were accepted as published, but it is clear that some cases of moderate to severe paresis were included in some papers that would have been excluded from others.

Another problem common to most of these papers was the relatively small number of subjects. Some of the papers included patients with vocal fold paralysis as well as patients with other diagnoses that had undergone the same treatment (e.g., vocal cord injection for UVFP or for vocal fold atrophy). In the summary tables, the numbers of patients listed include only the subgroups that had the diagnosis of vocal fold paralysis. Also, most of the studies included no untreated patients or other control groups.

The studies that compared two different general approaches to treating UVFP, such as medialization versus reinnervation, comprise the most interesting papers in this chapter, but they share a common shortcoming: they are *not randomized*. Instead, the patients were assigned to one group or the other by the surgeon(s), based on some typically undefined criteria. Typically this was done because the surgeon believed the patient would be better treated by a particular procedure; for example, some surgeons use injection to medialize the vocal folds of patients with small glottal gaps, and use an open implant technique for patients with larger gaps. Thus, the two patient groups could be fundamentally different because of a very strong selection bias.

A potential confounder common to several of these studies relates to the use of speech therapy. Some of the publications indicate that speech therapy was used in some cases during the follow-up period to augment the result. This creates a significant problem, as it then cannot be determined how much of any measured benefit should be attributed to the primary surgical intervention, and how much to the speech therapy. Furthermore, speech therapy tends to be highly individualized and thus very difficult to standardize; it may be best to hold any speech therapy until after the observation period and exclude any patient that violates this restriction. Most of the studies do not specifically state that speech therapy during the observation period was prohibited or regulated.

24 Unilateral Vocal Cord Paralysis

Vocal fold injection: Impact on subjective and objective measures of voice

Randall C. Paniello

METHODS

A computerized PubMed search of MEDLINE listings from 1966 to 2005 was performed, using keywords "vocal," "fold" or "cord," "paralysis" or "paresis" or "immobility" or "movement impairment," and "treatment." This process yielded 1930 publications. Papers were reviewed to identify those that met the following inclusion criteria: 1) adult patient population with unilateral vocal cord paralysis, 2) intervention with injectable material to medialize the paralyzed cord, 3) results reported in terms of subjective or objective measures of voice. The search was then further limited by excluding single case reports, papers on the incidence or etiology of vocal fold paralysis, review articles with no new patient data (except meta-analyses), duplicate or follow-up reports, and papers focusing on nonvoice outcomes such as swallowing. The bibliographies of the selected papers were reviewed to determine whether any additional studies had been missed in the search, and these were added. A total of 42 papers met the search criteria [1–42].

RESULTS

Outcome Measures. The goal of injection laryngoplasty is to move the vocal fold toward the midline by injecting a selected material lateral to the vocal fold. All of the studies attempted to report both subjective and objective data regarding the functional effect of this procedure. The subjective data were most frequently a qualitative rating provided by the patient, or by one or more "expert" judges that listened to recordings of the patients' voices. The judges' training or qualifications for rendering these evaluations was usually not given, except to state what professional training they had (speech pathologist, otolaryngology resident, etc.); the basis criteria for such judgments was not reported. The objective data were usually measurements of the maximum phonation time (MPT), the fundamental frequency range (F0r), or computerized analyses of a sustained vowel sample, for the frequently cited relevant waveform measurements. Videostroboscopy was often described either qualitatively, or more quantitatively by a measure of open quotient or membranous contact quotient. In addition to MPT, other aerodynamic measures such as airway pressure were often reported.

Potential Confounders. There is significant potential variation in the technique of vocal fold injection: location (anterior–posterior, medial–lateral, intramuscular or paraglottic), volume, transcervical/transoral, etc. This problem could potentially be overcome by using a prospective study design in which the injection site and method are prespecified.

Study Designs. Within the 42 relevant studies identified, the injectable materials studied included autologous fat (14), collagen (5), acellular dermis (3), fascia (5), Teflon (4), silicone (5), and others/mixed (6). The injection material and evidence level provided by these studies are summarized in tabular format below. Eight of the studies are highlighted in additional detail in an adjoining table [2–9].

The study by Hertegard et al. [6] is one of only two prospective randomized controlled trials (RCTs) in the unilateral vocal fold paralysis (UVFP) literature. The injectable material (bovine collagen versus hyaluronan) was randomized and the patient (but not the surgeon) remained blinded to the assignment. The patients were all evaluated by a speech pathologist preoperatively, and those judged appropriate received voice therapy before entry in the study. One problem with this study is that both study arms included equal numbers of patients with paralysis and with glottal insufficiency because of vocal fold bowing, and the data were not formally segregated by diagnosis (although it is stated that there was no difference in results between these two groups). It is not stated in the article how many patients with UVFP were randomized into each arm.

The remaining studies lacked a separate control group. In these studies, patients received the intervention and their postoperative results were reported in either a prospective or retrospective manner. A wide variety of injection techniques were analyzed, such as transoral, transnasal, and transcutaneous approaches. Specific aspects of the technique of injection were nonuniformly reported.

Highest Level of Evidence. Among these papers, only two studies were prospective RCTs, providing level 1 evidence. Hertegard et al. reported a significantly better result with hyaluronan than with collagen; hyaluronan resorbed less and lasted longer over a period of 1 year. There were also 16 level 2 studies, 13 level 3 studies, and

11 level 4 studies. All 42 studies reported favorable voice outcomes with cord injection and their details are shown in the adjoining tables. Similar results were found using all of the different materials reported. Overall, the results supported the use of injection laryngoplasty for patients needing 6 weeks to 12+ months of benefit, or for patients willing to undergo repeat injections as needed for longer-term benefit.

Applicability. The patients in these studies were all adults with unilateral vocal fold paralysis with diverse etiologies, and the results are applicable to this patient population.

Morbidity/Complications. There were very few complications in any of the studies. The bovine collagen injection studies used a subcutaneous test injection to verify that the patients did not have an allergy. All of the injection materials, given transorally or transcutaneously, seemed to have been well tolerated by the patients. Long-term problems from the injected materials (e.g., granulomas) were not observed, although the follow-up periods were 1 year or less.

CLINICAL SIGNIFICANCE AND FUTURE RESEARCH

The role of injection laryngoplasty is not yet fully defined, and continues to evolve. These studies demonstrate, mostly with level 2 or 4 evidence, that voice improvement can be expected if the vocal fold is moved toward the midline, irrespective of which material is used. The timeframe of that effect, however, is variable. The continued search for an ideal injection material relates to the duration of effect. Initial publications focused on Teflon, collagen, and liquid silicone papers, whereas later papers moved toward autologous fat, micronized acellular dermis, and calcium hydroxylapatite injectables. Overall, the roles of injection laryngoplasty at present seem to be 1) a temporizing maneuver for patients with acute UVFP who need immediate improvement, but in whom some recovery or compensation is considered likely; or 2) a reasonable minimally invasive option for terminal patients (frequently, with UVFP as a result of lung cancer) or for other patients whose medical condition precludes an open procedure such as thyroplasty.

The RCT by Hertegard et al. demonstrates that randomized trials can be successfully performed in this patient population. If an injectable material is found that offers longer-lasting benefit, it would be reasonable and valuable to perform a prospective RCT comparing that injection to an open procedure such as type I thyroplasty. (Thyroplasty is discussed in the following section.) The ease of performing vocal fold injections in an outpatient setting has led some to conclude that the injection approach may be preferable to an open procedure, even if it needs to be repeated periodically. A longitudinal randomized study, focusing on quality of life issues, would be the best way to weigh the "hassle factor" of returning to the clinic for repeat injections against the simplicity of avoiding an open neck procedure. Such a comparison may be the most feasible, because accumulating untreated control groups willing to remain untreated for long follow-up times may be difficult; most patients do present to the clinic requesting some treatment and thus may be unlikely to agree to a prolonged untreated period.

Future studies should also increase the number of patients enrolled. Only one paper in this group had more than 30 patients in the study. None of the papers reported a formal power analysis, but clearly the statistical power of these studies can be a critical issue.

Vocal fold injection: Data overview

	Evidence level				
Injection material	1	2	3	4	Total
Fat	0	1	6	7	14
Collagen	0	0	3	2	5
Acellular dermis	0	3	0	0	3
Fascia	0	5	0	0	5
Teflon	0	1	2	1	4
Silicone	0	3	2	0	5
Other/mixed	2	3	0	1	6
Total	2	16	13	11	42

Publications meeting criteria

First author, year	Level (design)	Sample size	Material used
Pearl 2002	2 (prospective)	n = 14	AlloDerm
Milstein 2005	2 (prospective)	n = 20	AlloDerm
Karpenko 2003	2 (prospective)	n = 10	AlloDerm
Ford 1986	3 (retrospective)	n = 54	Collagen
Anderson 2004	4 (retrospective)	n = 2	Collagen
Remacle 1999	3 (retrospective)	n = 8	Collagen
Remacle 1999	3 (retrospective)	n = 13	Collagen
Sagawa 1999	4 (retrospective)	n = 17	Collagen
Rihkanen 1998	2 (prospective)	n = 9	Fascia
Rihkanen 1999	2 (prospective)	n = 18	Fascia
Saarinen 2000	2 (prospective)	n = 10	Fascia
Reijonen 2002	2 (prospective)	n = 14	Fascia
Rihkanen 2004	2 (prospective)	n = 14	Fascia
Shaw 1997	2 (prospective)	n = 22	Fat
Hsiung 2000	3 (retrospective)	n = 9	Fat
McCulloch 2002	3 (retrospective)	n = 44	Fat
Brandenburg 1996	4 (retrospective)	n = 10	Fat
Brandenburg 1992	3 (retrospective)	n = 11	Fat
Mikaelian 1991	4 (retrospective)	n = 3	Fat
Umeno 2005	3 (retrospective)	n = 41	Fat
Havas 2003	4 (retrospective)	n = 45	Fat
Tucker 2001	3 (retrospective)	n = 23	Fat
Oluwole 1996	4 (retrospective)	n = 14	Fat
Shindo 1996	4 (retrospective)	n = 21	Fat
Laccourreye 1998	4 (retrospective)	n = 3	Fat
Laccourreye 1999	3 (retrospective)	n = 20	Fat
Laccourreye 2003	4 (prospective case series)	n = 80	Fat
Belafsky 2004	2 (prospective)	n = 14	Calcium hydroxyapatite
Rosen 2004	2 (prospective)	n = 11	Calcium hydroxyapatite
Harries 1998	2 (prospective)	n = 8	Teflon
Chu 1997	3 (retrospective)	n = 20	Teflon
McCaffrey 1989	4 (retrospective)	n = 19	Teflon
Weber 1985	3 (retrospective)	n = 111	Teflon
Duruisseau 2004	3 (retrospective)	n = 19	Silicone
Iwatake 1996	3 (retrospective)	n = 30	Silicone
Hirano 1995	2 (prospective)	n = 240	Silicone
Hirano 1990	2 (prospective)	n = 42	Silicone
Hirano 1988	2 (prospective)	n = 10	Silicone
Hallen 2001	2 (prospective)	n = 6	Other
Sittel 2000	4 (retrospective)	n = 7	Other
Hertegard 2004	1 (randomized)	n = 70	Other
Hertegard 2002	1 (randomized)	n = 83	Other

THE EVIDENCE CONDENSED: Vocal fold injection for unilateral vocal fold paralysis

Reference	Hertegard, 2002		Hirano, 1995	Harries, 1998	Rihkanen, 2004
Level (design)	1 (randomized controlled trial)		2 (prospective comparative)	2 (prospective comparative)	2 (prospective comparative)
Sample size	29 with unilateral paralysis, 83 total		240	8	12
Material(s)	Hyaluronan	Collagen	Silicone	Teflon	Fascia
OUTCOMES					
Objective variables, results	MPT 9.3 → 11.7, MCQ 0.52 → 0.73	MPT 9.6 → 9.5, MCQ 0.38 → 0.66	MPT 4.3 → 10.6, F0r 15.2 → 18.6, SPL 20.8 → 29.2	MPT 3 → 8, SPLmax 79 → 96, SNR 4.7 → 11.1	Gap index 7.2 → 1.7, MPT 5.8 → 11.4, Grade 3.3 → 7.6, NHR 0.48 → 0.19
Subjective variables, results	Self-rated 100-pt VAS: H 38 → 61	Self-rated 100-pt VAS: 35 → 59	Self-eval. 100-pt scale 23.8 → 68.8	Self-rating voice 2.4 → 6.7	Listener panel: better roughness and breathiness
Duration of effect	12+ mo	12+ mo	12+ mo	6+ wk	12+ mo
Control	None	None	None	None	None
p Value	<0.05 vs baseline NS vs collagen	<0.05 vs baseline NS vs hylan B	<0.01	<0.05	<0.001 to <0.002
Conclusion	Hylan B better result than collagen, resorbs less and lasts longer		Highly effective	Good short-term result	Safe and effective
Follow-up time	1 y		1 d–9 y, mean 8 mo	6 wk	Mean 13 mo
STUDY DESIGN					
Inclusion criteria	UVFP		UVFP	UVFP, terminal	UVFP, failed voice therapy
Exclusion criteria	<18 y old; prior Rx; allergy to Rx; pregnant; inflammatory disease		NR	NR	Age <10 or >80 y, revisions
Intervention regimen details	Transoral, transnasal, or suspension DL		Transcutaneous injection with FOE monitor	Transcutaneous injection with FOE monitor	Suspension DL
Age range (mean)	23–90 y (66 y)		17–86 y (59 y)	41–72 y (67 y)	42–73 y (59 y)
Masking	Patients blinded to study arm		NR	NR	NR
Morbidity/ complications	3: local inflammation at 1 wk	None	7: dyspnea, 1: granuloma	None	NR

NR = not reported, DL = direct laryngoscopy, NS = not significant, VAS = visual analog scale, MPT = maximum phonation time, F0r = fundamental frequency range, MCQ = membranous contact quotient, SPL = sound pressure level, SNR = signal-to-noise ratio, NHR = noise-to-harmonic ratio, FOE = fiberoptic examination, UVFP = unilateral vocal fold paralysis, pt = point.

When a study reported a change in a parameter from pretreatment to posttreatment, this is indicated in the table by the two values separated by an arrow (e.g., 4.1 → 11.5).

THE EVIDENCE CONDENSED: Vocal fold injection for unilateral vocal fold paralysis

Reference	Shaw, 1997	Ford, 1986	Pearl, 2002	Belafsky, 2004
Level (design)	2 (prospective comparative)	3 (retrospective comparative)	2 (prospective comparative)	2 (prospective comparative)
Sample size	11	56	14	14
Material(s)	Fat	Collagen	AlloDerm	CaHA
OUTCOMES				
Objective variables, results	F0r 102 → 168, OQ 0.887 → 0.690, closure 1.8 → 4.0, Grade 4.7 → 2.9	MPT 16 → 22, V. intensity 70 → 74, F0 160 → 160	MPT 3.8 → 6.7, jitter 5.14 → 2.31, shimmer 10.86 → 3.74	Videostrobe—good mucosal waves
Subjective variables, results	Self-rating effort 3.7 → 1.5, sound 4.3 → 1.7, function 4.3 → 1.8	Improved subjective parameters	VHI 62.8 → 37.5	Glottic closure index 15 → 5
Duration of effect	12–18+ mo	12+ mo	3+ mo	TBD
Control	None	None	None	None
p Value	<0.05	NR	<0.01 to <0.05	<0.0001
Conclusion	Highly effective	Good results are technique-related	Safe, good short-term results	Likely safe and effective
Follow-up time	1 y	1 y	3 mo	mean 20 wk
STUDY DESIGN				
Inclusion criteria	UVFP with gap <5 mm	UVFP with GI	"Permanent" UVFP	UVFP
Exclusion criteria	NR	DNRTC; positive skin test	NR	NR
Intervention regimen details	Suspension DL	Transoral injection	Suspension DL	Suspension DL
Age range (mean)	28–81 y (55 y)	26–77 y (55 y)	39–87 y (58 y)	(62 y)
Masking	NR	NR	NR	NR
Morbidity/complications	NR	NR	2/14 p-op stridor	2: resorption at 3 mo

NR = not reported, GI = glottic insufficiency, DL = direct laryngoscopy, VHI = voice handicap index, NS = not significant, MPT = maximum phonation time, F0r = fundamental frequency range, OQ = open quotient, SPL = sound pressure level, CaHA = calcium hydroxylapatite, TBD = to be determined, UVFP = unilateral vocal fold paralysis, DNRTC = did not return to clinic.
When a study reported a change in a parameter from pretreatment to posttreatment, this is indicated in the table by the two values separated by an arrow (e.g., 4.1 → 11.5).

REFERENCES

1. Pearl AW, Woo P, Ostrowski R, Mojica J, Mandell DL, Costantino P. A preliminary report on micronized Allo-Derm injection laryngoplasty. Laryngoscope 2002;112(6): 990–996.
2. Milstein CF, Akst LM, Hicks MD, Abelson TI, Strome M. Long-term effects of micronized AlloDerm injection for unilateral vocal fold paralysis. Laryngoscope 2005;115(9): 1691–1696.
3. Karpenko AN, Dworkin JP, Meleca RJ, Stachler RJ, Priestley KJ. Cymetra injection for unilateral vocal fold paralysis. Ann Otol Rhinol Laryngol 2003;112(11):927–934.
4. Ford CN, Bless DM. Clinical experience with injectable collagen for vocal fold augmentation. Laryngoscope 1986; 96(8):863–869.
5. Anderson TD, Sataloff RT. Complications of collagen injection of the vocal fold: report of several unusual cases and review of the literature. J Voice 2004;18(3):392–397.
6. Remacle M, Lawson G, Delos M, Jamart J. Correcting vocal fold immobility by autologous collagen injection for voice rehabilitation. A short-term study. Ann Otol Rhinol Laryngol 1999;108(8):788–793.
7. Remacle M, Lawson G, Keghian J, Jamart J. Use of inject-able autologous collagen for correcting glottic gaps: initial results. J Voice 1999;13(2):280–288.
8. Sagawa M, Sato M, Fujimura S, et al. Vocal fold injection of collagen for unilateral vocal fold paralysis caused by chest diseases. J Cardiovasc Surg 1999;40:603–605.
9. Rihkanen H. Vocal fold augmentation by injection of autologous fascia. Laryngoscope 1998;108(1 Pt 1):51–54.
10. Rihkanen H, Lehikoinen-Soderlund S, Reijonen P. Voice acoustics after autologous fascia injection for vocal fold paralysis. Laryngoscope 1999;109(11):1854–1858.
11. Saarinen A, Rihkanen H, Lehikoinen-Soderlund S, Sovi-jarvi AR. Airway flow dynamics and voice acoustics after autologous fascia augmentation of paralyzed vocal fold. Ann Otol Rhinol Laryngol 2000;109(6):563–567.
12. Reijonen P, Lehikoinen-Soderlund S, Rihkanen H. Results of fascial augmentation in unilateral vocal fold paralysis. Ann Otol Rhinol Laryngol 2002;111(6):523–529.

13. Rihkanen H, Reijonen P, Lehikoinen-Soderlund S, Lauri ER. Videostroboscopic assessment of unilateral vocal fold paralysis after augmentation with autologous fascia. Eur Arch Otorhinolaryngol 2004;261(4):177–183.

14. Shaw GY, Szewczyk MA, Searle J, Woodroof J. Autologous fat injection into the vocal folds: technical considerations and long-term follow-up. Laryngoscope 1997;107(2):177–186.

15. Hsiung MW, Woo P, Minasian A, Schaefer Mojica J. Fat augmentation for glottic insufficiency. Laryngoscope 2000;110(6):1026–1033.

16. McCulloch TM, Andrews BT, Hoffman HT, Graham SM, Karnell MP, Minnick C. Long-term follow-up of fat injection laryngoplasty for unilateral vocal cord paralysis. Laryngoscope 2002;112(7 Pt 1):1235–1238.

17. Brandenburg JH, Unger JM, Koschkee D. Vocal cord injection with autogenous fat: a long-term magnetic resonance imaging evaluation. Laryngoscope 1996;106(2 Pt 1):174–180.

18. Brandenburg JH, Kirkham W, Koschkee D. Vocal cord augmentation with autogenous fat. Laryngoscope 1992;102(5):495–500.

19. Mikaelian DO, Lowry LD, Sataloff RT. Lipoinjection for unilateral vocal cord paralysis. Laryngoscope 1991;101(5):465–468.

20. Umeno H, Shirouzu H, Chitose S, Nakashima T. Analysis of voice function following autologous fat injection for vocal fold paralysis. Otolaryngol Head Neck Surg 2005;132(1):103–107.

21. Havas TE. Autologous fat injection laryngoplasty for unilateral vocal fold paralysis. ANZ J Surg 2003;73(11):938–943.

22. Tucker HM. Direct autogenous fat implantation for augmentation of the vocal folds. J Voice 2001;15(4):565–569.

23. Oluwole M, Mills RP, Davis BC, Blair RL. The management of unilateral vocal cord palsy by augmentation using autologous fat. Clin Otolaryngol Allied Sci 1996;21(4):357–359.

24. Shindo ML, Zaretsky LS, Rice DH. Autologous fat injection for unilateral vocal fold paralysis. Ann Otol Rhinol Laryngol 1996;105(8):602–606.

25. Laccourreye O, Crevier-Buchman L, Le Pimpec-Barthes F, Garcia D, Riquet M, Brasnu D. Recovery of function after intracordal autologous fat injection for unilateral recurrent laryngeal nerve paralysis. J Laryngol Otol 1998;112(11):1082–1084.

26. Laccourreye O, Paczona R, Ageel M, Hans S, Brasnu D, Crevier-Buchman L. Intracordal autologous fat injection for aspiration after recurrent laryngeal nerve paralysis. Eur Arch Otorhinolaryngol 1999;256(9):458–461.

27. Laccourreye O, Papon JF, Kania R, Crevier-Buchman L, Brasnu D, Hans S. Intracordal injection of autologous fat in patients with unilateral laryngeal nerve paralysis: long-term results from the patient's perspective. Laryngoscope 2003;113(3):541–545.

28. Belafsky PC, Postma GN. Vocal fold augmentation with calcium hydroxylapatite. Otolaryngol Head Neck Surg 2004;131(4):351–354.

29. Rosen CA, Thekdi AA. Vocal fold augmentation with injectable calcium hydroxylapatite: short-term results. J Voice 2004;18(3):387–391.

30. Harries ML, Morrison M. Management of unilateral vocal cord paralysis by injection medialization with teflon paste. Quantitative results. Ann Otol Rhinol Laryngol 1998;107(4):332–336.

31. Chu PY, Chang SY. Transoral Teflon injection under flexible laryngovideostroboscopy for unilateral vocal fold paralysis. Ann Otol Rhinol Laryngol 1997;106(9):783–786.

32. McCaffrey TB, Lipton R. Transcutaneous Teflon injection for paralytic dysphonia. Laryngoscope 1989;99(5):497–499.

33. Weber RS, Neumayer L, Alford BR, Weber SC. Clinical restoration of voice function after loss of the vagus nerve. Head Neck Surg 1985;7(6):448–457.

34. Duruisseau O, Wagner I, Fugain C, Chabolle F. Endoscopic rehabilitation of vocal cord paralysis with a silicone elastomer suspension implant. Otolaryngol Head Neck Surg 2004;131(3):241–247.

35. Iwatake H, Iida J, Minami S, Sugano S, Hoshikawa T, Takeyama I. Transcutaneous intracordal silicon injection for unilateral vocal cord paralysis. Acta Otolaryngol Suppl 1996;522:133–137.

36. Hirano M, Mori K, Tanaka S, Fujita M. Vocal function in patients with unilateral vocal fold paralysis before and after silicone injection. Acta Otolaryngol 1995;115(4):553–559.

37. Hirano M, Tanaka S, Tanaka Y, Hibi S. Transcutaneous intrafold injection for unilateral vocal fold paralysis: functional results. Ann Otol Rhinol Laryngol 1990;99(8):598–604.

38. Hirano M, Hibi S, Yoshida T, Hirade Y, Kasuya H, Kikuchi Y. Acoustic analysis of pathological voice. Some results of clinical application. Acta Otolaryngol 1988;105(5–6):432–438.

39. Hallen L, Testad P, Sederholm E, Dahlqvist A, Laurent C. DiHA (dextranomers in hyaluronan) injections for treatment of insufficient closure of the vocal folds: early clinical experiences. Laryngoscope 2001;111(6):1063–1067.

40. Sittel C, Thumfart WF, Pototschnig C, Wittekindt C, Eckel HE. Textured polydimethylsiloxane elastomers in the human larynx: safety and efficiency of use. J Biomed Mater Res 2000;53(6):646–650.

41. Hertegard S, Hallen L, Laurent C, Lindstrom E, Olofsson K, Testad P, Dahlqvist A. Cross-linked hyaluronan versus collagen for injection treatment of glottal insufficiency: 2-year follow-up. Acta Otolaryngol 2004;124(10):1208–1214.

42. Hertegard S, Hallen L, Laurent C, et al. Cross-linked hyaluronan used as augmentation substance for treatment of glottal insufficiency: safety aspects and vocal fold function. Laryngoscope 2002;112(12):2211–2219.

24 Unilateral Vocal Cord Paralysis

24.C.i.

Open medialization with implant: Impact on subjective and objective measures of voice

Randall C. Paniello

Laryngeal framework surgery for unilateral vocal cord paralysis includes two complementary but different approaches to achieving vocal fold medialization. The first approach comprises medialization procedures involving an implant, similar to Isshiki's type I thyroplasty. In medialization laryngoplasty (ML), the vocal fold is pushed toward the midline by placing an implant between the vocal fold and the inner aspect of the thyroid cartilage. An additional approach (arytenoid adduction) is discussed in the subsequent section.

METHODS

A computerized PubMed search of MEDLINE listings from 1966 to 2005 was performed, using keywords "vocal," "fold" or "cord," "paralysis" or "paresis" or "immobility" or "movement impairment," and "treatment." This process yielded 1930 publications. Papers were reviewed to identify those that met the following inclusion criteria: 1) adult patient population with unilateral vocal cord paralysis, 2) intervention with ML (i.e., placing a solid implant between the vocal fold and the inner aspect of the thyroid cartilage to medialize the paralyzed cord), 3) outcome measured in terms of subjective or objective measures of voice. The search was then further limited by excluding isolated case reports of single patients, papers on the incidence or etiology of vocal fold paralysis, review articles with no new patient data (except meta-analyses), duplicate or follow-up papers, and papers focusing on nonvoice outcomes such as swallowing. In addition, articles that focused on bilateral vocal cord paralysis were excluded. The bibliographies of the selected papers were reviewed to determine whether any additional studies had been missed in the search, and these were added. A total of 52 papers met the search criteria [1–52].

RESULTS

Outcome Measures. Several of these studies used Hirano's GRBAS scale (Grade, Roughness, Breathiness, Asthenia, Strain), a perceptual rating system that can be taught and standardized. Also frequently reported were other objective measures based on computerized waveform analysis of sustained vowels, especially noise-to-harmonic ratio (NHR), jitter percent, and shimmer percent. The NHR is directly related to the amount of random

vibration that occurs from a flaccid, paralyzed fold that is not making good contact with the opposite side (i.e., it is a measure with high sensitivity for the condition under study). Maximum phonation time was used as an indirect measure of the glottal gap in some studies. Most studies did not directly measure glottic gap by videostroboscopy.

Potential Confounders. Potential confounders are multiple, as described in the initial overview in this chapter. For example, the use of concomitant voice therapy should ideally be taken into account. The additional variable of voice therapy may influence results in addition to the implant that is the focus of the study. More than half of the patients in the Schneider study had preoperative and postoperative speech therapy, whereas the authors of the McLean-Muse study specifically noted that none of their patients underwent voice therapy between preoperative and postoperative evaluations.

Study Designs. Within the 52 relevant studies, the types of implant material included silastic (20), the Montgomery implant (silicone) (5), GORE-TEX (expanded polytetrafluoroethylene, or ePTFE) (6), titanium/metallic (6), and others (6). Ten of the reports did not specifically state which implant type was used. There were 20 level 2 studies, 24 level 3 studies, and 9 level 4 studies, which were categorized by the type of implant and study design as shown in the table below.

Seven studies (selected by the criteria described in the overview to this chapter) are highlighted in additional detail in the adjoining table [10–16]. The paper by Plant et al. is presented in detail because it was the only study to use an untreated control group. For this "observation" group, voice recordings were made at two separate points in time (interval not reported) with no treatment performed between recordings. Nouwen et al. compared two types of ML (Montgomery implant versus GORE-TEX implant), but it is noted in the paper that "the decision of which technique to choose was left to the surgeon's discretion." This discretion, which may have favored the use of one implant in more affected patients, as well as the difference in the pretreatment voice severity scores between the two groups, must be taken into account with the direct comparison of the two implants.

The majority of studies regarding this topic compared preoperative to postoperative results. In the Haijoff study, 27 patients underwent silastic implantation; they completed preoperative and postoperative vocal performance questionnaires; the Nottingham Health Profile (NHP); instrumental analyses of jitter, shimmer, and NHR; and perceptual analyses of GRBAS. The McCulloch paper compared preoperative and postoperative voice scores with expanded polytetrafluoroethylene (GORE-TEX) ML in 16 patients. In the Lu study, 53 patients with unilateral vocal fold paralysis (UVFP) underwent vocal-function evaluation preoperatively and up to 6 months postoperatively. Vocal-function assessment included videostrobolaryngoscopic examination, acoustical and aerodynamic analysis, and perceptual judgment of voice characteristics. In the McLean-Muse study, 43 patients who were treated with the Montgomery Thyroplasty Implant System underwent preoperative and postoperative videostroboscopic, acoustic, aerodynamic, and clinical evaluations. Schneider reported the results with a titanium medialization implant in 28 patients; perceptive voice sound analysis, voice range profile measurements, videostroboscopy, and pulmonary function tests were performed. Most studies in this group had relatively short follow-up periods, with most patients followed for only 1–4 months, although follow-up was as long as 30 months in selected reports.

Highest Level of Evidence. Among these studies, nearly all showed improvement after this procedure. There were some patients in most studies that had little benefit and a rare patient that was worse, but the vast majority were better after medialization in every study.

The level 2 studies highlighted in this section showed that ML was an effective treatment for patients with UVFP. In the Plant study, the observation group showed a very slight deterioration in voice rating, compared with a significant improvement in rating in the postoperative group. In the Haijoff study, significant improvements were found in instrumental, perceptual and self-assessment of voice and the energy, social, and emotional dimensions of the NHP. Three patients had initially poor results but were successfully revised. The Lu study showed significant improvements in glottic-gap size, maximum phonation time, glottic-flow rate, jitter, NHP, breathiness, hoarseness, loudness, and phrasing after thyroplasty and remained stable as early as 1 month postoperatively, with only slight fluctuations over a 6-month period. The McLean-Muse team reported improvements in postoperative glottal closure, vocal fold amplitude, mucosal wave activity, average intensity, maximum intensity range, maximum phonation time, glottal airflow, average sound pressure, and subglottal pressure. They also noted that a majority of patients expressed satisfaction with the surgery and resulting voice quality. In the Schneider study, all voice-related parameters showed a significant improvement after titanium implantation.

Applicability. These studies included only adult patients with UVFP. A minority of subjects had undergone previous vocal fold injection or arytenoid adduction.

Morbidity/Complications. The complication rate in these studies was small. The most significant complication was the need to place a tracheotomy in one patient. Among 236 patients in seven publications, there were five cases of implant extrusion (2.1%), and three cases of implant malpositioning (1.3%). Occasional minor medical complications, consistent with UVFP patients' underlying disease processes, were also reported.

CLINICAL SIGNIFICANCE AND FUTURE RESEARCH

There are 52 studies that focus on patients who underwent ML for adult UVFP. All papers showed that the majority of patients improved after medialization. Also, one study (Plant et al.) showed that patients who were implanted had significantly better voice outcomes than those who underwent observation alone. One additional study compared two types of ML (Montgomery implant versus GORE-TEX implant), but differences in the pretreatment voice severity scores between the two groups temper interpretation of their results.

Some authors have reported that the initial benefit from ML may diminish with time, because of late vocal fold atrophy (up to 2 years post-onset). In considering future research, longer follow-up periods would be helpful in determining whether any of the ML implants is more robust against the effects of atrophy. Future studies may follow the example of Plant et al. by including an untreated observation group. In addition, potential confounders such as the concomitant use of voice therapy could be strictly controlled. In addition, there are multiple validated instruments to measure voice outcomes that could be utilized further in prospective studies.

Open medialization with implant: Data overview

Implant type	Evidence level				Total
	1	2	3	4	
Silastic	0	6	11	3	20
Not stated	0	6	0	4	10
Montgomery	0	2	2	1	5
GORE-TEX	0	3	3	0	6
Titanium/metal	0	0	6	0	6
Other	0	3	2	1	6
Total	0	20	24	9	52

Composite total is not additive because one study used both GORE-TEX and Montgomery implants.

Publications meeting criteria

First author, year	Level (design)	Sample size	Material used
Gray 1992	2 (prospective)	n = 15	Not specified
Harries 1995	2 (prospective)	n = 10	Not specified
Adams 1996	2 (prospective)	n = 9	Not specified
Plant 1997	2 (prospective)	n = 16	Not specified
Hajioff 2000	2 (prospective)	n = 27	Not specified
Sridhara 2003	2 (prospective)	n = 15	Not specified
Hamdan 2004	4 (retrospective)	n = NA	Not specified
Rosingh 1995	4 (retrospective)	n = 29	Not specified
Kumar 2001	4 (retrospective)	n = 10	Not specified
Bryant 1996	4 (retrospective)	n = 4	Not specified
Ramadan 1996	3 (retrospective)	n = 29	Silastic
Gorham 1998	3 (retrospective)	n = 38	Silastic
Lundy 2000	3 (retrospective)	n = 26	Silastic
Lu 1996	2 (prospective)	n = 49	Silastic
Lundy 2004	2 (prospective)	n = 20	Silastic
Billante 2001	2 (prospective)	n = 28	Silastic
Billante 2002	2 (prospective)	n = 40	Silastic
Billante 2002	4 (prospective)	n = 35	Silastic
Sasaki 1990	2 (prospective)	n = 13	Silastic
Koufman 1986	3 (retrospective)	n = 11	Silastic
Mori 1994	3 (retrospective)	n = 21	Silastic
Omori 1996	3 (retrospective)	n = 20	Silastic
Omori 1996	3 (retrospective)	n = 22	Silastic
Omori 2000	3 (retrospective)	n = 18	Silastic
Hogikyan 2000	3 (retrospective)	n = 30	Silastic
Shin 2002	2 (prospective)	n = 20	Silastic
Kraus 1996	4 (retrospective)	n = 48	Silastic
LaBlance 1992	3 (retrospective)	n = 8	Silastic
Abraham 2002	4 (retrospective)	n = 11	Silastic
Abdel-Aziz 1998	3 (retrospective)	n = 12	Silastic
Gliklich 1999	2 (prospective)	n = 56	Montgomery
Mclean-Muse 2000	3 (retrospective)	n = 43	Montgomery
Laccourreye 2005	3 (retrospective)	n = 96	Montgomery
Montgomery 1997	4 (retrospective)	n = 176	Montgomery
Nouwen 2004	2 (prospective)	n = 57	GORE-TEX or Montgomery
McCulloch 1998	2 (prospective)	n = 16	GORE-TEX
Selber 2003	2 (prospective)	n = 14	GORE-TEX
Cohen 2004	3 (retrospective)	n = 16	GORE-TEX
Giovanni 1999	3 (retrospective)	n = 13	GORE-TEX
Stasney 2001	3 (retrospective)	n = 26	GORE-TEX
Dulguerov 1999	3 (prospective)	n = 22	Other
Hong 2001	2 (prospective)	n = 6	Other
Nishiyama 2002	2 (prospective)	n = 8	Other
Alves 2002	2 (prospective)	n = 16	Other
Tanaka 2004	4 (retrospective)	n = 9	Other
Sakai 1996	3 (retrospective)	n = 10	Other
Schneider 2003	3 (retrospective)	n = 14	Titanium/metallic
Schneider 2003	3 (retrospective)	n = 28	Titanium/metallic
Schneider 2003	3 (retrospective)	n = 28	Titanium/metallic
Schneider 2003	3 (retrospective)	n = 30	Titanium/metallic
Dean 2001	3 (retrospective)	n = 53	Titanium/metallic
Friedrich 1999	3 (retrospective)	n = 20	Titanium/metallic

THE EVIDENCE CONDENSED: Medialization laryngoplasty for unilateral vocal fold paralysis

Reference	McLean-Muse, 2000	Nouwen, 2004		Schneider, 2003
Level (design)	3 (retrospective comparative)	2 (prospective comparative)		2 (retrospective comparative)
Implant type	Montgomery	GORE-TEX	Montgomery	Titanium
Sample size	43	24	33	28
OUTCOMES				
Objective variables, results	MPT 7.5 → 15.7, MIR 34.5 → 43.4, MW nl 13 → 31	Shimmer % 12.5 → 8.6, NHR 0.26 → 0.2, SR 116 → 130	Shimmer % 8.9 → 5.3, NHR 0.17 → 0.14, SR 129 → 149	s/z 3.4 → 1.7, VDI 2.6 → 1.3
Subjective variables, results	80% of voices judged improved 80% of patients satisfied	Self-assessment: "improved" 100%		Grade 2.7 → 1.0, rough 2.6 → 1.0, breathy 2.4 → 0.7
Untreated control	None	None		None
p Value	<0.05	<0.05		<0.001
Conclusion	Implant system works as well as other methods	Montgomery implant better results than GORE-TEX; study limited by certain biases		Easy, worked well, all parameters improved
Follow-up time	1.5–30 mo	1 mo		6–30 mo
STUDY DESIGN				
Inclusion criteria	UVFP	UVFP		UVFP
Exclusion criteria	NR	NR		NR
Age range (mean)	19–83 y (59 y)	35–86 y (53 y)	32–84 y (57 y)	19–84 y (57 y)
Masking	Panel blinded to pre- or postoperative	NR		Not specified
Morbidity/complications	NR	n = 3: unable to insert Montgomery, used GORE-TEX n = 2: late—implant extruded/dislodged		n = 7: small hematoma n = 1: repositioned

UVFP = unilateral vocal fold paralysis, NHR = noise-to-harmonic ratio, MPT = maximum phonation time, MW = mucosal wave, MIR = maximum intensity range, SR = speech rate (words/min), VDI = voice dysfunction index, NR = not reported.
When a study reported a change in a parameter from pretreatment to posttreatment, this is indicated in the table by the two values separated by an arrow (e.g., 4.1 → 11.5).

THE EVIDENCE CONDENSED: Medialization laryngoplasty for unilateral vocal fold paralysis

Reference	Hajioff, 2000	Plant, 1997	Lu, 1996	McCullough, 1998
Level (design)	2 (prospective comparative)	2 (prospective comparative)	2 (prospective comparative)	2 (prospective comparative)
Implant type	Silastic	Not specified	Not specified	GORE-TEX
Sample size	27	16	49	16
OUTCOMES				
Objective variables, results	Jitter %, shimmer %, NHR, GRBAS improved	Pitch amplitude +1.51	GGap 3.3 → 1.2, MPT 6 → 11, jitter % 70 → 5	NR
Subjective variables, results	VPQ 35 → 18, NHPE 61 → 24, NHPS 10 → 0	Perceptual rating −1.01 units	Loud 2.4 → 3.7, breathy 2.5 → 0.75, hoarse 2.0 → 1.2	Grade 2.3 → 1.1, breathy 2.0 → 0.4
Untreated control	None	Untreated UVFP	None	None
p Value	<0.001	<0.01	<0.05	<0.01
Conclusion	Quality of life improvement because of voice improvement	Pitch amplitude best correlate to perceptual rating	Benefit at 1 mo lasts to 6 mo but never normal	Works well, easy, can be combined with other procedures
Follow-up time	1–14 mo (mean 4)	1–10 wk (mean 3)	6 mo	1–12 mo (mean 6)
STUDY DESIGN				
Inclusion criteria	UVFP	UVFP	UVFP	UVFP
Exclusion criteria	NR	NR	Revisions	NR
Age range (mean)	44–91 y (66 y)	(58 y)	16–81 y (52 y)	13–83 y (62 y)
Masking	NR	Panel blinded to study group	Treating SLP nonblinded ratings	NR
Morbidity/complications	n = 1: pneumonia, n = 1: stridor	NR	n = 3: late implant extrusion	n = 1: late trach n = 2: revisions

UVFP = unilateral vocal fold paralysis, NHR = noise-to-harmonic ratio, GGap = glottal gap, NR = not reported, VPQ = vocal performance questionnaire, NHPE = Nottingham Health Profile/Energy, NHPS = Nottingham Health Profile/Social Isolation, SLP = speech language pathologist. When a study reported a change in a parameter from pretreatment to posttreatment, this is indicated in the table by the two values separated by an arrow (e.g., 4.1 → 11.5).

REFERENCES

1. Gray SD, Barkmeier J, Jones D, Titze I, Druker D. Vocal evaluation of thyroplastic surgery in the treatment of unilateral vocal fold paralysis. Laryngoscope 1992;102(4): 415–421.
2. Harries ML, Morrison M. Short-term results of laryngeal framework surgery: thyroplasty type I—a pilot study. J Otolaryngol 1995;24(5):281–287.
3. Adams SG, Irish JC, Durkin LC, Wong DL, Brown DH. Evaluation of vocal function in unilateral vocal fold paralysis following thyroplastic surgery. J Otolaryngol 1996;25(3):165–170.
4. Plant RL, Hillel AD, Waugh PF. Analysis of voice changes after thyroplasty using linear predictive coding. Laryngoscope 1997;107(6):703–709.
5. Hajioff D, Rattenbury H, Carrie S, Carding P, Wilson J. The effect of Isshiki type 1 thyroplasty on quality of life and vocal performance. Clin Otolaryngol Allied Sci 2000; 25(5):418–422.
6. Sridhara SR, Ashok KG, Raghunathan M, Mann SB. To study voice quality before and after thyroplasty type 1 in patients with symptomatic unilateral vocal cord paralysis. Am J Otolaryngol 2003;24(6):361–365.
7. Hamdan AL, Mokarbel R, Dagher W. Medialization laryngoplasty for the treatment of unilateral vocal cord paralysis: a perceptual, acoustic and stroboscopic evaluation. J Med Liban 2004;52(3):136–141.
8. Rosingh HJ, Dikkers FG. Thyroplasty to improve the voice in patients with a unilateral vocal fold paralysis. Clin Otolaryngol Allied Sci 1995;20(2):124–126.
9. Kumar VP, Reddy SR. Medialisation laryngoplasty: a new surgical frontier in the management of vocal cord paralysis. J Indian Med Assoc 2001;99(11):638–639.
10. Bryant NJ, Gracco LC, Sasaki CT, Vining E. MRI evaluation of vocal fold paralysis before and after type I thyroplasty. Laryngoscope 1996;106(11):1386–1392.
11. Ramadan HH. Medialization laryngoplasty for the treatment of unilateral vocal cord paralysis. W V Med J 1996; 92(5):268–270.
12. Gorham MM, Avidano MA, Crary MA, Cotter CS, Cassisi NJ. Laryngeal recovery following type I thyroplasty. Arch Otolaryngol Head Neck Surg 1998;124(7):739–742.
13. Lundy DS, Casiano RR, Xue JW, Lu FL. Thyroplasty type I: short-versus long-term results. Otolaryngol Head Neck Surg 2000;122(4):533–536.
14. Lu FL, Casiano RR, Lundy DS, Xue JW. Longitudinal evaluation of vocal function after thyroplasty type I in the

treatment of unilateral vocal paralysis. Laryngoscope 1996;106(5 Pt 1):573–577.

15. Lundy DS, Casiano RR, Xue JW. Can maximum phonation time predict voice outcome after thyroplasty type I? Laryngoscope 2004;114(8):1447–1454.

16. Billante CR, Spector B, Hudson M, Burkard K, Netterville JL. Voice outcome following thyroplasty in patients with cancer-related vocal fold paralysis. Auris Nasus Larynx 2001;28(4):315–321.

17. Billante CR, Clary J, Childs P, Netterville JL. Voice gains following thyroplasty may improve over time. Clin Otolaryngol Allied Sci 2002;27(2):89–94.

18. Billante CR, Clary J, Sullivan C, Netterville JL. Voice outcome following thyroplasty in patients with longstanding vocal fold immobility. Auris Nasus Larynx 2002; 29(4):341–345.

19. Sasaki CT, Leder SB, Petcu L, Friedman CD. Longitudinal voice quality changes following Isshiki thyroplasty type I: the Yale experience. Laryngoscope 1990;100(8):849–852.

20. Koufman JA. Laryngoplasty for vocal cord medialization: an alternative to Teflon. Laryngoscope 1986;96(7):726–731.

21. Mori K, Blaugrund SM, Yu JD. The turbulent noise ratio: an estimation of noise power of the breathy voice using PARCOR analysis. Laryngoscope 1994;104(2):153–158.

22. Omori K, Kacker A, Slavit DH, Blaugrund SM. Quantitative videostroboscopic measurement of glottal gap and vocal function: an analysis of thyroplasty type I. Ann Otol Rhinol Laryngol 1996;105(4):280–285.

23. Omori K, Slavit DH, Kacher A, Blaugrund SM. Quantitative criteria for predicting thyroplasty type I outcome. Laryngoscope 1996;106(6):689–693.

24. Omori K, Slavit DH, Kacker A, Blaugrund SM, Kojima H. Effects of thyroplasty type I on vocal fold vibration. Laryngoscope 2000;110(7):1086–1091.

25. Hogikyan ND, Wodchis WP, Terrell JE, Bradford CR, Esclamado RM. Voice-related quality of life (V-RQOL) following type I thyroplasty for unilateral vocal fold paralysis. J Voice 2000;14(3):378–386.

26. Shin JE, Nam SY, Yoo SJ, Kim SY. Analysis of voice and quantitative measurement of glottal gap after thyroplasty type I in the treatment of unilateral vocal paralysis. J Voice 2002;16(1):136–142.

27. Kraus DH, Ali MK, Ginsberg RJ, et al. Vocal cord medialization for unilateral paralysis associated with intrathoracic malignancies. J Thorac Cardiovasc Surg 1996;111(2):334–339; discussion 339–341.

28. LaBlance GR, Maves MD. Acoustic characteristics of post-thyroplasty patients. Otolaryngol Head Neck Surg 1992;107(4):558–563.

29. Abraham MT, Bains MS, Downey RJ, Korst RJ, Kraus DH. Type I thyroplasty for acute unilateral vocal fold paralysis following intrathoracic surgery. Ann Otol Rhinol Laryngol 2002;111(8):667–671.

30. Abdel-Aziz MF, el-Hak NA, Carding PN. Thyroplasty for functional rehabilitation of the incompetent larynx. J Laryngol Otol 1998;112(12):1172–1175.

31. Gliklich RE, Glovsky RM, Montgomery WW. Validation of a voice outcome survey for unilateral vocal cord paralysis. Otolaryngol Head Neck Surg 1999;120(2):153–158.

32. McLean-Muse A, Montgomery WW, Hillman RE, et al. Montgomery thyroplasty implant for vocal fold immobility: phonatory outcomes. Ann Otol Rhinol Laryngol 2000;109(4):393–400.

33. Laccourreye O, El Sharkawy L, Holsinger FC, Hans S, Menard M, Brasnu D. Thyroplasty type I with Montgomery implant among native French language speakers with unilateral laryngeal nerve paralysis. Laryngoscope 2005;115(8):1411–1417.

34. Montgomery WW, Montgomery SK. Montgomery thyroplasty implant system. Ann Otol Rhinol Laryngol Suppl 1997;170:1–16.

35. Nouwen J, Hans S, De Mones E, Brasnu D, Crevier-Buchman L, Laccourreye O. Thyroplasty type I without arytenoid adduction in patients with unilateral laryngeal nerve paralysis: the Montgomery implant versus the Gore-Tex implant. Acta Otolaryngol 2004;124(6):732–738.

36. McCulloch TM, Hoffman HT. Medialization laryngoplasty with expanded polytetrafluoroethylene. Surgical technique and preliminary results. Ann Otol Rhinol Laryngol 1998;107(5 Pt 1):427–432.

37. Selber J, Sataloff R, Spiegel J, Heman-Ackah Y. Gore-Tex medialization thyroplasty: objective and subjective evaluation. J Voice 2003;17(1):88–95.

38. Cohen JT, Bates DD, Postma GN. Revision Gore-Tex medialization laryngoplasty. Otolaryngol Head Neck Surg 2004;131(3):236–240.

39. Giovanni A, Vallicioni JM, Gras R, Zanaret M. Clinical experience with Gore-Tex for vocal fold medialization. Laryngoscope 1999;109(2 Pt 1):284–288.

40. Stasney CR, Beaver ME, Rodriguez M. Minifenestration type I thyroplasty using an expanded polytetrafluoroethylene implant. J Voice 2001;15(1):151–157.

41. Dulguerov P, Schweizer V, Caumel I, Esteve F. Medialization laryngoplasty. Otolaryngol Head Neck Surg 1999;120(2):275–278.

42. Hong KH, Kim JH, Kim HK. Anterior and posterior medialization (APM) thyroplasty. Laryngoscope 2001;111(8):1406–1412.

43. Nishiyama K, Hirose H, Iguchi Y, Nagai H, Yamanaka J, Okamoto M. Autologous transplantation of fascia into the vocal fold as a treatment for recurrent nerve paralysis. Laryngoscope 2002;112(8 Pt 1):1420–1425.

44. Alves CB, Loughran S, MacGregor FB, Dey JI, Bowie LJ. Bioplastique medialization therapy improves the quality of life in terminally ill patients with vocal cord palsy. Clin Otolaryngol Allied Sci 2002;27(5):387–391.

45. Tanaka S, Asato R, Hiratsuka Y. Nerve-muscle transplantation to the paraglottic space after resection of recurrent laryngeal nerve. Laryngoscope 2004;114(6):1118–1122.

46. Sakai N, Nishizawa N, Matsushima J, et al. Thyroplasty type I with ceramic shim. Artif Organs 1996;20(8):951–954.

47. Schneider B, Bigenzahn W, End A, Denk DM, Klepetko W. External vocal fold medialization in patients with recurrent nerve paralysis following cardiothoracic surgery. Eur J Cardiothorac Surg 2003;23(4):477–483.

48. Schneider B, Denk DM, Bigenzahn W. Functional results after external vocal fold medialization thyroplasty with the titanium vocal fold medialization implant. Laryngoscope 2003;113(4):628–634.

49. Schneider B, Denk DM, Bigenzahn W. Acoustic assessment of the voice quality before and after medialization thyroplasty using the titanium vocal fold medialization implant (TVFMI). Otolaryngol Head Neck Surg 2003;128(6):815–822.

50. Schneider B, Kneussl M, Denk DM, Bigenzahn W. Aerodynamic measurements in medialization thyroplasty. Acta Otolaryngol 2003;123(7):883–888.

51. Dean CM, Ahmarani C, Bettez M, Heuer RJ. The adjustable laryngeal implant. J Voice 2001;15(1):141–150.

52. Friedrich G. Titanium vocal fold medializing implant: introducing a novel implant system for external vocal fold medialization. Ann Otol Rhinol Laryngol 1999;108(1):79–86.

24 Unilateral Vocal Cord Paralysis

Medialization laryngoplasty alone versus medialization with arytenoid adduction: Comparative voice outcomes

Randall C. Paniello and Jennifer J. Shin

Arytenoid adduction (AA) procedures reposition the arytenoid cartilage to move the vocal fold toward the midline; traction on a suture passed through the muscular process rotates the arytenoid so that the vocal process moves medially.

METHODS

A computerized PubMed search of MEDLINE listings from 1966 to 2005 was performed, using keywords "vocal," "fold" or "cord," "paralysis" or "paresis" or "immobility" or "movement impairment," and "treatment." This process yielded 1930 publications. Papers were reviewed to identify those that met the following inclusion criteria: 1) adult patient population with unilateral vocal cord paralysis, 2) intervention with medialization laryngoplasty (ML) alone versus AA with ML, 3) outcome measured in terms of subjective or objective measures of voice. Studies that reported combined data (i.e., pooled data from AA + ML combined with ML alone) from which comparative data could not be extrapolated were excluded. Also excluded were isolated case reports of single patients, papers on the incidence or etiology of vocal fold paralysis, review articles with no new patient data (except meta-analyses), duplicate or follow-up papers, and papers focusing on nonvoice outcomes such as swallowing. The bibliographies of the selected papers were reviewed to determine whether any additional studies had been missed in the search, and these were added. A total of three papers met the inclusion/exclusion criteria [1–3].

RESULTS

Outcome Measures. The Abraham report focused on laryngoscopic estimates of the glottal gap and patient report of symptomatic improvement. The McCullough study measured patient ratings of voice discomfort and quality of life. Measures of voice effort and GRBAS (Grade, Roughness, Breathiness, Asthenia, Strain) scale ratings were also used. Thompson used trained observer evaluations of videostroboscopy recordings.

Potential Confounders. In these retrospective studies, key confounders include the potential factors that would prompt a surgeon to choose AA + ML instead of AA alone. Even when some pretreatment group differences are acknowledged, there may be other intrinsic pretreatment differences of which the deciding surgeon is unaware. Such pretreatment differences make it difficult to determine whether posttreatment differences are attributable to different treatments or to a preexisting condition. In addition, the type of material and individual methods of medialization thyroplasty or adduction could influence results. Also, the use of speech therapy in one or both groups could alter outcomes.

Study Designs. There were three studies that provided comparative data, all from retrospective case series. The Abraham study was the largest; it compared symptom improvement and glottic gap outcomes in nearly 200 patients. Patients who underwent ML alone were more likely to have had a previous procedure. Having more distortions from previous laryngeal surgeries in one group could impact comparative results. Also, the group treated with ML alone had been paralyzed longer than the combined group, possibly affecting the degree of atrophy present. Most of the patients in the study had been treated for lung cancer, and about half of the patients in each study arm had been previously treated with radiation therapy to the chest (and possibly the neck), making the results less generalizable to the noncancerous population.

McCulloch also reported retrospective comparative data. In this study, the combined ML + AA group were younger and had wider pretreatment glottal gaps, with >50% paralyzed from skull base surgery (high vagal injuries). These investigators attempted to address these discrepancies in noting that the preoperative voice parameters were very similar. The McCulloch study also included several patients who had already had prior injections (58% of the ML-only patients versus 32% of the ML + AA group). Follow-up times were approximated to be one year or more.

The Thompson study provided additional retrospective comparative data from 12 patients regarding ML versus ML + AA. They reported a trend toward better voice outcomes with ML + AA, but no statistical analysis was reported and sample sizes were small. Follow-up times ranged from 5 weeks to 15 months.

Highest Level of Evidence. There were three studies that directly compared ML alone with ML + AA. All three studies suggested that both procedures resulted in improvements in patient symptoms and glottic closure. McCulloch and Thompson reported a trend toward more improvement with AA, but none of the three studies demonstrated a statistically significant difference between the two groups. Power calculations were not reported. One study did not comment on group comparison before treatment, but two studies noted that there were differences in the groups even before treatment. As noted above, such pretreatment differences make it difficult to determine whether posttreatment differences are attributable to the treatment or a preexisting condition.

Applicability. All of the patients in these studies were adults with unilateral vocal fold paralysis, from diverse etiologies. Most of the Abraham et al. study patients had a history of lung cancer; in fact, 47% of their study population was dead of disease within 1 year of implantation. Thus, their data are more applicable to the patient population with cancer as compared to other data.

Morbidity/Complications. Two of the papers [17, 19] included data on complications. There were five tracheotomies needed following combined AA + ML procedures (4.3%), but no tracheotomies in the ML-only groups. The Abraham et al. study reported complication rates of 14% and 19% for the ML-only and AA + ML groups, respectively, with about half of these complications "significant enough to warrant intervention." There were three implant extrusions, all in the ML-only group.

CLINICAL SIGNIFICANCE AND FUTURE RESEARCH

There were three retrospective studies comparing voice outcomes with medialization alone versus medialization with AA. Both approaches result in voice improvement by repositioning the paralyzed vocal fold in the midline. Overall, no statistically significant differences have been uncovered comparing the two procedures. To determine what magnitude of study would be needed to uncover such a difference, the data from these studies can be used to calculate the sample size needed to uncover a clinically meaningful difference between groups. Using the postoperative McCulloch patient quality of life data for calculations, 220 patients would be required to achieve a 90% power. Using the postoperative hoarseness data from the Thompson study, >300 patients would be required to achieve a 90% power. Thus, large sample sizes are needed. The Abraham study numbers approached these sample sizes and found no significant difference between groups.

Future research may focus on providing prospective data with larger sample sizes. In addition, there are multiple validated instruments that assess the impact of a treatment on vocal quality of life. Treatment of vocal fold paralysis confers not only a change in voice, but also a change in swallowing. Such swallowing outcomes are worthy of further analysis.

Reference	Abraham, 2001	McCulloch, 2000
Level (design)	3 (retrospective comparative study)	3 (retrospective comparative study)
Sample size*	n = 98 type 1 thyroplasty alone n = 96 thyroplasty with AA	n = 72 procedures, 44 of which had preoperative and postoperative video/stroboscopic data

OUTCOMES

	Symptom improvement	Mean postoperative vocal fold gap	Preoperative	Postoperative
Medialization thyroplasty	94%	0.2 mm	Patient rating: 4.5 ± 1.4 QOL: 4.4 ± 1.4 MPT: 8.3 ± 5.0	Patient rating: 2.8 ± 1.3 QOL: 1.9 ± 1.6 MPT: 9.9 ± 5.6
Medialization and AA	93%	0.1 mm	Patient rating: 4.2 ± 1.5 QOL: 3.8 ± 1.6 MPT: 6.9 ± 4.1	Patient rating: 1.6 ± 1.4 QOL: 1.2 ± 1.8 MPT: 16.7 ± 9.1
p Value	NS	NS	Not reported	Not reported
Conclusion	Both groups improved postoperatively. No difference noted between groups	Postoperatively, both groups trended toward improvement. Trend toward more improvement with adduction	
Follow-up time	Not specified. 47% of patients were dead of disease within 1 y of implantation	"Mean follow up time for nearly all patient data sets approximates or exceeds 1 year"	

STUDY DESIGN

Inclusion criteria	All patients who underwent unilateral vocal cord medialization surgery with type 1 thyroplasty with or without AA at Memorial Sloan Kettering Cancer Center 1991–1999	Patients who had undergone previous GOR-TEX medialization with or without AA with preoperative and postoperative voice data
Exclusion criteria	Not specified	Patients undergoing medialization for nonparalysis laryngeal problems
Comparison of groups before treatment	Baseline characteristics similar between the 2 groups, except for history of previous vocal fold medialization (more in thyroplasty-alone group) and timing of operation relative to sacrifice of recurrent laryngeal nerve	Preoperative voice evaluations of the 2 groups were nearly identical. AA group younger and more with surgically induced paralysis. Revisions: 15 medialization alone, 6 adduction and medialization
Age	Mean 62 y	Average age with medialization 66 y, AA and medialization 52 y
Outcome measurements	Percent of patients who reported improvement in symptoms. Glottic gap as measured by flexible fiberoptic examination	Voice dysfunction severity was rated by patient on a scale of 0 (normal voice) to 6 (worst voice you can imagine). Vocal QOL was rated by patient on a scale of 0 (no quality of life impact) to 6 (voice quality affecting everything in life). Voice effort was evaluated as percent required to produce sound for speech (i.e., 100 normal effort, 200 twice normal effort). Subjective voice rating was measured with GRBAS scale: 0 normal to 3 severely abnormal. Maximum phonation time measured in seconds
Consecutive patients?	Not specified	Not specified
Morbidity/ complications	Mean time of surgery and mean hospital stay was increased with AA (p < 0.0001). Overall complication rates (wound hematoma or infections, implant extrusion) were 14% with thyroplasty, 19% with added adduction	2 patients with episodic dyspnea, one of which had later tracheotomy, after GOR-TEX thyroplasty with AA

AA = arytenoid adduction, QOL = quality of life, NS = not significant, GRBAS = Grade, Roughness, Breathiness, Asthenia, Strain, MPT = maximum phonation time.
* Sample size: numbers shown for those not lost to follow-up and those (initially recruited).

THE EVIDENCE CONDENSED: Medialization laryngoplasty alone versus medialization and arytenoid adduction

Reference	Thompson, 1995	
Level (design)	3 (retrospective comparative study)	
Sample size*	n = 12 patients	

OUTCOMES

	% Resolved hoarseness	% Consistent complete glottic closure
Medialization thyroplasty	75% (n = 3/4)	0% (n = 0/4)
Medialization and AA	87.5% (n = 7/8)	62.5% (n = 5/8)
p Value	Not reported	Not reported
Conclusion	Trend toward more improvement with adduction. No significant difference noted between groups	
Follow-up time	5 wk–15 mo (mean 5 mo)	

STUDY DESIGN

Inclusion criteria	Unilateral vocal cord paralysis undergoing type 1 thyroplasty with or without AA with sufficient clinical information, preoperative and postoperative videotape recordings
Exclusion criteria	Paralysis previously treated by Teflon, collagen, or thyroplasty, or the nonparalyzed vocal cord had been previously traumatized either chemically or surgically
Comparison of groups before treatment	Not specified
Age	36–72 y
Outcome measurements	Videostroboscopy recordings were randomized and evaluated separately by 3 judges (2 otolaryngologists, 1 speech pathologist). Judges were blinded to the identity of the patient but preoperative and postoperative data were reviewed consecutively for each patient. Each judge individually rated the vibratory patterns of each vocal fold: mucosal wave, amplitude, phasic timing, glottic closure, closure consistency. Concordance rate was 94%
Consecutive patients?	Not specified
Morbidity/ complications	Not specified

AA = arytenoid adduction, QOL = quality of life, NS = not significant, GRBAS = Grade, Roughness, Breathiness, Asthenia, Strain.
* Sample size: numbers shown for those not lost to follow-up and those (initially recruited).

REFERENCES

1. Abraham MT, Gonen M, Kraus DH. Complications of type I thyroplasty and arytenoid adduction. Laryngoscope 2001; 111(8):1322–1329.

2. McCulloch TM, Hoffman HT, Andrews BT, Karnell MP. Arytenoid adduction combined with Gore-Tex medialization thyroplasty. Laryngoscope 2000;110(8):1306–1311.

3. Thompson DM, Maragos NE, Edwards BW. The study of vocal fold vibratory patterns in patients with unilateral vocal fold paralysis before and after type I thyroplasty with or without arytenoid adduction. 1995;105(5 Pt 1):481–486.

24 Unilateral Vocal Cord Paralysis

24.D.

Laryngeal reinnervation for unilateral vocal cord paralysis: Impact on voice outcomes

Randall C. Paniello

Laryngeal reinnervation procedures seek to restore some neural input to the paralyzed hemilaryngeal muscles, increasing the chronic tonicity and causing the vocal fold to drift toward the midline using the natural vectors of muscle action on the arytenoid cartilage.

METHODS

A computerized PubMed search of MEDLINE listings from 1966 to 2005 was performed, using keywords "vocal," "fold" or "cord," "paralysis" or "paresis" or "immobility" or "movement impairment," and "treatment." This process yielded 1930 publications. Papers were reviewed to identify those that met the following inclusion criteria: 1) adult patient population with unilateral vocal cord paralysis, 2) intervention with reinnervation of the paralyzed cord, 3) results reported in terms of subjective or objective measures of voice. The search was then further limited by excluding single case reports, papers on the incidence or etiology of vocal fold paralysis, review articles with no new patient data (except meta-analyses), and papers focusing on nonvoice outcomes such as swallowing. The bibliographies of the selected papers were reviewed to determine whether any additional studies had been missed in the search, and these were added. A total of 11 papers met the search criteria [1, 11].

RESULTS

Outcome Measures. Most of the reports included frequently cited voice parameters similar to the papers on laryngeal framework surgery in the preceding sections, such as maximum phonation time, noise-to-harmonic ratio, and GRBAS (Grade, Roughness, Breathiness, Asthenia, Strain) scores. Videostroboscopic assessment of atrophy and glottal gap was also included. In one report, the author's subjective evaluation of the patients' voice results was reported as the only data.

Potential Confounders. When considering the impact of reinnervation, multiple variables must be considered that could impact the speed and efficacy of restoration of muscle function and/or tone. For example, the time elapsed since paralysis, the age of the patient, and the length of recurrent nerve that was sacrificed could all impact results. In addition, results could vary according to the multiple methods of reinnervation that have been reported: direct anastomosis to the ansa cervicalis, anas-

tomosis to the hypoglossal, and transfer of nerve-muscle pedicle (i.e., ansa with omohyoid). In addition, because the effect of reinnervation may not be appreciated for several months after the procedure, concomitant procedures are also often performed; the effects of such concomitant procedures may confound the results of the reinnervation process.

Study Designs. There were 11 studies that reported voice outcomes after reinnervation procedures. One study was prospective, although it reported on a noncomparative cohort. There were three retrospective comparative studies, as well as seven retrospective case series. Several methods of reinnervation were studied, including transfer of nerve-muscle pedicle (i.e., ansa with omohyoid), as well as direct anastomosis to the hypoglossal or ansa cervicalis nerves. For all of the studies, the selection criteria for choosing reinnervation over other procedures for cord paralysis were not stated. Follow-up times ranged from 2 months to 5 years.

Highest Level of Evidence. Overall, the results showed either a statistically significant improvement or a trend toward improvement in voice parameters after reinnervation.

Applicability. These data are applicable to adults with unilateral vocal cord paralysis, with individual studies' more specific applicability varying according to the inclusion/exclusion criteria tabulated for the reader.

Morbidity/Complications. No complications were reported in three of the studies. Tucker reported one delayed tracheotomy (2%) and two late implant extrusions (4%); the extrusions, however, were likely related to the medialization laryngoplasty (ML) component of the combined procedure, not the reinnervation component.

CLINICAL SIGNIFICANCE AND FUTURE RESEARCH

There were 11 studies that suggested that reinnervation procedures offer voice improvement for patients with unilateral cord paralysis. Improvement has been reported with anastomosis to the ansa cervicalis or hypoglossal, as well as with nerve-muscle transfer.

A number of clinical questions remain unanswered:

- Are the voice results from reinnervation better than those from the best framework procedure? If the answer

depends on the specific clinical scenario, what guidelines should be followed?

- If reinnervation results are better than medialization
  results, is the additional benefit worth waiting a few
  extra months to achieve? What degree of additional
  benefit would be considered clinically significant?
- If ML gives a better short-term benefit, and reinnervation a better long-term benefit, should both procedures
  be performed in every patient? If not all patients, which
  ones (i.e., is there some criterion such as electromyography that would indicate that reinnervation is unlikely
  to result in more innervation than that which has
  already occurred spontaneously?)

Each of these questions would ideally be answered by a
randomized clinical trial (RCT). To perform an RCT on
this subject, however, a large number of patients would
be needed. Patients must be asked to forego speech
therapy until after the observation period, which should
be at least 1 year, and they must be willing to be randomized among two or more surgical options. The patients
must also be willing to return to the medical center for
data collection at the prescribed intervals. A project of
this nature requires significant support in this era of
ever-shrinking grant availability.

This author recently attempted to lead a multicenter,
prospective RCT comparing reinnervation (using ansa
cervicalis) to medialization (participating surgeon's
choice of technique). A grant from NIH-NIDCD
(National Institutes of Health–National Institute on
Deafness and Other Communication Disorders) was
awarded, and several subsites were recruited to enroll
patients. After 3 years of accrual, the study had enrolled
only about 20% of the accrual target. There were many
reasons for this shortfall, but the primary reason was that
patients were frequently unwilling to be randomized
between the two surgical approaches. They were told that
both approaches give good results, that we do not pres-
ently have any scientific rationale for choosing one procedure over the other, and that if they did not get the
results they were hoping for, with either approach a revision would be possible. But many patients presented with
a bias toward one approach (some wanted reinnervation,
some wanted medialization) and were unwilling to risk
being randomized to the opposite procedure. Because of
low accrual and some other administrative issues, this
study has been closed and the limited data obtained are
undergoing analysis.

This experience should not deter investigators
from pursuing additional RCTs on this topic, however.
Some of the research questions above may be more
acceptable to patients. For example, the question of
ML versus ML + reinnervation could be successfully
randomized; in either arm the patient would obtain
the early result from the ML. There are also nonrandomized study designs that can yield useful results,
provided enough patients are enrolled and the data
are collected carefully and analyzed in a blinded
manner.

Reference	Miyauchi, 1998	Olson, 1998
Level (design)	3 (retrospective controlled)	3 (retrospective comparative)
Sample size	45	12
OUTCOMES		
No reinnervation	Maximum phonation time mean: men 10.1 ± 5.3 s, women 6.5 ± 4.5 s	Mean percent improvement postreinnervation compared with prereinnervation: dysphonia 28%, roughness 22%, breathiness 27%, asthenia 15%, strain 10%
Postreinnervation	Maximum phonation time mean: men 26.2 ± 13.0 s, women 17.2 ± 5.2 s	
Nonparalyzed control	Maximum phonation time mean: men 28.6 ± 10.8 s, women 16.7 ± 5.1 s	Not applicable
p Value	Postreinnervation vs no reinnervation: men < 0.02, women < 0.0001	Dysphonia <0.05, roughness NS, breathiness <0.05, asthenia <0.05, strain NS, respectively
Conclusion	Significant improvement in maximum phonation time with reinnervation	Significant improvement in dysphonia, breathiness, and asthenia with reinnervation
Follow-up time	Measurements were taken 12 mo postoperatively. Patients were followed for 1.1–10.7 y [mean (SD) 4.2 (2.3) y].	At least 8 mo
STUDY DESIGN		
Inclusion criteria	Reconstructed RLN in patients who had unilateral vocal cord paralysis or whose unilateral RLN or vagus was to be sacrificed because of various diseases	With exception of clear cases of traumatic transection of RLN, a minimum of 1 y had elapsed since the onset of vocal cord paralysis, with a maximum of 6 y
Exclusion criteria	Not reported	Lack of preoperative vocal analysis
Intervention regimen details	The reconstruction was done at the time of surgery for primary or recurrent thyroid cancer. The ends of the severed RLN were anastomosed directly if possible. If the defect was long, a free nerve graft taken from the transverse cervical nerve, supraclavicular nerves, or ansa cervicalis was used to fill the defect. In cases in which both the RLN and vagus nerves were to be sacrificed, the proximal end of the vagus was anastomosed to the distal end of the RLN. When there was no distal portion of the RLN left below the Berry's ligament, the inferior pharyngeal constrictor muscle was divided along the lateral edge of the thyroid cartilage to find the distal stump of the RLN. The thyroid cartilage was retracted, and the cricothyroid joint opened, if necessary. The most posterior branch was not used for the anastomosis because it could innervate the posterior cricoarytenoid muscle, which is the abductor of the vocal cord	Gelfoam injection into paralyzed fold concomitantly with reinnervation. Ansa cervicalis to RLN anastomosis
Method of voice evaluation	Maximum phonation time [the duration of sustained phonation of the vowel (a) after maximum inspiration] was measured at 12 mo postoperatively and periodically	The voice samples from the patients were randomized with age- and sex-matched samples from normal subjects and judged by trained listeners for overall dysphonia, roughness, breathiness, asthenia, and strain
Age	23–73 y (mean 52 y)	25–73 y (46 y)
Masking	None	Voice samples from patients randomized with age- and sex-matched samples
Consecutive patients?	No	No
Morbidity/ complications	Not reported	Not reported

RLN = recurrent laryngeal nerve, NS = not significant.

Reference	Tucker, 1989	Tucker, 1997	Tucker, 1981	Zheng, 1996
Level (design)	4 (retrospective review)	4 (retrospective review)	4 (retrospective review)	4 (retrospective review)
Sample size	70	52	31	8
OUTCOMES				
Postreinnervation vs prereinnervation	25% normal 58% greatly improved 5% somewhat improved 12% not improved	72% normal/great improvement	84% normal/great improvement	88% return to normal/great improvement
p Value	Not reported	Not reported	Not reported	Not reported
Conclusion	Voice in the majority of patients with unilateral cord paralysis improved after reinnervation	Voice in the majority of patients undergoing combined nerve-muscle pedicle reinnervation and surgical medialization improved	Nerve-muscle pedicle reinnervation may be used as a means of reanimation of unilaterally paralyzed vocal cords with good-to-excellent results within 4 mo in carefully selected patients	Voice in the majority of patients with unilateral cord paralysis improved after reinnervation
Follow-up time	2–6 mo, 1 y	At least 2 y	At least 6 mo	At least 1 y
STUDY DESIGN				
Inclusion criteria	Unilateral vocal cord paralysis, patients chosen for reinnervation only if voices were critical to livelihood	Unilateral vocal fold paralysis >6 mo	Unilateral vocal cord paralysis, indicated interest in nerve-muscle pedicle reinnervation, counseling by surgeon and speech pathologist preoperatively	Minimum 6 mo after paralysis Minimum follow-up of 1 y
Exclusion criteria	Not reported	Fixation or limitation of motion of vocal fold, adequate voice return after compensation or speech therapy, health problems preventing surgery	Not reported	Multiple cranial nerve deficits
Intervention regimen details	Nerve-muscle pedicle transfer: obtained from anterior belly of omohyoid muscle and transferred to lateral thyroarytenoid muscle bed	Surgical medialization of the paralyzed vocal cord with simultaneous nerve-muscle pedicle reinnervation under local anesthesia	Nerve-muscle pedicle transfer: obtained from anterior belly of omohyoid muscle and transferred to lateral thyroarytenoid muscle bed	Main branch of ansa adductor of RLN anastomosis for unilateral vocal cord paralysis
Method of voice evaluation	Voice graded subjectively at 1 y by surgeon, speech pathologist, and patient as normal, greatly improved, somewhat improved, or not improved	Voice graded subjectively when compared with preoperative voice by speech pathologist, 1 otolaryngologist, and 1 resident as normal, greatly improved, somewhat improved, unchanged, or worse	Voice graded subjectively by surgeon, speech pathologist, and patient as normal, greatly improved, somewhat improved, or not improved	3 speech pathologists and 3 doctors listened to each audio tape and rated each for perceived voice quality (breathy, hoarse, harsh, strained) using a 4-point scale from normal to severe dysfunction
Age	Not reported	Not reported	Not reported	21–62 y
Masking	None	None	None	No
Consecutive patients?	No	No	No	No
Morbidity/complications	No complications of surgery	1 delayed tracheotomy 2 extrusions	No complications of surgery	No complications

RLN = recurrent laryngeal nerve.

THE EVIDENCE CONDENSED: Reinnervation versus no reinnervation for unilateral vocal cord paralysis

Reference	Sato, 1985	Maronian, 2003		Crumley, 1986
Level (design)	4 (retrospective review)	4 (retrospective review)		4 (retrospective review)
Sample size	5	9		2
OUTCOMES				
Reinnervation	Maximum phonation time postreinnervation 11.5–22.2 s. Vocal cord atrophies were not seen. Obvious adduction of the operated vocal fold at phonation was obtained only in 2 cases and other 2 cases showed slight adduction	Preoperatively: dysphonia 1.9, hoarseness 1.8, breathiness 1.4, loudness 1.2, strain 0.2	Postoperatively: dysphonia 0.9, hoarseness 1, breathiness 0.5, loudness 0.5, strain 0	No apparent aperiodicity, roughness, or residual breathiness. Voice range 100–392 Hz. Restoration of fundamental tone, increase in acoustic power, near-normal pitch, tone, and spectral analysis
p Value	Not reported	Dysphonia <0.05, hoarseness <0.05, breathiness <0.06, loudness NS, strain NS		Not reported
Conclusion	Reinnervation may improve voice	Reinnervation resulted in significantly better dysphonia, hoarseness, breathiness. There was a trend toward improvement in loudness, strain		Trend toward synchronous and symmetrical oscillations of the vocal fold during phonation resulting in normal/near-normal voice with reinnervation
Follow-up time	8–15 mo	At least 8 mo		4 mo, 5 y
STUDY DESIGN				
Inclusion criteria	Unilateral RLN paralysis caused by thyroid cancer	Unilateral RLN paralysis, reinnervation procedure conducted at University of Washington Medical center, preoperative awake electromyography, perceptual analysis of voice and videostroboscopy		Proximal transactions of vagus nerve with hoarseness and aspiration, preference for reinnervation over Teflon injection
Exclusion criteria	Not specified	Cricoarytenoid joint fixation		Not reported
Intervention regimen details	The abductor branch was cut selectively in 4 cases, followed by free nerve grafting of the ansa cervicalis and pedicle nerve muscle graft of the thyrohyoid muscle implanted in 1 case	Preference given to performing direct neurorrhaphy between the distal RLN and the ansa cervicalis branch. If the distal stump was disrupted or unable to be identified, a nerve-muscle pedicle was used		Ansa hypoglossi-RLN anastomosis
Method of voice evaluation	Maximum phonation time was measured in seconds. GRBAS scale was used to measure voice quality	3 speech pathologists performed preoperative and postoperative voice assessment using a perceptual rating scale for voice quality and characteristics. The ratings were accomplished in a blinded manner with patient voice samples arranged randomly. Grade for overall dysphonia, hoarseness, loudness, breathiness, and strain (0 = normal, 1 = mild, 2 = moderate, 3 = severe)		The data were analyzed by subjective and objective means, including acoustics and electroglottography
Age	41–75 y	37–54 y		30, 37 y
Masking	Not reported	Speech pathologists were blinded		No
Consecutive patients?	Not specified	No		No
Morbidity/ complications	Not reported	No complications		Not reported

RLN = recurrent laryngeal nerve, NS = not significant, GRBAS = Grade, Roughness, Breathiness, Asthenia, Strain.

THE EVIDENCE CONDENSED: Reinnervation versus no reinnervation for unilateral vocal cord paralysis

Reference	Paniello, 2000	Crumley, 1991
Level (design)	4 (prospective noncomparative cohort)	3 (retrospective comparative)
Sample size	5	12
OUTCOMES		
Postreinnervation vs prereinnervation	100% excellent voice quality, resolution of any preoperative aspiration, and minimal morbidity	42% returned to normal voice. 92% were thought to be far superior to results with Teflon injection and Isshiki thyroplasty
Control	Preoperative voice	Preoperative voice and patient voices who had undergone Teflon injection or Isshiki thyroplasty
p Value	Not reported	Not reported
Conclusion	Voice in the majority of patients with unilateral cord paralysis improved after reinnervation via the hypoglossal nerve	Ansa cervicalis to RLN anastomosis is the procedure of choice in younger patients or those who use their voice professionally because phonatory quality is superior to Teflon injection or Isshiki thyroplasty
Follow-up time	1 y	Minimum 6 mo
STUDY DESIGN		
Inclusion criteria	Unilateral vocal cord paralysis; known transaction of RLN within the past year or electromyographic evidence of denervation of the thyroarytenoid muscle, with no evidence of recovery at both 4 mo and 6 mo after the onset of paralysis	Unilateral vocal cord paralysis, desired improvement of voice, or prevention of aspiration
Exclusion criteria	Not reported	Not reported
Intervention regimen details	Hypoglossal to RLN reinnervation	In patients with intracranial, cervical, vagal injuries, or intrathoracic injuries (those patients with an intact cervical portion of the RLN), the infrathyroid technique is used: RLN anastomosed to distal portion of ansa's branches. More distal lesions of the RLN such as those that might occur during thyroidectomy, carotid endarterectomy, or cervical spine disk procedures require that the RLN be identified higher, in a more distal location
Method of voice evaluation	The patients were followed monthly with voice recordings, videolaryngoscopy, subjective voice evaluation, and careful questioning regarding aspiration. Voice analysis was performed using a sustained /a/ with the Multidimensional Voice Program for jitter percentage, shimmer percentage, noise-to-harmonic ratio, and voice turbulence index	Postoperative voice studies unless distance prevented return visits. These latter patients were telephoned and asked several questions. They were also asked to submit recorded audiocassettes for completion of vocal studies. It is not stated who conducted the voice analysis.
Age	30–76 y	Not reported
Masking	No	None
Consecutive patients?	No	No
Morbidity/ complications	1 patient died during first perioperative month from a myocardial infarction. Patients showed mild tongue deviation to ipsilateral side and mild to moderate atrophy during the first year. 2 patients complained about biting their tongue which improved in 6 mo. No other complication reported	1 failure, no morbidity or complications reported. This patient had an idiopathic subglottic stenosis and had several prior laryngeal procedures; the RLN was small and its identity could not be confirmed

RLN = recurrent laryngeal nerve.

REFERENCES

1. Miyauchi A, Matsusaka K, Kihara M, et al. The role of ansa-to-recurrent-laryngeal nerve anastomosis in operations for thyroid cancer. Eur J Surg 1998;164(12):927–933.

2. Olson DE, Goding GS, Michael DD. Acoustic and perceptual evaluation of laryngeal reinnervation by ansa cervicalis transfer. Laryngoscope 1998;108(12):1767–1772.

3. Tucker HM. Combined surgical medialization and nerve-muscle pedicle reinnervation for unilateral vocal fold paralysis: improved functional results and prevention of long-term deterioration of voice. J Voice 1997;11(4):474–478.

4. Tucker HM. Long-term results of nerve-muscle pedicle reinnervation for laryngeal paralysis. nn Otol Rhinol Laryngol 1989;98(9):674–677.

5. Tucker HM, Rusnov M. Laryngeal reinnervation for unilateral vocal cord paralysis: long-term results. Ann Otol Rhinol Laryngol 1981;90(5 Pt 1):457–459.

6. Zheng H, Li Z, Zhou S, Cuan Y, Wen W. Update: laryngeal reinnervation for unilateral vocal cord paralysis with the ansa cervicalis. Laryngoscope 1996;106(12 Pt 1):1522–1527.

7. Sato F, Saito H. Functional reconstruction for unilateral recurrent laryngeal nerve paralysis caused by thyroid cancer. Auris Nasus Larynx 1985;12 Suppl 2:S210–216.

8. Crumley RL, Izdebski K. Voice quality following laryngeal reinnervation by ansa hypoglossi transfer. Laryngoscope 1986;96(6):611–616.

9. Maronian N, Waugh P, Robinson L, Hillel A. Electromyographic findings in recurrent laryngeal nerve reinnervation. Ann Otol Rhinol Laryngol 2003;112(4):314–323.

10. Paniello RC. Laryngeal reinnervation with the hypoglossal nerve. II. Clinical evaluation and early patient experience. Laryngoscope 2000;110(5 Pt 1):739–748.

11. Crumley RL. Update: ansa cervicalis to recurrent laryngeal nerve anastomosis for unilateral laryngeal paralysis. Laryngoscope 1991;101(4 Pt 1):384–387; discussion 388.

24 Unilateral Vocal Cord Paralysis

24.E.

Vocal fold injection versus medialization laryngoplasty: Impact on subjective and objective measures of voice

Randall C. Paniello and Shivan Amin

METHODS

A computerized PubMed search of MEDLINE listings from 1966 to 2005 was performed, using textwords "vocal," "fold" or "cord," "paralysis" or "paresis" or "immobility" or "movement impairment," and "treatment." This process yielded 1930 publications. Papers were reviewed to identify those that met the following inclusion criteria: 1) adult patient population with unilateral vocal cord paralysis, 2) intervention with injectable material in comparison to a solid preconstructed implant to medialize the paralyzed cord, 3) results reported in terms of subjective or objective measures of voice. The search was then further limited by excluding single case reports, papers on the incidence or etiology of vocal fold paralysis, review articles with no new patient data (except meta-analyses), papers focusing on nonvoice outcomes such as swallowing. Articles in which mathematical models were extrapolated without comparative clinical data were excluded. The bibliographies of the selected papers were reviewed to determine whether any additional studies had been missed in the search, and these were added. A total of four papers met these search criteria [1, 4].

RESULTS

Outcome Measures. Outcomes were measured in terms of flexible fiberoptic nasendoscopy, including measurements of glottic gap and glottic closure. In addition, electroglottography, auditory perceptual evaluations, acoustics morphology, aerodynamics, and self-assessment were used. More specifically described were jitter rate, noise-to-harmonic ratio, and maximum phonation time (MPT). The voice handicap index (VHI) was also used, an instrument composed of 30 questions or statements with responses scored from 0 to 4 for individual items. At the completion of the VHI, the score can be totaled for a VHI score ranging from 0 to 120, with higher numbers corresponding to a greater amount of disability because of a voice-related problem. A VHI score of 0–30 represents a low score, with a minimal amount of associated handicap. A score of 31–60 suggests a moderate impact, but a score from 60 to 120 represents a significant and serious amount of handicap.

Potential Confounders. There are multiple potential confounders, as described in the introductory overview to this chapter. Such confounders include the selection biases inherent to retrospective reviews; because patients were treated according to surgeon preference, there may be differences in the two groups even before treatment has occurred, making it fairly difficult to compare the two treatment groups after intervention. In addition, the use of speech therapy, the presence of concomitant neurologic or cervical disorders, the distribution of nerve lesion site (i.e., high versus low vagal lesions), patient age, and capacity for compensatory function may all influence results.

Study Designs. There were four studies comparing medialization laryngoplasty (ML) to vocal fold injection. One study analyzed a prospective cohort of patients undergoing vocal fold injection with a retrospective control group of age- and sex-matched patients that had undergone ML. This study by Lundy [4] asked a worthwhile question, and the findings were interesting, but the limitations of the study must be considered. Although the ML group was age- and sex-matched, it cannot be discerned whether there were any important differences related to their vocal pathology. The group sizes were small. The follow-up period of 1 month is the shortest among all of the studies.

The other three studies relied on retrospective data alone. When considering such retrospective data, it is important to remember the inherent potential for selection bias; more severe symptoms or glottal gaps may have prompted the choice of one surgery over the other, making one group inherently clinically worse at the outset and thus more likely to have a worse outcome.

Additional aspects of the study designs included the use of consecutive patients, a range of follow-up times, and somewhat limited sample sizes. Consecutive patients were reported in one of the four studies [1]. Such reporting of consecutive patients helps minimize bias. Follow-up times ranged from 1 month to 17 years. One study reported results at an early and late follow-up period, and the timing of the follow-up may notably impact the results. Sample sizes were small, but still statistically significant differences were found in multiple comparisons.

A variety of medialization methods were used in these four studies. Injectable materials included Teflon, Cymetra (homologous cadaveric collagen), and liquid silicone. ML was performed with a solid implant, typically specified as silicone.

Highest Level of Evidence. Overall, results were mixed, supporting either no difference between results with ML versus injection, or showing better results with ML. Two studies [3, 4] showed no significant difference between ML versus injection. One study [1] showed that ML was associated with significantly less strain, hoarseness, and severity of voice, as well as a trend toward more complete glottic closure. The fourth study [2] showed a trend toward better late results with ML. The comparative voice result may simply be dependent on the follow-up time, as the two studies with the longest follow-up times showed better results with ML, whereas the two studies with the shortest follow-up times showed no difference between ML and injection. Multiple studies confirm the significant improvement postprocedure, as compared with preprocedure.

Only one publication included any prospective data. These results from Lundy, et al. [4] showed that both procedures significantly improved the voice. Comparing the two groups, there were no statistically significant differences (at the $p < 0.05$ level). A closer look at the data suggests that this may have been in part because of the small sample size. The VHI scores were better for the ML group than for the injection group by 10% or more, but this did not reach statistical significance with only eight patients in each group. In contrast, the MPT for the injection group was 11% longer than the ML group, but this was not significant.

Applicability. The results of these studies are applicable to adults with unilateral vocal fold paralysis.

Morbidity/Complications. Only one of the four studies reported any adverse outcomes. Complications of thyroplasty included implant extrusion, hematomas, extreme persistent local pain, and "inesthetic wound healing."

Complications of injection included three small granulomas with slight to moderate repercussion on vocal cord vibration.

CLINICAL SIGNIFICANCE AND FUTURE RESEARCH

There were four studies that provided a direct comparison between voice outcomes after ML versus injection in patients with unilateral vocal fold paralysis. Overall, results were mixed, with two studies supporting either no difference between results with ML versus injection, and two studies showing better results with ML. There are issues regarding limited sample size and power that make the studies showing no difference refutable. Meanwhile, there are also issues regarding potential inherent biases (selection and otherwise) in retrospective studies that allow one to challenge the results showing ML is better. It may also be that the comparative voice result is dependent on the follow-up time only, as the two studies with the longest follow-up times showed better results with ML, whereas the two studies with the shortest follow-up times showed no difference between ML and injection.

Future research may focus on developing more prospective comparative data with larger sample sizes with regimented, timed follow-up points before 6 months and after 1 year. In addition, it would be useful to study the long-term impact of ML versus sequential repeated injections. A quality of life parameter measuring the "hassle factor" could be included in studies evaluating injection laryngoplasty, and the data should be collected prospectively for 1 year or longer to answer this question.

THE EVIDENCE CONDENSED: Injection versus type I thyroplasty for unilateral vocal fold paralysis treatment

Reference	Lundy, 2003	Tsuzuki, 1991
Level (design)	3 (prospective cohort with retrospective control)	3 (retrospective comparative)
Sample size	8 injection, 8 thyroplasty	18 patients untreated, 15 injection, 18 thyroplasty
OUTCOMES		
Outcome measures	Glottal closure, jitter rate, NHR, MPT, GFR, patient perception—VHI	MPT
Medialization laryngoplasty	Glottal gap size 1.00, jitter rate 2.00%, NTHR 0.21, MPT 10.75, GFR 199.38, VHI 34.3	n = 13/17 with "remarkable improvement" of MPT between visits 1 and 2 n = 13/18 "somewhat improved" between visits 2 and 3
Injection	Glottal gap size 1.00 (=minimal posterior gap), jitter rate 1.90%, NTHR 0.24, MPT 11.94, GFR 231.25, VHI 38.5	n = 13/15 patients had improved MPT at visit 2 n = 6/15 with "significant improvement" between visits 2 and 3 (n = 3 had little improvement, n = 6 worsened)
p Value	<0.05, pre-ML vs post-ML <0.05, pre- vs postinjection NS, post-ML vs postinjection	Not reported
Conclusion	No difference in glottal closure, NHR, MPR, GFR, VHI post-ML vs postinjection	Both silicone injection and implant improved MPT. Trend toward better late results with ML
Follow-up time	1 mo postoperatively	Visit 1 preoperatively, visit 2 postoperatively, visit 3 4–17 y postoperatively.
STUDY DESIGN		
Inclusion criteria	Unilateral vocal fold paralysis	Unilateral recurrent laryngeal nerve paralysis
Exclusion criteria	None specified	None specified
Medialization laryngoplasty details	Thyroplasty type I	Liquid silicone treated with catalyst injected into vocal fold before solidification
Injection details	For majority injection transcervical through cricothyroid membrane. Injected with Cymetra (injectable homologous cadaveric collagen)	Injection of viscous silicone into vocal fold (3000 centistokes viscosity, 21-gauge needle for injection)
Voice and video measurements	Videostroboscopy for assessment of glottal closure. Acoustical analysis using MDVP. Aerodynamics measured with Multi-Spiro Sensor computer-interfaced system	None performed
Age	Injection 65.9 y, thyroplasty 65.6 y	Liquid silicone 51.1 y, solid silicone 56.3 y
Masking	None	None
Diagnostic criteria for cord paralysis	Not specified	Not specified
Consecutive patients?	No. Thyroplasty group used as controls, retrospectively analyzed from surgical database to match injection group	No
Morbidity/ complications	None reported	None reported

NTHR = noise-to-harmonic ratio, GFR = glottal flow rate, VHI = voice handicap index, ML = medialization laryngoplasty, MPT = maximum phonation time, NS = not significant, MDVP = multidimensional voice profile.

THE EVIDENCE CONDENSED: Injection versus type I thyroplasty for unilateral vocal fold paralysis treatment

Reference	Dejonckere, 1998
Level (design)	3 (retrospective comparative)
Sample size	28 patients with UVFP: 19 Teflon injection, 9 thyroplasty
OUTCOMES	
Outcome measures	Perceptual evaluation, acoustics morphology, aerodynamics, self-assessment All graded on 1–100 scale (0 = normal) here pre- and postoperative median values included test (range): preop, postop
Medialization laryngoplasty	Perceptual evaluation (0–100): 60, 40 Jitter (0–12): 8, 4 Shimmer (0–25): 11, 6 Main cepstrum peak (0–500): 70, 190 Mucosal wave (0–100): 85, 68 Phonation flow (0–800): 620, 400 Self-assessment (0–100): 60, 45
Injection	Perceptual evaluation (0–100): 49, 30 Jitter (0–12): 6, 4 Shimmer (0–25): 9, 6 Main cepstrum peak (0–500): 110, 160 Mucosal wave (0–100): 88, 70 Phonation flow (0–800): 570, 360 Self-assessment (0–100): 60, 35
p Value	NS, Post-ML vs postinjection; NS, pre-ML vs preinjection <0.05, pre- vs post-ML for phonation flow, cepstrum peak, and jitter <0.05, pre- vs post-Teflon injection for self-assessment, phonation flow, cepstrum peak, jitter
Conclusion	No significant difference between ML vs injection Significant improvement post-vs pre-ML Significant improvement post-vs preinjection
Follow-up time	Evaluated before surgery, and 3–7 mo after surgery
STUDY DESIGN	
Inclusion criteria	Acquired UVFP for at least 1 y with follow-up of at least 3 mo
Exclusion criteria	None specified
Medialization laryngoplasty details	Isshiki thyroplasty type I Note: 1 patient underwent thyroplasty I after 2 prior Teflon injections
Injection details	Teflon injection
Voice and video measurements	Perception graded by phoniatrician or speech pathologist using G parameter in GRBAS scale. Acoustics measured as described by Dejonckere (1996). Morphology measured with videostroboscopy. Aerodynamics assessed by phonation flow mL/s with Gould pneumotachograph
Age	Not specified
Masking	None
Diagnostic criteria for cord paralysis	In all cases diagnosis of peripheral neurogenic lesion confirmed by electromyography
Consecutive patients?	No
Morbidity/complications	Thyroplasty: 1 extrusion, 2 hematomas, 1 extreme local pain ×1 wk, 1 "inesthetic wound healing" Injection: 3 small granulomas with slight to moderate repercussion on vocal cord vibration

UVFP = unilateral vocal fold paralysis, ML = medialization laryngoplasty, NS = not significant, GRBAS = Grade, Roughness, Breathiness, Asthenia, Strain.
* Sample size: numbers shown for those not lost to follow-up and those (initially recruited).

Reference	D'Antonio, 1995		
Level (design)	3 (retrospective comparative).		
Sample size	6 Teflon injection, 6 thyroplasty		
OUTCOMES			
Outcome measures	Auditory perception evaluations; values graded on 1–7 scale (1 = normal)	Aerodynamic evaluations: Ps, V for male, female	Flexible fiberoptic endoscopy: glottic closure pattern
Medialization laryngoplasty	Strain 2.8, hoarseness 1.9, severity 2.8	Ps (cm H_2O) 12.1, 7.6 V (cc/s) 350, 116	n = 2/4 complete, n = 1/4 incomplete n = 1/4 posterior chink pattern
Injection	Strain 4.4, hoarseness 3.4, severity 4.4	Ps (cm H_2O) 7.2, 7.7 V (cc/s) 344, 268	n = 2/6 complete n = 1/6 incomplete n = 3/6 irregular patterns
p Value	0.05 strain, 0.05 hoarseness, 0.03 severity	NS, subglottic pressure NS, laryngeal airflow velocity	Not reported
Conclusion	Significantly less strain, hoarseness, severity with ML	No significant difference in subglottic pressure, laryngeal airflow velocity	Trend toward more complete closure with ML
Follow-up time	4–417 wk postoperatively		
STUDY DESIGN			
Inclusion criteria	Subjects were drawn from a 2.5-y consecutive series of patients with UVFP. Paralysis was secondary to prior surgery in all cases		
Exclusion criteria	None specified		
Medialization laryngoplasty details	Isshiki thyroplasty type I with Silastic® implant, performed by 1 surgeon		
Injection details	Teflon injection was performed by multiple surgeons, without standardized operative technique		
Voice and video measurements	Conducted by masked speech pathologist evaluating videotape. 1 patient from thyroplasty group was omitted. Rating form assessed 9 voice-quality characteristics. 3 judges rated voice quality, 2 judges rated fiberoptic measurements		
Age	Thyroplasty: mean 33.3 y, Teflon: mean 54.2 y		
Masking	Observer masked study		
Diagnostic criteria for cord paralysis	Acquired UVFP. Location of vagal denervation not specified		
Consecutive patients?	Yes		
Morbidity/complications	None reported		

UVFP = unilateral vocal fold paralysis, ML = medialization laryngoplasty, Ps = subglottic pressure, V = laryngeal airflow, NS = not significant, GRBAS = Grade, Roughness, Breathiness, Asthenia, Strain.

REFERENCES

1. D'Antonio LL, Wigley TL, Zimmerman GJ. Quantitative measures of laryngeal function following Teflon injection or thyroplasty type I. Laryngoscope 1995;105:256–262.

2. Tsuzuki T, et al. Voice prognosis after liquid and solid silicone injection. Am J Otolaryngol 1991;12:165–169.

3. Dejonckere PH. Teflon injection and thyroplasty: objective and subjective outcomes. Rev Laryngol Otol Rhinol 1998;119(4):265–269.

4. Lundy DS, et al. Early results of transcutaneous injection laryngoplasty with micronized acellular dermis versus type-I thyroplasty for glottic incompetence dysphonia due to unilateral vocal fold paralysis. J Voice 2003;17(4):589–595.

5. Dejonckere PH, Rerracie M, Fresnel-Elbaz E, Woisard V, Crevier-Buchman L, Millet B. Differentiated perceptual, evaluation of pathological voice quality: reliability and correlations with acoustic measurements. Rev Laryngol Otol Rhinol (Bord) 1996;117(3):219–224.

24 Unilateral Vocal Cord Paralysis

24.F.

Reinnervation versus no reinnervation: Impact on subjective and objective measures of voice

Randall C. Paniello and Shivan Amin

METHODS

A computerized PubMed search of MEDLINE listings from 1966 to 2005 was performed, using textwords "vocal," "fold" or "cord," "paralysis" or "paresis" or "immobility" or "movement impairment," and "treatment." This process yielded 1930 publications. Papers were reviewed to identify those that met the following inclusion criteria: 1) adult patient population with unilateral vocal cord paralysis, 2) intervention with reinnervation versus no reinnervation, 3) results reported in terms of subjective or objective measures of voice. The search was then further limited by excluding single case reports, papers on the incidence or etiology of vocal fold paralysis, review articles with no new patient data (except meta-analyses), papers focusing on nonvoice outcomes such as swallowing. Articles in which mathematical models were extrapolated without comparative clinical data were excluded. Articles in which results from reinnervation were pooled with results from medialization procedures were excluded because procedure-specific data could not be extrapolated. The bibliographies of the selected papers were reviewed to determine whether any additional studies had been missed in the search, and these were added. A total of three papers met these search criteria [1–3].

RESULTS

Outcome Measures. Outcomes were measured in a variety of ways in these studies. In Tucker's study [1], audio tapes of voice samples from each patient were rated as normal, greatly improved, somewhat improved, no better, or voice worse, by a panel of "sophisticated" listeners, including at least one speech and language pathologist and one otolaryngologist other than the surgeon. In Chhetri's study [2], measurements were performed of glottal closure, mucosal wave, symmetry, laryngeal airflow, subglottic pressure, and perceptual analysis by a panel of voice professionals. Chou et al. [3] used the maximum phonation time, as well as the GRBAS (Grade, Roughness, Breathiness, Asthenia, Strain) scale, a Likert scale in which each category receives a rating of 0–4 (0 normal, 1 mild, 2 moderate, 3 severe, 4 complete).

Potential Confounders. As described in this chapter's introductory overview, there are multiple potential confounders to consider when studying this topic. Such confounders include the selection biases inherent to retrospective reviews, the use of speech therapy, the presence of concomitant neurologic or cervical disorders, the distribution of nerve lesion sites (i.e., high versus low vagal lesions), patient age, and capacity for compensatory function.

Study Designs. There were three studies that directly compared the impact of reinnervation versus no reinnervation. The first [3] was a prospective cohort study of 12 patients. Eight of the 12 had primary repair, whereas four did not because of cancer invasion of the distal stump. This malignant invasion may have further affected results, especially if it continued to progress, with gross recurrence in the cricoarytenoid joint or elsewhere in the larynx. It is, however, useful that they presented the decision-making algorithm that determined whether reinnervation was pursued or not. Perceptual voice quality was rated according to the GRBAS scale, which was measured along with maximum phonation times at 3 and 6 months after recurrent laryngeal nerve injury or neurorrhaphy.

This Chhetri study compared a series of adult patients with unilateral vocal fold paralysis (UVFP) that had undergone arytenoid adduction (AA) plus reinnervation (with ansa cervicalis, "combined" group, n = 10) to another group that had undergone AA alone (n = 9). The paper indicated that "no set protocol was used to randomly assign patients into the treatment arms," but noted that the combined procedure was used more frequently in the later years. No other details regarding patient selection for the addition of reinnervation were provided. Preoperative and postoperative data were collected, consisting of videolaryngoscopy, aerodynamic analysis, and a voice recording. The postoperative data collection interval varied from 2 weeks to 60 months, with the mean follow-up interval of the combined group about 4 months longer than the AA-alone group. Notably, the AA-only group had six patients with 3 months or less of follow-up, whereas only one patient in the combined group had less than 7 months of follow-up. The longer follow-up time for the combined group allowed for full reinnervation to occur, but the short time in the AA-only group likely did not allow for manifestation of atrophy effects. There were also two patients in each group that had previously undergone a medialization laryngoplasty procedure for their UVFP. Perceptual analysis was performed on seven samples in each group using blinded volunteer listeners that rated 2-second sustained vowel samples on a 7-point visual analog scale. The samples were randomly presented using a computer algorithm. (Previous work by this group had shown no difference between the 2-second samples and connected speech samples.) Test-retest reliability was examined and found to be acceptable.

The third study [1] was a retrospective analysis of 60 consecutive patients with unilateral vocal fold immobility who underwent direct electromyographic (EMG) studies of the exposed lateral thyroarytenoid muscle at the time of surgery to determine if there was retained or recovered innervation of the vocal fold. Patients who exhibited any residual innervation (i.e., cord fixation or partial recovery after paralysis) underwent surgical medialization only using an individually carved Silastic implant (n = 27). Patients who showed no EMG evidence of reinnervation underwent a combined procedure with nerve-muscle pedicle reinnervation combined with Silastic implant. It is useful that they presented a clear indication for determining whether reinnervation was performed or not. Reinnervation was performed with an ansa cervicalis pedicle. Results for consecutive patients were reported to minimize bias. Grading of voice was performed by a panel including at least one speech and language pathologist and one otolaryngologist other than the surgeon. Voices were rated as normal, greatly improved, somewhat improved, no better, or worse, when comparing preoperative to postoperative results. Voice assessment and ranking was conducted at 3 months, 6 months, and 2 years postoperatively.

Highest Level of Evidence. There were three studies that directly compared the impact of reinnervation versus no reinnervation, and results were mixed. The prospective study by Chou et al. showed a significantly better maximum phonation time and significantly less atrophy with reinnervation. This study also demonstrated significant improvement in the GRBAS scale between 3 and 6 months postoperatively with reinnervation, whereas there were no significant improvements in the GRBAS scale with no reinnervation. These positive results, however, must be taken in the context of how patients were selected to undergo reinnervation or not; no reinnervation was performed if there was malignant invasion of the distal nerve stump. Such invasion may have ultimately involved the cricoarytenoid joint or other laryngeal function, which could bias results against the nonreinnervated group. These results do, however, suggest that in a correctly selected patient population, reinnervation may result in superior results.

The results from the Chhetri group showed no significant differences between the two study groups. Both groups had significant improvement of most parameters from pretreatment to posttreatment, but the two posttreatment results did not differ from each other, with mean follow-up intervals averaging 4 months longer in

the reinnervation group. The concept of combining reinnervation with AA is that reinnervation counteracts the effects of vocal muscle atrophy, which are frequently seen up to 2 years after the onset of paralysis. The short follow-up of the AA-only group may have missed this effect, so the benefit of adding reinnervation may not have been realized.

The Tucker study, in which patients underwent reinnervation based on intraoperative EMG measurement, showed no significant differences between the two postoperative groups. The study did show multiple significant postoperative improvements in multiple objective voice parameters for both AA alone and for AA with reinnervation. Because both groups were unequal (based on different EMG results) at the outset, it is difficult to draw accurate conclusions regarding the specific impact of reinnervation. It is possible that the group who had no reinnervation potentials on EMG would have done worse than the group whose EMG showed reinnervation potentials. If such a bias toward worse results for the group EMG showing no reinnervation potential existed at the outset, then the ansa-reinnervation may have actually been beneficial as there was no difference between the two groups in the end.

Applicability. The results of these studies are applicable to patients with UVFP.

Morbidity/Complications. None of these studies reported any morbidity or complications of the procedures they analyzed.

CLINICAL SIGNIFICANCE AND FUTURE RESEARCH

There were three studies that directly compared voice outcomes with reinnervation with no reinnervation/neurorrhaphy. Results were mixed, with one study showing better results with reinnervation and two studies showing no difference. Closer examination of the details of these studies, however, showed that selection bias and timing of follow-up may have significantly influenced their results. In addition, sample sizes were small, conferring less power to uncover any differences that may truly exist.

Ideally, a large, prospective trial would be performed to provide a more definitive answer regarding the impact of reinnervation versus no reinnervation. In accordance with this goal, there was a recent attempt to lead a multicenter, prospective randomized controlled trial comparing reinnervation (using ansa cervicalis) to medialization. Although it was supported by funding from NIH-NIDCD (National Institutes of Health–National Institute on Deafness and Other Communication Disorders) and several sites were recruited to enroll patients, subject accrual was too low, and this study has been closed and the limited data obtained are undergoing analysis.

Because there are multiple studies that have concluded that postreinnervation results are better than pre- reinnervation results (see Section 24.D), future research may also focus on which patient populations may most benefit from reinnervation. In addition, it may be further studied as an adjunctive procedure to formal medialization laryngoplasty or AA, with particular attention on long-term results in a time frame when atrophy is likely to have occurred.

Reference	Tucker, 1999		
Level (design)	3 (retrospective comparative)		
Sample size	27 medialization, 33 combined medialization with reinnervation		
OUTCOMES			
Outcome measures	Voice assessment and rankings: high-quality audio tapes of voice samples from each patient were rated at 3 mo, 6 mo, and 2 y postoperatively		
No reinnervation	19% normal 56% improved 19% greatly improved 8% somewhat better 0% no worse	15% normal 63% improved 15% greatly improved 7% somewhat better 0% no worse	7% normal 41% improved 37% greatly improved 15% somewhat better 0% no worse
Reinnervation	21% normal 48% improved 21% greatly improved 6% somewhat better 3% no worse	36% normal 39% improved 18% greatly improved 3% somewhat better 3% no worse	39% normal 45% improved 12% greatly improved 3% somewhat better 3% no worse
Follow-up time	3 mo	6 mo	2 y
p Value	Not reported	Not reported	Not reported
Conclusion	Trend toward more normal voice with ML + reinnervation vs ML alone, especially at later follow-up times		
STUDY DESIGN			
Inclusion criteria	Persistent unilateral vocal fold immobility. At the time of surgery, direct EMG studies of the exposed lateral thyroarytenoideus muscle were performed to determine if there was retained or recovered innervation of the vocal fold. Patients with any residual innervation had medialization alone. Those with no EMG evidence of reinnervation received combined therapy		
Exclusion criteria	None specified		
Medialization details	Customized carved Silastic implant used for medialization. EMG performed to assess thyroarytenoid function during procedure		
Reinnervation details	Nerve muscle pedicle created from 1 of strap muscles. Pedicle placed in close proximity to exposed laryngeal muscle fibers		
Voice and video measurements	Videostroboscopic was not available for all patients, therefore results not reported in paper. Methods for recording of voice samples were not elaborated. All patients' voices were assessed by a panel of "sophisticated" listeners, including at least 1 speech and language pathologist and 1 otolaryngologist other than the surgeon. They ranked the voices heard on high-quality audio tapes as normal, greatly improved, somewhat improved, no better, or voice worse, when comparing preoperative to postoperative results		
Age	Not specified		
Masking	Not specified		
Diagnostic criteria for cord paralysis	Clinical diagnosis with intraoperative EMG evaluation		
Consecutive patients?	Yes		
Morbidity/complications	Not reported		

AA = arytenoid adduction, ML = medialization laryngoplasty, EMG = electromyographic.

Reference	Chhetri, 1999
Level (design)	3 (retrospective comparative)
Sample size	9 AA patients, 10 combined AA and reinnervation patients

OUTCOMES

Outcome measures	Glottal closure, mucosal wave, symmetry, laryngeal airflow, subglottic pressure, perceptual analysis by panel of voice professionals
No reinnervation	

Group 1: Arytenoid Adduction

Parameter	Pre		Post	P value
Closure	1.6		4.0	<0.05
Mucosal wave				
P	2.0		3.8	<0.05
NP	2.8		4.4	<0.05
Symmetry		x^2		>0.05
Pressure	8.0		7.7	>0.05
Airflow	586		326	<0.05
Resistance	14.8		35.3	<0.05
Perceptual	5.2		3.8	<0.05

Reinnervation	

Group 2: Combined Adduction and Reinnervation

Parameter	Pre		Post	P value
Closure	2.6		4.5	<0.05
Mucosal wave				
P	3.3		4.2	<0.05
NP	4.0		4.8	<0.05
Symmetry		x^2		>0.05
Pressure	8.6		8.2	>0.05
Airflow	445		298	>0.05
Resistance	22.3		31.5	>0.05
Perceptual	4.3		2.9	<0.05

Follow-up time	Follow-up voice recording 2–60 mo
p Value	Not reported
Conclusion	No significant difference noted in comparing AA + reinnervation vs AA + no reinnervation. Significant improvements in multiple parameters pre- vs post–AA + reinnervation and pre- vs post–AA + no reinnervation

STUDY DESIGN

Inclusion criteria	Unilateral vocal fold paralysis. Patients underwent aforementioned procedures for treatment of unilateral vocal fold paralysis. All patients with adequate preoperative evaluation were included in study
Exclusion criteria	Inadequate preoperative evaluation or inability to have postoperative evaluation
Medialization details	Arytenoid adduction as described by Isshiki et al. (1978) with modifications as described by Bielamowicz et al. (1995)
Reinnervation details	Ansa cervicalis to recurrent laryngeal nerve anastomosis as described by Crumley (1986)
Voice and video measurements	90-degree telescopic laryngoscope with camera and stroboscopic unit. Laryngeal airflow and subglottic pressure measured as described by Smitehran and Hixon (1981). 2-second voice samples excerpted from middle of sentence
Age	48.2 y medialization group, 40.1 y combined group
Masking	For voice sample recording
Diagnostic criteria for cord paralysis	Unilateral vocal fold paralysis
Consecutive patients?	No
Morbidity/complications	None reported

AA = arytenoid adduction, ML = medialization laryngoplasty, EMG = electromyographic.

Reference	Chou, 2002	
Level (design)	2 (prospective cohort study)	
Sample size	8 reinnervation, 4 medialization laryngoplasty	

OUTCOMES

Outcome measures	**GRBAS scale:** 0 normal, 1 mild, 2 moderate, 3 severe, 4 complete	**Maximum phonation time**

Grade — Neurorrhaphy (n = 8), Without neurorrhaphy (n = 4), p1 = 0.008, p = 0.317; Follow-up months (3 months, 6 months)

Roughness — Neurorrhaphy (n = 8), Without neurorrhaphy (n = 4), p2 = 0.023, p > 0.9; Follow-up months (3 months, 6 months)

With neurorrhaphy 4.9 ± 1.3 s, 10 ± 1.8 s
Without neurorrhaphy "No change"

Breathiness — Neurorrhaphy (n = 8), Without neurorrhaphy (n = 4), p3 = 0.038, p = 0.317; Follow-up months (3 months, 6 months)

Asthenia — Neurorrhaphy (n = 8), Without neurorrhaphy (n = 4), p4 = 0.014, p = 0.317; Follow-up months (3 months, 6 months)

Vocal fold atrophy
With neurorrhaphy 12.5% (n = 1/8)
Without neurorrhaphy 100% (n = 4/4)
All 4 required medialization laryngoplasty

Strain — Neurorrhaphy (n = 8), Without neurorrhaphy (n = 4), p5 = 0.034, p = 0.317; Follow-up months (3 months, 6 months)

p Value	As shown above, 3 mo vs 6 mo	**MPT** 0.011, with neurorrhaphy 3 mo vs 6 mo NS, without neurorrhaphy **Atrophy** 0.01, with neurorrhaphy vs without neurorrhaphy
Conclusion	Significant improvement between 3 and 6 mo with neurorrhaphy No significant change between 3 and 6 mo without neurorrhaphy	
Follow-up time	3 mo, 6 mo	

STUDY DESIGN

Inclusion criteria	UVFP in patients with complete RLN injury or resection caused by various diseases. 8 patients had primary repair, the other 4 had no repair secondary to cancer involvement of distal stump
Exclusion criteria	None specified
No reinnervation details	No reinnervation allowed only in patients with cancer invasion of distal stump of nerve not eligible for neurorrhaphy. Otherwise not specified
Reinnervation details	Primary repair of RLN under operating microscope. Anastomoses were usually made with two stitches of 10-0 nylon
Voice and video measurements	Laryngoscopy and laryngovideoscopy performed at 3 and 6 mo after RLN injury or neurorrhaphy. Stroboscopy performed with standard equipment
Age	Mean 45.9 y
Masking	No
Diagnostic criteria for cord paralysis	Endocrine surgeon judged completeness of nerve injury intraoperatively
Consecutive patients?	No
Morbidity/complications	None reported

Source: Figures from Chou et al. [3], reproduced with permission from Elsevier.
GRBAS = Grade, Roughness, Breathiness, Asthenia, Strain, RLN = recurrent laryngeal nerve, UVFP = unilateral vocal fold paralysis, NS = not significant.

REFERENCES

1. Tucker HM. Long-term preservation of voice improvement following surgical medialization and reinnervation for unilateral vocal fold paralysis. J Voice 1999;13(2):251–256.
2. Chhetri DK. Combined arytenoid adduction and laryngeal reinnervation in the treatment of vocal fold paralysis. Laryngoscope 1999;109:1928–1936.
3. Chou FF, Su CY, Jeng SF, Hsu KL, Lu KY. Neurorrhaphy of the recurrent laryngeal nerve. J Am Coll Surg 2003; 197(1). Presented at the Annual Meeting of the International College of Surgeons, Taipei, Taiwan, October 2002.
4. Isshiki N, Tanabe M, Sawada M. Arytenoid adduction for unilateral vocal cord paralysis. Arch Otolaryngol 1978 Oct; 104(10):555–558.
5. Biel amowicz S, Berke GS. An improved method of medialization laryngoplasty using a three-sided thyroplasty window. Laryngoscope 1995 May; 108(5 Pt 1):537–539.
6. Crumley RL, Izdebski K. Voice quality following laryngeal reinnervation by ansa hypoalossi transfer. Laryngoscope. 1986 Jun; 96(6):611–616.
7. Smitheran JR, Hixon TJ. A clinical method for estimating laryngeal airway resistance during vowel production. J Speech Hear Disord 1981 May; 46(2):138–146.

SECTION V

Systematic Reviews in Head and Neck Oncologic Surgery

Section Editors

Jonas Johnson, MD

Gregory Randolph, MD

25 Survival Analysis

Sandra S. Stinnett

Survival analysis is concerned with time to the occurrence of an *event*, such as death, recurrence or disease, or failure of an implanted medical device. Computing only the overall proportion surviving the event neglects the important aspect of time. We need a measure that accounts not only for *whether* patients die, but also for *when* they die. In other words, we want to look at the pattern of dying over time.

OVERVIEW

In survival analysis, patients are followed for a specified period of time or until the event has occurred. Some patients may not even experience the event during the follow-up period. Other patients may be lost to follow-up during the study period. Both of these types of patients have incomplete data for survival or "time-to-an-event" and are called "censored." The analysis of survival data requires special methods that account for censoring. These methods focus on the pattern of occurrences of the event which is displayed as a "survival curve." Survival patterns are summarized by survival probabilities at certain time points. The median time to reach the endpoint can also be reported. Often, two or more groups of patients are compared with respect to their survival patterns. The significance of the difference between survival curves can also be examined using statistical tests. In addition, the effect of other variables on the survival function can be modeled and assessed for significance.

There are three primary methods for analyzing these types of data that deal with the issue of censoring. The first method, called the life-table (LT) or actuarial method, was used primarily before the advent of computers because it is easy to compute by hand. In this method, follow-up times are divided into intervals and those dying (or experiencing the event) in that interval of time are counted. From this, the probability of surviving through that interval of time is computed. If you do not know the exact times of death, just intervals in which deaths occurred, you are limited to using this method. The second method is the Kaplan-Meier (KM) method, in which exact times of death (or other event) are used and a computer does all the work in computing the survival function. This method is preferred because it is more accurate. It is possible to use statistical tests to assess whether two or more survival curves differ from each other in their patterns of survival. The third method is the Cox proportional hazards model which includes the tests to assess differences in survival curves and also allows other variables to be added to the model. In an analysis, one might want to begin with the KM method, use tests to compare survival functions, and then proceed to examine additional variables with the Cox model. There are many statistical software packages that contain procedures for survival analysis. Computations for this chapter were performed using SAS® procedures LIFETEST (KM) and PHREG (Cox model) [1].

	Definitions
Survival methods	Techniques for analyzing time-to-event data that account for censoring
Status	Whether the individual experienced the event or not
Censored	Not experiencing the event during the follow-up time or lost to follow-up at a specific time
Survival function	The probability of an individual not experiencing the endpoint at specific times after the start of the study
Survival curves	Plots that display survival probabilities
Life-table method	The method of computing survival probabilities when the time to reach an endpoint or censored time is known only within an interval of time
Kaplan-Meier method	The method of computing survival probabilities when an endpoint occurs, displayed as a series of steps
Kaplan-Meier model	A regression model used to test the effect of potentially explanatory variables on survival
Logrank test	A test that assesses whether there are differences in the survival curves between groups being studied
Hazard function	The instantaneous potential per unit time for the event to occur, at a time t, given survival up to time t. For the LT method: $q_i = d_i/n_i'$. For the KM method: $q_t = d_t/n_t$. (See notation below.)
Hazard ratio	Over all time points, the ratio of the risk of the event in one group to the risk of the event in another group
Proportional hazard	The constancy of the hazard ratio over time

Notation

t	Time to the event or, if censored, duration of time observed as during an *interval* (t_i for LT) or at a given *time* (t_t for KM)
d	The number of deaths in the time interval (d_i for LT) or at a given time (d_t for KM)
c	The number of censored observations in the time interval (c_i for LT) or at a given time (c_t for KM)
n	The number of individuals who are alive and are at risk of death at the start of the interval (n_i for LT) or at a given time (n_t for KM)
n_i'	The average number of individuals who are at risk in a time interval (for LT), computed as the number entering the interval n_i minus half the number of censored observations c_i
q	The proportion *dying* in the interval (q_i for LT) or at a given time (q_t for KM), computed as $q_i = d_i/n_i'$ for LT and as $q_t = d_t/n_t$ for KM
p	The proportion *surviving* the interval (p_i for LT) or at a given time (p_t for KM), computed as $p = 1 - q$
S	Survivorship function or the probability of surviving to a given time interval (S_i for LT) or point (S_t for KM), given the survival of all previous time intervals or time points, computed by multiplying together all previous probabilities of survival: $S_i = p_i \, p_{(i-1)} \ldots p_2 p_1$ for LT and $S_t = p_t p_{(t-1)} \ldots p_2 p_1$ for KM

ASSUMPTIONS OF SURVIVAL ANALYSIS

Norman and Steiner [2] provide a good discussion of the assumptions of survival analysis:

1. *An identifiable starting point*, such as time since diagnosis or time since first treatment and it should be applied uniformly for all patients.
2. *A clear end point.* Death is usually clear; however, death attributable to other causes (not the one being investigated) will have to be classified as either death or withdrawal. How to handle this situation should be decided in advance. Recurrence may be problematic, especially if a condition or disease recurs many times. Usually time to first recurrence is used.
3. *Loss to follow-up should not be related to the outcome.* If those who dropped out of a study did so because they died of the disease in question and this was unknown to the investigator, the results of the study would be biased.
4. *No secular trend.* This means that during the trial period, nothing should change regarding the selection of patients, the treatment or other factors that would impact the outcome.

ILLUSTRATIVE EXAMPLE

We will consider a data set from a hypothetical clinical trial of two different treatments for laryngeal cancer. In this study, patients were treated with either radiation alone or with both radiation and surgery. Each group had 40 patients. The main purpose of this study was to determine whether patients treated with radiation and surgery survive longer than patients treated with radiation alone. Data for all patients are shown in Table 25.1. In addition to survival time in months (time since treatment), the data include sex and age of the patient at trial entry. The status at the end of the study is given as "Alive" or "Dead." If patients are alive at the end of the study or at the time of withdrawal from the study, they are "censored"(see definitions above), which means that they have not died yet. They were also censored if they were "lost" during the study. Dawson and Trapp [3] clearly illustrate the analysis of survival data with examples; the illustration of computations here is patterned after their presentation.

We can consider whether the two variables, sex and age, are related to survival. If they are, we can account for this in the comparison of survival of the two groups. Because these data are from a clinical trial in which patients were randomized to treatment groups, the groups should be similar in terms of demographics. If they are not, this difference may impact the survival times; this is another reason to account for them in the analysis.

In this study, there was a preponderance of males in both groups, 92.5% in the radiation group and 87.5% in the surgery + radiation group. These proportions were not significantly different. The average age of patients in the radiation group was 66.9 years. In the surgery + radiation group, the average age was 62 years. The difference in ages is significant ($p = 0.003$, two-sample *t*-test). The mean and median survival times were 12.8 and 9.9 months for the radiation group and 20.4 and 16.7 for the surgery + radiation group. From this preliminary analysis, we conclude that those in the surgery + radiation group survived longer than those receiving radiation alone. In the survival analysis, we will see how the patterns of survival differ in the two groups.

LIFE-TABLE METHOD OF SURVIVAL ANALYSIS

In the LT, or actuarial, method, the times to death are not known exactly, but are known within an interval of time.

TABLE 25.1. Survival times of laryngeal cancer patients in a hypothetical clinical trial to compare treatments

Patient no.	Treatment	Age (y)	Sex	Months Survival	Status	Patient no.	Treatment	Age (y)	Sex	Months Survival	Status
1	Surgery/radiation	61	Male	20.9	Alive	41	Surgery/radiation	68	Female	23.7	Dead
2	Surgery/radiation	51	Male	50.5	Alive	42	Surgery/radiation	63	Male	17.1	Dead
3	Radiation	72	Male	18.1	Dead	43	Surgery/radiation	66	Male	44.8	Dead
4	Radiation	69	Male	4.9	Dead	44	Radiation	71	Male	14.5	Dead
5	Surgery/radiation	72	Male	23.6	Dead	45	Radiation	70	Male	8.8	Dead
6	Radiation	70	Male	19.0	Alive	46	Radiation	71	Male	8.3	Alive
7	Surgery/radiation	62	Male	43.4	Alive	47	Surgery/radiation	67	Male	12.5	Alive
8	Radiation	65	Female	9.3	Alive	48	Surgery/radiation	62	Male	13.5	Alive
9	Radiation	70	Male	4.9	Alive	49	Radiation	64	Male	5.5	Alive
10	Radiation	72	Male	13.3	Dead	50	Radiation	70	Male	5.4	Alive
11	Surgery/radiation	50	Male	18.4	Alive	51	Radiation	63	Male	17.6	Alive
12	Surgery/radiation	53	Female	16.9	Alive	52	Surgery/radiation	69	Male	44.6	Alive
13	Radiation	71	Male	10.5	Dead	53	Surgery/radiation	70	Female	12.5	Alive
14	Surgery/radiation	71	Male	25.5	Dead	54	Surgery/radiation	46	Male	9.2	Alive
15	Surgery/radiation	52	Male	8.0	Alive	55	Surgery/radiation	72	Male	30.7	Alive
16	Radiation	70	Male	12.6	Alive	56	Surgery/radiation	73	Male	15.1	Alive
17	Radiation	66	Female	8.8	Dead	57	Surgery/radiation	34	Female	8.4	Alive
18	Radiation	54	Male	35.5	Alive	58	Radiation	68	Male	14.7	Alive
19	Radiation	72	Male	33.6	Alive	59	Radiation	74	Male	26.6	Dead
20	Surgery/radiation	53	Male	37.7	Alive	60	Radiation	62	Male	15.9	Dead
21	Surgery/radiation	61	Male	42.8	Alive	61	Radiation	63	Male	6.4	Dead
22	Radiation	71	Male	11.8	Alive	62	Radiation	61	Male	6.5	Dead
23	Surgery/radiation	66	Male	29.7	Dead	63	Radiation	71	Male	8.9	Dead
24	Surgery/radiation	65	Male	12.3	Alive	64	Surgery/radiation	60	Male	26.3	Dead
25	Surgery/radiation	54	Male	7.9	Alive	65	Surgery/radiation	72	Male	9.9	Alive
26	Radiation	58	Male	15.5	Dead	66	Surgery/radiation	69	Male	5.0	Alive
27	Radiation	61	Male	5.9	Alive	67	Radiation	66	Male	16.3	Alive
28	Surgery/radiation	56	Male	23.6	Alive	68	Radiation	73	Male	9.4	Alive
29	Radiation	69	Male	13.9	Alive	69	Radiation	69	Male	3.8	Alive
30	Radiation	70	Male	16.5	Alive	70	Surgery/radiation	55	Male	13.3	Alive
31	Radiation	63	Male	26.3	Alive	71	Surgery/radiation	69	Male	17.9	Dead
32	Radiation	55	Male	10.4	Alive	72	Radiation	73	Female	9.4	Alive
33	Surgery/radiation	56	Female	10.1	Alive	73	Surgery/radiation	51	Male	11.0	Dead
34	Surgery/radiation	73	Male	16.6	Dead	74	Surgery/radiation	71	Male	15.6	Alive
35	Surgery/radiation	60	Male	21.7	Alive	75	Surgery/radiation	65	Male	15.9	Alive
36	Surgery/radiation	69	Male	15.8	Dead	76	Radiation	73	Male	5.9	Dead
37	Radiation	58	Male	9.4	Dead	77	Radiation	66	Male	6.7	Dead
38	Radiation	68	Male	27.3	Dead	78	Surgery/radiation	59	Male	17.2	Alive
39	Surgery/radiation	71	Male	11.8	Dead	79	Radiation	65	Female	9.3	Dead
40	Surgery/radiation	62	Male	14.9	Alive	80	Radiation	60	Male	5.3	Alive

Therefore, the analysis focuses on the interval in which the death occurred. The information needed for computation of survival is displayed in Table 25.2 for the patients in the radiation group. Even though we know the actual number of months of survival, we have grouped them into time intervals here to illustrate the analysis.

In Table 25.2, d_i and c_i denote the number of deaths and the number that are censored, respectively, in the time interval. The number of individuals who are alive and are at risk of death at the start of the interval is n_i. Now, we assume that the censored individuals leave the study uniformly during the interval. So, the average number of individuals who are at risk, n_i', is computed as the number entering the interval, n_i, minus half the number of censored observations, c_i. The number at risk, n_i', is the denominator in the computation of the proportion dying, which is computed as $(q_i = d_i/n_i')$. The proportion surviving the interval is one minus the proportion dying, $(p_i = 1 - q_i)$.

The probability that an individual survives through a given time interval is the product of the probabilities that an individual survives through the start of that interval given that they had survived through each of the preceding intervals. This is called the LT estimate of survival, S, and is referred to as the survival function. The estimated probability of surviving until the start of the first interval is 1. In the example above, no events occur in the first interval, 0–3 months. So, the probability of survival until the start of the second interval is still 1. In the second interval, >3 to 6 months, there are two deaths and six withdrawals, or censored individuals. We compute the number at risk, n_i', as 40 minus half the censored individuals (3). So, the number at risk is 37 and the proportion dying is $2/37 = 0.0541$. Then, the proportion surviving is $1 - 0.0541 = 0.9459$. The survival function is computed as the product of the previous value of the survival function and the proportion surviving the current interval. For this interval, the survival function is $1.000 \times 0.9459 = 0.9459$. For the second interval, the survival function is computed as $0.9459 \times 0.8095 = 0.7658$. This procedure is repeated for the remaining intervals.

The survival function is usually presented in graphical form as a survival curve, as shown for these data in Figure 25.1.

The LT survival distribution for patients in the surgery + radiation group is shown in Table 25.3. For comparison, see Figure 25.2.

TABLE 25.2. Life-table survival distribution for patients in the radiation group

Time interval (mo) (i)	No. entering interval (n_i)	No. censored during interval (c_i)	No. at risk ($n_i' = n_i - 0.5c_i$)	No. of events (d_i)	Proportion dying ($q_i = d_i/n_i'$)	Proportion surviving ($p_i = 1 - q_i$)	Survival function ($S_i = p_i p_{(i-1)} \cdots p_2 p_1$)
0 to 3	40	0	40	0	0	1.000	1.000
>3 to 6	40	6	37	2	0.0541	0.9459	0.9459
>6 to 9	32	1	31.5	6	0.1905	0.8095	0.7658
>9 to 12	25	5	22.5	3	0.1333	0.8667	0.6637
>12 to 15	17	3	15.5	2	0.1290	0.8710	0.5780
>15 to 18	12	3	10.5	2	0.1905	0.8095	0.4679
>18 to 21	7	1	6.5	1	0.1538	0.8462	0.3959
>21	5	3	3.5	2	0.5714	0.4286	0.1697

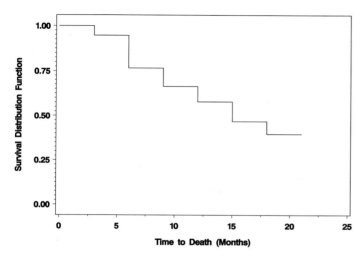

Figure 25.1. Life-table survival distribution for the radiation group.

TABLE 25.3. Life-table survival distribution for patients on surgery + radiation

Time interval (mo) (i)	No. entering interval (n_i)	No. censored during interval (c_i)	No. at risk ($n_i' = n_i - 0.5c_i$)	No. of events (d_i)	Proportion dying ($q_i = d_i/n_i'$)	Proportion surviving ($p_i = 1 - q_i$)	Survival function ($S_i = p_i p_{(i-1)} \cdots p_2 p_1$)
0 to 3	40	0	40	0	0	1.000	1.000
>3 to 6	40	1	39.5	0			
>6 to 9	39	3	37.5	0			
>9 to 12	36	3	34.5	2	0.0580	0.9420	0.9420
>12 to 15	31	6	28	0			
>15 to 18	25	5	22.5	4	0.1778	0.8222	0.7746
>18 to 21	16	2	15	0			
>21	14	8	10	6	0.6000	0.4000	0.3098

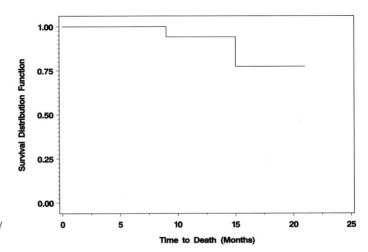

Figure 25.2. Life-table survival distribution for surgery/radiation group.

KAPLAN-MEIER PRODUCT LIMIT METHOD OF SURVIVAL ANALYSIS

In the KM method of survival analysis, survival is estimated as each event occurs (patient dies or has recurrence). Table 25.4 illustrates the computation of the survival function for the radiation group. The time at which an event occurs is denoted as t. The number at risk at the time of the event is (n_t). The number of events (d_t) and the proportion having an event ($q_t = d_t/n_t$) are shown in the next two columns. The proportion surviving ($p_t = 1 - q_t$) and the survival function ($S_t = p_t p_{(t-1)} \cdots p_2 p_1$) are given in the last two columns. Computations are similar to the LT method, but are performed each time an event (death) occurs. Before the first event, all 40 patients are alive and the value of the survival function is 1.000. In this example, one patient is lost to follow-up, or censored, at 3.80 months. The number at risk is now 39. The first patient dies at 4.86 months. We now compute mortality, proportion surviving, and the survival function at this point. The proportion dying is 1/39 = 0.0256; the proportion surviving is 1 − 0.0256 = 0.9744; the survival function is 1.000 × 0.9744 = 0.9744. One patient is subsequently censored at each of the following times: 4.90, 5.30, 5.36, and 5.52 months. These four patients, plus the

patient censored at 3.8 months and the one death comprise those who have left the study. There are now 34 patients remaining at risk when the next death occurs at 5.90 months. At this point, the proportion dying is 1/34 = 0.0294; the proportion surviving is 1 − 0.0294 = 0.9706; the survival function is 0.9744 × 0.9706 = 0.9457. The process is repeated for the remaining events.

The survival function estimates are presented in a graph, as shown in Figure 25.3 for the radiation group.

COMPARING TWO SURVIVAL CURVES

Often, investigators want to compare two or more groups of patients in terms of survival. The KM survival curves for both treatment groups are shown in Figure 25.4. A visual examination of the curves reveals that the survival was similar for the first 5 months of the study. At that point, the curves diverge rapidly. We see that those receiving radiation alone died more quickly and had lower survival rates. One patient in the surgery + radiation group survived more than 50 months, whereas the last patient in the radiation group survived approximately 35 months. Typically, the median survival time and the survival rate at a certain time, such as at 1 year or 5 years, are reported and compared for the two groups. Survival

TABLE 25.4. Survival distribution for patients on radiation

Event time (mo) (t)	No. at risk (n_t)	No. of events (d_t)	Proportion dying ($q_t = d_t/n_t$)	Proportion surviving ($p_t = 1 - q_t$)	Survival function ($S_t = p_t p_{(t-1)} \cdots p_2 p_1$)
0	40			1.0000	1.0000
3.80	40				
4.86	39	1	0.0256	0.9744	0.9744
4.90	38				
5.30	37				
5.36	36				
5.52	35				
5.90	34	1	0.0294	0.9706	0.9457
5.95	33				
6.37	32	1	0.0313	0.9688	0.9161
6.50	31	1	0.0323	0.9677	0.8866
6.67	30	1	0.0333	0.9667	0.8570
8.34	29				
8.80	28	1	0.0357	0.9543	0.8264
8.80	27	1	0.0370	0.9630	0.7958
8.90	26	1	0.0385	0.9615	0.7652
9.30	25	1	0.0400	0.9600	0.7346
9.30	24				
9.40	23				
9.43	22	1	0.0455	0.9545	0.7012
9.43	21				
10.40	20				
10.51	19	1	0.0526	0.9474	0.6643
11.80	18				
12.58	17				
13.27	16	1	0.0625	0.9375	0.6228
13.86	15				
14.50	14	1	0.0714	0.9286	0.5783
14.65	13				
15.50	12	1	0.0833	0.9167	0.5301
15.87	11	1	0.0909	0.9091	0.4819
16.26	10				
16.46	9				
17.61	8				
18.10	7	1	0.1429	0.8571	0.4131
18.99	6				
26.30	5				
26.60	4	1	0.2500	0.7500	0.3098
27.30	3	1	0.3333	0.6667	0.2065
33.60	2				
35.50	1				

rates can be read from computer output (similar to Table 25.4) which also contains confidence intervals around the survival estimates. In this example, the median survival times are 15.87 months for the radiation group and 29.70 months for the radiation + surgery group. The 1-year survival rate is 0.6643 for the radiation group and 0.9394 for the radiation + surgery group.

The Logrank Test. There are several methods for testing the significance of the difference in survival rates depicted by the two curves. The most frequently used statistic is the logrank test, which compares the number of *observed* deaths in each group with the number of deaths that would be *expected* based on the number of deaths in the combined groups, disregarding group membership.

Computer programs calculate the logrank statistic without dividing the data into intervals. The observed and expected number of failures or deaths is computed each time a patient dies or is censored. The computations for this method are intensive, though accurate. However, to illustrate how the statistic is calculated, we will divide the data into intervals as was done for the LT method.

In Table 25.5, the time intervals are listed in column 1. Columns 2 and 3 give the number "at risk" at the beginning of each interval (removing those who died or were censored in the previous interval). Column 4 gives the total number of patients at risk in the interval. Columns 5–7 give the *observed* number of deaths in each treatment group and the total number of deaths. Columns 8–10 give the *expected* number of deaths for each group and the total. The expected values are computed by multiplying the proportion in each group at each interval by the total number of deaths occurring in that interval. (Column 2/column 4) × column 7 = column 8. (Column 3/column 4) × column 7 = column 9. For a given time interval, the total number of observed deaths (column 7) is of course the same as the total number of expected deaths (column 10).

For example, in the interval >6 to 9 months, the proportion of patients in the radiation group is 32/71 = 0.4507. The total number of deaths occurring in that interval is 6. So, the expected number of deaths in the radiation group is 0.4507 × 6 = 2.70423. For the surgery + radiation group, the proportion of patients is 39/71 = 0.5493. The expected number of deaths in the surgery/radiation group is 0.5493 × 6 = 3.29577. This process is repeated for each interval. The total number of observed and expected deaths is computed as the sum of the values (rows) in columns 5 and 6 and columns 8 and 9, respec-

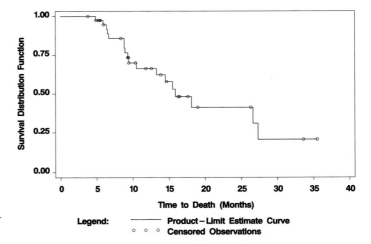

Figure 25.3. Kaplan-Meier survival distribution for radiation group.

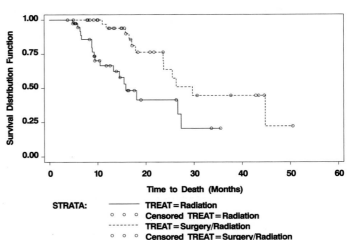

Figure 25.4. Kaplan-Meier survival distributions for both treatment groups.

tively. The totals are used in the computation of the logrank statistic which has a chi-square distribution (χ^2) with one degree of freedom. [The χ^2 distribution is a statistical distribution that is used to test differences between proportions and to test differences between observed and expected data. The χ^2 distribution has one parameter, its degrees of freedom (df). Its shape has a positive skew (longer tail on the right end of the distribution). The skew decreases as df increase.]

The following equation is used to assess whether the survival distributions are the same in each group.

$$\chi^2 = (O_1 - E_1)^2/E_1 + (O_2 - E_2)^2/E_2$$
$$= (18 - 10.8172959)^2/(10.8172959)$$
$$+ (12 - 19.1827041)^2/19.1827041$$
$$= 7.46$$

In this equation, O_1 and E_1 and O_2 and E_2 are the numbers of observed and expected deaths in group 1 (radiation) and group 2 (surgery/radiation), respectively. The χ^2 distribution with one df has a critical value of 3.841. Because our computed value of 7.46 exceeds 3.841, we conclude that there is a statistically significant difference between the two survival curves. The p value that corresponds to this value of the test statistic is 0.006.

The Hazard Ratio. The hazard function is the probability that a person will die (or fail or have a recurrence) in the next interval of time, given that the person has survived until the beginning of the interval. The hazard ratio is a measure that is frequently used to quantify the difference between survival distributions for two groups. It is computed as

$$\text{Hazard ratio} = (O_1/E_1)/(O_2/E_2).$$

For this study, the hazard ratio, or risk of death for patients in the radiation group compared to patients in the surgery/radiation group is

$$\text{Hazard ratio} = (18/10.8170)/(12/19.1830) = 2.66.$$

The risk of death in the radiation group is about 2.7 times greater than the risk in the surgery + radiation group. An assumption has been made that the hazard ratio remains the same through the study period. When this is not the case, other methods of comparing the two groups may be more appropriate.

Cox Proportional Hazards Model. Often, investigators would like to know the effect of certain variables on the length of survival. In this particular study, we might want to examine the effects of age and sex on survival. This is accomplished by using a statistical model that has some similarities to multiple linear regression. In multiple linear regression, the simultaneous effect of several independent variables on an outcome or dependent variable are calculated. The result of the analysis, provided by a statistical software program, is a series of coefficients or parameter estimates that comprise a linear combination of the variables. In a similar manner, the Cox proportional hazards model produces a set of coefficients for the variables in the model. However, in this case, the response or dependent variable is the time-to-event (death, recurrence, or device failure). The exponentials of these coefficients are the hazard ratios. Each ratio represents the risk of having the endpoint for a unit increase in the corresponding variable, adjusting for other variables in the model. For variables that are dichotomous (having two values such as yes or no), the hazard ratio gives the risk for one group relative to the other. To calculate the associated statistical test, the Wald χ^2 statistic, the parameter estimate (the coefficient of the variable) is divided by its standard error and then squared.

The computation involved in the Cox model is extensive and requires a computer program. Here, we simply present the results of running the procedure PHREG in SAS (statistics software). The SAS output for the first model containing only treatment (TREAT, where the variable is coded as 0 = surgery + radiation and 1 = radiation) is shown below.

TABLE 25.5. Computing the logrank statistic

Time interval (mo) (1)	Patients at risk			Observed deaths			Expected deaths		
	Rad (2)	Surgery/ radiation (3)	Total (4)	Radiation (5)	Surgery/ radiation (6)	Total(7)	Radiation (8)	Surgery/ radiation (9)	Total (10)
0 to 3	40	40	80	0	0	0	0	0	0
>3 to 6	40	40	80	2	0	2	1.00000	1.000	2
>6 to 9	32	39	71	6	0	6	2.70423	3.29577	6
>9 to 12	25	36	61	3	2	5	2.04918	2.95082	5
>12 to 15	17	31	48	2	0	2	0.70833	1.29167	2
>15 to 18	12	25	37	2	4	6	1.94595	4.05405	6
>18 to 21	7	16	23	1	0	1	0.30435	0.69565	1
>21	5	14	19	2	6	8	2.10526	5.89474	8
Totals				18	12	30	10.8170	19.1830	30

Model 1

Variable	df	Standard Estimate	Error	Hazard χ^2 Pr	$> \chi^2$	Variable Ratio	Label
TREAT	1	1.09127	0.38676	7.9612	0.0048	2.978	Treatment

The parameter estimate, 1.09127, is exponentiated ($e^{1.09127}$) to obtain the hazard ratio, 2.978. (Here, the data are not divided into intervals as it was when we computed this value by hand so the results differ slightly. This result is more accurate because it is computed each time a patient dies.) The hazard ratio means that the risk of dying in the radiation group is nearly 3 times greater than the risk of dying in the surgery + radiation group. The χ^2 statistic with a p value of 0.0048 indicates that there is a statistically significant difference between the treatment groups in their length of survival.

Model 2

Variable	df	Standard Estimate	Error	Hazard χ^2 Pr	$> \chi^2$	Variable Ratio	Label
TREAT	1	0.92063	0.39966	5.3062	0.0212	2.511	Treatment
AGE	1	0.04952	0.03162	2.4528	0.1173	1.051	

SAS output for models containing treatment (TREAT) and each covariable separately and jointly are shown below. The variable SEX is coded as 0 = males and 1 = females. For these models, the hazard ratio is "adjusted" for other variables in the model, meaning that these are the risk for that variable, given that treatment or other variables are in the model simultaneously.

Model 3

Variable	df	Standard Estimate	Error	Hazard χ^2 Pr	$> \chi^2$	Variable Ratio	Label
TREAT	1	1.16031	0.39349	8.6950	0.0032	3.191	Treatment
SEX	1	0.87696	0.64104	1.8715	0.1713	2.404	

Model 4

Variable	df	Standard Estimate	Error	Hazard χ^2 Pr	$> \chi^2$	Variable Ratio	Label
TREAT	1	0.98942	0.40546	5.9548	0.0147	2.690	Treatment
AGE	1	0.05235	0.03208	2.6624	0.1027	1.054	
SEX	1	0.95762	0.64124	2.2302	0.1353	2.605	

In these models, we see that treatment is the only variable that is significant. We can conclude that length of survival is not affected by age or by sex when in the presence of treatment. The interpretation of the hazard ratio for age in model 2 is that the risk of dying increases by 5% (1.051) for every year of age, after adjusting for treatment. The interpretation of the hazard ratio for sex in model 3 is that the risk of dying is 2.4 times greater in females that in males, after adjusting for treatment. However, these risks are not significant in the presence of the treatment variable. If the variables had been significant, we could have obtained new "adjusted" survival curves derived from the model with additional variables.

EXAMPLES OF SURVIVAL ANALYSIS IN OTOLARYNGOLOGY

A search of the journal *Otolaryngology–Head and Neck Surgery* over the years 2000–2004 revealed 16 articles and six abstracts of presentations at the AAO-HNS (American Academy of Otolaryngology–Head and Neck Surgery) annual meetings that utilized survival analysis. These are listed in the reference section. Applications of the analysis include:

- Determining staging characteristics and survival outcomes for primary malignancies of the trachea (Bhattacharyya [4])
- Determining if survival for second primary head and neck cancer is poorer than for first primaries (Bhyattacharyya and Nayak [5])
- Clarifying the importance of 16 possible prognostic factors for survival in patients with T3 NO MO laryngeal carcinoma treated with total laryngectomy (Gallo et al. [6])
- Determining the survival and prognostic factors for differentiated thyroid carcinoma (Bhattacharyya [7])
- Comparing the correlation of TANIS and TNM '97 with the survival rate in laryngeal cancer (Carinci et al. [8])

- Identifying factors influencing the outcome of post-operative radiotherapy in patients with advanced laryngeal cancer (Marshak et al. [9])
- Reporting the oncologic and functional outcome of patients undergoing near-total laryngectomy (Bernaldez et al. [10])
- Analyzing oncologic results, prognostic factors, and consideration of transglottic tumors as a separate entity in patients with T3 glottic carcinoma treated by surgery ± radiation therapy (Lassaletta et al. [11])
- Determining the prognostic importance of 8p23 loss in patients with head and neck squamous cell carcinoma (Bockmühl et al. [12])
- Assessing whether supracricoid laryngectomy with cricohyoidoepiglottopexy could successfully cure disease and preserve voice in glottic laryngeal cancer (Lima et al. [13])
- Analyzing the clinical and histologic features and follow-up of a series of patients with extra thyroid spread undergoing surgery for papillary carcinoma of the thyroid (Ortiz et al. [14])
- Evaluating the impact on survival achieved with the combination of surgical and postoperative radiotherapy in patients with advanced head and neck carcinomas and identifying the prognostic value of several host- and tumor-related factors (DeStefani et al. [15])
- Determining the cure rate and prognostic factors in patients who underwent endoscopic CO_2 laser excision for previously untreated early glottic cancer (Peretti et al. [1])
- Determining whether human papillomavirus type 16 affects survival in oral squamous cell carcinoma (Schwartz et al. [17]).

SUMMARY

Survival analysis provides a means of examining patterns of experiencing an event such as death, recurrence, or device failure. The methods used in survival analysis are special in that they use information from individuals who have not experienced the event by the end of the study or who have been lost during the course of the study. The survival patterns of one or more groups can be plotted for a visual examination of differences and tested for a statistical assessment of differences. Explanatory variables that may be related to the survival patterns may be included in additional analyses and tested for their significance. Adjusted survival curves resulting from these analyses can be compared and tested after accounting for these variables. Use of these methods in otolaryngology allows physicians to determine the patterns of survival after diagnosis of malignancy and other conditions, and also to compare and test the relative effects of treatments for these diseases among their patients.

REFERENCES

1. SAS/STAT® User's Guide. Version 8. Cary, NC: SAS Institute; 1999 (Procedures LIFETEST and PHREG).
2. Norman GR, Streiner DL. Biostatistics: The Bare Essentials. Hamilton, Ontario: BC Decker; 2000: Chapter 24.
3. Dawson B, Trapp RG. Basic and Clinical Biostatistics. 4th ed. New York: McGraw-Hill; 2004: Chapters 9 and 10.
4. Bhattacharyya N. Contemporary staging and prognosis for primary tracheal malignancies: a population-based analysis. Otolaryngol Head Neck Surg 2004;131(5):639–642.
5. Bhattacharyya N, Nayak VK. Survival outcomes for second primary head and neck cancer: a matched analysis. Otolaryngol Head Neck Surg 2004;131(2):P62–P63.
6. Gallo O, Sarno A, Baroncelli R, Bruschini L, Boddi V. Multivariate analysis of prognostic factors in T3 N0 laryngeal carcinoma treated with total laryngectomy. Otolaryngol Head Neck Surg 2003;128(5):654–662.
7. Bhattacharyya N. A population-based analysis of survival factors in differentiated and medullary thyroid carcinoma. Otolaryngol Head Neck Surg 2003;128(1):115–123.
8. Carinci F, Farina A, Pulicchi S, et al. Stage grouping reliability: TNM '97 versus TANIS in laryngeal cancer. Otolaryngol Head Neck Surg 1999;120(4):499–501.
9. Marshak G, Rakowsky E, Schachter J, et al. Is the delay in starting postoperative radiotherapy a key factor in the outcome of advanced (T3 and T4) laryngeal cancer? Otolaryngol Head Neck Surg 2004;131(4):489–493.
10. Bernaldez R, García-Pallarés M, Morera E, Lassaletta L, del Palacio A, Gavilán J. Oncologic and functional results of near-total laryngectomy. Otolaryngol Head Neck Surg 2003;128(5):700–705.
11. Lassaletta L, García-Pallarés M, Morera E, Bernáldez R, Gavilan J. T3 glottic cancer: oncologic results and prognostic factors. Otolaryngol Head Neck Surg 2001;124(5):556–560.
12. Bockmühl U, Ishwad CS, Ferrell RE, Gollin SM. Association of 8p23 deletions with poor survival in head and neck cancer. Otolaryngol Head Neck Surg 2001;124(4):451–455.
13. Lima RA, Freitas EQ, Kligerman J, et al. Supracricoid laryngectomy with CHEP: functional results and outcome. Otolaryngol Head Neck Surg 2001;124(3):258–260.
14. Ortiz S, Rodríguez JM, Soria T, et al. Extrathyroid spread in papillary carcinoma of the thyroid: clinicopathological and prognostic study. Otolaryngol Head Neck Surg 2001; 124(3):261–265.
15. De Stefani A, Magnano M, Cavalot A, et al. Adjuvant radiotherapy influences the survival of patients with squamous carcinoma of the head and neck who have poor prognoses. Otolaryngol Head Neck Surg 2000;123(5):630–636.
16. Peretti G, Nicolai P, de Zinis LOR, et al. Endoscopic CO laser excision for Tis, T1, and T2 glottic carcinomas: cure rate and prognostic factors. Otolaryngol Head Neck Surg 2000;123(1):124–131.
17. Schwartz SR, Yueh B, McDougall JK, Daling JR, Schwartz SM. Human papillomavirus infection and survival in oral squamous cell cancer: a population-based study. Otolaryngol Head Neck Surg 2001;125(1):1–9.

FOR FURTHER STUDY

1. Kirkwood BR, Sterne AC. Essential Medical Statistics. 2nd ed. Oxford UK: Blackwell Science; 2003: Chapter 26.

2. Banerjee A. Medical Statistics Made Clear: An Introduction to Basic Concepts. London: Royal Society of Medicine Press; 2003: Chapter 10.

3. Rosner B. Fundamentals of Biostatistics. 5th ed. Pacific Grove, CA: Duxbury; 2000: Chapter 14.

4. Aviva P, Sabin C. Medical Statistics at a Glance. Oxford, UK: Blackwell Science; 2000: Chapter 41.

5. Chang KP, Hao SP, Tsang NM. The 30-bp deletion from LMP-1 gene in the clinicopathological manifestation of NPC tumors. Otolaryngol Head Neck Surg 2004;131(2): P113–P114.

6. Ow TJ, Lin SJ, Mittal B, et al. Adenoid cystic carcinoma in the head and neck: an updated survival analysis. Otolaryngol Head Neck Surg 2004;131(2):P242–P243.

7. Ozdek A, Sarac S, Akyol MU, Sungur A, Yilmaz T. c-myc and bcl-2 expression in supraglottic squamous cell carcinoma of the larynx. Otolaryngol Head Neck Surg 2004; 131(1):77–83.

8. Nathan CAO, Amirghahari N, Rong X, Zhou H, Harrison L. EIF4E overexpression may confer radioresistance in a head and neck cancer cell line. Otolaryngol Head Neck Surg 2004;131(2):P178–P179.

9. Arora A, Mutairy AA, Harmer C, Rhys-Evans P. Comparison of surgery versus combined modality treatment in pt4 thyroid cancer. Otolaryngol Head Neck Surg 2004;131(2): P182.

10. Arora A, Powles J, Vini L, et al. The long-term outcome of patients with locally advanced thyroid carcinoma. Otolaryngol Head Neck Surg 2004;131(2):P183.

11. Kazi RA, Rhys Evans PH. A retrospective analysis of surgery for the oral cavity and oropharyngeal squamous cell carcinoma. Otolaryngol Head Neck Surg 2004;131(2):P234.

12. Ozdek A, Sarac S, Akyol MU, Sungur A, Yilmaz T. c-myc and bcl-2 expression in supraglottic squamous cell carcinoma of the larynx. Otolaryngol Head Neck Surg 2004; 131(1):77–83.

13. Paleri V, Pearson JP, Bulmer D, Jeannon JP, Wight RG, Wilson JA. Expression of mucin gene products in laryngeal squamous cancer. Otolaryngol Head Neck Surg 2004; 131(1):84–88.

26 Head and Neck Quality of Life Assessment and Outcomes Research

Richard Gliklich

Head and neck cancer and its treatment can be both debilitating and disfiguring. There is an undeniable impact on function, appearance, and pain, with potentially devastating consequences for nutrition, communication, and social interaction. Because of this impact, head and neck cancer treatment outcomes must center not only on survival, but also on quality of life (QOL). Whereas survival or disease-free survival can be mathematically straightforward measurements, QOL is more difficult to characterize and to measure. A QOL outcomes monitoring system for head and neck cancer and treatment requires tools that are valid and reliable, and that also address broad constructs of general health as well as those specific to the head and neck region.

QOL measurements can be global or disease-specific. Global QOL refers to a general assessment of patient functioning and well-being and may be affected by multiple disease processes. General health measures, such as the Medical Outcomes Study Short Form 36-item Survey (SF-36), allow comparisons across disease entities, and provide a gauge to understand side effects and tradeoffs of different therapies. Disease-specific QOL, in contrast, refers to the impact of one disease only. Head and neck–specific measures are less affected by comorbid illness, may be more precise, and are usually more sensitive to clinical change. Theoretically, the combination of specific and general measures provides the most comprehensive assessment strategy. The current approaches to measuring QOL center on utilizing either two measure batteries (general and disease-specific) or a single battery which combines elements of the two [1–10]. There are currently at least nine well-validated measures for QOL assessment in the head and neck, and probably others that have been less widely utilized [11–35].

To limit burden for the patient, it is necessary to determine which health dimensions are important in head and neck disease and which are truly specific to the head and neck. Gotay and Moore [8] conducted a systematic review of the published literature on head and neck cancer and grouped all the dimensions of QOL that were assessed using a standard categorization scheme. These included emotional well-being, spirituality, sexuality/intimacy, social functioning, occupational functioning, physical functioning, physical status including pain,

treatment satisfaction, global ratings, speech/communication, and eating/swallowing. Most of these health dimensions are assessed by several current, well-tested, general health measures such as the Medical Outcomes Study SF-36 Health Survey. Domains that may be considered specific to the head and neck include eating/swallowing, speech/communication, and appearance. Other studies have suggested that pain reporting differs between general and regional specific questions in head and neck cancer patients and head and neck pain may be an important specific domain.

Gliklich and Goldsmith [36] performed a comprehensive assessment to determine if head and neck–specific domains are truly different from those assessed by general health measures alone and found that health status domains considered relevant to the head and neck are not routinely evaluated by a general health measure alone. Comprehensive assessment of QOL in patients undergoing head and neck surgery requires both a general health survey and a head and neck–specific measure. The latter should include domains that reflect eating/swallowing, speech/communication, and appearance-related issues. Head and neck pain might also be considered for distinct measurement in both this report and others.

In reviewing QOL measures, it is important to understand the performance characteristics of the measurement systems. Performance characteristics include validity, reliability, and sensitivity to clinical change. Validity refers to whether or not the tool is measuring what it is intended to measure. In addition to "face" validity, questionnaires are developed from item banks and tested using standard assessments against predetermined hypotheses such as whether or not the measures converge or diverge from similar or different measures in terms of what they assess. Reliability refers to whether or not the measure gives repeatable results, such as when the same patient is retested without known interval clinical change (test–retest reliability) or when different raters are asked to rate the same patients (inter-rater reliability). Sensitivity to clinical change measures the extent to which the measure is likely to detect real clinical change. This is typically reported as a standardized response mean (SRM) or effect size (ES). These standardized performance characteristics provide the reviewer or selector of these instruments common parameters to compare one measure to another. However, before determining whether or not a particular measure is suitable for a particular use, the measure or tool should also be reviewed for other relevant parameters expected in actual use. These include using the measure in accordance with its intended purpose and selecting a measure with a reasonable level of respondent burden (e.g., how long it takes to complete the instrument) as well as other suitability parameters specific to each situation.

INDIVIDUAL INSTRUMENTS

The European Organization for Research and Treatment of Cancer (EORTC) is a modular instrument designed to bridge the roles of disease-specific and global QOL scales. It is patient-based, self-administered, and multidimensional. The EORTC QLQ-C30 core questionnaire (version 3.0) consists of 30 questions organized into five domains: physical, role, cognitive, emotional, and social; three symptom scales: fatigue, pain, nausea, and vomiting; two global scales (global health and QOL); and six single items (dysphagia, appetite loss, sleep disturbance, constipation, diarrhea, and financial impact). The head and neck module consists of 35 questions organized into seven domains (pain, swallowing, senses, speech, social eating, social contact, and sexuality), as well as 11 single items (problems with teeth, problems opening mouth, dry mouth, sticky saliva, coughed, felt ill, painkillers, nutritional supplements, feeding tube, lost weight, gained weight). Items for the core or general questionnaire were adapted from the literature.

The EORTC QLQ-H&N35 is intended for use in patients with head and neck cancer in all stages. Some issues, such as shoulder dysfunction and acute radiotherapy skin reactions, are not assessed. The questionnaire is self-administered. The mean completion time is 18 minutes. Cronbach's alpha (a standard measure of reliability) is above 0.70 for most scales in most patient groups. However, the "social eating" and "speech" subscales are not considered reliable. The scales do demonstrate responsiveness to changes over time.

The Functional Assessment of Cancer Therapy—Head & Neck (FACT-H&N) comprises a core questionnaire called FACT-G, and a disease-specific subscale (Figure 26.1). It was designed for descriptive, discriminative, and evaluative use. The FACT instruments are self-administered multiitem indices using category-rating scales. FACT-G consists of 27 questions in four domains—physical, social/family, emotional, and functional. The 38-item FACT-H&N also includes an 11-item head and neck cancer specific subscale. Each response is rated

from 0 to 4 on a Likert index, considering the past 7 days. Scores are calculated separately for each domain, and an unweighted summary score is calculated for the FACT-G and the total FACT-H&N. A scoring guide is available.

Whereas the FACT-G has been broadly developed, the H&N module utilized fewer than the recommended 50 patients for item generation. FACT-H&N is self-administered and easy to read, with clear instructions and consistent response options. The stated completion time is 5 minutes. Cronbach's alpha ranges from 0.4 to 0.75 for various subscales, demonstrating acceptable internal consistency, and 0.75 to 1 for the total physical and functional subscales corresponding to excellent consistency. In summary, the FACT-H&N is a modular, disease-specific QOL instrument with reasonable internal consistency. Test–retest reliability has not been reported. It has been shown to demonstrate longitudinal change. It is relatively short to administer.

The Head and Neck Radiotherapy Questionnaire (HNRQ) is a 22-item interviewer-administered questionnaire that was developed as an evaluative instrument to measure radiation-induced acute morbidity and QOL in patients with locally advanced head and neck cancer (stage III and IV). It presents six Likert scale dimensions (skin, throat, oral stomatitis, digestion, energy, psychosocial). Higher scores reflect better function. It has a summary scale. The completion time is 10 minutes per patient. Twenty-two questions were piloted in eight patients undergoing combined radiochemotherapy. Certain content issues are not addressed such as appearance, head and neck pain (e.g., throat irritation). Reliability (but not test–test reliability) and validity have been assessed. In summary, the HNRQ is a QOL instrument intended for acute assessment of advanced-stage patients undergoing radiotherapy or chemoradiotherapy. Although it has been tested appropriately for reliability and validity, it is unclear whether the initial development included adequate patient input. It does not seem to have the same broad applicability across disease stages and treatment modalities as other measures. Its correlation to other measures is fair.

Quality of Life Instrument for Head and Neck Cancer (QL-H&N) has been developed and tested by Morton et al. in New Zealand as a short, sensitive disease-specific questionnaire with an emphasis on psychological factors. The self-administered questionnaire consists of grouping of existing generic scales, with added disease-specific questions. It uses individual physical, social, and psychological domains that are scored separately, without the use of a summary score. The details of its development, degree of patient input, and item selection and reduction criteria are not published. Several issues relevant to patients with head and neck cancer are not covered by the questionnaire. Test–retest reliability was assessed in a 10-patient sample. Correlation coefficients on this small sample were 0.57 for the GHQ, 0.94 for the LS-10,

The FACT-G Scale

FACT-G (version 2)

Name: _____

Date: _____

Below is a list of statements that other people with your illness have said are important. By filling in one circle per line, please indicate how true each statement has been for you during the past 7 days.

During the past 7 days: PHYSICAL WELL-BEING	not at all	a little bit	some-what	quite a bit	very much
1. I have a lack of energy	0	1	2	3	4
2. I have nausea	0	1	2	3	4
3. I have trouble meeting the needs of my family	0	1	2	3	4
4. I have pain	0	1	2	3	4
5. I am bothered by side effects of treatment	0	1	2	3	4
6. In general, I feel sick	0	1	2	3	4
7. I am forced to spend time in bed	0	1	2	3	4

8. How rouch does your **PHYSICAL WELL-BEING** affect your quality of life?
   Not at all 0 1 2 3 4 5 6 7 8 9 10 Very much so

During the past 7 days: SOCIAL/FAMILY WELL-BEING	not at all	a little bit	some-what	quite a bit	very much
9. I feel distant from my friends	0	1	2	3	4
10. I get emotional support from my family	0	1	2	3	4
11. I get support from my friends and neighbors	0	1	2	3	4
12. My family has accepted my illness	0	1	2	3	4
13. Family communication about my illness is poor	0	1	2	3	4

If you have a spouse/partner, or are sexually active, please answer #14-15, Otherwise, go to #16.

	not at all	a little bit	some-what	quite a bit	very much
14. I feel close to my partner (for main suppout)	0	1	2	3	4
15. I am satisfied with my sex life	0	1	2	3	4

16. How much does your **SOCIAL/FAMILY WELL-BEING** affect your quality of life?
   Not at all 0 1 2 3 4 5 6 7 8 9 10 Very much so

During the past 7 days: RELATIONSHIP WITH DOCTOR	not at all	a little bit	some-what	quite a bit	very much
17. I have confidence in my doctor(s)	0	1	2	3	4
18. My doctor is available to answer my questions	0	1	2	3	4

19. How much does your **RELATIONSHIP WITH THE DOCTOR** affect your quality of life?
   Not at all 0 1 2 3 4 5 6 7 8 9 10 Very much so

During the past 7 days: EMOTIONAL WELL-BEING	not at all	a little bit	some-what	quite a bit	very much
20. I feel sad	0	1	2	3	4
21. I am proud of how I'm coping with my illness	0	1	2	3	4
22. I am losing hope in the fight against my illness	0	1	2	3	4
23. I feel nervous	0	1	2	3	4
24. I worry about dying	0	1	2	3	4

25 How much does your **EMOTIONAL WELL-BEING** affect your quality of life?
   Not at all 0 1 2 3 4 5 6 7 8 9 10 Very much so

During the past 7 days: FUNCTIONAL WELL-BEING	not at all	a little bit	some-what	quite a bit	very much
26. I am able to work (include work in home)	0	1	2	3	4
27. My work (include work in home) is fulfilling	0	1	2	3	4
28. I am able to enjoy life "in the moment"	0	1	2	3	4
29. I have accepted my illness	0	1	2	3	4
30. I am sleeping well	0	1	2	3	4
31. I am enjoying my usual leisure pursuits	0	1	2	3	4
32. I am content with the quality of my life right now	0	1	2	3	4

33. How much does your **FUNCTIONAL WELL-BEING** affect your quality of life?
   Not at all 0 1 2 3 4 5 6 7 8 9 10 Very much so

©Copyright 1988. 1991 by David F. Cclla. PhD.

Figure 26.1. FACT-G instrument. (Courtesy of David F. Cella, PhD)

0.61 for the global life-satisfaction measure, and 0.90 for the disease-specific questions. Internal consistency yielded an excellent Cronbach's alpha of 0.83 for the GHQ-12 and LS-10, and was not measured for other components of the questionnaire. In summary, this composite measure of QOL really utilizes validated general scales from other measures combined with added head and neck–specific questions. The instrument itself has not been published.

Quality of Life Questionnaire for Advanced Head and Neck Cancer (QLQ) was designed and used in a United Kingdom study to discriminate between patients with advanced head and neck cancer randomized to either radiation alone or surgery and radiation. It utilizes four domains: physical, functional/mood, psychological, and attitude to treatment. It was developed using only 11 head and neck cancer patients within 2 years of their treatment. It does not cover some areas of appearance and eating/swallowing. Speech/communication is covered with a single item describing how other people might have difficulty understanding what the patient may have said. No reliability data are currently available. Until validity, reliability, and responsiveness to longitudinal change have been carefully evaluated and published, this instrument is less recommended for effectiveness research.

Quality of Life–Radiation Therapy Instrument Head & Neck Module (QOL-RTI/H&N) is a general QOL instrument with a disease-specific companion module. The head and neck module was designed to address the specific issues of the head and neck radiotherapy patient but the generation and reduction of items was done by expert consensus rather than a patient panel. The current QOL-RTI/H&N is a 39-item self-assessed questionnaire, with all questions using a 10-item Likert response scale. The general portion consists of four domains: functional, emotional, family and socioeconomic, and general. The disease-specific module has 14 items. A summary score is calculated for the QOL-RTI, and the H&N module is scored separately. The H&N module is currently available. Both internal consistency and test–retest reliability have been assessed for this instrument. One-week test–retest reliability (a relatively short interval) produced a Pearson correlation coefficient of 0.79. Internal consistency measured by Cronbach's alpha is 0.87. The domains were not assessed separately. In summary, the QOL-RTI/H&N is a very specific instrument for the measurement of QOL in head and neck cancer patients undergoing radiotherapy. The QOL-RTI/H&N would be applicable to the same population as the HNRQ, and although it may have advantages in broader coverage of general QOL issues and nonphysical symptoms, it has not been extensively evaluated.

The University of Michigan Head and Neck Quality of Life (HNQOL) instrument includes 21 items intended for the overall assessment of outcome for patients with head and neck cancer (Figure 26.2). It is an interviewer-administered questionnaire assessing four domains: pain, emotion, communication, and eating. Each item is rated on a five-point Likert scale, and each domain generates a score of 0–100, with higher scores reflecting better QOL. In addition, a single item assesses "overall disturbance or bother" as a result of head and neck cancer. A summary score is not calculated. The interviewer-administered design is a disadvantage for convenient administration. Methods for item generation and reduction were not fully reported. The authors recommend that the HNQOL be administered in combination with a general QOL instrument. The average completion time was 11.2 minutes for the 37-item version. Intraclass correlation coefficient values were excellent, ranging from 0.73 for communication to 0.92 for emotion. Similarly, internal consistency was high, with Cronbach's alpha ranging from 0.79 (for pain) to 0.93. Convergent validity was tested by concurrent administration of the Medical Outcomes Study Short Form 12 (SF-12) mental (MCS) and physical (PCS) scales. Pearson correlations were only moderate, ranging from 0.44 for the eating domain versus the PCS, to 0.60 for the emotion domain versus the MCS. In summary, the HNQOL is a valid and reliable tool although experience outside of the institution is somewhat limited.

University of Washington Quality of Life Questionnaire (UW QOL), developed at the institution whose name it bears, was intended as a discriminative instrument for a variety of head and neck cancer sites and stages but it has been used primarily for patients undergoing surgery (Figure 26.3). It is a self-administered instrument consisting of 12 questions: nine disease-specific items (pain, chewing, swallowing, speech, shoulder disability, appearance, activity, recreation, and employment), plus three general items measuring global health-related QOL, change in health-related QOL since diagnosis, and overall QOL. Each question has 3–6 response options, using a Likert-type scale. Each item is scored from 0 to 100, with higher scores indicating better QOL. There is a summary score. The general items are scored individually. Information on the generation of the items has not been published. The addition of an importance scale improved its patient centricity. The UW QOL is short and has been demonstrated to be preferred to the longer Sickness Impact Profile (SIP). Test–retest reliability was very strong (0.94). Internal consistency was assessed and in the acceptable range, from 0.74 to 0.83. Concurrent validity was also assessed, correlation with the SIP (coefficients 0.82–0.96) and the Karnofsky score (coefficients 0.79–0.85) were high. Responsiveness to change was large. In summary, the UW QOL is a short instrument best suited to patients undergoing surgery.

The Head and Neck Survey (H&NS) was developed at Harvard and intended to be used with the generic SF-12 or -36 as a brief, focused, disease-specific form (Figure

INSTRUCTIONS: This survey is designed to assess how much you are bothered by your Head and Neck condition and/or treatment.
Please answer every question by marking one box. If you are unsure about how to answer, please give the best answer you can.

1. As a result of your head and neck condition or treatment, over the past FOUR WEEKS how much have you been BOTHERED by your…

	Not at all	Slightly	Moderately	A lot	Extremely
A. Ability to talk to other people	❑	❑	❑	❑	❑
B. Ability to talk on the phone	❑	❑	❑	❑	❑

2. As a result of your head and neck condition or treatment, over the past FOUR WEEKS how much have you been BOTHERED by problems with…

	Not at all	Slightly	Moderately	A lot	Extremely
A. Volume of your voice	❑	❑	❑	❑	❑
B. Clarity of your voice	❑	❑	❑	❑	❑
C. Difficulty opening your mouth	❑	❑	❑	❑	❑
D. Dryness in your mouth while eating	❑	❑	❑	❑	❑
E. Chewing food (For example, pain, difficulty opening or closing your mouth, moving food in your mouth, or teeth or denture problems)	❑	❑	❑	❑	❑
F. Swallowing liquids	❑	❑	❑	❑	❑
G. Swallowing soft foods and/or solids	❑	❑	❑	❑	❑
H. Your ability to taste food (For example, loss of taste, and/or loss of appetite due to poor tasta)	❑	❑	❑	❑	❑
I. Pain, burning, and/or discomfort in your mouth, jaw, or throat	❑	❑	❑	❑	❑
J. Shoulder or neck pain	❑	❑	❑	❑	❑

3. Over the past FOUR WEEKS, how often did you take pain medication?…

Never	Rarely	Sometimes	Frequently	Always
❑	❑	❑	❑	❑

4. Over the past FOUR WEEKS, how much have you been bothered by …

	Not at all	Slightly	Moderately	A lot	Extremely
A. Concerns or worries about your appearance related to your head and neck condition or treatment	❑	❑	❑	❑	❑
B. Emotional problems related to your head and neck condition or treatment	❑	❑	❑	❑	❑
C. Embarrassment about your symptoms	❑	❑	❑	❑	❑
D. Frustration about your condition	❑	❑	❑	❑	❑
E. Financial worries due to medical problems	❑	❑	❑	❑	❑
F. Worries that your condition will get worse	❑	❑	❑	❑	❑
G. Physical problems related to your head and neck condition	❑	❑	❑	❑	❑

5. Were you working (employed) prior to being diagnosed with cancer?

Yes	No	
❑	❑	If no, go to question 6

5A. If yes, did your doctor declare you unable to work due to your head and neck condition or treatment?

Yes	No
❑	❑

6. Have there been other problems related to your head and neck condition that were not mentioned? If so please write them in the spaces below and tell us how much this problem has bothered you. (For instanse, if your treatment included surgical transfer of tissue from a donor site to the head and seck, does the donor site bother you)

	Not at all	Slightly	Moderately	A lot	Extremely
A. _____	❑	❑	❑	❑	❑
B. _____	❑	❑	❑	❑	❑
C. _____	❑	❑	❑	❑	❑

7. For the past FOUR WEEKS, please rate your OVERALL amount of disturbance or BOTHER as a result of your head and neck cancer condition.

Not at all	Slightly	Moderately	A lot	Extremely
❑	❑	❑	❑	❑

8. Overall how satisfied are you with your Head and Neck cancer treatment at this hospital?

❑	❑	❑	❑	❑

9. Overall how would you rate your response to treatment?

Poor	Fair	Good	Very Good	Excellent
❑	❑	❑	❑	❑

10. Approximately how long did it take you to answer this questionnaire? _____ Minutes

11. How difficult was it to complete this questionnaire?

Not at all	Slightly	Moderately	Very	Extremely
❑	❑	❑	❑	❑

Figure 26.2. University of Michigan Head and Neck Quality of Life Instrument. (From [30]. Reprinted with permission. © 1997, American Medical Association. All rights reserved.)

Pain
  I have no pain.
  There is mild pain not needing medication.
  I have moderate pain—requires regular medication (codeine or non-narcotic).
  I have severe pain controlled only by narcotics.
  I have severe pain not controlled by medication.
Disfigurement
  There is no change in my appearance.
  The change in my appearance is minor.
  My appearance bothers me but I remain active.
  I feel significantly disfigured and limit my activities due to my appearance.
  I cannot be with people due to my appearance.
Activity
  I am as active as I have ever been.
  There are times when I can't keep up my old pace, but not often.
  I am often tired and I have slowed down my activities although I still get out.
  I don't go out because I don't have the strength.
  I am usually in a bed or chair and don't leave home.
Recreation/entertainment
  There are no limitations to recreation home and away from home.
  There are a few things I can't do but I still get out and enjoy life.
  There are many times when I wish I could get out more but I'm not up to it.
  There are severe limitations to what I can do, mostly I stay home and watch TV.
  I can't do anything enjoyable.
Employment
  I work full time.
  I have a part-time but permanent job.
  I only have occasional employment.
  I am unemployed.
  I am retired (circle one below)
    Not related to cancer treatment.
    Due to cancer treatment.
Eating
  Chewing
    I can chew as well as ever.
    I can eat soft solids but cannot chew some foods.
    I cannot even chew soft solids.
  Swallowing
    I can swallow as well as ever.
    I cannot swallow certain solid foods.
    I can only swallow liquid food.
    I cannot swallow because it "goes down the wrong way" and chokes me.
Speech
  My speech is the same as always.
  I have difficulty with saying some words but I can be understood over the phone.
  Only my family and friends can understand me.
  I cannot be understood.
Shoulder disability
  I have no problem with my shoulder.
  My shoulder is stiff but it has not affected my activity or strength.
  Pain or weakness in my shoulder has caused me to change my work.
  I cannot work due to problems with my shoulder.

Figure 26.3. University of Washington Quality of Life Instrument. (Courtesy of E. Weymuller.)

26.4). The H&NS is an 11-item questionnaire that generates a total index and three head and neck–specific domain scores. It was formulated by an expert panel (including patients) with the goal of evaluating potentially unique dimensions of head and neck–specific health. Total score is determined from all 11 questions. The eating/swallowing (ES) scale contains five items, the speech/communication (SC) scale has two items, and the appearance (AP) scale has four items. A head and neck pain (HNP) scale includes two items. The HNP items and scale are not included in the H&NS total score. Overall internal consistency for the H&NS is very high (0.89) and compared favorably with the UW QOL (0.85) in the same population. Test–retest reliability was excellent for the H&NS total score (0.88). Convergent validity of the disease-specific measures is stronger with each other than with the general health score. The head and neck pain scale correlates strongly with the bodily pain scale of the SF-36 and the appearance scale correlates strongly with the social functioning scale of the same instrument. The H&NS overall score correlates strongly with the UW QOL and with the Performance Status Scale Head and Neck. The H&NS was developed primarily with stage III and IV patients. Although both the UW QOL and the H&NS are brief and easy to administer with strong reliability characteristics, the H&NS uses multi-item domains whereas the UW QOL uses single-item domains and this translates to potentially higher precision for the H&NS in small populations (fewer than 150 patients).

The information in Table 26.1 is provided in lieu of making broad generalized comparisons between the various instruments because it is highly likely that one or another instrument will be more suitable to one or another purpose. In making determinations of which instrument to use for a research study or in clinical practice, potential users of these QOL instruments should consider the reliability, sensitivity, and other standardized performance characteristics of the instrument as one factor, but should also consider other information such as the reported respondent burden and the populations in which the particular instrument has been developed and utilized as other equally important factors. In some cases, one instrument will not suffice.

The importance of QOL measurement in head and neck cancer cannot be overstated. Selection of appropriate measurement tools requires defining the right tool for the specific purpose. Key considerations include:

- Measurement includes domains of interest
- Use is matched to that intended for the QOL instruments
- Performance characteristics (validity, reliability, sensitivity to change)
- Burden of administering or completing the surveys is minimized

1. In the past 4 weeks I have been able to eat:
   nothing at all, almost nothing, very few of the things that I want to, some of the things that I want to, anything I want to.
2. When I speak (by any form) I am understood:
   by no one at all, rarely-even by people who know me well, only by people who know me well, by most of the people around me but not all, by almost everyone around me.
3. I am able to eat food that I want to:
   none of the time, a little of the time, some of the time, most of the time, all of the time.
4. I have trouble with food going down the wrong pipe when I eat, or I find myself coughing after eating or drinking:
   all of the time, most of the time, some of the time, a little of the time, none of the time.
5. When I swallow, food tends to stick in my throat:
   all of the time, most of the time, some of the time, a little of the time, none of the time.
6. When I speak in a crowded or noisy room, I am understood:
   none of the time, a little of the time, some of the time, most of the time, all of the time.
7. My appearance affects my willingness to work or participate in recreational activities:
   all of the time, most of the time, some of the time, a little of the time, none of the time.
8. My appearance affects how often I see family or friends:
   all of the time, most of the time, some of the time, a little of the time, none of the time.
9. Because of difficulty with eating, I avoid eating in restaurants or other people's homes:
   definitely true, mostly true, don't know, mostly false, definitely false.
10. My appearance has affected my self esteem:
    definitely true, mostly true, don't know, mostly false, definitely false.
11. My appearance prevents me from participating in social activities:
    definitely true, mostly true, don't know, mostly false, definitely false.

Head and Neck Pain Items
   A. In the past 4 weeks, pain from my head and neck has been:
      very severe, severe, moderate, mild, very mild, I have no pain.
   B. In the past 4 weeks, pain from my head and neck has been present:
      all of the time, most of the time, some of the time, a little of the time, none of the time.

Figure 26.4. Head and Neck Survey (H&NS) (© Massachusetts Eye and Ear Infirmary. Used with permission.)

Scoring algorithms: each response is graded from 1 to 5. Total score = (sum (Q1 to Q11) − 11)/44 • 100; Domain scores: eating/swallowing (ES) = (Sum (Q1,3,4,5,9) − 5)/20 • 100; speech/communication (SC) = (Sum (Q2,6) − 2)/8 • 100; appearance (AP) = (Sum (Q7,8,10,11) − 4)/16 • 100. Head and neck pain (HNP) = (Sum (QA,B) − 2)/8 • 100.

TABLE 26.1. Representative validated instruments used in head and neck cancer

Instrument	Type	No. items/domains	Comments	Performance characteristics reported?
EORTC QLQ-C30	General with head/neck module	General: 30:5 Head/neck: 35:7	Intended for all stages of cancer	Yes
FACT-H&N	General (FACT-G) with head/neck module	General: 27:4 Head/neck: 38:5	Intended for all stages of cancer	Yes
HNRQ	Head/neck radiotherapy specific	Combined: 22:6	Very specific to radiotherapy	Yes
QL-H&N	Combined	Combined: 29:3	Several issues relevant to head/neck cancer not presented	Partial
QLQ	Combined	Combined: 19:4	No reliability data available	Limited
QOL-RTI/H&N	General and specific	General: 39:4 Specific: 14:summary score	Relatively specific for radiotherapy	Yes
HNQOL	Combined	General: 21	Interviewer-administered design	Yes
UW QOL	Combined	Combined: 12:9	Surgical focus	Yes
H&NS	Specific (intended to be combined with generic such as SF-12)	Specific: 11:4	Higher precision	Yes

REFERENCES

1. Cronbach LJ. Coefficient alpha and the internal structure of tests. Psychometrika 1951;16:297–334.
2. Drettner B, Ahlbom A. Quality of life and state of health for patients with cancer in the head and neck. Acta Otolaryngol 1983;96:307–314.
3. Dropkin MJ, Malgady RG, Oberst MT, Strong EW. Scaling of disfigurement and dysfunction in postoperative head and neck patients. Head Neck 1983;6:559–570.
4. Pruyn JFA, deJong PC, Bosman LJ, et al. Psychosocial aspects of head and neck cancer—a review of the literature. Clin Otolaryngol 1986;11:469–474.
5. Nunnally JC. Psychometric Theory. New York: McGraw Hill; 1978:245–246.
6. Guyatt G, Walter S, Norman G. Measuring change over time: assessing the usefulness of evaluative instruments. J Chronic Dis 1987;40:171–178.
7. Aaronson NK, Bullinger M, Ahmedzai S. A modular approach to quality of life assessment in cancer clinical trials. Rec Results Cancer Res 1988;111:231–249.
8. Gotay CC, Moore TD. Assessing quality of life in head and neck cancer. Qual Life Res 1992;1:5–17.
9. Gliklich RE. Prospective study of quality of life after intraoral tumor surgery: discussion. J Oral Maxillofac Surg 1996;54:669–670.

10. Ware JE Jr, Sherbourne CD. The MOS 36-Item Short-Form Health Survey (SF-36). I. Conceptual framework and item selection. Med Care 1992;30:473–483.

11. List MA, Ritter-Sterr C, Lansky SB. A performance status scale for head and neck cancer patients. Cancer 1990;66:564–569.

12. Gliklich RE, Goldsmith TA, Funk GF. Are head and neck specific quality of life measures necessary? Head Neck 1997;19:474–480.

13. Bjordal K, Ahlner-Elmqvist M, Tollesson E, et al. Development of a European Organization for Research and Treatment of Cancer (EORTC) questionnaire module to be used in quality of life assessments in head and neck cancer patients. Acta Oncol 1994;33:879–885.

14. Aaronson NK, Ahmedzai S, Bullinger M, et al. The EORTC core quality of life questionnaire: interim results of an international field study. In: Osoba D, ed. Effect of Cancer on Quality of Life. Boston: CRC Press; 1991:185–203.

15. Hammerlid E, Bjordal K, Ahlner-Elmqvist M, et al. Prospective longitudinal quality of life study of patients with head and neck cancer: a feasibility study including the EORTC QLQ-C30. Otolaryngol Head Neck Surg 1997;116:666–673.

16. Jones E, Lund VJ, Howard DJ, et al. Quality of life of patients treated surgically for head and neck cancer. J Laryngol Otol 1992;106:238–242.

17. Bjordal K, Kaasa S. Psychometric validation of the EORTC core quality of life questionnaire, 30-item version and a diagnosis-specific module for head and neck cancer patients. Acta Oncol 1992;31(3):311–321.

18. Bjordal K, Freng A, Thorvik J, et al. Patient self-reported and clinician-rated quality of life in head and neck cancer patients: a cross-sectional study. Eur J Cancer B Oral Oncol 1995;31B(4):235–241.

19. Bjordal K, Kaasa S, Mastekaasa A. Quality of life in patients treated for head and neck cancer: a follow-up study 7 to 11 years after radiotherapy. Int J Radiat Oncol Biol Phys 1994;28(4):847–856.

20. Cella DF, Tulsky DS. Measuring quality of life today: methodological aspects. Oncology 1990;4:29–38.

21. Cella DF, Tulsky DS, Gray G, et al. The functional assessment of cancer therapy scale: development and validation of the general measure. J Clin Oncol 1993;11(3):570–579.

22. List MA, D'Antonio LL, Cella DF, et al. The performance status scale for head and neck cancer patients and the functional assessment of cancer therapy-head and neck scale. Cancer 1996;77(11):2294–2300.

23. D'Antonio LL, Zimmerman GJ, Cella DF, et al. Quality of life and functional status measures in patients with head and neck cancer. Arch Otolaryngol Head Neck Surg 1996;122:482–487.

24. Browman GP, Levine MN, Hodson ID, et al. The head and neck radiotherapy questionnaire: a morbidity/quality of life instrument for clinical trials of radiation therapy in locally advanced head and neck cancer. J Clin Oncol 1993;11(5):863–872.

25. Morton RP, Witterick IJ. Rationale and development of a quality-of-life instrument for head-and-neck cancer patients. Am J Otolaryngol 1995;16(5):284–293.

26. Morton RP. Quality-of-life and cost-effectiveness. Head Neck 1997;19:243–250.

27. Rathmell AJ, Ash DV, Howes M, et al. Assessing quality of life in patients treated for advanced head and neck cancer. Clin Oncol 1991;3:10–16.

28. Johnson DL, Casey L, Noriega B. A pilot study of patient quality of life during radiation therapy treatment. Qual Life Res 1994;3:267–272.

29. Trotti A, Johnson DL, Gwede C, et al. Development of a head and neck companion module for the Quality of Life-Radiation Therapy Instrument (QOL-RTI). Int J Radiat Oncol Biol Phys 1998;4292:257–261.

30. Terrell JE, Nanavati KA, Esclamado RM, et al. Head and neck cancer-specific quality of life. Arch Otolaryngol Head Neck Surg 1997;123:1125–1132.

31. Terrell JE, Fisher SG, Wolf GT, et al. Long-term quality of life after treatment of laryngeal cancer. Arch Otolaryngol Head Neck Surg 1998;124:964–971.

32. Hassan SJ, Weymuller EA. Assessment of quality of life in head and neck cancer patients. Head Neck 1993;15:485–496.

33. Deleyiannis FW, Weymuller EA, Coltera MD. Quality of life of disease-free survivors of advanced (stage III or IV) oropharyngeal cancer. Head Neck 1997;19:466–473.

34. Deleyiannis FW-B, Weymuller EA, Coltera MD. Quality of life after laryngectomy: are functional disabilities important? Head Neck 1999;21:319–324.

35. Weymuller EA, Yueh B, Deleyiannis FW-B, Kuntz AL, Alsarraf R, Coltrera MD. Quality of life in patients with head and neck cancer. Arch Otolaryngol Head Neck Surg 2000;126:329–335.

36. Gliklich RE, Goldsmith TA, Funk GF. Are head and neck specific quality of life measures necessary? Head Neck 1997 Sep; 19(6):424–480.

27 Prophylaxis in Head and Neck Surgery

27.A.

One-day versus longer-course perioperative antibiotics: Impact on postoperative surgical-site infections

Jennifer J. Shin and Jonas T. Johnson

METHODS

A computerized PubMed search of MEDLINE 1966–December 2005 was performed. Articles that mapped to the medical subject headings "antibiotic prophylaxis," "anti-bacterial agents," "lactams," "fluoroquinolones," "macrolides," or "clindamycin" were collected into one group. A second group was created by identifying articles that mapped to the medical subject heading "head and neck neoplasms," cross-referenced with those mapping to the medical subject heading "perioperative care" or the subheading "surgery." These articles were then reviewed to identify those that met the following inclusion criteria: 1) patient population undergoing clean-contaminated surgery for head and neoplasm, 2) intervention with 1-day versus longer-course systemic antibiotic therapy, 3) outcome measured in terms of surgical-site wound infections, 4) randomized controlled trials (RCTs). Excluded were data from articles in which only clean, noncontaminated wounds, distant infections, and non–head and neck surgery were evaluated. Also excluded were articles that compared one dose of antibiotics to a 1-day course, as well as reports comparing two longer durations of antibiotic use. The bibliographies of the articles that met these inclusion/exclusion criteria were manually checked to ensure no further relevant articles could be identified. Two articles were identified that reported similar results from the same ongoing clinical trial [1,2], so only the more detailed report was included in this review. This process overall yielded 7 RCTs [1–7].

RESULTS

Herein, we describe results of individual studies. In the subsequent section, please find results for the related meta-analysis.

Outcome Measures. The basis for the diagnosis of wound infection varied among studies. Wound infections were defined by purulent drainage or development of mucocutaneous fistula in four studies. In another study, wound infections were defined by an erythematous edematous wound or a pink wound with purulent drainage. The remaining two studies defined wound infection in terms of erythema, tenderness, purulent drainage, necrosis, wound dehiscence, and bacterial recovery of possible pathogens.

Potential Confounders. The antibiotic choice itself, extent of procedure, preoperative radiation, nutritional status, immune status, or predisposing comorbidities such as diabetes mellitus may all affect infectious outcomes. In addition, the type of reconstruction used (primary closure, pedicled flap, free flap) and the duration (hours) of surgery are both related to the observed incidence of postoperative infection. In many studies, the authors attempted to account for such potential confounders by either balancing them with randomization or eliminating them as a concern through exclusion criteria during subject selection. Another key issue is whether drains or other foreign bodies were still in place when antibiotics were discontinued. No reports comment on this issue.

Study Designs. All seven studies were RCTs which provided level 1 evidence comparing a 1-day course to a longer course of antibiotics. Four of these RCTs compared a 5-day course, whereas the other three compared a 3- to 4-day course. Blinded evaluation of outcomes was performed in the four RCTs that evaluated a 5-day therapy group. Antibiotic regimens evaluated included cefoperazone, clindamycin, cefazolin, carbenicillin, and gentamicin with clindamycin. Wounds were evaluated daily in most cases, with follow-up times between 5 and 20 days. One study reported an *a priori* power analysis, and one reported a *post hoc* power analysis. The one publication that did include an *a priori* power analysis stopped subject accrual when annual review disclosed that differences between study groups were much lower than projected, so that additional accrual would be meaningless.

Highest Level of Evidence. All seven studies concluded that there was no difference in postoperative surgical-site infections when a 1-day antibiotic course was compared with 5-, 4-, or 3-day therapy for a clean-contaminated head and neck wound. All of the studies were in agreement on this topic, although only two studies either had the sample size necessary to achieve an 80% power or determined that additional patient accrual would not alter the results of a statistical comparison. If a study's power is not high enough, it may not be able to identify a difference that truly exists.

With this power issue in mind, we have performed meta-analyses to increase sample size and thus increase the power of the overall data. These meta-analyses can be found immediately after the tables detailing the individual studies.

Applicability. The results of these studies apply to patients undergoing resection of head and neck neoplasms with creation of a clean-contaminated wound.

Morbidity/Complications. No instances of drug reactions were reported. There was a trend toward more hypokalemia in the longer-course group receiving carbenicillin in one study, but no significant difference was identified. One study also determined that 100% of patients who had been previously radiated developed fistulas once wound infection had occurred.

Please also see the associated meta-analysis after the adjoining tables which detail individual studies.

THE EVIDENCE CONDENSED: One- versus five-day perioperative antibiotics for clean-contaminated head and neck surgery

Reference	Johnson, 1986		
Level (design)	1 (randomized controlled trial)		
Sample size*	109 (142)		
OUTCOMES			
	Surgical-site infection without flap necrosis	**Flap necrosis preceding infection**	**Total surgical-site infections**
1 day	18.9% (n = 10/53)	5.7% (n = 3/53)	24.5% (n = 13/53)
5 days	25.0% (n = 14/56)	3.6% (n = 2/56)	28.6% (n = 16/56)
p Value	>0.05	Not specified	Not specified
Conclusion	No significant difference	No significant difference	No significant difference
Follow-up time	Until discharge		
STUDY DESIGN			
Inclusion criteria	Patients requiring pedicled myocutaneous flap reconstruction for oropharyngeal or laryngeal defects		
Exclusion criteria	Allergy to cephalosporin, antibiotic use within the 4 d before surgery		
Randomization effectiveness	Stratification to ensure equal numbers of patients with radiation, tubed reconstruction, and poor nutrition in each group		
Age	Not specified		
Masking	Double-blind design, with patients in the 1-d group receiving 4 d of placebo		
Antibiotic regimen details	Cefoperazone, beginning 1–2 h preoperatively and continuing for 24 h vs 120 h		
Wound evaluation	Wound was observed daily by the surgical team. Wound rated: 1+ = 1-cm erythema around wound, 2+ = <5-cm erythema, 3+ = diffuse erythema and induration, 4+ = purulent drainage (spontaneously or by incision and drainage), 5+ = mucocutaneous fistula		
Diagnostic criteria for wound infection	Wound score 4–5		
Management of infection while in study	Not specified		
Compliance	Not specified		
Surgery types	Pedicled myocutaneous flap		
Criteria for withdrawal from study	Intraoperative decision to use an alternative form of wound closure to create a wound that was not contaminated by saliva		
Intention to treat analysis	Not specified		
Power	Not reported		
Morbidity/complications	100% of previously irradiated patients who developed wound infection subsequently developed a myocutaneous fistula		

IV = intravenous, q = every.
* Sample size: numbers shown for those not lost to follow-up and those (initially recruited).

THE EVIDENCE CONDENSED: One- versus five-day perioperative antibiotics for clean-contaminated head and neck surgery

Reference	Carroll, 2003		
Level (design)	1 (randomized controlled trial)		
Sample size*	74 (74)		
OUTCOMES			
	Surgical-site infection	**Fistula**	**Flap necrosis**
1 day	11% (n = 4/35)	9% (n = 3/35)	0% (n = 0/35)
5 days	10% (n = 4/39)	8% (n = 3/39)	3% (n = 1/39)
p Value	0.99	0.99	0.99
Conclusion	No significant difference	No significant difference	No significant difference
Follow-up time	7 d or until discharge		
STUDY DESIGN			
Inclusion criteria	Surgical ablation of head and neck malignancies involving mucous membranes of the upper aerodigestive tract with immediate free flap reconstruction		
Exclusion criteria	Tumors that did not involve mucous membranes of the upper aerodigestive tract		
Randomization effectiveness	Not specified		
Age	21–88 y (mean 62 y)		
Masking	Wound infections were documented according to surgeons who were blinded to treatment group		
Antibiotic regimen details	Clindamycin 900 mg IV q 8 h for 3 or 15 doses (or until discharge), initiated preoperatively		
Wound evaluation	Wound was evaluated daily for 7 d or until discharge by faculty head and neck surgeon. Wound and donor sites were scored: wound color 1 = normal, 2 = pink, 3 = red or swollen; drainage 1 = none, 2 = serous, 3 = purulent		
Diagnostic criteria for wound infection	Red color or swollen, or pink wound with purulent drainage		
Management of infection while in study	Not specified		
Compliance	Not specified		
Surgery types	Free flaps: radial forearm 42%, jejunal 26%, rectus 20%, fibula 12%		
Criteria for withdrawal from study	Not specified		
Intention to treat analysis	Not specified, although all 74 patients completed the study in their original groups		
Power	110 patients to achieve 80% power to detect a 15% difference in infection rates between the two groups. Subject accrual was terminated early, when annual review disclosed that differences between study groups were much lower than projected, so that additional accrual would be meaningless		
Morbidity/complications	No adverse events		

IV = intravenous, q = every.
* Sample size: numbers shown for those not lost to follow-up and those (initially recruited).

THE EVIDENCE CONDENSED: One- versus five-day perioperative antibiotics for clean-contaminated head and neck surgery

Reference	Brand, 1982	
Level (design)	1 (randomized controlled trial)	
Sample size*	83 (83)	

OUTCOMES		
Surgical-site infection		
	Cefazolin	**Gentamicin/clindamycin**
1 day	35% (n = 7/20)	9% (n = 2/22)
5 days	18% (n = 4/22)	5% (n = 1/19)
p Value	0.05	Not reported
Conclusion	No significant difference	No significant difference
Follow-up time	POD 10	

STUDY DESIGN	
Inclusion criteria	Oncologic surgery involving transcervical entry into upper aerodigestive tract
Exclusion criteria	Allergy to test drugs, renal dysfunction (creatinine >2), immunodeficiency from unrelated disease, any disease that might predispose to infection, recent antibiotic therapy, hearing loss >45-dB speech reception threshold, symptomatic vestibular abnormality
Randomization effectiveness	Not specified
Age	Not specified
Masking	Placebo use for 4 d in the 1-d treatment group
Antibiotic regimen details	Cefazolin 500 mg IV q 8 h for 1 or 5 d or gentamicin + clindamycin 1.7 mg/kg + 300 mg IV q 8 h; placebo given for 4 d in 1-d treatment group
Wound evaluation	Wounds graded daily by 2 independent observers: 0 = normal, 1 = redness limited to 1 cm around incision or suture line, 2 = 1- to 5-cm erythema, 3 = >5-cm erythema/blanches on digital pressure, 4 = suppurative drainage either spontaneous or by incision, 5 = mucocutaneous fistula
Diagnostic criteria for wound infection	Wound score 4–5
Management of infection while in study	Not specified
Compliance	Not specified
Surgery types	50% flaps (these were prone to a 54% rate of infection)
Criteria for withdrawal from study	Not specified
Intention to treat analysis	Not specified, though all 83 patients completed the study in their original groups
Power	"Our numbers are too small to expect statistical significance in all 16 subgroups generated by the 4 stratifiers in each of the 4 treatment categories," no *a priori* calculation
Morbidity/complications	No instance of drug toxicity

IV = intravenous, q = every.
* Sample size: numbers shown for those not lost to follow-up and those (initially recruited).

THE EVIDENCE CONDENSED: One- versus five-day perioperative antibiotics for clean-contaminated head and neck surgery

Reference	Bhathena, 1998	
Level (design)	1 (randomized controlled trial)	
Sample size*	50 (50)	
OUTCOMES		
	Surgical-site infection	**Flap necrosis** (preceded surgical-site infection)
1 day	7.1% (n = 3/28)	3.6% (n = 1/28)
5 days	9.8% (n = 5/22)	13.6% (n = 3/22)
p Value	Not reported	Not reported
Conclusion	"No beneficial effect from administration of antibiotics for more than 24 h postoperatively"	
Follow-up time	POD 5	
STUDY DESIGN		
Inclusion criteria	Patients requiring major flap reconstruction after extensive ablative surgery for head and neck cancer in which clean-contaminated wounds were created. Patients with associated systemic problems such as diabetes or hypertension were also included in the study	
Exclusion criteria	Not specified	
Randomization effectiveness	Similar numbers of pectoralis major and pectoralis major with deltopectoral flaps	
Age	Not specified	
Masking	Double blind	
Antibiotic regimen details	Cefoperazone 2 g IV q 12 h ×3 doses versus cefotaxime 1g IV q 8 h ×5 d, starting 1 h before the onset of surgery. "Other drugs started simultaneously" in the 2 groups were "gentamicin 60 mg and metronidazole 100 cc IV q 8 h ×3 d and 5 d respectively"	
Wound evaluation	Wound scores ever 48 h: 0 = normal, 1 = redness limited to 1 cm around incision or suture line, 2 = 1- to 5-cm erythema, 3 = >5-cm erythema/blanches on digital pressure, 4 = suppurative drainage either spontaneous or by incision, 5 = mucocutaneous fistula	
Diagnostic criteria for wound infection	Wound score 4–5	
Management of infection while in study	Not specified	
Compliance	Not specified	
Surgery types	Either pectoralis major flap alone or with skin deltopectoral flap	
Criteria for withdrawal from study	Not specified	
Intention to treat analysis	Not specified, though all 140 patients completed the study in their original groups	
Power	Not reported	
Morbidity/complications	Not reported	

IV = intravenous, q = every.

* Sample size: numbers shown for those not lost to follow-up and those (initially recruited).

THE EVIDENCE CONDENSED: One- versus four/three-day perioperative antibiotics for clean-contaminated head and neck surgery

Reference	Piccart, 1983
Level (design)	1 (randomized controlled trial)
Sample size*	140 (140)
OUTCOMES	
	Combined surgical-site and respiratory-tract infections
1 day	14% (n = 10/72)
3–4 days	10% (n = 7/68)
p Value	0.52
Conclusion	No difference
Follow-up time	POD 14
STUDY DESIGN	
Inclusion criteria	Surgery for cancer of the oral cavity, pharynx, and larynx
Exclusion criteria	Not specified
Randomization effectiveness	Similar numbers of minor and major/extensive procedures in both groups
Age	Not specified
Masking	Not specified
Antibiotic regimen details	Carbenicillin 1 d vs 4 d, initiated with the induction of narcosis
Wound evaluation	An epidemiologist nurse reviewed the patient's chart daily for evidence of infection or other pertinent data
Diagnostic criteria for wound infection	Wound infections were documented by clinical criteria such as erythema and tenderness, purulent discharge, necrosis, wound dehiscence, and by bacterial recovery of possible pathogens
Management of infection while in study	Not specified
Compliance	Not specified
Surgery types	Minor (small tumors in oral cavity/oropharynx, partial glossectomy, pharyngoplasty); moderately extensive (total laryngectomy, resection of FOM, total glossectomy, resection of mandible, excision of lower lip, closure of pharyngostoma); very extensive (same with radical neck dissection)
Criteria for withdrawal from study	Not specified
Intention to treat analysis	Not specified
Power	Not reported
Morbidity/complications	Not reported

NS = not significant, IV = intravenous, q = every.
* Sample size: numbers shown for those not lost to follow-up and those (initially recruited).

THE EVIDENCE CONDENSED: One- versus four/three-day perioperative antibiotics for clean-contaminated head and neck surgery

Reference	Mombelli, 1981		Righi, 1995
Level (design)	1 (randomized controlled trial)		1 (randomized controlled trial)
Sample size*	140 (140)		126 (136)
OUTCOMES			
	Surgical-site infection	**Fever or elevated WBC**	**Surgical-site infection**
1 day	9.7% (n = 7/72)	20.6%	1.6% (n = 1/62)
3–4 days	5.9% (n = 4/68)	15.6%	4.7% (n = 3/64)
p Value	NS	NS	NS
Conclusion	No difference		No difference
Follow-up time	POD 14		Postoperative d 20
STUDY DESIGN			
Inclusion criteria	Surgery for cancer of the oral cavity, pharynx, and larynx		Clean-contaminated (skin to mucosa) surgery for cancer of the larynx, pharynx, or oral cavity through cervical skin incisions
Exclusion criteria	Not specified		Pedicled or microvascular reconstruction, surgery performed without skin incision
Randomization effectiveness	Both groups similar in age, sex, type of surgical procedure		No significant differences in demographics, type and severity of underlying disease, type of surgery
Age	62 y (mean) in 1-d group, 59 y (mean) in 4-day group		64.2 y (mean) in 1-d group, 63.8 y (mean) in 3-d group
Masking	Not specified		Not specified
Antibiotic regimen details	Carbenicillin 10 g ×4 doses (1 d) vs 12 doses (4 d)		Clindamycin 600 mg IV q 8 h, cefonicid 1 g IV q 12 h, starting from induction for 1 d vs 3 d
Wound evaluation	An epidemiologist nurse reviewed the patient's chart daily for evidence of infection or other pertinent data		Not specified
Diagnostic criteria for wound infection	Wound infections were documented by clinical criteria such as erythema and tenderness, purulent discharge, necrosis, wound dehiscence, and by bacterial recovery of possible pathogens		Purulent discharge from the wound (spontaneous or drainage) or mucocutaneous fistula during the first 20 d after surgery
Management of infection while in study	Not specified		Not specified
Compliance	Not specified		Not specified
Surgery types	Minor (small tumors in oral cavity/oropharynx, partial glossectomy, pharyngoplasty); moderately extensive (total laryngectomy, resection of FOM, total glossectomy, resection of mandible, excision of lower lip, closure of pharyngostoma); very extensive (same with radical neck dissection)		Partial or total laryngectomy, oral cavity/oropharyngeal surgery without mandibulectomy, "commando" operation, relapse after total laryngectomy
Criteria for withdrawal from study	Not specified		Protocol violation (n = 6), immediate postoperative complications (hemorrhage, pulmonary embolism, pneumothorax, suprapubic urinary catheterization)
Intention to treat analysis	Not specified		Not specified
Power	Not reported		Not reported
Morbidity/complications	Hypokalemia in 36% of 1-d group, 48% of 4-d group		No adverse effects of treatment regimen

WBC = white blood cell, NS = not significant, IV = intravenous, q = every.
* Sample size: numbers shown for those not lost to follow-up and those (initially recruited).

Methods of Meta-Analysis.
All of the studies included in this meta-analysis are RCTs (level 1) and they represent the highest level of evidence comparing the impact of 1-day versus longer-course therapy on the incidence of postoperative surgical-site infections in patients undergoing resection of head and neck neoplasms with resulting clean-contaminated wounds. Further details regarding the search and selection process are as noted in the initial methods of this review.

With multiple moderately sized studies showing negative results, the key question arises as to whether those studies have the statistical power to uncover any difference that might truly exist; if there is a real difference in outcome with 1-day versus longer therapy, then a study must have enough patients in order to say with confidence that it would uncover such a difference. To understand this concept, consider a coin flip example in which you are given a coin that has either two heads or one head and one tail. If you flip that coin twice and get heads twice, you have demonstrated no difference, but your confidence in saying that both sides are heads is quite attenuated by the fact that you only did two flips. This example is analogous to a low-power study; the low number of flips (i.e., low sample size) gives low confidence that you would have found a difference in the two sides of the coin. Instead, if you were to flip that coin 10,000 times and get heads every time, then you could say with great confidence that that there were heads on both sides, because it would be so unlikely to demonstrate no difference 10,000 times if one side was in fact different from the other. This example is analogous to a high-power study; the high number of coin flips (i.e., high sample size) gives high confidence that you would have found a difference in the two sides of the coin.

A meta-analysis is a way in which data from multiple studies are pooled together. The pooling creates an increased sample size, which in turn creates more statistical power to uncover any difference that could truly exist. We performed a meta-analysis of all seven RCTs (fixed effects, inverse variance), as well as a sensitivity analysis of subgroups of longer-duration therapy.

Results of Meta-Analysis.
When all data were considered together, there was no difference between surgical-site infections in the 1-day versus longer-course groups. In a more focused sensitivity analysis, when the data were considered in subgroups for 1 day versus 5 days or 1 day versus 3–4 days, there was still no significant difference in outcome.

Many surgeons consider patients undergoing flap reconstruction to be at increased risk for poorer outcome either in terms of infection or as a sequelae of infection. Because of this, we also considered the subgroup of data regarding patients undergoing flap reconstruction. Again, there was no significant difference between 1-day versus 5-day therapy.

These reports did not provide enough detail to allow meta-analyses of subgroups who had prior radiation therapy or potential risk factors for infection such as immunocompromise or diabetes mellitus.

There were two reports that compared 2-day therapy to 6- or 7-day therapy. Although these reports were not included in our main analysis, we did pool the data from these studies in order to ensure that we did not inadvertently exclude key data. Again, however, the combined data show no significant difference in surgical-site infection with the shorter- versus longer-course antibiotic therapy.

Overall, there was scant reported morbidity/complications associated with the use of antibiotics, whether as a long or short course.

CLINICAL SIGNIFICANCE AND FUTURE RESEARCH

There were seven RCTs that compared the outcome of surgical-site infections with 1-day versus longer perioperative antibiotic courses in patients undergoing resection of head and neck neoplasms with resulting clean-contaminated wounds. Whether the data are considered all together, or in subgroup analyses of 1 day versus 5 days or 3–4 days therapy, there is no difference between groups. Likewise, when flap patients are considered separately, there are still no differences between groups.

The combined sample sizes for our meta-analyses ranged from 233 to 722. If we estimate a 15% rate of infection, and want to determine a 10% difference in infection rate and accept the standard 0.05 error rate, then in order to achieve a 90% power, 532 patients would be required. We achieved this sample size when we pooled data from all seven trials, but not in the subgroup analyses. Also, as noted above, the individual reports did not provide enough detail to allow meta-analyses of subgroups that had prior radiation therapy or other risk factors for infection or worsened sequelae thereof. Overall, these data suggest that there is no overall decrease in surgical-site infection when all patients undergoing clean-contaminated head and neck surgery are treated with 1-day versus longer therapy. There is, however, not enough data to determine whether certain higher-risk groups may still benefit from longer therapy. Because there was minimal morbidity/complications reported with longer courses of antibiotics, longer therapy in high-risk groups may still be warranted.

Future studies may focus on the analysis of such groups at increased risk for infections and their complications. Given the associated high stakes such as flap failure and fistula, further study focusing on patients who have received preoperative radiation or who are undergoing free flap reconstruction would be useful.

One- versus five-day perioperative antibiotics for all types of clean-contaminated head and neck surgery

	One day	Five days
Johnson, 1986	18.9% (n = 10/53)	25.0% (n = 14/56)
Carroll, 2003	11.4% (n = 4/35)	10.2% (n = 4/39)
Brand, 1982	35.0% (n = 7/20)	18.2% (n = 4/22)
	9.1% (n = 2/22)	5.3% (n = 1/19)
Bhathana, 1998	7.1% (n = 3/28)	9.8% (n = 5/22)
Total	**16.5% (n = 26/158)**	**17.7% (n = 28/158)**

One-versus five-day perioperative antibiotics for all types of clean-contaminated head and neck surgery

Study name	Risk difference	Lower limit	Upper limit	p-Value	Risk difference and 95% CI
Johnson	-0.061	-0.216	0.093	0.437	
Carroll	0.012	-0.130	0.154	0.872	
Brand	0.092	-0.067	0.252	0.256	
Bhathana	-0.120	-0.329	0.089	0.261	
Total	-0.007	-0.088	0.074	0.863	

-0.50 -0.25 0.00 0.25 0.50
Favors one day   Favors five day

One-versus five-day perioperative antibiotics for all types of clean-contaminated head and neck surgery

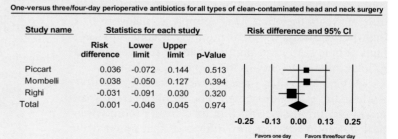

Study name	Odds ratio	Lower limit	Upper limit	p-Value	Odds ratio and 95% CI
Johnson	0.698	0.279	1.744	0.441	
Carroll	1.129	0.260	4.900	0.871	
Brand	1.964	0.597	6.460	0.267	
Bhathana	0.408	0.086	1.938	0.260	
Total	0.909	0.498	1.656	0.754	

0.1 0.2 0.5 1 2 5 10
Favors one day   Favors five day

One- versus three/four-day perioperative antibiotics for all types of clean-contaminated head and neck surgery

	One day	Three/four days
Piccart, 1983	13.9% (n = 10/72)	10.3% (n = 7/68)
Mombelli, 1981	9.7% (n = 7/72)	5.9% (n = 4/68)
Righi, 1995	1.6% (n = 1/62)	4.7% (n = 3/64)
Total	**8.7% (n = 18/206)**	**7.0% (n = 14/200)**

One-versus three/four-day perioperative antibiotics for all types of clean-contaminated head and neck surgery

Study name	Risk difference	Lower limit	Upper limit	p-Value	Risk difference and 95% CI
Piccart	0.036	-0.072	0.144	0.513	
Mombelli	0.038	-0.050	0.127	0.394	
Righi	-0.031	-0.091	0.030	0.320	
Total	-0.001	-0.046	0.045	0.974	

-0.25 -0.13 0.00 0.13 0.25
Favors one day   Favors three/four day

One-versus three/four-day perioperative antibiotics for all types of clean-contaminated head and neck surgery

Study name	Odds ratio	Lower limit	Upper limit	p-Value	Odds ratio and 95% CI
Piccart	1.406	0.503	3.931	0.517	
Mombelli	1.723	0.481	6.173	0.403	
Righi	0.333	0.034	3.294	0.347	
Total	1.291	0.606	2.749	0.508	

0.1 0.2 0.5 1 2 5 10
Favors one day   Favors three/four day

One- versus three/four/five-day perioperative antibiotics for all types of clean-contaminated head and neck surgery

	One day	Three/four/five days
Johnson, 1986	18.9% (n = 10/53)	25.0% (n = 14/56)
Carroll, 2003	11.4% (n = 4/35)	10.2% (n = 4/39)
Brand, 1982	35.0% (n = 7/20)	18.2% (n = 4/22)
	9.1% (n = 2/22)	5.3% (n = 1/19)
Bhathana, 1998	7.1% (n = 3/28)	9.8% (n = 5/22)
Piccart, 1983	13.9% (n = 10/72)	10.3% (n = 7/68)
Mombelli, 1981	9.7% (n = 7/72)	5.9% (n = 4/68)
Righi, 1995	1.6% (n = 1/62)	4.7% (n = 3/64)
Total	**12.1% (n = 44/364)**	**11.7% (n = 42/358)**

One-versus three/four/five-day perioperative antibiotics for all types of clean-contaminated head and neck surgery

Study name	Statistics for each study				Risk difference and 95% CI
	Risk difference	Lower limit	Upper limit	p-Value	
Johnson	-0.061	-0.216	0.093	0.437	
Carroll	0.012	-0.130	0.154	0.872	
Brand	0.092	-0.067	0.252	0.256	
Bhathana	-0.120	-0.329	0.089	0.261	
Piccart	0.036	-0.072	0.144	0.513	
Mombelli	0.038	-0.050	0.127	0.394	
Righi	-0.031	-0.091	0.030	0.320	
	-0.002	-0.042	0.037	0.910	

-0.25 -0.13 0.00 0.13 0.25
Favors one day   Favors three/four/five day

One-versus three/four/five-day perioperative antibiotics for all types of clean-contaminated head and neck surgery

Study name	Statistics for each study				Odds ratio and 95% CI
	Odds ratio	Lower limit	Upper limit	p-Value	
Johnson	0.698	0.279	1.744	0.441	
Carroll	1.129	0.260	4.900	0.871	
Brand	1.964	0.597	6.460	0.267	
Bhathana	0.408	0.086	1.938	0.260	
Piccart	1.406	0.503	3.931	0.517	
Mombelli	1.723	0.481	6.173	0.403	
Righi	0.333	0.034	3.294	0.347	
	1.041	0.650	1.666	0.868	

0.1 0.2 0.5 1 2 5 10
Favors one day   Favors three/four/five day

One- versus five-day perioperative antibiotics for clean-contaminated head and neck surgery with flaps

	One day	Five days
Johnson, 1986	18.9% (n = 10/53)	25.0% (n = 14/56)
Carroll, 2003	11.4% (n = 4/35)	10.2% (n = 4/39)
Bhathana, 1998	7.1% (n = 3/28)	9.8% (n = 5/22)
Total	**14.7% (n = 17/116)**	**19.7% (n = 23/117)**

One-versus five-day perioperative antibiotics for flaps

Study name	Statistics for each study				Risk difference and 95% CI
	Risk difference	Lower limit	Upper limit	p-Value	
Johnson	-0.061	-0.216	0.093	0.437	
Carroll	0.012	-0.130	0.154	0.872	
Bhathana	-0.120	-0.329	0.089	0.261	
	-0.041	-0.135	0.052	0.386	

-0.50 -0.25 0.00 0.25 0.50

Favors one day Favors five day

One-versus five-day perioperative antibiotics for flaps

Study name	Statistics for each study				Odds ratio and 95% CI
	Odds ratio	Lower limit	Upper limit	p-Value	
Johnson	0.698	0.279	1.744	0.441	
Carroll	1.129	0.260	4.900	0.871	
Bhathana	0.408	0.086	1.938	0.260	
Total	0.699	0.348	1.400	0.312	

0.1 0.2 0.5 1 2 5 10

Favors one day Favors five day

Two- versus six/seven-day perioperative antibiotics for clean-contaminated head and neck surgery

	Two day	Six/seven days
Sawyer, 1990	32.0% (n = 8/25)	20% (n = 5/25)
Gehanno, 1988	23.7% (n = 23/97)	17.0% (n = 17/100)
Total	**25.4% (n = 31/122)**	**17.6% (n = 22/125)**

Two-versus six/seven-day perioperative antibiotics for flaps

Study name	Statistics for each study				Risk difference and 95% CI
	Risk difference	Lower limit	Upper limit	p-Value	
Sawyer	0.120	-0.121	0.361	0.329	
Gehanno	0.067	-0.045	0.179	0.241	
Total	0.077	-0.025	0.178	0.140	

-0.50 -0.25 0.00 0.25 0.50

Favors two day Favors six/seven day

Two-versus six/seven-day perioperative antibiotics for flaps

Study name	Statistics for each study				Odds ratio and 95% CI
	Odds ratio	Lower limit	Upper limit	p-Value	
Sawyer	1.882	0.518	6.845	0.337	
Gehanno	1.517	0.753	3.058	0.243	
Total	1.594	0.861	2.951	0.138	

0.1 0.2 0.5 1 2 5 10

Favors two day Favors six/seven day

REFERENCES

1. Righi M, Manfredi R, Farneti G, Pasquini E, Romei Bugliari D, Cenacchi V. Clindamycin/cefonicid in head and neck oncoiogic surgery: one-day prophylaxis is as effective as a three-day schedule. J Chemother 1995;7(3):216–220.
2. Righi M, Manfredi R, Farneti G, Pasquini E, Cenacchi V. Short-term versus long-term antimicrobial prophylaxis in oncologic head and neck surgery. Head Neck. 1996 Sep-Oct;18(5):399–404. In head and neck oncologic surgery: one-day prophylaxis is as effective as a three-day schedule. J Chemother. 1995 Jun;7(3):216–220.
3. Johnson JT, Schuller DE, Silver F, et al. Antibiotic prophylaxis in high-risk head and neck surgery: one-day versus five-day therapy. Otolaryngol Head Neck Surg 1986;95:554.
4. Carroll WR, Rosenstiel D, Fix JR, et al. Three-dose vs extended-course clindamycin prophylaxis for free-flap reconstruction of the head and neck. Arch Otolaryngol Head Neck Surg 2003;129(7):771–774.
5. Brand B, Johnson JT, Myers EN, Thearle PB, Sigler BA. Prophylactic perioperative antibiotics in contaminated head and neck surgery. Otolaryngol Head Neck Surg 1982;90(3 Pt 1):315–318.
6. Bhathena HM, Kavarana NM. Prophylactic antibiotics administration head and neck cancer surgery with major flap reconstruction: 1-day cefoperazone versus 5-day cefotaxime. Acta Chir Plast 1998;40(2):36–40.
7. Piccart M, Dor P, Klastersky J. Antimicrobial prophylaxis of infections in head and neck cancer surgery. Scand J Infect Dis Suppl 1983;39:92–96.
8. Mombelli G, Coppens L, Dor P, Klastersky J. Antibiotic prophylaxis in surgery for head and neck cancer. Comparative study of short and prolonged administration of carbenicillin. J Antimicrob Chemother 1981;7(6):665–671.

27 Prophylaxis in Head and Neck Surgery

27.B.i.

Mechanical versus chemical prophylaxis in otolaryngologic surgery: Impact on thromboemboli

Jennifer J. Shin and Jonas T. Johnson

METHODS

A computerized PubMed search of MEDLINE 1966–December 2005 was performed. The medical subject headings "otolaryngology," "otorhinolaryngologic surgical procedures," or "otorhinolaryngologic diseases" were exploded and the resulting articles were cross-referenced with those obtained by exploding the medical subject headings, "pulmonary embolism," "thromboembolism," "thrombosis," or "venous thrombosis," yielding 589 publications. These articles were then reviewed to identify those that met the following inclusion criteria: 1) patient population undergoing otolaryngologic surgery, 2) intervention with mechanical or chemical prophylaxis (ideally with comparative data), 3) outcome measured in terms of deep vein thrombosis (DVT), pulmonary embolism (PE), and/or bleeding. Excluded were articles that had only nonperioperative data, isolated case reports, surveys of practice methods without thromboembolic or bleeding data. The bibliographies of the articles that met these inclusion/exclusion criteria were manually checked to ensure no further relevant articles could be identified. This process yielded two studies that also met such criteria [1,2]. In addition, two studies were identified that simply presented data regarding the incidence of DVT/PE after otolaryngologic surgery [2,3]. Two of the four studies were reported together in the same publication [2]. The two additional studies will be briefly discussed as they relate to determining the potential for future definitive studies on this topic in our field.

RESULTS

Outcome Measures. Bleeding outcomes were described in terms of bleeding at the wound and other sites, hemoglobin decrease, and intraoperative bleeding volume. Thromboembolic events were reported in terms of the number and percent of patients or limbs with DVT or PE.

Potential Confounders. When evaluating thromboembolic events, consideration of potential risk factors is key: age, body habitus, activity level, time of procedure, presence of malignancy. In addition, when considering both thromboembolic outcomes and bleeding, the use of heparin, nonsteroidal antiinflammatory agents, or warfarin therapy for comorbid conditions or surgical procedures could affect outcomes.

Study Designs. There was one prospective controlled (level 2) study of 40 patients, half of whom received no prophylaxis and half of whom received heparin followed by coumadin. This prospective study was not blinded. In addition, its small sample size limited its power, leaving its negative results open to question. The retrospective case control study (level 3) compared 20 cases (i.e., patients with DVT/PE) to 65 controls (i.e., patients without DVT/PE). Cases and controls were compared for age, weight, hours in the operating room, TNM (Tumor-Node-Metastasis) staging, malignant or benign disease, and use of DVT/PE prophylaxis. Data were examined by logistic regression analysis. This case control study was reported within a larger retrospective case series of 12,805 patients who were examined for incidence of DVT and PE.

Highest Level of Evidence. The prospective study found no significant difference in DVT and PE incidence whether a regimen of sequential heparin and coumadin was used or not. The power limitations associated with the small sample size, however, still leave the question open; there was a trend toward less PE with anticoagulation and it is unclear if such a difference could be demonstrated definitively with a larger sample size/greater statistical power. The case control study showed that thromboembolic phenomena in head neck surgery patients were correlated with age and inversely correlated with the use of compression devices. These data must be considered in the context of the potential inherent biases of a retrospective review, although regression analyses attempt to adjust for potential confounders.

Applicability. The results of these studies are applicable to patients undergoing head and neck surgery.

Morbidity/Complications. The bleeding outcomes as noted in the adjacent chart were the only morbidity/complications reported. There were no data provided on morbidity associated with the use of compressive devices.

CLINICAL SIGNIFICANCE AND FUTURE RESEARCH

There were two studies with comparative data regarding thromboembolic disease in otolaryngologic surgery. One study suggests no difference in postoperative rates of

DVT/PE with heparin/coumadin versus no prophylaxis, but interpretation of these results must be tempered by the limited power associated with the small sample size in this study. Limited power means that the study may not have been able to identify a difference that truly exists. The second study suggests that compression devices decrease the incidence of thromboembolic disease, but has the potential inherent biases of a retrospective study.

Up to 80% of pulmonary emboli may present without prior symptoms, so prevention is of paramount importance. Also, thromboembolic disease has been implicated in 5%–15% of acute care deaths, so decisions regarding the method of prophylaxis (mechanical, chemical, or otherwise) should be made with careful deliberation regarding their risks and benefits. Ideally, data from our own patients would guide these decisions. DVT/PE has been reported in 0.3%–17.5% of otolaryngology patients (see details in the second adjoining chart). Using the most recent incidence data for estimation, in order to identify a twofold difference in outcome with one regimen versus another, >15,000 otolaryngology patients would be required to achieve a 90% power. Such a study may not be feasible. In other surgical fields, however, DVT/PE is more common (up to 50% of postoperative patients in some studies), so higher-powered studies can be produced with smaller sample sizes. Reflecting this greater feasibility, there is rich literature in these other fields. Given the improbability of a highly powered study in otolaryngology patients that could definitively address this problem, we have elected to also examine the literature from other surgical specialties. Please see Section 27.B.ii, the second portion of the systematic reviews addressing this consequential topic.

Reference	Abraham-Inpijn, 1979	
Level (design)	2 (prospective controlled study)	
Sample size*	40: 20 heparin, 20 control (40)	

OUTCOMES		
	Bleeding measures (primary outcome)	**PE/DVT**
Heparin prophylaxis	Wound hematoma 5% (n = 1/20) GI bleed 5% (n = 1/20) Postoperative hemoglobin decrease: 1.2 mmol/L (SEM 0.2) Intraoperative bleeding effect was not observed EBL 871 cc (SEM 169)	PE 0% (n = 0/20) DVT 0% (n = 0/20)
No prophylaxis	Thyroid artery bleed 5% (n = 1/20) GI bleed 5% (n = 1/20) Postoperative hemoglobin decrease: 1.6 mmol/L (SEM 0.3) Intraoperative bleeding effect was not observed EBL: 656 cc (SEM 149)	PE 20% (n = 4/20) DVT 0% (n = 0/20)
p Value	>0.05	"Not proved"
Conclusion	No difference in bleeding	Trend toward less PE with heparin
Follow-up time	Not specified	

STUDY DESIGN	
Inclusion criteria	Patients with laryngeal carcinoma undergoing laryngectomy with or without neck dissection. All patients had physiotherapy before and after the operation, including breathing exercises. They were ambulant until the day of the procedure
Exclusion criteria	"No patient was excluded."
Group comparison before intervention	2 patients in each group had a history of venous thrombosis or PE. 1 patient in the heparin group and 2 patients in the control group had preoperative acenocoumarol (warfarin). Ages similar in both groups. Operations similar in both groups. Duration of operation was longer in the heparin group
Procedures	Each group had: 13 laryngectomy only, 6 laryngectomy with unilateral neck dissection, 1 laryngectomy with bilateral neck dissection
Age	63 y (mean) in heparin group 60 y (mean) in control group
Masking	None
Identification of DVT	"Diagnosed by clinical methods, including X-ray and scanning of the pulmonary vascular system with 99m Tc-labeled macroaggregated albumin"
Regimen details	Heparin 5000 U subcutaneously b.i.d., first dose given with premedication, continued until POD 7. Coumadin was given starting on POD 6
Monitoring for bleeding	Serum hemoglobin preoperatively and on POD 1–2. Urine and feces screened for hemoglobin. EBL was measured by the anesthetist.
Criteria for withdrawal	Not specified
Consecutive patients?	Not specified
Morbidity	Bleeding analysis as above

DVT = deep vein thrombosis, PE = pulmonary embolism, b.i.d. = two times per day, POD = postoperative day, GI = gastrointestinal, EBL = estimated blood loss.
*Sample size: numbers shown for those not lost to follow-up and those (initially recruited).

Reference	Moreano, 1998		
Level (design)	3 (retrospective case control)		
Sample size	85: 20 case (DVT/PE), 65 control (no DVT/PE)		
OUTCOMES			
	Pneumatic compression	Age	Other covariates
Association with DVT/PE	Correlation coefficient: −1.42 Odds ratio: 0.242 (95% Cl 0.077–0.755)	Correlation coefficient: +0.0518	Weight, hours in the operating room, TNM staging, malignant or benign disease were also examined in a regression model.
p Value	p = 0.0146	p = 0.0369	p = NS
Conclusion	Compression is significantly inversely correlated with DVT/PE.	Age is significantly positively correlated with DVT/PE.	These other covariates had no statistically significant effect on DVT/PE.
Follow-up time	Not specified		
STUDY DESIGN			
Inclusion criteria	Cases were identified from head and neck surgery cases among total operations by the Department of Otolaryngology in patients >18 y old at 1 institution 1987–1994 Controls were selected from a list of all patients undergoing head and neck surgery during the same time frame; systematic selection process included the first patient to have head and neck procedure each month until an adequate number was obtained		
Exclusion criteria	Not specified		
Group comparison before intervention	Not specified		
Procedures	Head and neck surgical procedures, not further specified		
Age	Not specified		
Masking	Not applicable		
Identification of DVT	Patients who had postoperative DVT/PE were identified with the use of an abstracting database that cross-referenced disease-specific codes for otolaryngologic procedures with codes for DVT/PE		
Regimen details	Pneumatic compression boots, further details not specified		
Monitoring for bleeding	Not specified		
Criteria for withdrawal	Not applicable		
Consecutive patients?	Not specified		
Morbidity	Not specified		

DVT = deep vein thrombosis, PE = pulmonary embolism, b.i.d. = two times per day, POD = postoperative day, GI = gastrointestinal, TNM = Tumor-Node-Metastasis, CI = confidence interval, EBL = estimated blood loss.

THE EVIDENCE CONDENSED: Incidence of postoperative thromboembolism in otolaryngologic procedures

Reference	Moreano, 1998		Graham, 1976	
Level (design)	4 (retrospective review)		4 (retrospective review)	
Sample size	12,805		103: 68 head and neck, 35 otology	
OUTCOMES				
	DVT	PE	DVT	PE
All procedures	0.3%	0.2%	17.5%	Not reported
Head and neck surgery	0.6%	0.4%	27.5%	Not reported
Otology/neurotology	0.3%	0.2%	0.0%	Not reported
Plastics/trauma	0.1%	0.1%	Not reported	Not reported
General otolaryngology	0.1%	0.04%	Not reported	Not reported
STUDY DESIGN				
Inclusion criteria	Total operations by the Department of Otolaryngology in patients >18 y old at 1 institution 1987–1994		Consecutive patients having major head and neck ("scale of operation ranged from external ethmoidectomy to total laryngectomy, radical neck dissection, and excision of the base of tongue") or ear operations	
DVT identification	Patients who had postoperative DVT/PE were identified with the use of an abstracting database that cross-referenced disease-specific codes for otolaryngologic procedures with codes for DVT/PE.		I^{125} fibrinogen isotope counts were made from the first POD until discharge or until the 14th POD, whichever was earlier. DVT was diagnosed with a sustained increase of 15% or a single site over a 24-h period. No attempt was made to confirm positive findings by phlebography	

DVT = deep vein thrombosis, PE = pulmonary embolism, POD = postoperative day.

REFERENCES

1. Abraham-Inpijn L. Critical evaluation of low-dose heparin in laryngectomy. Arch Chir Neerl 1979;31(1):9–15.
2. Moreano EH, Hutchison JL, McCulloch TM, Graham SM, Funk GF, Hoffman HT. Incidence of deep venous thrombosis and pulmonary embolism in otolaryngology-head and neck surgery. Otolaryngol Head Neck Surg 1998;118(6):777–784.
3. Graham JM, Robinson JM, Ashcroft PB, Glennie R. Deep vein thrombosis in ear, nose and throat surgery. J Laryngol Otol 1976;90(5):427–432.

27 Prophylaxis in Head and Neck Surgery

27.B.ii.

Compression versus subcutaneous heparin: Impact on postoperative or post-traumatic deep vein thrombosis, pulmonary emboli, and bleeding

Jennifer J. Shin and Jonas T. Johnson

METHODS

A computerized PubMed search of MEDLINE 1966–December 2005 was performed. The medical subject headings "heparin" or "low-molecular weight heparin" were exploded and the articles collected into a first group. Next, articles obtained by exploding the medical subject heading "intermittent pneumatic compression devices" and those which mapped to text words "boots" or "compression" were collected into a second group. Afterwards, the medical subject headings "pulmonary embolism" and "venous thrombosis" were exploded and the resulting articles were collected into a third group. Finally, the three groups were cross-referenced. The resulting 222 articles were reviewed to identify those that met the following inclusion criteria: 1) patient population undergoing surgery or admitted immediately post-trauma, 2) prophylaxis with mechanical compression versus subcutaneous heparin, 3) outcome measured in terms of deep vein thrombosis (DVT), pulmonary embolism (PE), or bleeding, 4) randomized controlled trials. Articles were excluded if: a) randomization occurred but the choice of compression versus heparin was not randomized, b) heparin was evaluated not alone but only in combination with other agents (such as dihydroergotamine), c) additive therapy with heparin and compression was examined in comparison to one agent alone. The bibliographies of the articles which met these inclusion/exclusion criteria were manually checked to ensure no further relevant articles could be identified. This process yielded 13 randomized controlled trials (RCTs). The outcome measures in these trials were similar enough so as to allow meta-analyses (i.e. statistical pooling of data) and these analyses are also further detailed in this systematic review [1–13].

RESULTS

Herein we describe results of individual studies. In the subsequent section, please find results for the related meta-analysis.

Outcome Measures. Thromboembolic outcomes were most consistently reported as the percent of patients who developed DVT or PE. Occasionally it was reported as the percent of limbs identified with thrombus. Some studies also distinguish between calf/distal and thigh/proximal thrombi. Bleeding outcomes were described as percent with major or minor bleeding, hematoma formation, transfusion requirement, oozing or ecchymosis at the wound.

Potential Confounders. Age, body habitus, duration of procedure, presence of malignancy, lower extremity and pelvic surgery/injuries, estrogen supplementation, and comorbid conditions (especially those interfering with ambulation) could all affect rates of DVT/PE. In addition, when considering both thromboemboli and bleeding, the use of non-steroidal anti-inflammatory agents or warfarin therapy for concomitant medical disease could potentially influence results. The majority of the RCTs confirmed that their randomization process resulted in similar rates of potential confounders in both groups.

Study Designs. These are all RCTs which provide level 1 data. Within each trial, patients were randomly allocated into treatment with either mechanical compression or heparin. Mechanical compression included either calf/thigh sleeves, foot pumps, and/or elastic stockings. Heparin therapy was either unfractionated or low molecular weight. The precise regimens of mechanical and chemical prophylaxis are detailed in the adjoining charts. In several studies, the radiologists who interpreted the DVT screening imaging were blinded as to the treatment group of the patient. Approximately one half of the reports included their own power calculations, although only one trial met their intended sample size. Another trial stopped patient accrual when they realized that even with extreme results from the additional subjects they were planning to enroll, they would not demonstrate a statistically significant difference between groups.

Highest Level of Evidence. The majority of the RCTs (10 of 13) reported no significant difference in the rate of DVT with compression versus subcutaneous heparin. In contrast, 2 trials reported significantly less DVTs with compression, while 1 other reported significantly less DVTs with heparin. We have attempted to explore and resolve this conflicting data by performing meta-analyses of all of their reported results, as well as an analysis of the individual reports to determine how the studies with differing results are distinct from the remaining trials.

In individual studies, the rate of PE was often too low to allow statistical analysis and therefore no comparative conclusions would be drawn. By combining data from the 12 studies that reported PE outcomes, we can increase the number of patients analyzed and allow more meaningful statistical analysis. Thus, we have also performed a meta-analysis of PE results for these trials.

In individual studies, the conclusions regarding bleeding were also varied. Three RCTs showed a significantly worse rate of bleeding with heparin than with compression. Four showed no significant difference. Two reported numbers but no statistical analysis. Again, we have attempted to resolve this conflicting data by performing meta-analyses of all of their reported results regarding major bleeding/hematoma, minor bleeding/oozing, and number of patients requiring transfusion.

The adjoining charts detail individual studies, and are followed by meta-analyses addressing the rate of DVT, PE, and bleeding with compression versus subcu-

taneous heparin. In addition, a risk/benefit analysis is given.

Applicability. These studies are most applicable to the type of patient that they study (i.e. orthopedic, gynecologic, urologic, abdominal surgery, trauma, or a combination). The studies most applicable to our otolaryngology patients are detailed in part 27.B.i. of these reviews (i.e. those performed on otolaryngology patients). As mentioned at the conclusion of that review, however, because of the logistical difficulty in executing level 1 studies on this topic within our field, we have carefully considered this data from other fields as well.

Morbidity/Complications. See the adjoining charts.

Reference	Ginzburg, 2003		
Level (Design)	1 (randomized controlled trial)		
Sample Size†	398 (442)		
	OUTCOMES		
	DVT	**PE**	**Total**
Compression	2.7% (n = 6/224)	0.5% (n = 1/224)	3.1% (n = 7/224)
Heparin	0.5% (n = 1/218)	0.5% (n = 1/218)	0.9% (n = 2/218)
p value	p = 0.122	P = NS	p = 0.176
Conclusion	No significant difference in rate of DVT or PE		
Follow-up time	Time of discharge or 30 days from admission		
	STUDY DESIGN		
Inclusion criteria	Adult patients with severe injuries (injury severity score ≥9) and at least one leg and one arm available for a intermittent pneumatic compression device		
Exclusion criteria	Need for systemic anticoagulation, contraindication to low molecular weight heparin therapy, <18 years old, patients who were unlikely to survive or remain in the hospital for ≥7 days, renal failure (serum creatinine >3.4 mg/dL), pregnant women, patients who were unable to undergo bilateral Doppler ultrasonography, morbid obesity (body mass index >26 kg/m2), coagulopathy, antiplatelet therapy except some NSAIDs given for analgesia		
Randomization effectiveness	Similar age, sex, other demographics, injury severity distribution, neurologic, pelvic, and extremity trauma rates (except for femur fractures), obesity, previous hip surgery, myocardial infarction, congestive heart failure, chronic obstructive pulmonary disease, and tobacco use. More femur fractures and shorter hospital stay in the enoxaparin group		
Age	>40 years old		
Masking	Not specified		
Screening regimen	Duplex imaging on both legs on admission, then weekly until discharge, at 30 days or when there was a thrombotic event (whichever occurred first). Clinical suspicion of PE was verified by spiral CT or ventilation-perfusion scintography		
Compression details	DVT10 Calf garment placed on both legs, unless leg trauma prevented (instead placed on one leg and one arm) until walking independently or discharged from hospital. Sleeve disuse tolerated for up to 8 h within the protocol. Elastic stockings were not used		
Heparin details	Enoxaparin (low molecular weight heparin) 30 mg subcutaneously Q12 hrs beginning within 24 hrs of the trauma until walking independently or discharged from hospital. Enoxaparin was held 12 h before any surgical procedure, but was resumed at the first postoperative dose, so that a maximum of 2 doses was missed		
Compliance	Compression noncompliance (>8 h without boots) 6.7% (n = 15/224) Enoxaparin noncompliance (>2 doses missed) 13.3% (n = 29/218)		
Criteria for withdrawal	Failure to comply with regimen: >8 hrs without boots, >2 doses heparin missed		
Intention to treat analysis	Patients who could not comply with protocol were excluded from analysis		
Power	900 patients needed for 80% power to detect a clinically significant 30% difference in treatment efficacy, with an anticipated dropout rate of 5%		
Morbidity/complications	No deaths		

† Sample Size: numbers shown for those not lost to follow up and those (initially recruited).
NSAID = nonsteroidal anti-inflammatory agents.

THE EVIDENCE: Compression versus subcutaneous heparin for thromboembolism prevention

Reference	Warwick, 1998			
Level (Design)	1 (randomized controlled trial)			
Sample Size†	274 (290)			
OUTCOMES				
	All DVT	**Proximal DVT**	**Calf DVT**	**PE**
Compression	18% (n = 24/136)	13% (n = 17/136)	5% (n = 7/136)	0.7% (n = 1/136)
Heparin	13% (n = 18/138)	8% (n = 11/138)	4% (n = 6/138)	0.0% (n = 0/1136)
p value	p = NS	p = NS	p = NS	p = NS
Conclusion	No significant difference in rate of DVT or PE			
Follow-up time	3 months postoperatively			
STUDY DESIGN				
Inclusion criteria	Primary total hip replacement 1995–1997			
Exclusion criteria	Refusal of consent, long-term anticoagulation therapy for reexisting cardiac or cerebrovascular disease, active malignant tumor, gastrointestinal ulceration, previous bleeding diatheses, wounds on or painful joints in the feet, enrollment in another trial necessitating planned early discharge form the hospital or modification of wound drainage			
Randomization effectiveness	Similar age, gender, weight, previous thromboembolism, osteoarthritis, rheumatoid arthritis, use of NSAIDs, method of fixation, regional anesthesia, opsterior operative approach in both groups			
Age	Mean 69 years old (standard deviation 11)			
Masking	Radiologists were blinded to treatment groups			
Screening regimen	Ascending venography on POD6,7,8. Clinical symptoms consistent with pulmonary embolism were investigated with ventilation-perfusion scanning			
Compression details	Foot pump was fitted in the recovery room, then kept activated whenever the patient was not bearing weight, through POD7			
Heparin details	Enoxaparin (low molecular weight heparin) 40 mg starting 12 hours before the operation then Q24 hrs through POD7			
Compliance	Foot pump noncompliance in 3% (n = 5), median use 15 hours per day			
Criteria for withdrawal	Refusal of venography, discharge prior to venography, refusal of foot pump, surgeon request because of wound hematoma or early dislocation			
Intention to treat analysis	Yes, patients who could not tolerate foot pump continued in the analysis			
Power	280 patients 80% power to detect a 15% difference with a prevalence of DVT or 10–20 percent in an equivalence trial			
Morbidity/complications	No deaths			

† Sample Size: numbers shown for those not lost to follow up and those (initially recruited).
NSAID = nonsteroidal anti-inflammatory agents.

THE EVIDENCE: Compression versus subcutaneous heparin for thromboembolism prevention

Reference	Nicolaides, 1980		Rasmussen, 1988	
Level (Design)	1 (randomized controlled trial)		1 (randomized controlled trial)	
Sample Size†	251 (271)		248 (248)	

	OUTCOMES			
	DVT	**PE**	**DVT**	**PE**
Compression	Single chamber 22.2% (n = 37/166 calves) Sequential compression 22.2% (n = 37/166)	Single 0.6% (n = 1/166) Sequential 0% (n = 0/166)	29.7% (n = 22/74)	0% (n = 0/74)
Heparin	11.7% (n = 20/170 calves)	(n = 1/170)	29.4% (n = 25/85)	0% (n = 0/85)
p value	Not specified	NS	p > 0.05 for all comparisons	
Conclusion	Trend toward less DVT with heparin		No difference between groups	
Follow-up time	Postoperative day 7		Postoperative day 4–5	

	STUDY DESIGN			
Inclusion criteria	Emergency or elective laparatomy or open operation on bladder or prostate		Major abdominal surgery >1 hr duration, age >40 years old	
Exclusion criteria	Not specified		Anticoagulant treatment, hemorrhagic diathesis	
Randomization effectiveness	Similar number of patients with malignancy, age >60 years old, prostatectomy, emergency cases		Similar age, duration of surgery in treatment groups, as well as presence of obesity, history of thrombosis, varicose veins, smoking	
Age	Not specified		41–87 years old	
Masking	Not specified		Not specified	
Screening regimen	I-fibrinogen injection immediately after operation with legs scanned on POD1, 3,5,7, or daily if raised counts detected		99mTc-plasmin test of the lower limbs on POD4 or 5. Differences in quotient units in calf, knee, and thigh of 13 units were diagnostic of DVT	
Compression details	Intermittent pneumatic compression with single chamber Flotronaire from induction of anesthesia until 16–24 hrs postoperatively versus intermittent pneumatic compression with multichamber devices		Bilateral graduated compression stockings from toes to knee (TED stockings)	
Heparin details	Heparin 5000 u SC Q12 hrs starting 2 hours before operation and continuing for a minimum of 7 days or until patient became fully ambulant		Heparin sodium 5000 u SC Q12 hrs	
Length of prophylaxis	16 hrs to 7 days		Began on the evening before operation and continued until complete mobilization or for not less than 5 days postoperatively	
Compliance	Not specified		Not specified	
Criteria for withdrawal from study	Failure to follow protocol (n = 5, no DVT), death before POD5 (n = 15, PE found at necrotopsy in n = 2 (1 compression, 1 heparin)		Not specified	
Intention to treat analysis	Patients were rejected from the analysis if they did not follow protocol		Not specified	
Power	Not reported		Not reported	
Morbidity/complications	2 deaths, both with PE at necrotopsy		Not reported	

† Sample Size: numbers shown for those not lost to follow up and those (initially recruited).
Hr = hours, POD = postoperative day, SC = subcutaneously, Q12h = every 12 hours. Preop = preoperatively.

THE EVIDENCE: Compression versus subcutaneous heparin for thromboembolism prevention

Reference	Maxwell, 2001	
Level (Design)	1 (randomized controlled trial)	
Sample Size†	211 (211)	

OUTCOMES		
	DVT	**PE**
Compression	0.9% (n = 1/106)	0% (n = 0/106)
Heparin	1.9% (n = 2/105)	0% (n = 0/105)
p value	Not specified	NS
Conclusion	No difference between groups	
Follow-up time	Postoperative day 30	

STUDY DESIGN		
Inclusion criteria	>40 years old, major procedure for gynecologic malignancy	
Exclusion criteria	DVT or PE in previous 6 months, contraindications to heparin therapy, conduction anesthesia, heparin sensitivity, pregnancy, coagulation abnormalities, PT or PTT >1.5 times normal, platelet count <100,000	
Randomization effectiveness	Similar pretreatment characteristics and thromboembolic risk factors between groups	
Age	35–87 years old	
Masking	Radiologist interpreting ultrasound was blinded	
Screening regimen	Doppler ultrasound lower extremities on POD3–5, interview 30 days after surgery to detect patients who developed DVT or PE after discharge	
Compression details	Venodyne external pneumatic compression sleeves placed with induction, continued through POD5. When the patients were ambulating independently, they were removed until return to bed	
Heparin details	Dalteparin (low molecular weight heparin) 2500 u SC 1–2 hrs preop and 12 hrs later then 5000 u daily though POD5, longer if not ambulatory	
Length of prophylaxis	Through postoperative day 5, longer if not yet ambulatory	
Compliance	Not specified	
Criteria for withdrawal from study	Not specified	
Intention to treat analysis	Yes	
Power	200 patients need for 80% power to detect a proportion of 0.34 in the heparin group compared with a 0.17 proportion in the compression group (alpha 0.05)	
Morbidity/complications	No symptomatic DVTs. 5 cases of thrombocytopenia in heparin group, 1 in compression group.	

† Sample Size: numbers shown for those not lost to follow up and those (initially recruited).
Hr = hours, POD = postoperative day, SC = subcutaneously, Q12h = every 12 hours. Preop = preoperatively.

THE EVIDENCE: Compression versus subcutaneous heparin for thromboembolism prevention

Reference	Clarke-Pearson, 1993	
Level (Design)	1 (randomized controlled trial)	
Sample Size†	208 (218)	
	OUTCOMES	
	DVT	**PE**
Compression	4.0% (n = 4/101)	0% (n = 0/101)
Heparin	6.5% (n = 7/107)	0% (n = 0/107)
p value	p = 0.54	NS
Conclusion	No difference between groups	
Follow-up time	Postoperative day 30	
	STUDY DESIGN	
Inclusion criteria	Surgery for gynecologic growths (benign and malignant)	
Exclusion criteria	History of bleeding diathesis, thromboembolism in previous 3 months, warfarin or heparin use in previoius 6 weeks, PTT or PT >1.2 times control, platelet <100,000/mL3	
Randomization effectiveness	Similar age, race, diagnoses, numbers and types of procedures, duration of anesthesia	
Age	22–89 years old	
Masking	Not specified	
Screening regimen	Iodine-125 fibrinogen uptake leg scans daily until discharge. DVT diagnosed if counts were >20% more than in same site in contralateral leg or adjacent site. If scan was positive then ascending venography used to confirm DVT. PE assessed by ventilation perfusion lung scan and pulmonary arteriography	
Compression details	Venodyne pneumatic calf compression initiated at induction of anesthesia and continued through POD5, longer if not full ambulatory by then, sooner if patient was discharged before then	
Heparin details	Heparin 5000 u subcutaneously Q8 h, starting with 3 doses preoperatively until POD7, longer if not full ambulatory by then, sooner if patient was discharged before then	
Compliance	1 patient discontinued compression because of minor discomfort	
Criteria for withdrawal from study	Cancellation of surgery	
Intention to treat analysis	Yes, only patients whose surgery was canceled were excluded (n = 10)	
Power	"would have required 1780 patients to have sufficient statistical power"	
Morbidity/complications	3 heparin discontinuation because of bleeding associated with prolonged PTT.	

† Sample Size: numbers shown for those not lost to follow up and those (initially recruited).
Hr = hours, POD = postoperative day, SC = subcutaneously, Q12h = every 12 hours. PTT = activated partial thromboplastin time. PT = prothrombin time.

THE EVIDENCE: Compression versus subcutaneous heparin for thromboembolism prevention

Reference	Pitto, 2004		Kosir, 1998		
Level (Design)	1 (randomized controlled trial)		1 (randomized controlled trial)		
Sample Size†	200 (216)		136 (160)		

OUTCOMES					
	DVT	PE	DVT	PE	Death
Compression	3% (n = 3/100)	(n = 0/100)	0.0% (n = 0/67)	(n = 1/67)	(n = 0/67)
Heparin	6% (n = 6/100)	(n = 0/100)	3.0% (n = 2/66)	(n = 1/66)	(n = 1/66)
p value	P < 0.05	NS	Not reported	NS	NS
Conclusion	Compression sig. better to prevent DVT		Trend toward less DVT with compression		
Follow-up time	Postoperative day 45		Postoperative day 30		

STUDY DESIGN		
Inclusion criteria	Osteoarthritis of hip requiring cemented total hip arthroplasty, age >18 and <80 years old	General surgical procedure (pelvic, abdominal, thoracic, inguinal, plastic, head and neck, peripheral vascular not involving both femoral regions) ≥1 hr with spinal or general anesthesia
Exclusion criteria	History of thromboembolic disease, heart disease, bleeding diathesis, patient refusal, active malignancy, gastrointestinal ulceration, superficial wounds or painful joints of in the feet	Anticoagulant treatment, nonambulatory patients
Randomization effectiveness	Similar gender, age, body mass index, duration of operation, intraoperative blood loss, and duration of hospitalization	Similar age, surgery type, procedure time, anesthetic method, diabetes, vascular disease, COPD, hypertension, cardiac disease, malignancy, estrogen supplement, immobility, obesity in the two groups
Age	18–80 years old	Mean 62.5 years old
Masking	Radiologist was blinded. Observers of wound for bleeding were not blinded	Not specified for DVT screening
Screening regimen	Serial duplex sonography on POD 3,10,45	Duplex venous studies on POD1,7,30
Compression details	A-V Impulse Foot pump starting in the recovery room. All patients received a single dose of fraxiparin 12 hrs prior to surgery	Athrombic 2500 Pneumatic compression devices applied before induction and used for 48 hrs postoperatively while the patient was at bedrest or overnight
Heparin details	Fraxiparin (low molecular weight heparin), dose adjusted to body weight (0.2–0.6 mL, 0.1 mL = 950 IU of anti-Xa) until discharge. All patients received a single dose of fraxiparin 12 hrs prior to surgery	Unfractionated heparin 5000 u SC Q12 hrs, starting 1 hour prior to surgery and for 48 hrs postoperatively
Compliance	13 discontinued compression	Measured but not specified
Criteria for withdrawal from study	Patients who did not tolerate continuous use of foot pump for >4 hrs (n = 16) or use of heparin	Canceled or short surgery, change in anesthetic methods, physician request due to complications, broken blood tubes, improper protocol prophylaxis method (n = 24)
Intention to treat analysis	Patients failing to complete protocol were excluded	Patients failing to complete protocol were excluded
Power	200 patients to achieve 80% power to detect a 20% difference	Not reported
Morbidity/complications	1 heparin induced thrombocytopenia	1 death from PE

† Sample Size: numbers shown for those not lost to follow up and those (initially recruited).
Hr = hours, POD = postoperative day, SC = subcutaneously, Q12h = every 12 hours. PTT = activated partial thromboplastin time. PT = prothrombin time.

THE EVIDENCE: Compression versus subcutaneous heparin for thromboembolism prevention

Reference	Kurtoglu, 2004		
Level (Design)	1 (randomized controlled trial)		
Sample Size†	120 (120)		

OUTCOMES

	DVT	PE	Mean time to mobilization
Compression	6.6% (n = 4/60)	3.3% (n = 2/60)	12.1 h (SD 2.1)
Heparin	5.0% (n = 3/60)	6.6% (n = 4/60)	13 h (SD 1.9)
p value	p = 0.04	p = 0.07	p = NS
Conclusion	"was not statistically significant"	Trend but no signif. diff.	No significant difference
Follow-up time	1 week after discharge		

STUDY DESIGN

Inclusion criteria	Severe head/spinal trauma (epidural hematoma 33.3%, contusion 23.3%, subdural hematoma 20%, subarachnoid hemorrhage 9.1%, intracerebral hemorrhage 5%, spinal fracture/dislocation 9.1%)
Exclusion criteria	<14 years old, hepatic or urinary dysfunction, spinal cord injury, history of DVT, high bleeding risk (platelets <100,000 or INR >1.5), use of anticoagulants, continuing hemorrhage on control scans within 24 h of admission, patients requiring craniotomy
Randomization effectiveness	Similar rates of intracranial injury, contusion, subdural hematoma, subarachnoid hemorrhage
Age	18–76 years old
Masking	Not specified
Screening regimen	Venous duplex ultrasound of lower extremities performed on admission to ICU, each week of hospitalization and 1 week after discharge, and if there was a 10% increase in calf diameter on daily measurements. Spiral computed tomography was used when there was a suspicion of pulmonary embolism
Compression details	Prophylactic DVT System below-knee intermittent pneumatic compression devices or AV Impulse system device
Heparin details	Enoxaparin (low molecular weight heparin) 40 mg/day. All patients began with compression devices, awaiting serial scans to ensure no continuing hemorrhage
Compliance	Not specified
Criteria for withdrawal from study	Not specified
Intention to treat analysis	120 patients analyzed in their original groups
Power	"when the alpha was set to 0.05 and the beta to 0.2, the power was about 0.20"
Morbidity/complications	deaths from PE: 3.33% (n = 2) compression group, 6.66% (n = 4) heparin group

† Sample Size: numbers shown for those not lost to follow up and those (initially recruited).
Kurtoglu: vena cava filters were placed in 3 patients who developed DVT while on LMWH prophylaxis.

THE EVIDENCE: Compression versus subcutaneous heparin for thromboembolism prevention

Reference	Santori, 1993			
Level (Design)	1 (randomized controlled trial)			
Sample Size†	132 (132)			

OUTCOMES

	DVT	Major thromboses	Minor thromboses	PE
Compression	13.4% (n = 9/67)	4.5% (n = 3/67)	9.0% (n = 6/67)	0.0% (n = 0/67)
Heparin	35.4% (n = 23/65)	24.6% (n = 16/65)	10.8% (n = 7/65)	3.1% (n = 2/65)
p value	$p < 0.005$	$p < 0.005$	Not specified	Not specified
Conclusion	Compression significantly better than heparin for DVT and major thromboses		Trend toward less PE and minor thrombosis with compression but no statistical comparison	
Follow-up time	6 weeks postoperatively			

STUDY DESIGN

Inclusion criteria	General anesthesia for primary total hip replacement by a lateral approach
Exclusion criteria	Previous history of thromboembolism, varicose veins, venous insufficiency, malignancy
Randomization effectiveness	Similar age, gender, indications for hip replacement, duration of operation, total blood loss
Age	Mean 72.4 (SD 6.65) in compression group, Mean 69.8 (SD 6.22) in heparin group
Masking	Not specified
Screening regimen	Doppler ultrasound and liquid crystal thermography on POD 8–10, 42 for screening. Phlebography if Doppler positive or if negative with convincing clinical exam. Major thrombi = iliac, femoral, or proximal veins or calf >5 cm. Minor thrombi = calf, <5 cm.
Compression details	AV Impulse foot pump to both feet immediately after the operation until POD7–10. All patients received non-pneumatic compression stockings after the completion of the surgery.
Heparin details	Heparin calcium 5000 IU SC TID ×10 days, starting on the day before the operation. All patients received non-pneumatic compression stockings after the completion of the surgery.
Compliance	Not specified
Criteria for withdrawal from study	Not specified
Intention to treat analysis	Not specified
Power	Not reported
Morbidity/complications	1 death from PE in the heparin group. 3 superficial skin abrasions from foot pump.

† Sample Size: numbers shown for those not lost to follow up and those (initially recruited).

THE EVIDENCE: Compression versus subcutaneous heparin for thromboembolism prevention

Reference	Blanchard, 1999		Nicolaides, 1983	
Level (Design)	1 (randomized controlled trial)		1 (randomized controlled trial)	
Sample Size†	130 (130)		100 (100)	
OUTCOMES				
	DVT	PE	DVT	PE
Compression	54.0% (n = 34/63)	0.0% (n = 0/63)	6.0% (n = 3/50 patients) (n = 4 thrombi/100 limbs—1 bilateral)	NR
Heparin	23.9% (n = 16/67)	0.0% (n = 0/67)	14.0% (n = 7/50 patients) (n = 9 thrombi/100 limbs—2 bilateral)	NR
p value	p < 0.001	p = NS	p = 0.05–0.10	p = NS
Conclusion	Heparin significantly better to prevent DVT		Trend toward less DVT with compression	
Follow-up time	Postoperative day 8–12		Postoperative day 20	
STUDY DESIGN				
Inclusion criteria	Elective total knee arthroplasty, >40 years old, weight between 40–100 kg		Major abdominal operations	
Exclusion criteria	Not specified		Not specified	
Randomization effectiveness	See chart		Randomization by risk stratification created similar ages, previous DVT, infection, malignancy	
Age	>40 years old		57.3 mean (13.4 SD) years old in compression group, 58.6 (13.3) in heparin group	
Masking	Radiologist was blinded		Not specified	
Screening regimen	Bilateral phlebography in 108 patients on POD 8–12 or earlier if symptoms occurred; venous compression ultrasound in 15 patients because phlebography was technically not possible or it was refused; both used in outcome measurement		I-fibrinogen injection immediately after operation with legs scanned on POD1, 3,5,7, or daily if raised counts detected	
Compression details	Because the traditional whole leg compression boots are not suited to knee surgery, the arteriovenous impulse foot system was developed		Sequential compression devices used continuously during the operation and for a minimum of 72 hrs during the postoperative period. Devices were discontinued and TED stockings were used when patient was ambulant	
Heparin details	Nadroparin calcium (low molecular weight heparin) daily dosage adapted to body weight, injected 12 hrs before and 12 hrs postop, then once daily for 10–12 days		Heparin 5000 u SC Q12 hrs from 2 hrs preop until discharge from hospital	
Compliance	25% discontinued use of foot pump because of local symptoms		Not specified	
Criteria for withdrawal	Not specified		Not specified (all patients completed the study)	
Intention to treat analysis	Yes		All patients completed the study	
Power	No *a priori* calculation		No *a priori* calculation	
Morbidity/ complications	No difference in platelet counts between the two groups		None reported	

† Sample Size: numbers shown for those not lost to follow up and those (initially recruited).
NR = Not reported, hrs = hours, POD = postoperative day, SC = subcutaneously, preop = preoperatively.

THE EVIDENCE: Compression versus subcutaneous heparin for thromboembolism prevention

Reference	Coe, 1978	
Level (Design)	1 (randomized controlled trial)	
Sample Size†	81 (83)	
OUTCOMES		
	DVT	PE
Compression	3.4% +scan, pos venogram (n = 1/29)* 3.4% +scan, no venogram (n = 1/29)** 6.8% +scan, neg venogram (n = 2/29)° 86% −scan, no venogram (n = 25/29)°°	0.0% (n = 0/21)
Heparin	21.4% + scan, pos venogram (n = 6/28)* 0.0% +scan, no venogram (n = 0/28)** 7.1% +scan, neg venogram (n = 2/28)° 71.4% −scan, no venogram (n = 20/28)°°	0.0% (n = 0/32)
p value	*+** vs °+°°: p = NS, * vs °+°°: p < 0.04	p = NS
Conclusion	Trend toward better DVT prevention with compression, possibly significant	No sig. diff.
Follow-up time	Postoperative day 30	
STUDY DESIGN		
Inclusion criteria	Open urological operations	
Exclusion criteria	Not specified in detail	
Randomization effectiveness	Similar age, anesthesia duration, malignancy, varicose veins, previous thrombophlebitis, prostatectomy, lithotomy, nephrectomy in both groups. More cystectomy in compression group	
Age	Heparin group mean 63 +/− 16 years old, compression group mean 55 +/−11	
Masking	Not specified	
Screening regimen	I-125 fibrinogen scan daily until discharge—judged as positive if any location was 20 percentage points higher than adjacent sites on the same leg or the same site on the opposite leg on the same or previous day. Positive fibrinogen scan prompted follow up phlebogram but several patients refused it. Suspicion of pulmonary embolism investigated by chest roentgenography, pulmonary angiography	
Compression details	External pneumatic compression of both calves by means of Anti-Em Extremity Pump inflatable boots, starting after the induction of anesthesia and continuing until discharge. "Short periods were allowed in which the boots were removed for patient comfort, nursing care, ambulation. Occasionally EPC was discontinued prematurely bc of patient discomfort"	
Heparin details	Heparin sodium 5000 u SC Q12 hrs, starting 2 hours before surgery and continuing until discharge	
Compliance	Heparin prophylaxis continued significantly longer than patients in EPC group (p < 0.005), primarily bc of discomfort caused by boots	
Criteria for withdrawal	Treatment with anticoagulant drugs in the postoperative period	
Intention to treat analysis	Yes	
Power	No *a priori* calculation	
Morbidity/ complications	Not specified in more detail	

† Sample Size: numbers shown for those not lost to follow up and those (initially recruited).

NR = Not reported, hrs = hours, POD = postoperative day, SC = subcutaneously, preop = preoperatively.

*, **, °, °° Symbols denote which data comparisons correspond to the referenced p values.

META-ANALYSES

Methods of Meta-Analyses. All of the studies included in this meta-analysis are randomized controlled trials (level 1) and they represent the highest level of evidence comparing DVT/PE and bleeding outcomes with compression versus heparin prophylaxis within all types of surgery and post-trauma patients. Further details regarding the search and selection process are as noted in the initial methods of this review. Overall, given the anticipated difficulties in performing a well-powered study addressing this issue in otolaryngology patients (see part B.i. of these reviews), the relevant literature from all types of post-surgical and post-trauma patients was considered. Because of the need to evaluate both benefits and risks, meta-analyses of DVT, PE, and bleeding outcomes were performed. Analysis was performed using a random effects model with inverse variance or Mantel-Haenszel weights.

Results of Meta-Analysis

Benefits: Thromboembolic Outcomes. First, a meta-analysis focusing on the outcomes of DVT was performed. Individual publications reported the gamut of conclusions: no difference, less DVT with compression, and less DVT with heparin. When the data from all of the studies were pooled, there was no significant difference in the rate of DVTs in subjects who received compression versus heparin. Likewise, when the rate of PE was compared, there was no significant difference between groups (See tables). With the large sample size from pooled data, 95% confidence intervals were very tight, reflecting the increased power of the combined data.

In a sensitivity analysis, neither the type of compression nor the type of heparin used affected the result. Whether calf/thigh boots, foot pump, or elastic stockings were analyzed separately, there was still no significant difference between compression and heparin. Likewise, whether unfractionated heparin or low molecular weight heparin was administered, there was still no distinction between groups (See tables). Thus, when considering all inpatient postoperative and post-trauma patients, the DVT/PE impact of mechanical compression and subcutaneous heparin was similar, regardless of the particular regimen used.

Risks: Bleeding Outcomes. Having considered the benefits, we also considered the risks involved. Individual papers reported a mix of results; some concluded that there was no increased risk of major or minor bleeding, while others found a greater risk of bleeding with subcutaneous heparin. In an attempt to resolve these heterogeneous results, we performed meta-analyses of 3 bleeding measures.

First, the rate of major bleeding and/or hematoma was considered. When the data from all papers that reported this outcome were pooled, there was a statistically significant worse outcome with subcutaneous heparin (p = 0.006). The associated odds ratio suggests that the rate of major bleeding/hematoma is nearly 4 times higher with heparin than with compression. Fortunately, the overall rate of major bleeding/hematoma is still low: 3.1% versus 0.8%. The rate difference between the two groups translates to a number needed to harm of 44, meaning that if 44 patients receive subcutaneous heparin, 1 of them will have a major bleed or hematoma who would not have otherwise. This number shows us that the risk is present, but not excessive.

Second, another meta-analysis was performed of all papers reporting results regarding minor bleeding and/or oozing from the wound. When all data from articles reporting this outcome were combined, there was significantly more minor bleeding and oozing from the wound in the group who received subcutaneous heparin. The odds of having minor bleeding/oozing with heparin are 2.6 times higher than if compression is used for prophylaxis. The data also suggests that if 6 patients receive subcutaneous heparin, 1 of them will have minor bleeding/oozing that would not have otherwise.

Third, a meta-analysis was performed of all data from publications reporting the number of patients who required transfusion. Similar to the other meta-analyses of bleeding results, a larger percent of patients required transfusion if they received subcutaneous heparin rather than compression prophylaxis.

Because of the variety of outcome measures reported, it is difficult to pool data to allow insight into whether bleeding rates differed with unfractionated versus low molecular weight heparin in comparison to compression, as well as to rigorously pool data from all studies at once.

CLINICAL SIGNIFICANCE AND FUTURE RESEARCH

Benefits versus Risks. The overall results of these meta-analyses suggest that when compression and subcutaneous heparin are compared, the benefits (thromboembolic restriction) are the same but the risks (bleeding) are increased with subcutaneous heparin. Therefore, the use of subcutaneous heparin instead of compression prophylaxis must be undertaken with the understanding that there is an associated increased risk. This understanding does not mean that heparin should never be used in our patients, but that it should be used either when additional heparin-associated benefits are anticipated or when compression is not a viable option.

Future studies may focus on the analysis of patients who receive compression alone versus compression combined with subcutaneous heparin. Such double coverage may be especially relevant for head and neck surgery patients who often have multiple risk factors (i.e. malignancy, longer time to ambulation, comorbid conditions) for thromboembolic disease.

META-ANALYSES: THROMBOEMBOLIC EVENTS

DVT (All)

	Compression	Heparin
Ginzburg, 2003	2.7% (n = 6/224)	0.5% (n = 1/218)
Warwick, 1998	18% (n = 24/136)	13% (n = 18/138)
Nicolaides, 1980*	22.2% (n = 37/166)	11.7% (n = 10/85)
Rasmussen, 1988	29.7% (n = 22/74)	29.4% (n = 25/85)
Maxwell, 2001	0.9% (n = 1/106)	1.9% (n = 2/105)
Clarke-Pearson, 1993	4.0% (n = 4/101)	6.5% (n = 7/107)
Pitto, 2003	3.0% (n = 3/100)	6.0% (n = 6/100)
Kosir, 1998	0.0% (n = 0/67)	3.0% (n = 2/66)
Kirtoglu, 2004	6.6% (n = 4/60)	5.0% (n = 3/60)
Santori, 1993	13.4% (n = 9/67)	35.4% (n = 23/65)
Blanchard, 1999	54.0% (n = 34/63)	23.9% (n = 16/67)
Nicolaides, 1983	6.0% (n = 3/50)	14.0% (n = 7/50)
Coe, 1978	6.8% (n = 2/29)	21.4% (n = 6/28)
Total	**12.0% (n = 149/1243)**	**10.7% (n = 126/1174)**

* number of patients extrapolated from number of calves as reported.

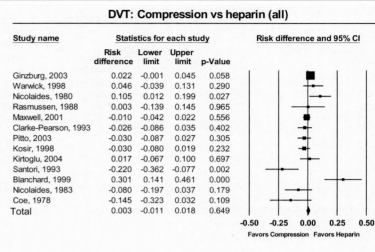

DVT: Compression vs heparin (all)

Study name	Statistics for each study				Risk difference and 95% CI
	Risk difference	Lower limit	Upper limit	p-Value	
Ginzburg, 2003	0.022	-0.001	0.045	0.058	
Warwick, 1998	0.046	-0.039	0.131	0.290	
Nicolaides, 1980	0.105	0.012	0.199	0.027	
Rasmussen, 1988	0.003	-0.139	0.145	0.965	
Maxwell, 2001	-0.010	-0.042	0.022	0.556	
Clarke-Pearson, 1993	-0.026	-0.086	0.035	0.402	
Pitto, 2003	-0.030	-0.087	0.027	0.305	
Kosir, 1998	-0.030	-0.080	0.019	0.232	
Kirtoglu, 2004	0.017	-0.067	0.100	0.697	
Santori, 1993	-0.220	-0.362	-0.077	0.002	
Blanchard, 1999	0.301	0.141	0.461	0.000	
Nicolaides, 1983	-0.080	-0.197	0.037	0.179	
Coe, 1978	-0.145	-0.323	0.032	0.109	
Total	0.003	-0.011	0.018	0.649	

-0.50 -0.25 0.00 0.25 0.50

Favors Compression Favors Heparin

SENSITIVITY ANALYSIS: DVT (Calf/Thigh Boots)

	Compression	Heparin
Ginzburg, 2003	2.7% (n = 6/224)	0.5% (n = 1/218)
Nicolaides, 1980*	22.2% (n = 37/166)	11.7% (n = 10/85)
Maxwell, 2001	0.9% (n = 1/106)	1.9% (n = 2/105)
Clarke-Pearson, 1993	4.0% (n = 4/101)	6.5% (n = 7/107)
Kosir, 1998	0.0% (n = 0/67)	3.0% (n = 2/66)
Kirtoglu, 2004	6.6% (n = 4/60)	5.0% (n = 3/60)
Nicolaides, 1983	6.0% (n = 3/50)	14.0% (n = 7/50)
Coe, 1978	6.8% (n = 2/29)	21.4% (n = 6/28)

* number of patients extrapolated from number of calves as reported.

DVT: Compression vs heparin (calf/thigh boots)

Study name	Statistics for each study				Risk difference and 95% CI
	Risk difference	Lower limit	Upper limit	p-Value	
Ginzburg, 2003	0.022	-0.001	0.045	0.058	
Nicolaides, 1980	0.105	0.012	0.199	0.027	
Rasmussen, 1988	0.003	-0.139	0.145	0.965	
Maxwell, 2001	-0.010	-0.042	0.022	0.556	
Clarke-Pearson, 1993	-0.026	-0.086	0.035	0.402	
Kosir, 1998	-0.030	-0.080	0.019	0.232	
Kirtoglu, 2004	0.017	-0.067	0.100	0.697	
Nicolaides, 1983	-0.080	-0.197	0.037	0.179	
Coe, 1978	-0.145	-0.323	0.032	0.109	
Total	0.004	-0.011	0.020	0.587	

-0.25 -0.13 0.00 0.13 0.25

Favors Compression Favors Heparin

SENSITIVITY ANALYSIS: DVT (Footpump)

	Compression	Heparin
Warwick, 1998	18% (n = 24/136)	13% (n = 18/138)
Pitto, 2003	3.0% (n = 3/100)	6.0% (n = 6/100)
Santori, 1993	13.4% (n = 9/67)	35.4% (n = 23/65)
Blanchard, 1999	54.0% (n = 34/63)	23.9% (n = 16/67)
Total	**19.1% (n = 70/366)**	**17.0% (n = 63/370)**

DVT: Compression vs heparin (footpump)

Study name	Statistics for each study				Risk difference and 95% CI
	Risk difference	Lower limit	Upper limit	p-Value	
Warwick, 1998	0.046	-0.039	0.131	0.290	
Pitto, 2003	-0.030	-0.087	0.027	0.305	
Santori, 1993	-0.220	-0.362	-0.077	0.002	
Blanchard, 1999	0.301	0.141	0.461	0.000	
Total	-0.004	-0.047	0.040	0.871	

-0.50 -0.25 0.00 0.25 0.50

Favors Compression   Favors Heparin

SENSITIVITY ANALYSIS: DVT (Compressive Stocking)

	Compression	Heparin
Rasmussen, 1988	29.7% (n = 22/74)	29.4% (n = 25/85)
Total	**(95% CI 20.5%–40.9%)**	**(95% CI 20.8%–39.8%)**

SENSITIVITY ANALYSIS: DVT (Unfractionated Heparin)

	Compression	Heparin
Nicolaides, 1980	22.2% (n = 37/166)	11.7% (n = 10/85)
Rasmussen, 1988	29.7% (n = 22/74)	29.4% (n = 25/85)
Clarke-Pearson, 1993	4.0% (n = 4/101)	6.5% (n = 7/107)
Kosir, 1998	0.0% (n = 0/67)	3.0% (n = 2/66)
Santori, 1993	13.4% (n = 9/67)	35.4% (n = 23/65)
Nicolaides, 1983	6.0% (n = 3/50)	14.0% (n = 7/50)
Coe, 1978	6.8% (n = 2/29)	21.4% (n = 6/28)
Total	**13.9% (n = 77/554)**	**16.5% (n = 80/486)**

DVT: Compression vs heparin (unfractionated heparin)

Study name	Statistics for each study				Risk difference and 95% CI
	Risk difference	Lower limit	Upper limit	p-Value	
Nicolaides, 1980	0.105	0.012	0.199	0.027	
Rasmussen, 1988	0.003	-0.139	0.145	0.965	
Clarke-Pearson, 1993	-0.026	-0.086	0.035	0.402	
Kosir, 1998	-0.030	-0.080	0.019	0.232	
Santori, 1993	-0.220	-0.362	-0.077	0.002	
Nicolaides, 1983	-0.080	-0.197	0.037	0.179	
Coe, 1978	-0.145	-0.323	0.032	0.109	
Total	-0.029	-0.060	0.003	0.078	

-0.50 -0.25 0.00 0.25 0.50

Favors Compression   Favors Heparin

SENSITIVITY ANALYSIS: DVT (Low Molecular Weight Heparin)

	Compression	Heparin
Ginzburg, 2003	2.7% (n = 6/224)	0.5% (n = 1/218)
Warwick, 1998	18% (n = 24/136)	13% (n = 18/138)
Maxwell, 2001	0.9% (n = 1/106)	1.9% (n = 2/105)
Pitto, 2003	3.0% (n = 3/100)	6.0% (n = 6/100)
Kirtoglu, 2004	6.6% (n = 4/60)	5.0% (n = 3/60)
Blanchard, 1999	54.0% (n = 34/63)	23.9% (n = 16/67)
Total	**10.4% (n = 72/689)**	**6.7% (n = 48/688)**

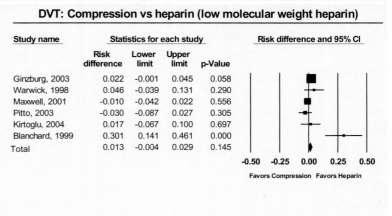

DVT: Compression vs heparin (low molecular weight heparin)

Study name	Risk difference	Lower limit	Upper limit	p-Value
Ginzburg, 2003	0.022	-0.001	0.045	0.058
Warwick, 1998	0.046	-0.039	0.131	0.290
Maxwell, 2001	-0.010	-0.042	0.022	0.556
Pitto, 2003	-0.030	-0.087	0.027	0.305
Kirtoglu, 2004	0.017	-0.067	0.100	0.697
Blanchard, 1999	0.301	0.141	0.461	0.000
Total	0.013	-0.004	0.029	0.145

META-ANALYSIS: PE (All)

	Compression	Heparin
Ginzburg, 2003	1/224	1/218
Warwick, 1998	1/136	0/138
Nicolaides, 1980	1/166	1/85
Rasmussen, 1988	0/74	0/74
Maxwell, 2001	0/106	0/105
Clarke-Pearson, 1993	0/101	0/107
Pitto, 2003	0/100	0/100
Kosir, 1998	1/67	1/67
Kirtoglu, 2004	2/60	4/60
Santori, 1993	0/67	2/65
Blanchard, 1999	0/63	0/67
Nicolaides, 1983	NR	NR
Coe, 1978	1/29	1/28
Total	**0.6% (n = 7/1193)**	**0.9% (n = 10/1114)**

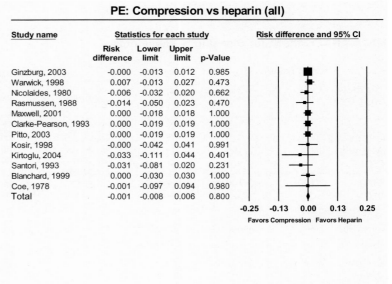

PE: Compression vs heparin (all)

Study name	Risk difference	Lower limit	Upper limit	p-Value
Ginzburg, 2003	-0.000	-0.013	0.012	0.985
Warwick, 1998	0.007	-0.013	0.027	0.473
Nicolaides, 1980	-0.006	-0.032	0.020	0.662
Rasmussen, 1988	-0.014	-0.050	0.023	0.470
Maxwell, 2001	0.000	-0.018	0.018	1.000
Clarke-Pearson, 1993	0.000	-0.019	0.019	1.000
Pitto, 2003	0.000	-0.019	0.019	1.000
Kosir, 1998	-0.000	-0.042	0.041	0.991
Kirtoglu, 2004	-0.033	-0.111	0.044	0.401
Santori, 1993	-0.031	-0.081	0.020	0.231
Blanchard, 1999	0.000	-0.030	0.030	1.000
Coe, 1978	-0.001	-0.097	0.094	0.980
Total	-0.001	-0.008	0.006	0.800

META-ANALYSES: BLEEDING EVENTS

INDIVIDUAL REPORTS: All Bleeding/Hematoma/Transfusion Outcomes

	Compression	Heparin	Measure	Statistical Analysis
Ginzburg, 2003	8/224	13/218	Bleeding (major and minor) from any site	NS
Warwick, 1998	16/136	69/138	Oozing from wound at Day 7	p < 0.001
Nicolaides, 1980	—	—	—	—
Rasmussen, 1988	—	—	—	—
Maxwell, 2001	0/106	1/105	Wound hematoma	NS
Clarke-Pearson, 1993	17/101	34/107	Number requiring transfusion	p = 0.03
Pitto, 2003	0/100, 41/100	3/100, 58/100	Bleeding from wound, Wound oozing POD3	p < 0.05
Kosir, 1998	—	—	—	—
Kirtoglu, 2004	1/60	1/60	Expanding hematoma	NS
Santori, 1993	0/67	9/65	Excess bleeding or wound hematoma	Not reported
Blanchard, 1999	0/63	1/67	Major bleeding from wound	NS
Nicolaides, 1983	—	—	—	—
Coe, 1978	9/29	14/28	Number requiring transfusion	Not reported

META-ANALYSIS: Major Bleeding or Hematoma

	Compression	Heparin	Measure
Ginzburg, 2003	4/224	4/218	Major bleeding from any site
Maxwell, 2001	0/106	1/105	Wound hematoma
Pitto, 2003	0/100	3/100	Bleeding from wound
Kirtoglu, 2004	1/60	1/60	Expanding hematoma
Santori, 1993	0/67	9/65	Excess bleeding or wound hematoma
Blanchard, 1999	0/63	1/67	Major bleeding from wound
Total	**0.8% (n = 5/620)**	**3.1% (n = 19/615)**	

Compression vs Heparin: Major Bleeding

Study name	Statistics for each study				risk difference and 95% CI
	MH risk difference	Lower limit	Upper limit	p-Value	
Ginzburg, 2003	-0.000	-0.025	0.024	0.969	
Maxwell, 2001	-0.010	-0.035	0.016	0.472	
Pitto, 2003	-0.030	-0.068	0.008	0.124	
Kirtoglu, 2004	0.000	-0.046	0.046	1.000	
Santori, 1993	-0.138	-0.226	-0.051	0.002	
Blanchard, 1999	-0.015	-0.056	0.026	0.476	
Total	-0.023	-0.039	-0.007	0.006	

-0.25 -0.13 0.00 0.13 0.25

Favors Compression Favors Heparin

META-ANALYSIS: Minor Bleeding, Oozing from Wound

	Compression	Heparin	Measure
Ginzburg, 2003	4/224	9/218	Minor bleeding from operative or other sites
Warwick, 1998	16/136	69/138	Oozing from wound on POD7
Pitto, 2003	41/100	58/100	Oozing from wound on POD3
Total	**13.3% (n = 61/460)**	**29.8% (n = 136/456)**	

Compression vs Heparin: Minor Bleeding

Study name	MH risk difference	Lower limit	Upper limit	p-Value
Ginzburg, 2003	-0.024	-0.064	0.016	0.238
Warwick, 1998	-0.382	-0.482	-0.283	0.000
Pitto, 2003	-0.170	-0.307	-0.033	0.015
Total	-0.163	-0.209	-0.117	0.000

risk difference and 95% CI

-0.50 -0.25 0.00 0.25 0.50

Favors Compression Favors Heparin

META-ANALYSIS: Number of Patients Requiring Transfusions

	Compression	Heparin
Clarke-Pearson, 1993	17/101	34/107
Coe, 1978	9/29	14/28
Total	**20.0% (n = 26/130)**	**35.6% (n = 48/135)**

Postoperative Transfusions: Compression vs Heparin

Study name	Risk difference	Lower limit	Upper limit	p-Value
Clark-Pearson, 1993	-0.149	-0.264	-0.035	0.011
Coe 1978	-0.190	-0.440	0.061	0.138
Total	-0.156	-0.261	-0.052	0.003

Risk difference and 95% CI

-0.50 -0.25 0.00 0.25 0.50

Favors Compression Favors Heparin

REFERENCES

1. Ginzburg E, Cohn SM, Lopez J, Jackowski J, Brown M, Hameed SM. "Deep Vein Thrombosis Study Group. "Randomized clinical trial of intermittent pneumatic compression and low molecular weight heparin in trauma." Br J Surg. 2003 Nov;90(11):1338–44.

2. Warwick D, Harrison J, Glew D, Mitchelmore A, Peters TJ, Donovan J. Comparison of the use of a foot pump with the use of low-molecular-weight heparin for the prevention of deep-vein thrombosis after total hip replacement. A prospective, randomized trial. J Bone Joint Surg Am. 1998 Aug;80(8):1158–66.

3. Nicolaides AN, Fernandes e Fernandes J, Pollock AV. "Intermittent sequential pneumatic compression of the legs in the prevention of venous stasis and postoperative deep venous thrombosis." Surgery. 1980 Jan;87(1): 69–76.

4. Rasmussen A, Hansen PT, Lindholt J, Poulsen TD, Toftdahl DB, Gram J, Toftgaard C, Jespersen J. "Venous thrombosis after abdominal surgery. A comparison between subcutaneous heparin and antithrombotic stockings, or both." J Med. 1988;19(3–4):193–201.

5. Maxwell GL, Synan I, Dodge R, Carroll B, Clarke-Pearson DL. "Pneumatic compression versus low molecular weight heparin in gynecologic oncology surgery: a randomized trial." Obstet Gynecol. 2001 Dec;98(6):989–95.

6. Clarke-Pearson DL, Synan IS, Dodge R, Soper JT, Berchuk A, Coleman RE. "A Randomized Trial of Low-Dose Heparin and Intermittent Pneumatic Calf Compression for the prevention of deep venous thrombosis after gynecologic oncology surgery. Am J Obstet Gynec. 1993; 168(4): 1146–1154.

7. Pitto RP, Hamer H, Heiss-Dunlop W, Kuehle J. Mechanical prophylaxis of deep-vein thrombosis after total hip replacement a randomised clinical trial. J Bone Joint Surg Br. 2004 Jul;86(5):639–42.

8. Kosir MA, Schmittinger L, Barno-Winarski L, Duddella P, Pone M, Perales A, Lange P, Brish LK, McGee K, Beleski K, Pawlak J, Mammen E, Sajahan NP, Kozol RA. "Prospective double-arm study of fibrinolysis in surgical patients." J Surg Res. 1998 Jan;74(1):96–101.

9. Kurtoglu M, Yanar H, Bilsel Y, Guloglu R, Kizilirmak S, Buyukkurt D, Granit V. "Venous thromboembolism prophylaxis after head and spinal trauma: intermittent pneumatic compression devices versus low molecular weight heparin." World J Surg. 2004 Aug;28(8):807–11. Epub 2004 Aug 3.

10. Blanchard J, Meuwly JY, Leyvraz PF, Miron MJ, Bounameaux H, Hoffmeyer P, Didier D, Schneider PA. "Prevention of deep-vein thrombosis after total knee replacement. Randomised comparison between a low-molecular-weight heparin (nadroparin) and mechanical prophylaxis with a

foot-pump system." J Bone Joint Surg Br. 1999 Jul;81(4): 654–9.

11. Nicolaides AN, Miles C, Hoare M, Jury P, Helmis E, Venniker R. "Intermittent sequential pneumatic compression of the legs and thromboembolism-deterrent stockings in the prevention of postoperative deep venous thrombosis." Surgery. 1983 Jul;94(1):21–5.

12. Coe NP, Collins RE, Klein LA, Bettmann MA, Skillman JJ, Shapiro RM, Salzman EW. "Prevention of deep vein thrombosis in urological patients: a controlled, randomized trial of low-dose heparin and external pneumatic compression boots." Surgery. 1978 Feb;83(2): 230–4.

13. Santori FS, Vitullo A, Stopponi M, Santori N, Ghera S. "Prophylaxis against deep-vein in total hip replacement. Comparison of heparin and foot impulse pump." J Bone Joint Surg Br. 1994 Jul; 76(4):579–583.

28 Selective Neck Dissection for Upper Aerodigestive Tract Squamous Cell Carcinoma

28.A.

Supraomohyoid neck dissection versus modified radical neck dissection (type 3) for N0 oral cavity carcinoma: Chance of recurrence, chance of survival at 5 years

Jennifer J. Shin and Gregory W. Randolph

METHODS

A computerized Ovid search of MEDLINE 1966–September 2003 was performed. The term "neck dissection" was exploded and cross-referenced with articles containing the keywords "selective" or "supraomohyoid." Next, these articles were cross-referenced with articles obtained by exploding the following terms: "head and neck neoplasms," "mouth neoplasms," "otorhinolaryngologic neoplasms," and "pharyngeal neoplasms." The resulting 141 articles were reviewed to determine if they met our inclusion criteria. We required: 1) a distinct population of patients with previous untreated oral cavity squamous cell carcinoma with N0 necks, 2) intervention with ipsilateral or bilateral supraomohyoid neck dissection (SND) compared with modified radical neck dissection (MRND), and 3) outcome measures of regional recurrence and survival. In addition, the reference lists of included articles and all review articles that were obtained were manually checked to ensure that all known relevant articles were included. Reports in which results for patients with oral cavity carcinoma could not be extracted from a report of data pooled from patients who also had oropharyngeal, laryngeal, or hypopharyngeal carcinoma were excluded. This process yielded just two controlled trials [1, 2].

RESULTS

Outcome measures. The outcome of histologically confirmed recurrence in the neck is described as occurring in the ipsilateral dissected neck, ipsilateral undissected neck, or the contralateral neck. The survival outcome is described as the actuarial overall survival or as mortality rates at 2 and 5 years.

Confounders. There may be subtle variability in the procedure that investigators refer to as a "supraomohyoid neck dissection." Also, the method that investigators use to determine whether a neck is N0 can influence the results; use of physical examination alone may stage a patient with a short thick neck as N0 when use of computed tomography (CT) could stage that same patient as N1. In addition, the primary subsites within the oral cavity can influence the results. For example, floor of mouth carcinoma is more likely than buccal carcinoma to metastasize to the neck. Also, oral tongue carcinoma may develop skip metastases to level IV, which may not be included in the standard SND. Likewise, a higher T stage or greater tumor thickness is associated with a higher incidence of neck disease. Differences in institutional adjuvant radiation therapy protocols may also confound results, as could the development of second primaries or the laterality of the dissection. Last, the final categorization of SNDs that were converted to MRND for intraoperative findings may affect results; these subjects are ideally included in the SND group with an intention to treat analysis, but some may assign them to the MRND group. All of these potential confounders have been cataloged for the reader in the adjoining table.

Study Designs. One randomized controlled trial (RCT) confirmed no significant pretreatment differences in the MRND and SND groups, carefully defined the N0 status and SND, and reported a strict intention to treat analysis [1]. The authors reported no significant difference in the neck or survival results, although no *a priori* power calculation was noted. The only other controlled trial was a his-torical cohort with the potential inherent bias of that retrospective study design [2]. Pretreatment differences between the SND and MRND groups were not addressed, and because multiple head and neck primary sites were included, there was no statistical analysis of the neck recurrence rates in a distinct group of patients with oral cavity primary lesions. There was, however, a survival analysis of a distinct group of N0 oral cavity carcinoma patients.

Highest Level of Evidence. One RCT and one historical cohort compared recurrence and survival rates in MRND versus SND in a distinct population of previously untreated patients with N0 oral cavity carcinoma. Where statistical analysis was reported, there was no difference in recurrence in the ipsilateral neck [1] or in 5-year survival [1, 2], although the issue of the studies' intended power was not addressed.

Applicability. These results apply to adults with N0 oral cavity squamous cell carcinoma who receive surgery at both the primary site and the neck as the initial intervention. In addition, the results of the RCT apply only to those with T2–4 N0 M0 primary lesions, no myocutaneous or free flap, no significant cardiopulmonary disease, and moderate activity levels.

Morbidity. The RCT reported significantly fewer complications with SND [1]. Complications included flap necrosis, wound infection, fistula, seroma, and postoperative death.

CLINCIAL SIGNIFICANCE AND FUTURE RESEARCH

Level 1 and 3 studies showed no significant difference in neck recurrence and 5-year survival after treatment of N0 oral cavity carcinoma with MRND versus SND concurrent with initial surgery at the primary site, but their power was limited. Using the data from the 1998 study for calculations, in order for a future study to achieve a 90% power[1] to detect a 5% rate difference (RD)[2] in overall survival, approximately 2000 patients would be necessary. An ambitious study such as this would also ideally occur in the context of an N0 neck with standardized evaluation for staging (i.e., with or without CT), an SND with clearly defined boundaries, a

primary lesion with defined thickness and subsite characterics, and standardized adjuvant radiation protocols. In the meantime, while there is no further directly controlled evidence to support or refute whether SND and MRND result in comparable control rates, physicians should incorporate the data in those prospective studies into their clinical decisions regarding which procedure will better serve individuals with N0 oral cavity carcinoma.

> **Supraomohyoid Neck Dissection:** Removal of lymph nodes contained in the submental and submandibular triangles (level I), the upper jugular lymph nodes (levels II), and the midjugular lymph nodes (level III). The posterior limit of the dissection is marked by a parallel plane defined by the cutaneous branches of the cervical plexus or the lateral border of the sternocleidomastoid muscle. The inferior limit is the junction between the superior belly of the omohyoid muscle and the internal jugular vein [3].
>
> **Modified Radical Neck Dissection, Type III:** Removal of all cervical lymph node groups extending from the inferior border of the mandible superiorly to the clavicle inferiorly, from the lateral border of the sternohyoid muscle, hyoid bone, and contralateral anterior belly of the digastric muscle medially, to the anterior border of the trapezius muscle laterally (levels I–V). It spares the spinal accessory nerve, internal jugular vein, and sternocleidomastoid muscle [3].

---

[1] Power is defined as the probability of finding a statistically significant difference (by convention defined as $p \leq 0.05$) if a difference actually exists. Power is a variable that is dependent on the sample size, the final results and their variability, and the effect size that is of clinical interest. For example, the power of the RCT to determine a RD of 10% is 77% but the same study has only a 36% power to determine a RD of 5%.

[2] The absolute RD is defined as the absolute difference in successful outcomes between the study group and the control group. For example, in the RCT, 67% of the SND patients versus 63% of the MRND patients were alive after 5 years. The RD in this scenario is 67% − 63% = 4%.

THE EVIDENCE CONDENSED: Modified radical neck dissection type 3 versus supraomohyoid neck dissection for N0 oral cavity squamous cell carcinoma

Reference	Brazilian Head and Neck Cancer Study Group, 1998				Majoufre, 1999			
Level (design)	1 (RCT: MRND type 3 vs SND)				3 (HC: MRND type 3 vs SND)			
Sample size	148 (148)				160 (161)			

OUTCOMES

Recurrence		MRND	SND	p Value		MRND	SND	p Value
	NID	9%	8%	0.8505	NID	0%	2.4%	NR
	NIU	—	NR	—	NIU	—	0%	—
	NCU	1%	6%	NR	NCU	NR	NR	NR
	DM	0%	1%	NR	DM	22%	6.3%	NR
Survival		MRND	SND	p Value		MRND	SND	p Value
					2 y	73.6%	85.8%	NR
	AOS 5 y	63%	67%	0.7159	5 y	57.2%	70.2%	0.071
Conclusion	No significant difference				No significant difference			
Follow-up time	5 y				Median 89 mo, 1 lost to follow-up			

STUDY DESIGN

Inclusion criteria	Resectable T2–4, N0; no prior treatment; histologic diagnosis of squamous cell carcinoma of the oral tongue, FOM, inferior gingiva, or RMT; no myocutaneous or free flap; Karnofsky score >60				No prior treatment; no delay to time of surgery; surgery at primary site and neck at same time as initial treatment			
Exclusion criteria	Significant cardiac, pulmonary disease; distant metastases; multiple primaries				NR			
Primary subsite	Oral tongue 42% FOM 33% RMT 17% Gingiva 8%				Oral tongue 37% FOM 32% RMT 12% Gingiva 11% Other 8%			
Initial T stage	T1 0% T2 62% T3 18% T4 20%				T1 4% T2 43% T3 33% T4 17% Tx 3%			
Tumor thickness	≤3 mm 14%; >3 mm 86%				NR			
N0 stage determination	"Clinically negative neck . . . pretreatment staging evaluations included physical exam, CXR, and roentgrams as indicated . . . imaging exams were not used for neck staging"				"Clinical status of the neck"; further details of physical examination or imaging NR			
SND performed	Levels I–III; with frozen section of suspicious nodes; if frozen section positive then conversion to MRND (n = 3)				Levels I–III, upper and middle V; use of frozen sections NR			
Pretreatment characteristics	No significant difference in age, sex, subsite of primary, T stage, primary tumor resection, laterality of neck, or continuity of specimen				NR			
Radiation therapy	Postoperative RT 50 Gy for positive margins or positive lymph nodes in specimen				RT 50 Gy for positive margins, T3–4 tumors, histologically positive neck specimen; 60–65 Gy for extracapsular spread			
Occult neck metastases	MRND	SND	p Value		29% of combined MRND and SND groups			
	32%	21%	0.099					
Laterality	MRND 85% unilateral, 15% bilateral; SND 93% unilateral, 7% bilateral				"Bilateral neck dissections were performed for whenever the primary site crossed the median line and systematically for the apex linguae"			
Complications of neck dissection	MRND	SND	p Value		NR			
	41%	25%	0.043					

RCT = randomized controlled trial, HC = historical cohort, NR = not reported, Karnofsky score is a measure of activity, SND = supraomohyoid neck dissection (levels I–III), MRND = modified radical neck dissection, RND = radical neck dissection, FOM = floor of mouth, RT = radiation therapy, RMT = retromolar trigone; neck recurrence site: NID = ipsilateral dissected, NIU = ipsilateral undissected, NCU = contralateral undissected, AOS = actuarial overall survival, DM = distant metastases.

REFERENCES

1. Anonymous. Results of a prospective trial on elective modified radical classical versus supraomohyoid neck dissection in the management of oral squamous carcinoma. Brazilian Head and Neck Cancer Study Group. Am J Surg 1998; 176(5):422–427.

2. Majoufre C, Faucher A, Laroche C, et al. Supraomohyoid neck dissection in cancer of the oral cavity. Am J Surg 1999;178(1):73–77.

3. Robbins KT, ed. Pocket Guide to Neck Dissection and TNM Staging of Head and Neck Cancer. 2nd ed. Committee for Neck Dissection Classification, American Head and Neck Society Committee for Head and Neck Surgery and Oncology: American Academy of Otolaryngology–Head and Neck Surgery. Alexandria, VA: American Academy of Otolaryngology–Head and Neck Surgery Foundation; 2001.

28 Selective Neck Dissection for Upper Aerodigestive Tract Squamous Cell Carcinoma

28.B.

Supraomohyoid neck dissection versus observation alone for stage I–II oral cavity carcinoma: Chance of recurrence, chance of survival at 2–3.5 years

Jennifer J. Shin and Gregory W. Randolph

METHODS

A computerized Ovid search of MEDLINE was performed as described in Section 12.A. For inclusion in this analysis, we required the following: 1) a distinct population of patients with previously untreated stage I–II oral cavity squamous cell carcinoma, 2) intervention with ipsilateral or bilateral supraomohyoid neck dissection (SND) compared with observation, and 3) outcome measures of regional recurrence and survival. Again, reports from which results for a distinct group of patients with T1–2 N0 oral cavity carcinoma could not be extracted from a report of data pooled from patients who also had oropharyngeal, laryngeal, or hypopharyngeal carcinoma were excluded. This process yielded just two articles [1, 2].

RESULTS

Outcome Measures, Confounders. As described in Section 28.A.

Study Designs. One study is a randomized controlled trial (RCT) [1], although the pretreatment characteristics of the selective neck versus observation groups, the means of determining the N0 status, and the adjuvant radiation protocol were not reported. Also, follow-up was limited to 3.5 years. Statistical significance was at the minimum accepted convention of $p = 0.05$, which means that there is a 5% chance that there was in fact no difference between the two groups. The second study was a historical cohort that compared observation alone with elective treatment, which included SND or radiation therapy (RT) [2]. The data for recurrence in this publication were reported in terms of a distinct population of stage I–II oral cavity carcinoma patients who underwent SND versus observation, but statistical analysis of data was not reported and follow-up was limited to a median of 2 years.

Highest Level of Evidence. One RCT with a 3.5-year follow-up period showed a borderline significant decrease ($p = 0.05$) in the ipsilateral neck recurrence and disease-free survival after SND for stage I–II oral cavity carcinoma [1]. One historical cohort showed a trend in the same direction, but without statistical analysis and after a shorter follow-up period [2]. Together, these results are clearly suggestive of improved survival with SND, but not undisputedly so. No other controlled studies are available for a distinct population of stage I–II oral cavity carcinoma patients, although the reader may refer to the uncontrolled studies on this topic for supplementary data (see Section 28.C).

Applicability. These results apply to adults with previously untreated T1–2 N0 carcinoma of the tongue and floor of mouth who receive surgical treatment at the primary site.

CLINICAL SIGNIFICANCE AND FUTURE RESEARCH DIRECTIONS

Currently, directly controlled evidence on this topic is limited to the results of these two trials, which suggest that selective neck dissection may result in fewer recurrences in the neck and improved survival at a relatively short follow-up period of 2–3.5 years.

Further study of this topic would still prove useful. Future research will preferably focus specifically on T1 oral cavity carcinoma with attention to tumor thickness, the method of determining the N0 status, and standardized adjuvant radiation protocols.

THE EVIDENCE CONDENSED: Observation alone versus supraomohyoid neck dissection for N0 stage I–II oral cavity squamous cell carcinoma

Reference	Kligerman, 1994				Yii, 1999			
Level (design)	1 (RCT: SND vs observation alone)				3 (HC: SND or RT vs observation alone)			
Sample size	67 (67)				71 (77)			
OUTCOMES								
Recurrence		**OBS**	**SND**	**p Value**	2 y	**OBS**	**SND**	**p Value**
	NIN	39%	12%	0.05	NIN	43, side	0%	NR
	NCU	0%	0%	—	NCU	NR	8%	NR
Survival	3.5 y	**OBS**	**SND**	**p Value**		**OBS**	**SND**	**p Value**
	OS	48%	82%	NR	Actuarial 5 y	65%	NR (75%)*	NR*
	DFS	49%	72%	0.05				
Follow-up time	3.5 y				Median 48 mo			
STUDY DESIGN								
Primary subsite	Oral tongue 61%, FOM 39%				Oral tongue 100%			
Initial T stage	T1 46%	T2 54%	T3 0%	T4 0%	T1 42%	T2 58%	T3 0%	T4 0%
Tumor thickness	≤4 mm 45%; >4 mm 55%				NR			
N0 staging method	NR				NR			
SND performed	Levels I–III; "plus resection of the submandibular gland, preserving the SCM, spinal accessory nerve, and IJ"				Details of the SND itself not reported; suspicious nodes found intraoperatively were analyzed by frozen section and if positive, procedure was converted to MRND			
Occult neck metastases	21%				23%			
Inclusion criteria	T1 N0 or T2 N0 oral cavity carcinoma				Previously untreated T1 N0 or T2 N0 SCCA of oral tongue			
Exclusion criteria	NR				Previous treatment			
Pretreatment characteristics	All patients received transoral resection of the lesion at the primary site; otherwise not reported				NR			
Radiation therapy	All 21 patients who underwent SND with "occult metastases were treated postoperatively with radiotherapy"; no further details reported				2 patients were treated with surgery and RT; no further details reported			

RCT = randomized controlled trial, HC = historical cohort, NR = not reported, SND = supraomohyoid neck dissection, MRND = modified radical neck dissection, FOM = floor of mouth, SCCA = squamous cell carcinoma; neck recurrence: NIU = ipsilateral undissected, NIN = ipsilateral but whether recurrences were in the dissected or undissected neck was not reported, NCU = contralateral undissected; survival: OS = overall survival, DFS = disease-free survival, RT = radiation therapy.

*Yii study reported "elective neck treatment" versus observation alone; the "elective neck treatment" group included 13 who received neck dissection and 14 who received XRT; in their reporting of survival, grouping of the data prevented extrapolation of the survival data meeting our inclusion criteria. (Value shown here is for the combined "elective neck treatment" group.)

REFERENCES

1. Kligerman J, Lima RA, Soares JR, et al. Supraomohyoid neck dissection in the treatment of T1/T2 squamous cell carcinoma of oral cavity. Am J Surg 1994;168(5):391–394.

2. Yii NW, Patel SG, Rhys-Evans PH, Breach NM. Management of the N0 neck in early cancer of the oral tongue. Clin Otolaryngol Allied Sci 1999;24(1):75–79.

28 Selective Neck Dissection for Upper Aerodigestive Tract Squamous Cell Carcinoma

28.C.

Supraomohyoid neck dissection for N0 oral cavity carcinoma: Chance of recurrence, chance of survival

Jennifer J. Shin and Gregory W. Randolph

METHODS

Because of the paucity of controlled studies on this topic, we also conducted a search to identify the uncontrolled studies regarding supraomohyoid neck dissection (SND) for N0 oral cavity carcinoma in order to supplement the controlled, site-specific, stage-specific data presented in 28.A and 28.B. A computerized Ovid search of MEDLINE 1966–September 2003 was performed as described in Section 28.A. We required: 1) a distinct population of patients with previous untreated oral cavity squamous cell carcinoma with N0 necks, 2) intervention with ipsilateral or bilateral supraomohyoid neck dissection, and 3) outcome measures of regional recurrence and survival. Reports in which results for patients with oral cavity carcinoma could not be extracted from a report of data pooled from patients with multiple primary carcinoma sites were excluded. Given the primary focus on determining whether SND directly improves subsequent clinical outcomes, reports in which a histologic analysis was the primary outcome were also excluded. This process yielded just four case series [1–4].

RESULTS

Study Designs. These additional studies are all level 4 retrospective case series, with the inherent biases of that study design. These data supplement the higher level controlled data presented previously (28.A., 28.B.). Three case series reported recurrence and survival rates after SND in a distinct population of previously untreated patients with N0 oral cavity carcinoma. Also, one review noted a small series of patients in tabular format and this is also referenced.

Additional Level of Evidence. The supplementary results from these case series suggest that the neck recurrence rate ranges from 0% to 16% after at least 1 year of follow-up. Survival results are also variable, ranging from approximately 50% to 80% at ≥1 year.

CLINICAL SIGNIFICANCE

Limited site-specific, stage-specific data from these retrospective case series which focus on the primary outcomes of survival and recurrence supplement the scarcity of site- and stage-specific controlled studies that exist on this topic. These additional studies help place the controlled studies that were previously presented in context. While there is a rich body of mixed-stage and mixed-primary site data, it is difficult but beneficial to focus on stage-specific and site-specific outcomes, since the biologic aggression of disease varies significantly according to these factors. Furthermore, it is also beneficial to clearly separate those patients with previously untreated versus recurrent disease. Such factors are key potential confounders in the ongoing study of this often controversial subject.

ADDITIONAL EVIDENCE: Supraomohyoid neck dissection for N0 oral cavity squamous cell carcinoma with no prior treatment

Reference	Hao, 2002	Manni, 1991; Van den Hoogen, 1992	Khafif, 2001
Level (design)	4 (RCS)	4 (RCS)	4 (RCS)
Sample size	140 (140)	57 (57)	50 (50)
Primary subsite	Oral tongue 29% Buccal 35% FOM 12% Hard palate 1.4% RMT 15% Gingiva 7%	Oral tongue 37% FOM 37% RMT 15% Alveolar ridge 11%	Oral tongue 100%
Initial T stage	T1 24%, T2 48%, T3 16%, T4 12%	T1 16%, T2 62%, T3 11%, T4 11%	T1 36%, T2 52%, T3 14%, T4 0%
Tumor thickness	NR	NR	Reported only in 4/50 patients
N0 stage determination	"Clinically negative neck"; further details NR	"Clinically classified as N0"; further details NR	"No clinically obvious lymph node metastases"; further details NR
SND performed	Levels I–III; upper neck nodes posterior to CN11 (IIB), nodes posterior to IJ but anterior to cervical plexus exiting at posterior border of SCM, omohyoid nodes	Levels I–III; suboccipital tissue lying on deep muscles of upper neck below trapezius; frozen section of most suspicious/largest jugulodigastric node, most distal juguloomohyoid node; if frozen positive then convert to MRND	Levels I–III; if >1.5 cm or hardened lymph nodes encountered in levels I–III at surgery then level IV also dissected (34%)
OUTCOMES			
Recurrence	NID 8%, NIU NR, NCN 1%, DM NR	NID 4%, NIU 2%, NCN 9%, DM 4%	NID 16%, NIU 0%, NCN 0%, DM NR
Survival	Not fully reported, although all patients with recurrence in NID died with disease within 1 y	5-y actuarial survival rate 84%; total 5-y survival rate 55%; 5 deaths <2 y with NED	At last follow-up 80% alive NED, 10% died NED, 6% died from disease, 2% alive with disease
Follow-up time	≥2 y	2–9 y	"Average" 4.1 y, ≥1 y if levels I–III dissected, ≥2 y if levels I–IV dissected
Occult metastases	24.3%	35%	26%
STUDY DESIGN			
Inclusion criteria	"Oral cavity carcinoma who presented with clinically negative neck and underwent SND"	Newly diagnosed with histologically proven SCCA of the oral cavity	SCCA of the oral tongue with clinically staged N0 neck
Exclusion criteria	Persistent or recurrent disease after any previous surgery, RT, or chemotherapy; those found to have positive LN on frozen section during SND that were converted to MRND	Ipsilateral MRND with contralateral SND	1 patient did not receive neck dissection because of severe comorbidities
Radiation	Postoperative RT ≥6000 rads for "advanced primary, close margins," pathologically node positive	Postoperative RT 60–70 Gy "based on nodal status and resection margins"	Postoperative RT when histopathology revealed ≥2 metastatic lymph nodes, extracapsular spread; primary tumor with perineural or perivascular invasion
Complications	NR	1 postoperative death, 1 "protracted complication"	3 wound infections, 0 chylous fistulas

RCS = retrospective case series, NR = not reported, SCCA = squamous cell carcinoma, FOM = floor of mouth, RMT = retromolar trigone, SND = supraomohyoid neck dissection (levels I–III), IJ = internal jugular vein, SCM = sternocleidomastoid muscle, MRND = modified radical neck dissection; Neck recurrence site: NID = ipsilateral dissected, NIU = ipsilateral undissected, NCN contralateral with dissection not reported, RT = radiation therapy, DM = distant metastases, NED = with no evidence of disease, LN = lymph nodes.
One additional study by Houck et al., 1995, reported in a single table in a review a personal experience of 51 cases in which SND was performed for oral cavity carcinoma with 2 years of follow-up. In all of these cases, the primary site was controlled, and there were 0 recurrences in the ipsilateral side of the neck. No other details were reported [4].

REFERENCES

1. Hao SP, Tsang NM. The role of supraomohyoid neck dissection in patients of oral cavity carcinoma. Oral Oncol 2002;38(3):309–312.

2. Manni JJ, van den Hoogen FJ. Supraomohyoid neck dissection with frozen section biopsy as a staging procedure in the clinically node-negative neck in carcinoma of the oral cavity. Am J Surg 1991;162(4):373–376.

3. Khafif A, Lopez-Garza JR, Medina JE. Is dissection of level IV necessary in patients with T1–T3 N0 tongue cancer? Laryngoscope 2001;111(6):1088–1090.

4. Houck JR, Medina JE. Management of cervical lymph nodes in squamous carcinomas of the head and neck. Semin Surg Oncol 1995;11(3):228–239.

5. Van den Hoogen FJ, Manni JJ. Value of the supraomohyoid neck dissection with frozen section analysis as a staging precedure in the clinically negative neck in squamous cell carcinoma of the oral cavity. Eur Arch Otorhinolaryngol 1992;249(3):144–148.

28 Selective Neck Dissection for Upper Aerodigestive Tract Squamous Cell Carcinoma

28.D.

Supraomohyoid neck dissection as a staging procedure for N0 oral cavity carcinoma: Chance of recurrence or survival at 2 or more years with a negative versus positive specimen

Jennifer J. Shin and Gregory W. Randolph

METHODS

A computerized Ovid search of MEDLINE was performed as described in Section 28.A. For inclusion in this analysis, we required the following: 1) a distinct population of patients with previous untreated N0 oral cavity squamous cell carcinoma, 2) intervention with ipsilateral or bilateral supraomohyoid neck dissection, and 3) outcome measures of regional recurrence and survival discussed in the context of pathologic nodal status. Again, reports in which results for patients with oral cavity carcinoma could not be extracted from a report of data pooled from patients who also had oropharyngeal, laryngeal, or hypopharyngeal carcinoma were excluded. This process yielded the two articles discussed below [1, 2] and a brief note in tabular format in a review that is also referenced [3].

RESULTS

Outcome Measures. As described in 28.A.

Confounders. As described in 28.A.

Study Designs. Both studies are retrospective case series with follow-up periods of at least 2 years. The larger study included consecutive patients to minimize bias [1]. Both reported the initial T stages, but did not provide details of tumor thickness or how the clinical N0 status was determined.

Highest Level of Evidence. Only two level 4 trials addressed the probability of neck recurrence with a positive versus negative specimen in a distinct population of patients with N0 oral cavity carcinoma [1, 2]. Both studies reported that subjects with pathologically positive nodes were approximately 2–3 times as likely to develop neck recurrence as those with negative nodes. Despite this, the positive predictive value of occult metastases for predicting neck recurrence at 2 years is relatively low (0.15–0.25, combined[1] 0.19). When the overall rate of recurrence (9–14%, combined[1] 10%) is considered, however, an approximately doubled likelihood of recurrence is corroborated; the positive predictive value of 0.19 suggests that 2 in 10 patients with positive pathology will have recurrence, which is twice the overall rate of 1 in 10. The negative predictive value of lack of occult metastases for nonrecurrence is comparatively high (0.92–0.93, combined[1] 0.93), suggesting that 9 of 10 subjects without occult metastases will remain free of neck disease and be alive at 2 years. When this value is considered relative to the overall probability of no recurrence (86%–91%, combined[1] 90%), it is less impressive. Overall, the odds of recurrence are low with negative pathology, but the additional information gained from that negative pathology is limited.

Only one study addressed the chance of death with a positive versus negative specimen in a distinct population of patients with N0 oral cavity carcinoma [2]. In this report, death at 2 years is almost 3 times as likely with pathologically positive nodes. The positive predictive value, however, is relatively low at 0.15. When this value is considered relative to the overall death rate at 2 years (9%), however, a limited but still increased likelihood of death is implied. The negative predictive value of a negative pathologic specimen for survival is quite high at 95%. When this value is contemplated relative to the overall survival rate at 2 years of 91%, a mild but still increased likelihood of survival with a negative specimen is also corroborated.

Applicability. These results apply to adults with previously untreated T1–2 N0 carcinoma of the tongue and floor of mouth who receive surgical treatment at the primary site.

Morbidity. One study reported a 3.5% complication rate from supraomohyoid neck dissection (SND) [2].

CLINICAL SIGNIFICANCE AND FUTURE RESEARCH DIRECTIONS

The data from these two trials suggest that SND may be used effectively as a staging procedure for N0 oral cavity carcinoma, given that the odds of neck recurrence and death at 2 years are 2–3 times as high if occult

---

[1]Pooled analysis: The number of true positives, true negatives, false positives, and false negatives from each study were added and used to calculate the point estimates of the positive and negative predictive values, as well as the overall recurrence rate, for the two studies combined.

metastases are identified. These positive and negative predictive values (combined[1] data 0.93 and 0.19, respectively) must be considered relative to the overall rates of neck recurrence and death at 2–3.5 years (see above).

Future studies may attempt to minimize confounders by presenting a predetermined protocol to define the clinically N0 (i.e. all confirmed by computed tomography), a clearly defined SND, a primary lesion with defined thickness and subsite characteristics, and standardized adjuvant radiation protocols. A prospective analysis would facilitate these efforts. In addition, longer minimum follow-up times of at least 5 years would be beneficial.

Shown here are the pooled data [1, 2] for neck recurrence and the calculations of predictive values and overall recurrence rate. Calculations were performed using Bayesian Analysis.		Neck recurrence	No neck recurrence	Totals	Calculations
	Pathology positive	n = 10	n = 44	n = 54	PPV = 0.19
	Pathology negative	n = 10	n = 133	n = 143	NPV = 0.93
	Totals	n = 20	n = 177	n = 197	Overall recurrence rate = 0.10

PPV = positive predictive value, NPV = negative predictive value.

THE EVIDENCE CONDENSED: Supraomohyoid neck dissection as a staging procedure for N0 oral cavity squamous cell carcinoma

Reference	Hao, 2002	Manni, 1991, Van den Hoogen, 1992
Level (design)	4 (RCS)	4 (RCS)
Sample size	140 (140)	57 (57)
Primary subsite	Oral tongue 29%, FOM 12%, RMT 15%, Gingiva 7%, Buccal 35%, Hard palate 1.4%	Oral tongue 37%, FOM 37%, RMT 15%, Alveolar ridge 11%
Initial T stage	T1 24% T2 48% T3 16% T4 12%	T1 16% T2 62% T3 11% T4 11%
Tumor thickness	NR	NR
N0 stage determination	"Clinically negative neck"; not further reported	"Clinically classified as N0"; not further reported
SND performed	Levels I–III; upper neck nodes posterior to CN11 (IIB), nodes posterior to IJ but anterior to cervical plexus exiting at posterior border of SCM, omohyoid nodes	Levels I–III; suboccipital tissue lying on deep muscles of upper neck below trapezius muscle; frozen section of most suspicious and largest jugulodigastric node, most distal juguloomohyoid node if present; if frozen section positive then convert to MRND

OUTCOMES

Histopathology	Negative for occult mets	Positive for occult mets	Odds	Negative for occult mets	Positive for occult mets	Odds
Neck recurrence	6.6%	14.7%	1:2.2	8.1%	25.0%	1:3.1
Distant metastases	NR	NR	—	NR	10.0%	—
Death at 2 y	NR	NR	—	5.4%	15.0%	1:2.8
PPV*	For neck recurrence 0.15			For neck recurrence 0.25; death at 2 y 0.15		
NPV*	For neck recurrence 0.93			For neck recurrence 0.92; death at 2 y 0.95		
Follow-up time	≥2 y			2–9 y		

STUDY DESIGN

Overall rate of neck recurrence	9%			14%		
Occult mets	24.3%			35%		
Inclusion criteria	"Oral cavity carcinoma who presented with clinically negative neck and underwent SND"			Newly diagnosed with histologically proven SCCA of the oral cavity		
Exclusion criteria	Persistent or recurrent disease after any previous surgery, RT, or chemotherapy; those found to have positive LN on frozen section during SND that were converted to MRND			Ipsilateral MRND with contralateral SND		
Radiation	Postoperative RT ≥6000 rads for "advanced primary, close margins," pathologically node positive			Postoperative RT 60–70 Gy "based on nodal status and resection margins"		
Complications	Not reported			1 postoperative death, 1 "protracted postoperative complication"		

RCS = retrospective case series, mets = metastases, SCCA = squamous cell carcinoma, SND = supraomohyoid neck dissection (levels I–III), FOM = floor of mouth, RMT = retromolar trigone, IJ = internal jugular vein, MRND = modified radical neck dissection, SCM = sternocleidomastoid muscle, PPV = positive predictive value, NPV = negative predictive value, NR = not reported, RT = radiation therapy, LN = lymph nodes.
* Calculated from reported data.
One additional study by Houck et al., 1995, reported in a single table in a review a personal experience of 51 cases in which SND was performed for oral cavity carcinoma with 2 years of follow-up. In all of these cases, the primary site was controlled, and there were 0 recurrences in the ipsilateral side of the neck. No other details were reported [3].

REFERENCES

1. Hao SP, Tsang NM. The role of supraomohyoid neck dissection in patients of oral cavity carcinoma (small star, filled). Oral Oncol 2002;38(3):309–312.
2. Manni JJ, van den Hoogen FJ. Supraomohyoid neck dissection with frozen section biopsy as a staging procedure in the clinically node-negative neck in carcinoma of the oral cavity. Am J Surg 1991;162(4):373–376.
3. Houck JR, Medina JE. Management of cervical lymph nodes in squamous carcinomas of the head and neck. Semin Surg Oncol 1995;11(3):228–239.
4. Van den Hoogen FJ, Manni JJ. Value of the supraomohyoid neck dissection with frozen section analysis as a staging precedure in the clinically negative neck in squamous cell carcinoma of the oral cavity. Eur Arch Otorhinolaryngol 1992;249(3):144–148.

28 Selective Neck Dissection for Upper Aerodigestive Tract Squamous Cell Carcinoma

28.E.

Lateral neck dissection versus type 3 modified radical neck dissection: Impact on survival, recurrence

Jennifer J. Shin and Gregory W. Randolph

METHODS

A computerized Ovid search of MEDLINE 1966–July 2003 was performed. The terms "laryngeal neoplasms" and "larynx" were exploded and the resulting articles were cross-referenced with those obtained by exploding "neck dissection." This process yielded 374 articles, which were reviewed for the following inclusion criteria: 1) a distinct population of patients with N0 laryngeal carcinoma, 2) intervention with lateral neck dissection (LND) (levels II–IV) versus modified radical neck dissection (MRND), and 3) outcome measures of regional recurrence and survival. Studies that included posterolateral dissections (levels II–V) or that reported only combined data from laryngeal carcinoma with pharyngeal or other primary sites were excluded. Given the primary focus on determining whether lateral neck dissection directly improves subsequent clinical outcomes, reports in which a histologic analysis was the primary outcome were likewise excluded. Studies that reported only combined data from N0 and N1 laryngeal disease or that did not strictly define the included levels of neck dissection were also excluded. Abstracts from meetings without an accompanying manuscript to specify relevant details were excluded. These criteria were set *a priori* in order to obtain purely site-specific data. This rigorous process yielded just one clinical trial [1].

RESULTS

Outcome Measures. The outcome of histologically confirmed recurrence in the neck is described as occurring in the ipsilateral or contralateral neck. The survival outcome is described as the actuarial overall survival.

Potential Confounders. Differences in primary tumor site, T stage, concurrent laryngectomy, or other procedures could alter results, but these factors are well balanced in the LND and the MRND groups through subject randomization. In addition, differential exposure to postoperative radiation could bias results but this exposure was also evenly distributed.

Study Designs. This study is a level 1 prospective controlled trial in which randomization effectively minimized the difference between the two pretreatment groups. The authors carefully defined how they determined N0 status and performed the LND. Follow-up time was relatively long, with a mean of 3–4 years. They did not report an *a priori* power calculation, but used their own results as pilot data to calculate the sample sizes necessary to achieve 90% power for subsequent trials on this topic.

Highest Level of Evidence. This trial shows no difference in neck recurrence, cancer-specific and actuarial overall survival, or complication rate with LND versus type III MRND for T2–4 N0 M0 supraglottic or transglottic squamous cell carcinoma.

Applicability. These results are applicable to patients with histologically proven supraglottic or transglottic squamous cell carcinoma that is previously untreated, resectable, stage T2–4 N0 M0. In addition, patients should have an activity level comparable to a Karnofsky score of at least 60. Also, this study included a majority of patients with transglottic or T3 disease, and therefore the results are most germane to this further specified subset of patients.

Morbidity. There was no significant difference in postoperative complications of wound infection, flap necrosis, fistula, hematoma, and perioperative death.

CLINICAL SIGNIFICANCE AND FUTURE RESEARCH DIRECTIONS

There is level 1 evidence to suggest that LND and MRND result in similar recurrence and survival rates for patients with N0 supraglottic or transglottic squamous cell carcinoma, but it is limited by the study's power. As the authors of this article note, future trials would have to include 483 patients to determine an 8% rate difference in 5-year actuarial overall survival to achieve 90% power. Such a trial would ideally focus on patients with previously untreated, subsite-specific, laryngeal squamous cell carcinoma with preset protocols for postoperative radiation. Awaiting the results of such a trial, there is no evidence to suggest that LND results in worse recurrence or survival than MRND for T2–4 N0 M0 supraglottic or transglottic carcinoma.

Reference	Brazilian Head and Neck Cancer Study Group, 1999			
Level (design)	1 (RCT)			
Sample size*	132 (132)			
Primary subsites	16% supraglottic, 92% transglottic			
Initial T stage	18% T2, 67% T3, 14% T4			
OUTCOMES				
Recurrence		**MRND**	**LND**	**p Value**
	Ipsilateral neck	5.6%	3.2%	p = 0.636 for all types of
	Contralateral neck	0.0%	4.9%	recurrence vs no recurrence
5-y survival		**MRND**	**LND**	**p Value**
	Cancer specific survival	81.3%	81.0%	0.778
	Actuarial overall survival	72.3%	62.4%	0.312
Occult neck metastases	25% MRND, 29% LND			
Follow-up time	Mean 42.9 mo			
STUDY DESIGN				
Inclusion criteria	Histologic diagnosis of SCCA, previously untreated, respectable, T2–4 N0 M0, supraglottic or transglottic carcinoma, Karnofsky score ≥60			
Exclusion criteria	Previous treatment, clinically N+ disease			
Randomization effectiveness	No difference in age, sex, primary tumor site, T stage, concurrent laryngectomy, laterality			
Radiation therapy	Postoperative radiation for positive margins, positive lymph nodes in the specimen, "huge T3" or T4 lesions: 50–60 Gy; 18 MRND and 16 LND			
Bilateral dissection	Indicated for tumor crossing the midline of the epiglottis: 13/71 bilateral MRND, 61/61 bilateral LND			
N0 stage determination	Imaging was not routinely used for neck staging, but computed tomography scans were obtained to determine resectability or planning extension of resection of some primary tumors			
LND details	Levels II–IV; all suspicious lymph nodes were evaluated by frozen section—if positive then conversion to MRND			
Morbidity/complications	No difference in wound infection, flap necrosis, fistula formation, hematoma, or postoperative death			

RCT = randomized controlled trial, LND = lateral neck dissection, MRND = modified radical neck dissection (type III), SCCA = squamous cell carcinoma.
* Sample size: numbers shown for those completing the trial and those (initially recruited).

REFERENCE

1. Brazilian Head and Neck Cancer Study Group. End results of a prospective trial on elective lateral neck dissection vs type III modified radical neck dissection in the management of supraglottic and transglottic carcinomas. Head Neck 1999;21(8):694–702.

28 Selective Neck Dissection for Upper Aerodigestive Tract Squamous Cell Carcinoma

28.F.

Sparing the spinal accessory nerve without versus with dissection of level V: Impact on postoperative quality of life

Jennifer J. Shin and Gregory W. Randolph

METHODS

Does a selective neck dissection (SND) sparing level V result in better head and neck or shoulder related quality of life than a modified radical neck dissection (MRND) that spares but skeletonizes the spinal accessory nerve in level V? A computerized Ovid search of MEDLINE 1966–December 2003 was performed to answer this question. The term "neck dissection" was exploded and the articles obtained were cross-referenced with those obtained by exploding "quality of life." Forty-three articles were obtained and reviewed to see which met the following inclusion criteria: 1) a distinct population of patients with head and neck malignancy, 2) treated with SND sparing level V versus MRND in which level V is dissected but the spinal accessory nerve is spared, 3) with outcome measured by a validated quality of life or functional instrument. Studies that evaluated only modified and standard radical neck dissection, as well as one study that evaluated patients' subjective responses without a validated instrument, were excluded. This screening process resulted in three studies which are discussed in detail below [1–3].

RESULTS

Outcome Measures. Quality of life is best measured by validated instruments, because they provide a standardized scoring mechanism, and have proven reproducibility and responsiveness. The University of Michigan Head and Neck Quality of Life Instrument contains 30 items that ask the responder to evaluate the previous 4 weeks. The University of Washington Head and Neck Quality of Life Instrument contains 15 items that assess the previous 7 days. Both of these instruments evaluate several head and neck–related domains, and these are tabulated for the reader. In contrast, Constant's shoulder scale focuses only on the shoulder and has both subjective and objective components.

Potential Confounders. The additional delivery of radiation therapy may worsen functional outcomes, as demonstrated by one study. In contrast, postoperative physical therapy may improve function. Likewise, age, the length of time postoperatively, site and staging of the

primary site and neck may contribute to head and neck quality of life, and all of these are tabulated for the reader in as much detail as the primary articles allow. The resection of certain neck structures (such as the sternocleidomastoid muscle) might also contribute to neck pain and shoulder disability but these are not discussed in detail in these studies.

Study Designs. All are level 2, prospective controlled studies. Two of these used head and neck–related quality of life instruments for evaluation, which assess multiple domains that may obviously or unexpectedly be affected by neck dissection [2, 3]. Using these instruments may introduce confounding effects from other regional procedures or disease, but it may also uncover effects that are not necessarily logical based on knowledge of physiology and anatomy (consider the effect of antibiotics on post-tonsillectomy pain or dexamethasone on post-tonsillectomy nausea). The third study used a validated scale that is specific to shoulder function [1]. Each study attempted to address potential confounders: One study assessed subjects specifically at 6 and 12 months postoperatively to account for potential changes in one patient over the course of the first postoperative year [2]. These authors also reported that preoperative quality of life scores were similar, even though a difference was noted after treatment. Two considered the impact of radiation therapy [1, 2] and two handled data from bilateral necks with a specific protocol [1, 3]. One study described a physical therapy regimen [2]. All reported the primary sites and stages. As might be expected, in all reports, there is a significant difference in N stage, with less disease in the SND groups than in the MRND groups. This disparity may serve to confound results, as the disease itself as well as more aggressive regional treatments may alter the related quality of life.

Highest Level of Evidence. One study reported significantly better scores regarding pain, physical problems, and eating with SND [3]. Another study showed significantly better scores for shoulder disability and pain with SND, but no difference in chewing or swallowing [2]. The third study also showed better subjective (including pain, recreation, sleep, and vocation), objective, and total shoulder function scores with SND [1]. Overall, there is consensus regarding better scores for pain and shoulder/physical problems with SND as compared with MRND. This did not, however, translate into significantly different scores in activity, recreation, employment, emotional impact, and overall bother in the two head and neck–related quality of life assessments. There were also no differences in speech or perceived appearance.

Applicability. These results are applicable to patients with head and neck carcinoma (mostly squamous cell carcinoma of the oral cavity, oropharynx, or larynx/hypopharynx) who undergo neck dissection.

CLINICAL SIGNIFICANCE AND FUTURE RESEARCH

There is level 2 evidence to suggest that SND sparing level V results in less pain and shoulder dysfunction than MRND in which the spinal accessory nerve is spared, although these results may be influenced by the lower N staging that was present in the SND groups in all of these studies. Awaiting studies that control for such variations in N stage, we can only conclude that patients with N0 disease that are treated with SND will report a higher postoperative head and neck–related quality of life than those with N2–3 disease that are treated with MRND.

Future research would ideally focus on randomized patients of similar stage who are eligible for either SND or MRND sparing the spinal accessory nerve, sternocleidomastoid, and internal jugular vein. It would evaluate both head and neck as well as shoulder specific quality of life at specified intervals over at least the first postoperative year. The frequency and regimen for radiation therapy and protocol for handling bilateral necks should also be standardized. Necessary sample sizes for these studies could be calculated by using the mean score results reported in these studies and by contacting these authors to determine the standard deviations around those means.

Reference	Terrell, 2000		
Level (design)	2 (PCT)		
Sample size	129		

OUTCOMES

QOL Instrument	University of Michigan Head and Neck Quality of Life instrument Medical Outcomes study SF-12 or SF-36 General Health Survey		
Instrument scale	UMHNQOL: 0 worst to 100 best SF-12 or SF-36: norm-based algorithm with mean 50, standard deviation 10		

QOL results		SND	MRND*	p Value
	n =	68	61 (44)	—
	HNQOL domains			
	Pain	70.8	61.3 (61.1)	0.03
	Speech	71.3	62.1 (61.9)	NS
	Eating	72.2	58.7 (58.4)	0.01
	Emotion	72.4	67.4 (67.4)	NS
	Overall bother	63.4	58.2 (57.9)	NS
	HNQOL items			
	Shoulder/neck pain	73.5	59.6 (59.3)	0.01
	Analgesic use	70.6	65.4 (65.7)	NS
	Physical problems	69.6	57.4 (57.1)	0.03
	SF-12 mental, physical	49.4, 42.8	47.1(46.9), 41.4(41.9)	NS, NS
Conclusions	SND better in some domains			

STUDY DESIGN

Inclusion criteria	Convenience sample of patients with major head and neck carcinoma requiring neck dissection
Exclusion criteria	Patients with skin cancer if resections did not include major structures or neck dissections
Comparison of SND and MRND sets	No difference in age, sex, primary, T stage, bilaterality between groups Less N2–3 disease in SND group
Time of evaluation	1 mo to >24 mo postoperatively
Radiation	NR
Bilateral necks analysis	Bilateral necks were placed in category of the most aggressive dissected side
Primary tumor	38% hypopharynx/larynx; 16% oral cavity; 23% oropharynx; 4% parotid, maxilla, nose, or orbit; 3% NP; 15% other/unknown
Staging	16% stage I, 17% stage II, 18% stage III, 30% stage IV; 19% incomplete/unknown
Physical therapy	NR

PCT = prospective controlled trial, QOL = quality of life, SF = Short Form, SND = selective neck dissection, MRND = modified radical neck dissection, ND = neck dissection, SCCA = squamous cell carcinoma, NR = not reported, NS = not significant as defined by p > 0.05, RT = radiation therapy.
* In Terrell 2000, comparative data were provided in terms of neck dissections that spared the spinal accessory nerve and spared level V (SND) versus neck dissections that spared the spinal accessory nerve but resected level V. The latter group included MRND and these data are shown in parentheses.

THE EVIDENCE CONDENSED: Sparing spinal accessory nerve without versus with level V dissection

Reference	Kuntz, 1999
Level (design)	2 (PCT)
Sample size	75

OUTCOMES

QOL Instrument	University of Washington Quality of Life Instrument
Instrument scale	0 greatest dysfunction to 100 normal function

QOL results		SND	MRND	p Value
	n =	41	34	—
	HNQOL domains			
	Shoulder	90	95	NS
	disability	84	60	0.004
		82	68	NS
	Pain	71	71	NS
		85	71	NS
		82	78	0.005
	Appearance	NR	NR	
	Activity	NR	NR	
	Recreation	NR	NR	
	Chewing	NR	NR	
	Swallowing	NR	NR	
	Speech	NR	NR	
	Employment	NR	NR	

Results are shown for preoperative, then 6 and 12 mo postoperative, as extrapolated from reported bar charts.

Conclusions	SND better than MRND in some domains

STUDY DESIGN

Inclusion criteria	Patients undergoing neck dissections for head and neck cancer
Exclusion criteria	Patients who declined participation, did not complete questionnaires, were lost to follow-up, or had recurrence or death before 12 mo
Comparison of SND and MRND sets	No difference in age More women, T4, N0 in SND group
Time of evaluation	All standardized at 6 and 12 mo postoperatively
Radiation	No difference in pain with or without additional RT preoperatively or at 6 or 12 mo postoperatively
Bilateral necks analysis	NR
Primary tumor	SCCA 100% of MRND, 83% of SND; "other types included papillary, mucoepidermoid, and adenoid cystic"; 41% oral cavity, 24% oropharynx, 17% larynx/hypopharynx, 4% sinus; 13% other/unknown
Staging	15% T1, 24% T2, 28% T3, 21% T4, 9% Tx; 43% N0, 24% N1, 33% N2–3
Physical therapy	No standardized physical therapy program, though all were encouraged to do independent strengthening and ROM exercises

PCT = prospective controlled trial, QOL = quality of life, SF = Short Form, SND = selective neck dissection, MRND = modified radical neck dissection, ND = neck dissection, SCCA = squamous cell carcinoma, NR = not reported, NS = not significant as defined by p > 0.05, RT = radiation therapy.

Reference	Chepeha, 2002		
Level (design)	2 (PCT)		
Sample size	54 patients, 64 ND		

OUTCOMES

QOL Instrument	Constant's Shoulder Scale weighted test of 35% subjective symptom scores (pain, sleep, recreation, vocation), 65% objective active function measure		
Instrument scale	0–100 total, from 0–35 subjective and 0–65 objective, with higher scores better		

QOL results		SND	MRND	p Value
	n =	32	32	—
	Subjective	29.1	22.0	0.002
	Objective	50.8	40.8	0.001
	Total	79.9	62.8	0.0002

Conclusions	SND better than MRND		

STUDY DESIGN

Inclusion criteria	Consecutive head and neck cancer patients, previously untreated and concurrently required SND (none with level V dissection and none without level II–III dissection) or MRND
Exclusion criteria	Patients with <11 mo of postoperative follow-up, with any history of unrelated neck or shoulder disease
Comparison of SND and MRND sets	No difference in age Lower weight, time of follow-up, N2 in SND group
Time of evaluation	Mean 34 mo postoperatively (range 11–120); mean 22.4 mo for SND, mean 42.9 mo for MRND
Radiation	87% received surgery and RT; subjective and total scores were reduced significantly with RT
Bilateral necks analysis	Each side was evaluated and scored independently
Primary tumor	92.5% SCCA; 43% oropharynx, 19% oral cavity, 19% larynx/hypopharynx, 19% other/unknown
Staging	28% T1–2, 47% T3–4, 8% Tx, 47% N0, 16% N1, 37% N2–3
Physical therapy	NR

PCT = prospective controlled trial, QOL = quality of life, SF = Short Form, SND = selective neck dissection, MRND = modified radical neck dissection, ND = neck dissection, SCCA = squamous cell carcinoma, NR = not reported, NS = not significant as defined by p > 0.05, RT = radiation therapy.

REFERENCES

1. Chepeha DB, Taylor RJ, Chepeha JC, et al. Functional assessment using Constant's Shoulder Scale after modified radical and selective neck dissection. Head Neck 2002;24(5):432–436.

2. Kuntz AL, Weymuller EA Jr. Impact of neck dissection on quality of life. Laryngoscope 1999;109(8):1334–1338.

3. Terrell JE, Welsh DE, Bradford CR, et al. Pain, quality of life, and spinal accessory nerve status after neck dissection. Laryngoscope 2000;110(4):620–626.

29 Oropharyngeal Squamous Cell Carcinoma

29.A.i.

Surgical resection with postoperative radiotherapy versus chemoradiation for stage III–IV oropharyngeal carcinoma: Impact on survival, recurrence

Richard Wein and Randal S. Weber

METHODS

A computerized PubMed search of MEDLINE April 1969–July 2005 was performed. The terms "oropharyngeal carcinoma," "combined modality therapy," "radiotherapy," "chemotherapy," and "surgical procedures, operative" were exploded and the resulting articles were cross-referenced with "survival," "prognosis," "recurrence," "stage 3," and "stage 4" yielding 237 trials. These articles were then reviewed to identify those that met the following inclusion criteria: 1) patient population undergoing treatment for stage III–IV oropharyngeal carcinoma, 2) intervention with primary surgical resection and postoperative radiation therapy (RT) versus concomitant chemoradiation, 3) outcome measured in terms of locoregional recurrence and disease-free/overall survival. Articles that included data combined from other head and neck primary sites in addition to the oropharynx were excluded. Reports of oropharyngeal carcinoma in which stage III–IV patients were grouped with stage I–II patients were also excluded. Chemoradiation was defined as concomitant delivery of treatment and excluded studies performing induction chemotherapy followed by radiation alone. However, studies using induction chemotherapy before concomitant chemoradiation were included within the reviewed sample. Studies using preoperative chemoradiation before surgical resection were also excluded from analysis. There were, unfortunately, no studies directly comparing surgery with postoperative RT versus chemoradiation. Because of this, search criteria were revised to include noncomparative studies. The bibliographies of the articles that met these criteria were manually checked to ensure no further relevant articles could be identified. This process yielded five articles [1–5].

RESULTS

Outcome Measures. Tumor staging was defined by AJCC (American Joint Committee on Cancer) criteria for stage III and IV oropharyngeal squamous cell carcinomas. Survival was reported in a variety of ways including actuarial overall survival (calculated from event-free survival statistics [1]), progression-free survival, and disease-free survival. The specific rates of locoregional and distant metastatic control for the different modalities of treatment were obtained for varying timeframes.

Kaplan-Meier estimates were used to generate actuarial statistics in all five studies.

Potential Confounders. The surgery-oriented studies focused on tongue base and tonsillar fossa primary lesions only [3–5] whereas the chemoradiation protocols included lateral pharyngeal wall and soft palate tumors in addition to tonsil and tongue base [1, 2]. The inclusion of a limited number of non–squamous cell carcinomas was noted in two of the studies [2, 5]. Although the distribution of overall tumor staging was comparable for most of the studies (3 : 1 to 4 : 1 for stage IV:III), the percentage of patients with T4 lesions did vary considerably per study (20%–56%) and could have impacted local control rates. Patients with evidence of mandibular invasion were not included in chemoradiation protocols. Specific histopathologic features of tumors, such as perineural invasion, that may be correlated with locoregional failure were only assessed with surgical protocols.

Study Designs. Five level 4 studies were identified and reviewed for this analysis. The two chemoradiation studies were prospective in design [1, 2]. The three studies evaluating surgery with postoperative radiation were retrospective. Median follow-up ranged from 31 months to 7 years among studies.

Highest Level of Evidence. No studies were identified that compared a matched population undergoing chemoradiation to surgery for the inclusion criteria stated. Among the noncomparative data, overall survival was similar between the surgical and chemoradiation protocols at 3 and 5 years posttreatment. The locoregional control rates were also comparable between treatment modalities. The rate of distant metastases (30% versus 46%) was generally higher in patients treated with surgery/radiation than it was with chemoradiation. The rate of response to induction chemotherapy (allowing a patient to proceed to concurrent chemoradiation) varied from 89% [1] to 65% [2] and may be related to the induction chemotherapeutic regimen used.

Applicability. The inclusion criteria apply primarily to advanced-stage (III/IV) lesions that are considered technically resectable. In patients with mandibular or maxillary bony spread, conclusions cannot be drawn concerning the feasibility of concomitant chemoradiation.

Morbidity/Complications. The complications experienced within the chemoradiation protocols were reported differently with acute and late-stage treatment toxicities defined in one study [1] or not otherwise specified in the other [2]. Treatment-related mortality was the most significant complication experienced. The method of reporting of mucositis and dermatitis grade rates experienced with radiation varied. Complications of surgical management were not specified in the studies reviewed.

CLINICAL SIGNIFICANCE AND FUTURE RESEARCH

Five level 4 studies addressed this issue, but there are no data directly comparing surgery with postoperative RT versus chemoradiation in a study of purely advanced oropharyngeal carcinoma. Comparable locoregional and survival rates were experienced for advanced-stage oropharyngeal carcinoma when treated with concomitant chemoradiation or primary surgery with postoperative radiation when surveying data from all studies. Surgical trials showed a distant metastatic rate nearly 2 times that of the chemoradiation protocols. The addition of chemotherapy to postoperative radiation was not utilized in the reviewed studies and would seem to be a topic for additional research.

Level 1 or 2 studies directly comparing chemoradiation to surgery with postoperative radiation are needed. The necessity of induction chemotherapy and its impact on survival and locoregional control compared with concurrent chemoradiation alone for carcinoma of the oropharynx also requires additional investigation.

THE EVIDENCE CONDENSED: Induction chemotherapy followed by chemoradiation for advanced oropharyngeal carcinoma

Reference	Machtay, 2002	Mantz, 2001
Level (design)	4 (prospective)	4 (prospective)
Sample size	53	61
OUTCOMES		
Survival	70%* at 3 y (overall) 59% at 3 y (event-free)	51%* at 5 y (overall) 64% at 5 y (event-free)
Locoregional control	82% at 3 y	70% at 5 y
No distant metastases	91% at 3 y	89% at 5 y
Response rates	Endoscopic evaluation: "major responders" (>50% reduction in size) 89%	Clinical assessment: complete 65%, partial 34%, no 1%
Follow-up time	34 mo (median) for survivors, 31 mo (median) for all patients	68 mo (median) for survivors, 39 mo for all patients
STUDY DESIGN		
Inclusion criteria	Resectable stage III/IV squamous cell carcinoma of the oropharynx, T3–4 N0 M0 or T2 N2–3 M0 staging, Karnofsky performance status between 70%–100%, WBC ≥4 × 10^9 cells/L, platelets ≥150 × 10^9 cells/L, Hb ≥11 g/dL, Cr ≤ 1.5 g/dL	Stage IV disease; cancer and leukemia group B performance status of 0–2; normal hematologic, renal, and hepatic function
Exclusion criteria	T1–2 N1 disease, mandible invasion	Not specified
Treatment plan	IC (2 cycles) followed by concomitant chemo RT	IC (3 cycles) followed by concomitant chemo RT
Chemotherapy regimen details	IC: 2 cycles of carboplatin (dosed at AUC = 6) and paclitaxel (200 mg/m^2) Concomitant chemotherapy: weekly paclitaxel (30 mg/m^2/wk) Additional chemotherapy at time of ND: 2 cycles of carboplatin and paclitaxel (induction dosing)	IC: 3 cycles of cisplatin (100 mg/m^2), 5-fluorouracil (640 mg/m^2/d), leucovorin (300 mg/m^2/d), and interferon α 2b (2 MU/m^2/d) Concomitant chemotherapy: 7–8 cycles of 5-fluorouracil and hydroxyurea
RT regimen	RT 200 cGy daily over 7 wk to 7000 cGy	RT 180–200 cGy daily, 6800–7500 cGy to gross disease, 5000–6000 cGy to draining lymphatics
Planned neck dissections	N2/3 disease: consolidative ND with additional chemotherapy	N2/3 disease: ND (timing varied)
Age	57% <60 y	62 y (median)
Population aspects	All patients with SCCa, organ preservation rate 77%	95% SCCa, 5% with non-SCCa pathology (epithelioma, mucoepidermoid carcinoma)
Predictors of failure	Lack of a pathologic CR in the neck was predictive of DM (p = 0.02)	Tumor stage was predictive of LRC (p = 0.02)
Compliance	89% of patients considered to have a "major response" (partial and complete) after IC 66% received full course of chemotherapy (7/7 doses) 82% received 6/7 doses 96% received 5/7 doses 78% of N2/3 patients underwent posttreatment ND 53% of N2/3 patients received additional 2 cycles of chemotherapy 3/6 nonresponders to IC underwent radical surgery	65% with complete response to IC (defined as disappearance of all clinically evident disease). Complete responders proceeded to concomitant chemo RT Partial responders (>50% response) underwent "organ-sparing" surgical performed (34%) Patients with no response (<50% response) or progression of disease with IC underwent radical resection (1%)
T4 lesions	40%	56%
Clinical stage	Stage III 13%, stage IV 87%	Stage III 3%, stage IV 97%
Enrollment of patients	Defined accrual period after offering enrollment to patients	Defined accrual period after offering enrollment to patients
Morbidity/ complications	Used RTOG acute morbidity scale for the first 6 mo after treatment. Used RTOG/EORTC late morbidity scale for events after 6 mo. 4% treatment-related mortality, 24% late grade 3 toxicity (chronic dysphagia, aspiration, soft tissue ulceration)	7% treatment-related mortality

CR = complete response, LRC = locoregional control, DM = distant metastasis, WBC = white blood cell, Hb = hemoglobin, Cr = serum creatinine, AUC = area under curve, ND = neck dissection, IC = induction chemotherapy, RT = radiation therapy, BOT = base of tongue, RTOG = Radiation Therapy Oncology Group, EORTC = European Organization for Research and Treatment of Cancer.

THE EVIDENCE CONDENSED: Surgery with postoperative radiation therapy for advanced stage oropharyngeal carcinoma

Reference	DeNittis, 2001	Zelefsky, 1992	Hansen, 2002
Level (design)	4 (retrospective review)	4 (retrospective review)	4 (retrospective review)
Sample size	51	51	43
OUTCOMES			
Survival*	51% at 3 y (overall)	52% at 7 y (overall) 64% at 7 y (disease free)	41%, 34% at 3, 5 y (overall)
Locoregional control*	73% at 3 y	81% at 7 y (tongue base) 83% at 7 y (tonsillar fossa)	80%, 80% at 3, 5 y
No distant metastases*	69% at 3 y	71% at 7 y (tongue base) 76% at 7 y (tonsillar fossa)	59%, 54% at 3, 5 y
Follow-up time (median)	34 mo for survivors, 23 mo for all patients	7 y (3 y minimum)	2 y (35 mo mean)
STUDY DESIGN			
Inclusion criteria	ECOG performance score (0–1), BOT (n = 20) and tonsil (n = 31) squamous cell carcinoma	TF (n = 20) and BOT (n = 31) SCCa, no prior treatment, no gross residual disease present at the start of RT	TF (n = 18) and BOT (n = 21) carcinoma (n = 42 SCCa, n = 1 mucoepidermoid carcinoma)
Exclusion criteria	T1–2 N1 disease History of adjuvant chemotherapy	Prior treatment Gross residual present at the start of RT	None specified
RT regimen details	1.8–2.0 Gy fractions to a median dose of 63.7 Gy to primary site and regional lymphatics, no adjuvant chemotherapy utilized	2 Gy fractions, 60 Gy to the primary site, 60 Gy to involved necks	1.8–2 Gy fractions to 63 Gy to the "tumor-bed"
Surgery regimen details	Complete oncologic resection and ipsilateral or bilateral lymph node dissection. Reconstruction with free flap, pectoralis flap, skin graft, or primary	Radical neck dissection for N1 disease, supraomohyoid or modified neck dissection for N0 disease; concomitant total or partial laryngectomy for disease extension into larynx (n = 9), hemimandibulectomy (n = 11)	Resection of the primary tumor with no gross residual disease at the initiation of RT. Neck dissection was performed for regional disease in n = 37/43.
Age	58 y (mean)	55 y (median)	58 y (mean)
Population aspects	All patients with SCCa Margin status not specified	All patients with SCCa 22% of BOT patients with positive margins 45% of TF patients with positive margins	42 patients with SCCa, 1 with mucoepidermoid carcinoma; 26% of patients with positive surgical margins
Predictors of failure	Number of pathologically involved nodes (3-y survival) 0–2 + nodes 70%; ≥3 + nodes 38% (p = 0.04); p < 0.001 for survival and DM; p = 0.003 for LRC	Treatment interruption had a negative impact on local control rates. Local control with break 64%. Local control without break 93% (p = 0.05)	Trend noted for nodal extracapsular extension and distant metastatic spread (p < 0.11)
Compliance	All patients received postoperative RT	42% with a 1-wk treatment interruption secondary to severe mucositis	2% of voluntary withdrawal from RT
T4 lesions Clinical stage	41% Stage III 14% Stage IV 86%	BOT 39%, TF 20% Stage II 4% Stage III 27% Stage IV 68%	35% Stage III 12% Stage IV 88%
Enrollment of patients	Reviewed consecutively treated patients during a defined timeframe	Reviewed consecutively treated patients during a defined timeframe	Reviewed consecutively treated patients during a defined timeframe
Morbidity/ complications	Not specified	Delayed wound healing 20% Osteoradionecrosis 6%	Grade 4 soft tissue radionecrosis 2% Grade 3 mucositis 2%

ECOG = Eastern Cooperative Oncology Group, BOT = base of tongue, TF = tonsillar fossa, DM = distant metastasis, LRC = locoregional control, RT = radiation therapy, SCCa = squamous cell carcinoma.
* Survival, local regional control, and freedom from distant metastases were measured as an actuarial rate in all three studies.

REFERENCES

1. Machtay M, Rosenthal DI, Hershock D, et al. Organ preservation therapy using induction plus concurrent chemoradiation for advanced resectable oropharyngeal carcinoma: a University of Pennsylvania Phase II Trial. J Clin Oncol 2002;20(19):3964–3971.
2. Mantz CA, Vokes EE, Stenson K, et al. Induction chemotherapy followed by concomitant chemoradiotherapy in the treatment of locoregionally advanced oropharyngeal cancer. Cancer J 2001;7(2):140–148.
3. DeNittis AS, Machtay M, Rosenthal DI, et al. Advanced oropharyngeal carcinoma treated with surgery and radiotherapy: oncologic outcome and functional assessment. Am J Otolaryngol 2001;22(5):329–335.
4. Zelefsky MJ, Harrison LB, Armstrong JG. Long-term treatment results of postoperative radiation therapy for advanced stage oropharyngeal carcinoma. Cancer 1992;70(10):2388–2395.
5. Hansen E, Panwala K, Holland J. Post-operative radiation therapy for advanced-stage oropharyngeal cancer. J Laryngol Otol 2002;116(11):920–924.

29 Oropharyngeal Squamous Cell Carcinoma

29.A.ii.

Surgical resection with postoperative radiotherapy versus chemoradiation for oropharyngeal carcinoma: Impact on quality of life

Richard Wein and Randal S. Weber

METHODS

A computerized PubMed search of MEDLINE April 1969–July 2005 was performed. The terms "oropharyngeal carcinoma," "combined modality therapy," "radiotherapy," "chemotherapy" and "surgical procedures, operative" were exploded and the resulting articles were cross-referenced with "survival," "prognosis," "recurrence," "stage 3," and "stage 4" yielding 237 trials. These articles were then reviewed to identify those that met the following inclusion criteria: 1) patient population was defined as individuals undergoing treatment for oropharyngeal carcinoma , 2) intervention with surgical resection with postoperative radiation therapy, ideally in comparison to concomitant chemoradiation, 3) outcome measured in terms of quality of life and posttreatment functional status. Articles that included primary sites other than the oropharynx were excluded from analysis. The bibliographies of the articles that met these inclusion criteria were manually checked to ensure no further relevant articles could be identified. This process yielded five articles [1–5].

RESULTS

Outcome Measures. Impact on quality of life was assessed through the use of validated instruments including the European Organization for Research and Treatment of Cancer Quality of Life Questionnaire 30 (EORTC QLQ-30) [1, 3, 5], EORTC QLQ–Head and Neck (H&N)35 [1, 5], Penetration-Aspiration Scale (PAS) [2], M.D. Anderson Dysphagia Inventory (MDADI) [2], Performance Status Scale for Head and Neck Cancer (PSSHN) [3, 4], and the General Health Questionnaire (GHQ)-12 [5]. Reports concerning the treatment of oropharyngeal carcinoma typically lacked uniformity concerning the use of chemotherapy (induction ± concurrent administration).

Potential Confounders. Quality of life assessments dependent on questionnaire information have the potential for selection and performance bias. In addition, varying lengths of follow-up may alter a patient's response to the impact of short- and long-term morbidities.

Study Designs. Three studies with level 3 evidence and two with level 4 evidence were identified. The structure of studies varied from simple questionnaire completion [1] to objective assessments utilizing blinding, masking, and matching for T stage and tumor site. [2] In the reviewed manuscripts, study populations were limited in size and thus temper the conclusions that can be drawn from their results. Three studies compared the functional results of surgical versus nonsurgical approaches. The format used by Gillespie et al. [2] addressed the potential for detection bias, but the overall number of enrolled patients was limited. Tschudi et al. [1] had an excellent completion percentage for their questionnaire with a sample size greater than most studies but their population represented three different treatment options with varying percentages of advanced-stage lesions per grouping. Allal et al. [3] included patients that received concomitant chemotherapy in their "radical" radiation group that was predominantly composed of radiation-alone patients.

Highest Level of Evidence. There are two retrospective studies that compared surgery/postoperative radiation with chemotherapy/radiation. Both studies found that function was better with chemoradiation. Patients undergoing treatment with a nonsurgical modality ("radical" radiation or chemoradiation) demonstrated better quality of life scores and had findings suggestive of a better swallowing function than patients treated with surgery and postoperative radiation [2]. One of these two studies found that early-stage tumors showed no significant difference in quality of life with treatment modality [3].

A third study by Tschudi et. al. compared patients who received surgery/postoperative radiation with patients who received radiation with or without cisplatin chemotherapy. This study found no difference in global or disease-specific quality of life. This third study also provided comparative data for surgery/postoperative radiation in comparison to radiation or surgery alone; these data are also provided in tables as background information. Individuals treated with surgery alone, when compared with those individuals treated with radiation alone or surgery with postoperative radiation, in general, faired the best in parameters such as swallowing-related functions and pain control [1]. Background data from noncomparative studies are also shown. These articles by DeNittis et al. [4] and Watkinson et al. [5] provide baseline information for populations with oropharyngeal carcinoma.

Applicability. Results are applicable to patients undergoing teatment for oropharyngeal carcinoma. More specifically, inclusion criteria for these studies required disease-free status and willingness to perform questionnaires and assessments. Exclusion criteria included criteria that could obscure the comparative results of speech and swallowing assessments such as patients that received triple therapy (chemotherapy, radiation, and surgery) in addition to individuals with a history of neurologic disorders. [2]

Morbidity/Complications. No complications were reported.

CLINICAL SIGNIFICANCE AND FUTURE RESEARCH

There are 2 level 3 studies that suggest that functional results are better with chemoradiation than surgery/postoperative radiation. One of these studies, as well as a third level 3 study, suggest that there is no difference in quality of life, however. These results are not only mixed, but also retrospective. Groups compared were not matched for potentially confounding factors. Overall, this means that if the correct patients are selected, then they may do better with chemoradiation. Unfortunately, it does not mean that this is true for all patients with oropharyngeal carcinoma.

Higher-level investigation is clearly necessary. Prospective data could minimize confounders and give a more generalizable result. Functional assessments that include both subjective and objective components to quantify quality of life parameters may provide better evidence than simple nonvalidated questionnaires, and require additional investigation.

OUTCOMES: Surgery/radiation therapy versus chemotherapy/radiation therapy

Study, year	Quality of life/functional measure	Comparative data	Conclusion
Allal, 2003	PSSHN	Eating in public, p = 0.08	Chemo/RT better
		Speech understandability, p = 0.0025	Chemo/RT better
		Normalcy of diet, p = 0.25	No difference
	EORTC QLQ	Global, p = NS	No difference
		Physical, p = NS	No difference
		Role, p = NS	No difference
		Emotional, p = NS	No difference
		Cognitive, p = NS	No difference
		Social, p = NS	No difference
Gillespie, 2005	Penetration aspiration score	5 mL swallow, p = 0.02	Chemo/RT better
		10 mL swallow, p = 0.04	Chemo/RT better
		20 mL swallow, p = 0.04	Chemo/RT better
	M.D. Anderson Dysphagia Inventory	Swallow score, p = 0.02	Chemo/RT better
Tschudi, 2003*	EORTC QLQ-QTC	Global, p = NS	No difference
		Physical, p = NS	No difference
		Role, p = NS	No difference
		Emotional, p = NS	No difference
		Cognitive, p = NS	No difference
		Social, p = NS	No difference
	EORTC QLQ-H&N35	Dysphagia, p = NS	No difference
		Social eating, p = NS	No difference
		Social contact, p = NS	No difference
		Dry mouth, p = NS	No difference
		Sticky saliva, p = NS	No difference
		Mouth opening, p = NS	No difference
		Pain, p = NS	No difference
		Senses problems, p = NS	No difference
		Speech problems, p = NS	No difference
		Less sexuality, p = NS	No difference
		Teeth, p = NS	No difference
		Coughing, p = NS	No difference
		Pain killers, p = NS	No difference
		Feeding tube, p = NS	No difference
		Weight loss/gain, p = NS	No difference

PSSHN = Performance Status Scale for Head and Neck Cancer, EORTC QLQ = European Organization for Research and Treatment of Cancer Quality of Life Questionnaire, chemo = chemotherapy, NS = not significant, H&N = head and neck, RT = radiation therapy.
* In this study, some but not patients in the RT group received cisplatin.

OUTCOMES: Surgery versus radiation therapy ± chemotherapy: Quality of life and functional outcome

Tschudi, 2003*	EORTC QLQ-C30	Global, p = NS	No difference
		Physical, p = NS	No difference
		Role, p = NS	No difference
		Emotional, p = NS	No difference
		Cognitive, p = NS	No difference
		Social, p = NS	No difference
	EORTC QLQ-H&N35	Dysphagia, p = 0.006	Surgery better than RT
		Social eating, p = 0.007	Surgery better than RT
		Social contact, p = 0.008	Surgery better than RT
		Dry mouth, p < 0.0001	Surgery better than RT
		Sticky saliva, p = 0.0001	Surgery better than RT
		Mouth opening, p = 0.001	Surgery better than RT
		Pain, p = NS	No difference
		Senses problems, p = NS	No difference
		Speech problems, p = NS	No difference
		Less sexuality, p = NS	No difference
		Teeth, p = NS	No difference
		Coughing, p = NS	No difference
		Pain killers, p = NS	No difference
		Feeding tube, p = NS	No difference
		Weight loss/gain, p = NS	No difference

EORTC QLQ = European Organization for Research and Treatment of Cancer Quality of Life Questionnaire, NS = not significant, H&N = head and neck, RT = radiation therapy.
* In this study, some but not patients in the RT group received cisplatin.

OUTCOMES: Surgery versus Surgery/RT: Quality of life and functional outcome

Tschudi, 2003*	EORTC QLQ-QTC	Global, p = NS	No difference
		Physical, p = NS	No difference
		Role, p = NS	No difference
		Emotional, p = NS	No difference
		Cognitive, p = NS	No difference
		Social, p = NS	No difference
	EORTC QLQ-H&N35	Mouth opening, p = 008	Surgery better than Surgery/RT
		Dry mouth, p < 0.0001	Surgery better than Surgery/RT
		Sticky saliva, 0.0005	Surgery better than Surgery/RT
		Pain, p = NS	No difference
		Swallowing, p = NS	No difference
		Senses problems, p = NS	No difference
		Speech problems, p = NS	No difference
		Social eating, p = NS	No difference
		Social contact, p = NS	No difference
		Less sexuality, p = NS	No difference
		Teeth, p = NS	No difference
		Coughing, p = NS	No difference
		Pain killers, p = NS	No difference
		Nutritional supplements, p = NS	No difference
		Feeding tube, p = NS	No difference
		Weight loss/gain, p = NS	No difference

EORTC QLQ = European Organization for Research and Treatment of Cancer Quality of Life Questionnaire, NS = not significant, H&N = head and neck, RT = radiation therapy.
* In this study, some but not patients in the RT group received cisplatin.

Reference	Tschudi, 2003	Gillespie, 2005	Allal, 2003
Level (design)	3 (retrospective)	3 (retrospective)	3 (retrospective)
Sample size	99 (217 treated)	21	60 (177 treated)
OUTCOMES			
	Please see preceding tables	Please see preceding tables	Please see preceding tables
Timing of assessment	71 mo (median)	Minimum of 12 mo posttreatment Mean follow-up Surgery/RT group 4.7 y ChemoXRT group 3.8 y	Minimum of 12 mo posttreatment Median follow-up RT group 27 mo Surgery/RT group 78 mo
STUDY DESIGN			
Inclusion criteria	Disease-free survivors that completed the questionnaires	Stage III/IV OP SCCa ≥18 y of age	Disease-free 1 y posttreatment Patients treated with accelerated RT
Exclusion criteria	None specified	Triple therapy (chemotherapy, surgery, and RT) History of neurologic condition (stroke, neurodegenerative disease)	None specified
Intervention regimen details	89% questionnaire completion rate	Attempts made to match for tumor site and T stage Masking of patient identifiers for video swallows performed for MDADI Blinding of speech-language pathologists scoring swallowing trials for PAS data	Existing patients solicited during a scheduled clinic visit
Age	Surgery 56 y (median) RT 59 y (median) Surgery/RT 55 y (median)	59 y (mean) ChemoXRT group 62 y (mean) surgery/RT group	61 y (median) RT group 61 y (median) surgery/RT group
Compliance	217 patients treated for curative intent during defined timeframe 111 disease-free survivors identified 99 completed survey	No compliance issues reported	117/177 not included in analysis 53/93 RT group 44 survivors identified 1 lost to follow-up 3 with active disease 64/84 surgery/RT group 27 survivors identified 4 refused to participate 3 with active disease
Clinical stage	Surgery: overall staging I (35.5%), II (16.1%), III (29%), IV (19.4%) RT alone: overall staging II (10.5%), III (15.8%), IV (73.7%) Surgery/RT: overall staging III (16.3%), IV (83.7%)	Surgery/RT T staging T1/2 (73%), T3 (18%), T4 (9%) ChemoXRT T staging T1/2 (50%), T3 (30%), T4 (20%)	RT group staging I (5%), II (30%), III (25%), IV (40%) Surgery/RT group staging I (10%), II (15%), III (20%), VI (50%)
Enrollment of patients	Reviewed consecutively treated patients during a defined timeframe	Eligible patients identified based on inclusion criteria and contacted for enrollment	Reviewed consecutively treated patients during a defined timeframe

RT = radiation therapy, OS = overall survival, H&N = head and neck, PSS = Head and Neck Performance Status Scale, SCCa = squamous cell carcinoma, ECOG = Eastern Cooperative Oncology Group, OP = oropharyngeal, PAS = Penetration-Aspiration Scale, MDADI = M.D. Anderson Dysphagia Inventory, QOL = quality of life, EORTC QLQ-C30 = European Organization for Research and Treatment of Cancer Core QOL questionnaire.

THE EVIDENCE CONDENSED: Oropharyngeal carcinoma posttreatment quality of life

Reference	DeNittis, 2001		Watkinson, 2002	
Level (design)	4 (retrospective)		4 (retrospective)	
Sample size	29 (51 treated)		18	
OUTCOMES				
Intervention	Surgery with postoperative RT		Surgery with postoperative RT	
Functional assessment	**H&N PSS** (0–25) normal (25–50) mild (50–75) moderate (75–100) severe decrease in function	3 parameters Normalcy of diet: 48 Ability to eat in public: 53 Understandability of speech: 75 (mean scores)	**EORTC QLQ** 25% scored poorly in the global health section	**GHQ-12 QOL-Q** 75% with high healthy level of general functioning
Conclusion	Suboptimal results for functional outcome		Conservation surgery with postoperative RT produce minimal functional deficit and do not negatively impact QOL	
Timing of assessment	Minimum of 12 mo posttreatment		3.8 y (median), 1.5 y minimum	
STUDY DESIGN				
Inclusion criteria	ECOG performance score: (0–1) BOT (20) and tonsil (31) SCCa Patients that maintained LRC were eligible for PSS assessment		Disease-free survivor that completed questionnaire T1/T2 oropharyngeal SCCa	
Exclusion criteria	T1–2 N1 disease History of adjuvant chemotherapy		None specified	
Intervention regimen details	Medical record review with phone interviews, patients and/ or family members assessed PSS scores		66% questionnaire completion rate	
Age	58 y (mean)		54 y (mean)	
Specific results of functional performance	PSS speech understandability score was associated with T stage (T1/2 vs T3/4) (p = 0.01) No factors were found correlated with PSS eating in public scores Relationship of PSS normalcy of diet scores to advancing T stage and age suggested (p = 0.06, 0.07 respectively)		EORTC QLQ Specific symptoms section Problems reported with: mouth opening (25%), dry mouth (50%), sticky saliva (42%), had significant weight loss (33%), required pain medication (33%) p values not reported	
Compliance	22/51 not included in PSS analysis 10 locoregional failure 10 early death from disease 2 inability to contact		Individuals (3) with poor scores on the global health EORTC section 2 patients with mental health and financial issues 1 patient smoked during treatment and continued to smoke at the time of testing	
Clinical stage	Stage III 14% Stage IV 86%		Stage I (5%), II (5%), III (5%), IV (85%)	
Enrollment of patients	Reviewed consecutively treated patients during a defined timeframe		Reviewed consecutively treated patients during a defined timeframe	

QOL = quality of life, PSS = Head and Neck Performance Status Scale, SCCa = squamous cell carcinoma, EORTC QLQ-C30 = European Organization for Research and Treatment of Cancer QOL Core questionnaire, EORTC QLQ-H&N35 = EORTC QOL Core Head and Neck Cancer Module questionnaires, PSS = Performance Status Scale, GHQ = General Health Questionnaire, RT = radiation therapy.

REFERENCES

1. Tschudi D, Stoeckli S, Schmid S. Quality of life after different treatment modalities for carcinoma of the oropharynx. Laryngoscope 2003;113:1949–1954.
2. Gillespie MB, Brodsky MB, Day TA, Sharma AK, Lee F, Martin-Harris B. Laryngeal penetration and aspiration during swallowing after the treatment of advanced oropharyngeal cancer. Arch Otolaryngol Head Neck Surg 2005;131: 615–619.
3. Allal AS, Nicoucar K, Mach N, Dulguerov. Quality of life in patients with oropharynx carcinomas: assessment after accelerated radiotherapy with or without chemotherapy versus radical surgery and postoperative radiotherapy. Head Neck 2003;25:833–840.
4. DeNittis AS, Machtay M, Rosenthal DI, et al. Advanced oropharyngeal carcinoma treated with surgery and radiotherapy: oncologic outcome and functional assessment. Am J Otolaryngol 2001;22(5):329–335.
5. Watkinson JC, Owen C, Thompson S, Das Gupta AR, Glaholm J. Conservation surgery in the management of T1 and T2 oropharyngeal squamous cell carcinoma: the Birmingham UK experience. Clin Otolaryngol Allied Sci 2002; 27(6):541–548.

29 Oropharyngeal Squamous Cell Carcinoma

29.B.

Computed tomography scan versus orthopantomogram (Panorex) to assess mandibular invasion by oral cavity or oropharyngeal carcinoma: Positive and negative predictive values with respect to surgical or histologic confirmation

Richard Wein and Randal S. Weber

METHODS

A computerized PubMed search of MEDLINE July 1986–February 2005 was performed. The terms "head and neck," "oral cavity," "oropharyngeal and pharyngeal carcinomas/neoplasms" were exploded and cross-referenced with the terms "tomography," "X-ray/CT scan," and "mandibular/jaw neoplasm, bony invasion" yielding 144 articles. These articles were then reviewed to identify those that met the following inclusion criteria: 1) patients with oral cavity or oropharyngeal squamous cell carcinoma with potential mandibular invasion, 2) evaluation with pretreatment computed tomography (CT) scan or Panorex (ideally comparing both modalities), 3) outcome measured in terms of correlation of imaging modality findings with histopathologic evidence of mandibular involvement. Articles focusing primarily on alternative imaging modalities or modifications of standard CT scanning were excluded. The bibliographies of the articles that met these inclusion criteria were manually checked to ensure no additional relevant articles could be identified. This process yielded five publications [1–5].

RESULTS

Outcome Measures. Mandibular invasion was defined by histopathologic evidence of neoplastic involvement of cortical bone.

Potential Confounders. Inclusion criteria based on the investigators' degree of clinical suspicion of mandibular involvement can affect the ultimate outcome of a study. Patient factors that were reported to affect imaging study quality include amalgam artifact and patient movement. The selected CT scan section thickness (1.5–6 mm) and imaging techniques (bone algorithms or coronal imaging) varied within studies. Patients undergoing nonsurgical treatment options were excluded from analysis. Surgical techniques varied and did not always require bony resection if the periosteal aspect of surgical specimens were considered negative for tumor extension [1, 4]. The average period of time from imaging to surgical resection was specified in only one study [5].

Study Designs. The studies examining this topic represent the range of level 2 to 4 evidence (prospective and retrospective controlled studies and case series). Patient enrollment was often limited in number and was frequently defined by a set period of time at a single institution. Most studies limited enrollment to patients without history of treatment. Imaging techniques that were evaluated and compared varied widely. Only three studies actually compared CT scan to Panorex [1–3]. Many of the studies controlled for observational bias by using radiologists unaware of the patient's clinical examination or histopathologic results [2–5]. Numerical analyses within the studies was limited to assessing estimated sensitivity, specificity, positive and negative predictive values (PPV, NPV), without 95% confidence intervals for statistical comparison of the two modalities. Means of evaluation of surgical specimens for tumor extension were standard and similar among studies.

Highest Level of Evidence. Studies examining this topic were prospective and retrospective. Retrospective studies tended to lack uniformity in the imaging techniques used within a patient population. Only two prospective trials comparing CT and Panorex imaging were identified in which patients were imaged preoperatively with both modalities [1, 2]. In these studies, sensitivities ranged from 64% to 80% for Panorex and 78% to 100% with CT scanning [1, 2]. One of prospective studies reported enough data to allow for a *post hoc* analysis [1] (see below). Acton et al. noted a sensitivity of 81% when both imaging modalities were used in combination to assess for invasion [2]. The retrospective studies demonstrated a wide range of sensitivities for CT imaging that relate to primary site location. In one study, a sensitivity of 50% was noted for tumors of the retromolar trigone [4]. Meanwhile, another study showed a sensitivity of 96% in a population composed of primarily floor of mouth and gingivobuccal carcinomas clinically fixed to the mandible [5].

Applicability. The results of these studies pertain to patients with clinically extensive oral (excluding hard palate) and oropharyngeal (including primarily base of tongue) primary lesions. However, the results for selected subsites, such as the retromolar trigone, may not be applicable to other specific primary sites within the oral cavity and oropharynx.

Morbidity/Complications. The associated morbidity of the various imaging techniques is minimal. Special provisions for patients with renal insufficiency undergoing CT scan with contrast were acknowledged.

CLINICAL SIGNIFICANCE AND FUTURE RESEARCH

There are two level 2, one level 3, and two level 4 studies that addressed this topic. There is a trend toward CT appearing more sensitive than Panorex in assessing for mandibular invasion, but statistical differences have not been demonstrated. In addition, the level of sensitivity may be dependent on the primary site of the lesion in question. Although Panorex and CT may be used to assess for mandibular involvement, these techniques are also obtained preoperatively for other indications. Panorex imaging can guide the need for dental extraction whereas CT scan can assess the extent of a primary lesion and also determine the regional lymphatic spread.

Future research should focus on obtaining prospective data comparing emerging imaging techniques to existing modalities for specific primary sites within the oral cavity while accruing larger overall patient numbers. Magnetic resonance imaging has been shown to have a high sensitivity for detecting mandibular invasion but has been criticized for a low specificity and a tendency to overestimate extent of involvement [3]. Single photon emission computed tomography bone scanning and DentaScan (assessment of CT imaging) have been described as improvements over existing means of assessment and require additional study [2, 6].

THE EVIDENCE CONDENSED: Computed tomography scan versus Panorex for preoperative identification of mandibular involvement

Reference	Close, 1986		Acton, 2000		Van den Brekel, 1998	
Level (design)	2 (prospective controlled study)		2 (prospective controlled study)		3 (retrospective controlled study)	
Sample size	43		67		29	

			OUTCOMES			
Intervention	CT scan	Panorex and dental occlusive views	CT scan	Panorex	CT scan	Panorex
Sensitivity	100%	64%	78%	80%	50%	63%
Specificity	97%	97%	83%	72%	91%	90%
PPV	92%	88%	82%	75%		
NPV	100%	89%	79%	75%		
Comparative statistics	Not reported		Not reported		Not reported	
Conclusion	CT is better than Panorex at detecting mandibular involvement		Current assessment modalities may fail to accurately detect bone invasion		The inaccuracy of imaging modalities reinforces the importance of clinical examination	
Additional studies performed	Clinical evaluation: PPV 60%, NPV 93%		SPECT bone scans: 60% sensitivity, 67% specificity, 50% PPV, 75% NPV. Clinical evaluation: 94% sensitivity, 25% specificity, 57% PPV, 80% NPV		MRI: 94% sensitivity, 73% specificity. Clinical evaluation: 39% sensitivity, 100% specificity	

			STUDY DESIGN			
Inclusion criteria	Previously untreated, T2 or greater primary squamous carcinoma of the FOM, buccal mucosa, lower lip, alveolar ridge, RMT, tonsillar fossa, and BOT		Previously untreated, squamous carcinoma of the FOM, inferior alveolus, and RMT with clinical suspicion of mandible invasion		Previously untreated squamous carcinoma of the FOM and RMT	
Exclusion criteria	Not specified		CT scans that were uninterpretable because of dental amalgam, patient movement, and poor compliance		Not specified	
Surgical intervention	Resection to the level of periosteum, "inner table" of mandible, or segmental mandibulectomy		Surgical resection of the primary tumor, procedures unspecified		Marginal (15) or segmental (14) mandibulectomy performed in all patients	
CT scan specifics	Axial CT with contrast with bone and soft tissue windows and overlapping 5-mm-thick sections		Axial and coronal CT with bone windows		Axial CT scan with contrast and 5- to 6-mm-thick sections (bone windows obtained in 24/29 patients)	
Assessment of imaging studies	Not specified		By a single radiologist before surgical intervention		By 2 independent experienced observers blinded to the results of other modalities; in cases of disagreement, consensus would be reached	
Mean age	Not specified		61.8 y		57 y	
Average time from imaging to surgery	1 wk from imaging to biopsy and endoscopy, resection not specified		Not specified		Not specified	

CT = computed tomography, PPV = positive predictive value, NPV = negative predictive value, SPECT = single photon emission computed tomography, MRI = magnetic resonance imaging, FOM = floor of mouth, RMT = retromolar trigone, BOT = base of tongue.

THE EVIDENCE CONDENSED: Computed tomography scan versus Panorex for preoperative identification of mandibular involvement

Reference	Lane, 2000	Mukherji, 2001
Level (design)	4 (retrospective case series)	4 (retrospective case series)
Sample size	29	49
OUTCOMES		
Intervention	CT scan	CT scan
Sensitivity	50%	96%
Specificity	91%	87%
PPV	61%	89%
NPV	91%	95%
Conclusion	CT is less accurate in assessing RMT carcinoma bone invasion in this series	Thin-section (3 mm) CT is an accurate technique to assess mandible invasion by tumors of the oral cavity
Additional studies performed	None reported	None reported
STUDY DESIGN		
Inclusion criteria	Squamous carcinoma of the RMT treated with surgical excision	Squamous carcinoma of FOM, gingival/buccal mucosa, alveolar ridge, and RMT with clinical evidence of fixation of tumor to the mandible
Exclusion criteria	Lesions not clearly centered over the RMT were excluded	Freely mobile tumor to bimanual examination; primary oral tongue carcinoma; previous surgery involving the mandible
Surgical intervention	Resection to the level of periosteum or marginal/segmental mandibulectomy	Marginal (34) or segmental (15) mandibulectomy performed in all patients
CT scan specifics	Axial CT with contrast and 5-mm-thick sections (bone algorithm and coronal sections excluded because of lack of uniformity)	Axial CT scan with contrast and 3-mm-thick sections, soft tissue and bone algorithms used, angling technique for patients with amalgam
Assessment of imaging studies	By a single radiologist unaware of the pathologic findings	By a neuroradiologist unaware of histopathologic status
Mean age	Not specified	59 y
Average time from imaging to surgery	Not specified	Resection performed within 14.3 d

CT = computed tomography, PPV = positive predictive, NPV = negative predictive value, FOM = floor of mouth, RMT = retromolar trigone, BOT = base of tongue.

A *post hoc* analysis was performed on the data provided by Close et al. (There was not enough raw data specified in the second prospective report to perform a definitive *post hoc* analysis.) Within their results, they provided enough raw data to form the basis for the analysis below. The raw data are shown in the tables of imaging findings versus histologic findings below. The estimated values for PPV, NPV, sensitivity, and specificity are as reported in the original publications. Based on the number of patients included in the study, the results of the study, and statis-tical factors, 95% confidence intervals surrounding those estimated values can be calculated. The upper and lower limits of these 95% confidence intervals are shown below. Analysis of the 95% confidence intervals shows overlap in the data for sensitivity, specificity, PPV, and NPV of CT versus Panorex. This overlap suggests that although there is a trend toward more accuracy with CT, it is not statistically demonstrated in a conclusive way.

Computed tomography

	Histologic invasion		
	Positive	Negative	Totals
Positive	11	1	12
Negative	0	31	31
Totals	11	32	43

	Estimated value	95% confidence interval	
		Lower limit	Upper limit
PPV	91.7%	59.8%	99.5%
NPV	100%	86.2%	100%
Sensitivity	100%	67.9%	100%
Specificity	96.9%	82.0%	99.8%

Panorex

	Histologic invasion		
	Positive	Negative	Totals
Positive	7	1	8
Negative	4	31	35
Totals	32	11	43

	Estimated value	95% confidence interval	
		Lower limit	Upper limit
PPV	87.5%	46.7%	99.3%
NPV	88.5%	72.3%	96.3%
Sensitivity	63.6%	31.6%	87.6%
Specificity	96.8%	82.0%	99.8%

REFERENCES

1. Close LG, Merkel M, Burns DK, Schaefer SD. Computed tomography in the assessment of mandibular invasion by intraoral carcinoma. Ann Otol Rhinol Laryngol 1986;95(4 Pt 1):383–388.
2. Acton CHC, Layt C, Gwynne R, Cooke R, Seaton D. Investigative modalities of mandibular invasion by squamous cell carcinoma. Laryngoscope 2000;110:2050–2055.
3. Van den Brekel MWM, Runne RW, Smeele LE, Tiwari RM, Snow GB, Castelijns JA. Assessment of tumour invasion into the mandible: the value of different imaging techniques. Eur Radiol 1998;8(9):1552–1557.
4. Lane AP, Buckmire RA, Mukherji SK, Pillsbury HC III, Meredith SD. Use of computed tomography in the assessment of mandibular invasion in carcinoma of the retromolar trigone. Otolaryngol Head Neck Surg 2000;122:673–677.
5. Mukherji SK, Isaacs DL, Creager A, Shockley W, Weissler M, Armao D. CT detection of mandibular invasion by squamous cell carcinoma of the oral cavity. AJR Am J Roentgenol 2001;177(1):237–243.
6. Brockenbrough JM, Petruzzelli GJ, Lomasney L. DentaScan as an accurate method of predicting mandibular invasion in patients with squamous cell carcinoma of the oral cavity. Arch Otolaryngol Head Neck Surg 2003;129:113–117.

30 Laryngeal Squamous Cell Carcinoma: Early-Stage Disease

30.A.i.

Endoscopic resection versus radiation therapy for stage I–II glottic carcinoma: Impact on survival and local recurrence

Yen-Lin Chen and Kian Ang

METHODS

A computerized PubMed search of MEDLINE from 1966 to 2005 was performed. The diagnosis terms "larynx," "glottic," or "true vocal cord" were exploded and combined. The terms "cancer," "carcinoma," or "squamous cell carcinoma" were exploded and combined. The above two searches were then limited to "early stage," "T1," "T2," "stage I," or stage II" to yield articles focused on early-stage I–II glottic cancer. These articles were then subjected to the PubMed Clinical Queries using Research Methodology Filters [1] optimized for sensitive/broad search for articles in the category of "therapy," yielding 311 articles. These articles were then cross-referenced with the headings "radiation," "radiotherapy," "laser excision," "endoscopic surgery," "endolaryngeal resection," "transoral surgery," "CO_2 cordectomy," "laser cordectomy," or "microsurgery," yielding a total of 250 publications, whose titles and abstracts were reviewed to identify those that met the following inclusion criteria: 1) patient population with primary newly diagnosed, biopsy-proven T1 or T2 larynx carcinoma, 2) intervention with radiation or endoscopic resection (with or without laser), 3) outcome measured in terms of survival, local recurrence, and/or larynx preservation. There were no published prospective randomized controlled trials comparing endoscopic resection versus radiation for stage I–II glottic carcinoma. There were 46 retrospective, uncontrolled case series of a single modality reporting similar survival outcomes for radiation or endoscopic resection [1–47]. One systematic review was identified that compared open surgery versus radiation but did not address endoscopic surgery [6]. A total of three nonrandomized, comparative cohort studies were identified that compared primary radiation versus endoscopic resection that met the above inclusion criteria. Articles comparing conventional versus altered radiation dose fractionation or open versus endoscopic surgery were excluded. The bibliographies of the articles that met these inclusion criteria were manually checked to ensure no further relevant articles could be identified. This process yielded three articles which are reviewed below [36, 44, 48].

RESULTS

Outcome Measures. The primary outcome measures for the three retrospective cohort studies reported were survival (overall or disease-specific survival) and locoregional control.

Potential Confounders. As nonrandomized, uncontrolled studies, these three studies have a number of potential confounders. In two of the studies, the endoscopic laser resection group participants were from a significantly later time period compared with radiation and were more likely to have smaller disease (T1a), be younger (potentially biasing survival), and have shorter follow-up. The most significant confounding factor in one study is that 11 of the 31 patients treated with endoscopic laser surgery had positive margins on pathology and of those 10 went on to receive postoperative radiotherapy [48]. In one study, radiation doses were different in two different decades, reflecting two different eras of radiation technique, machine, fields, and daily fractionation [44].

Study Designs. All three studies are single institutional cohort studies of patients with T1 and/or T2 larynx cancer treated with radiation or endoscopic resection. Two studies are retrospective chart review or tumor registry data extraction [44, 48]. One is a prospective database starting in 1963 capturing unselected, sequentially treated early larynx cancer patients at a single institution. Study periods span two to three decades in all three studies, beginning from 1963 to 2004. Two of the studies reported increasing numbers of endoscopically treated patients in more recent times, reflecting the relatively new development of endoscopic resection techniques [44, 48]. One study included all subsites of larynx (supraglottic, glottic, and subglottic) [36] whereas the other two studies focused on stage I (T1 N0 M0) glottic cancers [44, 48]. Radiation total doses ranged from 50 to 70 Gy. One study divided patients into low-dose radiation (total dose 55–65 Gy at 1.5–1.8 Gy per fraction) versus high-dose radiation (65–70 Gy at 2–2.25 Gy per fraction). Field sizes and treatment duration were similar in all studies. Endoscopic resection ranged from CO_2 laser resection to microlaryngoscopic surgery.

Highest Level of Evidence. There is insufficient evidence to show whether radiation or endoscopic surgery is better for patients with early glottic cancer. These three retrospective/prospective nonrandomized, uncontrolled cohort studies provide limited level 3 evidence that endoscopic resection and radiation may result in comparable outcomes. Both modalities result in 5-year survival rates ranging from 74% to 95% and locoregional control rates ranging from 80% to 91% for stage I/II glottic cancer. One study suggests that low-dose radiation therapy (RT) (55–65 Gy at 1.5–1.8 Gy per fraction) or endoscopic resection result in worse locoregional control compared with higher total dose and higher dose per fraction (65–75 at 2–2.5 Gy per fraction). After salvage, the ultimate locoregional control and cause-specific survival did not differ. These studies are, however, limited by small number of patients, potential selection biases favoring upfront radiation or adjuvant radiation for larger tumors, anterior commissure involvement, or other high-risk features, and shorter follow-up for patients treated with endoscopic surgery or higher radiation dose because of changing practices over time.

Applicability. These results are applicable for patients with mainly T1 glottic carcinoma treated with endoscopic resection or primary radiation.

Morbidity/Complications. Radiation and endoscopic surgery for early glottic cancer are both well tolerated. Although there does not seem to be significant difference in voice quality between radiation and endoscopic surgery, these three studies were not primarily designed to assess voice quality.

CLINICAL SIGNIFICANCE AND FUTURE RESEARCH

Well-designed prospective randomized controlled clinical trials are needed to guide decision making for patients with early glottic cancer. There are insufficient data to suggest endoscopic or radiation is better for survival or local control of early glottic carcinoma. Management decisions must encompass not only survival data, but also patient preference and quality of life. The next section provides evidence from studies more specifically designed to compare the quality of voice as the primary outcome.

THE EVIDENCE CONDENSED: Endoscopic resection versus radiation therapy for stage I–II glottic carcinoma: Impact on survival and local recurrence

Reference	Rosier, 1998	
Level (design)	3 (retrospective cohort)	
Sample size	72* (of total of 106 in the study): RT 41, E 31	

OUTCOMES		
Survival	OS 5	OS 10
Radiation	74%	58.6%
Surgery	74%	NR
p Value	>0.05	
Recurrence	LRC 5	LRC 10
Radiation	0.90 (0.97)§	0.90 (0.97)§
Endoscopic surgery	0.88 (1.00)§	NR (NR)§
p Value	>0.05	
Conclusion	No difference in overall survival or LRC	
Follow-up time	Median 63.5 mo	

STUDY DESIGN	
Inclusion criteria	T1 N0 M0 glottic cancer treated from 1979 to 1995 at 1 institution
Exclusion criteria	NR
RT details	Parallel opposed fields, cobalt-therapy (88%), or linear accelerator (12%). Field sizes: 4×4 to 6×6 cm. Doses: 50–70 Gy (median 64 Gy) at 2 Gy per fraction. Wedge filters
Endoscopic procedure	SHARPLAN 1055 CO_2 laser
Therapy decision	Therapy dependent on referring physician
Period biases	Laser not introduced until 1988 so follow-up was shorter for E (33 mo) than RT (74 mo), $p < 0.01$
Selection biases	Selection bias: T1b, anterior commissure involvement, or younger patients less likely to get E ($p < 0.01$)
Postoperative RT	11 patients with E had positive margins: 10 received postoperative RT
Morbidity/ complications	RT: 7.7% grade II or more grade II RTOG toxicity. RT and E had comparable perceptual voice rating by patient and therapists ($p = 0.06$)

RT = radiation therapy, E = endoscopic surgery (laser and/or microlaryngoscopic surgery), NR = not reported, OS 5/10 = overall survival at 5 or 10 years, respectively, CSS 5/10 = cause-specific survival at 5 or 10 years, respectively, LRC 5/10 = locoregional control at 5 or 10 years, respectively, NS = not significant.

* Sample size: numbers shown for those RT vs E (results for open partial laryngectomy in 34 patients not included for this comparison).

† Of 448 patients, 56 had glottic cancer and of those, 32 had RT and 24 had surgery (not further subdivided into open partial laryngectomy versus laser). All 69 surgery patients (supraglottic, glottic, and subglottic) were reported together in the paper. Although glottic patients were more likely to receive radiotherapy than surgery compared with other subsites, there was also no further categorization into endoscopic versus open partial laryngectomy because of small numbers.

‡ 659 patients total T1 N0 M0 patients: 404 had open partial laryngectomy, 90 had low-dose RT, 104 had high-dose RT, and 61 had endoscopic resection.

§ LRC before salvage laryngectomy (LRC after salvage).

THE EVIDENCE CONDENSED: Endoscopic resection versus radiation therapy for stage I–II glottic carcinoma: Impact on survival and local recurrence

Reference	Jones, 2004		Spector, 1999	
Level (design)	3 (prospective database)		3 (retrospective cohort)	
Sample size	56† (glottic carcinoma of total of 488 in the study): RT 32, S 24		255‡ RT low dose 90. RT high dose 104, E 61	
OUTCOMES				
Survival	CSS 5	CSS 10	CSS 5	OS 5
Radiation	87%	84%	Low-dose RT: 0.92 High dose: 0.95	0.72 0.83
Surgery	77%	77%	E: 0.95	
p Value	0.102		0.68	0.004
Recurrence	LF 5	LF 10	Primary LRC 5	LRC 5 after salvage
Radiation	0.20	0.22	Low-dose RT: 0.78 High dose: 0.89	Low dose: 0.97 High dose: 0.96
Endoscopic surgery	0.22	0.23	E: 0.77	0.98
p Value	0.7205		0.02	NS
Conclusion	No difference in cause-specific survival or local failure		No difference in cause-specific survival. Worse outcome in low-dose RT group. Worse initial (not ultimate) LRC with E or low-dose RT compared with high-dose RT	
Follow-up time	Median 16.6 y		At least 3 y. Median NR	
STUDY DESIGN				
Inclusion criteria	T1–2 N0 M0 larynx cancer (supraglottic, glottic, and subglottic) 1963–2004		T1 N0 M0 glottic cancer treated between 1971 and 1990 at 1 institution	
Exclusion criteria	1 lost to follow-up after only 6 mo. 4 excluded because of incomplete data		At least 3 y	
RT details	5 or 6 MeV linear accelerator. Doses: 60–66 Gy at 2 Gy per fraction. Wedge filters		Low-dose RT: 55–65 Gy at 1.5–1.8 Gy per fraction using Cobalt or 4-MV High-dose RT: 65–70 Gy at 2–2.25 Gy per fraction using 4- or 6-MV photons. Fields 5×5 to 6×6 cm. Wedges	
Endoscopic procedure	12 had endoscopic laser surgery. 13 had endoscopic microlaryngoscopic surgery		Endoscopic resection with CO_2 laser or KTP laser	
Therapy decision	Therapy dependent on referring physician, patient mandate		Therapy dependent on referring physician or patient mandate	
Period biases	Period bias: radiation more likely used in the 1980s and 1990s. Surgery more likely used in the 1960s and 1970s		Period bias: low RT was given from 1971 to 1985 whereas high RT was given from 1986 to 1995	
Selection biases	No separation of endoscopic vs open partial laryngectomy or by larynx subsite because of small numbers		Selection: endoscopic resection only for superficial lesions confined to membranous vocal cords	
Postoperative RT	Only 2 patients in the surgery group had postoperative RT		None of the E group had immediate postoperative RT	
Morbidity/ complications	RT: 2 moderate dysphagia and 2 mild dysphagia. 2 cartilage necrosis. S: (not clear if open or endoscopic) 4 fistula and 2 stenosis. 4 with medical complications (1 died). Voice quality worse with S than RT (p = 0.0017)		0.1% complication deaths and 6% intercurrent disease associated with use of tobacco and second primary malignancies	

RT = radiation therapy, E = endoscopic surgery (laser and/or microlaryngoscopic surgery), NR = not reported, OS 5/10 = overall survival at 5 or 10 years, respectively, CSS 5/10 = cause-specific survival at 5 or 10 years, respectively, LRC 5/10 = locoregional control at 5 or 10 years, respectively, NS = not significant.

* Sample size: numbers shown for those RT vs E (results for open partial laryngectomy in 34 patients not included for this comparison).

† Of 448 patients, 56 had glottic cancer and of those, 32 had RT and 24 had surgery (not further subdivided into open partial laryngectomy versus laser). All 69 surgery patients (supraglottic, glottic, and subglottic) were reported together in the paper. Although glottic patients were more likely to receive radiotherapy than surgery compared with other subsites, there was also no further categorization into endoscopic versus open partial laryngectomy because of small numbers.

‡ 659 patients total T1 N0 M0 patients: 404 had open partial laryngectomy, 90 had low-dose RT, 104 had high-dose RT, and 61 had endoscopic resection.

§ LRC before salvage laryngectomy (LRC after salvage).

REFERENCES

1. Haynes RB, et al. Optimal search strategies for retrieving scientifically strong studies of treatment from Medline: analytical survey. BMJ 2005;330(7501):1179.
2. Ansarin M, et al. Endoscopic CO2 laser surgery for early glottic cancer in patients who are candidates for radiotherapy: results of a prospective nonrandomized study. Head Neck 2006;28(2):121–125.
3. Brandenburg JH. Laser cordotomy versus radiotherapy: an objective cost analysis. Ann Otol Rhinol Laryngol 2001;110(4):312–318.
4. Cellai E, et al. Radical radiotherapy for early glottic cancer: results in a series of 1087 patients from two Italian radiation oncology centers. I. The case of T1N0 disease. Int J Radiat Oncol Biol Phys 2005;63(5):1378–1386.
5. Csanady M, Czigner J, Savay L. Endolaryngeal CO2 laser microsurgery of early vocal cord cancer. A retrospective study. Adv Otorhinolaryngol 1995;49:219–221.
6. Dey P, et al. Radiotherapy versus open surgery versus endolaryngeal surgery (with or without laser) for early laryngeal squamous cell cancer. Cochrane Database Syst Rev 2002(2):CD002027.
7. Eckel HE. Local recurrences following transoral laser surgery for early glottic carcinoma: frequency, management, and outcome. Ann Otol Rhinol Laryngol 2001;110(1):7–15.
8. Fein DA, et al. T1-T2 squamous cell carcinoma of the glottic larynx treated with radiotherapy: a multivariate analysis of variables potentially influencing local control. Int J Radiat Oncol Biol Phys 1993;25(4):605–611.
9. Franchin G, et al. Radiotherapy for patients with early-stage glottic carcinoma: univariate and multivariate analyses in a group of consecutive, unselected patients. Cancer 2003;98(4):765–772.
10. Frata P, et al. Radical radiotherapy for early glottic cancer: results in a series of 1087 patients from two Italian radiation oncology centers. II. The case of T2N0 disease. Int J Radiat Oncol Biol Phys 2005;63(5):1387–1394.
11. Gallo A, et al. CO2 laser cordectomy for early-stage glottic carcinoma: a long-term follow-up of 156 cases. Laryngoscope 2002;112(2):370–374.
12. Garden AS, et al. Results of radiotherapy for T2N0 glottic carcinoma: does the "2" stand for twice-daily treatment? Int J Radiat Oncol Biol Phys 2003;55(2):322–328.
13. Hirano M, Hirade Y, Kawasaki H. Vocal function following carbon dioxide laser surgery for glottic carcinoma. Ann Otol Rhinol Laryngol 1985;94(3):232–235.
14. Keilmann A, et al. Vocal function following laser and conventional surgery of small malignant vocal fold tumours. J Laryngol Otol 1996;110(12):1138–1141.
15. Krespi YP, Meltzer CJ. Laser surgery for vocal cord carcinoma involving the anterior commissure. Ann Otol Rhinol Laryngol 1989;98(2):105–109.
16. Maurizi M, et al. Laser carbon dioxide cordectomy versus open surgery in the treatment of glottic carcinoma: our results. Otolaryngol Head Neck Surg 2005;132(6):857–861.
17. McGuirt WF, et al. Comparative voice results after laser resection or irradiation of T1 vocal cord carcinoma. Arch Otolaryngol Head Neck Surg 1994;120(9):951–955.
18. Medini E, et al. Radiation therapy in early carcinoma of the glottic larynx T1N0M0. Int J Radiat Oncol Biol Phys 1996;36(5):1211–1213.
19. Mendenhall WM, et al. T1-T2N0 squamous cell carcinoma of the glottic larynx treated with radiation therapy. J Clin Oncol 2001;19(20):4029–4036.
20. Motta G, et al. T1-T2-T3 glottic tumors: fifteen years experience with CO2 laser. Acta Otolaryngol Suppl 1997;527:155–159.
21. Ossoff RH, Sisson GA, Shapshay SM. Endoscopic management of selected early vocal cord carcinoma. Ann Otol Rhinol Laryngol 1985;94(6 Pt 1):560–564.
22. Peretti G, et al. Endoscopic CO2 laser excision for tis, T1, and T2 glottic carcinomas: cure rate and prognostic factors. Otolaryngol Head Neck Surg 2000;123(1 Pt 1):124–131.
23. Pradhan SA, et al. Transoral laser surgery for early glottic cancers. Arch Otolaryngol Head Neck Surg 2003;129(6):623–625.
24. Rebeiz EE, et al. Preliminary clinical results of window partial laryngectomy: a combined endoscopic and open technique. Ann Otol Rhinol Laryngol 2000;109(2):123–127.
25. Sigston E, et al. Early-stage glottic cancer: oncological results and margins in laser cordectomy. Arch Otolaryngol Head Neck Surg 2006;132(2):147–152.
26. Smith JC, Johnson JT, Myers EN. Management and outcome of early glottic carcinoma. Otolaryngol Head Neck Surg 2002;126(4):356–364.
27. Steiner W. Results of curative laser microsurgery of laryngeal carcinomas. Am J Otolaryngol 1993;14(2):116–121.
28. Wolfensberger M, Dort JC. Endoscopic laser surgery for early glottic carcinoma: a clinical and experimental study. Laryngoscope 1990;100(10 Pt 1):1100–1105.
29. Zeitels SM. Phonomicrosurgical treatment of early glottic cancer and carcinoma in situ. Am J Surg 1996;172(6):704–709.
30. Akine Y, et al. Radiotherapy of T1 glottic cancer with 6 MeV X rays. Int J Radiat Oncol Biol Phys 1991;20(6):1215–1218.
31. Barton MB, et al. The effect of treatment time and treatment interruption on tumour control following radical radiotherapy of laryngeal cancer. Radiother Oncol 1992;23(3):137–143.
32. Harwood AR, et al. Radiotherapy of early glottic cancer—I. Int J Radiat Oncol Biol Phys 1979;5(4):473–476.
33. Harwood AR, Tierie A. Radiotherapy of early glottic cancer—II. Int J Radiat Oncol Biol Phys 1979;5(4):477–482.
34. Hendrickson FR. Radiation therapy treatment of larynx cancers. Cancer 1985;55(9 Suppl):2058–2061.
35. Howell-Burke D, et al. T2 glottic cancer. Recurrence, salvage, and survival after definitive radiotherapy. Arch Otolaryngol Head Neck Surg 1990;116(7):830–835.
36. Jones AS, et al. The treatment of early laryngeal cancers (T1-T2 N0): surgery or irradiation? Head Neck 2004;26(2):127–135.
37. Karim AB, et al. Heterogeneity of stage II glottic carcinoma and its therapeutic implications. Int J Radiat Oncol Biol Phys 1987;13(3):313–317.
38. Kelly MD, et al. Definitive radiotherapy in the management of stage I and II carcinomas of the glottis. Ann Otol Rhinol Laryngol 1989;98(3):235–239.

39. Klintenberg C, et al. Primary radiotherapy of T1 and T2 glottic carcinoma—analysis of treatment results and prognostic factors in 223 patients. Acta Oncol 1996; 35(Suppl 8):81–86.

40. Le QT, et al. Influence of fraction size, total dose, and overall time on local control of T1-T2 glottic carcinoma. Int J Radiat Oncol Biol Phys 1997;39(1):115–126.

41. Olszewski SJ, et al. The influence of field size, treatment modality, commissure involvement and histology in the treatment of early vocal cord cancer with irradiation. Int J Radiat Oncol Biol Phys 1985;11(7):1333–1337.

42. Pellitteri PK, et al. Radiotherapy. The mainstay in the treatment of early glottic carcinoma. Arch Otolaryngol Head Neck Surg 1991;117(3):297–301.

43. Schwaab G, et al. Surgical salvage treatment of T1/T2 glottic carcinoma after failure of radiotherapy. Am J Surg 1994;168(5):474–475.

44. Spector JG, et al. Stage I (T1 N0 M0) squamous cell carcinoma of the laryngeal glottis: therapeutic results and voice preservation. Head Neck 1999;21(8):707–717.

45. Van den Bogaert W, Ostyn F, van der Schueren E. The significance of extension and impaired mobility in cancer of the vocal cord. Int J Radiat Oncol Biol Phys 1983;9(2): 181–184.

46. Wiggenraad RG, et al. The importance of vocal cord mobility in T2 laryngeal cancer. Radiother Oncol 1990;18(4): 321–327.

47. Yu E, et al. Impact of radiation therapy fraction size on local control of early glottic carcinoma. Int J Radiat Oncol Biol Phys 1997;37(3):587–591.

48. Rosier JF, et al. Comparison of external radiotherapy, laser microsurgery and partial laryngectomy for the treatment of T1N0M0 glottic carcinomas: a retrospective evaluation. Radiother Oncol 1998;48(2):175–183.

30 Laryngeal Squamous Cell Carcinoma: Early-Stage Disease

30.A.ii.

Endoscopic resection versus radiation therapy for stage I–II glottic carcinoma: Impact on voice and quality of life

Yen-Lin Chen and Kian Ang

METHODS

A computerized PubMed search of MEDLINE from 1966 to 2005 was performed. The terms "larynx," "glottic," or "true vocal cord" were exploded and combined. The terms "cancer," "carcinoma," or "squamous cell carcinoma" were exploded and combined. The above two searches were then limited to "early stage," "T1," "T2," "stage I," or "stage II" to yield articles focused on early-stage I–II glottic cancer. These articles were then subjected to the PubMed Clinical Queries using Research Methodology Filters [1] optimized for sensitive/broad search for articles in the category of "therapy," yielding 311 articles. These articles were then cross-referenced with the headings "radiation," "radiotherapy," "laser excision," "endoscopic surgery," "endolaryngeal resection," "transoral surgery," "CO_2 cordectomy," "laser cordectomy," or "microsurgery," yielding a total of 308 articles. These publications were then further limited to "human" and "English language," resulting in 250 publications, whose titles and abstracts were reviewed to identify those that met the following inclusion criteria: 1) patient population with primary newly diagnosed, biopsy-proven T1 or T2 larynx carcinoma, 2) intervention with radiation or endoscopic resection (with or without laser), 3) outcome measured in terms of voice quality. There were no published prospective randomized controlled trials comparing voice and quality of life (QOL) outcomes for endoscopic resection versus radiation for stage I–II glottic cancer. There were 47 retrospective cohort or retrospective series on radiation or endoscopic resection in the management of T1 to T2 larynx cancer [2–48]. The bibliographies of the articles that met these inclusion criteria were manually checked to ensure no further relevant articles could be identified. Of these articles, a total of three nonrandomized patient or clinician questionnaire-based cohort studies were identified that compared the voice quality and/or QOL after radiation versus endoscopic resection using validated QOL or voice-quality instruments. Studies that used nonvalidated subjective or objective patient/physician rated scales or mainly focused on videolaryngostroboscopy findings were not included for this analysis [5, 8, 21, 30, 40, 49–52].

RESULTS

Outcome Measures. The primary outcome measures for the three retrospective cohort studies were self-reported voice quality, expert voice rating, and QOL [53–55]. One study used several well-validated instruments [53] and other studies used one or more of these instruments [54, 55]:

1. University of Washington Quality of Life Questionnaire (UW-QOL): 17 self-reported questions on QOL in head and neck patients including pain, appearance, activity, recreation, swallowing, chewing, speech, shoulder disability, taste, saliva production, dryness, and employment [56]. Dryness and employment were removed from the revised version (UW-QOL-R) because of poor correlation with the other 10 domains [57]. Scale is 0 to 100 per domain: 100 is totally functional and 0 is completely incapacitated. Total score ranges from 0 up to 1000 points for all 10 domains.

2. Performance Status Scale for Head and Neck (PSS-HN): Three-question clinician-rated instrument on eating in public, understandability of speech, and normalcy of diet score from 0 to 100 [58].

4. Voice Handicap Index (VHI): 30 multiple choice questions of patients' perception of voice quality in functional, physical, and emotional domains [59–66].

5. Vocal Performance Questionnaire (VPQ): 12 physician-reported questions on patient voice quality from normal (score of 12) to severely abnormal (score of 60), used for patients with dysphonia [60, 67].

6. Voice Symptom Score (VoiSS): 44 patient self-reported questions on voice impairment, emotional reaction, and physical symptoms derived from a British-based noncancer population [65, 68].

7. Functional Assessment of Cancer Therapy Head and Neck Questionnaire (FACT-HN): 38 self-reported questions on QOL with nine items specifically on head and neck cancer in four domains—physical, social/family, emotional, and functional [69].

8. Hospital Anxiety and Depression Scale (HADS): seven questions in two subscales (anxiety and depression) [70].

Potential Confounders or Limitations. There may be potential selection bias in recruitment of patients. It is possible that patients who have worse QOL may not be as likely to participate as patients who experience minimal impact and therefore more eager to participate in the surveys. A limitation for all studies is that there is no baseline evaluation before treatment to determine the degree of change after treatment. Also, the length of follow-up from completion of treatment is not clearly stated in all of the studies. A single time point may not capture the temporal characteristics of these outcomes. There is also the potential for recall bias.

Study Designs. All three series were retrospective cohort studies that compared the voice quality and/or QOL after radiation versus endoscopic resection using validated QOL or voice-quality instruments. Sequentially treated patients at single institutions were identified and contacted by telephone for voluntary participation in filling out questionnaires.

Highest Level of Evidence. All three studies showed no significant difference in voice and QOL outcomes between endoscopic resection and radiation for T1–2 larynx cancer using a number of validated instruments. The studies were limited by small and imbalanced sample sizes between the treatment arms and insufficient power to detect subtle changes.

Applicability. These results are applicable for patients with mainly Tis or T1 glottic carcinoma treated with endoscopic resection or primary radiation.

CLINICAL SIGNIFICANCE AND FUTURE RESEARCH

Currently, there are few studies using validated instruments comparing the QOL and voice-quality outcomes between endoscopic resection and radiation for early glottic cancer. The three studies presented here show comparable QOL and voice-quality results for both modalities. A well-designed prospective randomized controlled clinical trial comparing endoscopic resection and radiation for early glottic cancer would require sufficient power and utilize validate QOL and voice-related quality of life instruments. Such a trial would prove to be very challenging to pursue.

THE EVIDENCE CONDENSED: Endoscopic resection versus radiation therapy for stage I–II glottic carcinoma: Impact on voice and quality of life

Reference	Stoeckli, 2001			
Level	3 (retrospective cohort)			
Patients	T1 or T2 larynx cancer (not divided by subsites)			
General methods	Validated EORTC QOL questionnaires			
Response rate	56/62	E (n = 40)	RT (n = 16)	
Time from treatment		NR	NR	

	RESULTS			
Instrument		**E score:** (p value)	**RT score**	(p value)
EORTC QLQ-C30		Scale: 0 = incapacitated; 100 = normal		
	Functional	81–90	82–86	(NS)
	Global health	71.9	73.9	(NS)
Symptom scales		Scale: worse if higher		
	Financial difficulties	19.2	4.8	(<0.05)
	Other items			(NS)
EORTC QLQ H&N 35		Scale: worse if higher		
	Pain	7.7	13.5	(NS)
	Swallowing	5.0	24.4	(<0.05)
	Solid food Other food	6.0	12.7	(NS)
	Social eating	30	56.3	(<0.05)
	Dry mouth	8.3	28.9	(<0.05)
	Teeth Other	10.2	23.4	(NS)
	Senses	9.9	19.4	(NS)
	Speech	32.8	21.4	(NS)
	Social contact	5.0	8.0	(NS)
	Sexuality	25.6	31.1	(NS)
Conclusions	No significant difference between surgery or radiation in global QOL or most head and neck–specific QOL except for solid food swallowing, dry mouth, and tooth problems were worse in RT. Voice quality comparable			

	STUDY DESIGN			
Inclusion criteria	Sequential patients with T1 or T2 larynx cancer (no detail on field of RT or degree of endoscopic surgery). Patients were sent a letter of introduction. Nonresponders followed up with telephone contact. 90% of 62 alive patients returned the questionnaires. No information on patient or pathology characteristics			
Exclusion criteria	Patients lost to follow-up, did not return questionnaire, and refused to participate were excluded. No details on whether salvage was given or status of disease			
Confounders	Potential participation bias (patients who did not participate may have worse QOL)			

EORTC = European Organization for Research and Treatment of Cancer, E = endoscopic resection, RT = radion therapy, UW-QOL-R = revised University of Washington Quality of Life questionnaire (speech and saliva domain slightly modified by author) [54], NS = not significant, VHI = Voice Handicap Index, VoiSS = Voice Symptom Scale, VPQ = Vocal Performance Questionnaire, GRBAS = expert rating of patient recording of a phonetically balanced passage in five domains—grade, rough, breathy, asthenic, and strained, HADS = Hospital Anxiety and Depression Scale, UW-QOL = University of Washington Quality of Life questionnaire, FACT = Functional Assessment of Cancer Therapy head and neck questionnaire, NR = not reported.

THE EVIDENCE CONDENSED: Endoscopic resection versus radiation therapy for stage I–II glottic carcinoma: Impact on voice and quality of life

Reference	Smith, 2003		
Level	3 (retrospective cohort)		
Patients	Patients with Tis and T1 invasive glottic cancer		
General methods	Validated patient questionnaires and institutional hidden cost analysis		
Response rate	55/101	E (n = 30)	RT (n = 10)
Time from treatment		NR	NR

		RESULTS	
Instrument		**E mean Score**	**RT mean score**
UW-QOL-R		Scale: 0 = incapacitated; 100 = complete normal	p values NR
	Pain	100	100
	Appearance	100	98
	Activity	100	100
	Recreation	100	100
	Swallowing	100	100
	Chewing	100	100
	Speech*	91	88
	Shoulder	100	100
	Taste	99	**100**
	Saliva*	99	100
PSS-HN	PSS-HN Eating	100	100
	PSS-HN Speech	98	100
	PSS-HN Diet	100	100
Conclusions	No significant difference between surgery or radiation in both QOL questionnaires. Patients who underwent more than 1 modality (not shown above) had decreased score in most domains. Hidden cost analysis (nonvalidated) also included in the study showed cost of travel, distance, and hours of work missed were higher with RT		

	STUDY DESIGN	
Inclusion criteria	Sequential patients with Tis (22) or T1 (79) glottic cancer treated with surgery (total responders 44: 38 E, 4 hemilaryngectomy, and 1 total laryngectomy) or radiation (66–70.2 Gy at 1.8–2 Gy per fraction). Stages were well balanced between the 2 groups of responders. Subjects invited by telephone to participate in the study. No difference in response rate between arms	
Exclusion criteria	Patients lost to follow-up, died, did not own a phone, or return calls. 23% endoscopic patients who had additional salvage therapy were not excluded. One radiation patient who required endoscopic salvage was not excluded	
Confounders	Potential participation bias (patients who did not participate may have worse QOL)	

EORTC = European Organization for Research and Treatment of Cancer, E = endoscopic resection, RT = radion therapy, UW-QOL-R = revised University of Washington Quality of Life questionnaire (speech and saliva domain slightly modified by author) [54], NS = not significant, VHI = Voice Handicap Index, VoiSS = Voice Symptom Scale, VPQ = Vocal Performance Questionnaire, GRBAS = expert rating of patient recording of a phonetically balanced passage in five domains—grade, rough, breathy, asthenic, and strained, HADS = Hospital Anxiety and Depression Scale, UW-QOL = University of Washington Quality of Life questionnaire, FACT = Functional Assessment of Cancer Therapy head and neck questionnaire, NR = not reported.

THE EVIDENCE CONDENSED: Endoscopic resection versus radiation therapy for stage I–II glottic carcinoma: Impact on voice and quality of life

Reference	Loughran, 2005			
Level	3 (retrospective cohort)			
Patients	T1a glottic cancer with no evidence of tumor recurrence			
General methods	Validated patient and physician questionnaires and expert speech pathologist voice rating			
Response rate	36/55	E (n = 18)	RT (n = 18)	
Time from treatment	>2 y	>2 y	>2 y	

RESULTS

Instrument		E mean score	RT mean score	(p value)
UW-QOL		89.9	89.1	(0.21)
VHI		22.2	25.4	(0.70)
VPQ		20.9	18.5	(0.56)
VoiSS	VoiSS total	27.5	20.4	(0.35)
	VoiSS impairment	16.1	12.6	(0.36)
	VoiSS physical	6.8	6.3	(0.74)
	VoiSS emotional	4.6	1.4	(0.04)
GRBAS		6.6	5.1	(0.29)
HADS		9.1	8.6	(0.78)
FACT	FACT emotion	4.4	4.5	(0.35)
	FACT function	21.3	21.7	(0.75)
	FACT physical	3	2.8	(0.54)
	FACT social	21.9	21.1	(0.27)
	FACT head neck	23.8	23.7	(0.68)
Conclusions	E and RT were similar in voice self-report scores, which were similar to patients with other dysphonia (chronic laryngitis or nodules), except for VoiSS emotional impact was less for RT. VHI <30 (minimal handicap) in both arms. Expert voice rating was no different. QOL decreased slightly after both treatments			

STUDY DESIGN

Inclusion criteria	Sequential patients with Tis or T1a glottic cancer treated by either E or external beam RT. Subjects invited by telephone and if interested sent questionnaires. Completed questionnaires reviewed in a clinic appointment. Patients consented to audio recording for expert rating of voice using GRBAS
Exclusion criteria	Patients who received salvage surgery after radiation were excluded
Confounders	Potential participation bias (patients who did not participate may have worse QOL)

EORTC = European Organization for Research and Treatment of Cancer, E = endoscopic resection, RT = radion therapy, UW-QOL-R = revised University of Washington Quality of Life questionnaire (speech and saliva domain slightly modified by author) [54], NS = not significant, VHI = Voice Handicap Index, VoiSS = Voice Symptom Scale, VPQ = Vocal Performance Questionnaire, GRBAS = expert rating of patient recording of a phonetically balanced passage in five domains—grade, rough, breathy, asthenic, and strained, HADS = Hospital Anxiety and Depression Scale, UW-QOL = University of Washington Quality of Life questionnaire, FACT = Functional Assessment of Cancer Therapy head and neck questionnaire, NR = not reported.

REFERENCES

1. Haynes RB, et al. Optimal search strategies for retrieving scientifically strong studies of treatment from Medline: analytical survey. BMJ 2005;330(7501):1179.

2. Akine Y, et al. Radiotherapy of T1 glottic cancer with 6 MeV X rays. Int J Radiat Oncol Biol Phys 1991;20(6): 1215–1218.

3. Ansarin M, et al. Endoscopic CO2 laser surgery for early glottic cancer in patients who are candidates for radiotherapy: results of a prospective nonrandomized study. Head Neck 2006;28(2):121–125.

4. Barton MB, et al. The effect of treatment time and treatment interruption on tumour control following radical radiotherapy of laryngeal cancer. Radiother Oncol 1992; 23(3):137–143.

5. Brandenburg JH. Laser cordotomy versus radiotherapy: an objective cost analysis. Ann Otol Rhinol Laryngol 2001;110(4):312–318.

6. Cellai E, et al. Radical radiotherapy for early glottic cancer: results in a series of 1087 patients from two Italian radiation oncology centers. I. The case of T1N0 disease. Int J Radiat Oncol Biol Phys 2005;63(5):1378–1386.

7. Csanady M, Czigner J, Savay L. Endolaryngeal CO2 laser microsurgery of early vocal cord cancer. A retrospective study. Adv Otorhinolaryngol 1995;49:219–221.

8. Delsupehe KG, et al. Voice quality after narrow-margin laser cordectomy compared with laryngeal irradiation. Otolaryngol Head Neck Surg 1999;121(5):528–533.

9. Eckel HE. Local recurrences following transoral laser surgery for early glottic carcinoma: frequency, management, and outcome. Ann Otol Rhinol Laryngol 2001; 110(1):7–15.

10. Fein DA, et al. T1-T2 squamous cell carcinoma of the glottic larynx treated with radiotherapy: a multivariate analysis of variables potentially influencing local control. Int J Radiat Oncol Biol Phys 1993;25(4):605–611.

11. Franchin G, et al. Radiotherapy for patients with early-stage glottic carcinoma: univariate and multivariate analyses in a group of consecutive, unselected patients. Cancer 2003;98(4):765–772.

12. Frata P, et al. Radical radiotherapy for early glottic cancer: results in a series of 1087 patients from two Italian radiation oncology centers. II. The case of T2N0 disease. Int J Radiat Oncol Biol Phys 2005;63(5):1387–1394.

13. Gallo A, et al. CO2 laser cordectomy for early-stage glottic carcinoma: a long-term follow-up of 156 cases. Laryngoscope 2002;112(2):370–374.

14. Garden AS, et al. Results of radiotherapy for T2N0 glottic carcinoma: does the "2" stand for twice-daily treatment? Int J Radiat Oncol Biol Phys 2003;55(2):322–328.

15. Harrison LB, et al. Prospective computer-assisted voice analysis for patients with early stage glottic cancer: a preliminary report of the functional result of laryngeal irradiation. Int J Radiat Oncol Biol Phys 1990;19(1):123–127.

16. Harwood AR, et al. Radiotherapy of early glottic cancer—I. Int J Radiat Oncol Biol Phys 1979;5(4):473–476.

17. Harwood AR, Tierie A. Radiotherapy of early glottic cancer—II. Int J Radiat Oncol Biol Phys 1979;5(4):477–482.

18. Hendrickson FR. Radiation therapy treatment of larynx cancers. Cancer 1985;55(9 Suppl):2058–2061.

19. Hirano M, Hirade Y, Kawasaki H. Vocal function following carbon dioxide laser surgery for glottic carcinoma. Ann Otol Rhinol Laryngol 1985;94(3):232–235.

20. Howell-Burke D, et al. T2 glottic cancer. Recurrence, salvage, and survival after definitive radiotherapy. Arch Otolaryngol Head Neck Surg 1990;116(7):830–835.

21. Jones AS, et al. The treatment of early laryngeal cancers (T1-T2 N0): surgery or irradiation? Head Neck 2004;26(2): 127–135.

22. Karim AB, et al. Heterogeneity of stage II glottic carcinoma and its therapeutic implications. Int J Radiat Oncol Biol Phys 1987;13(3):313–317.

23. Keilmann A, et al. Vocal function following laser and conventional surgery of small malignant vocal fold tumours. J Laryngol Otol 1996;110(12):1138–1141.

24. Kelly MD, et al. Definitive radiotherapy in the management of stage I and II carcinomas of the glottis. Ann Otol Rhinol Laryngol 1989;98(3):235–239.

25. Klintenberg C, et al. Primary radiotherapy of T1 and T2 glottic carcinoma—analysis of treatment results and prognostic factors in 223 patients. Acta Oncol 1996;35(Suppl 8): 81–86.

26. Krespi YP, Meltzer CJ. Laser surgery for vocal cord carcinoma involving the anterior commissure. Ann Otol Rhinol Laryngol 1989;98(2):105–109.

27. Le QT, et al. Influence of fraction size, total dose, and overall time on local control of T1-T2 glottic carcinoma. Int J Radiat Oncol Biol Phys 1997;39(1):115–126.

28. Lustig RA, et al. The Patterns of Care Outcome Studies: results of the national practice in carcinoma of the larynx. Int J Radiat Oncol Biol Phys 1984;10(12):2357–2362.

29. Maurizi M, et al. Laser carbon dioxide cordectomy versus open surgery in the treatment of glottic carcinoma: our results. Otolaryngol Head Neck Surg 2005;132(6):857–861.

30. McGuirt WF, et al. Comparative voice results after laser resection or irradiation of T1 vocal cord carcinoma. Arch Otolaryngol Head Neck Surg 1994;120(9):951–955.

31. Medini E, et al. Radiation therapy in early carcinoma of the glottic larynx T1N0M0. Int J Radiat Oncol Biol Phys 1996;36(5):1211–1213.

32. Mendenhall WM, et al. T1-T2N0 squamous cell carcinoma of the glottic larynx treated with radiation therapy. J Clin Oncol 2001;19(20):4029–4036.

33. Motta G, et al. T1-T2-T3 glottic tumors: fifteen years experience with CO2 laser. Acta Otolaryngol Suppl 1997;527: 155–159.

34. Olszewski SJ, et al. The influence of field size, treatment modality, commissure involvement and histology in the treatment of early vocal cord cancer with irradiation. Int J Radiat Oncol Biol Phys 1985;11(7):1333–1337.

35. Ossoff RH, Sisson GA, Shapshay SM. Endoscopic management of selected early vocal cord carcinoma. Ann Otol Rhinol Laryngol 1985;94(6 Pt 1):560–564.

36. Pellitteri PK, et al. Radiotherapy. The mainstay in the treatment of early glottic carcinoma. Arch Otolaryngol Head Neck Surg 1991;117(3):297–301.

37. Peretti G, et al. Endoscopic CO2 laser excision for tis, T1, and T2 glottic carcinomas: cure rate and prognostic factors. Otolaryngol Head Neck Surg 2000;123(1 Pt 1): 124–131.

38. Pradhan SA, et al. Transoral laser surgery for early glottic cancers. Arch Otolaryngol Head Neck Surg 2003;129(6):623–625.

39. Rebeiz EE, et al. Preliminary clinical results of window partial laryngectomy: a combined endoscopic and open technique. Ann Otol Rhinol Laryngol 2000;109(2):123–127.

40. Rosier JF, et al. Comparison of external radiotherapy, laser microsurgery and partial laryngectomy for the treatment of T1N0M0 glottic carcinomas: a retrospective evaluation. Radiother Oncol 1998;48(2):175–183.

41. Schwaab G, et al. Surgical salvage treatment of T1/T2 glottic carcinoma after failure of radiotherapy. Am J Surg 1994;168(5):474–475.

42. Sigston E, et al. Early-stage glottic cancer: oncological results and margins in laser cordectomy. Arch Otolaryngol Head Neck Surg 2006;132(2):147–152.

43. Smith JC, Johnson JT, Myers EN. Management and outcome of early glottic carcinoma. Otolaryngol Head Neck Surg 2002;126(4):356–364.

44. Spector JG, et al. Stage I (T1 N0 M0) squamous cell carcinoma of the laryngeal glottis: therapeutic results and voice preservation. Head Neck 1999;21(8):707–717.

45. Steiner W. Results of curative laser microsurgery of laryngeal carcinomas. Am J Otolaryngol 1993;14(2):116–121.

46. Van den Bogaert W, Ostyn F, van der Schueren E. The significance of extension and impaired mobility in cancer of the vocal cord. Int J Radiat Oncol Biol Phys 1983;9(2):181–184.

47. Verdonck-de Leeuw IM, et al. Multidimensional assessment of voice characteristics after radiotherapy for early glottic cancer. Laryngoscope 1999;109(2 Pt 1):241–248.

48. Verdonck-de Leeuw IM, et al. Consequences of voice impairment in daily life for patients following radiotherapy for early glottic cancer: voice quality, vocal function, and vocal performance. Int J Radiat Oncol Biol Phys 1999;44(5):1071–1078.

49. Epstein BE, et al. Stage T1 glottic carcinoma: results of radiation therapy or laser excision. Radiology 1990;175(2):567–570.

50. Krengli M, et al. Voice quality after treatment for T1a glottic carcinoma—radiotherapy versus laser cordectomy. Acta Oncol 2004;43(3):284–289.

51. Rydell R, et al. Voice evaluation before and after laser excision vs. radiotherapy of T1A glottic carcinoma. Acta Otolaryngol 1995;115(4):560–565.

52. Tamura E, et al. Voice quality after laser surgery or radiotherapy for T1a glottic carcinoma. Laryngoscope 2003;113(5):910–914.

53. Loughran S, et al. Quality of life and voice following endoscopic resection or radiotherapy for early glottic cancer. Clin Otolaryngol 2005;30(1):42–47.

54. Smith JC, et al. Quality of life, functional outcome, and costs of early glottic cancer. Laryngoscope 2003;113(1):68–76.

55. Stoeckli SJ, et al. Quality of life after treatment for early laryngeal carcinoma. Eur Arch Otorhinolaryngol 2001;258(2):96–99.

56. Hassan SJ, Weymuller EA Jr. Assessment of quality of life in head and neck cancer patients. Head Neck 1993;15(6):485–496.

57. Weymuller EA, et al. Quality of life in patients with head and neck cancer: lessons learned from 549 prospectively evaluated patients. Arch Otolaryngol Head Neck Surg 2000;126(3):329–335; discussion 335–336.

58. List MA, et al. The Performance Status Scale for Head and Neck Cancer Patients and the Functional Assessment of Cancer Therapy-Head and Neck Scale. A study of utility and validity. Cancer 1996;77(11):2294–2301.

59. Bogaardt HC, et al. Validation of the Voice Handicap Index Using Rasch Analysis. J Voice 2006;Feb 24.

60. Deary IJ, et al. Short, self-report voice symptom scales: psychometric characteristics of the voice handicap index-10 and the vocal performance questionnaire. Otolaryngol Head Neck Surg 2004;131(3):232–235.

61. Hsiung MW, Pai L, Wang HW. Correlation between voice handicap index and voice laboratory measurements in dysphonic patients. Eur Arch Otorhinolaryngol 2002;259(2):97–99.

62. Kandogan T, Sanal A. Quality of life, functional outcome, and voice handicap index in partial laryngectomy patients for early glottic cancer. BMC Ear Nose Throat Disord 2005;5(1):3.

63. Kandogan T, Sanal A. Quality of life, functional outcome, and voice handicap index in partial laryngectomy patients for early glottic cancer. BMC Ear Nose Throat Disord 2006;6:1.

64. Portone CR, et al. Correlation of the Voice Handicap Index (VHI) and the Voice-Related Quality of Life Measure (V-RQOL). J Voice 2006.

65. Wilson JA, et al. The Voice Symptom Scale (VoiSS) and the Vocal Handicap Index (VHI): a comparison of structure and content. Clin Otolaryngol Allied Sci 2004;29(2):169–174.

66. Woisard V, et al. The Voice Handicap Index: correlation between subjective patient response and quantitative assessment of voice. J Voice 2006.

67. Carding PN, Horsley IA, Docherty GJ. The effectiveness of voice therapy for patients with non-organic dysphonia. Clin Otolaryngol Allied Sci 1998;23(4):310–318.

68. Deary IJ, et al. VoiSS: a patient-derived Voice Symptom Scale. J Psychosom Res 2003;54(5):483–489.

69. D'Antonio LL, et al. Quality of life and functional status measures in patients with head and neck cancer. Arch Otolaryngol Head Neck Surg 1996;122(5):482–487.

70. Zigmond AS, Snaith RP. The hospital anxiety and depression scale. Acta Psychiatr Scand 1983;67(6):361–370.

30 Laryngeal Squamous Cell Carcinoma: Early-Stage Disease

Open partial laryngectomy versus endoscopic laryngectomy for T1–2 glottic carcinoma: Impact on recurrence, salvage surgeries, and survival

Ramon Franco and Jennifer J. Shin

METHODS

A computerized Ovid search of MEDLINE from 1966 to July 2006 was performed. The subject headings "laryngectomy," "laser," "laryngeal cancer," and "endoscopic" were exploded and the resulting articles were cross-referenced. These articles were then reviewed to identify those that met the following inclusion criteria: 1) patient population with primary laryngeal (glottal) carcinoma, 2) intervention with open partial laryngectomy versus endoscopic laryngectomy, 3) outcome measured in terms of recurrence, salvage surgeries, and survival. Case reports or manuscripts in which results for either endoscopic laryngectomy alone or partial laryngectomy alone were reported, without comparative data, were also excluded. The bibliographies of the articles meeting these inclusion criteria were manually checked to ensure no further relevant articles could be identified. This process yielded just three retrospective articles [1–3].

RESULTS

Outcome Measures. Outcome measures included survival (disease-specific and disease-free), local recurrence, locoregional nodal metastases, and measures of salvage treatment. The number of patients undergoing salvage surgery based on the primary surgical treatment chosen (endoscopic versus open surgery), as well as what fraction of them were successfully salvaged or inoperable were reported.

Potential Confounders. Potential confounders included any disease factors or concomitant treatment that could alter responses: initial stage of the primary lesion, extent of neck disease, type (if any) of neck dissection, radiation therapy, type/extent of partial laryngectomy, experience of the operating surgeon. In any study comparing treatment modalities, there may be a bias toward including patients with more disease burden in one group because it is considered the "standard" treatment regimen. In this case, patients who were treated with open procedures may have had more disease burden than those who were chosen for endoscopic treatment. The variety of open (cordectomy, frontolateral laryngectomy, horizontal glottic laryngectomy) and endoscopic techniques (cordectomy, glottectomy, cordo-commissurectomy) introduces more bias because disease location, burden, and surgeon comfort all may have influenced who would undergo which procedure. It is true that extent of disease should dictate the procedure being performed, but it also makes comparisons very tricky because of the inherent bias the choice of procedure imposes.

Study Designs. All three studies were retrospective studies based on chart reviews. None were case control studies. The largest study [1] considered 573 partial laryngectomies performed for T1a or small T2 glottic disease. Of these, 315 were open and 258 were endoscopic. The criteria that led surgeons to choose the endoscopic approach versus the open approach were not reported. There were 325 T1a glottic lesions, 185 T1b, and 63 T2 lesions. Because of the variety of procedures used to treat the patients (both open and endoscopic), this study attempted to compare in a head-to-head manner the three main open and endoscopic techniques: 1) external cordectomy versus laser endoscopic cordectomy, 2) frontolateral partial laryngectomy versus laser endoscopic cordo-commissurectomy, and 3) horizontal glottectomy versus laser endoscopic glottectomy. In group 1, 388 surgeries were performed (196 external cordectomies for T1a lesions, 129 laser cordectomies for T1a lesions, and 63 widened laser cordectomies for T2 lesions.) In group 2, 147 procedures were performed (110 external frontolateral partial laryngectomies and 37 laser endoscopic cordo-commissurectomies). All of these patients were considered to have T1 disease. In group 3, 38 procedures were performed (9 external horizontal glottectomies and 29 laser glottectomies). All patients were also considered to have T1 disease. The mismatch in number between the open and laser groups in groups 2 and 3 may be attributable to recruitment bias from the location of disease or surgeon preference.

The next largest study [2] looked at 198 patients treated via open surgery (66 patients) versus laser cordectomy (132 patients). Assignment to open or endoscopic groups was random. There were 66 patients treated by open resection (60 were T1 and 6 were T2). In the endoscopic group (132 patients), 118 were considered to have T1 disease whereas 14 were classified as having T2 lesions. The fact that the patients were randomly selected improves this study's design and decreases the selection bias.

The smallest study [3] reviewed 83 patients treated by simple or enlarged open cordectomy (30 patients, 22 T1a, 8 T2), horizontal glottectomy (22 patients, 3 T1a, 10 T1b, 9 T2), or endoscopic laser resection (31 patients, 23 T1a, 4 T1b, 4 T2). The T stage breakdown included 48 T1a, 14 T1b, and 21 selected cases of T2 with impaired vocal fold mobility. The criteria that led surgeons to choose the endoscopic approach versus the open approach were not reported. As evidenced by the lower numbers of T2 lesions (4 for the laser group versus 8 for open cordectomy and 9 for the open horizontal glottectomy) there seems to be a bias toward lower disease burden (lower T stage) for those patients who underwent laser endoscopic procedures.

None of these articles reported an *a priori* power calculation. Follow-up time was long, ranging from 2 to 16 years after surgery. In addition, patients were followed at regular intervals to evaluate for evidence of recurrences. Those patients who developed recurrences underwent salvage surgery that consisted of endoscopic resections, radiation therapy, total laryngectomy, or a combination of the preceding options. The actual protocol varied by study.

Highest Level of Evidence. There were three retrospective reviews that compared results with open versus endoscopic partial laryngectomy. Results must be considered with the limitations of the retrospective study in mind.

First survival was compared. Among the eight direct comparisons made in the three studies, there were no significant differences between open versus endoscopic techniques in seven comparisons. In one study, however, they did report that disease-specific survival was significantly better with endoscopic cordectomy than with external cordectomy (94% versus 84%, p = 0.04).

Second, local recurrence was compared. There was a trend toward fewer recurrences with endoscopic management in some cases (e.g., endoscopic versus external cordectomy for T1a disease [2]) but the opposite trend existed in other comparisons (e.g., endoscopic versus open cordectomy for T2 disease [3]). Overall, no statistically significant differences were reported in any of the studies.

Third, neck metastases were reported. These were delayed cervical neck metastases that were discovered during patient follow-up examinations. There were very few cases of cervical disease, just 1%–2% in all three studies. Again, no significant differences were reported.

Fourth, salvage therapy was compared. There seemed to be better salvage rates in the endoscopic group versus the open group (de Campora, laser 70.8% versus 53.5% open; Maurizi, laser 63% versus 44% open; Puxeddu, laser 100% versus 29% open) but statistical analyses were not performed.

Fifth, no formal statistical comparisons were made between the lengths of stay after laser endoscopic procedures versus open procedures. Maurizi et al. was the only study to not mention length of stay. In the de Campora study, endoscopic cordectomy required 1–3 days whereas external cordectomy required 4–10 days in the hospital. Endoscopic cordo-commissurectomy patients stayed an average of 1.3 days whereas the frontolateral partial laryngectomy patients required 7 days. The endoscopic glottectomy patients were in the hospital a mean of 3 days whereas the horizontal glottectomy patients had a 12-day stay (mean). In the Puxeddu study, endoscopic cordectomy required 2.1 days, whereas open cordectomy and horizontal glottectomy required an average of 7.3 days and 9.8 days, respectively.

Applicability. These results are applicable to patients with T1 or T2 glottic carcinoma, with the caveats of potential confounders and study design.

Morbidity. Comparison of morbidity and postoperative complications revealed less for those patients undergoing endoscopic treatment in the de Campora and Puxeddu studies. This was not reported in the Maurizi study.

CLINICAL SIGNIFICANCE AND FUTURE RESEARCH

There were three retrospective comparative trials that compared survival, local recurrence, neck metastases, salvage therapy, and hospital stay with open partial versus endoscopic laryngectomy for the treatment of glottic carcinoma. Overall, the vast majority of results showed no significant difference between endoscopic and open resection, although two comparisons showed a difference between groups (survival and salvage better in the endoscopic group [2]). These results must be viewed with the limitations of retrospective studies and sample size in mind. As discussed in more detail above, all retrospective studies may be especially subject to selection bias. Such bias results when subjects in two compared groups are not similar at the outset; for example, patients who received endoscopic intervention may have been more likely to have lesser disease and thus a better prognosis, which would bias toward better results with endoscopic surgery. Such potential bias is inherent to the retrospective study design.

If one were to design a prospective study to compare these two approaches, it would ideally focus on specific subsites and stages of disease to allow for the most direct comparison; a comparison of patients with a T1 epiglottic carcinoma (who could be treated with epiglottectomy or supraglottic horizontal laryngectomy) to patients with a T3 false cord carcinoma extending into the glottis (who could be treated with supracricoid laryngectomy) is somewhat irrelevant, but a focused study of endoscopic versus open intervention for the former group alone or the latter group alone would be very useful. It may be challenging to perform a prospective study with an adequate sample size, because in order to have a 90% power to detect a 10% difference in survival rate (i.e., 85% versus 95%, based on the retrospective data described here), a total of 416 patients would need to complete the study. Such numbers would likely prove difficult to recruit, especially given the large number of patients who choose radiation as a preferential treatment for early-stage laryngeal carcinoma.

The retrospective data published to date suggest that there may be advantages to the endoscopic approach over the open approach, and this viewpoint has been championed in Europe by Steiner and Eckel. There is, however, much controversy with respect to endoscopic treatment of T2 glottic carcinoma. There is some evidence that suggests that supracricoid laryngectomy may result in higher local control rates in T2 carcinoma, but at present there are no head to head trials of endoscopic versus this type of open partial laryngectomy. None of the comparative data discussed in this systematic review included any patients who underwent supracricoid laryngectomy. Ideally, future prospective trials will help address these controversial issues further.

Reference	de Campora, 2001
Level (design)	3b (retrospective)
Sample size	573 operations: 196 external cordectomies, 129 laser cordectomies, 63 widened laser cordectomies, 110 external frontolateral partial laryngectomies, 37 laser endoscopic cordo-commissurectomies, 9 external horizontal glottectomies, 29 laser glottectomies

OUTCOMES

	Endoscopic cordectomy	External cordectomy	p Value	Endoscopic cordo-commissurectomy	Frontolateral partial laryngectomy	p Value	Endoscopic glottectomy	Horizontal glottectomy	p Value
Survival	T1a: 122/129 (95%) T2: 59/63 (94%)	T1a: 184/196 (94%) at 2 y	NR	36/37 (97%)	101/110 (92%)	NR	27/29 (93%) at 25 mo	8/9 (88%) at 29 mo	NR
Local recurrence	T1a: 23/129 (18%) T2: 10/63 (16%)	T1a: 24/196 (12%)	NR	5/37 (14%)	11/110 (10%)	NR	6/29 (21%)	2/9 (24%)	NR
Neck metastases	T1a: 1/129 (<1%) T2: 1/63 (2%)	4/196 (2%)	NR	None	2/110 (2%)	NR	None	None	NR
Salvage therapy	T1a: 17/23 (73.9%) successful salvage 17/23 supracricoid 6/23 XRT alone 1/1 neck dissection with postoperative XRT T2: 6/10 (60%) successful salvage 5/10 total laryngectomy with postoperative XRT 5/10 XRT alone 1/1 neck dissection with postoperative XRT	14/24 (62.5%) successful salvage 18/24 total laryngectomy with postoperative XRT 6/24 XRT alone 2/4 neck dissection 2/4 neck dissection with postoperative XRT	NR	4/5 (80%) successful salvage 3/5 total laryngectomy with postoperative XRT 2/5 XRT alone	4/11 (36.3%) successful salvage 3 patients had too extensive disease to salvage 7/11 total laryngectomy with postoperative XRT 1/11 XRT alone	NR	4/6 (66.6%) successful salvage 4/6 total laryngectomy with postoperative XRT 2/6 XRT alone	1/2 (50%) successful salvage 1/2 total laryngectomy with postoperative XRT 1/2 too extensive spread to have salvage	NR
Hospital stay	1–3 d	6 d (range 4–10) Add 2 d for those with tracheotomy	NR	1.3 d (maximum of 4)	7 d	NR	3 d	12 d	NR

STUDY DESIGN

Inclusion criteria	Cordectomy or widened cordectomy for the treatment of T1a and T2 (limited involvement of the ventricle floor) glottic tumors
Exclusion criteria	T3 or T4
Staging details	Preoperative classification of the tumor was performed by endoscopy (direct laryngoscopy, strobolaryngoscopy) in the case of T1a and by endoscopy and CT/NMR in the case of T2
Decision for endoscopic vs open surgery	Factors NR
Endoscopic surgery details	NR
Open partial laryngectomy details	NR
Extent of partial laryngectomy	Cordectomy, frontolateral, horizontal glottectomy
Age	NR
Consecutive patients?	NR
Morbidity/ complications	More frequent in open vs endoscopic. Open: 35% subQ emphysema, 9% prelaryngeal infection, 9% anterior webs, 2% dysphagia from hypopharyngeal hematoma. Endoscopic: 6% anterior webs

NR = not reported, CT = computed tomography, NMR = nuclear magnetic resonance.

Reference	Maurizi, 2005		
Level (design)	3b (retrospective)		
Sample size	198 cases (132 endoscopic, 66 open partial)		

OUTCOMES

	Endoscopic cordectomy	External cordectomy	p Value
Survival	DSS 94% (5 y)	DSS 84% (5 y)	0.04
	DFS 85% (5 y)	DFS 77% (5 y)	NS
Local recurrence	T1a 13/118 (11%)	T1a 16/60 (27%)	NS
	T2 3/14 (21%)	T2 2/6 (33%)	NS
Neck metastases	3/132 (2%)	5/66 (8%)	NR
Salvage therapy	16 cases	18 cases	NR
	10/16 (63%) successful salvage	8/18 (44%) successful salvage	NR
	1/16 (6%) inoperable	4/18 (22%) inoperable	<0.05
Hospital stay	NR	NR	NR

STUDY DESIGN

Inclusion criteria	Consecutive, untreated primary glottic squamous cell carcinoma, T1a or T2 without involvement of anterior commissure, underwent cordectomy
Exclusion criteria	T3 or T4
Staging details	Preoperative staging with indirect laryngoscopy, videolaryngoscopy, strobolaryngoscopy, and phoniatric evaluation in T1a cases and by the same endoscopy with imaging (CT/MR) in T1b and T2 cases. All patients were restaged retrospectively according to 1997 TNM system
Decision for endoscopic vs open surgery	"The assignation to surgical procedure of the patients was random." Endoscopic group: 118 patients were cT1a N0 M0, 14 cT2 N0 M0. External group: 60 cT1a N0 M0, 6 cT2 N0 M0
Endoscopic surgery details	Transoral surgery was performed with a CO_2 laser. The excised tissue was whole-mounted on a slide and oriented, with the anterior and medial margins marked. If the frozen sections revealed a positive margin, resections were extended
Open partial laryngectomy details	External cordectomy was performed through a laryngofissure as described by Buck (a vertical incision is created through the thyroid cartilage off of midline on the contralateral side to gain access to the larynx. The diseased vocal fold is removed under direct visualization)
Extent of partial laryngectomy	Frontolateral
Age	Average 63 y (range, 34–88 y)
Consecutive patients?	Yes
Morbidity/complications	Anterior commissure involvement was not a factor in achieving locoregional control ($p > 0.05$)

NR = not reported, NS = not significant, DSS = disease specific survival, DFS = disease-free survival, CT = computed tomography, MR = magnetic resonance, TNM = Tumor-Node-Metastasis.

Reference	Puxeddu, 2000			
Level (design)	3b (retrospective)			
Sample size	83 cases (31 endoscopic, 30 open cordectomy, 22 horizontal glottectomy)			

OUTCOMES

	Endoscopic cordectomy	Open cordectomy	Horizontal glottectomy	p value
Survival	DSS 92% (3 y) DFS 88% (3 y)	DSS 93% (3 y) DFS 86% (3 y)	DSS 90% (3 y) DFS 85% (3 y)	NR
Local recurrence	T1a 1/23 (4%) T1b 1/4 (25%) T2 1/4 (25%)	T1a 3/22 (14%) None treated T2 1/8 (13%)	T1a 1/3 (33%) T1b 1/10 (10%) T2 1/9 (11%)	NR
Neck metastases	0/31 (0%)	Open procedures 1/52 (2%)		NR
Salvage therapy	3 cases 3/3 (100%) successful salvage	7 cases 2/7 (29%) successful salvage		NR
Hospital stay	2.1 d 0 feeding tube 0 tracheotomy	7.3 d 0 feeding tube 0 tracheotomy	9.8 d 7–23 d to remove feeding tube, 6–27 d to decannulate	NR

STUDY DESIGN

Inclusion criteria	Glottic cancer, T1 or T2
Exclusion criteria	T3 or T4, massive involvement of anterior commissure
Staging details	Preoperative staging with preoperative and intraoperative endoscopic evaluation in the endoscopic group. CT scanning was added preoperatively in cases in which tumor involved the anterior commissure or for clinically stage II tumors
Decision for endoscopic vs open surgery	Not specified
Endoscopic surgery details	Transoral surgery was performed with the aid of the CO_2 laser. 5 types of procedures were performed depending on the depth of invasion: 1) superficial cordectomy—up to vocal ligament (5 patients), 2) partial cordectomy—removal of medial vocalis (15 patients), 3) total cordectomy—not involving inner perichondrium (4 patients), 4) total cordectomy with inner perichondrium (3 patients), 5)extended cordectomy—false vocal fold or contralateral true vocal fold (4 patients)
Open partial laryngectomy details	Horizontal glottectomy involves creating 2 horizontal incisions, the lower through the cricothyroid membrane, and the upper one across the wings of the thyroid. The gap is then closed by approximating the cricoid to the thyroid remnants (cricothyropexy). The entire region of the glottis and its cartilaginous elements are removed
Extent of partial laryngectomy	Cordectomy, horizontal glottectomy
Age	Mean age 60.6 y (range, 42–80 y)
Consecutive patients?	Not specified
Morbidity/complications	Mild aspiration, subQ emphysema, minor stenosis not affecting breathing

NR = not reported, NS = not significant, DSS = disease specific survival, DFS = disease-free survival, CT = computed tomography, MR = magnetic resonance, TNM = Tumor-Node-Metastasis.

REFERENCES

1. de Campora E, Radici M, de Campora L. External versus endoscopic approach in the surgical treatment of glottic cancer. Eur Arch Otorhinolaryngol 2001;258(10):533–536.
2. Maurizi M, et al. Laser carbon dioxide cordectomy versus open surgery in the treatment of glottic carcinoma: our results. Otolaryngol Head Neck Surg 2005;132(6):857–861.
3. Puxeddu R, et al. Surgical therapy of T1 and selected cases of T2 glottic carcinoma: cordectomy, horizontal glottectomy and CO2 laser endoscopic resection. Tumori 2000; 86(4):277–282.

30 Laryngeal Squamous Cell Carcinoma: Early-Stage Disease

30.C.

Open partial laryngectomy with/without radiation therapy versus radiation therapy alone for T1–2 N0 supraglottic laryngeal carcinoma: Impact on survival and recurrence

Yen-Lin Chen and Kian Ang

METHODS

A computerized PubMed search of MEDLINE 1966–2005 was performed. First, articles mapping to the terms "supraglottis" or "supraglottic larynx" were cross-referenced with those mapping to the terms "cancer" or "squamous cell carcinoma." Second, articles mapping to the terms "supraglottic laryngectomy," "hemilaryngectomy," or "partial laryngectomy" were obtained. Third, publications mapping to the terms "radiotherapy" or "external beam radiation" were obtained. These three searches were cross-referenced, yielding 106 articles on partial laryngectomy and/or radiation for supraglottic cancer. These articles were then reviewed to identify those that met the following inclusion criteria: 1) patient population with newly diagnosed, previously untreated T1–2 supraglottic larynx squamous cell carcinoma, 2) intervention with open partial laryngectomy (hemilaryngectomy, supraglottic laryngectomy, or supracricoid laryngectomy) with or without postoperative radiation versus definitive external beam radiation, 3) outcome measured in terms of local control and survival. Articles on treatment of recurrent supraglottic cancer after radiation failure or surgical failure were excluded. Articles in which the majority of patients had T3, T4, N+, or M+ disease, near-total laryngectomy, total laryngectomy, nonsquamous histology, endoscopic resection, or single modality only were excluded for this analysis [1–49]. Articles that used nonstandard staging were also excluded. Articles that had n<20 per treatment modality, pre-partial laryngectomy radiation, unclear stage separation for analysis, or chemotherapy were also excluded [22, 40, 50–53]. The bibliographies of the articles that met these inclusion criteria were manually checked to ensure no further relevant articles could be identified. This process yielded a total of three articles with retrospective cohort comparisons between open partial laryngectomy versus primary radiation for early supraglottic cancer [54–56].

RESULTS

Outcome Measures. The outcome measures for the three retrospective cohort studies were initial local control, ultimate local control after salvage therapy, voice preservation, and survival (overall or disease-specific).

Potential Confounders. All three studies were single institution, retrospective analyses of consecutive patients treated for supraglottic larynx cancer. Patients were not balanced in terms of comorbidities, smoking, age, pathologic staging, performance status, or other risk factors that may have impacted outcome except in one study [56]. In one study [55], downstaging of the surgical cohort may have been a potential confounder; patients with cN0 disease who were found to have pN+ disease requiring postoperative radiation were excluded from analysis. This exclusion may have resulted in a bias toward more favorable results in the surgery cohort. However, the studies that included patients receiving postoperative radiation after surgery may have masked potential inadequacy of surgery in the primary management of patients who may have had occult nodal disease [54, 56].

Study Designs. All three studies were single institutional retrospective cohort studies of patients with supraglottic larynx cancer. There was significant variation in the radiation therapy (RT) delivered (daily versus b.i.d. radiation, ^{60}Co up to 17 MV, with or without elective neck or low anterior neck radiation). There was also significant variation in the degree of partial laryngectomy performed. Patient treatment with conservative surgery depended on a variety of considerations including anatomic location as well as the medical condition. However, no objective guidelines for pulmonary function were reported in the studies. Both RT and surgery policies also changed over time.

Highest Level of Evidence. These three retrospective nonrandomized, uncontrolled cohort studies provided limited level 3 evidence that open partial laryngectomy and radiation yield comparable ultimate local control, voice preservation, and five-year survival rates. These studies were, however, limited by the small number of patients in subgroups, as well as potential selection biases favoring pathologic N0, healthier, and younger patients for surgical resection. Thus, there is insufficient definitive evidence to show whether radiation or open partial laryngectomy endoscopic surgery is better for patients with early supraglottic cancer.

Applicability. These results are applicable for patients with T1–2 N0 supraglottic carcinoma treated with partial laryngectomy or primary radiation.

Morbidity/Complications. Radiation had a different set of acute reactions (mucositis, radiation dermatitis, or dry mouth) compared with surgery (broncho-aspiration). Chondronecrosis (from RT) or severe aspiration (from partial laryngectomy) were both unusual events ranging from 0% to 4% in all three studies. Radiotherapy patients who needed nonlaryngectomy salvage surgery had more frequent and severe complications, with wound infection being the most common reason for prolonged hospitalization [56]. The complication rate was also related to the extent of conservative surgery [55]. Cricohyoidopexy or extended supraglottic laryngectomy both resulted in more swallowing, respiration, and phonation problems compared with horizontal supraglottic laryngectomy [55]. One study reported higher rates of morbidity when radiation was given pre- or postsurgery [54], with two fatal carotid blowouts (the stage or burden of neck disease for these two patients was not reported).

CLINICAL SIGNIFICANCE AND FUTURE RESEARCH

Well-designed prospective randomized controlled clinical trials would be useful to guide decision making for patients with early supraglottic cancer. Because there are insufficient data to suggest whether open partial laryngectomy or radiation is better for survival or local control of early supraglottic carcinoma, management decisions must be individualized as to patient preference, suitability for surgery versus radiation, comorbidities, and physician expertise. Unfortunately, these studies did not compare quality of life or quality of voice between the two approaches using validated instruments. Prospective studies addressing the impact of supraglottic laryngectomy versus radiation should address quality of life and quality of voice to help guide treatment decisions, especially if there is no local control or survival difference found.

Reference	Weems, 1987*	
Level (design)	3 (retrospective comparative)	
Study population	19 T1 N0 and 32 T2 N0	
RT	RT n = 27	
Surgery	TL or PL n = 24	

OUTCOME MEASURES

Initial LC	T1 N0	T2 N0
RT	90%	76%
Surgery ± RT	100%	87%
p Value	0.526	0.392
Ultimate LC after salvage	**T1 N0**	**T2 N0**
RT	100%	94%
Surgery ± RT	100%	93%
p Value	1.00	0.726
LC with voice preservation	**T1 (all N)**	**T2 (all N)**
RT	94%	84%
Surgery ± RT	89%	39%
p Value	0.6	<0.001
Survival	**OS5 T1 N0**	**OS5 T2 N0**
RT	100%	100%
Surgery ± RT	100%	89%
p Value	1.00	0.562
Conclusions	No difference between RT TL/PL ± RT for LRC, OS, or voice preservation (except T2)	

STUDY DESIGN

% requiring surgery or laryngectomy for complications	None needed laryngectomy but % needing some form of surgery: RT 5%, surgery alone 23% Preoperative RT + SGY 21% SGY + postoperative RT 17%
Inclusion criteria	All patients with supraglottic carcinoma treated from 1964 to 1994 at a single institution
Exclusion criteria	Patients lost to follow-up
RT methods	RT: ^{60}Co or 2, 8, or 17 MV photons with 1.8–2 Gy per fraction to 56–75 Gy q.d. or 1.2 Gy b.i.d. to 69.6–76.8 Gy. Small number treated using split-course schedule
Surgery methods	Total or partial laryngectomy (horizontal supraglottic laryngectomy), not further separated for analysis. Elective neck dissection levels II–V
Follow-up	At least 2 y (76% had 5 y follow-up). Median NR
Selection bias	No comparison between groups in age, smoking status, performance status, comorbidities, stage, other risk factors. >2/3 of patients treated with surgery had adjuvant RT: difficult to separate impact of surgery from RT

TL = total laryngectomy, PL = partial laryngectomy, RT = radiation therapy, NR = not reported, q.d. = every day, b.i.d. = twice a day.
* Results combined for TL and PL (30 patients total had supraglottic laryngectomy, but the article does not separate by TL vs supraglottic laryngectomy for each stage); LC = local control [except in Weems et al., the results above represent local and regional control above the clavicle for AJCC (American Joint Committee on Cancer) stage I (T1 N0) and stage II (T2 N0). Control of the primary was reported by T stage only but not by AJCC stages or nodal status and therefore not presented above]; # = reported for all patients (all stages): breakdown as follows 1) preoperatively: 1 fatal carotid blowout, 2) postoperative: 1 fatal carotid blowout and 1 severe laryngeal edema needing tracheostomy, and 3) RT: 4 severe laryngeal edema or chondronecrosis needing tracheostomies, 1 spinal cord myelitis, 1 MI, 1 pharyngocutaneous fistula and esophageal stricture.

Reference	Spriano, 1997	Orus, 2000
Level (design)	3 (retrospective comparative)	3 (retrospective comparative)
Study population	166 T1–2 N0 supraglottic carcinoma cases	115 T1–2 N0
RT	RT n = 100	RT n = 90
Surgery	PL n = 66	PL n = 25
OUTCOME MEASURES		
Initial LC	**T1–2 N0**	**T1–2 N0**
RT	75%	79%
Surgery ± RT	95%	84%
p Value	NR	>0.5
Ultimate LC after salvage	**T1–2 N0**	**T1–2 N0**
RT	87%	87%
Surgery ± RT	98%	88%
p Value	NR	NS
LC with voice preservation	**T1–2 N0**	**T1–2 N0**
RT	72%	83%
Surgery ± RT	95%	80%
p Value	NR	NS
Survival	**DFS5 T1 + T2**	**OS**
RT	76.4% ± 6.1	71%
Surgery ± RT	88.4% ± 4.5	78%
p Value	NR	0.4
Conclusions	Both approaches yield reasonable results. Direct comparison not possible because of selection bias	No difference between RT and need to individualize according to suitability for either modality
STUDY DESIGN		
Complications % requiring surgery or laryngectomy for complications	% requiring total laryngectomy RT 0% (2 had chondronecrosis requiring hyperbaric oxygen) PL 3% (for aspiration; both had >horizontal supraglottic laryngectomy)	% requiring laryngectomy RT 0% PL 1/25 (for aspiration)
Inclusion criteria	All T1 T2 N0 supraglottic carcinoma treated from 1983 to 1992 at a single institution	All clinically staged T1 T2 N0 supraglottic larynx cancers treated from 1984 to 1996 at a single institution
Exclusion criteria	Non-squamous cell, prior or synchronous tumors, lost to follow-up, Tx-Nx,T3–4, N+ (or N0 but path N+), M1, TL, no neck RT	No exclusions reported
RT methods	RT: ^{60}Co or 6 MV photons parallel opposed portals to primary and upper and mid-neck nodes. LAN field added in T2 N0 patients. 1.5 Gy b.i.d. or 2 Gy q.d. to total of 64–72 Gy	RT: ^{60}Co parallel opposed portals to primary and upper and mid-neck nodes plus low anterior neck field. 65–70 Gy to primary and 50 Gy electively to neck
Surgery methods	Horizontal supraglottic laryngectomy in 38, extended horizontal supraglottic laryngectomy in 16, and cricohyoidopexy in 12. Neck dissection levels II–V	Horizontal supraglottic laryngectomy + elective bilateral neck dissection of areas II, III, and IV
Follow-up	Median 80 mo	All >29 mo. Median NR
Selection bias	RT patients do not have histologically proven negative pN, may be sicker, or have other risk factors. Surgery group excluded cN0 pN+ and may have had more favorable disease. Patients who required postoperative RT were excluded	Both groups well balanced except for age (older in RT group compared with PL). Otherwise no difference in stage, grade, and location. 7/25 patients had postoperative RT: difficult to separate impact of surgery from RT

TL = total laryngectomy, PL = partial laryngectomy, RT = radiation therapy, NR = not reported, q.d. = every day, b.i.d. = twice a day.
* Results combined for TL and PL (30 patients total had supraglottic laryngectomy, but article does not separate by TL vs supraglottic laryngectomy for each stage); LC = local control [except in Weem et al., the results above represent local and regional control above the clavicle for AJCC (American Joint Committee on Cancer) stage I (T1 N0) and stage II (T2 N0). Control of the primary was reported by T stage only but not by AJCC stages or nodal status and therefore not presented above]; # = reported for all patients (all stages): breakdown as follows 1) preoperatively: 1 fatal carotid blowout, 2) postoperative: 1 fatal carotid blowout and 1 severe laryngeal edema needing tracheostomy, and 3) RT: 4 severe laryngeal edema or chondronecrosis needing tracheostomies, 1 spinal cord myelitis, 1 MI, 1 pharyngocutaneous fistula and esophageal stricture.

REFERENCES

1. Adamopoulos G, et al. Supraglottic laryngectomy—series report and analysis of results. J Laryngol Otol 1997;111(8):730–734.
2. Akbas Y, Demireller A. Oncologic and functional results of supracricoid partial laryngectomy with cricohyoidopexy. Otolaryngol Head Neck Surg 2005;132(5):783–787.
3. Bataini JP, et al. Treatment of supraglottic cancer by radical high dose radiotherapy. Cancer 1974;33(5):1253–1262.
4. Biller HF, Lawson W. Partial laryngectomy for transglottic cancers. Ann Otol Rhinol Laryngol 1984;93(4 Pt 1):297–300.
5. Bocca E. Limitations of supraglottic laryngectomy and conservative neck dissection. Can J Otolaryngol 1975;4(3):403–419.
6. Bocca E, Pignataro O, Oldini C. Supraglottic laryngectomy: 30 years of experience. Ann Otol Rhinol Laryngol 1983;92(1 Pt 1):14–18.
7. Burstein FD, Calcaterra TC. Supraglottic laryngectomy: series report and analysis of results. Laryngoscope 1985;95(7 Pt 1):833–836.
8. Chevalier D, et al. Supraglottic hemilaryngopharyngectomy plus radiation for the treatment of early lateral margin and pyriform sinus carcinoma. Head Neck 1997;19(1):1–5.
9. Clippe S, et al. Role of brachytherapy in treatment of epidermoid carcinomas of the vallecula after conservative supraglottic laryngectomy followed by irradiation. Int J Radiat Oncol Biol Phys 2002;53(1):29–35.
10. Deffebach RR, Phillips TL. Role of radiation therapy in the treatment of supraglottic carcinoma. Cancer 1972;30(5):1159–1163.
11. DeSanto LW. Radiation in the treatment of early supraglottic cancer. Arch Otolaryngol 1984;110(3):208.
12. Devineni VR, et al. Supraglottic carcinoma: impact of radiation therapy on outcome of patients with positive margins and extracapsular nodal disease. Laryngoscope 1991;101(7 Pt 1):767–770.
13. Esposito E, Motta S, Motta G. Exclusive surgery versus postoperative radiotherapy for supraglottic cancer. ORL J Otorhinolaryngol Relat Spec 2002;64(3):213–218.
14. Ferlito A, et al. The role of partial laryngeal resection in current management of laryngeal cancer: a collective review. Acta Otolaryngol 2000;120(4):456–465.
15. Fletcher GH, et al. Reasons for irradiation failure in squamous cell carcinoma of the larynx. Laryngoscope 1975;85(6):987–1003.
16. Greisen O, Carl J, Pedersen M. A consecutive series of patients with laryngeal carcinoma treated by primary irradiation. Acta Oncol 1997;36(3):279–282.
17. Haffty BG, Hurley RA, Peters LG. Carcinoma of the larynx treated with hypofractionated radiation and hyperbaric oxygen: long-term tumor control and complications. Int J Radiat Oncol Biol Phys 1999;45(1):13–20.
18. Harwood AR, et al. Management of early supraglottic laryngeal carcinoma by irradiation with surgery in reserve. Arch Otolaryngol 1983;109(9):583–585.
19. Hinerman RW, et al. Carcinoma of the supraglottic larynx: treatment results with radiotherapy alone or with planned neck dissection. Head Neck 2002;24(5):456–467.
20. Hoekstra CJ, Levendag PC, van Putten WL. Squamous cell carcinoma of the supraglottic larynx without clinically detectable lymph node metastases: problem of local relapse and influence of overall treatment time. Int J Radiat Oncol Biol Phys 1990;18(1):13–21.
21. Johansen LV, Grau C, Overgaard J. Supraglottic carcinoma: patterns of failure and salvage treatment after curatively intended radiotherapy in 410 consecutive patients. Int J Radiat Oncol Biol Phys 2002;53(4):948–958.
22. Jones AS, et al. The treatment of early laryngeal cancers (T1-T2 N0): surgery or irradiation? Head Neck 2004;26(2):127–135.
23. Jorgensen K, et al. Cancer of the larynx—treatment results after primary radiotherapy with salvage surgery in a series of 1005 patients. Acta Oncol 2002;41(1):69–76.
24. Laccourreye H, et al. Supracricoid laryngectomy with cricohyoidopexy: a partial laryngeal procedure for selected supraglottic and transglottic carcinomas. Laryngoscope 1990;100(7):735–741.
25. Lutz CK, et al. Supraglottic carcinoma: patterns of recurrence. Ann Otol Rhinol Laryngol 1990;99(1):12–17.
26. MacKenzie RG, et al. Comparing treatment outcomes of radiotherapy and surgery in locally advanced carcinoma of the larynx: a comparison limited to patients eligible for surgery. Int J Radiat Oncol Biol Phys 2000;47(1):65–71.
27. Makeieff M, et al. Supraglottic hemipharyngolaryngectomy for the treatment of T1 and T2 carcinomas of laryngeal margin and piriform sinus. Head Neck 2004;26(8):701–705.
28. Marks JE, et al. Carcinoma of the supraglottic larynx. AJR Am J Roentgenol 1979;132(2):255–260.
29. Mendenhall WM, et al. Radiotherapy for carcinoma of the supraglottis. Otolaryngol Clin North Am 1997;30(1):145–161.
30. Mendenhall WM, et al. Carcinoma of the supraglottic larynx: a basis for comparing the results of radiotherapy and surgery. Head Neck 1990;12(3):204–209.
31. Mukherji SK, et al. The ability of tumor volume to predict local control in surgically treated squamous cell carcinoma of the supraglottic larynx. Head Neck 2000;22(3):282–287.
32. Ogura JH, Marks JE, Freeman RB. Results of conservation surgery for cancers of the supraglottis and pyriform sinus. Laryngoscope 1980;90(4):591–600.
33. Ogura JH, Sessions DG, Ciralsky RH. Supraglottic carcinoma with extension to the arytenoid. Laryngoscope 1975;85(8):1327–1331.
34. Prgomet D et al. Videofluoroscopy of the swallowing act after partial supraglottic laryngectomy by CO(2) laser. Eur Arch Otorhinolaryngol 2002;259(8):399–403.
35. Rebeiz EE, et al. Preliminary clinical results of window partial laryngectomy: a combined endoscopic and open technique. Ann Otol Rhinol Laryngol 2000;109(2):123–127.
36. Robbins KT, et al. Conservation surgery for T2 and T3 carcinomas of the supraglottic larynx. Arch Otolaryngol Head Neck Surg 1988;114(4):421–426.
37. Rudert HH, Werner JA, Hoft S. Transoral carbon dioxide laser resection of supraglottic carcinoma. Ann Otol Rhinol Laryngol 1999;108(9):819–827.
38. Schweinfurth JM, Silver SM. Patterns of swallowing after supraglottic laryngectomy. Laryngoscope 2000;110(8):1266–1270.

39. Seiden AM, et al. Advanced supraglottic carcinoma: a comparative study of sequential treatment policies. Head Neck Surg 1984;7(1):22–27.

40. Sessions DG, Lenox J, Spector GJ. Supraglottic laryngeal cancer: analysis of treatment results. Laryngoscope 2005; 115(8):1402–1410.

41. Shimm DS, Coulthard SW. Radiation therapy for squamous cell carcinoma of the supraglottic larynx. Am J Clin Oncol 1989;12(1):17–23.

42. Suarez C, et al. Supraglottic laryngectomy with or without postoperative radiotherapy in supraglottic carcinomas. Ann Otol Rhinol Laryngol 1995;104(5):358–363.

43. Succo G, et al. Twenty years of experience with Marullo's supraglottic laryngectomy. Eur Arch Otorhinolaryngol 1999;256(10):496–500.

44. Tu GY, Tang PZ, Jia CY. Horizontovertical laryngectomy for supraglottic carcinoma. Otolaryngol Head Neck Surg 1997;117(3 Pt 1):280–286.

45. Wang CC, Montgomery WW. Deciding on optimal management of supraglottic carcinoma. Oncology (Williston Park) 1991;5(4):41–46; discussion 46, 49, 53.

46. Wang CC, et al. Role of accelerated fractionated irradiation for supraglottic carcinoma: assessment of results. Cancer J Sci Am 1997;3(2):88–91.

47. Wang CC, Schulz MD, Miller D. Combined radiation therapy and surgery for carcinoma of the supraglottis and pyriform sinus. Am J Surg 1972;124(4):551–554.

48. Weinstein GS, et al. Laryngeal preservation with supracricoid partial laryngectomy results in improved quality of life when compared with total laryngectomy. Laryngoscope 2001;111(2):191–199.

49. Wendt CD, et al. Hyperfractionated radiotherapy in the treatment of squamous cell carcinomas of the supraglottic larynx. Int J Radiat Oncol Biol Phys 1989;17(5):1057–1062.

50. Fu KK, et al. A Radiation Therapy Oncology Group (RTOG) phase III randomized study to compare hyperfractionation and two variants of accelerated fractionation to standard fractionation radiotherapy for head and neck squamous cell carcinomas: first report of RTOG 9003. Int J Radiat Oncol Biol Phys 2000;48(1): 7–16.

51. Gregor RT, et al. Supraglottic laryngectomy with postoperative radiation versus primary radiation in the management of supraglottic laryngeal cancer. Am J Otolaryngol 1996;17(5):316–321.

52. Coates HL, et al. Carcinoma of the supraglottic larynx. A review of 221 cases. Arch Otolaryngol 1976;102(11):686–689.

53. Goepfert H, et al. Treatment of laryngeal carcinoma with conservative surgery and postoperative radiation therapy. Arch Otolaryngol 1978;104(10):576–578.

54. Weems DH, et al. Squamous cell carcinoma of the supraglottic larynx treated with surgery and/or radiation therapy. Int J Radiat Oncol Biol Phys 1987;13(10):1483–1487.

55. Spriano G, et al. Conservative management of T1-T2N0 supraglottic cancer: a retrospective study. Am J Otolaryngol 1997;18(5):299–305.

56. Orus C, et al. Initial treatment of the early stages (I, II) of supraglottic squamous cell carcinoma: partial laryngectomy versus radiotherapy. Eur Arch Otorhinolaryngol 2000;257(9):512–516.

30 Laryngeal Squamous Cell Carcinoma: Early-Stage Disease

30.D.

Hyperfractionated versus conventional radiotherapy for T2 N0 laryngeal carcinoma: Impact on recurrence and survival

Yen-Lin Chen and Kian Ang

METHODS

A computerized PubMed search of MEDLINE 1966–2005 was performed. First, articles mapping to the textwords "larynx," "glottis," "supraglottis," or "subglottis," were combined with "cancer," "carcinoma," or "squamous cell carcinoma" and cross-referenced with those containing the terms "early stage" or "T2." Second, articles mapping to the terms "radiotherapy," "external beam," "radiation," "fractionation," "hyperfractionation," "accelerated fractionation," "altered fractionation," and "BID" were combined. Results from the above two sets of searches were then cross-referenced, yielding 178 articles. The remaining articles were then reviewed to identify those that met the following inclusion criteria: 1) patient population with predominantly T2 larynx cancer, 2) intervention with conventional versus hyperfractionated external beam radiation only, without chemotherapy, 3) outcome measured in terms of survival, local recurrence, and quality of life. Articles regarding locally advanced (T3–4 or N+) larynx cancer [1, 2], comparing T2 versus T1 [3], a split-course regimen [4], chemotherapy, or only once-daily radiation were excluded. Also, articles that analyzed only T1 disease were excluded [5], as well as articles in which results of T2 disease were reported only as a conglomerate with stage III–IV disease [6]. The bibliographies of the articles that met these inclusion criteria were manually checked to ensure no further relevant articles could be identified. This process yielded a total of three retrospective cohort comparisons between conventional versus altered fractionation in T2 larynx cancer [7–9].

RESULTS

Outcome Measures. The primary outcome measure for the three retrospective cohort studies reported was local control.

Potential Confounders. The main confounder in all three studies was the potential for patient bias: patients who had larger disease burden may have been more likely to receive twice-daily radiation instead of once-daily radiation, potentially adversely impacting the outcome of the hyperfractionation group, resulting in no apparent benefit to hyperfractionation. However, patients who were not able to come for twice-daily radiation (socioeconomic reasons, inconvenience, transportation, comorbidities that make twice-daily radiation difficulty to tolerate) may not have received hyperfractionation even if they had other features that may have benefited. Additional confounders that make interpretation of the results difficult in all three studies included changing radiation techniques, dose fractionation, and total dose over time.

Study Designs. All three studies were single institutional cohort studies of patients with T1 and/or T2 larynx cancer treated with conventional versus hyperfractionation.

Highest Level of Evidence. There was insufficient evidence to show whether hyperfractionation or conventional fractionation radiation was better for patients with T2 larynx cancer. These three retrospective nonrandomized, uncontrolled cohort studies provided conflicting results on the benefit of hyperfractionation over conventional fractionation in local control. Two of the studies showed no significant difference in local control between the two fractionation regimens [7, 8] whereas one study showed a trend toward better local control with hyperfractionation over conventional fractionation and significantly better local control over daily fraction size of <2 Gy [9]. However, there was no benefit of hyperfractionation over daily fraction size of >2 Gy. The optimal dose fractionation, therefore, remains controversial.

Applicability. These results are applicable for patients with T2 larynx cancer.

Morbidity/Complications. Conventional and hyperfractionated radiation for T2 larynx cancer are both well tolerated. There may be more acute mucositis with hyperfractionation but no significant difference in late effects has been reported. None of the studies used validated instruments for comparing quality of life and voice quality.

CLINICAL SIGNIFICANCE AND FUTURE RESEARCH

There were three retrospective comparative studies that compared the recurrence/survival impact of hyperfractionated versus conventional radiotherapy. Overall, results were mixed, with two studies showing no difference and one study showing a better result with hyperfractionation.

Well-designed, prospective randomized controlled clinical trials are needed to guide decision making regarding the optimal radiation dose fractionation for patients with T2 larynx cancer. The Radiation Therapy Oncology Group is currently testing this question in a randomized prospective trial of hyperfractionation given in twice-daily doses versus conventional fractionation for T2 N0 glottic carcinoma. Furthermore, studies comparing the two fractionation schedules need to assess cost effectiveness, patient convenience, acute and late side effects, voice quality, and quality of life measures to help guide decision making between the two fractionation schedules.

THE EVIDENCE CONDENSED: Hyperfractionated versus conventional radiotherapy for T2 N0 larynx carcinoma: Impact on recurrence and survival

Reference	Sakata, 2000		Mendenhall, 2001	
Level (design)	3 (retrospective cohort)		3 (retrospective cohort)	
Sample size	CF n = 17 HF n = 33		CF n = 151 HF n = 67	

OUTCOMES

Disease control	LC	OS	LC for T2A	LC for T2B
CF	62.7% ± 12.2%	80.3% ± 7.3%	82%	71%
HF	74.7% ± 7.8%	82.4% ± 9.2%	83%	69%
p Value	NS	NS	0.88	0.80
Complications	Confluent mucositis		Confluent mucositis	
CF	1.9%		0	
HF	97.6%		1/67	
p Value	NR (no severe late complications)		NR (3 patients required permanent tracheostomy for persistent laryngeal edema but fractionation NR)	
Factors associated with higher risk of local failure	Patients Ki-67 of <50% receiving CF vs HF RT		Long overall treatment time and pathology were the most significant factors on LC. Fractionation marginally affected LC (p = 0.07) and did not significantly affect larynx preservation rate, cause-specific survival, or overall survival	
Conclusion	HF does not significantly improve LC or OS in T2 larynx cancer		HF is marginally significant for LC. Overall treatment time is more important than fractionation	

STUDY DESIGN

Inclusion criteria	Patients with T2 N0 glottic cancer treated with RT only. Minimum follow-up at 2 y Median of 69 mo Excluded N+ or M+ patients		Patients with T1 N0 or T2 N0 glottic cancer treated with RT only. Minimum follow-up of 2 y. Median follow-up of 9.87 y. HF started in 1978	
Exclusion criteria	Patients lost to follow-up		Patients with N+ neck, synchronous head and neck primary, split course technique, or lost to follow-up	
CF	64 Gy at 2 Gy per fraction q.d. from 1984 to 1989		54–77.5 Gy at 1.74–2.57 Gy/fraction	
HF	55–58 Gy at 1.72 Gy per fraction b.i.d. from 1990 onward		74–76.8 Gy at 1.2–1.25 Gy per fraction	
Radiation technique	^{60}Co γ-ray using parallel opposed lateral fields with most field sizes 6 × 6 cm. Minimum of 6 h between b.i.d. fractions		^{60}Co γ-ray or 2-MV (more ^{60}Co in recent years). Lateral decubitus position with single field initially and subsequently parallel-opposed fields. Minimum of 6 h between b.i.d. fractions	
Selection biases	Patients with smaller disease tend to be treated with q.d. fractionation. Patients who can come for b.i.d. treatment are more likely to receive b.i.d. treatment		Patients with smaller disease tend to be treated with q.d. fractionation. Patients who can come for b.i.d. treatment are more likely to receive b.i.d. treatment	
Period bias	Improved techniques over time may impact outcome		Improved techniques over time may impact outcome.	

T2 glottic cancer = vocal cord tumor that extends to supraglottis or subglottis with or without impairment of vocal cord mobility, RC = retrospective cohort, RT = radiation therapy, CF = Conventional fractionation, HF = hyperfractionation, NS = not significant, NR = not reported, q.d. = every day, b.i.d. = twice a day, T2A = without vocal cord immobility, T2B = with vocal cord immobility.

THE EVIDENCE CONDENSED: Hyperfractionated versus conventional radiotherapy for T2 N0 larynx carcinoma: Impact on recurrence and survival

Reference	Garden, 2003	
Level (design)	3 (retrospective cohort)	
Sample size	CF n = 146 HF n = 81	

OUTCOMES		
Disease control	LC	LC by fraction size
CF	67%	80% if >2.06 Gy q.d. 59% if <2 Gy q.d.
HF	79%	79%
p Value	0.06	0.01
Complications	Rate of larynx dysfunction	
CF	2/146	
HF	3/81	
p Value	NR None resulted in laryngectomy	
Factors associated with higher risk of local failure	Subglottic extension did worse overall (63% vs 81%; p < 0.01) and if treated with daily ≤2 Gy vs >2 Gy (51% vs 74%). Supraglottic extension, impaired vocal cord mobility, and involvement of bilateral vocal cord/anterior commissure had no impact to LC	
Conclusion	HF resulted in a trend toward better LC compared with CF and significantly better LC compared with CF with daily dose <2 Gy, particularly in patients with subglottic extension. However, q.d. hypofractionation (>2 Gy per fraction) had equivalent LC to HC	

STUDY DESIGN		
Inclusion criteria	Patients with clinically staged T2 N0 glottic cancer treated with RT only with minimum follow-up of 20 mo	
Exclusion criteria	10 patients excluded: 6 with nodal involvement; 2 had induction chemotherapy; and 2 did not complete treatment	
CF	89 treated with 32–75 Gy at 2 Gy per fraction q.d.; 57 had 66–70 Gy at 2.06–2.26 Gy per fraction q.d.; 1 had 1.8 Gy per fraction	
HF	68 had 1.2 Gy/fraction b.i.d. 13 had 1.1 Gy/fraction b.i.d.	
Radiation technique	78% of patients had parallel opposed lateral fields. 20% had single appositional field. 3 patients had three-field technique. 85% had 6 × 6 cm field sizes. Minimum of 6 h between b.i.d. fractions	
Selection biases	Patients with smaller disease tend to be treated with q.d. fractionation. Patients who can come for b.i.d. treatment are more likely to receive b.i.d. treatment	
Period bias	Improved techniques over time may impact outcome	

T2 glottic cancer = vocal cord tumor that extends to supraglottis or subglottis with or without impairment of vocal cord mobility, RC = retrospective cohort, RT = radiation therapy, CF = Conventional fractionation, HF = hyperfractionation, NS = not significant, NR = not reported, q.d. = every day, b.i.d. = twice a day, T2A = without vocal cord immobility, T2B = with vocal cord immobility.

REFERENCES

1. Fu KK, et al. A Radiation Therapy Oncology Group (RTOG) phase III randomized study to compare hyperfractionation and two variants of accelerated fractionation to standard fractionation radiotherapy for head and neck squamous cell carcinomas: first report of RTOG 9003. Int J Radiat Oncol Biol Phys 2000;48(1):7–16.
2. Horiot JC, et al. Present status of EORTC trials of hyperfractionated and accelerated radiotherapy on head and neck carcinoma. Recent Results Cancer Res 1994;134:111–119.
3. Haugen H, Johansson KA, Mercke C. Hyperfractionated-accelerated or conventionally fractionated radiotherapy for early glottic cancer. Int J Radiat Oncol Biol Phys 2002; 52(1):109–119.
4. Wang CC, Blitzer PH, Suit HD. Twice-a-day radiation therapy for cancer of the head and neck. Cancer 1985;55(9 Suppl):2100–2104.
5. Overgaard J, Hansen HS, Specht L, et al., on behalf of the Danish Head and Neck Cancer Study Group. Five compared with six fractions per week of conventional radiotherapy of squamous-cell carcinoma of head and neck: DAHANCA 6&7 randomised controlled trial. Lancet 2003;362:933–940.
6. Yamazaki H, Nishiyama K, Tanaka E, Koizumi M, Chatani M. Radiotherapy for early glottic carcinoma (T1N0M0): results of prospective randomized study of radiation fraction size and overall treatment time. Int J Radiat Oncol Biol Phys 2006;64(1):77–82.
7. Sakata K, et al. Accelerated radiotherapy for T1, 2 glottic carcinoma: analysis of results with KI-67 index. Int J Radiat Oncol Biol Phys 2000;47(1):81–88.
8. Mendenhall WM, et al. T1-T2N0 squamous cell carcinoma of the glottic larynx treated with radiation therapy. J Clin Oncol 2001;19(20):4029–4036.
9. Garden AS, Forster K, Wong PF, Morrison WH, Schechter NR, Ang KK. Results of radiotherapy for T2N0 glottic carcinoma: does the "2" stand for twice-daily treatment? Int J Radiat Oncol Biol Phys 2003;55(2):322–328.

31 Laryngeal Squamous Cell Carcinoma: Advanced Disease

31.A.i.

Open partial laryngectomy versus total laryngectomy: Impact on disease-specific quality of life

Ramon Franco, Jennifer J. Shin, and James Netterville

METHODS

A computerized Ovid search of MEDLINE from 1966 to May 2004 was performed. The subject headings "laryngectomy" and "quality of life" were exploded and the resulting articles were cross-referenced, yielding 122 publications. These articles were then reviewed to identify those that met the following inclusion criteria: 1) patient population with primary laryngeal carcinoma, 2) intervention with open partial laryngectomy versus total laryngectomy, 3) outcome measured in terms of validated instruments measuring disease-specific quality of life (QOL). (Global QOL is addressed in the subsequent section, 31.A.ii.) Articles in which data from patients with laryngeal carcinoma were pooled with data from patients with oropharyngeal carcinoma were excluded. The one paper in which only two patients with hypopharyngeal carcinoma were pooled with 29 patients with purely laryngeal carcinoma was included. Articles in which results for either total laryngectomy alone or partial laryngectomy alone were reported, without comparative/controlled data, were also excluded. Reports using instruments that had not been validated (i.e., untested questionnaires) were excluded. The bibliographies of the articles meeting these inclusion criteria were manually checked to ensure no further relevant articles could be identified. This process yielded just three articles [1–3].

RESULTS

Outcome Measures. Five disease-specific instruments were used in these trials: 1) The European Organization for Research and Treatment of Cancer Quality of Life Core Questionnaire Head and Neck 35 is a diagnosis-specific instrument with 35 items about symptoms attributable to head and neck cancer or its treatment. 2) The University of Michigan Head and Neck Quality of Life (UM HNQOL) instrument is a validated 30-item instrument that measures four domains: communication, eating, pain, and emotion. Scores range from 0 to 100, with higher scores corresponding to better QOL. 3) The University of Michigan Voice Related Quality of Life instrument generates physical, social, emotional, and total scores for voice-related disorders. Scores also range from 0 (worst) to 100 (best). 4) The Performance Status

Scale for Head and Neck Cancer Patients is a clinician-rated instrument with three subscales assessing normalcy of diet, understandability (not quality or type) of speech, and eating in public; scores range from 0 to 100 with higher scores meaning better performance. 5) The Functional Assessment of Cancer Therapy with Head and Neck additional concerns subscale (FACT-H&N) is a comprehensive instrument developed specifically for use with cancer patients; it yields a total score and six subscale scores—physical, social, relationship with doctor, emotional, functional, head and neck. Higher scores represent better QOL.

Potential Confounders. Potential confounders include any disease factors or concomitant treatment that could alter responses: initial stage of the primary lesion, extent of neck disease, type (if any) of neck dissection, radiation therapy and its timing relative to evaluation, type/extent of partial laryngectomy, concomitant resection of tongue base or tracheoesophageal puncture.

Study Designs. All three studies were prospective controlled studies. Sample sizes were unclear in one study, as this particular clinical question was addressed in only a subset of their larger reported patient number. The other two studies had 14 and 31 subjects. None of these articles reported an *a priori* power calculation. Retrospective power calculations are reported where global scores were not significantly different between the two groups. Using the global mean scores and standard deviations for the UM HNQOL as prerequisite data, it is estimated that a sample size of 98 patients would be required to achieve a 90% power to detect a significant difference with $p < 0.05$. Using the FACT-H&N total score as prerequisite data, it follows that a sample size of 77 patients would be required to achieve a similar power. All studies were controlled, although the initial tumor stage was either not reported or not evenly matched or between the partial and total laryngectomy groups; patients undergoing partial laryngectomy had lower disease burden at the outset, which could bias results toward a better outcome in this group. In addition, radiation therapy was systematically separated in only one report. Follow-up time was long, ranging from 6 months to 10.7 years after surgery. In addition, patients were followed at regular intervals in one study.

Highest Level of Evidence. All three studies provided level 2 data, although power was somewhat limited and potential confounders were partially unbalanced between the two study groups at the outset. Results showed better pain control with partial laryngectomy in two studies. In addition, swallowing/eating was better in two studies, but a third study showed no difference in public eating. Surprisingly, speech and communication were no different in the longest-term follow-ups in each study. Social and emotional outcomes were mixed, with one study showing better results with partial laryngectomy but two showing no difference.

Applicability. These results are applicable to patients undergoing treatment for laryngeal carcinoma, with the caveats of potential confounders and study design.

Morbidity. Morbidity and postoperative complications beyond QOL were not reported in these articles.

CLINICAL SIGNIFICANCE AND FUTURE RESEARCH

There are three level 2 trials comparing disease-specific QOL with partial versus total laryngectomy. Overall, results showed that partial laryngectomy resulted in better pain control, better swallowing/eating, and sometimes better social and emotional scores in head and neck–specific outcomes. The interspersed negative findings in these studies are partially tainted by sample sizes less than that required to achieve 90% power to detect any difference that truly exists. Among these negative findings, it is interesting to note that speech/communication scores were so comparable among the two groups, which suggests that esophageal speech or the use of an electrolarynx was eventually comparable to speech with a partially intact larynx.

Current data are limited by potential confounders and sample sizes. Attempting to accurately examine QOL data on limited data sets may result in flawed conclusions. Larger patient populations are needed to accurately demonstrate true QOL after total laryngectomy versus partial laryngectomy. Also, future research will ideally focus on stage-specific, site-specific outcomes. That is, because glottic carcinoma progresses differently than supraglottic carcinoma, an ideal study would focus specifically on one site or the other, rather than combining data from the two. Likewise, patients with stage 2 disease are predisposed to a better QOL outcome than patients with stage 4 disease, so an ideal study might either focus on just one stage or ensure that stages of disease are balanced at the outset in two groups being compared. In addition, preoperative data regarding pretreatment QOL may prove helpful in serving as a baseline for comparison in future studies.

THE EVIDENCE CONDENSED: Disease-specific quality of life after total laryngectomy versus open partial laryngectomy

Reference	Muller, 2001	Weinstein, 2001	
Level (design)	2 (prospective controlled)	2 (prospective controlled)	
Sample size*	2 of 5 groups which had a total of 124 patients (137)	31 (31)	

	OUTCOMES		
	EORTC QLQ-H&N35 Mean (SD)	UM HNQOL Mean (SD)	UM VRQOL Mean (SD)
Partial laryngectomy	Pain 4.73 (0.98) Swallowing 4.90 (1.35) Speech 6.84 (2.51) Social contact 6.48 (1.95)	Communication 68.8 (24.0) Eating 91.9 (10.4) Emotion 90.1 (12.0) Pain 93.0 (7.9) Global 85.9 (18.2)	Physical 71.1 (22.4) Social 85.2 (20.4) Total 76.8 (20.4)
Total laryngectomy	Pain 5.67 (2.11) Swallowing 5.81 (1.97) Speech 6.84 (2.21) Social contact 9.00 (4.68)	Communication 52.9 (26.3) Eating 80.8 (16.5) Emotion 73.6 (32.0) Pain 76.7 (22.3) Global 68.3 (34.7)	Physical 48.1 (34.4) Social 63.2 (40.7) Total 54.2 (34.4)
p Value	Pain <0.05 Swallowing <0.01 Speech NS Social contact <0.001	Communication NS Eating 0.032 Emotion NS Pain 0.010 Global NS	Physical 0.026 Social NS Total 0.032
Conclusion	Better pain, swallowing, and social contact with partial laryngectomy. No difference in speech problems	Better eating, pain with partial. No difference in communication, emotion, or global	Better physical function, total scores. No difference in social, emotional
Follow-up time	10 mo–10.7 y	29 mo mean	

	STUDY DESIGN		
Inclusion criteria	Treatment for laryngeal cancer	Treatment with supracricoid partial laryngectomy with either cricohyoidoepiglottopexy or cricohyoidopexy, or total laryngectomy with primary or secondary tracheoesophageal puncture	
Exclusion criteria	Failure to complete questionnaire	Not specified	
Primary site details	Not reported	71% glottis, 23% supraglottic, 6% hypopharynx Partial laryngectomy: 0% T1, 75% T2, 19% T3, 6% T4 Total laryngectomy: 13% T1, 20% T2, 27% T3, 40% T4	
Extent of partial laryngectomy	Not reported	Supracricoid partial laryngectomy: 88% with cricohyoidoepiglottopexy, 22% with cricohyoidopexy	
Procedures associated with total laryngectomy	Not reported	47% primary tracheoesophageal puncture 53% secondary tracheoesophageal puncture	
RT	Total laryngectomies also treated with radiation were reported separately; RT for partial laryngectomies not reported	Partial laryngectomy: 63% none, 31% radiation failure, 6% postoperative Total laryngectomy: 0% none, 53% radiation failure, 47% postoperative	
Neck dissection	Not reported	Not reported	
Age	66.7 y average	61.9 y mean (11.2 SD)	
Masking	None	None	
Consecutive patients?	Random sample, 71% response rate to questionnaire	Not reported	
Power	Not reported but identified significant differences	Not reported. Calculated at 73% using global HNQOL scores and variances	
Morbidity/complications	Not reported	Not reported	

EORTC QLC-H&N35 = The European Organization for Research and Treatment of Cancer Quality of Life Core Questionnaire Head and Neck 35 instrument, UM HNQOL = University of Michigan Head and Neck Quality of Life instrument, UM VRQOL = The University of Michigan Voice Related Quality of Life instrument, PSS-HN = Performance Status Scale for Head and Neck Cancer Patients, FACT-H&N = Functional Assessment of Cancer Therapy with Head and Neck additional concerns subscale, SD = standard deviation, SE = standard error, NS = not significant, RT = radiation therapy.
*Sample size: numbers shown for those not lost to follow-up and those (initially recruited).

THE EVIDENCE CONDENSED: Disease-specific quality of life after total laryngectomy versus open partial laryngectomy

Reference	List, 1996	
Level (design)	2 (prospective controlled)	
Sample size‡	14 (14)	

OUTCOMES

	PSS-HN Median (minimum to maximum)	FACT-H&N Mean (SE)
Partial laryngectomy	Diet *50 (0–100), †100 (60–100) Speech *100 (75–100), †100 (100–100) Public eating *62.5 (0–100), †100 (75–100)	H&N 21.5 (1.9) Total 87 (5.5)
Total laryngectomy	Diet *50 (20–100),†100 (30–100) Speech *0 (0–25), †100 (0–100) Public eating *50 (0–100), †100 (50–100)	H&N 18.3 (1.8) Total 83.3 (5.1)
p Value	Diet *NS, †NS Speech *p < 0.05, †NS Public eating *NS, †NS	H&N NS Total NS
Conclusion	Partial laryngectomy with better speech at 6 wk. No differences by 6 mo	No difference in pooled scores
Follow-up time	2 wk, *6 wk, 12 wk, †6 mo	0–6 mo

STUDY DESIGN

Inclusion criteria	Newly diagnosed, previously untreated laryngeal carcinoma
Exclusion criteria	Patients receiving radiation as part of a concomitant chemoradiotherapy protocol
Primary site details	Partial laryngectomy stage I–III Total laryngectomy stage III–IV
Extent of partial laryngectomy	Hemilaryngectomy, not further described; 1/7 involved anterior commissure
Procedures associated with total laryngectomy	2/5 had partial pharyngectomies
RT	Not reported
Neck dissection	Not reported
Age	Not reported
Masking	None
Consecutive patients?	Not reported
Power	Not reported. Calculated at 40% for FACT-H&N total scores and variances
Morbidity/complications	Not reported

EORTC QLC-H&N35 = The European Organization for Research and Treatment of Cancer Quality of Life Core Questionnaire Head and Neck 35 instrument, UM HNQOL = University of Michigan Head and Neck Quality of Life instrument, UM VRQOL = The University of Michigan Voice Related Quality of Life instrument, PSS-HN = Performance Status Scale for Head and Neck Cancer Patients, FACT-H&N = Functional Assessment of Cancer Therapy with Head and Neck additional concerns subscale, SD = standard deviation, SE = standard error, NS = not significant, RT = radiation therapy.

‡Sample size: numbers shown for those not lost to follow-up and those (initially recruited).

*, ‡ Symbols denote which data comparisons correspond to the referenced p values and follow-up times.

REFERENCES

1. Weinstein GS, El-Sawy MM, Ruiz C, et al. Laryngeal preservation with supracricoid partial laryngectomy results in improved quality of life when compared with total laryngectomy. Laryngoscope 2001;111(2):191–199.
2. List MA, Ritter-Sterr CA, Baker TM, et al. Longitudinal assessment of quality of life in laryngeal cancer patients. Head Neck 1996;18(1):1–10.
3. Muller R, Paneff J, Kollner V, Koch R. Quality of life of patients with laryngeal carcinoma: a post-treatment study. Eur Arch Otorhinolaryngol 2001;258(6):276–280.

31 Laryngeal Squamous Cell Carcinoma: Advanced Disease

Open partial laryngectomy versus total laryngectomy: Impact on global quality of life

Ramon Franco, Jennifer J. Shin, and James Netterville

METHODS

A computerized PubMed search of MEDLINE 1966–May 2004 was performed. The terms "laryngectomy" and "quality of life" were exploded and the resulting articles were cross-referenced, yielding 122 publications. These articles were then reviewed to identify those that met the following inclusion criteria: 1) patient population with primary laryngeal carcinoma, 2) intervention with open partial laryngectomy versus total laryngectomy, 3) outcome measured in terms of validated instruments measuring global quality of life (QOL) and overall functional status. (Disease-specific QOL is addressed in the preceding section, 31.A.i.) Articles in which data from patients with laryngeal carcinoma were pooled with data from patients with oropharyngeal carcinoma were excluded. Articles in which results for either total laryngectomy alone or partial laryngectomy alone were reported, without comparative/controlled data, were also excluded. Reports using instruments that had not been validated (i.e., untested questionnaires) were excluded. The bibliographies of the articles meeting these inclusion criteria were manually checked to ensure no further relevant articles could be identified. This process yielded the six articles discussed here [1–6].

RESULTS

Outcome Measures. Outcomes were measured using validated instruments that measure global QOL and/or overall performance: 1) the Psychosocial Adjustment to Illness Scale (PAIS) has 46 items, through which ratings are given from 1 (no problem) to 4 (total problem). The items are grouped into seven domains of health attitudes, work or school, relationship with spouse, sexuality, family relationship other than spouse, hobbies and activities, and psychologic. Patients are asked to complete the instrument with reference to the 30 days prior. A T score is generated for each domain, with 50 representing an average score, and 1 standard deviation being 10 greater or less than the mean. For the PAIS, lower scores mean better adjustment. Validated English and Spanish versions were used in two of these studies. 2) The European Organization for Research and Treatment of Cancer Quality of Life Core Questionnaire C30 (EORTC QLQ-C30) consists of 30 items comprising functional and symptom scales. The six functional scales are: physical, role, emotional, cognitive, social, and global health status. For these functional scales, a higher score is better. The symptom scales measure: fatigue, nausea/vomiting, pain, dyspnea, insomnia, appetite loss, constipation, diarrhea, and financial difficulties. In all, there are 30 questions. The patients answer each question with yes/no, or by indicating four steps (1 = not at all, 2 = not much, 3 = moderate, 4 = very much), or about a visual analogous scale (1 = very bad, 7 = excellent). For the symptom items, a higher score corresponds to a higher level of symptoms. 3) The Medical Outcomes Study Short Form 36 (SF-36) is a general health measure that generates scores from 0 (worst) to 100 (best) in eight physical and mental health domains. Scores are summarized with a physical component summary and mental component summary. 4) The Karnofsky Performance Status Rating Scale is a clinician-rated measure of a patient's global functioning in terms of degree of mobility and ability to maintain employment, live at home, and care for oneself; ratings range from 0 to 100 with higher scores indicating better performance.

Potential Confounders. The initial stage of the primary lesion, extent of neck disease, type (if any) of neck dissection, radiation therapy and its timing relative to evaluation, type/extent of partial laryngectomy, concomitant resection of tongue base or tracheoesophageal puncture, preoperative functional status, and response rate to surveys may all potentially influence results.

Study Designs. These six studies were prospective controlled studies in which patients who had partial or total laryngectomy were evaluated with validated instruments that measured global QOL and/or overall functional status. In five studies, patients had previously undergone surgery and were subsequently evaluated at a wide range of intervals. In the List study [5], patients were evaluated at the time of entry into the trial, as well as at specified uniform postoperative intervals. The Moscini publication [2] reported all consecutive patients, whereas the DeSanto publication [1] reported mostly consecutive patients. The Muller study [6] attempted to address the potential confounder of radiation by considering these patients separately. Likewise, the Moscini study attempted to address the potential confounder of concomitant radical neck dissection by considering these patients separately. Although these were all prospective trials, *a priori* power calculations were not in abundance, even in studies in which no difference was identified between groups; thus, it is unclear whether studies with negative findings were adequately powered to demonstrate a difference that might truly exist.

Highest Level of Evidence. There were six level 2 studies that compared global QOL and/or overall functional status in patients after partial versus total laryngectomy. Five of these six publications reported a significantly better outcome with partial laryngectomy. In particular, SF-36 physical component summaries, Karnofsky scores, EORTC QLQ-C30 global health scores, and fatigue, pain, and financial difficulty scores were significantly better with more conservative surgery. PAIS scores were likewise significantly better in the Weinstein study [4], although the Ramirez study [3] did not come to the same conclusion. Mental component SF-36 summary scores showed no difference in any study.

Applicability. These results are applicable to patients undergoing either partial or total laryngectomy for laryngeal cancer.

Morbidity. Morbidity and postoperative complications beyond QOL were not reported in these articles.

CLINICAL SIGNIFICANCE AND FUTURE RESEARCH

There were six prospective controlled trials that compared global QOL and/or overall performance in patients who had undergone either partial or total laryngectomy for laryngeal malignancy. The preponderance of the data suggests better global performance after partial rather than total laryngectomy. Better SF-36 physical component summaries, Karnofsky scores, PAIS scores, EORTC QLQ-C30 global health scores, and fatigue, pain, and financial difficulty scores were seen with more conservative surgery. There were, however, no significant differences in SF-36 mental component scores and certain EORTC QLQ-C30 symptom scores. With appropriate care, patients after total laryngectomy can fit well into society and have excellent QOL, but their overall performance may always be burdened with alaryngeal speech and transstomal ventilation. Partial laryngectomy patients, however, still enjoy transoral ventilation and transoral handsfree communication.

Future research should have better control of confounders and large patient populations. In addition, evaluations that further test general acceptance back into society could help accurately demonstrate QOL after total laryngectomy versus partial laryngectomy.

THE EVIDENCE CONDENSED: Global quality of life after total laryngectomy versus open partial laryngectomy

Reference	DeSanto, 1995	Mosconi, 2000		Ramirez, 2003
Level (design)	2 (prospective controlled)	2 (prospective controlled)		2 (prospective controlled)
Sample size*	172 (172)	134 (134) consecutive surgical treatments among 165 total patients		62 (response rate not specified)

OUTCOMES

	PAIS	SF-36 PCS Mean (SD NR)	SF-36 MCS Mean (SD NR)	PAIS (Spanish version) Lower scores mean better adjustment
		Score 0 = worst, 100 = best		
Partial laryngectomy	The partial laryngectomy group reported better psychosocial adjustment in all domains (health, work, spouse, sexual, family, activities, psychologic) than the total laryngectomy and near-total laryngectomy groups	51.2	46.2	*Horiz. supraglottic* Mean T score 51 (SD† 26) Return to work 50% *Partial vertical* Mean T score 40 (SD† 25) Return to work 85%
Total laryngectomy		41.9 with radical neck dissection 46.8 without radical neck dissection	42.1 with radical neck dissection 44.4 without radical neck dissection	T score 54.9 (SD† 20) Return to work 15%
p Value	p = 0.05 for partial vs total or near total	Treatment extent: p < 0.01 for PCS, p = NS for MCS Multivariate regression: p < 0.0001 partial vs total with radical neck, p = 0.4 for total without vs with radical neck		p = NS for total and individual domain scores Not specified for work scores
Conclusion	Significantly better adjustment with partial laryngectomy	Significantly better PCS with partial laryngectomy	Trend toward better MCS with partial, but no significant difference	Trend toward better adjustment with partial laryngectomy, but no significant difference
Follow-up time	3–48 mo postoperatively	Up to 262 mo		>36 mo

STUDY DESIGN

Inclusion criteria	Total, near-total, partial vertical, or horizontal laryngectomy in the preceding 3–48 mo	Histologically confirmed diagnosis of laryngeal cancer at any stage but without distant metastases, willingness to cooperate		Patients undergoing surgery for laryngeal or hypopharyngeal cancer who responded to mail questionnaire at Dr Peset University Hospital, Spain
Exclusion criteria	"There were no exclusions"	None specified		None specified
Primary site	Laryngeal	Laryngeal		Laryngeal or hypopharyngeal
Extent of partial laryngectomy	Excluded near-total laryngectomies	Excluded partial laryngectomies requiring tracheotomy		Horizontal supraglottic laryngectomy (n = 12) or partial vertical laryngectomy (n = 9)
Additional treatments	15% of 60 had failed RT previously	"Treatment extent" derived from primary and salvage treatment descriptions, ranging from least aggressive to most aggressive. Also divided data for total laryngectomies into those that did and did not require radical neck dissection		Not specified
Age	26–84 y	Mean age 64 y		41–85 y, mean 63.8 y
Additional instrument reference groups	None specified	None specified		Control group: patients with cancer of lung, breast, lymphoma, head and neck other than larynx—most treated by surgery and/or chemotherapy: T score of 50 is reference value for control group
Consecutive patients?	121 consecutive patients, with the remainder from attendance at voice institute or support group	165 consecutive patients		Not specified
Morbidity/ complications	Not otherwise specified	Not otherwise specified		Not otherwise specified

PAIS, Psychosocial Adjustment to Illness Scale, SF-36 = (Medical Outcomes Study) Short Form 36, SD NR = standard deviations not reported, horiz. = horizontal, PCS = physical component summary, MCS = mental component summary, NS = not significant, RT = radiation therapy.
* Sample size: numbers shown for those not lost to follow-up and those (initially recruited).
† Extrapolated from bar graph.

Reference	Weinstein, 2001	
Level (design)	2 (prospective controlled)	
Sample size*	31 (31)	

OUTCOMES

	SF-36 PCS Mean (SD)	SF-36 MCS Mean (SD)
Partial laryngectomy	52.6 (6.5)	53.8 (7.3)
Total laryngectomy	45.3 (10.2)	46.8 (13.8)
p Value	$p < 0.023$	$p < 0.084$
Conclusion	Physical function significantly better with partial	No difference in mental function
Follow-up time	29 mo mean	

STUDY DESIGN

Inclusion criteria	Treatment with supracricoid partial laryngectomy with either cricohyoidoepiglottopexy or cricohyoidopexy, or total laryngectomy with primary or secondary tracheoesophageal puncture
Exclusion criteria	Not specified
Primary site	71% glottis, 23% supraglottic, 6% hypopharynx Partial laryngectomy: 0% T1, 75% T2, 19% T3, 6% T4 Total laryngectomy: 13% T1, 20% T2, 27% T3, 40% T4
Extent of partial laryngectomy	Supracricoid partial laryngectomy: 88% with cricohyoidoepiglottopexy, 22% with cricohyoidopexy
Procedures associated with total laryngectomies	47% primary tracheoesophageal puncture 53% secondary tracheoesophageal puncture
RT	Partial laryngectomy: 63% none, 31% radiation failure, 6% postoperative Total laryngectomy: 0% none, 53% radiation failure, 47% postoperative
Neck dissection	Not reported
Age	61.9 y mean (11.2 SD)
Masking	None
Consecutive patients?	Not reported
Morbidity/complications	Not reported

SF-30 = (Medical Outcomes Study) Short Form 30, EORTC QLQ-C30 = European Organization for Research and Treatment of Cancer Quality of Life Core Questionnaire C30, SD = standard deviation, signif. = significantly, PCS = physical component summary, MCS = mental component summary, RT = radiation therapy.
* Sample size: numbers shown for those not lost to follow-up and those (initially recruited).

Reference	List, 1996				Muller, 2001	
Level (design)	2 (prospective controlled)				2 (prospective controlled)	
Sample size*	14 (14)				2 of 5 groups which had a total of 124 patients (137)	
OUTCOMES						
	% scoring >50 on Karnofsky score† (Karnofsky score, 0 = worst, 100 = best)				**EORTC QLQ-C30** Health status lower score worse Symptom scale lower score better	
	Entry	6 wk	12 wk	6 mo	Global health	Symptom scales
Partial laryngectomy	29%	85%	100%	100%	10.07 (2.50)	Fatigue 4.89 (2.04) Pain 2.54 (0.96) Financial difficulty 1.52 (0.77)
Total laryngectomy	55%	98%	88%	100%	8.53 (2.01)	Fatigue 6.47 (2.65) Pain 3.58 (1.81) Financial difficulty 2.38 (1.20)
p Value	"Significant differences in Karnofsky scores across all assessment points"				$p < 0.01$	Fatigue, $p < 0.05$ Pain, $p < 0.05$ Financial difficulty, $p < 0.001$
Conclusion	Total laryngectomy group with "slower and less complete recovery of overall function as indicated by . . . Karnofsky scores"				Global health signif. better with partial	Signif. less fatigue, pain, and financial difficulty with partial
Follow-up time	2 wk, 6 wk, 12 wk, 6 mo				10 mo–10.7 y after surgery	
STUDY DESIGN						
Inclusion criteria	Newly diagnosed, previously untreated laryngeal carcinoma				Treatment for laryngeal cancer	
Exclusion criteria	Patients receiving radiation as part of a concomitant chemoradiotherapy protocol				Failure to complete questionnaire	
Primary site	Partial laryngectomy stage I–III Total laryngectomy stage III–IV				Not reported	
Extent of partial laryngectomy	Hemilaryngectomy, not further described; 1/7 involved anterior commissure				Not reported	
Procedures associated with total laryngectomies	2/5 had partial pharyngectomies				Not reported	
RT	Not reported				Total laryngectomies also treated with radiation were reported separately; RT for partial laryngectomies not reported	
Neck dissection	Not reported				Not reported	
Age	Not reported				66.7 y average	
Masking	None				None	
Consecutive patients?	Not reported				Random sample, 71% response rate to questionnaire	
Morbidity/complications	Not reported				Not reported	

SF-30 = (Medical Outcomes Study) Short Form 30, EORTC QLQ-C30 = European Organization for Research and Treatment of Cancer Quality of Life Core Questionnaire C30, SD = standard deviation, signif. = significantly, PCS = physical component summary, MCS = mental component summary, RT = radiation therapy.
* Sample size: numbers shown for those not lost to follow-up and those (initially recruited).
† Extrapolated from line graph.

REFERENCES

1. DeSanto LW, Olsen KD, Perry WC, Rohe DE, Keith RL. Quality of life after surgical treatment of cancer of the larynx. Ann Otol Rhinol Laryngol 1995;104(10 Pt 1):763–769.
2. Mosconi P, Cifani S, Crispino S, Fossati R, Apolone G. The performance of SF-36 health survey in patients with laryngeal cancer. Head and Neck Cancer Italian Working Group. Head Neck 2000;22(2):175–182.
3. Ramirez MJ, Ferriol EE, Domenech FG, Llatas MC, Suarez-Varela MM, Martinez RL. Psychosocial adjustment in patients surgically treated for laryngeal cancer. Otolaryngol Head Neck Surg 2003;129(1):92–97.
4. Weinstein GS, El-Sawy MM, Ruiz C, et al. Laryngeal preservation with supracricoid partial laryngectomy results in improved quality of life when compared with total laryngectomy. Laryngoscope 2001;111(2):191–199.
5. List MA, Ritter-Sterr CA, Baker TM, et al. Longitudinal assessment of quality of life in laryngeal cancer patients. Head Neck 1996;18(1):1–10.
6. Muller R, Paneff J, Kollner V, Koch R. Quality of life of patients with laryngeal carcinoma: a post-treatment study. Eur Arch Otorhinolaryngol 2001;258(6):276–280.

31 Laryngeal Squamous Cell Carcinoma: Advanced Disease

Total laryngectomy with postoperative radiation therapy versus induction chemotherapy with radiation therapy for stage III–IV laryngeal carcinoma: Impact on survival, recurrence

Babar Sultan, Lori Wirth, and Merrill S. Kies

METHODS

A computerized PubMed search of MEDLINE 1966–May 2006 was performed. The medical subject headings "laryngeal neoplasms" and "radiotherapy" were exploded and the resulting articles were cross-referenced, yielding 1622 publications. Given the richness of the literature, these studies were then limited to randomized controlled trials (RCTs) and meta-analyses, yielding 40 trials. These articles were then reviewed to identify those that met the following inclusion criteria: 1) patient population with laryngeal carcinoma, 2) intervention with chemotherapy and radiation therapy (RT) versus surgery and RT, 3) outcome measured in terms of survival and recurrence. Articles in which RT alone, surgery alone, or chemotherapy alone was considered were excluded. Studies that combined populations of laryngeal carcinoma with head and neck cancers of different primary sites were likewise excluded. The bibliographies of the articles that met these inclusion criteria were manually checked to ensure no further relevant articles could be identified. This process yielded two articles [1, 2].

RESULTS

Outcome Measures. The Veterans Affairs (VA) Laryngeal Cancer Study [1] measured overall survival (OS) at 2 years, disease-free survival (DFS), patterns of recurrence (primary, regional, distant), response to chemotherapy (complete: disappearance of clinically evident tumor; partial: 50% reduction), and larynx preservation (LP) rate. Richard et al. [2] measured similar outcomes, although a different scale was used to determine response to chemotherapy (>80% reduction in tumor size was considered a good response).

Potential Confounders. Both trials were randomized and controlled to minimize bias. Blinding to treatment assignments was not possible with these designs but the comparisons in terms of survival and recurrences between arms should not be affected. More subjective outcomes, however, such as chemotherapy toxicities could be affected. Because the treatment in the chemotherapy arm was longer than that given in the surgical arm, a direct comparison of DFS and OS from the time of randomization rather than completion of therapy minimizes bias caused by therapy timing differences.

Study Designs. In the VA Study, patients were randomized to one of two arms: surgery then postoperative RT or induction chemotherapy then definitive RT. Surgery was dictated by the extent of the tumor. Classic wide-field laryngectomy was performed for nearly all primaries. Regional neck dissections were performed in all surgical patients, except those with T3 N0 tumors or those with midline supraglottic T4 N0 tumors for whom the side at risk could not be determined. The postoperative RT dose varied. Tissue volumes assumed to be at normal risk for microscopic disease received 50–50.4 Gy. Volumes at high risk for a local recurrence received an additional 10 Gy. Target volumes presumed to contain residual disease received an additional 15–23.8 Gy. The induction chemotherapy regimen consisted of cisplatin 100 mg/m^2 on day 1 + 5-fluorouracil (5-FU) 1000 mg/m^2/d by continuous infusion for 5 days, on days 1, 22, and 43. After the second cycle, patients with at least a partial response received a third cycle, then definitive RT. Partial response was defined as >50% tumor regression in this study. Patients without a partial response underwent immediate surgical resection and postoperative RT. The median follow-up of all patients was 33 months. Seven patients (2%) were lost to follow-up. Intention to treat analysis was conducted appropriately. Randomization was effective in that there were no significant differences between treatment groups with respect to age, sex, or known prognostic factors, including performance status, T class, N class, tumor stage, tumor site, tumor grade, cartilage involvement, or vocal cord fixation. Power analysis was not reported but the sample size was large.

Richard et al. randomized their patients to similar treatment arms: total laryngectomy followed by RT versus chemotherapy followed by RT if tumor regression was >80% or total laryngectomy if <80% response. Chemotherapy consisted of cisplatin (100 mg/m^2) on day 1 followed by continuous IV infusion of fluorouracil (1000 mg/m^2/d) for 5 days, repeated on day 22 and optionally on day 43. If the tumor had not progressed after the second cycle, then the third cycle was administered. Surgeries performed were classic total laryngectomy, modified neck dissection (if N0) and radical neck dissection (if palpable nodes). The trial was interrupted prematurely when the majority of patients refused entry because they wished to receive chemotherapy. The median follow-up was 8.3 years. Intention to treat analysis was conducted appropriately. Randomization was effective in that there were no significant differences between the treatment groups with respect to age, nodal status, tumor site, and performance status. Power analysis was not conducted, and of note, this trial was closed prematurely, after only 68 subjects were enrolled, because of poor accrual attributed to a strong patient preference to receive chemotherapy and radiation instead of surgery followed by radiation.

Highest Level of Evidence. These two RCTs which compared survival/recurrence with chemoradiotherapy (CRT) versus surgery/RT, suggested differing results. The VA Study concluded that induction chemotherapy and definitive radiotherapy could be effective in preserving the larynx, without compromising OS. 2-year OS was 68% in both treatment arms. In addition, DFS was similar in both groups (p = 0.1195). Overall rates of tumor relapse also did not differ, but differences in the pattern of recurrence were seen. Recurrences in the 1° site were less frequent with surgery compared with chemotherapy (2% versus 12%, p = 0.001). The rates of regional recurrence were similar (5% and 8%, respectively). Distant metastases were more common in the surgery group (17% and 11%, respectively, p = 0.001). Seventy-one percent of patients in the chemotherapy group received a third cycle of chemotherapy. The combined overall response rate in the 1° site and involved nodes after 2 or 3 cycles of chemotherapy was 85% and 98%, respectively. The larynx was, notably, preserved in 64% of patients assigned to induction chemotherapy. Risk factors for salvage laryngectomy were T4 and glottic primary tumors, fixed vocal cord, gross cartilage invasion, and stage IV disease.

Richard et al. concluded that LP for patients, selected on the basis of having responded to induction chemotherapy, could not be considered a standard treatment. The PF-RT group (cisplatin/5-FU, then RT) had a 2-year OS of 69% compared with the 84% of the surgery–RT group (p value not stated nor significance mentioned). The OS was higher in the surgery group (p = 0.0006). In addition, DFS was lower in chemotherapy group (p = 0.02). The specific value was not reported. There were more total recurrences in the CRT group (53% versus 34%, p value not reported) and more locoregional recurrences in the CRT group (17% versus 9%, p value not reported). The larynx was preserved in 42% of patients assigned to the induction chemotherapy treatment arm. Thirty-nine percent of tumors had >80% regression after chemotherapy and 43% of positive nodes had >80% regression after chemotherapy.

Some important differences exist between the studies that may explain the contradicting conclusions:

1) With regard to the initial stage of disease, 9% of patients enrolled in the VA study had T1 or T2 disease, whereas all of the Richard et al. patients had T3 disease. One hundred percent of patients in the latter study had vocal cord fixation at presentation, whereas approxi-

mately 60% of patients enrolled in the VA study presented with vocal cord fixation. This is an important difference, because vocal cord fixation is widely recognized as an important negative prognostic factor. As a result of these differences, the patient population in the VA larynx study had a better prognosis than those enrolled in the study by Richard et al.

2) There were also differences in the treatment regimens. Every patient was given identical chemotherapy for the first two cycles in both studies. However, in deciding whether to proceed to the third cycle and definitive RT, the VA study required >50% tumor regression whereas Richard et al. required >80% tumor regression. This may explain the higher rate of LP seen in the VA study compared with Richard et al. Also, to assess tumor status, the VA study used indirect laryngoscopy whereas Richard et al. used direct laryngoscopy. Classic wide-field total laryngectomy was used in all of the relevant Richard et al. patients whereas in the VA study, some supraglottic primary tumors were resected adequately with horizontal partial laryngectomy and regional neck dissections were performed in all surgical patients except those with T3 N0 tumors or those with midline supraglottic T4 N0 tumors for whom it could not be determined which side of the neck was chiefly at risk. In the study by Richard et al., all N0 patients underwent modified neck dissection and patients with palpable nodes underwent radical neck dissection. In the VA study, definitive radiotherapy was defined as 66–76 Gy whereas in the Richard et al. study, this was defined as 65–70 Gy.

3) Lastly, the outcome measures were slightly different between the two studies. The median follow-up in the VA study was shorter than the Richard et al. study (33 months versus 8.3 years). Both trials used an intention to treat analysis; neither conducted a power analysis.

Applicability. These data apply primarily to patients with untreated stage III or IV squamous cell carcinoma of the larynx with adequate bone marrow and renal function without previous cancer, distant metastasis, and previous RT to head and neck.

Morbidity/Complications. In the Richard et al. study, 45% (15 patients) experienced chemotherapy-related toxicity ranging in type and grade. Two postsurgical hematomas, three postsurgical pharyngostomies, and one radiation-related skin toxicity were encountered, as well. In the VA larynx study l, eight patients died during treatment, five in the chemotherapy group and three in the surgery group. Only one death from septicemia/leukopenia was considered directly a result of chemotherapy. The other four deaths in the chemotherapy group were attributed to tumor and unrelated causes. The three deaths in the surgery group were attributed to surgical complications. Twelve patients had complications from chemotherapy that required its discontinuation. The frequency and severity of RT complications (dermatitis, dehydration, anemia, and pain) were similar, except for grade 2 mucositis and severe laryngitis, which were slightly higher in the chemotherapy group (38%) versus the surgery group (24%); p value not reported.

CLINICAL SIGNIFICANCE AND FUTURE RESEARCH

The VA study is considered a landmark clinical trial that set the stage for organ preservation therapy in laryngeal carcinoma, and ultimately in other head and neck malignancy as well. This study showed that induction chemotherapy and definitive radiotherapy can preserve the larynx, without compromising OS. However, Richard et al. came to a different conclusion.

Important differences exist between the two studies that affect the clinical significance of each conclusion. For example, the VA study enrolled patients with less advanced disease on the whole, compared with Richard et al. Tumor response criteria differed, a higher dose of definitive radiation was used, and follow-up time was shorter. Some argue that induction chemotherapy remains investigational and may actually induce radio-resistant clonal populations [3]. This concept may argue for more RCTs with diverse, well-defined patient populations with more treatment arms, such as only RT or concurrent CRT. The Radiation Therapy Oncology Group study, 91-11 does address the comparison of induction therapy to RT alone and CRT. The initial report by Forastiere et al. [4] favored CRT, however updated data suggest that CRT and induction yield equivalent laryngectomy-free survival and OS [5].

Appropriate selection of patients for organ preservation is a subject of particular interest. Urba et al. [6] have recently reported results with 97 patients with stage III or IV larynx cancers entered into a phase II clinical trial with induction PF administered in a single cycle. Patients who achieved a partial response ($\geq$50%) went on to receive concurrent CRT. Nonresponders and those with evidence of persistent disease following induction therapy and CRT had planned salvage surgery. The outcomes are promising. Of the entire group, 75% went on to CRT. OS at 3 years is 85%, with LP in 70% of patients. Thus, the authors posit that response to PF may be useful as a selection factor that predicts a favorable outcome following CRT. More study is needed to determine the therapeutic effect of induction chemotherapy, and whether induction chemotherapy should be administered as a single cycle or several cycles before CRT. If chemotherapy is to have an effect on distant metastasis, more may be better. Large phase III RCTs that explore the value of adding highly active three-drug induction chemotherapy (i.e., a taxane plus cisplatin/5-FU) to CRT for the treatment of locally advanced squamous cell carcinoma of the head and neck, including cancers of the larynx, are now underway [7]. There is also great interest in the incorporation of targeted therapies, such as the monoclonal anti-epidermal growth factor receptor, cetuximab, to effective CRT, as a potential means of enhancing treatment effect without increasing toxicity [8].

Reference	Wolf, 1991 (VA Larynx Cancer Study)		
Level (design)	1 (RCT)		
Sample size	332		

OUTCOMES

Outcome measure	*1° Outcome* 2-y OS	*2° Outcomes* DFS Patterns of recurrence Response to chemo LP rate	
Chemo/RT	2-y OS = 68%		
Surgery/RT	2-y OS = 68%		
p Value	0.9846		
Conclusion	Induction chemo and definitive radiotherapy can be effective in preserving the larynx, without compromising OS		
Follow-up time	Median: 33 mo		

STUDY DESIGN

Inclusion criteria	Untreated stage III or IV squamous cell carcinoma of the larynx; Karnofsky PS ≥50; Adequate bone marrow and renal function; Adequate auditory, nutritional, pulmonary, and cardiac status; Written informed consent
Exclusion criteria	T1 N1 carcinoma, Unresectable cancer, DM, Previous cancer, Previous RT to head and neck
Patient characteristics	Median age 62 y, 97% male, 80% white, 76% Karnofsky PS ≥80, 1° site: 63% supraglottis and 37% glottis, 57% stage III, 43% stage IV, TN stage, T1 and 2: 9%, T3: 65%, T4: 26%, N0: 54%, N1: 18%, N2–3: 28%, 9% cartilage invasion, 57% fixed cord
Randomization Effectiveness	Patients stratified according to PS, T stage, N stage, and 1° site. There were no significant differences between treatment groups with respect to age, sex, or prognostic factors, i.e., PS, TN stage, 1° site, cartilage involvement, and vocal cord paralysis
Study regimens	Classic wide-field laryngectomy was performed for nearly all primaries. Regional neck dissections were performed in all surgical patients, except those with T3 N0 tumors or those with midline supraglottic T4 N0 tumors for whom the side at risk could not be determined. Postoperative RT administered depending on risk of remaining disease (5000 + 1000–2380 cGy) PF-RT = cisplatin 100 mg/m^2 on day 1 + 5-FU 1000 mg/m^2/d by continuous infusion for 5 d, on days 1, 22, and 43. After the 2nd cycle, patients with ≥PR received a 3rd cycle, then definitive RT. Patients without a PR underwent immediate surgical resection and postoperative RT. Definitive RT was administered as above, except to a total dose of 6600–7600 cGy
Outcome measurements in detail	Survival times were estimated by the Kaplan-Meier method, and differences were determined by logrank testing. Survival times were measured from the date of randomization. The chi-square test and Student's *t*-test were used for analysis of categorical and continuous variables. All p values were two-sided
Potential confounders	Because the treatment on the chemo arm was longer than that given on the surgical arm, a direct comparison of DFS from the time of randomization rather than the time of completing therapy minimizes the introduction of bias caused by therapy timing differences Blinding to treatment assignment is not possible with this design, but the comparisons in terms of survival and recurrences between arms made should not be affected
Intention to treat analysis	Performed appropriately
Power	NR
Other secondary endpoints	DFS was similar in both groups (p = 0.1195). Overall rates of tumor relapse also did not differ, but differences in the pattern of recurrence were seen. Recurrences in the 1° site were less frequent with surgery compared with chemo (2% vs 12%, p = 0.001). The rates of regional recurrence were similar (5% and 8%, respectively). DM were more common in the surgery group (17% and 11%, respectively, p = 0.001). 71% of patients in the chemo group received a 3rd cycle of chemo. The combined ORR in the 1° site and involved nodes after 2 or 3 cycles of chemo were 85% and 98%, respectively The larynx was preserved in 64% of patients assigned to induction chemo. Risk factors for salvage laryngectomy were T4 and glottic 1° tumors, fixed vocal cord, gross cartilage invasion, and stage IV disease
Morbidity/ complications	8 patients died during treatment, 5 in the chemo group and 3 in the surgery group. Only 1 death from septicemia/ leukopenia was considered directly caused by chemo. The other 4 deaths in the chemo group were attributed to tumor and unrelated causes. The 3 deaths in the surgery group were attributed to surgical complications 12 patients had complications from chemo that required discontinuation of chemo. The frequency and severity of RT complications (dermatitis, dehydration, anemia, and pain) were similar, except for grade 2 mucositis and severe laryngitis, which were slightly higher in the chemo group (38%) vs the surgery group (24%)

VA = Veterans Affairs, RCT = randomized controlled trial, LP = larynx preservation, OS = overall survival, DFS = disease-free survival, RT = radiation therapy, PF-RT = cisplatin/5-FU then radiotherapy, PS = performance status, DM = distant metastasis, 5-FU = 5-fluorouracil, PR = partial response, ECOG = Eastern Cooperative Oncology Group, Gy = Gray, NR = not reported, ORR = overall response rate, chemo = chemotherapy, CT = computed tomography.

Reference	Richard, 1998
Level (design)	1 (RCT)
Sample size	68

OUTCOMES

Outcome measure	1° Outcome OS	2° Outcomes DFS Patterns of recurrence Response to chemo LP rate

Chemo/RT	Lower OS (at 2 y = 69%)
Surgery/RT	Higher OS (at 2 y = 84%)
p Value	0.0006
Conclusion	LP for patients, selected on the basis of having responded to induction chemo, had less favorable outcomes
Follow-up time	Median: 8.3 y

STUDY DESIGN

Inclusion criteria	Squamous cell carcinoma of larynx: T3, N0, N1, N2a, or N2b, considered for total laryngectomy; ECOG PS >2; Adequate bone marrow and renal function; Adequate auditory and cardiac status
Exclusion criteria	Tumor of supralarynx, Unresectable cancer, DM, Previous treatment, Previous cancer
Patient characteristics	Mean age 56 y; 98.5% male; 87% ECOG PS <2; 1° site: 31% supraglottis, 41% glottis, 28% unspecified; T3: 100%; N0 78%, N1 15%, N2 or N3 7%; 100% fixed cord; 37% had CT scan
Randomization Effectiveness	No stratification, 36 assigned to induction chemo group, 32 to no chemo group, no significant differences in age, nodal status, tumor site, and performance status
Study regimens	Total laryngectomy followed by RT vs chemo followed by RT if regression >80% or total laryngectomy. Chemo: cisplatin (100 mg/m^2) on day 1 followed by 24-h IV infusion of fluorouracil (1000 mg/m^2/d) for 5 d. Repeated on day 22 and optionally on day 43. Surgery: classic total laryngectomy, N0 underwent modified neck dissection and palpable nodes underwent radical neck dissection RT: postsurgery 50–70 Gy, postresponse to chemo 65–70 Gy
Outcome measurements in detail	Patient distribution compared using Pearson chi-square test. Survival curves compared with logrank test in the univariate analysis. All survival curves are Kaplan-Meier plots. Median follow-up computed using inverse Kaplan-Meier method
Potential confounders	Because the treatment on the chemo arm was longer than that given on the surgical arm, a direct comparison of DFS from the time of randomization rather than the time of completing therapy minimizes the introduction of bias caused by therapy timing differences. Blinding to treatment assignment is not possible with this design, but the comparisons in terms of survival and recurrences between arms made should not be affected
Intention to treat analysis	Performed appropriately
Power	NR
Other secondary endpoints	DFS lower in chemo group (p = 0.02). More total recurrences in chemo group (53% vs 34%) More locoregional recurrences in chemo group (17% vs 9%). The larynx was preserved in 42% of patients assigned to induction chemo. 39% of tumors >80% regression after chemo, 43% of positive nodes >80% regression after chemo
Morbidity/ complications	45% (15 patients) experienced chemo toxicity ranging in type and grade, 2 postsurgical hematomas, 3 postsurgical pharyngostomies, 1 patient had RT discontinued in chemo group because of skin toxicity

VA = Veterans Affairs, RCT = randomized controlled trial, LP = larynx preservation, OS = overall survival, DFS = disease-free survival, RT = radiation therapy, PF-RT = cisplatin/5-FU then radiotherapy, PS = performance status, DM = distant metastasis, 5-FU = 5-fluorouracil, PR = partial response, ECOG = Eastern Cooperative Oncology Group, Gy = Gray, NR = not reported, ORR = overall response rate, chemo = chemotherapy, CT = computed tomography.

REFERENCES

1. Wolf GT, Hong WK, Fisher SG et al. Induction chemotherapy plus radiation compared with surgery plus radiation in patients with advanced laryngeal cancer. N Engl J Med 1991;324(24):1685–1690.

2. Richard JM, Sancho-Garnier H, Pessey JJ, et al. Randomized trial of induction chemotherapy in larynx carcinoma. Oral Oncol 1998;34(3):224–228.

3. Jaulerry C, Rodriguez J, Brunin F, et al. Induction chemotherapy in advanced head and neck tumors: results of two randomized trials. Int J Radiat Oncol Biol Phys 1992; 23(3):483–489.

4. Forastiere AA, Goepfert H, Maor M, et al. Concurrent chemotherapy and radiotherapy for organ preservation in advanced laryngeal cancer. N Engl J Med 2003;349(22): 2091–2098.

5. American Society of Clinical Oncology; Pfister DG, Laurie SA, Weinstein GS, et al. American Society of Clinical Oncology clinical practice guideline for the use of larynx-preservation strategies in the treatment of laryngeal cancer. J Clin Oncol 2006;24(22):3693–3704.

6. Urba S, Wolf G, Eisbruch A, et al. Single-cycle induction chemotherapy selects patients with advanced laryngeal cancer for combined chemoradiation: a new treatment paradigm. J Clin Oncol 2006;24(4):593–598.

7. Posner MR, Haddad RI, Wirth L, et al. Induction chemotherapy in locally advanced squamous cell cancer of the head and neck: evolution of the sequential treatment approach. Semin Oncol 2004;31(6):778–785.

8. Bonner JA, Harari PM, Giralt J, et al. Radiotherapy plus cetuximab for squamous-cell carcinoma of the head and neck. N Engl J Med 2006;354(6):567–578.

31 Laryngeal Squamous Cell Carcinoma: Advanced Disease

31.B.ii.

Total laryngectomy with postoperative radiation therapy versus induction chemotherapy with radiation therapy for stage III–IV laryngeal carcinoma: Impact on quality of life, functionality

Babar Sultan, Lori Wirth, and Merrill S. Kies

METHODS

A computerized PubMed search of MEDLINE 1966–May 2006 was performed. The medical subject headings "laryngeal neoplasms" and "radiotherapy" were exploded and the resulting articles were cross-referenced, yielding 26 publications. These articles were then reviewed to identify those that met the following inclusion criteria: 1) patient population with laryngeal carcinoma, 2) intervention with chemotherapy and radiation therapy versus surgery and radiation therapy, 3) outcome measured with validated quality of life (QOL) instruments and/or functionality measures. Articles in which radiation therapy alone, surgery alone, or chemotherapy alone was considered were excluded. Studies that combined populations of laryngeal carcinoma with head and neck cancers of multiple different primary sites were likewise excluded. The bibliographies of the articles that met these inclusion criteria were manually checked to ensure no further relevant articles could be identified. This process yielded five articles [1–5].

RESULTS

Outcome Measures. Several different QOL instruments exist, some specific to head and neck cancer, some not. Hillman et al. attempted to assess communication-related function, swallowing and eating-related function, and employment status. Communication-related function was measured using intelligibility of speech, reading rate (syllables per minute), number of speech therapy sessions needed, and a Communication Profile Score (CPS). The CPS is based on 24 statements which represent a patient's reactions to various communication situations, scored 0 (worst)–5 (best). Swallowing and eating-related function as well as employment status were based on subjective self-report by the patient.

Terrell et al. used the Medical Outcomes Studies Short Form 36 (SF-36) as a general health measure and the University of Michigan Head and Neck Quality of Life instrument (HNQOL), which is specific to head and neck cancer. The SF-36 generates scores for eight different domains: physical functioning, role limitations attributable to physical problems, role limitations because of emotional problems, bodily pain, general health perception, vitality, social functioning, and mental health. Scores range from 0 to 100, with a higher score corresponding to a better QOL. HNQOL scores for four specific domains: communication, eating, head and neck pain, and emotional factors. Again, a higher score corresponds to a higher QOL. This study also used the Beck Depression Inventory, a 13-item instrument used to assess symptoms of depression, with a higher score corresponding to more severe depression.

Fung et al. used the Voice-Related Quality of Life (V-RQOL) and Performance Status Scale for Head and Neck cancer patients (PSS-HN) as their measurement tools. The V-RQOL is a 10-item self-administered voice outcomes measure of two domains (social–emotional and physical functioning) with higher scores indicating better voice-related QOL. PSS-HN includes three observer-rated items: eating in public, normalcy of diet, and understandability of speech, with higher scores relating to higher function.

Hanna et al. used the European Organization for Research and Treatment of Cancer Quality of Life Core Questionnaire C30 (EORTC QLQ-C30), as well as the Quality of Life Questionnaire Head and Neck Module 35 (QLQ-H&N35). EORTC QLQ-C30 has 30 items including six functional scales (physical, role, cognitive, emotional, social functioning, and global QOL), three symptom scales (fatigue, pain, and emesis), and six individual items (dyspnea, sleep disturbance, appetite, constipation, diarrhea, and financial impact). EORTC QLQ-H&N35 has seven multiple-item scales (pain, swallowing, senses, speech, social eating, social contact, and sexuality) and 10 single items relating to problems with teeth, dry mouth, cough, opening the mouth wide, sticky saliva, weight loss, weight gain, use of nutritional supplements, feeding tubes, and painkillers. Higher scores on the functional scales represent better QOL, whereas higher scores on symptom and individual item scales indicate greater difficulty.

LoTempio et al. used the University of Washington Head and Neck Quality of Life Instrument, version 4 (UW QOL v 4), which is composed of three parts. Part 1 has 12 domains: pain, appearance, activity, recreation, swallowing, chewing, speech, shoulder function, taste, saliva, mood, and anxiety. Part 2 asks, "Which of 12 domains was the most important in last 7 days?" and part 3 contains general questions. This scale is scored 0–100, with a higher score relating to better QOL.

Study Designs. The five studies cited vary in their design. Hillman et al. (level 1) presented a prospective companion study of the Veterans Affairs Laryngeal Cancer Study, a prospective randomized controlled trial (RCT) that compared survival of patients randomized to surgery plus radiotherapy versus chemotherapy plus radiotherapy [6] with follow-up after initial randomization at 1 month, 6 months, 12 months, 18 months, and 24 months. The authors used several methods to control data collection bias. They used identical sets of recording equipment of voices for analysis, standardized training of speech pathologists, and ongoing quality control. The swallowing function data in the study were based on patients' subjective reports instead of an objective measure.

Terrell et al. (level 1) reported a follow-up study of the Veterans Affairs Laryngeal Cancer study cited above. This study also benefited from the initial randomization but had limited power to detect differences because of the small sample size of patients from the original study who were available to participate in the follow-up QOL study. There was also potential selection bias because only a fraction of the originally randomized group was included. In addition, there was potential for statistical error because of the comparison of multiple mean QOL scores.

Fung et al. (level 2) presented a prospective companion study to a nonrandomized phase II trial in which patients were given a single course of induction chemotherapy [7]. Those who had a response >50% were given combination chemoradiotherapy, whereas those with <50% response were managed surgically with appropriate postoperative adjuvant therapy. This study only looked at patients who were free of disease and the authors did not conduct a statistical analysis to detect differences between the two groups. Moreover, the surgery group had a higher percentage of T3 patients.

Hanna et al. (level 3) reported a retrospective cross-sectional study. The choice of treatment was not controlled, rather based on patient preference and there were differences in the timing of evaluation between the two groups. The postoperative radiation was not detailed and the cycles of chemotherapy not controlled.

LoTempio et al. (level 3) also reported a retrospective cross-sectional study in which few details were provided regarding the protocols of surgery, chemotherapy, and radiation therapy. Thus, there were different chemoradiation protocols among patients and they were given the choice of treatment to pursue. Also, there were differences in the time elapsed from treatment to when questionnaire was completed.

Highest Level of Evidence. The Hillman, Terrell, and Fung studies offered the highest level of evidence because they presented prospective data. Hillman et al. reported that patients with advanced laryngeal cancer fared better in the speech communication component if they could be treated without laryngectomy (intelligibility, communication profile score). Few significant differences for other non–speech-related measures were found. Terrell et al. reported better QOL for chemotherapy plus radiation versus surgery plus radiotherapy, mainly because of freedom from pain, better emotional well-being, and lower levels of depression. Fung et al. also reported better voice-related QOL in the chemotherapy plus radiation therapy group. The Hanna and LoTempio studies, in which patients controlled the therapy they received, showed no overall difference in QOL between the two groups. These two studies also had smaller sample sizes, granting them less power to identify differences between populations. However, there were some differences in the individual domains. Hanna et al. reported that surgery plus radiotherapy produced significantly fewer complaints of dry mouth than chemoradiotherapy. LoTempio et al. showed that chemoradiation patients experienced greater pain, difficulty swallowing, and problems chewing compared with laryngectomy patients. Laryngectomy patients had greater impairment of speech and shoulder function.

Applicability. Based on the inclusion/exclusion criteria for these papers, the majority of the results can be applied to patients with stage III–IV laryngeal squamous cell carcinoma receiving either chemotherapy plus radiotherapy or surgery plus radiation therapy.

CLINICAL SIGNIFICANCE AND FUTURE RESEARCH

The studies that provide the highest level of evidence indicate a better QOL after treatment with chemoradiation therapy (rather than surgery with postoperative radiation) for advanced laryngeal carcinoma. Smaller, retrospective studies show equivocal results. Along with data regarding survival and recurrence, QOL is an important factor in guiding patient choice of therapy. Moreover, in the era of highly effective combined modality treatments for head and neck cancer, QOL issues are emerging as significant concerns in the surviving patient population. It is hoped that as targeted therapies are incorporated into the curative treatment of head and neck cancer, not only will therapeutic efficacy be improved, but so will QOL. High-quality prospectively obtained QOL studies will be necessary to evaluate this potential.

Future research could significantly improve the QOL information available as further instruments are developed. An ideal study would be a companion study to an adequately powered prospective, RCT comparing one treatment strategy for laryngeal cancer to another. This companion study would use an accepted, validated QOL instrument, with baseline measurements, measurements during and immediately after treatment, and measurements taken after a period of time to allow for full recovery from the acute and long-term toxicities of therapy.

Reference	Hillman, 1998
Level (design)	1 (prospective follow-up of RCT)
Sample size	332

OUTCOMES

Outcome measure	1° Outcomes Speech outcomes: intelligibility (%), reading rate (syllables per min), CPS [24 statements about a patient's reactions to various communication situations, scored 0 (worst)–5 (best)], amount of speech therapy, and swallowing and eating-related function, employment status at 1, 6, 12, 18, and 24 mo after treatment

	Intelligibility (%): 1, 6, 12, 18, 24 mo	Reading rate: 1, 6, 12, 18, 24 mo	CPS: 1, 6, 12, 18, 24 mo	Mean therapy sessions/ patient: 1, 6, 12, 18, 24 mo	Normal swallowing (%): 1, 6, 12, 18, 24 mo	Diet texture normal (%): 1, 6, 12, 18, 24 mo	Employment status, disabled (%): 1, 6, 12, 18, 24 mo
Chemo/RT	93.2, 88.9, 90.0, 90.5, 90.8	190.3, 177.4, 179.7, 186.4, 182.1	73.5, 71.3, 73.8, 73.1, 75.9	2.2, 1.8, 0.9, 0.1, 0.8	60.58, 59.32, 59.05, 60.67, 70.83	62.04, 63.87, 74.29, 80.90, 80.82	33.58, 35.83, 30.48, 30.34, 30.14
Surgery/RT	76.8, 79.2, 84.5, 85.4, 84.9	154.6, 157.5, 159.6, 171.2, 169.0	63.3, 65.9, 66.9, 66.6, 71.5	15.1, 3.6, 2.6, 0.9, 0.6	48.28, 50.39, 64.42, 59.30, 68.00	50.34, 61.42, 71.15, 65.12, 76.00	25.52, 29.92, 29.81, 30.23, 33.33
p Value	Over time, p = 0.0012	Over time, p = 0.0894	Over time, p = 0.0119	Over time, p = 0.0001	NR	NR	NR
Conclusion	Patients with advanced laryngeal cancer fare better in speech communication if they can be treated without removal of the larynx. Few significant differences for other non–speech-related measures						
Follow-up time	Median 60 mo						

STUDY DESIGN

Inclusion criteria	Biopsy-proven, previously untreated stage III or IV SCC of larynx
Exclusion criteria	1. T1 N1 carcinomas 2. Pyriform sinus lesions 3. Unresectable cancers 4. Distant metastasis 5. Prior head and neck RT 6. Prior malignancy with exception of non-melanoma skin cancer
Patient characteristics	1. 63% supraglottic, 37% glottic 2. Median age 62 y 3. 80% white 4. 99% used tobacco 5. 85% consumed alcohol 6. 321 men, 11 women
Baseline group comparison	No significant differences between treatment groups with respect to age, sex, tumor size, or site of lesion
Surgery/RT details	Surgery was dictated by the extent of the tumor. Classic wide-field laryngectomy was performed for nearly all primaries. Regional neck dissections were performed in all surgical patients, except those with T3 N0 tumors or those with midline supraglottic T4 N0 tumors for whom the side at risk could not be determined. Postoperative RT administered depending on risk of remaining disease (5000 cGy + 1000–2380 cGy)
Chemo/RT details	Cisplatin 100 mg/m^2 on day 1 + 5-FU 1000 mg/m^2/d by continuous infusion for 5 d, on days 1, 22, and 43. After the 2nd cycle, patients with ≥50% response received a 3rd cycle, then definitive RT. Patients without a PR underwent immediate surgical resection and postoperative RT. Definitive RT was administered to a total dose of 6600–7600 cGy
Intention to treat analysis	Done appropriately
Power	NR
Compliance	7 patients (2%) lost to medical follow-up, occurring between 11 and 33 mo

5-FU = 5-fluorouracil, CPS = Communication Profile Score, NR = not reported, RCT = randomized control trial, RT = radiation therapy, SCC = squamous cell carcinoma, PR = partial response.

THE EVIDENCE CONDENSED: Quality of life after chemoradiation therapy versus surgery with postoperative radiation

Reference	Terrell, 1998		
Level (design)	1 (follow-up of RCT)		
Sample size	65		

<table>
<tr><th></th><th colspan="3">OUTCOMES</th></tr>
<tr><td>Outcome measure</td><td>1° Outcome
SF-36: 0 (worst) to 100 (best)</td><td colspan="2">2° Outcomes
UM HNQOL: 0 (worst) to 100 (best)
BDI: 0 (best) to 63 (worst)</td></tr>
<tr><td></td><td>Mental health</td><td>Pain domain</td><td>BDI >8</td></tr>
<tr><td>Chemo/RT</td><td>76</td><td>81.3</td><td>15%</td></tr>
<tr><td>Surgery/RT</td><td>63</td><td>64.3</td><td>28%</td></tr>
<tr><td>p Value</td><td><0.05</td><td><0.05</td><td>NR</td></tr>
<tr><td>Conclusion</td><td colspan="3">Better QOL scores in the CRT group seem to be related to more freedom from pain, better emotional well-being, and lower levels of depression than to preservation of speech function</td></tr>
<tr><td>Follow-up time</td><td colspan="3">10.4 y (mean)</td></tr>
</table>

<table>
<tr><th colspan="2">STUDY DESIGN</th></tr>
<tr><td>Inclusion criteria</td><td>Surviving member of Veterans Affairs Laryngeal Cancer Study No. 268 on CRT vs TL + RT</td></tr>
<tr><td>Exclusion criteria</td><td>NR</td></tr>
<tr><td>Patient characteristics</td><td>Mean age 58.3 y
Men 91.3%,
T1–2: 11%
T3: 61%
T4: 28%
N0–1: 71%
N2–3: 29%
Stage III: 50%
Stage IV: 50%
Mean Karnofsky performance status: 85.4</td></tr>
<tr><td>Baseline group comparison</td><td>Baseline demographic and clinical characteristics similar except CRT group slightly older, with mean age 61.2 y vs 55.7 y, p < 0.05</td></tr>
<tr><td>Surgery/RT details</td><td>Surgery was dictated by the extent of the tumor. Classic wide-field laryngectomy was performed for nearly all primaries. Regional neck dissections were performed in all surgical patients, except those with T3 N0 tumors or those with midline supraglottic T4 N0 tumors for whom the side at risk could not be determined. Postoperative RT administered depending on risk of remaining disease (5000 cGy + 1000–2380 cGy)</td></tr>
<tr><td>Chemo/RT details</td><td>Cisplatin 100 mg/m^2 on day 1 + 5-FU 1000 mg/m^2/d by continuous infusion for 5 d, on days 1, 22, and 43. After the 2nd cycle, patients with ≥50% response received a 3rd cycle, then definitive RT. Patients without a PR underwent immediate surgical resection and postoperative RT. Definitive RT administered to a total dose of 6600–7600 cGy</td></tr>
<tr><td>Compliance</td><td>46/65 (71%) patients responded</td></tr>
<tr><td>Intention to treat analysis</td><td>NR</td></tr>
<tr><td>Power</td><td>NR</td></tr>
</table>

5-FU = 5-fluorouracil, BDI = Beck Depression Inventory, CRT = chemoradiotherapy, Gy = Gray, =PSS-HN = Performance Status Scale for Head and Neck cancer patients, QOL = quality of life, RCT = randomized controlled trial, RT = radiotherapy, SF-36 = (Medical Outcomes Studies) Short Form 36, SCC = squamous cell carcinoma, TL = total Laryngectomy, UM HNQOL = University of Michigan Head and Neck Quality of Life instrument, V-RQOL = Voice-Related Quality of Life, NR = not reported.

Reference	Fung, 2005			
Level (design)	2 (prospective nonrandomized trial)			
Sample size	97			

OUTCOMES

Outcome measure	1° Outcome **V-RQOL:** 0 (worst) to 100 (best)		2° Outcomes **PSS-HN:** includes 3 observer-rated items: eating in public (1–5), normalcy of diet (0–10), and understandability of speech (1–5), higher score relates to higher function **Nutritional Mode**	
	Social–emotional	**Physical functioning**	**Understandability of speech**	**Oral intake alone**
Chemo/RT	85.5	76.9	4.52	90%
Surgery/RT	68.1	63.6	3.43	65%
p Value	0.007	0.03	0.001	0.09
Conclusion	Voice-related QOL is better in patients after CRT compared with salvage TL			
Follow-up time	40 mo (median)			

STUDY DESIGN

Inclusion criteria	Stage III or IV SCC of larynx or hypopharynx that was previously untreated, surgically resectable, and curable with conventional surgery and radiotherapy
Exclusion criteria	Prior head and neck malignancy Metastatic disease Prior head and neck RT Prior chemotherapy
Patient characteristics	Mean age 58.4 y 78.6% male T2: 8.9% T3: 55.4% T4: 35.7%
Baseline group comparison	Larynx preserved vs laryngectomy: male 70.3% vs 94.7%, T2 10.8% vs 5.3%, T3 51.4% vs 63.2%, T4 37.8% vs 31.5%
Surgery/RT details	Every patient given single course of induction chemotherapy (cisplatin 100 mg/m^2 on day 1 and 5-FU 1000 mg/m^2/d ×5 d). If <50% response, then TL. Appropriate postoperative therapy given according to surgical outcomes
Chemo/RT details	Every patient given single course of induction chemotherapy (cisplatin 100 mg/m^2 on day 1 and 5-FU 1000 mg/m^2/d ×5 d). If >50% response then 72 Gy and cisplatin 100 mg/m^2 on days 1, 22, 43 followed by 2 cycles of adjuvant chemotherapy every 21 d 8 wk after completion of RT
Compliance	58% completed V-RQOL survey, 42% completed PSS-HN data
Intention to treat analysis	NR
Power	NR

5-FU = 5-fluorouracil, BDI = Beck Depression Inventory, CRT = chemoradiotherapy, Gy = Gray, =PSS-HN = Performance Status Scale for Head and Neck cancer patients, QOL = quality of life, RCT = randomized controlled trial, RT = radiotherapy, SF-36 = (Medical Outcomes Studies) Short Form 36, SCC = squamous cell carcinoma, TL = total Laryngectomy, UM HNQOL = University of Michigan Head and Neck Quality of Life instrument, V-RQOL = Voice-Related Quality of Life, NR = not reported.

Reference	Hanna, 2004
Level (design)	3 (nonrandomized, retrospective, cross-sectional study)
Sample size	42

OUTCOMES

Outcome measure	1° Outcomes
	EORTC QLQ-C30: 30 items comprising 6 functional scales (physical, role, cognitive, emotional, social functioning, and global QOL), 3 symptom scales (fatigue, pain, and emesis), and 6 individual items (dyspnea, sleep disturbance, appetite, constipation, diarrhea, and financial impact)
	EORTC QLQ-H&N35: 7 multiple-item scales (pain, swallowing, senses, speech, social eating, social contact, and sexuality) and 10 single items (problems with teeth, dry mouth, cough, opening the mouth wide, sticky saliva, weight loss, weight gain, use of nutritional supplements, feeding tubes, and painkillers) Scale 0–100 (higher scores represent better functioning, higher scores on symptom and individual item scales indicate greater difficulty)

	C30; QOL	H&N35; senses	H&N35; painkillers	H&N35; cough	H&N35; dry mouth
Chemo/RT	63.6	20	26.7	37.8	37.8
Surgery/RT	65.8	59.3	59.3	69.2	18.5
p Value	NS	0.001	0.049	0.004	0.02
Conclusion	The overall QOL scores of both groups seem similar, but individual symptom scores differ				

Follow-up time	Mean: 36 mo

STUDY DESIGN

Inclusion criteria	1. Stage III or IV laryngeal cancer 2. Previously treated with either TL or concurrent CRT
Exclusion criteria	Completion of therapy <3 mo before study
Patient characteristics	TL + RT: Median age: 65.6 y Male: 87% Married: 61% White: 78% CRT: Median age: 60.8 y Male: 68% Married: 53% White: 90%
Baseline group comparison	Did not differ significantly with respect to age, sex, marital status, or ethnicity
Surgery/RT details	TL: TL + neck dissection, plus postoperative RT, further details not provided
Chemo/RT details	At least 2 cycles of cisplatin and fluorouracil concurrently with RT; RT: total dose of 66–72 Gy
Intention to treat analysis	Done appropriately
Power	NR

5-FU = 5-fluorouracil, CRT = chemoradiotherapy, EORTC QLQ-C30 = European Organization for Research and Treatment of Cancer Quality of Life Questionnaire C30, EORTC QLQ-H&N35 = European Organization for Research and Treatment of Cancer Quality of Life Questionnaire head and neck module 35, Gy = Gray, NR = not reported, NS = not significant, QOL = quality of life, RT = radiotherapy, SCC = squamous cell carcinoma, TL = total Laryngectomy, UW QOL = University of Washington Head and Neck Quality of Life instrument.

Reference	LoTempio, 2005
Level (design)	3 (nonrandomized, retrospective cross-sectional study)
Sample size	49

OUTCOMES

Outcome measure	*1° Outcome* **UW QOL instrument version 4:** composed of 3 parts. Part 1: 12 domains: pain, appearance, activity, recreation, swallowing, chewing, speech, shoulder function, taste, saliva, mood, and anxiety. Part 2: which of 12 domains most important in last 7 d. Part 3: general questions; Scale 0–100, higher score relates to higher QOL

	1; pain: 25	1; swallowing: 0	1; chewing: 0	1; speech: 0	2; shoulder function problems	3; general questions
Chemo/RT	20%	27%	20%	0%	7%	NR
Surgery/RT	3%	6%	3%	9%	26%	NR
p Value	0.079	0.061	0.027	0.001	0.018	NS
Conclusion	Pain, swallowing, chewing, speech, and shoulder function recorded as significant factors affecting their lives, varies depending on TL + RT vs CRT					
Follow-up time	Median: 6 mo for CRT and 40 mo for TL + RT					

STUDY DESIGN

Inclusion criteria	1. Stage II–IV SCC of larynx and had completed CRT or TL + RT
Exclusion criteria	NR
Patient characteristics	Median age: 69 y Male: 92% Diverse ethnic backgrounds
Baseline group comparison	CRT vs TL + RT: 1 female vs 3 females, 14 males vs 31 males, 62 y vs 71 y
Surgery/RT details	No further details provided
Chemo/RT details	No further details provided
Intention to treat analysis	NR
Power	NR

5-FU = 5-fluorouracil, CRT = chemoradiotherapy, EORTC QLQ-C30 = European Organization for Research and Treatment of Cancer Quality of Life Questionnaire C30, EORTC QLQ-H&N35 = European Organization for Research and Treatment of Cancer Quality of Life Questionnaire head and neck module 35, Gy = Gray, NR = not reported, NS = not significant, QOL = quality of life, RT = radiotherapy, SCC = squamous cell carcinoma, TL = total Laryngectomy, UW QOL = University of Washington Head and Neck Quality of Life instrument.

REFERENCES

1. LoTempio MM, Wang KH, Sadeghi A, Delacure MD, Juillard GF, Wang MB. Comparison of quality of life outcomes in laryngeal cancer patients following chemoradiation vs. total laryngectomy. Otolaryngol Head Neck Surg 2005;132(6): 948–953.

2. Fung K, Lyden TH, Lee J, et al. Voice and swallowing outcomes of an organ-preservation trial for advanced laryngeal cancer. Int J Radiat Oncol Biol Phys 2005;63(5):1395–1399.

3. Hanna E, Sherman A, Cash D, et al. Quality of life for patients following total laryngectomy vs chemoradiation for laryngeal preservation. Arch Otolaryngol Head Neck Surg 2004;130(7):875–879.

4. Terrell JE, Fisher SG, Wolf GT. Long-term quality of life after treatment of laryngeal cancer. The Veterans Affairs Laryngeal Cancer Study Group. Arch Otolaryngol Head Neck Surg 1998;124(9):964–971.

5. Hillman RE, Walsh MJ, Wolf GT, Fisher SG, Hong WK. Functional outcomes following treatment for advanced laryngeal cancer. Part I. Voice preservation in advanced laryngeal cancer; Part II. Laryngectomy rehabilitation: the state of the art in the VA System. Research Speech-Language Pathologists. Department of Veterans Affairs Laryngeal Cancer Study Group. Ann Otol Rhinol Laryngol Suppl 1998; 172:1–27. Review.

6. Urba S, Wolf G, Eisbruch A, et al. Single-cycle induction chemotherapy selects patients with advanced laryngeal cancer for combined chemoradiation: a new treatment paradigm. J Clin Oncol 2006;24(4):593–598.

7. Wolf GT, Hong WK, Fisher SG et al. Induction chemotherapy plus radiation compared with surgery plus radiation in patients with advanced laryngeal cancer. N Engl J Med 1991;324(24):1685–1690.

31 Laryngeal Squamous Cell Carcinoma: Advanced Disease

31.C.

Chemoradiation therapy versus radiation therapy alone for stage III–IV laryngeal carcinoma: impact on survival, recurrence

Lori Wirth, Babar Sultan, and Merrill S. Kies

METHODS

A computerized OVID search of MEDLINE 1966-May, 2006 was performed. The terms "laryngeal carcinoma," "organ preservation therapy" and "chemotherapy radiotherapy and squamous cell carcinoma" were exploded and the resulting articles were cross referenced, yielding 117 articles limited to "human" and "English language." These articles or abstracts were then reviewed to identify randomized controlled trials that met the following inclusion criteria: 1) patient population with laryngeal carcinoma, 2) intervention with a platinum-based chemoradiation arm versus a standard radiotherapy arm, and 3) primary outcome measured in terms laryngeal preservation, overall survival or locoregional control. The references of these articles were reviewed and manually cross-checked to ensure all applicable literature was included. Publications which focused on other chemotherapeutic agents, such as mitcomycin, were excluded. Publications which reported only pooled data from patients with laryngeal carcinoma combined with those with carcinomas of other head and neck sites were also excluded. This process yielded 2 publications [1–2]. The literature is summarized below, with a detailed analysis of these randomized controlled trials (RCTs) presented.

SUMMARY

Induction chemotherapy with cisplatin and 5-fluorouracil (PF) has long been recognized as active therapy in SCCHN [3–5]. Clinical partial and complete responses were observed in 80% to 90% of previously untreated patients. It was postulated that a substantial response to initial treatment with chemotherapy could lead to an improvement in therapeutic efficacy for surgery or radiotherapy in SCCHN [6]. This early experience with PF led to the Department of Veterans Affairs (VA) Laryngeal Cancer Study reported by Wolf et al [7]. This landmark study demonstrated that induction chemotherapy followed by radiotherapy, with salvage laryngectomy reserved for failures only, is effective treatment for larynx cancer, and thus established organ preservation as a realistic goal for nonsurgical treatment of larynx cancer. Lefebvre, et al. later reported similar outcomes in a Euro-

pean Organization for Research and Treatment of Cancer trial (EORTC 24891) involving patients with cancers of the hypopharynx [8]. The success of these studies prompted further investigations of chemotherapy and radiation for the treatment of intermediate stage larynx cancer, using 1) induction PF followed by RT (PF-RT), 2) concurrent cisplatin chemotherapy plus radiation (CRT), or 3) radiation alone (RT) in the Radiation Therapy Oncology Group study RTOG 91-11 reported by Forastiere et al. At 2 years, 80% of patients on the concurrent CRT achieved local control, versus 65% with PF-RT, and 58% with RT alone. Weber et al went on further to analyze the salvage laryngectomy patients from the three treatment arms of the Forastiere et al study. Locoregional control for these patients was excellent and survival following salvage total laryngectomy was not influenced by the initial organ preservation treatment. Thus, for patients with intermediate stage squamous cell carcinoma of the larynx, a program of concurrent CRT, with the objectives of tumor eradication and laryngeal preservation, is often appropriate.

RESULTS

Outcome Measures. Forastiere et al analyzed the rate of larynx preservation (LP) at 2 years following randomization as the primary outcome. LP was determined by cumulative incidence. Secondary outcomes included overall survival (OS), laryngectomy-free survival, disease-free survival (DFS), patterns of recurrence and treatment toxicity. Beyond the gold standard endpoint of OS, the outcome of LP is of great interest; even if survival is not improved by the experimental therapy, natural speech, voice and swallowing may be preserved, leading to major quality of life benefits. As a note of caution, LP does not necessarily mean that function is also preserved. In Forastiere et al, moderate speech impairment, defined as difficulty pronouncing some words and being understood on the telephone, or worse, was found in 6% of those enrolled on the PF-RT arm, 11% of those on the CRT arm, and 13% on the RT alone arm. Weber et al analyzed OS, recurrence, post-surgery complications (major: significantly prolong hospitalization, life threatening; minor: self-limited, hospitalization not significantly prolonged), DFS, and loco-regional control for patients undergoing salvage total laryngectomy.

Potential Confounders. Potential bias exists in comparing survival times in subjects treated on protocol due to differences between arms in treatment duration. Forastiere et al described measures to control such bias. Weber et al analyzed OS and DFS from the point of randomization due to varying times of receiving a total laryngectomy. The inability to blind study subjects and staff to treatment arm assignment may also have introduced some bias into the evaluation of study outcomes, particularly in interpreting more subjective information, such as toxicity. The lack of blinding should have not or just minimally biased the interpretation of surgical complications in Weber et al.

Study Designs. These 2 studies provide level 1 evidence from randomized clinical trials. Forastiere et al randomized 547 patients with untreated stage III or IV glottic or supraglottic larynx cancers (except T4 primaries invading cartilage or the base of tongue) to one of three arms: PF-RT, CRT or RT alone. Induction chemotherapy consisted of 2 cycles of cisplatin/5-FU. Those with at least a partial response in the primary site and no progression in the neck received a third cycle, then radiotherapy. In the CRT arm, cycles of cisplatin were administered during radiation on days 1, 22 and 43. Radiotherapy was the same in all study arms, to a total dose of 70 Gy in 35 2-Gy fractions over 7 weeks, except for those with a poor response to PF induction therapy after 2 cycles. These patients underwent laryngectomy, then adjuvant radiotherapy to a minimum dose of 50 Gy. The sample size and power calculations were outlined in detail by Forastiere, et al., with the sample size designed to detect an improvement of 15% above the expected 2-year LP rate of 65% with the control arm, PF-RT, with type I and II error rates of 0.05 and 0.20.

Weber et al. analyzed 129 patients who had undergone one of the randomized treatment arms in the Forastiere et al study, and had a salvage total laryngectomy for disease progression after two cycles of chemotherapy in PF-RT, biopsy proven disease at the primary site at least 8 weeks after RT, or laryngeal dysfunction with aspiration or laryngeal necrosis.

Highest Level of Evidence. Forastiere et al demonstrated that the 2-year LP rate was superior with concurrent CRT 88%, compared to RT alone (70%, $p < 0.001$) or PF-RT (75%, $p = 0.005$). The rate of LR control at 2-years was also significantly better with CRT. Both chemotherapy arms resulted in fewer distant metastases and better disease-free survival (DFS), however OS was unchanged, with estimated 5-year OS 55% with PF-RT, 54% with CRT and 56% with RT alone. A composite endpoint of laryngectomy-free survival (LFS) was also considered. Estimated LFS at 5 years was 43%, 45% and 38%, respectively. Pair-wise comparisons of PF-RT to RT alone and CRT to RT alone yielded p values of 0.08 and 0.01, respectively.

Weber et al demonstrated that OS at 24 months after a salvage laryngectomy for CRT: 71%, RT: 76%, and PF-RT: 75% did not differ significantly. Recurrence rates after surgery for CRT: 28%, RT: 31%, and PF-RT: 44% also did not differ significantly. Loco-regional control was excellent for all three groups after surgery; CRT: 74%, RT: 90%, PF-RT: 74% with no significance reported. Distant failure with above clavicle control was reported as CRT: 8%, RT: 20%, PF-RT: 18%, no significance reported.

Applicability. These results can be best applied to patients with intermediate stage laryngeal squamous cell carcinomas for which surgical treatment would require total laryngectomy. Both the Forstiere et al and Weber et al studies contained more stage III than stage IV patients, and thus the patient populations best represented in these studies are those with intermediate stage disease more so than bulky locoregionally advanced disease. Patients with more bulky stage IV disease, without DM, were eligible to participate in the trials, but were in the minority, compared to patients with stage III disease. Finally, Forastiere et al also excluded patients with T4 primaries invading cartilage or base of tongue, so results are not applicable to patients with that extent of disease.

Morbidity/Complications. Deaths related to treatment were rare. The treatment arms involving chemotherapy resulted in the expected toxicities, such as neutropenia, nausea, vomiting and renal dysfunction. Concurrent CRT, compared to PF-RT or RT alone in Forastiere et al was associated with more ≥grade 3 stomatitis and dermatitis, as expected, however the incidence of late toxicities was similar in all 3 groups. In the Weber et al study, overall incidence of major and minor surgical complications was CRT: 59%, RT: 52%, PF-RT: 58%. Systemic complications included 1 perioperative death (myocardial infarction), non fatal cardiovascular events in 7 patients, and 1 cerebrovascular accident. No significant differences in frequency of systemic complications among the three groups. Pharyngocutaneous fistula occurred in CRT: 30%, RT: 15%, PF-RT: 25%, $p > 0.05$. Incidence of complications across the 3 arms was independent of the time from the end of treatment to laryngectomy ($p = 0.86$)

CLINICAL SIGNIFICANCE AND FUTURE RESEARCH

These trials indicate that for patients with intermediate stage squamous cell carcinoma of the larynx, a concurrent CRT program may be more beneficial than RT or PF-RT, with the objectives of tumor eradication and laryngeal preservation. It is important to recognize that patients with locally advanced destructive primary laryngeal cancers were not included in the two studies.

Future research could further examine the role of concurrent CRT in the setting of more advanced laryngeal disease. Also, the type of and duration of chemotherapy agents can be varied to find the most efficacious protocol with minimal toxicities. In addition with further breakthroughs in radiation technology, the question of CRT vs. RT can be re-evaluated using advanced delivery systems for radiation therapy.

Reference	Forastiere, 2003
Level (Design)	1 (RCT)
Sample Size	547

OUTCOMES

Outcomes measured	1° Outcome, LP rate	2° Outcomes, OS, DFS, LFS, LR control, Distant metastasis, Toxicity
Specific results	LP rate at 2 yrs	
CRT	88%	
RT	70%	
PF-RT	75%	
***p* value**	<0.001, 0.005	
Conclusion	Radiotherapy with concurrent cisplatin is superior to induction chemotherapy followed by radiotherapy or radiotherapy alone for LP and LR control.	
Follow-up time	3.8 yrs	

STUDY DESIGN

Inclusion criteria	1. Untreated stage III or IV squamous cell carcinoma of the glottic or supraglottic larynx; 2. Surgical treatment would require total laryngectomy; 3. Disease that is considered curable with surgery and post-op radiotherapy; 4. Karnofsky PS ≥ 60; 5. Adequate bone marrow and renal function, normal serum calcium; 6. Written informed consent
Exclusion criteria	1. T1 primary; 2. Large-volume T4 primary (tumor penetrating through cartilage or extending >1 cm into base of tongue)
Patient Characteristics	Median age 59; 77% male; 96% Karnofsky PS ≥ 80; 1° site—69% supraglottis, 31% glottis, 65% stage III, 35% stage IV, TN stage—T2—12%, T3 w. fixed cord—46%, T3 no fixed cord—32%, T4—10%, N0—50%, N1—21%, N2–3—29%
Randomization Effectiveness	The groups were well balanced with regard to the patient characteristics noted above. There were minor differences, such as the RT alone arm had slightly more unfavorable prognosis patients with more advanced nodal disease and supraglottic *vs.* glottic tumors, but these differences are unlikely to account for statistically significant differences in study outcomes.
Study regimens	RT alone = 70 Gy in 35 fractions of 2-Gy fractions, 5 d/wk over 7 wks. CRT = RT as above + concurrent cisplatin 100 mg/m² on days 1, 22 and 43. PF-RT = cisplatin 100 mg/m² on day 1 + 5FU 1000 mg/m²/d by continuous infusion for 120 hrs, every 3 wks for 2 cycles. If restaging showed ≥ PR, a 3rd cycle was given, followed by RT, as above. If < PR, laryngectomy and post-op RT was recommended. All patients with ≥ N2A disease were required to undergo neck dissection 8 wks after the completion of RT. Laryngectomy was performed as above, and in any patient with biopsy-proven persistent or recurrent 1° tumor.
Outcome measurements in detail	All events were measured from the date of randomization to their occurrence or last follow-up. NCI Common Toxicity Criteria, v. 1.0 and RTOG toxicity criteria for toxicities during RT were used. Because the study compared 2 experimental arms to 1 standard arm, Dunnett's two-sided test was used to adjust for multiple comparisons. Survival rates were estimated by the Kaplan-Meier method and compared by the log-rank test. Rates of LP, LR control and DM were compared by Gray's method.
Potential Confounders	Differences in the timing of therapy between arms could bias the measured time outcomes because therapy on the PF-RT arm was longer than the other study arms. To minimize bias, all laryngectomies performed within the 1st 6 months of the start of treatment were considered early treatment failures and were analyzed as if they occurred at the same time. Other potential confounders were minimized by randomization and stratification according to 1° site, T and N stage. Observation of toxicities may have been influenced by inability to blind investigators and patients to treatment arm, whereas the recording of hard data points, such as laryngectomy and survival should not be affected by lack of blinding.
Compliance	93% of patients on the PF-RT arm who had ≥ PR after the 2nd cycle of PF received the 3rd cycle. 70% of patients on the CRT arm received all 3 cycles of concurrent cisplatin. 84% of the PF-RT patients received ≥ 95% of the recommended RT dose (i.e., ≥67 Gy), whereas 91% and 94% of the CRT and RT arms, respectively, received ≥ 95% of the recommended RT dose.
Power	The study was designed to detect an improvement of 15% above the expected LP rate of 65% at 2 yrs, with a power of 80% and type I error of 0.05. The sample size was inflated by 10% to account for patients deemed ineligible or lost to follow-up.
Morbidity/Complications	PF chemotherapy toxicity was primarily neutropenia, stomatitis, nausea and vomiting. Toxicity during radiation was nearly identical in the PF-RT and RT arms, consisting of ≥ grade 3 stomatitis (24% and 24%, respectively) and dermatitis (10% and 9%, respectively). In the CRT arm, ≥ grade 3 stomatitis was 43% and dermatitis was 7%. The incidence of late ≥ grade 3 toxicities was 24% in the PF-RT arm, 30% in the CRT arm, and 36% in the RT alone arm. There were no differences between the 3 arms with regard to speech. At 2 yrs, <10% had moderate speech impairment, defined as difficulty pronouncing some words and being understood on the telephone. Swallow function at 2 yrs was also very similar, with about 15% of patients reporting difficulty.
Other Secondary Endpoints	Estimated 5-yr OS did not differ significantly between groups, and was 55% with PF-RT, 54% with CRT and 56% with RT alone. Patients who received chemotherapy had improved DFS, with 5-yr DFS rates of 38% (p = 0.02), 36% (p = 0.006) and 27%, respectively. 5-yr LFS (composite endpoint of laryngectomy or death) rates were 43% (p = 0.08), 45% (p = 0.01) and 38%, respectively. LR control was significantly better with CRT. 2-yr LR control rates were 61% (p = 0.16), 78% (p < 0.001) and 56%, respectively. The 5-yr DM rates were 15% (p N/A), 12% (p = 0.03) and 22%, respectively. Results after 5 yrs of follow-up have been presented in abstract form. While the rate of LP remained significantly better with CRT (83.6%) compared to PF-RT (70.5%, p = 0.0029) or RT (65.7%, p = 0.00017), the rate of LFS is not better with CRT *vs.* PF-RT (44.6% *vs.* 46.6%, p = 0.98), but LFS with RT alone is inferior (33.9%). This implies that more patients in the CRT arm are dying compared to PF-RT, to account for the lack of difference in this composite endpoint. OS remains flat across all 3 groups (CRT 54.6%, PF-RT 59.2%, RT 53.5%).[11]

Abbreviations: RCT, randomized controlled trial; LP, larynx preservation; OS, overall survival; LFS, laryngectomy-free survival; DFS, disease-free survival; LR, locoregional; CRT, chemoradiotherapy; RT, radiotherapy; PF-RT, cisplatin/5FU, then radiotherapy; WHO, World Health Organization; PS, performance status; DM, distant metastasis; 5FU, 5-fluorouracil; PR, partial response; PD, progressive disease; Gy, Gray; CR, complete response; NCI, National Cancer Institute; RTOG, Radiation Therapy Oncology Group; CIs, confidence intervals; NR, information not available; HR, hazard ratio; ORR, overall response rate.

Reference	Weber, 2003
Level (Design)	1 (RCT)
Sample Size	129

OUTCOMES

Outcomes measured	OS, Recurrence, Post-surgery complications (major: significantly prolonged hospitalization, life threatening; minor: self-limited, hospitalization not significantly prolonged), DFS, LR

Specific results	OS at 24 months	Recurrence	Minor/Major Complications	Pharyngocutaneous fistula
CRT	71%	28%	59%	30%
RT	76%	31%	52%	15%
PF-RT	69%	44%	58%	25%
p value	NS	NS	NS	p > 0.05

Conclusion	Survival following salvage TL was not influenced by the initial organ preservation treatment. Perioperative mortality is low but one third of patients will develop a pharyngocutaneous fistula
Follow-up time	Mean CRT: 39.0 months, RT: 36.5 months, PF-RT: 35.4 months

STUDY DESIGN

Inclusion criteria	1. Initially had to meet the inclusion criteria listed in Forastiere et al then undergo either CRT, RT, or PF-RT; 2. Undergo salvage total laryngectomy because of disease progression after two cycles of chemotherapy in PF-RT, biopsy proven disease at the primary site at least 8 weeks after RT, or laryngeal dysfunction with aspiration or laryngeal necrosis
Exclusion criteria	Initially had to pass exclusion criteria listed in Forastiere et al.
Patient Characteristics	+Salvage Total Laryngectomy; Age > 60: CRT: 44% RT: 43% PF-RT: =46%; Male: CRT: 96%, RT: 81%, PF-RT: 75%; Karnofsky PS ≥ 80: CRT: 70%, RT: 61%, PF-RT: 46% (1° site—supraglottis: CRT: 59% RT: 67% PF-RT: 54%; glottis: CRT: 41% RT: 33% PF-RT: 46%; stage III CRT: 78%, RT: 67% PF-RT: 69%; stage IV CRT: 22% RT: 33% PF-RT: 31%; TN stage—T2—CRT: 11%, RT: 9%, PF-RT: 19%); T3 w. fixed cord—CRT: 56%, RT: 44%, PF-RT: 29%; T3 no fixed cord—CRT: 26%, RT: 35%, PF-RT: 17%; T4—CRT: 7%, RT: 11%, PF-RT: 4%; N0—CRT: 59%, RT: 53%, PF-RT: 52%; N1—CRT: 26%, RT: 20%, PF-RT: 21%; N2-3—CRT: 15%, RT: 14%, PF-RT: 27%
Randomization Effectiveness	Please refer to randomization effectiveness of Forastiere et al prior to salvage total laryngectomy.
Study regimens	RT alone = 70 Gy in 35 fractions of 2-Gy fractions, 5 d/wk over 7 wks. CRT = RT as above + concurrent cisplatin 100 mg/m² on days 1, 22 and 43. PF-RT = cisplatin 100 mg/m² on day 1 + 5FU 1000 mg/m²/d by continuous infusion for 120 hrs, every 3 wks for 2 cycles. If restaging showed ≥ PR, a 3rd cycle was given, followed by RT, as above. If <PR, laryngectomy and post-op RT was recommended. All patients with ≥ N2A disease were required to undergo neck dissection 8 wks after the completion of RT. Laryngectomy was performed as above, and in any patient with biopsy-proven persistent or recurrent 1° tumor, laryngeal dysfunction with aspiration or laryngeal necrosis.
Outcome measurements in detail	OS and DFS were measured from randomization rather than time from surgery because salvage TL was performed at different time points. OS and DFS were estimated using the Kaplan-Meier method. Statistical testing was done by both the log rank and Wilcoxon tests. Multivariate analysis was performed using the Cox proportional hazards model. Categorical variables were examined by chi-squared analysis.
Potential Confounders	Initial randomization and stratification minimize confounders. Differences in timing of laryngectomies negated by measuring survival from initial randomization. Observation of surgical complications unlikely to be influenced by inability to blind investigators. Comparisons by assigned treatment limited only to patients needing salvage TL for disease are biased because whether a patient would require salvage TL was unknown at time of randomization. Comparisons not invalid but may not reflect overall treatment results among entire group of randomized patients.
Compliance	Seven patients required a laryngectomy for necrosis or dysfunction, and one patient had a laryngectomy prior to protocol treatment. These cases were included in assessment of complications but not in analysis of overall survival or recurrence.
Power	Not reported
Morbidity/ Complications	Overall incidence of major and minor surgical complications was CRT: 59%, RT: 52%, PF-RT: 58%. Systemic complications included 1 perioperative death (myocardial infarction), non fatal cardiovascular events in 7 patients, and 1 cerebrovascular accident. No significant differences in frequency of systemic complications among the three groups. Pharyngocutaneous fistula occurred in CRT: 30%, RT: 15%, PF-RT: 25%, p > 0.05. Incidence of complications across the 3 arms was independent of the time from the end of treatment to laryngectomy (p = 0.86)
Other Secondary Endpoints	LR control: CRT: 74%, RT: 90%, PF-RT: 74% Distant failure with above clavicle control: CRT: 8%, RT: 20%, PF-RT: 18% Minor complication: CRT: 41%, RT: 28%, PF-RT: 38% Major complication: CRT: 19%, RT 24%, PF-RT: 21% DFS: CRT: 52%, RT: 51%, PF-RT: 40%, p = 0.50

Abbreviations: RCT, randomized controlled trial; LP, larynx preservation; OS, overall survival; LFS, laryngectomy-free survival; DFS, disease-free survival; LR, locoregional; CRT, chemoradiotherapy; RT, radiotherapy; PF-RT, cisplatin/5FU, then radiotherapy; WHO, World Health Organization; PS, performance status; DM, distant metastasis; 5FU, 5-fluorouracil; PR, partial response; PD, progressive disease; Gy, Gray; CR, complete response; NCI, National Cancer Institute; RTOG, Radiation Therapy Oncology Group; CIs, confidence intervals; NR, information not available; HR, hazard ratio; ORR, overall response rate.

REFERENCES

1. Weber RS, Berkey BA, Forastiere A, Cooper J, Maor M, Goepfert H, Morrison W, Glisson B, Trotti A, Ridge JA, Chao KS, Peters G, Lee DJ, Leaf A, Ensley J. Outcome of salvage total laryngectomy following organ preservation therapy: the Radiation Therapy Oncology Group trial 91-11. Arch Otolaryngol Head Neck Surg. 2003 Jan;129(1): 44–9.

2. Forastiere AA, Goepfert H, Maor M, Pajak TF, Weber R, Morrison W, et al. Concurrent chemotherapy and radiotherapy for organ preservation in advanced laryngeal cancer. N Engl J Med 2003;349(22):2091–8

3. Ensley JF, Jacobs JR, Weaver A, Kinzie J, Crissman J, Kish JA, et al. Correlation between response to cisplatinum-combination chemotherapy and subsequent radiotherapy in previously untreated patients with advanced squamous cell cancers of the head and neck. Cancer 1984;54(5):811–4.

4. Kies MS, Gordon LI, Hauck WW, Krespi Y, Ossoff RH, Pecaro BC, et al. Analysis of complete responders after initial treatment with chemotherapy in head and neck cancer. Otolaryngol Head Neck Surg 1985;93(2):199–205.

5. Ervin TJ, Clark JR, Weichselbaum RR, Fallon BG, Miller D, Fabian RL, et al. An analysis of induction and adjuvant chemotherapy in the multidisciplinary treatment of squamous-cell carcinoma of the head and neck. J Clin Oncol 1987;5(1):10–20.

6. Spaulding MB, Fischer SG, Wolf GT. Tumor response, toxicity, and survival after neoadjuvant organ-preserving chemotherapy for advanced laryngeal carcinoma. The Department of Veterans Affairs Cooperative Laryngeal Cancer Study Group. J Clin Oncol 1994;12(8):1592–1599.

7. Induction chemotherapy plus radiation compared with surgery plus radiation in patients with advanced laryngeal cancer. The Department of Veterans Affairs Laryngeal Cancer Study Group. N Engl J Med 1991;324(24):1685–90.

8. Lefebvre JL, Chevalier D, Luboinski B, Kirkpatrick A, Collette L, Sahmoud T. Larynx preservation in pyriform sinus cancer: preliminary results of a European Organization for Research and Treatment of Cancer phase III trial. EORTC Head and Neck Cancer Cooperative Group. J Natl Cancer Inst 1996;88(13):890–9.

32 Advanced Head and Neck Malignancy

32.A.

Adjuvant chemoradiotherapy versus adjuvant radiation therapy for high-risk head and neck cancer: Impact on survival, recurrence

Lori Wirth, Babar Sultan, and Merrill S. Kies

METHODS

A computerized Ovid search of MEDLINE 1966–January 2006 was performed. The terms "postoperative therapy," "adjuvant therapy," and "head and neck cancer" were exploded and the resulting articles were cross-referenced, yielding 7643 articles limited to "human" and "English language." These articles or abstracts were then reviewed to identify those that met the following inclusion criteria: 1) patient population with operable squamous cell carcinoma of the head and neck (SCCHN) with high-risk features, 2) intervention with a postoperative experimental arm (postoperative cisplatin with radiotherapy) versus a standard therapy arm (postoperative radiotherapy alone), 3) primary outcome measured in terms of progression- or disease-free survival, overall survival (OS), or locoregional (LR) control. The references of these articles were reviewed and manually cross-checked to ensure all applicable literature was included. This process yielded three randomized controlled trials (RCTs), a detailed analysis of which is presented below.

SUMMARY

LR recurrence is common after surgical treatment of stage III or IV SCCHN. Risk factors for recurrence and death include positive surgical margins, extranodal extension, and multiple involved nodes [1–4]. Several strategies to improve the outcome of resectable locally advanced SCCHN have been studied since the 1970s. The benefit of adding radiotherapy to surgery has been consistently demonstrated, though not in the preoperative setting, only postoperatively [5–7]. Attempts were made to improve upon conventional radiotherapy by shortening the overall radiation treatment time without reducing the dose by accelerated fractionation by a twice-daily concomitant boost schedule. Two RCTs, however, failed to yield better outcomes over conventional radiotherapy [8, 9]. Similar disappointing results were seen with postoperative chemotherapy. When explored alone and added sequentially to postoperative radiotherapy, chemotherapy did not improve LR control or OS [10–12]. Because concurrent chemotherapy plus radiotherapy was shown to be superior to radiotherapy alone in other settings, this strategy was explored in several studies for postoperative treatment of locally advanced SCCHN [13–17]. Several regimens have been examined, including mitomycin and cisplatin. The RCTs that focused on cisplatin therapy are reviewed in detail below [13, 16, 17].

RESULTS

Outcome Measures. The primary outcome of the European Organization for Research and Treatment of Cancer (EORTC) 22931 trial was progression-free survival (PFS), defined as the time from randomization to progression of disease or death from any cause. OS was defined as the time from randomization to death from any cause. Both endpoints were estimated using the Kaplan-Meier method. The primary outcome measured in Radiation Therapy Oncology Group (RTOG) 9501 was LR control, defined as absence of disease recurrence in the original tumor bed and/or cervical node metastasis. OS was measured as described for the EORTC study, and the Kaplan-Meier method was used. The smaller Bachaud study measured LR control as the primary endpoint, with secondary endpoints including OS and disease-free survival (DFS). Although primary outcomes measured in these studies were slightly different, all are good indicators of the risk of treatment failure for patients in one treatment group relative to the other.

Potential Confounders. EORTC 22931 and RTOG 9501 enrolled similar, but not uniform patient populations, in part because of the different criteria used to define postoperative SCCHN patients at high risk for recurrence. The EORTC eligibility criteria included: 1) tumor (T) stage of T3 or T4 and any nodal (N) stage, except T3 N0 of the larynx with negative margins, 2) stage T1 or 2, N0 or 1 with an unfavorable pathologic finding [extracapsular spread (ECS), positive resection margin, perineural involvement, or vascular tumor embolism], or 3) oral cavity or oropharyngeal tumors with involved level IV or V cervical nodes. The RTOG high-risk eligibility criteria included: 1) involvement of ≥2 regional nodes, 2) ECS, or 3) positive resection margin. Table 32.A.1 summarizes the major differences in patients enrolled in the two studies in terms of primary site, stage, and high-risk pathologic features.

TABLE 32.A.1. Differences in EORTC 22931 and RTOG 9501 studies

Characteristic	EORTC 22931 (%)	RTOG 9501 (%)
1° site		
Oral cavity	26	27
Oropharynx	30	42
Larynx	22	21
Hypopharynx	20	10
Other	1	<1
T stage		
T1–2	33	39
T3–4	66	61
Unknown	1	0
N stage		
N0–1	43	6
N2–3	57	94
High-risk path		
ECS alone	41	49
+margin alone	13	6
+margin and ECS	16	4

In contrast to the later EORTC and RTGO studies, Bachaud et al. required ECS in all subjects as a sole high-risk factor for study entry. In retrospect, ECS seems to be one of the most potent risk factors for recurrence. Thus, its requirement in all subjects may in part explain the positive results in such a small sample size.

Study Designs. All three studies provide level 1 evidence from randomized phase III designs comparing the addition of concurrent cisplatin chemotherapy to postoperative radiotherapy with radiotherapy alone in patients with high-risk SCCHN. Chemotherapy in two studies was the same, with cisplatin given during radiotherapy at 100 mg/m^2 on days 1, 22, and 43. The radiotherapy administered was slightly different, with 60 Gy ± a 6-Gy boost in the RTOG study, versus 66 Gy administered to all patients in the EORTC study. In Bachaud et al., cisplatin 50-mg bolus was given once a week in 7–9 cycles plus postoperative radiation (54 Gy in 32 fractions ± 20-Gy boost). The boost was dependent on the burden of disease after surgery. Given the obvious treatment differences in study arms, assignments were not blinded, nor was placebo given. The EORTC trial enrolled 334 patients, 459 patients were enrolled in RTOG, and 88 patients in Bachaud et al. Median follow-up times were 60 months, 46 months, and minimum 60 months, respectively. Sample size calculations differed, with EORTC 22931 powered to detect a 15% increase in absolute PFS

from 40% to 55% at 3 years, with a power of 0.80 and two-sided level of significance of 0.05. RTOG 9501 was powered to detect a 15% improvement in the 2-year rate of LR recurrence expected from radiotherapy alone (38%), using the same significance level and power. The Bachaud study was not powered for a particular sample size. Investigators initially hoped to accrue 200 patients, but because of a growing use of neoadjuvant chemotherapy at the time, the study closed early because of poor accrual.

Highest Level of Evidence. EORTC 22931 demonstrated significant improvement in PFS with concurrent postoperative chemoradiotherapy compared with radiotherapy alone. The estimated 5-year PFS rates were, respectively, 47% and 36% (p = 0.04). Overall 5-year survival rate was also better in the chemoradiotherapy arm, with the rates of 53% and 40%, respectively (p = 0.02). This study further demonstrated improved LR control with chemoradiotherapy at 5 years (18% versus 31%). With chemoradiotherapy, severe mucositis (41% versus 21%), neutropenia, and nausea/vomiting were more frequent. Late adverse effects, including xerostomia, dysphagia, and serious complications such as mucosal necrosis, bone and laryngeal complications were similar.

RTOG 9501 also showed an improvement in the study's primary endpoint, LR control, with postoperative chemoradiotherapy compared with radiotherapy alone, with a hazard ratio for LR recurrence of 0.62 [95% confidence interval (CI) 0.41–0.91, p = 0.01]. The estimated 2-year LR control was 82% with chemoradiotherapy, versus 72% with radiotherapy. Despite this improvement in disease control, OS was not better with chemoradiotherapy, as reflected in the hazard ratio of 0.84 (95% CI 0.65–1.09, p = 0.19). As expected, adverse effects were greater in the chemoradiotherapy arm, with more hematologic, mucosal, and gastrointestinal side effects. Four patients on the chemoradiotherapy arm died from protocol-related events, compared with none on the radiotherapy arm. Late effects encountered were not significantly different.

Bachaud et al. also showed a trend toward improvement in the study's primary endpoint, LR control, when comparing postoperative chemoradiotherapy to radiotherapy alone, although the difference was not statistically significant (77% versus 59%, p = 0.08). OS and DFS were better in the chemoradiotherapy group compared with radiotherapy alone with statistically significant differences; at 2 years OS was 72% versus 46%, respectively, whereas at 5 years OS was 36% and 13% (p < 0.01). DFS at 2 years and 5 years was 68% and 45% versus 44% and 23% (p < 0.02).

A retrospective subgroup analysis using data pooled from the RTOG and EORTC trials has been performed in order to further explore the characterization of risk factors that might warrant intense postoperative chemoradiotherapy [18]. As shown in Table 32.A.1, the proportion of patients with N2–3 disease was substantially higher in the RTOG study, which also had more patients with oropharyngeal primaries and fewer patients with hypopharyngeal primaries. Also of note, when the high-risk pathologic features common to both studies (ECS and positive margins) were considered, fewer RTOG patients than EORTC patients (59% versus 70%) had common high-risk features. The impact of these common high-risk features on OS was examined in the pooled data, and results showed that patients with ECS and/or positive margins had significantly poorer survival than those without these risk factors. Moreover, OS in this subset of patients in both studies was improved with cisplatin plus radiotherapy compared with radiotherapy alone. This was, however, not the case when the subset of patients without ECS and/or positive margins was examined. The benefit of chemotherapy added to radiotherapy was also seen in terms of LR control and DFS in the pooled subset of patients with the common high-risk features of ECS and/or positive margins. Conclusions drawn from this retrospective unplanned analysis should be made with caution and taken only as exploratory in nature. Nonetheless, this retrospective subgroup analysis suggests that the superiority of postoperative chemoradiotherapy, regardless of which endpoint is considered, is accounted for primarily by the subset of patients that possessed one or more of the high-risk features common to both studies (i.e., ECS and/or positive margins). The magnitude of benefit of intensive postoperative concurrent chemoradiotherapy in patients at risk by virtue of stage III–IV disease, ≥2 involved nodes, perineural invasion, tumor vascular embolism, or involved level IV or V nodes in patients with oral cavity or oropharyngeal cancers is less clear.

Applicability. The results of EORTC 22931 and RTOG 9501 are applicable to patients with high-risk SCCHN who have undergone complete resection. The definition of high-risk disease differed between the two studies, although the high-risk features common to both studies (ECS and/or positive margins) clearly define a patient population that will have better outcomes with cisplatin plus radiotherapy compared with radiotherapy alone. Other high-risk factors that should be taken into account when planning postoperative therapy are: 1) T stage of T3 or T4 and any N stage, except T3 N0 of the larynx with negative margins, 2) stage T1 or 2, N0 or 1 with perineural involvement or vascular tumor embolism, 3) oral cavity or oropharyngeal tumors with involved level IV or V cervical nodes, or 4) involvement of ≥2 regional nodes. The Bachaud study supports the inclusion of ECS as a high-risk feature that obligates the addition of chemotherapy to radiotherapy in the postoperative setting.

Morbidity/Complications. Treatment intensification by adding chemotherapy to postoperative radiotherapy for SCCHN comes at a price of increased toxicity. In the EORTC study, 41% of the combined therapy group experienced acute grade ≥3 adverse effects, versus 21% of the radiotherapy-alone group. In RTOG 9501, 77% of combined therapy versus 34% of radiotherapy patients experienced acute grade ≥3 adverse effects, and notably, there were four treatment-related deaths in the former group. However, the long-term toxicities studied did not differ between treatment groups in either study. In Bachaud et al., 15% of the radiotherapy group and 20% of the chemoradiotherapy group, respectively, experienced >grade 2 late toxicity on RTOG/EORTC scale. Serious complications also included osteoradionecrosis and pharyngeal stenosis.

CLINICAL SIGNIFICANCE AND FUTURE RESEARCH

Until recently, the standard of care has been to administer radiotherapy in the postoperative setting to decrease the risk of LR recurrence in patients with advanced, resectable head and neck cancer. Now, with the publication of two large, well-run RCTs and another smaller but similar older study, a new standard of care is established, supporting the use of adjuvant chemoradiotherapy for postoperative high-risk SCCHN. Chemoradiotherapy decreases the risk of LR recurrence, and may also improve OS. Unfortunately, the addition of bolus cisplatin to radiotherapy does not seem to decrease the risk of distant metastasis (DM). With improved ability to achieve LR control, DM is becoming the most common site of recurrent disease. Studies aimed at improving systemic therapies for SCCHN are thus needed. Strategies now under investigation include the addition of targeted therapies, such as EGFR (epidermal growth factor receptor) monoclonal antibodies and tyrosine kinase inhibitors, to postoperative chemoradiotherapy. Beyond the potential for improved disease control, targeted therapy is an appealing addition because of non-overlapping toxicities that may allow for enhanced efficacy without significantly increasing the acute and long-term toxicity of intensive chemoradiotherapy.

Given the intensity of postoperative chemoradiotherapy, especially the potential for late adverse effects including dysphagia and xerostomia that can have lifelong impact on quality of life, it is imperative that we have a better understanding of the high-risk factors that distinguish between patients who will benefit from an aggressive postoperative chemoradiotherapy approach, and those who might do as well with less toxic therapy.

THE EVIDENCE CONDENSED: Adjuvant chemoradiotherapy versus adjuvant radiotherapy alone for high-risk squamous cell carcinoma of the head and neck

Reference	Bernier, 2004 (EORTC 22931)	
Level (design)	1 (RCT)	
Sample size	334	

OUTCOMES

Outcome measure	1° Outcome PFS	2° Outcomes OS LR recurrence Distant metastasis 2nd primary tumor Toxicity (acute and late)
Results of intervention	5-y PFS 47%	5-y OS 53%
Results of control	5-y PFS 36%	5-y OS 40%
p Value	0.04	0.02
Conclusion	Postoperative concurrent cisplatin and RT CRT improves PFS and OS in high-risk SCCHN, without substantial increase in toxicity, compared with RT alone	
Follow-up time	60 mo	

STUDY DESIGN

Inclusion criteria	1. SCCHN of oral cavity, oropharynx, hypopharynx, or larynx, and 2. T3 or 4 (except T3 N0 of larynx) 3. OR T1 or 2 with ECS, +margin, or perineural involvement, OR vascular tumor embolism, OR oral cavity or oropharyngeal tumor with involved level IV or V nodes 4. Age ≥18 y, ≤70 y, KPS ≥60, adequate renal, liver, and bone marrow function
Exclusion criteria	1. No concurrent cancer, except nonmelanoma skin cancer 2. Previous chemotherapy 3. Known CNS disease
Randomization effectiveness	Well balanced in terms of sex, age, T & N stage, 1° site, margin status, degree of differentiation, ECS, perineural involvement, and vascular embolism
Age	53 y (median)
Masking	Not done
Study regimens	Postoperative radiation (66 Gy in 33 fractions) + concurrent cisplatin (100 mg/m^2 on days 1, 22, and 43) vs RT alone
Potential confounders	The impact of potential confounders in the 3 studies is minimized because of randomization. The inability to blind patients and investigators should have little impact on the hard endpoints of PFS, OS, and LR control. Awareness of treatment assignment, however, has potential to influence assessment of secondary toxicity endpoints
Compliance	28% of patients started treatment >6 wk after surgery. 4% did not receive specified RT dose. 25% had RT breaks leading to treatment lasting >7 wk. 64% of intervention group completed all 3 cycles of chemotherapy
Intention to treat analysis	Performed appropriately
Power	Designed to detect a 15% absolute increase in 3-y PFS from 40% to 55%, with a 2-sided significance level of 0.05 and power of 0.80
Morbidity/complications	Severe ≥grade 3 mucosal toxicity (according to NCI CTC v. 2.0 and RTOG/EORTC criteria) occurred in 41% of patients with CRT vs 21% with RT (p = 0.001). Severe leukopenia, neutropenia, and vomiting occurred in 16%, 13%, and 11% of patients with CRT, respectively. Other severe toxicities were similar in both groups No protocol-related deaths were reported
Other secondary endpoints	5-y LR recurrence 18% vs 31% (p = 0.007) (CRT vs RT) 5-y distant metastasis 21% vs 25% (p = 0.61) 5-y second primary tumor rate 12% vs 13% (p = 0.83)

EORTC = European Organization for Research and Treatment of Cancer, RTOG = Radiation Therapy Oncology Group, RCT = randomized controlled trial, PFS = progression-free survival, OS = overall survival, LR = locoregional, DFS = disease-free survival, HR = hazard ratio, CI = confidence interval, CRT = chemoradiotherapy, SCCHN = squamous cell carcinoma of the head and neck, RT = radiotherapy, ECS = extracapsular spread, KPS = Karnofsky performance score, CNS = central nervous system, N/A = not available, Gy = Gray, NCI = National Cancer Institute, CTC = common toxicity criteria.

THE EVIDENCE CONDENSED: Adjuvant chemoradiotherapy versus adjuvant radiotherapy alone for high-risk squamous cell carcinoma of the head and neck

Reference	Cooper, 2004 (RTOG 9501)	
Level (design)	1 (RCT)	
Sample size	459	

OUTCOMES

Outcome measure	1° Outcome LR control	2° Outcomes DFS OS Toxicity (acute and late)
Results of intervention	2-y LR control 82%	HR for OS 0.84 (95% CI 0.65–1.09)
Results of control	2-y LR control 72%	
p Value	0.01	0.19
Conclusion	Postoperative concurrent cisplatin and RT improves LR control in high-risk SCCHN. A statistically significant improvement in OS was not demonstrated. CRT was not substantially more toxic than RT	
Follow-up time	46 mo	

STUDY DESIGN

Inclusion criteria	1. SCCHN of oral cavity, oropharynx, hypopharynx, or larynx 2. Macroscopically complete resection 3. Any high-risk feature: ≥2 involved nodes, ECS, +margin 4. KPS ≥60
Exclusion criteria	1. Creatinine clearance <50 mL/min 2. White count <3500/m^3 3. Platelets <100,000/m^3
Randomization effectiveness	Well balanced in terms of sex, age, high-risk characteristic (margin status, ECS, or ≥2 nodes), racial or ethnic group, KPS, degree of differentiation, and 1° site. Of note, distribution of ECS and ≥2 nodes was not provided separately, allowing for possible imbalance between 2 groups in this important regard
Age	55 y (median) 24–80 y (range)
Masking	Not done
Study regimens	Postoperative radiation (60 Gy in 30 fractions ± 6-Gy boost) + concurrent cisplatin (100 mg/m^2 on days 1, 22, and 43) vs RT alone
Potential confounders	The impact of potential confounders in the 3 studies is minimized because of randomization. The inability to blind patients and investigators should have little impact on the hard endpoints of PFS, OS, and LR control. Awareness of treatment assignment, however, has potential to influence assessment of secondary toxicity endpoints
Compliance	<1% began treatment >62 d after surgery. The specified RT was delivered in 80%. 61% of intervention group completed all 3 cycles of chemotherapy
Intention to treat analysis	Performed appropriately
Power	Designed to detect a 15% decrease in 2-y LR recurrence rate, expected to be 38%, based on previous RTOG postoperative RT trials, with 0.80 power using 2-sided significance level of 0.05
Morbidity/complications	Acute ≥grade 3 toxicities (acc. to NCI CTC v. 2.0) occurred in 77% of patients with CRT vs 34% with RT (p < 0.001). Patients with CRT had more mucosal, hematologic, and gastrointestinal toxicities. ≥grade 3 late toxicities (acc. to RTOG criteria) occurred in 21% of patients with CRT vs 17% with RT (p = 0.29). 4 (2%) CRT patients died as a result of protocol-related events
Other secondary endpoints	HR for DFS 0.78 (95% CI 0.61–0.99, p = 0.04) Distant metastasis 20% vs 23% (p = 0.46) (CRT vs RT)

EORTC = European Organization for Research and Treatment of Cancer, RTOG = Radiation Therapy Oncology Group, RCT = randomized controlled trial, PFS = progression-free survival, OS = overall survival, LR = locoregional, DFS = disease-free survival, HR = hazard ratio, CI = confidence interval, CRT = chemoradiotherapy, SCCHN = squamous cell carcinoma of the head and neck, RT = radiotherapy, ECS = extracapsular spread, KPS = Karnofsky performance score, CNS = central nervous system, N/A = not available, Gy = Gray, NCI = National Cancer Institute, CTC = common toxicity criteria.

THE EVIDENCE CONDENSED: Adjuvant chemoradiotherapy versus adjuvant radiotherapy alone for high-risk squamous cell carcinoma of the head and neck

Reference	Bachaud, 1996	
Level (design)	1 (RCT)	
Sample size	88	

OUTCOMES

Outcome measure	1° Outcome LR control	2° Outcomes OS DFS Late toxicity
Results of intervention	LR control 77%	OS 2 y 72% 5 y 36%
Results of control	LR control 59%	OS 2 y 46%, 5 y 13%
p Value	0.08	<0.01
Conclusion	Concurrent cisplatin at 50 mg weekly and postoperative radiation improved LR control and survival. Although the difference in LR control did not meet statistical significance, the differences in survival were statistically significant	
Follow-up time	Minimum 60 mo or death	

STUDY DESIGN

Inclusion criteria	1. Stage III or IV SCC of oral cavity, oropharynx, hypopharynx, larynx, or unknown primary site, with cervical metastatic nodes 2. Histologic evidence of nodal ECS on surgically obtained specimen
Exclusion criteria	1. KPS <60 2. Gross residual disease following surgery 3. Concurrent or previous primary cancer except nonmelanoma skin cancer 4. Poor renal, bone marrow function 5. Treatment other than prior surgery
Randomization effectiveness	No significant differences in patient and tumor characteristics reported
Age	N/A
Masking	Not done
Study regimens	Cisplatin 50 mg weekly for 7–9 wk + postoperative cobalt radiation (54 Gy in 32 fractions ± 20-Gy boost) vs RT alone
Potential confounders	The impact of potential confounders in the 3 studies is minimized because of randomization. The inability to blind patients and investigators should have little impact on the hard endpoints of PFS, OS, and LR control. Awareness of treatment assignment, however, has potential to influence assessment of secondary toxicity endpoints
Compliance	5 patients excluded after inclusion (1 from RT, 4 from CRT group), 3 CRT patients lost to follow-up at 14, 21, and 52 mo
Intention to treat analysis	Not done
Power	Not done
Morbidity/ complications	Late toxicity: 15% RT group, 20% CRT group had >grade 2 on RTOG/EORTC scale. 5 patients (3 from RT, 2 from CRT) experienced pharyngeal stenosis, 1 RT patient died during mechanical dilation, 1 CRT patient had mandibular radionecrosis
Other secondary endpoints	RT vs CRT 2-y and 5-y DFS 44% and 23% vs 68% and 45% (p < 0.02), 2-y and 5-y survival without LR recurrence 59% and 55% vs 84% and 70% (p = 0.05), 2-y and 5-y survival without distant metastasis 81% and 49% vs 73% and 58% (p not significant)

EORTC = European Organization for Research and Treatment of Cancer, RTOG = Radiation Therapy Oncology Group, RCT = randomized controlled trial, PFS = progression-free survival, OS = overall survival, LR = locoregional, DFS = disease-free survival, HR = hazard ratio, CI = confidence interval, CRT = chemoradiotherapy, SCCHN = squamous cell carcinoma of the head and neck, RT = radiotherapy, ECS = extracapsular spread, KPS = Karnofsky performance score, CNS = central nervous system, N/A = not available, Gy = Gray, NCI = National Cancer Institute, CTC = common toxicity criteria.

REFERENCES

1. Johnson JT, Barnes EL, Myers EN, Schramm VL Jr, Borochovitz D, Sigler BA. The extracapsular spread of tumors in cervical node metastasis. Arch Otolaryngol 1981;107(12):725–729.

2. Snow GB, Annyas AA, van Slooten EA, Bartelink H, Hart AA. Prognostic factors of neck node metastasis. Clin Otolaryngol Allied Sci 1982;7(3):185–192.

3. Vikram B, Strong EW, Shah JP, Spiro R. Failure at the primary site following multimodality treatment in advanced head and neck cancer. Head Neck Surg 1984;6(3):720–723.

4. Cooper JS, Pajak TF, Forastiere A, et al. Precisely defining high-risk operable head and neck tumors based on RTOG #85-03 and #88-24: targets for postoperative radiochemotherapy? Head Neck 1998;20(7):588–594.

5. Vandenbrouck C, Sancho H, Le Fur R, Richard JM, Cachin Y. Results of a randomized clinical trial of preoperative irradiation versus postoperative in treatment of tumors of the hypopharynx. Cancer 1977;39(4):1445–1449.

6. Strong MS, Vaughan CW, Kayne HL, et al. A randomized trial of preoperative radiotherapy in cancer of the oropharynx and hypopharynx. Am J Surg 1978;136(4):494–500.

7. Tupchong L, Scott CB, Blitzer PH, et al. Randomized study of preoperative versus postoperative radiation therapy in advanced head and neck carcinoma: long-term follow-up of RTOG study 73-03. Int J Radiat Oncol Biol Phys 1991;20(1):21–28.

8. Ang KK, Trotti A, Brown BW, et al. Randomized trial addressing risk features and time factors of surgery plus radiotherapy in advanced head-and-neck cancer. Int J Radiat Oncol Biol Phys 2001;51(3):571–578.

9. Sanguineti G, Richetti A, Bignardi M, et al. Accelerated versus conventional fractionated postoperative radiotherapy for advanced head and neck cancer: results of a multicenter phase III study. Int J Radiat Oncol Biol Phys 2005;61(3):762–771.

10. Rentschler RE, Wilbur DW, Petti GH, et al. Adjuvant methotrexate escalated to toxicity for resectable stage III and IV squamous head and neck carcinomas—a prospective, randomized study. J Clin Oncol 1987;5(2):278–285.

11. Laramore GE, Scott CB, al-Sarraf M, et al. Adjuvant chemotherapy for resectable squamous cell carcinomas of the head and neck: report on Intergroup Study 0034. Int J Radiat Oncol Biol Phys 1992;23(4):705–713.

12. Pignon JP, Bourhis J, Domenge C, Designe L. Chemotherapy added to locoregional treatment for head and neck squamous-cell carcinoma: three meta-analyses of updated individual data. MACH-NC Collaborative Group. Meta-Analysis of Chemotherapy on Head and Neck Cancer. Lancet 2000;355(9208):949–955.

13. Bachaud JM, Cohen-Jonathan E, Alzieu C, David JM, Serrano E, Daly-Schveitzer N. Combined postoperative radiotherapy and weekly cisplatin infusion for locally advanced head and neck carcinoma: final report of a randomized trial. Int J Radiat Oncol Biol Phys 1996;36(5):999–1004.

14. Smid L, Budihna M, Zakotnik B, et al. Postoperative concomitant irradiation and chemotherapy with mitomycin C and bleomycin for advanced head-and-neck carcinoma. Int J Radiat Oncol Biol Phys 2003;56(4):1055–1062.

15. Haffty BG, Wilson LD, Son YH, et al. Concurrent chemo-radiotherapy with mitomycin C compared with porfiromycin in squamous cell cancer of the head and neck: final results of a randomized clinical trial. Int J Radiat Oncol Biol Phys 2005;61(1):119–128.

16. Bernier J, Domenge C, Ozsahin M, et al. Postoperative irradiation with or without concomitant chemotherapy for locally advanced head and neck cancer. N Engl J Med 2004;350(19):1945–1952.

17. Cooper JS, Pajak TF, Forastiere AA, et al. Postoperative concurrent radiotherapy and chemotherapy for high-risk squamous-cell carcinoma of the head and neck. N Engl J Med 2004;350(19):1937–1944.

18. Bernier J, Cooper JS, Pajak TF, et al. Defining risk levels in locally advanced head and neck cancers: a comparative analysis of concurrent postoperative radiation plus chemotherapy trials of the EORTC (#22931) and RTOG (#9501). Head Neck 2005;27(10):843–850.

32 Advanced Head and Neck Malignancy

32.B.

Standard versus experimental cisplatin regimens for recurrent and/or metastatic head and neck squamous cell carcinoma: Impact on survival, response rate

Lori Wirth and Merrill S. Kies

METHODS

A computerized Ovid search of MEDLINE from 1966 to January 2006 was performed. The terms "chemotherapy," "squamous cell carcinoma," and "recurrent metastatic head and neck cancer" were entered, and the resulting articles were cross-referenced, yielding 1158 articles limited to "human" and "English language." These articles or abstracts were then reviewed to identify those that met the following inclusion criteria: 1) patient population with recurrent and/or metastatic (R/M) squamous cell carcinoma of the head and neck (SCCHN), 2) intervention with comparative cisplatin-based regimens (experimental arm versus a standard therapy arm) in a phase III study, and 3) primary outcome measured in terms of response rate or progression-free survival, or overall survival (OS). The references of these articles were reviewed and manually cross-checked to ensure all applicable literature was included. Two hundred thirty-six articles were reviewed in detail, yielding the five relevant randomized controlled trials (RCTs) presented below [1–5].

SUMMARY

Despite advances in the upfront treatment of SCCHN, recurrent and metastatic SCCHN remains a significant problem. This is a result of the frequency of advanced disease at presentation. Ten percent of patients have incurable distant metastatic disease at presentation, and two-thirds of patients will present with locoregionally advanced stage III or IV disease. With current upfront treatments, at least half of these patients will eventually develop R/M disease. A potentially curative approach with salvage surgery or reirradiation is the preferred treatment for recurrent disease, yet not all patients will have disease that is amenable to these options. Therefore in R/M SCCHN, palliative chemotherapy may be the mainstay of treatment. A number of single-agent chemotherapies have activity in SCCHN, as demonstrated in phase II and phase III clinical trials. See Table 32.B.1 for a representative list of active drugs.

Attempts to improve outcomes have included investigating combination chemotherapy in phase III studies. These studies have, in general, shown increased response rates with combination chemotherapy, but have thus far failed to show a clear improvement in OS compared with single-agent therapy. Despite this, for patients who are able to tolerate more aggressive therapy, cisplatin-based combination chemotherapy is considered by many to be a standard therapy for patients with R/M SCCHN. Detailed analysis of five phase III RCTs which evaluated comparative cisplatin regimens is presented below.

RESULTS

Outcome Measures. The earlier studies [3–5] used overall response rate (ORR) as the primary endpoint, with time to progression, OS and toxicity as secondary endpoints. More recent studies [1, 2] have turned to survival endpoints, which may yield more clinically meaningful results than ORR.

Potential Confounders. The RCTs presented were randomized studies with stratification to ensure balance across study arms. Because blinding is difficult in intravenous chemotherapy studies that incorporate widely variable dosing and treatment schedules, these studies were not masked. The lack of blinding may, to a minor extent, influence perception of endpoints, such as clinical evaluation of response and toxicity, but should have little effect on determination of radiographic response and survival.

Study Designs. Level 1 evidence is provided in five RCTs examining the experimental chemotherapy arms to a standard therapy arm. Comparative regimens included: 1) cisplatin paclitaxel versus cisplatin 5-fluorouracil (5-FU), 2) cisplatin low-dose paclitaxel versus cisplatin high-dose paclitaxel granulocyte colony-stimulating factor, 3) cisplatin 5-FU versus methotrexate bleomycin vincristine cisplatin, 4) cisplatin 5-FU versus carboplatin 5-FU methotrexate, 5) cisplatin versus 5-FU versus both. In general, the RCTs presented showed effective randomization, with study arms well balanced for important prognostic factors, such as performance status, prior therapy, and age. Follow-up, even if short, was adequate because of the brief event-free and OS times seen in R/M SCCHN. All study designs were developed *a priori*, although as the small numerical differences in OS and absence of statistically significant survival differences suggest, these studies may have been underpowered to detect small survival benefits that might be obtained with combination chemotherapy.

TABLE 32.B.1. Single-agent chemotherapies

Single agents with activity in SCCHN
Cisplatin
Carboplatin
5-Fluorouracil
Paclitaxel
Docetaxel
Methotrexate
Pemetrexed
Vinorelbine
Irinotecan
Cetuximab

Highest Level of Evidence. Taken together, these five studies provide solid evidence that cisplatin-based combination chemotherapy is efficacious in R/M SCCHN. The response rates with cisplatin-based combination chemotherapy are higher than seen with single-agent therapy alone, but come at the cost of increased toxicity without clear survival benefit. The mainstay of therapy has become cisplatin plus 5-FU (CF). Attempts to improve upon outcomes with CF, such as with high-dose paclitaxel plus cisplatin [1], lower-dose paclitaxel plus cisplatin [2], combined methotrexate, bleomycin, vincristine and cisplatin [3], and carboplatin plus 5-FU [4], have failed to yield higher response or survival rates.

Applicability. These five studies enrolled a similar patient population of advanced unresectable SCCHN. Of note, a minority of patients were previously treated with chemotherapy. Now that many of the patients with SCCHN will receive organ preservation therapy with combined radiation and chemotherapy, more patients with R/M SCCHN in the future will have been previously treated with platinum-based chemotherapy in the upfront setting. Studies completed to date offer few data on this previously treated patient population.

Morbidity/Complications. Combination chemotherapy is associated with increased toxicity compared with single-agent therapy. The rate of treatment-related deaths ranges from 1–2% to 10%. Cisplatin-based combination therapy also seems to increase toxicities that may impact considerably on quality of life (QOL), such as nausea, vomiting, stomatitis, infection. If in combined therapy, 5-FU is replaced by a taxane (paclitaxel or docetaxel), stomatitis, diarrhea nausea, and serious infection may be improved.

CLINICAL SIGNIFICANCE AND FUTURE RESEARCH

CF has been established as a mainstay of treatment for R/M SCCHN. This is primarily based on superior response rates than seen with single-agent therapy. Unfortunately, improved responses have not translated into statistically significant improvements in OS. Therefore, cisplatin-based combination chemotherapy is frequently used in chemotherapy-naïve R/M SCCHN in the absence of serious comorbid conditions. Phase II study has shown impressive efficacy of cisplatin plus docetaxel, with an ORR of 40% and median survival of 9.6 months [6]. Single-agent therapy is, however, considered reasonable choice of therapy, particularly in patients with other illness or recurrent disease following combined chemoradiotherapy.

Several important studies are currently underway in the R/M disease setting. These include an RCT investigating docetaxel plus cisplatin compared with CF, and a phase II study investigating docetaxel, cisplatin, and erlotinib [an oral epidermal growth factor receptor (EGFR) tyrosine kinase inhibitor]. EGFR targeted therapy with cetuximab has also been shown in the phase II to have activity in R/M SCCHN. A randomized comparison to cisplatin plus cetuximab versus cisplatin alone has completed accrual, with the final results pending at the time of this writing. Additional ongoing and future studies will investigate other targeted therapies in head and neck cancer, and hold promise for improving on antitumor activity without increasing toxicity of therapy. Future studies are also expected to incorporate more QOL data that will more fully explore clinical benefits of therapy for R/M SCCHN.

Reference	Gibson, 2005
Level (design)	1 (RCT)
Sample size	218

OUTCOMES

Outcome measure	1° Outcome OS	2° Outcomes ORR, Toxicity, QOL
Results of experimental therapy	CP: 1-y survival 32.4%	
Results of standard therapy	CF: 1-y survival 41.4%	
p Value	0.49	
Conclusion	This RCT showed no improvement in survival with CP compared with CF	
Follow-up time	8.3 mo	

STUDY DESIGN

Inclusion criteria	1. Measurable SCCHN not curable with surgery or radiation, 2. Previously untreated extensive LR disease OR previously treated disease with LR recurrence or DM, 3. ECOG PS of 0 or 1, 4. Adequate renal, liver, and bone marrow function, 5. Written informed consent
Exclusion criteria	1. Nasopharyngeal primary, 2. Prior chemotherapy for recurrent disease, 3. Prior paclitaxel or 5-FU within 12 mo, 4. Prior cisplatin within 6 mo, 5. Concurrent malignancy, 6. Heart disease within 1 y, 7. Brain metastasis
Patient characteristics	81% male; 78% white; Median age 61 y; 26% PS = 0; 73% PS = 1; 12% newly diagnosed; 88% recurrent disease; 56% DM; 1° site: 25% larynx, 25% OP, 22% oral cavity, 13% HP
Randomization effectiveness	Well balanced in terms of sex, race, age, PS, new diagnosis vs recurrence. CF arm had slightly more patients with DM and HP primaries, both representing worse prognosis
Study regimens	CP = cisplatin 75 mg/m^2 day 1, paclitaxel 175 mg/m^2 over 3 h day 1, every 3 wk CF = cisplatin 100 mg/m^2 day 1, 5-FU 1000 mg/m^2 daily continuous IV infusion days 1–4, every 3 wk Carboplatin AUC 6 substituted for cisplatin in case of renal toxicity or neurotoxicity
Outcome measurements in detail	Survival data analysis used Kaplan-Meier method. Comparison between 2 groups by logrank test. Response determined according to ECOG criteria: CR = complete disappearance of all disease lasting ≥4 wk, PR = ≥50% decrease in tumor size lasting ≥4 wk, PD = ≥25% increase. QOL measured by FACT-H&N measured at baseline and wk 7 and 16, and at 6 mo. Brief Pain Inventory assessed at same intervals
Potential Confounders	Impact of potential confounders minimized by randomization and stratifying for newly diagnosed disease vs recurrent disease, and ECOG PS of 0 vs 1. Study not blinded to investigators or patients, but should have little effect on determination of hard endpoints such as survival and response. May have greater influence on perception of toxicities, QOL, and pain
Compliance	N/A
Intention to treat analysis	Performed appropriately
Power	80% power to detect a 15% difference in 1-y OS (from 20% to 35%), with type I error of 0.05, and 2-sided logrank test
Morbidity/ complications	12 deaths (6%) occurred, 5 in CP arm, 7 in CF arm. No difference between 2 arms in ≥grade 3 toxicities by Kruskal-Wallis test. Hematologic adverse events, stomatitis, and diarrhea numerically more frequent in CF arm. Nausea, vomiting, and neurotoxicity roughly equivalent
Other 2° endpoints	ORR = 26.0% (CP), 29.8% (CF) (p = 0.84) Multivariate analysis showed only ECOG PS predictive of survival. HR for death with PS ≥1 vs 0 = 1.47 (95% CI, 10.01–2.12) QOL and pain analysis published only in abstract form as of this writing, but suggest CP slightly better than CF in terms of QOL

RCT = randomized controlled trial, OS = overall survival, ORR = overall response rate, QOL = quality of life, EFS = event-free survival, TTP = time to progression, CABO = methotrexate/bleomycin/vincristine/cisplatin, CF = cisplatin/5-fluorouracil, CP = cisplatin/paclitaxel, SCCHN = squamous cell carcinoma of the head and neck, LR = locoregional, DM = distant metastasis, ECOG = Eastern Cooperative Oncology Group, PS = performance status, OP = oropharynx, HP = hypopharynx, 5-FU = 5-fluorouracil, AUC = area under the curve, G-CSF = granulocyte colony-stimulating factor, CR = complete response, PR = partial response, WHO = World Health Organization, PD = progressive disease, FACT-H&N = Functional Assessment of Cancer Therapy in Head and Neck Cancer, N/A = not available, HR = hazard ratio, CI = confidence interval.

THE EVIDENCE CONDENSED: Chemotherapy for recurrent and metastatic head and neck carcinoma

Reference	Forastiere, 2001
Level (design)	1 (RCT)
Sample size	210

OUTCOMES

Outcome measure	1° Outcome 2° Outcomes EFS OS, ORR, Toxicity
Results of experimental therapy	Arm A: median EFS 4.1 mo
Results of standard therapy	Arm B: median EFS 4.0 mo
p Value	N/A
Conclusion	There is no advantage with high-dose paclitaxel over low-dose paclitaxel with cisplatin. Excessive hematologic toxicity is associated with both regimens.
Follow-up time	N/A

STUDY DESIGN

Inclusion criteria	1. Measurable SCCHN not curable with surgery or radiation, 2. Newly diagnosed disease with DM or LR disease so extensive that cure not possible with surgery or radiation OR recurrent or metastatic disease after initial surgery or radiation, 3. ECOG PS of 0 or 1, 4. Adequate renal, liver, and bone marrow function, 5. Written informed consent
Exclusion criteria	1. Nasopharyngeal primary, 2. Prior chemotherapy for recurrent/metastatic disease, 3. Chemotherapy for initial treatment within 6 mo, 4. Significant cardiac disease
Patient characteristics	80% male; 80% white; Median age 59 y; 33% PS = 0; 67% PS = 1; 13% newly diagnosed; 87% recurrent disease; 63% DM; 1° site: 26% larynx, 35% OP, 21% oral cavity, 11% HP
Randomization effectiveness	Well balanced in terms of age, PS, new diagnosis vs recurrence, and DM. CF arm had slightly more patients with DM and 1° sites. Slightly more women in low-dose arm, and slightly more nonwhites in high-dose arm
Study regimens	Arm A = paclitaxel 200 mg/m^2 over 24 h day 1, cisplatin 75 mg/m^2 day 1, G-CSF, every 3 wk Arm B = paclitaxel 135 mg/m^2 over 24 h day 1, cisplatin 75 mg/m^2 day 1, every 3 wk
Outcome measurements in detail	Survival data analysis used Kaplan-Meier method. Comparison between 2 groups by logrank test. Response determined according to ECOG criteria
Potential Confounders	Impact of potential confounders minimized by randomization and stratifying for newly diagnosed disease vs recurrent disease, and ECOG PS of 0 vs 1. Study not blinded to investigators or patients, but should have little effect on determination of hard endpoints such as survival and response. May have greater influence on perception of toxicities
Compliance	N/A
Intention to treat analysis	N/A
Power	80% power to detect a 50% improvement in EFS (from 4 to 6 mo) with arm A compared with arm B, with alpha level of 0.05
Morbidity/complications	Weighted analysis showed no significant difference in grade 3–5 toxicities in both arms 22 deaths (10%), 13 from infection, 2 from renal failure, 2 for myocardial infarction, 5 from unknown cause Weighted analysis of grade 3–5 toxicities showed no difference between 2 arms Myelosuppression most common ≥grade 3 toxicity; 70% (arm A), 78% (arm B); hospitalization for febrile neutropenia 27% (arm A), 39% arm B Nausea, vomiting, and neurotoxicity were the most common nonhematologic toxicities
Other 2° endpoints	Median OS 7.6 mo (arm A) vs 6.8 mo (arm B) (p = 0.759) ORR = 35% (arm A) (95% CI, 25.5–44.8) vs 36% (arm B) (95% CI, 26.3–46.0) Multivariate analysis showed HR for EFS with following factors • Weight loss >5%, HR = 1.58 (p = 0.0083) • Recurrent disease vs new diagnosis, HR = 1.96 (p = 0.0236) • DM, HR = 1.62 (p = 0.0052)

RCT = randomized controlled trial, OS = overall survival, ORR = overall response rate, QOL = quality of life, EFS = event-free survival, TTP = time to progression, CABO = methotrexate/bleomycin/vincristine/cisplatin, CF = cisplatin/5-fluorouracil, CP = cisplatin/paclitaxel, SCCHN = squamous cell carcinoma of the head and neck, LR = locoregional, DM = distant metastasis, ECOG = Eastern Cooperative Oncology Group, PS = performance status, OP = oropharynx, HP = hypopharynx, 5-FU = 5-fluorouracil, AUC = area under the curve, G-CSF = granulocyte colony-stimulating factor, CR = complete response, PR = partial response, WHO = World Health Organization, PD = progressive disease, FACT-H&N = Functional Assessment of Cancer Therapy in Head and Neck Cancer, N/A = not available, HR = hazard ratio, CI = confidence interval.

Reference	Clavel, 1994
Level (design)	1 (RCT)
Sample size	382

OUTCOMES

Outcome measure	1° Outcome ORR	2° Outcomes TTP, OS, Toxicity
Results of experimental therapy	ORR of CABO = 34% ORR of CF = 31%	
Results of standard therapy	ORR of cisplatin = 15%	
p Value	<0.001 (CABO compared with cisplatin) 0.003 (CF compared with cisplatin)	
Conclusion	CF and CABO have higher ORRs than cisplatin alone, but toxicities are greater and OS is not better with either regimen.	
Follow-up time	N/A	

STUDY DESIGN

Inclusion criteria	1. Recurrent SCCHN with no suitable local treatment OR DM, 2. Age 18–75 y, 3. Karnofsky PS ≥50%, 4. Evaluable disease, 5. Normal renal, liver, and bone marrow function, 6. Witnessed informed consent
Exclusion criteria	1. Prior chemotherapy, 2. Serious concomitant disease, 3. Uncontrolled infection
Patient characteristics	88% male, Median age 58 y, 88% PS ≥70%, 69% locoregional disease, 31% DM, 63% prior surgery + radiation
Randomization effectiveness	Well balanced for characteristics noted above
Study regimens	CABO = methotrexate 40 mg/m^2 days 1, 15, bleomycin total dose of 10 mg/m^2 and vincristine total dose of 2 mg/m^2 days 1, 8, 15, plus cisplatin 50 50 mg/m^2 day 4, every 3 wk. Vincristine deleted after cycle 2 CF = cisplatin 100 mg/m^2 day 1, 5-FU 1000 mg/m^2 daily continuous IV infusion days 1–4, every 3 wk Cisplatin = 50 mg/m^2 days 1, 8, every 4 wk
Outcome measurements in detail	Response and toxicities determined according to WHO criteria. Response assessed before each cycle. Patients with early death or treatment held for toxicity considered PD. TTP and survival determined by Kaplan-Meier method, and compared by logrank and Breslow test
Potential Confounders	Impact of potential confounders minimized by randomization and stratifying for institution, PS, primary site, and prior treatment. Study not blinded to investigators or patients, but should have little effect on determination of hard endpoints such as survival and response. May have greater influence on perception of toxicities
Compliance	N/A
Intention to treat analysis	Not performed per se, however patients considered inevaluable (for treatment refusal, major protocol violation, development of a 2nd primary cancer, intercurrent disease, or loss to follow-up) were categorized as treatment failures
Power	N/A
Morbidity/ complications	4 toxic deaths reported, all in combination-chemotherapy arms Hematologic toxicity worse with combination chemotherapy; ≥grade 3 leukopenia seen in 12%, 13%, and 3% with CABO, CF, and cisplatin, respectively; infection seen in 7%, 13%, and <1%, respectively Alopecia, stomatitis, and diarrhea more frequent in combination arms vs cisplatin
Other 2° endpoints	Median TTP = 19 wk (CABO), 17 wk (CF), and 12 wk (cisplatin) (logrank p = 0.2, Breslow p = 0.01) Median OS 29 wk for all arms (logrank p = 0.35, Breslow p = 0.11)

RCT = randomized controlled trial, OS = overall survival, ORR = overall response rate, QOL = quality of life, EFS = event-free survival, TTP = time to progression, CABO = methotrexate/bleomycin/vincristine/cisplatin, CF = cisplatin/5-fluorouracil, CP = cisplatin/paclitaxel, SCCHN = squamous cell carcinoma of the head and neck, LR = locoregional, DM = distant metastasis, ECOG = Eastern Cooperative Oncology Group, PS = performance status, OP = oropharynx, HP = hypopharynx, 5-FU = 5-fluorouracil, AUC = area under the curve, G-CSF = granulocyte colony-stimulating factor, CR = complete response, PR = partial response, WHO = World Health Organization, PD = progressive disease, FACT-H&N = Functional Assessment of Cancer Therapy in Head and Neck Cancer, N/A = not available, HR = hazard ratio, CI = confidence interval.

Reference	Forastiere, 1992
Level (design)	1 (RCT)
Sample size	277

OUTCOMES

Outcome measure	1° Outcome 2° Outcomes ORR Duration of response, OS, Toxicity
Results of standard therapy	ORR of CF = 32% ORR of carbo/5-FU = 21%
Results of experimental therapy	ORR of MTX = 10%
p Value	<0.001 (CF compared with MTX) 0.05 (CF compared with carbo/5-FU)
Conclusion	Combination chemotherapy results in improved response rates in SCCHN, but toxicity is increased, and survival is not improved
Follow-up time	N/A

STUDY DESIGN

Inclusion criteria	1. Measurable SCCHN recurrent after attempted cure with surgery and radiation OR newly diagnosed disease with DM, 2. SWOG PS ≤2, 3. Life expectancy ≥12 wk, 4. Adequate renal, liver, and bone marrow function. Normal calcium, 5. Informed consent
Exclusion criteria	1. Prior chemotherapy for recurrent disease, 2. Prior induction chemotherapy ≤6 mo
Patient characteristics	84% male, 79% white, Median age 61 y, 72% PS = 0 or 1, 28% PS = 2, 7% newly diagnosed with DM, 93% recurrent disease, 11% prior cisplatin, 89% prior radiation
Randomization effectiveness	Well balanced in terms of sex, age, PS, new diagnosis vs recurrence. Carbo/5-FU arm had slightly more white patients, which may be associated with better prognosis than other races
Study regimens	CF = cisplatin 100 mg/m^2 day 1, 5-FU 1000 mg/m^2 daily continuous IV infusion days 1–4, every 3 wk Carbo/5-FU = carboplatin 300 mg/m^2 day 1, 5-FU 1000 mg/m^2 daily continuous IV infusion days 1–4, every 4 wk MTX = 40 mg/m^2 weekly, increased to 50 mg/m^2, if no mucositis or myelosuppression
Outcome measurements in detail	CR = disappearance of all disease lasting ≥4 wk, PR = ≥50% decrease in tumor size (sum of product of diameters of lesions measured) lasting ≥4 wk, PD = ≥25% increase. Survival measured from randomization to death. Survival curves determined by Kaplan-Meier method. Chi-square tests used to compare response and toxicity
Potential confounders	Impact of potential confounders minimized by randomization and stratifying for PS, prior cisplatin, prior radiation, and newly diagnosed vs recurrent disease. Study not blinded to investigators or patients, but should have little effect on determination of hard endpoints such as survival and response. May have greater influence on perception of toxicities
Compliance	N/A
Intention to treat analysis	Not performed per se, but all eligible patients included in analysis for response and survival
Power	N/A
Morbidity/ complications	3 treatment-related deaths occurred, 1 in each arm Overall maximum hematologic toxicity worse for CF and carbo/5-FU vs MTX. Thrombocytopenia most frequent with carbo/5-FU The most frequent nonhematologic toxicities were stomatitis, nausea, and vomiting. Chi-square tests showed CF associated with significantly more overall toxicity than MTX. Comparison between carbo/5-FU and MTX was nonsignificant
Other 2° endpoints	Median duration of response = 4.2 mo (CF), 5.1 mo (carbo/5-FU), and 4.1 mo (MTX) Median OS = 6.6 mo (CF), 5.0 mo (carbo/5-FU), and 5.6 mo (MTX) (p values not significant) Cox proportional hazards analysis showed of all variables considered, only PS significantly associated with survival

RCT = randomized controlled trial, ORR = overall response rate, OS = overall survival, TTP = time to progression, CF = cisplatin/5-fluorouracil, carbo = carboplatin, MTX = methotrexate, 5-FU = 5-fluorouracil, QOL = quality of life, N/A = not available, SCCHN = squamous cell carcinoma of the head and neck, DM = distant metastasis, SWOG = Southwest Oncology Group, PS = performance status, WHO = World Health Organization, OP = oropharynx, HP = hypopharynx, CR = complete response, PR = partial response, PD = progressive disease.

Reference	Jacobs, 1992
Level (design)	1 (RCT)
Sample size	249

OUTCOMES

Outcome measure	1° Outcome ORR	2° Outcomes TTP, OS, Toxicity
Results of standard therapy	ORR of CF = 32% ORR of cisplatin = 17%	
Results of experimental therapy	ORR of 5-FU = 13%	
p Value	0.035 (CF compared with cisplatin) 0.005 (CF compared with 5-FU)	
Conclusion	CF is superior to single-agent chemotherapy with regard to ORR, but not survival	
Follow-up time	N/A	

STUDY DESIGN

Inclusion criteria	1. SCCHN recurrent after primary therapy OR metastatic at diagnosis, 2. WHO PS <4, 3. Life expectancy ≥8 wk, 4. Adequate renal and bone marrow function, 5. Signed informed consent
Exclusion criteria	1. Prior chemotherapy, 2. Concurrent serious illness, 3. Prior malignancy
Patient characteristics	92% male; Mean age 58 y; 62% PS = 0 or 1; 38% PS = 2 or 3; 69% prior surgery; 49% prior radiation; 11% no prior treatment; 1° site: 42% oral cavity, 24% larynx, 15% OP, 6% nasal cavity, 5% nasopharynx, 4% HP, 2% other
Randomization effectiveness	Well balanced in terms of age, PS, prior treatment, and primary site
Study regimens	CF = cisplatin 100 mg/m^2 day 1, 5-FU 1000 mg/m^2 daily continuous IV infusion days 1–4, every 3 wk Cisplatin given at 100 mg/m^2 day 1, every 3 wk 5-FU given at 1000 mg/m^2 daily continuous IV infusion days 1–4, every 3 wk
Outcome measurements in detail	Tumor response measured at 3-wk intervals. CR = disappearance of all disease lasting ≥4 wk, PR = ≥50% decrease in tumor size (sum of product of diameters of lesions measured) lasting ≥4 wk. Definition of PD N/A. Survival data analysis used Kaplan-Meier method. Comparison between 2 groups by logrank test
Potential confounders	Impact of potential confounders minimized by randomization and stratifying for prior radiation, PS, and treatment center. Study not blinded to investigators or patients, but should have little effect on determination of hard endpoints such as survival and response. May have greater influence on perception of toxicities
Compliance	Noncompliance was increased in combination arm
Intention to treat analysis	Performed appropriately
Power	N/A
Morbidity/ complications	No deaths were reported. CF was associated with more vomiting, alopecia, nephrotoxicity, leukopenia, and infection, compared with both single therapy arms. 5-FU as a single agent and in combination caused more mucositis than cisplatin alone
Other 2° endpoints	TTP was 2 mo for cisplatin, 1.7 mo for 5-FU, and 2.4 mo for CF (p = 0.023) There was no survival difference among the 3 arms, with median OS of 5.7 mo for the entire group (p = 0.489)

RCT = randomized controlled trial, ORR = overall response rate, OS = overall survival, TTP = time to progression, CF = cisplatin/5-fluorouracil, carbo = carboplatin, MTX = methotrexate, 5-FU = 5-fluorouracil, QOL = quality of life, N/A = not available, SCCHN = squamous cell carcinoma of the head and neck, DM = distant metastasis, SWOG = Southwest Oncology Group, PS = performance status, WHO = World Health Organization, OP = oropharynx, HP = hypopharynx, CR = complete response, PR = partial response, PD = progressive disease.

REFERENCES

1. Forastiere AA, Leong T, Rowinsky E, et al. Phase III comparison of high-dose paclitaxel + cisplatin + granulocyte colony-stimulating factor versus low-dose paclitaxel + cisplatin in advanced head and neck cancer: Eastern Cooperative Oncology Group Study E1393. J Clin Oncol 2001; 19(4):1088–1095.

2. Gibson MK, Li Y, Murphy B, et al. Randomized phase III evaluation of cisplatin plus fluorouracil versus cisplatin plus paclitaxel in advanced head and neck cancer (E1395): an intergroup trial of the Eastern Cooperative Oncology Group. J Clin Oncol 2005;23(15):3562–3567.

3. Clavel M, Vermorken JB, Cognetti F, et al. Randomized comparison of cisplatin, methotrexate, bleomycin and vincristine (CABO) versus cisplatin and 5-fluorouracil (CF) versus cisplatin (C) in recurrent or metastatic squamous cell carcinoma of the head and neck. A phase III study of the EORTC Head and Neck Cancer Cooperative Group. Ann Oncol 1994;5(6):521–526.

4. Forastiere AA, Metch B, Schuller DE, et al. Randomized comparison of cisplatin plus fluorouracil and carboplatin plus fluorouracil versus methotrexate in advanced squamous-cell carcinoma of the head and neck: a Southwest Oncology Group study. J Clin Oncol 1992;10(8):1245–1251.

5. Jacobs C, Lyman G, Velez-Garcia E, et al. A phase III randomized study comparing cisplatin and fluorouracil as single agents and in combination for advanced squamous cell carcinoma of the head and neck. J Clin Oncol 1992;10(2):257–263.

6. Glisson BS, Murphy BA, Frenette G, Khuri FR, Forastiere AA. Phase II trial of docetaxel and cisplatin combination chemotherapy in patients with squamous cell carcinoma of the head and neck. J Clin Oncol 2002;20(6):1593–1599.

32 Advanced Head and Neck Malignancy

32.C.

Chemoradiotherapy versus radiotherapy alone for locally advanced head and neck squamous cell carcinoma: Impact on locoregional response, disease control, overall survival

Lori Wirth and Merrill S. Kies

METHODS

A computerized Ovid search of MEDLINE from 1966 to May 2006 was performed. The terms "chemotherapy," "radiotherapy," "squamous cell carcinoma," and "head and neck cancer" were exploded and the resulting articles were cross-referenced, yielding 2371 articles limited to "human" and "English language." These articles or abstracts were then reviewed to identify those that met the following inclusion criteria: 1) patient population with locally advanced squamous cell carcinoma of the head and neck (SCCHN), 2) intervention with an experimental arm of concurrent chemotherapy plus radiation therapy (RT) versus a standard therapy arm of RT, and 3) primary outcome measured in terms of response, disease control, or overall survival (OS). The references of these articles were reviewed and manually cross-checked to ensure all applicable literature was included. This process yielded 12 publications, all randomized controlled trials (RCTs). Detailed analysis of these phase III RCTs is presented in the results section below.

BACKGROUND AND SUMMARY

Meta-analyses and randomized trials have demonstrated that the concurrent administration of chemotherapy and radiation leads to improved local control and/or OS in patients with locally advanced SCCHN [1–16]. Most trials included patients with a mix of primary sites. Scrutiny of these manuscripts is advised, however, because the percentage of patients with oral cavity, pharyngeal, and laryngeal primary sites varies. Most often, oropharynx is the predominant primary site reported. Patients with unknown primary SCCHN and nasopharyngeal cancers are typically studied separately.

Mobile tongue, floor of mouth, and buccal SCCHNs are most often approached surgically. Depending on tumor histology, size, pathologic margins, and extent of nodal involvement, postoperative therapy is often administered. (See 32.A.) In unresectable SCCHN, and other sites in which organ preservation is considered achievable, selected prospective RCTs have investigated the value of concurrent chemoradiotherapy (CRT) compared with RT alone. Although virtually all patients entered into these trials had stage III or IV locally advanced disease, there was much variability among studies regarding primary site, T and N stages, and the definition of resectability. Patients were uniformly free of known distant metastasis (DM).

There has also been variability in treatment regimens. Cisplatin has been the drug most often used in a variety of schedules. RT has also been somewhat inconsistent from study to study. Most frequently, RT has been administered in a once-daily fractionation sequence, but, alternatively, RT has been investigated in a hyperfractionated twice-daily schedule, or the M.D. Anderson "concomitant boost" schedule with once-daily fractions in the initial phase of treatment, and twice-daily fractions in the last weeks of RT.

Overall, review of the data indicates that concurrent CRT reduces the risk of locoregional (LR) recurrence compared with RT alone. This can lead to an OS improvement. In general, the data have not, however, demonstrated an improvement in DM or second primary tumors with concurrent CRT. These improvements may come at a price of increased toxicity. A brisk mucocutaneous reaction typically occurs with CRT, and long-term xerostomia, fibrosis, and swallowing dysfunction can occur. The current standard approach for patients with stage III or IV locally advanced SCCHN who are not candidates for surgery is concurrent CRT.

RESULTS

Outcome Measures. Primary endpoints varied among studies, but mainly involved either OS or LR control. Other secondary endpoints included complete response rates, DM and other patterns of recurrence, progression-free survival, and toxicity. These outcome measures are all valuable indicators of clinical outcomes in SCCHN. Unfortunately, data regarding the side effects of therapy are primarily limited to toxicity data using standard criteria, such as the World Health Organization criteria for acute toxicity and the National Cancer Institute criteria, or Radiation Therapy Oncology Group/European Oncology Organization for Research and Treatment of Cancer (RTOG/EORTC) radiation toxicity guidelines for late toxicity. Thus, only limited information is available regarding the impact of therapy on quality of life and organ functional status. Data on outcomes with neck dissection are also limited, and only presented in one study [11].

Potential Confounders. These RCTs varied significantly in populations studied and chemotherapy/radiation regimens used. For example, some studies required unresectable disease for study entry [3, 8, 12–14, 16] whereas other studies allowed entry to patients who had technically resectable disease or did not specify [3, 6–11, 15, 17]. Primary tumor site inclusion criteria also differed; some studies allowed oropharynx, hypopharynx, and larynx primaries, whereas others limited the study to oropharynx primaries only. Other studies even included nasopharyngeal and paranasal sinus primary tumors [10, 11]. Further variability was introduced by differences in the role of surgery. Thus, broad interpretations of results should be made cautiously. These RCTs were, however, all of high quality, with study designs incorporating stratification for risk factors and randomization to minimize potential confounders. The study endpoints, such as OS and LR control, are readily determined and should not be affected by inability to blind study participants and investigators to treatment assignment, as is impossible to do in CRT versus RT studies.

Study Designs. All studies outlined provide level 1 evidence from randomized controlled designs comparing the concurrent CRT with RT alone in patients with locally advanced SCCHN. Chemotherapy regimens added to RT typically involved cisplatin, although dosing schedules varied considerably from study to study. Several studies also incorporated 5-fluorouracil (5-FU) chemotherapy. RT regimens were also variable, though the total dose delivered was similar across the different RCTs, and, in general, ranged from a total dose of 69.9 to 77.6 Gy. The altered fractionation regimens tended to treat to a higher dose than the dose of 70 Gy common to once-daily regimens.

Highest Level of Evidence. Taken together, these RCTs comparing CRT to RT alone for locally advanced SCCHN indicate that outcomes are generally improved by the addition of cisplatin-based concurrent chemotherapy to RT. Three-year OS with CRT ranged from 37% to 55%, versus 19% to 45% with RT alone. The average improvement in 3-year OS was 15%. AT 5 years, OS with CRT ranged from 23% to 49%, versus 16% to 32% with RT alone, with an average improvement of 12%.

LR control was significantly improved in all studies. At 3 years, LR control with CRT ranged from 47% to 70%, versus 34% to 44% with RT alone, with an average improvement of 21%. Five-year LR control rates ranged from 16% to 50% with CRT, versus 13% to 37% with RT. The average improvement in 5-year LR control was 12%. Superior results regarding DM are less convincing. The 3-year rates of DM-free survival with CRT ranged from 73% to 89%, versus 82% to 89% with RT. At 5 years, the DM-free survival with CRT ranged from 61% to 86%, versus 40% to 57% with RT.

Morbidity/Complications. Overall, acute and late toxicities were not as different between the CRT and RT groups as might be expected. The most frequent radiation-related acute toxicities of serious mucositis and dysphagia were determined in all studies. With CRT, serious mucositis was encountered in 40%–77% of patients treated, versus 32%–76% of patients receiving RT alone. Serious dysphagia occurred in 26%–72%, and 30%–72%, respectively. Serious long-term xerostomia occurred in 5%–43%, and 3%–67%, respectively.

Applicability. The results of these RCTs comparing CRT to RT alone are applicable to patients with locally advanced SCCHN, without DM, who are not appropriate candidates for surgical resection of their disease as a primary treatment modality. The definition of this patient population varies among the RCTs performed to date, but it is reasonable to consider this population to include patients with technically unresectable disease and those in whom there is potential for meaningful organ preservation, such as oropharynx and hypopharynx primary tumors. Toxicities are significant with organ preservation therapy, and thus patients with comorbid illness should be treated with caution. The toxicities of treatment necessitate aggressive support with analgesics, oral rinses for hygiene, attention to fluid and caloric intake, and speech and swallowing rehabilitation.

CLINICAL SIGNIFICANCE AND FUTURE RESEARCH

The body of evidence represented by the RCTs presented here clearly demonstrates that concurrent CRT is superior to RT alone in the nonsurgical treatment of locally advanced SCCHN, and constitutes the current standard approach to treatment in this patient population.

The recent report by Bonner and colleagues [6] is the first to demonstrate a survival benefit in SCCHN with the use of "molecularly targeted" therapy. In this case, cetuximab, a chimeric human-murine monoclonal antibody directed against epidermal growth factor receptor, added to RT improved survival compared with RT alone, from 44% to 57% at 3 years. This exciting report is, however, unlikely to lead to the replacement of cisplatin-based CRT with cetuximab–RT in the absence of a direct comparison between the two approaches in an RCT setting. Nonetheless, cetuximab–RT may be a reasonable choice for treatment in select patient populations. Ongoing studies are investigating the incorporation of cetuximab into CRT regimens (e.g., RTOG 05-22), as well as the role of other molecularly targeted therapies in SCCHN. The promise of targeted therapies in the curative approach to SCCHN is twofold: 1) targeted therapies may enhance cure rates by acting as radiation sensitizers;

and 2) the incorporation of targeted therapies may allow for modification of CRT regimens to improve on the substantial degree of treatment-related toxicity seen with current approaches.

A number of studies are also underway investigating the role of induction chemotherapy added to CRT regimens, in the "sequential therapy" model. These studies are based on the high response rates seen with induction chemotherapy, particularly taxane–cisplatin–5-FU combinations [18, 19]. Such effective induction chemotherapy preceding CRT has the potential to reduce initial tumor bulk to allow for CRT to be more effective for LR control, as well as improve the chance of decreasing the rate of DM, a goal that has yet to be clearly realized by current treatment strategies. If successful in one or both of these aims, induction chemotherapy is likely to further improve upon survival in this disease.

THE EVIDENCE CONDENSED: Chemoradiotherapy versus radiotherapy alone for locally advanced malignancy

Reference	Adelstein, 2003
Level (design)	1 (RCT)
Sample size	271

OUTCOMES

Outcome measure	1° Outcome 3-y survival rate	2° Outcomes Disease-specific survival CRR Recurrence patterns Toxicity
Results of chemo/RT	3-y survival 37% (CRT arm B) 3-y survival 27% (split-course arm C)	
Results of RT alone	3-y survival 23% (RT alone arm A)	
p Value	0.014, CRT (daily fractionated) vs RT not significant, CRT(split course) vs RT	
Conclusion	The addition of concurrent high-dose cisplatin to single daily fractionated radiation improves survival, and also increases toxicity, compared with radiation alone. Split-course radiation with chemotherapy does not improve outcomes	
Follow-up time	41 mo	

STUDY DESIGN

Inclusion criteria	1. Confirmed squamous cell or undifferentiated carcinoma of the head and neck, 2. Stage III or IV disease, without DM, 3. Unresectable disease, 4. ECOG PS of 0 or 1, 5. Adequate renal, liver, and bone marrow function. Normal calcium, 6. Written informed consent
Exclusion criteria	1. Nasopharynx, paranasal sinus or parotid primaries, 2. Unknown primary SCCHN, 3. Prior treatment for SCCHN, 4. Prior SCCHN, lung cancer, or other cancer (except squamous or basal cell skin cancer, or carcinoma *in situ* of the skin) within 5 y, 5. Pregnant or lactating women
Patient characteristics	87.8% male; 62.4% white; Median age 57 y; 33.6% PS = 0; 66.4% PS = 1; 96.3% stage IV; 85% T4 or N3; 1° site: 59.0% OP, 18.5% HP, 13.2% oral cavity, 9.2% larynx
Randomization effectiveness	There were no differences between arms in age, sex, race, PS, primary or degree of tumor differentiation
Study regimens	Arm A: **RT alone** (70 Gy in single daily 2-Gy fractions). Arm B: **RT + cisplatin** (70 Gy in 2-Gy fractions + cisplatin, 100 mg/m^2 days 1, 22, and 43 of radiation). Arm C: **split course RT + cisplatin/5-FU** (5-FU 1000 mg/ m^2/d for 4 d + cisplatin, 75 mg/m^2 day 1, every 4 wk + RT 2 Gy/d between 1st and 3rd chemotherapy cycles to total dose of 60–70 Gy. RT break used to allow for surgery in patients rendered resectable). Salvage surgery considered in all arms in case of residual disease. Planned ND encouraged with initial N2 or 3 disease
Outcome measurements in detail	"Conventional" definitions of response were used. Survival data analysis used Kaplan-Meier method. Significance tested by logrank tests. One-sided tests used to compare the 2 experimental arms to the control RT alone arm. Fisher's exact test used to analyze response rates
Potential confounders	Impact of potential confounders minimized by randomization and stratification for primary site, tumor extent, and nodal status. Study not blinded to investigators or patients, but may have little effect on determination of hard endpoints such as survival and response. Lack of blinding may have influenced perception of some toxicities
Compliance	Compliance was greatest in arm A (92.6%), with rates of 85.1% in arm B and 73% in arm C
Intention to treat analysis	NR
Power	Original accrual goal was 462 patients, powered to detect a 50% increase in survival with 80% power, and type I error or 0.025. Because of slow accrual, target accrual was reduced
Morbidity/complications	8 toxic deaths (3%) occurred, 2 in arm A, 4 in arm B, 2 in arm C. More nausea and vomiting occurred in arm B. Myelosuppression was increased in the 2 chemotherapy-containing arms. When all ≥grade 3 toxicities were considered, toxicity in arm B was the worst, with 85 patients in arm B experiencing ≥grade 3 toxicities, vs 51 patients in arm A (p = 0.0001) and 72 patients in arm C
Other 2° endpoints	CR = 27.4% (arm A), 40.2% (arm B), and 49.4% (arm C), with p values between arms A and B, and A and C, respectively 0.07 and 0.002. Median survival (with p values) in arms A, B, and C were, respectively, 12.6 mo, 19.1 mo (0.014), and 13.8 mo (>0.05). 3-y disease-specific survival (with p values) in arms A, B, and C were, respectively, 33%, 51% (0.01), and 41% (>0.05). There were no significant differences between arms in site of 1st recurrence, with DM as 1st recurrence in 17.9% (arm A), 21.8% (arm B), and 19.1% (arm C)

RCT = randomized controlled trial, CRR = complete response rate, DFS = disease-free survival, LR = locoregional, OS = overall survival, PFS = progression-free survival, ORR = overall response rate, CRT = chemoradiotherapy, RT = radiation therapy, DM = distant metastasis, PS = performance status, ECOG = Eastern Cooperative Oncology Group, SCCHN = squamous cell carcinoma of the head and neck, OP = oropharynx, HP = hypopharynx, EGFR = epidermal growth factor receptor, Gy = Gray, ND = neck dissection, CTX = cetuximab, NR = not reported, HR = hazard ratio, CI = confidence interval, 5-FU = 5-fluorouracil.

Reference	Calais, 1999
Level (design)	1 (RCT)
Sample size	226

OUTCOMES

Outcome measure	1° Outcome 3-y survival rate	2° Outcomes DFS LR control Recurrence patterns Toxicity (acute and late)
Results of chemo/RT	3-y survival 51% (CRT arm)	
Results of RT alone	3-y survival 31% (RT alone arm)	
p Value	0.02	
Conclusion	Concomitant CRT, compared with radiation alone, improves OS alone in carcinoma of the OP	
Follow-up time	35 mo	

STUDY DESIGN

Inclusion criteria	1. Stage III or IV squamous cell carcinoma of the OP, without DM, 2. Age < 75 y, 3. Karnofsky PS ≥ 60, 4. Adequate renal and bone marrow function, 5. Written informed consent
Exclusion criteria	1. Loss of >20% of body weight, 2. Previous treatment for this disease or other cancer (except basal cell skin cancer), 3. Synchronous primary lesions
Patient characteristics	90% male, Median age 55 y, 68% stage IV, 59% PS 90–100, 27% PS 80, 37% T4, 12% N3
Randomization effectiveness	Well balanced in terms of age, PS, stage, degree of tumor differentiation, extent of tumor involvement. The CRT arm had slightly more N3 patients, which might slightly skew the study in favor of RT alone
Study regimens	**RT alone** = 70 Gy in single daily 2-Gy fractions, 5 d/wk **CRT** = same RT + 3 cycles of chemotherapy (carboplatin 70 mg/m^2/d × 4 d and 5-FU 600 mg/m^2/d as continuous 24-h infusion × 4 d) in wk 1, 4, and 7
Outcome measurements in detail	Survival analysis used the Kaplan-Meier method, with comparison between the 2 groups by logrank test. p values 2-sided
Potential confounders	Impact of potential confounders minimized by randomization. No stratification was performed. Had this been done for major prognostic factors, including nodal status, there would not have been a difference between study arms in this regard. Study not blinded to investigators or patients, but may have little effect on determination of hard endpoints such as survival and response. Lack of blinding may have influenced perception of some toxicities. Information on ND not provided. Differences in approach to ND between study arms could skew outcomes
Compliance	Median duration of treatment breaks = 6.2 d (RT) and 8.9 (CRT). Radiation stopped before completion in 5% of patients in both arms. 65% of patients in the CRT arm received all 3 cycles
Intention to treat analysis	Performed appropriately
Power	80% power to detect an improvement in 3-y survival from 25% with RT alone to 40% with CRT, with a type I error of 0.05
Morbidity/ complications	1 patient died in the CRT arm because of febrile neutropenia and sepsis. Hematologic toxicity was greater with CRT, as expected. The incidence of grade 3 or 4 mucositis was higher with CRT (71% vs 39%, p = 0.005), associated with more weight loss and more need for feeding tube
Other 2° endpoints	Median survival = 15.4 mo (RT) and 29.2 mo (CRT). 3-y DFS = 20% (95% CI, 10%–33%) with RT and 42% (95% CI, 30%–57%) with CRT. LR control at 3-y = 42% (RT) and 66% (CRT) (p = 0.03). DM occurred in 11% of both arms There were no statistically significant differences in late toxicities. Neither bone necrosis nor radiation myelitis was encountered. Grade 3 or 4 xerostomia and severe cervical fibrosis were more numerically frequent with CRT

RCT = randomized controlled trial, CRR = complete response rate, DFS = disease-free survival, LR = locoregional, OS = overall survival, PFS = progression-free survival, ORR = overall response rate, CRT = chemoradiotherapy, RT = radiation therapy, DM = distant metastasis, PS = performance status, ECOG = Eastern Cooperative Oncology Group, SCCHN = squamous cell carcinoma of the head and neck, OP = oropharynx, HP = hypopharynx, EGFR = epidermal growth factor receptor, Gy = Gray, ND = neck dissection, CTX = cetuximab, NR = not reported, HR = hazard ratio, CI = confidence interval, 5-FU = 5-fluorouracil.

Reference	Bonner, 2006
Level (design)	1 (RCT)
Sample size	424

OUTCOMES

Outcome measure	1° Outcome LR control	2° Outcomes OS PFS ORR Toxicity
Results of chemo/RT	Median duration of LR control = 24.4 mo	
Results of RT alone	Median duration of LR control = 14.9 mo	
p Value	0.005	
Conclusion	Treatment of locoregionally advanced SCCHN with concomitant RT plus cetuximab improves LR control and mortality without increasing toxicities associated with RT	
Follow-up time	54 mo	

STUDY DESIGN

Inclusion criteria	1. Stage III or IV, nonmetastatic squamous cell carcinoma of the OP, HP, or larynx, 2. Medical suitability for RT, 3. Karnofsky PS $\geq$ 60, 4. Measurable disease, 5. Normal renal, liver, and bone marrow function, 6. Written informed consent
Exclusion criteria	1. Prior chemotherapy within 3 y, 2. Previous cancer, 3. Prior surgery or RT for SCCHN
Patient characteristics	80% male; Median age 57 y; 75% stage IV; 67% PS 90–100; 22% PS 80; 30% T4; 9% N3; 1° site: 60% OP, 15% HP, 25% larynx; EGFR staining: >50% = 37%, ≤50% = 42%, unknown = 20%
Randomization effectiveness	Well balanced for all characteristics noted above
Study regimens	**RT** = investigators allowed to select 1 of 3 regimens: 1) Once daily (70-Gy, 2.0-Gy fractions, 5 d/wk for 7 wk) 2) Twice daily (72–76.8 Gy, 1.2-Gy fractions, 10 fractions/wk for 6–6.5 wk) 3) Concomitant boost (1.8-Gy fractions, 5 d/wk for 3.6 wk, then 1.8 Gy 5 mornings/wk + 1.5 Gy 5 afternoons/wk for 2.4 wk) **CTX-RT** = investigators allowed to select 1 of 3 RT regimens above, + CTX, 400 mg/m^2 loading dose 1 wk before RT, then 250 mg/m^2 weekly during RT
Outcome measurements in detail	The Kaplan-Meier method was used to determine survival, with comparisons made by stratified logrank testing. 3-y rates compared by Z test, and Cox regression used to estimate HRs. CR was considered complete disappearance of disease, and PR was 50% reduction in cross products of measurements of all lesions
Potential confounders	Impact of potential confounders minimized by randomization and stratification for PS, tumor extent, nodal status, and radiation regimen selected. Study not blinded to investigators or patients, but the investigator-generated data were submitted for blinded review by independent committee of experts. Lack of blinding may have influenced perception of some toxicities.
Compliance	No differences in compliance with RT were detected. 44% treated as stipulated, with 12% "acceptable major variations" and 5% "unacceptable major variations." 90% of CTX-RT patients received all planned doses of CTX
Intention to treat analysis	Performed appropriately
Power	90% power to detect LR control at 1 y, from 44% to 57%, with a two-sided 5% significance level
Morbidity/complications	23 patients (5.4%) died within 60 d from the completion of RT. No death was known to be secondary to CTX. Toxicities were similar between the 2 groups, except for acneiform rash (≥grade 3, 8%) and infusion reactions (≥grade 3, 1.4%) attributed to CTX. CTX was stopped in 6.3% because of acneiform rash or infusion reaction. CTX did not increase mucositis, xerostomia, dysphagia, pain, weight loss, or decline in PS
Other 2° endpoints	3-y rates for CTX-RT vs RT (p values)—LR control: 47% vs 34% (<0.001); OS: 55% vs 45% (0.05); PFS: 42% vs 31% (0.04) Median survival times for CTX-RT vs RT (p values)—OS: 49.0 mo vs 29.3 mo (0.03); PFS: 17.1 mo vs 12.4 mo (N/A); ORR with CTX-RT vs RT = 74% vs 64% (0.04) HRs (95% CIs)—LR control: 0.68 (0.52–0.89); death: 0.74 (0.57–0.97); disease progression: 0.70 (0.54–0.90) Subgroup analysis showed almost all HRs seemed to favored CTX-RT, except for the once-daily radiation subgroup, with HR = 1.01. HR for HP subgroup was 0.92, also close to 1 (no 95% CI provided)

RCT = randomized controlled trial, CRR = complete response rate, DFS = disease-free survival, LR = locoregional, OS = overall survival, PFS = progression-free survival, ORR = overall response rate, CRT = chemoradiotherapy, RT = radiation therapy, DM = distant metastasis, PS = performance status, ECOG = Eastern Cooperative Oncology Group, SCCHN = squamous cell carcinoma of the head and neck, OP = oropharynx, HP = hypopharynx, EGFR = epidermal growth factor receptor, Gy = Gray, ND = neck dissection, CTX = cetuximab, NR = not reported, HR = hazard ratio, CI = confidence interval, 5-FU = 5-fluorouracil.

Reference	Budach, 2005
Level (design)	1 (RCT)
Sample size	384

OUTCOMES

Outcome measure	1° Outcome LR control	2° Outcomes OS PFS Freedom from DM Toxicity

Results of chemo/RT	5-y LR control 49.9% (C-HART arm)
Results of RT alone	5-y LR control 37.4% (HART arm)
p Value	0.001
Conclusion	Chemotherapy and hyperfractionated RT (C-HART) is superior to dose-escalated hyperfractionated RT, without increased toxicity.
Follow-up time	N/A

STUDY DESIGN

Inclusion criteria	1. Previously untreated inoperable stage III or IV head and neck carcinoma of the OP, HP, or oral cavity, 2. Squamous or undifferentiated histology, 3. Age between 18 and 70 y, 4. Karnofsky PS ≥ 70, 5. Written informed consent
Exclusion criteria	1. Nasopharyngeal lymphoepithelioma, 2. Other cancer, except skin cancer, 3. Surgery exceeding biopsy, 4. Prior chemotherapy or RT, 5. Severe vascular disease, HIV, insulin-dependent diabetes, cirrhosis, pregnancy, or renal disease
Patient characteristics	83.9% male; Median age 54.5 y; 65.6% PS 90–100; 19.5% PS 80; 94.0% stage IV; 71.6% T4; 14.8% N3; 1° site: 59.4% OP, 32.3% HP, 8.3% oral cavity
Randomization effectiveness	There were no noteworthy differences between arms in age, sex, PS, primary site, stage, or degree of tumor differentiation
Study regimens	**C-HART: RT** (2-Gy fractions/d to 30.0 Gy, then 1.4 Gy twice daily to 70.6 Gy) + chemotherapy (5-FU 600 mg/m^2/d days 1–5 + mitomycin 10 mg/m^2 days 5, 36) **HART:** 2-Gy fractions/d to 14.0 Gy, then 1.4 Gy twice daily to 77.6 Gy
Outcome measurements in detail	Survival curves estimated using Kaplan-Meier method. Compared by logrank statistics and Cox proportional hazards regression. Chi-square and exact tests used to evaluate potential toxicity differences between arms
Potential confounders	Impact of potential confounders minimized by randomization and stratification for primary site, stage, and participating center. Study not blinded to investigators or patients, but may have little effect on determination of hard endpoints such as survival and response. Lack of blinding may have influenced perception of some toxicities
Compliance	4% of patients deemed noncompliant with treatment or refused chemotherapy
Intention to treat analysis	Results included "per protocol population," excluding subjects who were found eligible because of detection of DM or second primary tumor, death, incorrect treatment, or noncompliance
Power	Designed with 85% power to detect a 15% difference in LR control between C-HART and HART
Morbidity/ complications	6 patients died during treatment, 1 on C-HART and 5 on HART. Causes of death were PD, MI, ventricular tachycardia, and PE. C-HART patients experienced significantly less ≥grade 3 mucositis, moist desquamation, and erythema. There was no difference in other acute toxicities. Hematologic toxicity with C-HART was minimal. There was no difference in late morbidity between arms, including xerostomia, dysphagia, radionecrosis, or fibrosis
Other 2° endpoints	5-y OS = 28.6% (C-HART) vs 23.7% (HART) (p = 0.023). 5-y PFS = 29.3% (C-HART) vs 26.6% (HART) (p = 0.009). 5-y freedom from DM = 51.9% (C-HART) vs 54.7% (HART) (p = 0.575)

RCT = randomized controlled trial, CRR = complete response rate, LR = locoregional, OS = overall survival, DM = distant metastasis, G-CSF = granulocyte colony-stimulating factor, PFS = progression-free survival, CRT = chemoradiotherapy, RT = radiation therapy, PS = performance status, C-HART = continuous hyperfractionated accelerated radiation therapy, OP = oropharynx, HP = hypopharynx, HIV = human immunodeficiency virus, Gy = Gray, ND = neck dissection, HR = hazard ratio, CI = confidence interval, SLC = survival with local control, WHO = World Health Organization, 5-FU = 5-fluorouracil, PD = progressive disease, MI = myocardial infarction, PE = pulmonary embolus.

Reference	Staar, 2001
Level (design)	1 (RCT)
Sample size	240

OUTCOMES

Outcome measure	1° Outcome SLC	2° Outcomes CRR LR control OS Toxicity Effect of G-CSF on mucositis

Results of chemo/RT	1-y SLC 58% (CRT arm)
Results of RT alone	1-y SLC 44% (RT alone arm)
p Value	0.05
Conclusion	There was a significantly better 1-y SLC after CRT with accelerated RT compared with RT alone, however the efficiency of chemotherapy with accelerated RT may not be as great as expected
Follow-up time	22.3 mo

STUDY DESIGN

Inclusion criteria	1. LR advanced stage III or IV squamous cell carcinoma of the OP or HP, without DM, 2. Unresectable disease, 3. WHO PS 0–2, 4. Adequate renal and bone marrow function, 5. Written informed consent
Exclusion criteria	1. No prior malignancy, 2. No prior chemotherapy or radiation
Patient characteristics	85% male; Median age 57 y; 96% stage IV; 37% T4; 10% N3; 1° site: 74% OP, 26% HP
Randomization effectiveness	Well balanced in terms of age, sex, stage, and 1° site
Study regimens	Arm A (**RT**): RT = daily doses of 1.8 and 1.5 Gy over 38 d to 69.9 Gy total dose, using concomitant boost in last 2.5 wk Arm B (**CRT**): RT as above + carboplatin 70 mg/m^2 and 5-FU 600 mg/m^2/d on days 1–5 and 29–33 Half of patients in arms A and B were randomized to prophylactic G-CSF injections, 263 µg s.c. on days 15–19
Outcome measurements in detail	Disease control and survival data estimated by the Kaplan-Meier method, with comparison between groups by logrank test. SLC defined as time from start of therapy to local progression of disease or death. Cox proportional hazards used to analyze risk factors, and HRs with 95% CIs were estimated
Potential confounders	Impact of potential confounders minimized by randomization. The period of 1 y for the primary endpoint was brief. Outcomes after longer follow-up were recently published, as detailed below
Compliance	9% of patients randomized did not start therapy. The median time of treatment was 41 d (38 d per protocol), and median RT dose 69.9 Gy (69.9 Gy per protocol). There were no differences in treatment breaks between the 2 arms
Intention to treat analysis	Performed appropriately
Power	Powered to detect an improvement in 1-y SLC from 40% to 65% between RT and CRT, with power >80% and 5% significance level
Morbidity/ complications	5 deaths occurred during treatment, 2 on CRT, and 3 on RT. Causes of death were tumor bleeding, heart failure, and pneumonia. Acute ≥ grade 3 toxicities observed were mucositis (68% vs 52%, p = 0.01), dermatitis (30% vs 28%, p > 0.05), and vomiting (8.2% vs 1.6%, p = 0.02) with CRT vs RT, respectively
Other 2° endpoints	The CRRs for RT vs CRT were 34% vs 40% (p = 0.3375). 2-y LR control rates were 45% vs 51% (p = 0.1379). 2-y OS rates were 39% (CI: 30%–48%) vs 48% (CI: 38%–58%). For OP 1° tumors, there was a significant improvement in 1-y SLC from 40% to 60% (p = −0.0091) and improvement in 1-y OS from 57% to 68% (p = −0.0468), whereas there were no significant differences in these 2 parameters in patients with HP 1° tumors Prophylactic G-CSF resulted in an unexpected reduction in LR control in both treatment arms (p = 0.0072). This was detected at the 1st interim analysis. Subsequently, G-CSF was no longer given prophylactically An update of this study with median follow-up of 57 mo was published by Semrau 2006 [12]. This showed a continued benefit from CRT in terms of SLC, with a median of 17 mo with CRT vs 11 mo with RT (p = 0.01). Median OS was also improved (23 vs 16 mo, p = 0.016). Subset analysis of 1° sites showed the improvements were statistically significant only in OP cancers, but not HP 1° tumors

RCT = randomized controlled trial, CRR = complete response rate, LR = locoregional, OS = overall survival, DM = distant metastasis, G-CSF = granulocyte colony-stimulating factor, PFS = progression-free survival, CRT = chemoradiotherapy, RT = radiation therapy, PS = performance status, C-HART = continuous hyperfractionated accelerated radiation therapy, OP = oropharynx, HP = hypopharynx, HIV = human immunodeficiency virus, Gy = Gray, ND = neck dissection, HR = hazard ratio, CI = confidence interval, SLC = survival with local control, WHO = World Health Organization, 5-FU = 5-fluorouracil, PD = progressive disease, MI = myocardial infarction.

Reference	Huguenin, 2004
Level (design)	1 (RCT)
Sample size	224

OUTCOMES

Outcome measure	1° Outcome TTF	2° Outcomes Time to local failure Time to nodal failure Time to DM OS Toxicity
Results of chemo/RT	Median TTF = 19 mo	
Results of RT alone	Median TTF = 16 mo	
p Value	>0.05	
Conclusion	There was no significant benefit with regard to TTF, although LR control and DM were improved in the CRT arm	
Follow-up time	39.5 mo	

STUDY DESIGN

Inclusion criteria	1. SCCHN of the oral cavity, OP, HP, or larynx, stage III–IV without DM, 2. WHO PS ≤2, 3. Age 20–75 y, 4. Adequate renal, liver, bone marrow function, cardiac and neurologic function, 5. Informed consent
Exclusion criteria	1. DM, 2. Other cancer, except nonmelanoma skin cancer and CIS of the cervix
Patient characteristics	89% male; Median age 57 y; 95% PS = 0 or 1; 69% stage IV; 36% T4; 57% N2–3; 1° site: 53% OP, 25% HP, 15% larynx, 8% oral cavity, 65% technically resectable
Randomization effectiveness	There were no differences between groups in terms of PS, primary site, staging, or resectability. The authors did not break down the numbers of patients between groups in terms of sex and age
Study regimens	**Hfx RT** = 72–76.8 Gy over 7 wk in 1.2-Gy fractions twice daily **CRT** = RT delivered as above + cisplatin 20 mg/m^2 IV on 5 consecutive days during wk 1 and 5 or 6 of RT
Outcome measurements in detail	Treatment failure was defined as tumor recurrence at any site, salvage surgery, 2nd primary tumor, or death resulting from any cause. Time-to-event endpoints were calculated from the time of randomization. Kaplan-Meier curves were used for time measurements. Differences between groups were analyzed by logrank test. Multivariate Cox regression was performed to analyze variables that impacted on outcomes
Potential confounders	The impact of potential confounders was minimized by randomization and stratification for institution, primary site, and nodal status. The study was not blinded to investigators or patients, but this may have little impact on the determination of hard endpoints such as TTF and survival. Lack of blinding has some potential for influencing perception of toxicities
Compliance	7% and 4% of patients did not complete the full RT in the Hfx RT and CRT groups, respectively. Unplanned RT interruptions occurred in 18% and 23% of the Hfx RT and CRT groups, respectively. The full dose of cisplatin was administered in 80% of CRT patients. Reasons for dose reduction were toxicity, patient refusal, or other
Intention to treat analysis	Analysis was done according to the intention to treat principle and included all patients, irrespective of the treatment received
Power	The study was initially designed to have 80% power to detect an improvement of 10% in TTF at 2.5 y. After the 1st interim analysis, the study was recalculated because of accrual that was slower than expected based on the actual accrual rate
Morbidity/ complications	There were no treatment-related deaths Maximum acute toxicity of RT was comparable in both groups, with grade 3 mucositis in 61% and 59% Hfx RT and CRT, respectively. Dysphagia requiring feeding tube placement occurred in 31% and 34%, respectively. Late toxicities were also comparable, with the most common being ≥ grade 3 dysphagia (17% and 12%, respectively) and ≥grade 3 xerostomia (24% and 21%, respectively)
Other 2° endpoints	OS at 2.5 and 5 y was 49% and 32% in the Hfx RT arm, and 59% and 46% in the CRT arm (logrank test, p = 0.15). 33 patients in the Hfx RT arm experienced local, regional, or LR relapse, compared with 18 patients in the CRT arm. DM-free survival at 5 y was 40% and 61%, with Hfx RT and CRT respectively

RCT = randomized controlled trial, DM = distant metastasis, CRR = complete response rate, DFS = disease-free survival, LR = locoregional, OS = overall survival, PFS = progression-free survival, CRT = chemoradiotherapy, RT = radiation therapy, PS = performance status, ECOG = Eastern Cooperative Oncology Group, SCCHN = squamous cell carcinoma of the head and neck, OP = oropharynx, HP = hypopharynx, Gy = Gray, ND = neck dissection, NR = not reported, SLC = survival with local control, WHO = World Health Organization, 5-FU = 5-fluorouracil, TTF = time to treatment failure, Hfx = hyperfractionated.

Reference	Jeremic, 2000
Level (design)	1 (RCT)
Sample size	130

OUTCOMES

Outcome measure	1° Outcome OS	2° Outcomes Progression-free survival Locoregional progression-free survival Distant metastases-free survival Complete response rate Toxicity

Results of chemo/RT	OS at 2 and 5 y = 68% and 49%
Results of RT alone	OS at 2 and 5 y = 46% and 25%
p Value	0.0075
Conclusion	Concurrent low-dose daily cisplatin plus Hfx RT offered a survival advantage, as well as improved LR-PS and DMFS, as compared with Hfx RT
Follow-up time	79 mo

STUDY DESIGN

Inclusion criteria	1. SCCHN of the nasopharynx, oral cavity, OP, HP, or larynx, stage III–IV without DM, 2. Karnofsky PS ≥50%, 3. Adequate renal, liver, and bone marrow function, 4. Measurable disease, 5. Written informed consent
Exclusion criteria	1. Primary tumors of the nasal cavity or paranasal sinuses, 2. Prior chemotherapy for recurrent/metastatic disease, 3. Other cancer, except nonmelanoma skin cancer, in the past 5 y
Patient characteristics	83% male; Median age 61 y; 95% PS ≥ 70%; 82% stage IV; 1° site: 37% OP, 21% oral cavity, 17% larynx, 16% HP, 9% nasopharynx
Randomization effectiveness	The arms were well balanced with regard to sex, age, PS, stage, and primary site
Study regimens	**Hfx RT** = 77 Gy in 70 1.1-Gy fractions over 7 wk (35 d) **CRT** = Hfx RT as above + cisplatin 6 mg/m² IV daily 3–4 h after 1st fraction of RT, 1–2 h before the 2nd fraction
Outcome measurements in detail	Survival outcomes were measured by the Kaplan-Meier method and compared by the logrank test. Response rates and toxicities were compared by Fisher's exact test
Potential confounders	The impact of potential confounders was minimized by randomization and stratifying for newly diagnosed disease vs recurrent disease, and ECOG PS of 0 vs 1. Study not blinded to investigators or patients, but may have little effect on determination of hard endpoints such as survival and response. May have greater influence on perception of toxicities
Compliance	All patients in both arms received 100% of planned RT and chemotherapy
Intention to treat analysis	NR
Power	Power to detect a 25% improvement in the 2-y OS rate, with an alpha level of 0.05 and power of 80%
Morbidity/ complications	There were no treatment-related deaths There were no statistical differences in the rates of ≥grade 3 acute toxicities, including stomatitis (42% and 49% RT and CRT, respectively), nausea/ vomiting (0% and 6%, respectively), and nephrotoxicity (0% and 5%, respectively). Leukopenia and thrombocytopenia were seen only in the CRT group at respective rates of 12% and 8%. Late toxicities were also comparable. The most frequent ≥ grade 3 late toxicity was xerostomia (15% and 22% RT and CRT, respectively). Other late toxicities that occurred infrequently were subcutaneous, bone, and skin toxicities
Other 2° endpoints	PFS was improved by the addition of cisplatin to Hfx RT (5-y PFS, 46% vs 25%, p = 0.0068). LRPFS and DMFS were also improved (5-y LRPFS, 50% vs 36%, p = 0.041; 5-y DMFS, 86% vs 57%, p = 0.0013). The CR rate favored CRT, as well (75% vs 48%, p = 0.002)

RCT = randomized controlled trial, DM = distant metastasis, CRR = complete response rate, DFS = disease-free survival, LR = locoregional, OS = overall survival, PFS = progression-free survival, CRT = chemoradiotherapy, RT = radiation therapy, PS = performance status, ECOG = Eastern Cooperative Oncology Group, SCCHN = squamous cell carcinoma of the head and neck, OP = oropharynx, HP = hypopharynx, Gy = Gray, ND = neck dissection, NR = not reported, SLC = survival with local control, WHO = World Health Organization, 5-FU = 5-fluorouracil, TTF = time to treatment failure, Hfx = hyperfractionated.

Reference	Brizel, 1998	
Level (design)	1 (RCT)	
Sample size	116	

OUTCOMES

Outcome measure	1° Outcome CRR	2° Outcomes 3-y LR control 3-y RFS 3-y OS Results ND Toxicity
Results of chemo/RT	CRR = 88%	
Results of RT alone	CRR = 73%	
p Value	0.52	
Conclusion	Although the primary endpoint was not met, the addition of chemotherapy to Hfx RT improved OS, without increasing mucositis or other severe complications. Thus CRT is more efficacious and not more toxic than Hfx alone	
Follow-up time	41 mo	

STUDY DESIGN

Inclusion criteria	1. Untreated SCCHN, ≥T3, or ≥T2 for base of tongue primary, 2. Age 18–75 y, 3. Karnofsky PS ≥ 60%, 4. Normal renal and bone marrow function, 5. Written informed consent
Exclusion criteria	1. Other cancer within 5 y, 2. Pregnancy, 3. History of other SCCHN
Patient characteristics	83% male; Median age 59 y; Mean PS = 80%; 41% T4; 54% N2–3; 1° site: 45% OP, 20% HP, 16% larynx, 6% nasopharynx, 5% oral cavity, 5% paranasal sinus, 3% other
Randomization effectiveness	Well balanced for characteristics noted above, except CRT arm had slightly more HP primaries, whereas the Hfx RT arm had slightly more advanced nodal disease
Study regimens	**Hfx RT** = 75 Gy in 1.25-Gy fractions twice daily over 6 wk **CRT** = Hfx RT as above + cisplatin 12 mg/m^2 IV bolus/d for 5 d/5-FU 600 mg/m^2 IV continuous infusion/d for 5 d during wk 1 and 6 of RT. 2 additional cycles of chemotherapy were planned after the completion of RT: cisplatin 80–100 mg/m^2 divided into 5 daily boluses for 5 d/5-FU 600 mg/m^2 IV continuous infusion/d for 5 d Neck management: patients with ≥N2 disease were evaluated 4–6 wk after RT. Elective ND was planned in patients who had a CR at the primary site, even if they also had CR in the neck
Outcome measurements in detail	The primary outcome was CR, though the method used to determine response was not described. RFS was considered survival free of relapse at any site, and OS included death from any cause. The Kaplan-Meier method was used to estimate survival times, and stratified logrank tests were used to test for differences in the distribution of events
Potential confounders	The impact of potential confounders was minimized by randomization and stratifying for resectability and hemoglobin concentration in block sizes of 6. The study was not blinded to investigators or patients, but this may have little effect on determination of hard endpoints such as survival and response, but may have some influence on the perception of toxicities
Compliance	The mean dose of RT was 7400 ± 273 cGy with Hfx RT, and 7050 ± 160 cGy with CRT. The average numbers of days over which RT was administered was 42 ± 6 and 47 ± 5, respectively (p < 0.001). There were no unplanned treatment breaks 98% of patients in the CRT arm received 2 cycles of concurrent chemo. 57% received the 3rd and 4th cycles of chemo (17 patients refused, and chemo was not offered to 7 patients who did not have a CR at the 1° site
Intention to treat analysis	NR
Power	Sample size determined for a power of 80% to detect an improvement in CRR by 20%, from 60% to 80%, with an alpha level of 0.05. This design would allow for a power of 80% to detect a difference in LR control of 25%
Morbidity/ complications	1 patient died of sepsis in the CRT arm. Sepsis was more frequent in the CRT arm. The incidence of confluent mucositis was the same in both arms (75% and 77% with Hfx RT and CRT, respectively), except that the mucositis lasted longer with CRT. There were no significant differences in weight loss (8% and 10%, respectively), but the CRT group required greater feeding tube support (29% and 44%, respectively).Long-term effects of osteonecrosis and soft-tissue necrosis were rare in both groups (2% and 0%; 7% and 11%, respectively)
Other 2° endpoints	3-y LRC with Hfx compared with CRT was 44% and 70%, respectively (p = 0.01). 3-y RFS was 41% and 61%, respectively (p = 0.08). 3-y OS was 34% and 55%, respectively (p = 0.07). After adjusting for differences in the nodal stage at baseline, the respective p values for these 3 endpoints were 0.01, 0.11, and 0.12 In the Hfx arm, the 1st site of recurrence was at the 1° site in 64%. Lymph nodes were involved in 45% and DM were seen in 18%. In the CRT arm, the 1st site of recurrence was at the 1° site in 73% ad DM were seen in 27% ND was performed in 16 Hfx patients, with 6 (38%) showing residual cancer. ND was performed in 14 CRT patients, with 3 (21%) showing residual cancer (p value NR)

RCT = randomized controlled trial, DM = distant metastasis, CRR = complete response rate, DFS = disease-free survival, LR = locoregional, OS = overall survival, PFS = progression-free survival, CRT = chemoradiotherapy, RT = radiation therapy, PS = performance status, ECOG = Eastern Cooperative Oncology Group, SCCHN = squamous cell carcinoma of the head and neck, OP = oropharynx, HP = hypopharynx, Gy = Gray, ND = neck dissection, NR = not reported, SLC = survival with local control, WHO = World Health Organization, 5-FU = 5-fluorouracil, TTF = time to treatment failure, Hfx = hyperfractionated.

Reference	Salvajoli, 1992		
Level (design)	1 (RCT)		
Sample size	90 patients		

OUTCOMES

Outcome measure	1° Outcome CR	2° Outcomes PR OS Toxicity	
Results of chemo/RT	Induction chemotherapy-RT CR: 30% CRT CR: 23.3%		
Results of RT alone	CR: 10%		
p Value	0.099		
Conclusion	An increased frequency of CR was seen in patients treated with the 2 different combinations of chemotherapy and irradiation compared with irradiation alone. However, toxicity was more common in patients treated with the 2 modalities of combined treatment and there were no differences in OS rate.		
Follow-up time	Median: 28 mo		

STUDY DESIGN

Inclusion criteria	1. Stage IV SCC, 2. Unresectable lesions, 3. Patients < 65 y, 4. No prior treatment, 5. No pulmonary or cardiac disease, 6. Histologic diagnosis of SCC of oral cavity, oropharynx, or hypopharynx, 7. Karnofsky PS > 50%		
Exclusion criteria	1. Inadequate bone marrow or renal function		
Patient characteristics	Age < 50 y: 36%, Male: 93.93%, SCC (grades I, II): 96%, Oral cavity: 47%, Oropharynx: 30%, Hypopharynx: 23%, T4: 84 %, N2–3: 54%		
Randomization effectiveness	NR		
Study regimens	**RT:** 2-Gy fractions once daily to a total dose of 70 Gy; **Induction chemotherapy-RT:** vinblastine (4 mg/m^2 on day 1), mitomycin (8 mg/m^2 on day 1), cisplatin (30 mg/m^2 on days 2 and 4), and bleomycin (10 mg/m^2 on days 2 and 4). Repeated 3 wk later to those with PR, then RT of 70 Gy. **CRT:** Combination of bleomycin (5 mg) on days 1 and 5, and cisplatin (20 mg/m^2) on days 2 and 3. Chemotherapy repeated every 21 d. Concomitant RT of 70 Gy		
Outcome measurements in detail	Toxicities were evaluated according to WHO scale and recorded as present if level III or IV. OS time was defined as the interval between the date of the beginning of treatment and the date of last consultation or date of death. CR: disappearance of all objective evidence of disease. PR: Tumor regression > 50% but <100%. Responses to treatment and complication compared by Fisher test. Logrank test used to assess differences among survival curves		
Potential confounders	The impact of potential confounders was minimized by randomization. The study was not blinded to investigators or patients, but this may have little impact on the determination of hard endpoints such as TTF and survival. Lack of blinding has some potential for influencing perception of toxicities		
Compliance	16 patients with residual tumor were lost to follow-up. 14 RT, 24 induction chemotherapy-RT, and 22 CRT did not receive irradiation in the scheduled time. 63.3% of induction chemotherapy-RT and 66.7% of CRT patients completed the planned irradiation treatment. Reasons for noncompliance were not specified		
Intention to treat analysis	Done appropriately		
Power	NR		
Morbidity/complications	No serious skin, pulmonary, neurologic, or otologic toxicity occurred. Irradiation alone as a single treatment did not result in any major complications. Induction chemotherapy-RT vs CRT: mucositis 16.7% vs 40%, hematologic 33% vs 23.3%, renal 33% vs 23.3%		
Other 2° endpoints	Logrank test of the actuarial survival curves of the 3 different treatment arms showed no significant difference (p = 0.706). RT vs induction chemotherapy vs CRT: PR + CR overall: 67% vs 60% vs 60%, p value NR; PR + CR primary site: 80% vs 60% vs 57%, p value NR		

CR = complete response, CRT = chemoradiotherapy, DFS = disease-free survival, DM = distant metastasis, Gy = Gray, NR = not reported, PS = performance status, OS = overall survival, PR = partial response, RCT = randomized control trial, RT = radiation therapy, SCC = squamous cell carcinoma, WHO = World Health Organization, RTOG/EORTC = Radiation Therapy Oncology Group/European Oncology Organization for Research and Treatment of Cancer, TTF = time to treatment failure.

Reference	Zakotnik, 1998
Level (design)	1 (RCT)
Sample size	64 patients

OUTCOMES

Outcome measure	1° Outcome CR rate	2° Outcomes DFS OS Toxicity
Results of chemo/ RT	CR rate: 59%	
Results of RT alone	CR rate: 31%	
p Value	0.04	
Conclusion	Concomitant treatment significantly improved CR rate, DFS, and OS in patients with inoperable oropharyngeal carcinoma in comparison with RT alone	
Follow-up time	Median: 42 mo	

STUDY DESIGN

Inclusion criteria	1. Histologically proven, inoperable SCC of head and neck, 2. WHO PS < 3, 3. Adequate lung, bone marrow, liver, and renal function
Exclusion criteria	1. DM, 2. Previous malignancy except cured skin cancer, 3. Psychotic or senile patients, 4. Refusal of proposed treatment
Patient characteristics	Median age: 51 y, Stage IV: 94%, Paranasal sinus: 9%, Oral cavity: 16%, Oropharynx: 64%, Hypopharynx: 11%
Randomization effectiveness	NR
Study regimens	**RT:** 2-Gy fractions once daily to a total dose of 66–70 Gy. **CRT:** IM Bleomycin 5 U twice a week for total 70 U, mitomycin C 15 mg/m^2 given IV after delivery of 10 Gy of irradiation. Mitomycin repeated on last day of RT at dose of 10 mg/m^2. Nicotinamide (650 mg/d) and Chlorpromazine (200 mg with bleomycin). Dicoumarol (300 mg) applied on the evening and morning before mitomycin C. Plus RT as above. Patients with residual disease rendered operable after completing treatment underwent surgery.
Outcome measurements in detail	Response to treatment: 2 months after last RT dose. Acute toxicity and response to therapy defined according to WHO criteria. Late toxicity according to the criteria of the RTOG/EORTC. Differences in response rate tested with chi-squared test, survival calculated from start of treatment using method of Kaplan-Meier, and logrank test used to calculate differences
Potential confounders	Initial randomization should minimize bias, however initial group characteristics not mentioned nor significance of differences. Not blinded, could affect analysis of toxicities
Compliance	Because of significantly better results achieved in CRT arm for patients with inoperable oropharyngeal carcinoma, the study was closed and such patients after December 1993 were routinely treated with CRT, 48 patients were treated like such. 1 patient from each treatment arm refused further irradiation. 1 patient from RT group had RT stopped because of hypotension from heart metastasis
Intention to treat analysis	NR
Power	Conducted power analysis with alpha = 0.05, beta = 0.80, need 100 patients
Morbidity/ complications	There was no treatment-related death. Acute toxicity was more severe in CRT arm so dose of bleomycin and/or mitomycin C had to be reduced in some patients (CRT vs RT grade 4 mucositis: 44% vs 6 %, p value NR). 3/4 survivors from RT group and 7/9 survivors from CRT group needed thyroid hormone replacement therapy
Other 2° endpoints	RT vs CRT: 4-y DFS 8% vs 37% (p = 0.01), 4-y OS 7% vs 26% (p = 0.08), CR rate for oropharyngeal site 29% vs 75% (p = 0.007), DFS oropharyngeal site 10% vs 48% (p = 0.001), OS oropharyngeal site 10% vs 38%, (p = 0.019)

CR = complete response, CRT = chemoradiotherapy, DFS = disease-free survival, DM = distant metastasis, Gy = Gray, NR = not reported, PS = performance status, OS = overall survival, PR = partial response, RCT = randomized control trial, RT = radiation therapy, SCC = squamous cell carcinoma, WHO = World Health Organization, RTOG/EORTC = Radiation Therapy Oncology Group/European Oncology Organization for Research and Treatment of Cancer, TTF = time to treatment failure.

Reference	Olmi, 2003		
Level (design)	1 (RCT)		
Sample size	192 patients		

OUTCOMES

Outcome measure	1° Outcome OS (2 y)	2° Outcomes Event-free survival (2 y) DFS (2 y) Toxicity	
Results of chemo/RT	OS (2 y) 51%		
Results of RT alone	S-AHF OS (2 y) 37% RT OS (2 y) 40%		
p Value	0.129		
Conclusion	The combination of simultaneous chemotherapy and RT with the regimen of this trial is better than RT alone in advanced oropharyngeal SCCs by increasing DFS		
Follow-up time	24 mo		

STUDY DESIGN

Inclusion criteria	1. Stage III or IV epidermoid carcinoma of the oropharynx, 2. Patients < 70 y, 3. Karnofsky PS > 70, 4. Adequate bone marrow, renal, cardiac, pulmonary function, 5. No previously treated tumors except basal cell skin cancer and appropriately treated *in situ* cervical cancer, 6. No infectious disease, 7. No psychosis		
Exclusion criteria	1. T1 N1, T2 N1, 2. DM, 3. Previous surgery to tumor, 4. Previous RT or chemo		
Patient characteristics	Male 88.5%, Median age 56.1 y, KPS: >90 91.1%, Stage IV: 73%, T3/T4: 84%, N > 0: 78.5%		
Randomization effectiveness	Distribution in terms of sex, age, histology type and grading, performance status, presence of comorbidities, and T and N stage was well balanced among the 3 arms		
Study regimens	**RT:** 66–70 Gy in 33–35 fractions, 5 d a week, 6.5–7 wk **S-AHF:** 64–67.2 Gy, 1.6-Gy fractions twice daily with ≥4 h between fractions, 5 d a week. At 38.4 Gy, a 2-wk break was planned. After the break, RT was resumed with the same schedule **CRT:** carboplatin (75 mg/m^2) days 1–4; 5-FU 1,000 mg/m^2 IV over 96 h, days 1–4 every 28 d in the 1st, 5th, and 9th weeks of RT Neck dissection was suggested for residual disease or nodal relapse; the choice of a surgical intervention for persistence or progression of primary tumor was left to physician's discretion		
Outcome measurements in detail	Survival estimates were performed by the Kaplan-Meier method and compared using logrank test and Cox proportional hazards models. OS was calculated from the date treatment was started to the date of death or last day patient was known to be alive. Event-free survival was calculated from the date when treatment was started to the date of any relapse or death from any cause, whichever came first, or occurrence of a second tumor		
Potential confounders	Bias was minimized because of effective randomization and stratification. Lack of blinding should not affect objective endpoints as survival and DFS but could affect assessment of toxicities		
Compliance	RT: 98.3% completed RT treatment S-AHF: 96.7% completed RT treatment CRT: 83.3% completed RT treatment CRT: 3 patients refused chemotherapy, 8 patients had only 1 cycle, 15 patients had 2 cycles. 62% of patients received the 3rd cycle with delay 1+ wk		
Intention to treat analysis	Done appropriately		
Power	A sample size of 260 patients was determined necessary to show difference between 30% and 55% in survival, with an alpha level of 0.05 and power of 80%. The study closed before enrolling this number of patients		
Morbidity/complications	RT vs S-AHF vs CRT: grade 3+ mucositis 14.7% vs 40.3% vs 44%, grade 3+ skin reaction 3.7% vs 7.6% vs 16%. 1 case of fatal nephrotoxicity occurred in the CRT arm, with leukopenia and thrombocytopenia occurring in 22.7%, and 4.5%, respectively. Late toxicity: CRT arm showed more grade 2+ skin, subcutaneous tissue, and mucosal side effects although significant late sequelae were uncommon. The occurrence of persistent grade 3 xerostomia was comparable in all 3 treatment arms		
Other 2° endpoints	RT vs S-AHF vs CRT: event-free survival at 24 mo 20% vs 19% vs 37% (p = 0.196), DFS at 2 y 23% vs 20% vs 42% (p = 0.022)		

CRT = chemoradiotherapy, DFS = disease-free survival, DM = distant metastasis, Gy = Gray, NR = not reported, NS = not significant OS = overall survival, RCT = randomized control trial, RT = radiation therapy, S-AHF = split-course accelerated hyperfractionated RT, PS = performance status, SCC = squamous cell carcinoma, 5-FU = 5-fluorouracil, KPS = Karnofsky Performance Scale.

Reference	Bensadoun, 2006
Level (design)	1 (RCT)
Sample size	171 patients

OUTCOMES

Outcome measure	1° Outcome OS (24 mo)	2° Outcomes DFS (24 mo) Specific survival (24 mo) Toxicity
Results of chemo/RT	OS (24 mo): 37.8%	
Results of RT alone	OS (24 mo): 20.1%	
p Value	0.038	
Conclusion	For unresectable carcinomas of the oropharynx and hypopharynx, chemoradiation provides better outcome than radiation alone, even with an "aggressive" dose-intensity radiotherapy schedule	
Follow-up time	40–50 mo	

STUDY DESIGN

Inclusion criteria	1. Age < 75 y, 2. Unresectable stage IV (T4 or large pan-pharyngeal T3), not previously treated SCC of the oropharynx or hypopharynx, 3. Karnofsky PS > 60, 4. Adequate hematologic, renal, and liver functions
Exclusion criteria	1. DM
Patient characteristics	88% male, Median age 54 y, PS: <2 94%, Oropharynx: 75%, Hypopharynx: 25%, T4: 67%, N0: 14%, N1: 10%, N2b: 21%, N2c: 37%, N3: 18%
Randomization effectiveness	Patients were evenly distributed between the 2 arms, no further analysis provided
Study regimens	**RT:** 1.2 Gy twice daily 5 d per week for 7 wk with ≥6 h between fractions. Total dose was 80.4 Gy to the oropharynx, and 75.6 Gy to hypopharynx **CRT:** 3 chemotherapy cycles of carboplatin–5-FU on days 1, 22, and 43 were given concurrently with RT. Doses were carboplatin 100 mg/m^2 on day 1 plus 5-FU 750 mg/m^2 per day by 5-d continuous infusion for cycle 1, and 430 mg/m^2 per day for cycles 2 and 3
Outcome measurements in detail	Survival analysis was performed by the Kaplan-Meier method. Durations of survival were calculated from the start of treatment to the most recent follow-up contact or date of known disease recurrence or death. Differences were evaluated using stratified logrank test
Potential confounders	Bias was minimized because of effective randomization and stratification. Lack of blinding should not affect objective endpoints as survival and DFS but could affect assessment of toxicities
Compliance	4 patients died between enrollment and the beginning of treatment. 2 patients were erroneously included but ineligible because of having resectable disease. 2 patients refused any treatment. Treatment compliance was otherwise satisfactory for most patients in both groups. No statistically significant differences between RT dose was seen between the 2 treatment arms. Of note, only 30% of patients received all 3 cycles of chemotherapy
Intention to treat analysis	Done appropriately
Power	A sample size of 80 patients per arm was determined to be necessary to detect a gain in OS at 2 y of 20%, with an alpha level of 0.05, and power of 80%, taking into account patients that might drop out or be lost to follow-up
Morbidity/ complications	No patients were hospitalized throughout treatment. RT vs CRT grade 3–4 mucositis was 69.5% vs 82.6% (p value NS), grade 3–4 neutropenia 2% vs 33% (p < 0.05). No interruption of twice-daily RT related to acute toxicity lasted >3 d and no break for neutropenia was >5 d. Early death occurred in 17 patients (10.4%), 6 in RT group and 11 in CRT group. The difference between the 2 arms for late toxicities did not reach significance at 1 or 2 y. Enteral nutrition gastrostomy tube was more frequent in CRT arm before treatment and at 6 m (p < 0.01)
Other 2° endpoints	RT vs CRT DFS at 24 mo 48.2% vs 25.2% (p = 0.002), disease-specific survival at 24 mo 44.5% vs 30.2% (p = 0.021)

CRT = chemoradiotherapy, DFS = disease-free survival, DM = distant metastasis, Gy = Gray, NR = not reported, NS = not significant OS = overall survival, RCT = randomized control trial, RT = radiation therapy, S-AHF = split-course accelerated hyperfractionated RT, PS = performance status, SCC = squamous cell carcinoma, 5-FU = 5-fluorouracil.

Reference	Semrau, 2006
Level (design)	1 (RCT)
Sample size	263 patients

OUTCOMES

Outcome measure	1° Outcome Survival under LRC	2° Outcomes OS Toxicity

Results of chemo/RT	Median LRC = 17 mo
Results of RT alone	Median LRC = 11 mo

p Value	0.01
Conclusion	Hyperfractionated-accelerated CRT is superior to hyperfractionated-accelerated RT in oropharyngeal carcinomas
Follow-up time	57 mo

STUDY DESIGN

Inclusion criteria	1. Stage III or IV histologically proven inoperable head and neck cancer located in oropharynx or hypopharynx., 2. No DM, 3. No prior malignant neoplasm, 4. No prior chemo or RT
Exclusion criteria	1. Inadequate bone marrow or renal function, 2. PS > 2
Patient characteristics	85% male, Median age 57 y, Oropharynx: 74%, Hypopharynx: 26%, T3: 16%, T4: 81%, N0: 10%, N1: 6%, N2: 74%, N3: 10%, Stage IV: 96%
Randomization effectiveness	The 2 treatment arms were well balanced for tumor site, T N stage, grading, and pretherapeutic hemoglobin levels
Study regimens	**RT:** In both arms was hyperfractionated and accelerated using concomitant boost. Total radiation dose was 69.9 Gy with daily doses of 1.8 Gy and 1.5 Gy for concomitant boost. The boost was applied ≥ 6 h after the morning dose during the last 2.5 wk of treatment. **CRT:** carboplatin (daily 70 mg/m^2) and 5-FU (daily 600 mg/m^2 per continuous infusion) in weeks 1 (days 1–5) and 5 (days 29–33). The report was an update of the Staar 2001 trial [8]
Outcome measurements in detail	Survival with LRC was calculated from the start of RT and to the date of the first occurrence of locoregional relapse or death from any cause. Death from all causes was the endpoint for OS. The Kaplan-Meier method was used for survival analyses. Point estimates of cumulative 5-y survival rates were provided, with 95% confidence intervals
Potential confounders	Bias was minimized because of effective randomization and stratification. Lack of blinding should not affect objective endpoints as survival and DFS but could affect assessment of toxicities
Compliance	NR
Intention to treat analysis	Analyses were based on as-treated population
Power	The study was powered to detect an improvement of 15% (45%–60%) in 1-y survival with LRC with a power > 80%, and alpha level of 0.05
Morbidity/ complications	7.1% of patients developed osteoradionecrosis. Xerostomia was the most common toxicity (89.2%). 14.3% of patients remained dependent on a gastric feeding tube. There were no statistically significant differences between the CRT and RT arms
Other 2° endpoints	OS was improved with CRT, with a median survival of 23 mo for CRT and 16 mo for RT (p = 0.016). However, the benefit of survival with locoregional control and OS was not seen in hypopharyngeal carcinomas. Pretherapeutic hemoglobin levels < 12.7 g/dL were associated with lower survival with LRC

CRT = chemoradiotherapy, DFS = disease-free survival, DM = distant metastasis, Gy = Gray, NR = not reported, NS = not significant OS = overall survival, RCT = randomized control trial, RT = radiation therapy, S-AHF = split-course accelerated hyperfractionated RT, PS = performance status, SCC = squamous cell carcinoma, 5-FU = 5-fluorouracil.

REFERENCES

1. Budach W, Hehr T, Budach V, Belka C, Dietz K. A meta-analysis of hyperfractionated and accelerated radiotherapy and combined chemotherapy and radiotherapy regimens in unresected locally advanced squamous cell carcinoma of the head and neck. BMC Cancer 2006;6:28.

2. Pignon JP, Bourhis J, Domenge C, Designe L. Chemotherapy added to locoregional treatment for head and neck squamous-cell carcinoma: three meta-analyses of updated individual data. MACH-NC Collaborative Group. Meta-Analysis of Chemotherapy on Head and Neck Cancer. Lancet 2000;355(9208):949–955.

3. Adelstein DJ, Li Y, Adams GL, et al. An intergroup phase III comparison of standard radiation therapy and two schedules of concurrent chemoradiotherapy in patients with unresectable squamous cell head and neck cancer. J Clin Oncol 2003;21(1):92–98.

4. Calais G, Alfonsi M, Bardet E, et al. Randomized trial of radiation therapy versus concomitant chemotherapy and radiation therapy for advanced-stage oropharynx carcinoma. J Natl Cancer Inst 1999;91(24):2081–2086.

5. Wendt TG, Grabenbauer GG, Rodel CM, et al. Simultaneous radiochemotherapy versus radiotherapy alone in advanced head and neck cancer: a randomized multicenter study. J Clin Oncol 1998;16(4):1318–1324.

6. Bonner JA, Harari PM, Giralt J, et al. Radiotherapy plus cetuximab for squamous-cell carcinoma of the head and neck. N Engl J Med 2006;354(6):567–578.

7. Budach V, Stuschke M, Budach W, et al. Hyperfractionated accelerated chemoradiation with concurrent fluorouracil-mitomycin is more effective than dose-escalated hyperfractionated accelerated radiation therapy alone in locally advanced head and neck cancer: final results of the Radiotherapy Cooperative Clinical Trials Group of the German Cancer Society 95-06 Prospective Randomized Trial. J Clin Oncol 2005;23(6):1125–1135.

8. Staar S, Rudat V, Stuetzer H, et al. Intensified hyperfractionated accelerated radiotherapy limits the additional benefit of simultaneous chemotherapy—results of a multicentric randomized German trial in advanced head-and-neck cancer. Int J Radiat Oncol Biol Phys 2001;50(5):1161–1171.

9. Huguenin P, Beer KT, Allal A, et al. Concomitant cisplatin significantly improves locoregional control in advanced head and neck cancers treated with hyperfractionated radiotherapy. J Clin Oncol 2004;22(23):4665–4673.

10. Jeremic B, Shibamoto Y, Milicic B, et al. Hyperfractionated radiation therapy with or without concurrent low-dose daily cisplatin in locally advanced squamous cell carcinoma of the head and neck: a prospective randomized trial. J Clin Oncol 2000;18(7):1458–1464.

11. Brizel DM, Albers ME, Fisher SR, et al. Hyperfractionated irradiation with or without concurrent chemotherapy for locally advanced head and neck cancer. N Engl J Med 1998;338(25):1798–1804.

12. Semrau R, Mueller RP, Stuetzer H, et al. Efficacy of intensified hyperfractionated and accelerated radiotherapy and concurrent chemotherapy with carboplatin and 5-fluorouracil: updated results of a randomized multicentric trial in advanced head-and-neck cancer. Int J Radiat Oncol Biol Phys 2006;64(5):1308–1316.

13. Salvajoli JV, Morioka H, Trippe N, Kowalski LP. A randomized trial of neoadjuvant vs concomitant chemotherapy vs radiotherapy alone in the treatment of stage IV head and neck squamous cell carcinoma. Eur Arch Otorhinolaryngol 1992;249(4):211–215.

14. Zakotnik B, Smid L, Budihna M, et al. Concomitant radiotherapy with mitomycin C and bleomycin compared with radiotherapy alone in inoperable head and neck cancer: final report. Int J Radiat Oncol Biol Phys 1998;41(5):1121–1127.

15. Olmi P, Crispino S, Fallai C, et al. Locoregionally advanced carcinoma of the oropharynx: conventional radiotherapy vs. accelerated hyperfractionated radiotherapy vs. concomitant radiotherapy and chemotherapy—a multicenter randomized trial. Int J Radiat Oncol Biol Phys 2003;55(1):78–92.

16. Bensadoun RJ, Benezery K, Dassonville O, et al. French multicenter phase III randomized study testing concurrent twice-a-day radiotherapy and cisplatin/5-fluorouracil chemotherapy (BiRCF) in unresectable pharyngeal carcinoma: Results at 2 years (FNCLCC-GORTEC). Int J Radiat Oncol Biol Phys 2006;64(4):983–994.

17. Denis F, Garaud P, Bardet E, et al. Late toxicity results of the GORTEC 94-01 randomized trial comparing radiotherapy with concomitant radiochemotherapy for advanced-stage oropharynx carcinoma: comparison of LENT/SOMA, RTOG/EORTC, and NCI-CTC scoring systems. Int J Radiat Oncol Biol Phys 2003;55(1):93–98.

18. Hitt R, Lopez-Pousa A, Martinez-Trufero J, et al. Phase III study comparing cisplatin plus fluorouracil to paclitaxel, cisplatin, and fluorouracil induction chemotherapy followed by chemoradiotherapy in locally advanced head and neck cancer. J Clin Oncol 2005;23(34):8636–8645.

19. Posner MR, Haddad RI, Wirth L, et al. Induction chemotherapy in locally advanced squamous cell cancer of the head and neck: evolution of the sequential treatment approach. Semin Oncol 2004;31(6):778–785.

33 Papillary Thyroid Carcinoma

33.A.

Unilateral versus total thyroidectomy for low-risk papillary thyroid carcinoma: Impact on survival, recurrence

Cristian Slough and Gregory W. Randolph

METHODS

A computerized PubMed search of MEDLINE 1966–May 2006 was performed. The terms "thyroid," "papillary," and "thyroidectomy" were exploded and the resulting articles were cross-referenced, yielding 2203 trials. An additional search was performed to identify those that mapped to the medical subject headings "thyroid neoplasms" and "thyroidectomy," as well as the text word "papillary," which yielded 1139 studies. These articles were then reviewed to identify those that met the following inclusion criteria: 1) patient population with "low risk papillary thyroid carcinoma," 2) intervention with total thyroidectomy versus unilateral lobectomy, 3) outcome measured in terms of survival (cause specific, overall, or otherwise) and disease recurrence. Articles were excluded if they included mixed follicular and papillary groups or did not specifically analyze low-risk groups. Many related papers pooled papillary and follicular cancers together. Although these two cancers are similar, they are also separate entities with clearly different natural histories and patterns of spread. We attempted to eliminate this potential confounder by focusing only on papers with a purity of low-risk papillary carcinomas. This very specific search strategy identified two papers that met the inclusion/exclusion criteria. The bibliographies of the articles that met the stated criteria were manually checked to ensure no further relevant articles could be identified. This process yielded one more article for a total of three retrospective studies. No prospective controlled studies were identified. The three criteria-meeting studies are discussed here [1–13]

RESULTS

Outcome Measures. The two main outcome measures used by these studies were survival and recurrence. Survival was measured as cause-specific and non–cause-specific data. Recurrence was measured as local, nodal, distant, or overall return of disease.

Potential Confounders. A major potential confounder within these publications was inherent to differing definitions of total/bilateral thyroidectomy versus unilateral thyroidectomy. This definition was often surgeon-specific despite attempts to clearly define the exact degree of resection. There was inclusion in several studies of total, near-total, and subtotal thyroidectomy as "total/

bilateral" procedures. In others, subtotal thyroidectomy, partial lobectomy, and complete lobectomy were included in the conservative "unilateral" group. The exact definitions of recurrence (thyroid bed, regional nodal vs distant metastasis) were also variable or unspecified. It was also not clear in several of these studies if patients receiving total thyroidectomy initially also had more aggressive initial nodal treatment than those with unilateral surgery. This variable could significantly affect the rates of subsequent nodal recurrence. The surgeon's bias toward a given procedure also could further bias results.

Study Designs. All of the studies were comparative case series. All three papers made attempts to match the two groups being compared but were restricted to a retrospective analysis with surgeon bias and current practice bias inherent to the study design. Because of the retrospective nature of the studies, only correlations can be drawn, making it difficult to establish a true cause and effect.

Only one of the papers mentioned the specific statistical method of analysis. The two papers by Hay et al. used the same patient group, reporting on this set of patients at different points in time. The Haigh paper, the one that was the most recent and had the largest patient group, did not clearly specify the length of follow-up or how total thyroidectomy versus a partial thyroidectomy was defined. The Hay 1998 paper had the most clearly defined study parameters and most clearly defined outcomes.

Highest Level of Evidence. The data from these retrospective studies overall favored no difference in survival but a lesser recurrence rate with total/bilateral thyroidectomy. All three papers (retrospective comparative reviews) did not find a statistically significant difference in survival when performing a head-to-head comparison of total thyroidectomy to partial thyroidectomy. Haigh et al., however, found an increased hazard ratio (strength of associations between predictor variables and estimated survival) for a total thyroidectomy compared with the unilateral thyroidectomy group. In addition, a significantly increased recurrence rate associated with unilateral thyroidectomy was seen in two of the three studies.

Applicability. Based on the inclusion/exclusion criteria for these trials, these results can be applied to 13- to 84-year-old patients with low-risk papillary thyroid carcinoma. The low-risk group definition for the different studies varied in terms of the AMES (age, metastasis, extent, size score), MACIS (metastasis, patient age, completeness of resection, local invasion, and tumor size), and TNM (Tumor-Node-Metastasis) classification. All three have somewhat similar definitions, however.

Morbidity/Complications. The papers did not specifically mention the complication rate from operation. The risks of bilateral versus unilateral thyroidectomy have been clearly delineated elsewhere in the literature.

CLINICAL SIGNIFICANCE AND FUTURE RESEARCH

There is retrospective evidence comparing the impact of total/bilateral versus unilateral thyroidectomy on survival and recurrence in patients with low-risk papillary thyroid carcinoma. The head-to-head comparisons show that total thyroidectomy may not significantly improve survival over unilateral thyroidectomy in patients with low-risk papillary thyroid carcinoma. One study, however, did report hazard ratios suggestive of better survival outcomes with total thyroidectomy. Two reports from Hay et al. also suggested that the risk of recurrence (local nodal, or overall) was greater for patients undergoing partial/unilateral thyroidectomy.

The indolent nature of this disease and subsequent long follow-up times required to determine meaningful differences in rates of recurrence and mortality makes a prospective controlled randomized study on this topic unlikely. Thus, retrospective data should be analyzed in a way that minimizes bias and confounders. For example, variations in radioactive iodine treatment and thyroid hormone suppression, which could further complicate the ability to delineate the effect of the extent of thyroidectomy on survival and recurrence, should be addressed in future formal case control studies. Larger sample sizes may be achieved by combining data for patients with low-risk papillary and follicular disease, but will provide less pure data as these two disease processes propagate by distinct routes.

THE EVIDENCE CONDENSED: Unilateral versus total thyroidectomy for low-risk papillary thyroid carcinoma

Reference	Haigh, 2005	
Level (design)	3 (retrospective comparative study)	
Sample size*	5432 (4402)	

OUTCOMES

Outcome measures	Cause nonspecific mortality rates HR was the strength of associations between predictor variables and estimated survival	
Intervention	Total thyroidectomy	Unilateral thyroidectomy
Survival	10-y 89%	10-y 91%
Additional outcome measure	HR (univariate): 1.32 HR (multivariate): 1.73	1.0 1.0
p Value	Survival: 0.07 HR univariate: 0.07 HR multivariate: <0.001	
Conclusion	No significant difference in survival but significant increased HR for total thyroidectomies	
Follow-up time	Up to 12 y (median 7.4 y)	

STUDY DESIGN

Database	SEER database
Inclusion criteria	Patients older than 20 y in the SEER database who were diagnosed with thyroid cancer in the 12 SEER regions between 1988 and 1995. Only those with papillary histologic subtypes were included
Exclusion criteria	Patients younger than 20 y and patients in whom the data were missing
Age	Patients >20 y old
Surgical intervention	Total thyroidectomy or partial thyroidectomy
Low-risk group definition	Low risk was defined as younger patients (≤40 y of age for men and ≤50 y for women) with intrathyroidal cancers and older patients with intrathyroidal cancers <5 cm without distant metastasis
High-risk group definition	High-risk group included all younger patients who had cancers with extrathyroidal extension and all older patients who had cancers at least 5 cm in size, any cancer with extrathyroidal extension, or intrathyroidal follicular cancers with major tumor capsular involvement or any patient with distant metastasis
Total thyroidectomy definition	Not clearly defined
Partial thyroidectomy definition	Not clearly defined

HR = hazard ratio, SEER = surveillance, epidemiology, and end results, AMES = age, metastasis, extent, size score.
* Sample size: numbers shown for those in the whole study (number of those in low-risk group).

THE EVIDENCE CONDENSED: Unilateral versus total thyroidectomy for low-risk papillary thyroid carcinoma

Reference	Hay, 1998		Hay, 2002	
Level (design)	3 (retrospective comparative study)		3 (retrospective comparative study)	
Sample size*	1913 (1656)		2174 (1835)	
OUTCOMES				
Outcome measures	30-y cause-specific mortality rates. Recurrence at 20 y: 1) regional nodal metastases, 2) local recurrences, 3) distant metastases		20-y cause-specific mortality rates. Recurrence at 20 y	
Intervention	Total thyroidectomy	Unilateral thyroidectomy	Total thyroidectomy	Unilateral thyroidectomy
Survival	20-y 99.3%. CSM 2.4%	20-y 97.3% CSM 2.6%	20-y 99.1%. CSM 0.9%	20-y 98.5% CSM 1.5%
Additional outcome measure	Recurrence Local: 0.4% Nodal: 0.7% Distant: 0.5%	Recurrence Local: 2.9% Nodal: 3.1% Distant: 1.4%	Recurrence rate: 7%	Recurrence rate: 26%
p Value	Survival: 0.21 Local: <0.001 Nodal: <0.001 Distant: 0.91		Survival: 0.31 Recurrence: <0.001	
Conclusion	No difference in survival but increased local and nodal recurrence in unilateral thyroidectomy group		No difference in survival but increased recurrence in unilateral thyroidectomy group	
Follow-up time	Up to 17 y for totals and 27 y for unilateral		Up to 60 y	
STUDY DESIGN				
Database	Patients treated at the Mayo Clinic during the 1940–1991 period		Patients treated at the Mayo Clinic during the 1940–2000 period	
Inclusion criteria	Papillary thyroid patients with a low AMES risk classification who had disease confined to the neck and who had undergone complete resection of the cancer with curative intent		Papillary thyroid patients with a low MACIS risk classification who had disease confined to the neck and who had undergone complete resection of the cancer with curative intent	
Exclusion criteria	Patients who had incomplete tumor resection and in whom gross residual disease persisted after resection		Patients who had incomplete tumor resection and in whom gross residual disease persisted after resection	
Age	Age 4–87 y, median 43 y		Not specifically mentioned	
Surgical intervention	Total thyroidectomy or partial thyroidectomy		Total thyroidectomy or partial thyroidectomy	
Low-risk group definition	Low risk was defined as younger patients (≤40 y of age for men and ≤50 y for women) with intrathyroidal cancers and older patients with intrathyroidal cancers <5 cm without distant metastasis		Low risk was defined as patients with MACIS score of <6	
High-risk group definition	High-risk group included all younger patients who had cancers with extrathyroidal extension and all older patients who had cancers at least 5 cm in size, any cancer with extrathyroidal extension, or intrathyroidal follicular cancers with major tumor capsular involvement or any patient with distant metastasis		High-risk group included all patients with MACIS score of 6+	
Total thyroidectomy definition	Total, near-total, or subtotal thyroidectomy		Total, near-total, or subtotal thyroidectomy	
Partial thyroidectomy definition	Total lobectomy with or without isthmusectomy		Total lobectomy with or without isthmusectomy	

HR = hazard ratio, SEER = surveillance, epidemiology, and end results, AMES = age, metastasis, extent, size score, CSM = cause-specific mortality, MACIS = metastasis, patient age, completeness of resection, local invasion, and tumor size.
* Sample size: numbers shown for those in the whole study (number of those in low-risk group).

REFERENCES

1. Haigh PI, Urbach DR, Rotstein LE. Extent of thyroidectomy is not a major determinant of survival in low- or high-risk papillary thyroid cancer. Ann Surg Oncol 2005;12(1):81–89.

2. Hay ID, Grant CS, Bergstralh EJ, Thompson GB, van Heerden JA, Goellner JR. Unilateral total lobectomy: is it sufficient surgical treatment for patients with AMES low-risk papillary thyroid carcinoma? Surgery 1998;124(6):958–964.

3. Hay ID, Thompson GB, Grant CS, et al. Papillary thyroid carcinoma managed at the Mayo Clinic during six decades (1940–1999): temporal trends in initial therapy and long-term outcome in 2444 consecutively treated patients. World J Surg 2002;26(8):879–885.

33 Papillary Thyroid Carcinoma

33.B.

Radioactive iodine versus no radioactive iodine as adjunctive treatment for low-risk papillary thyroid carcinoma: Impact on survival, recurrence

Cristian Slough and Gregory W. Randolph

METHODS

A computerized PubMed search of MEDLINE 1966–May 2006 was performed. Articles mapping to the medical subject headings "iodine radioisotopes" and "thyroid neoplasms" as well as the textword "papillary" were identified, yielding 948 papers. These articles were then reviewed to identify those that met the following inclusion criteria: 1) distinct patient population with "low risk differentiated thyroid carcinoma," 2) intervention with radioactive iodine (RAI) versus no RAI treatment, 3) outcome measured in terms of cause-specific survival, or death rate and disease recurrence.

Articles that included both low- and high-risk patients overall, but reported results for a distinct low-risk population were included. Articles that reported only lumped low-risk and high-risk data, however, were excluded. Many related papers pooled papillary and follicular cancers together. Although these two cancers are similar, they are also separate entities with clearly different natural histories and patterns of spread. We attempted to eliminate this potential confounder by focusing only on papers with a purity of low-risk papillary carcinomas. Three trials were identified that met these specific inclusion/exclusion criteria in the initial search. The bibliographies of the articles that met these inclusion criteria were manually checked to ensure no further relevant articles could be identified. This overall process yielded three relevant articles [1–3].

RESULTS

Outcome Measures. The main outcome measures used by these studies were cause-specific survival or death rate and recurrence. All of the studies used cause-specific survival (two at 10 years [1, 2] and one at 20 years [3]) as an outcome measure. Two of the studies also used recurrence rate as an added outcome measure [1, 2].

Potential Confounders. A major factor when comparing these studies was the differing definitions of "low-risk" papillary thyroid carcinoma. Although all the papers had similar definitions, there was no apparent universal definition used among all study groups. Another potential confounder was the differing additional therapies the patients received in conjunction with RAI treatment;

variations occurred in the degree of surgery and degree of T4 suppressive therapy which could affect outcome. Also the lack of prospective input or randomization resulted in probable selection bias in terms of which patients were chosen to receive I^{131} treatment. Another major confounding factor was the lack of clearly defined parameters for I^{131} treatment in any of the studies; it is inherently difficult to determine such parameters in retrospective studies. The exact dose of RAI used differed in all three of the studies.

Study Designs. All of the studies were retrospective in nature. Groups who had received RAI were compared with those who had not. A variety of RAI regimens were used. Patients were classified as low risk based on either the American Joint Committee on Cancer staging or stratification based on the AMES (age, metastasis, extent, size score) system [4, 5].

Highest Level of Evidence. All reports described were retrospective studies comparing results with versus without RAI therapy. The three papers from Brierley, Chow, and Sanders showed no differences in survival or recurrence with versus without RAI in low-risk differentiated thyroid carcinoma. Brierley's work showed a trend toward improved survival with RAI but no formally statistically significant difference. Chow's work showed no difference in survival but showed favorable numbers for control of local recurrence, although again numbers did not reach formal statistical significance.

Applicability. Based on the inclusion/exclusion criteria for these trials, the results can be applied to TNM (Tumor-Node-Metastasis) stage I patients with low-risk differentiated thyroid carcinoma. The low-risk group definition for the different studies varied in terms of the AMES, and TNM classification; but all three had agreed that stage I TNM constituted a low-risk group.

Morbidity/Complications. These papers did not specifically mention the complication rate from the RAI treatment. They all recognized that the morbidity of treatment is low. The common complications of RAI include salivary gland dysfunction, radiation sickness, and bone marrow depression. Although understated in the endocrine literature, some questions do exist with respect to the development of secondary malignancies relative to I^{131} treatment. These questions are among the concerns that generally result in restricted use of I^{131} in younger adults and children.

CLINICAL SIGNIFICANCE AND FUTURE RESEARCH

There is retrospective evidence that RAI treatment does not improve survival in patients with low-risk differentiated thyroid carcinoma. There was a trend toward reduc-

tion with RA1, but no statistically significant differences demonstrated. The indolent nature of this disease process makes a prospective study with adequate follow-up and power very challenging.

Future studies should concentrate on the effect of RAI on local, nodal, and distant metastasis in a prospective manner in a distinct group of either low-risk or high-risk patients.

THE EVIDENCE CONDENSED: Radioiodine for low-risk papillary thyroid carcinoma patients

Reference	Brierley, 2005		Chow, 2002		Sanders, 1998	
Level (design)	3 (retrospective comparative study)		3 (retrospective comparative study)		3 (retrospective comparative study)	
Sample size*	729 (324)		842 (97)		1019 (790)	
OUTCOMES						
Outcome measures	Cause-specific survival and local-regional relapse-free rate		Cause-specific survival, locoregional control, and freedom from distant metastasis		Cause-specific survival at 20 y	
Intervention	RAI treatment N = 228	Non-RAI N = 96	RAI treatment N = 54	Non-RAI N = 43	RAI treatment	Non-RAI
CSS	10 y 97%	10 y 100%	10 y 100%	10 y 100%	20 y 99.2%.	20 y 97.2%
Recurrence	LRFR 90%	LRFR 85%	Local: 100% Distant: 100%	Local: 91.7% Distant: 97.7%%	NR	NR
p Value	Survival: 0.35 LRFR: 0.52		Local: NS Distant: not reported		Survival: not significant	
Conclusion	Cause-specific survival and local recurrence rates were not significantly different between the 2 groups		No difference in survival but increased local and distant recurrence in non-RAI group but not statistically significant		No difference in survival in the 2 groups	
Follow-up time	Median 11.3 y		Median 9.2 y		Up to 13 y	
STUDY DESIGN						
Database	Patients with a new diagnosis of differentiated thyroid cancer seen at the Department of Radiation Oncology, Endocrine Oncology Clinic of the Prince Margaret Hospital between 1958 and 1985		Patients with differentiated thyroid cancer treated at the Queen Elizabeth Hospital, Hong Kong from 1960 to 1997		Patients treated at the Lahey Hitchcock Medical Center and the New England Deaconess Hospital during the 1940–1990 period	
Inclusion criteria	Only patients with newly diagnosed well-differentiated thyroid cancer treated at the above center but the criteria not clearly specified		Patients with differentiated papillary thyroid cancer treated at the Queen Elizabeth Hospital, Hong Kong from 1960 to 1997		Patients treated at the Lahey Hitchcock Medical Center and the New England Deaconess Hospital during the 1940–1990 period with differentiated thyroid carcinoma	
Exclusion criteria	Recurrent-disease patients		Not specified		Patients who were initially treated at other than 2 primary institutions were not included because of incompleteness of data	
Age	Age range not specified		Age 8.6–91.6 y, mean 45.1 y		Not specifically mentioned	
Intervention	RAI treatment vs no RAI treatment		RAI treatment vs no RAI treatment		RAI treatment vs no RAI treatment	
Low-risk group definition	Low risk was defined as patients younger than 45 y and AJCC stage I		Low risk was defined as patients with T1 N0 M0 disease		Low risk was defined according to the AMES scoring system	
High-risk group definition	High-risk group included all older patients and those with AJCC stages >I		Not clearly defined		All patients with distant metastases and older patients with either tumors >5 cm or extrathyroidal extension	
RAI treatment dose	30–100 mCi		80 mCi		Not specified	
Statistical analysis	Cox model analysis		Outcome measures were studied by using the Kaplan-Meier method and Cox regression models for multivariate analysis		Actuarial curves generated using life tables and differences measured using multivariate analysis and Cox regression analysis	

LRFR = local relapse free rate, RAI = radioactive iodine, NR = not reported, AMES = age, metastasis, extent, size score, AJCC= American Joint Committee on Cancer CSS = cause specific survival.
* Sample size: numbers shown for those in the whole study (number of those in low-risk group).

REFERENCES

1. Brierley J, Tsang R, Panzarella T, Bana N. Prognostic factor and the effect of treatment with radioactive iodine and external beam radiation on patients with differentiated thyroid cancer seen at a single institution over the 40 years. Clin Endocrinol 2005;63:418–427.

2. Chow SM, Law SCK, Mendenhall WM, et al. Papillary thyroid carcinoma: prognostic factors and the role of radio-iodine and external radiotherapy. Int J Radiat Oncol Biol Phys 2002;52:784–795.

3. Sanders LE, Cady B. Differentiated thyroid cancer: re-examination of risk groups and outcome of treatment. Arch Surg 1998;133:419–425.

4. Greene FL, Page DL, Fleming ID, et al. AJCC Cancer Staging Manual. 6th ed. New York: Springer; 2002.

5. Cady B, Rossi R. An expanded view of risk-group definition in differentiated thyroid carcinoma. Surgery 1988;104:947–953.

Index

Printed in the United States of America